PROCEDURES

P9-EGB-134

Today's MEDICAL ASSISTANT

learning system

REGISTER TODAY!

To access your Student Resources, visit:

http://evolve.elsevier.com/Bonewit/today/

Register today and gain access to:

- **Apply Your Knowledge**
  Interactive Review Questions that serve as a valuable study tool

- **Content Updates**
  Continually updated information to provide the latest updates
  on relevant issues for medical assistants

- **Prepare for Certification**
  Interactive exercises to help you prepare for success

ELSEVIER

Today's MEDICAL ASSISTANT

Clinical & Administrative Procedures

Kathy Bonewit-West, BS, MEd

Coordinator and Instructor
Medical Assistant Technology
Hocking College
Nelsonville, Ohio
Former Member, Curriculum Review Board of the
American Association of Medical Assistants

Sue A. Hunt, MA, RN, CMA (AAMA)

Former Professor and Coordinator
Medical Assisting Program
Middlesex Community College
Lowell, Massachusetts

Edith Applegate, MS

Professor of Biological Sciences
Kettering College of Medical Arts
Kettering, Ohio

SAUNDERS

ELSEVIER

SAUNDERS
ELSEVIER

11830 Westline Industrial Drive
St. Louis, Missouri 63146

TODAY'S MEDICAL ASSISTANT: CLINICAL AND   ISBN: 978-1-4160-4432-1
ADMINISTRATIVE PROCEDURES
Copyright © 2009 by Saunders, an imprint of Elsevier Inc.

All rights reserved. No part of this publication may be reproduced or transmitted in any form or by any means, electronic or mechanical, including photocopying, recording, or any information storage and retrieval system, without permission in writing from the publisher. Permissions may be sought directly from Elsevier's Rights Department: phone: (+1) 215 239 3804 (US) or (+44) 1865 843830 (UK); fax: (+44) 1865 853333; e-mail: healthpermissions@elsevier.com. You may also complete your request on-line via the Elsevier website at http://www.elsevier.com/permissions.

Some material was previously published.

Notice

Knowledge and best practice in this field are constantly changing. As new research and experience broaden our knowledge, changes in practice, treatment and drug therapy may become necessary or appropriate. Readers are advised to check the most current information provided (i) on procedures featured or (ii) by the manufacturer of each product to be administered, to verify the recommended dose or formula, the method and duration of administration, and contraindications. It is the responsibility of the practitioner, relying on their own experience and knowledge of the patient, to make diagnoses, to determine dosages and the best treatment for each individual patient, and to take all appropriate safety precautions. To the fullest extent of the law, neither the Publisher nor the Authors assume any liability for any injury and/or damage to persons or property arising out of or related to any use of the material contained in this book.

The Publisher

Library of Congress Cataloging-in-Publication Data
Bonewit-West, Kathy.
  Today's medical assistant : clinical and administrative procedures / Kathy Bonewit-West, Sue A. Hunt, Edith Applegate.—1st ed.
    p. ; cm.
  Includes index.
  ISBN 978-1-4160-4432-1
  1. Medical assistants.   2. Clinical medicine.   I. Hunt, Sue A.   II. Applegate, Edith J.   III. Title.
  [DNLM: 1. Physician Assistants.   2. Clinical Medicine–methods.   3. Office Management–organization & administration.   4. Patient Care–methods.   5. Professional Competence.   W 21.5 B712t 2009]
  R728.8.B664 2009
  610.73'7069–dc22

                                                                                            2008019307

Publisher: Michael S. Ledbetter
Associate Developmental Editor: Jennifer Bertucci
Publishing Services Manager: Patricia Tannian
Senior Project Manager: Kristine Feeherty
Design Direction: Charlie Seibel

Working together to grow
libraries in developing countries

www.elsevier.com | www.bookaid.org | www.sabre.org

ELSEVIER   BOOK AID International   Sabre Foundation

Printed in the United States of America
Last digit is the print number: 9 8 7 6 5 4 3

For Dave and Caitie
You are the wind beneath my wings
KBW

For Stan—my best friend and husband for 50 years
You are the GPS in my life
EA

Editorial Review Board

Gerry A. Brasin, AS, CMA (AAMA), CPC
Education Coordinator
Premiere Education Group
Springfield, Massachusetts

Jennifer Claire, AA, BA, MSHS, CMA (AAMA)
Instructor; Course Lead
Health Sciences Department
Kaplan University
Fort Lauderdale, Florida

Bethany Conquest, RN, BSN, MA-Ed
Director of Curriculum Development
Ross Education, LLC
Saint Clair, Michigan

Christy Gee, MSN, RN, RMA
Medical Assistant Program Department Chair
AAS in Medical Assisting Program
South College-Asheville
Asheville, North Carolina

Margie J. Goble, RHIA, CBCS
Medical Assisting and Medical Billing Specialist Instructor
Adult Health Occupations Programs
Pickaway-Ross Joint Vocational School District
Chillicothe, Ohio

Julie K. Pepper, BS, CMA (AAMA)
Instructor, Medical Assisting Program
Chippewa Valley Technical College
Eau Claire, Wisconsin

Theresa A Rieger, CMA (AAMA), CPC
Manager
Mercy Health Network Northwest Family Clinic
Oklahoma City, Oklahoma

Preface

Medical assistants, for many years an integral part of most physicians' staff, now fulfill an ever-expanding and varied role in the medical office, both clinically and administratively. With increased responsibilities, however, comes a greater need for professional knowledge and skills. This text has been designed to provide the basics of administrative and clinical competency combined with background knowledge of anatomy and physiology.

The underlying principle of this book is to provide a format for the achievement of professional competency in skills performed in the medical office, and the understanding of their application to real-life or on-the-job situations. When professional competency is achieved in the classroom, less of a gap should exist between the academic world and the real world, and thus the transition from student to practicing medical assistant is made more easily.

Although the book's usefulness to students in medical assisting educational programs has been emphasized, the practicing medical assistant will also find this text helpful as a learning and reference source. The organization of the text lends itself well to individualized instruction and convenient reference use.

FEATURES IN THIS TEXTBOOK

This textbook provides up-to-date information in both the administrative and clinical areas, and it incorporates current trends in technology.

Important Features Include the Following:

- Information about compliance to all aspects of HIPAA in the medical office
- Introduction to anatomy and physiology by body system
- Current information on the OSHA Bloodborne Pathogens Standard
- The theory and step-by-step procedure for measuring temperature using a temporal artery thermometer
- The theory and step-by-step procedure for performing pulse oximetry
- The theory of intravenous therapy
- The A_{1c} blood glucose test
- Comprehensive updated pharmacology drug table of medications commonly administered and prescribed in the medical office
- Use of the electronic medical record as it applies to the medical office
- Use of the revised CMS-1500 insurance form

- Information about obtaining an entry-level position as a medical assistant after graduation

STANDARD PEDAGOGICAL FEATURES IN THIS TEXTBOOK

Other very important features include valuable learning aids:

- **On the Web Resources** allow students to access websites containing additional information relating to the chapter.

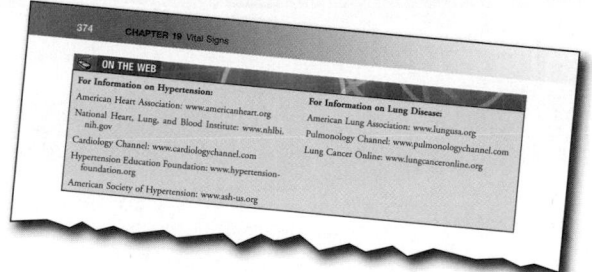

- The organizational format of this textbook facilitates the learning process by providing students and educators with detailed objectives and an in-depth study of the most current and up-to-date administrative and clinical procedures performed in the medical office. Presented at the beginning of each chapter are **Learning Objectives** and related **Procedures,** a **Chapter Outline, National Competencies,** and **Key Terms.** The learning objectives address the cognitive knowledge required to perform the procedures. Procedures coincide with the objectives to delineate the task or skill to be mastered by the student. (In the student Study Guide, most procedures are expanded into detailed performance objectives, including outcomes, and conditions and standards of acceptable performance.) The chapter outline provides a quick reference of the cognitive knowledge included in that chapter. National competencies indicate both the CAAHEP competencies and ABHES competencies met by both the theory and procedures in the chapter. The Key Terms list designates the terms and definitions that should be mastered for each chapter.

the level of competency required on the job. Each procedure is presented in an organized step-by-step format, with underlying principles and illustrations accompanying the techniques. A charting example follows each clinical procedure to provide the student with a guide for charting his or her own procedure. Students should find it much easier to acquire competency in charting with these examples.

- The **knowledge** or **theory** that the student must acquire to perform each skill is presented in a clear and concise manner. **Numerous illustrations** accompany the theory section to aid the student in acquiring the knowledge relating to each skill.
- **Procedures** for each skill follow the theory section and are designed to help the student perform the skill with

- The unique and memorable medical assistant biographical profiles (**Memories from Externship** and **Putting It All into Practice**) help students "connect" with their future beyond the classroom. The medical assistants featured are real people sharing their fears, likes, hopes, and aspirations, providing a "real-world" feel to the book and an inspiration for the student.

- **Case Studies** are designed to assist the student in responding to "real-life" situations that occur in the medical office. A practitioner's response is given for each case study too, as a means of comparison for the student.

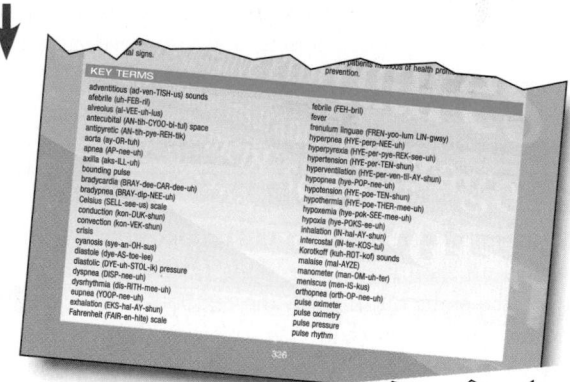

- **Key Terms** identified at the beginning of the chapter are defined at the end of the chapter in the **Terminology Review**, providing students with a valuable terminology overview for each chapter.

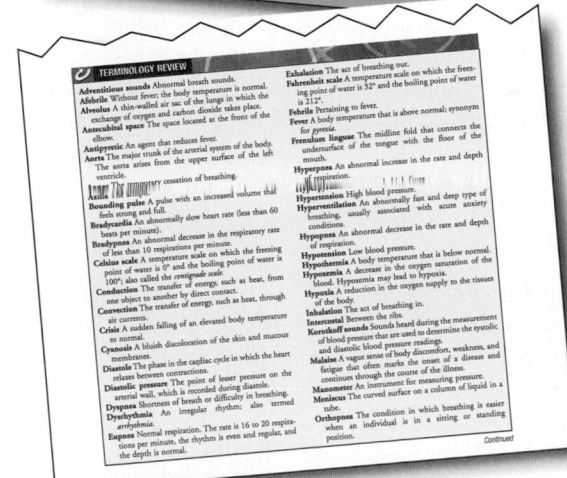

- **Patient Teaching** boxes emphasize this important aspect of the medical assistant's job and present it in context to make it more relevant, thereby making it more memorable.

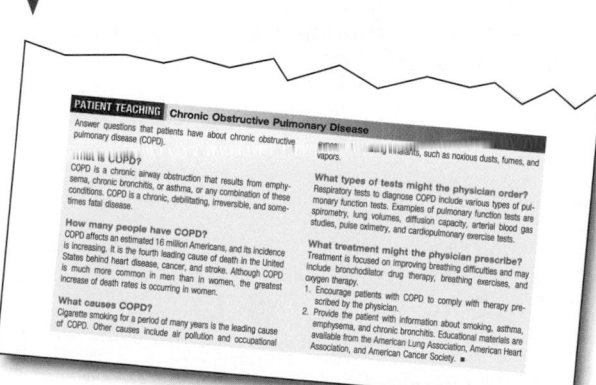

• Legal issues are important for medical assisting students to understand; it is damage control for the medical practice for which they will eventually work. **Medical Practice and the Law** boxes at the end of each chapter provide the student with current legal information pertaining to the chapter.

Continuing education is of utmost importance in such a rapidly changing profession. New techniques and developments in the field of medicine have a direct influence on the medical assisting profession. Continuing education helps the medical assistant maintain and improve existing skills and learn new skills. A list of helpful community resources for the medical assistant is found in Appendix C of this text.

The authors hope that individuals who use this approach to medical assisting will view this text not as a stopping place but as a means of opening doors to new paths to be explored in the medical assisting profession.

EXTENSIVE SUPPLEMENTAL RESOURCES
Student DVDs and CD-ROM

The most impressive feature of this textbook is the inclusion of clinical and administrative skills DVDs, which present many of the skills outlined in the textbook. An icon ● is placed next to the procedures in this text that are included on the DVDs. Students will have the invaluable opportunity to watch these procedures at home, on their own DVD players or computers. This should greatly enhance the learning of these clinical and administrative skills and provide the medical assistant graduate with competence and confi-

dence to perform clinical and administrative skills in the medical office.

A CD-ROM also accompanies the textbook and is designed for students to apply the theory and skills learned throughout the textbook. Organized by chapter, the CD includes Apply Your Knowledge questions and several games (i.e., "Quiz Show" and "Road to Recovery") to provide entertainment while learning important concepts related to selected chapters, matching exercises, labeling exercises, identification exercises, and other helpful activities for the student. An icon ● is placed at the end of each chapter to prompt students to access this CD.

Study Guide

The student *Study Guide* that accompanies the textbook greatly enhances the learning value of the textbook. In addition, its outcome-based approach meets the criteria required for outcome-based program accreditation as stipulated by the Commission on Accreditation of Allied Health Educational Programs (CAAHEP) and the Curriculum Review Board of the American Association of Medical Assistants (AAMA). Included are extensive exercises for each chapter, performance checklists, and a color board game, providing students with a fun way to refine their knowledge and skills. The study guide includes pretests and posttests, which help better prepare students for chapter tests, a textbook and student Study Guide assignment sheet for documenting completion of assignments and calculating points earned for each assignment, and a laboratory assignment sheet to keep track of student procedure performance.

Evolve Resources

The Evolve site includes all instructors' materials (for instructors only), content updates, **Apply Your Knowledge** review questions, **Prepare for Certification** exercises, a link to Clinical Medical Assisting Online, and more.

Clinical Medical Assisting Online

Clinical Medical Assisting Online is a complete online course that can stand alone as a distance education course (when combined with an on-site lab component) or provide additional reinforcement to a traditional classroom course. It covers all key accredited clinical competencies in an exciting, interactive format.

Clinical Medical Assisting Online

■ Module Outline ■ Lesson Outline Ⓖ Glossary ■ Clinic Floorplan   ◄ Previous ■ Screen 14 of 21 ■ Next ►

Lesson 1.1 Sanitizing Hands for Patient Safe Glossary

One important aspect of handwashing is turning on the water. Sounds easy, right? It is, but there are a few things that need to be considered, one of which is proper water temperature. Let's see if you can turn the water on to the correct temperature. Adjust the faucet below to the temperature needed to wash hands for Ⓖ medical asepsis.

Ms. Jenny Lee
Medical Assistant

Very Hot   Hot   Lukewarm   Cool   Cold

Once you've determined the correct water temperature, click **Next** to learn other things you need to consider when performing hand sanitization.

▲ Return to Top

Terms and Conditions | Privacy Policy | Contact Us | Copyright © 2007 Elsevier Inc. All rig
Evolve® is a registered trademark of Elsevier Inc. in the United States and/or other juris

Clinical Medical Assisting Online

■ Module Outline ■ Lesson Outline ■ Glossary ■ Clinic Floorplan   ◄ Previous ■ Screen 22 of 26 ■ Next ►

Lesson 1.2 Using Standard Precautions for Patient Safety

Well, that just about takes care of everything I wanted to make sure you understood before you learn the correct procedure for putting on, removing, and disposing of gloves, using standard precautions. Keep in mind everything Dr. Lopez and I have gone over with you when you are trying out the procedure for yourself, because this information can help protect you from exposure to disease and infection on the job.

The Training Activity includes a Guided Practice, which will introduce you to each step in the procedure for applying and removing gloves, as well as an Application Activity in which you will be expected to apply what you've learned. Click the Training Activity icon when you are ready to begin.

Ms. Jenny Lee
Medical Assistant

Practicing Standard Precautions

After you complete the Training Activity, click **Next** to continue.

▲ Return to Top   ◄ Previous ■ Next ►

Terms and Conditions | Privacy Policy | Contact Us | Copyright © 2007 Elsevier Inc. All rights reserved.
Evolve® is a registered trademark of Elsevier Inc. in the United States and/or other jurisdictions.

Acknowledgments

The completion of this text permits the opportunity to relay appreciation to the medical assisting educators who so eagerly and enthusiastically use and enjoy this text. To them the authors are also indebted for their helpful assistance and suggestions for this new text.

The photographs in the textbook were taken by Brian Blauser and Jack Foley, professional photographers. We are indebted to them for their careful precision and patience in taking and editing the photographs, thus greatly enhancing the learning value of this text.

We would like to gratefully acknowledge the following practicing medical assistants for contributing many hours to be photographed for demonstration of the clinical procedures in the text: Megan Baer, Dawn Bennett, Trudy Browning, Janet Canterbury, Theresa Cline, Marlyne Cooper, Hope Fauber, Dori Glover, Jennifer Hawk, Kevin Hickey, Cammie Lindner, Judy Markins, Korey McGrew, Natalie Morehead, Traci Powell, Linda Proffitt, Latisha Sharpe, Michelle Shockey, Kara Van Dyke, Michelle Villers, and Huang Ying.

We would also like to acknowledge the following individuals who portrayed patients in the text: Brian Adevc, Travis Allman, Jessica Bennett, Kim Bingham, Pamela Bitting, Caitlin Brennan, David Brennan, Hollie Bonewit, Phillip Carr, Chloe Cline, Angie Coffin, Chad Cron, Dawn Decaminada, Aja Fox, Markly Georges, Connie Hazlett, Gary Hazlett, Isabella Ipacs, Joey Ipacs, Susan Ipacs, Charles Larimer, Pam Larimer, Christopher Mace, Deborah Murray, Delaney Murray, Michael Nkrumah, Heather Pike, Jan Six,

Megan Skidmore, Colton Smith, Sydney Smith, Clinton Swart, Tristen West, and Lynn Witkowski.

We would like to extend our appreciation to the authors, publishers, and equipment companies who have granted us permission to use their illustrations.

The publication of this text was accomplished through the capable guidance of many talented individuals at Elsevier. Many thanks to Kristine Feeherty for her outstanding production work. This book could not have attained this level of excellence without the exceptional capabilities of Jennifer Bertucci, Associate Developmental Editor. Julia Dummitt created these beautiful interior and cover designs. And, finally, we want to relay a very special thank you to Michael Ledbetter, Publisher, for his dedication to quality medical assisting education and his encouragement in helping us achieve our very best in this edition.

With warm regard, we would like to recognize those very important individuals—the medical assisting students, graduates, and practicing medical assistants—who continually strive for excellence in meeting the demands and ever-increasing requirements of such a challenging profession. A quote by an unknown author really says it better: "Celebrate your talents, for they are what make you unique."

Kathy Bonewit-West, BS, MEd
Sue A. Hunt, MA, RN, CMA (AAMA)
Edith Applegate, MS

CAAHEP competencies used on chapter and section openers with permission from the American Association of Medical Assistants, Chicago, Illinois; and the Commission on Accreditation of Allied Health Education Programs, Clearwater, Florida.
ABHES competencies used on chapter and section openers with permission from the Accrediting Bureau of Health Education Schools, Falls Church, Virginia.

Clinical Procedure Icons

The OSHA Bloodborne Pathogens Standard must be followed when performing many of the clinical procedures presented in this text. To assist the student in following the OSHA Standard, icons have been incorporated into the procedures. An illustration of each icon along with its description is outlined below.

HAND HYGIENE is an important medical aseptic practice and is crucial in preventing the transmission of pathogens in the medical office. The medical assistant should sanitize the hands frequently, using proper technique. When performing clinical procedures, the hands should always be sanitized before and after patient contact, before applying gloves and after removing gloves, and after contact with blood or other potentially infectious materials.

CLEAN DISPOSABLE GLOVES should be worn when it is reasonably anticipated that you will have hand contact with the following: blood and other potentially infectious materials, mucous membranes, non-intact skin, and contaminated articles or surfaces.

BIOHAZARD CONTAINERS are closable, leakproof, and suitably constructed to contain the contents during handling, storage, transport, or shipping. The containers must be labeled or color coded and closed before removal to prevent the contents from spilling.

APPROPRIATE PROTECTIVE CLOTHING such as gowns, aprons, and laboratory coats should be worn when gross contamination can reasonably be anticipated during performance of a task or procedure.

FACE SHIELDS OR MASKS IN COMBINATION WITH EYE-PROTECTION DEVICES must be worn whenever splashes, spray, spatter, or droplets of blood or other potentially infectious materials may be generated, posing a hazard through contact with your eyes, nose, or mouth.

Contents

Section 3: Clinical Component

1

The Health Care System

LEARNING OBJECTIVES

Instructional Objectives
1. Describe the role of medical office care in the health care system.
2. Describe the historical development of managed care.
3. Identify the flow of activity in ambulatory care.
4. Identify the various types of health care professionals, and describe the job responsibilities of each professional.
5. State the educational requirements for physicians.
6. List and describe the parts of the medical office.
7. Identify and describe the various types of medical specialties.
8. Identify three medical practice types.
9. Compare and contrast various complementary and traditional medical treatments.

CHAPTER OUTLINE

Introduction to Health and the Health Care System
Shift from Hospital-Based to Community-Based Health Care
Managed Care versus Patient Care: Competing Forces
  Facing the Medical Office in the Twenty-First Century
    Fee-for-Service Insurance Plans
    Government Insurance Plans
    Managed Care
Ambulatory Care
    Flow of Activity in Ambulatory Care
    The Health Care Team
Parts of the Medical Office
    Reception Area and Waiting Room
    Examination Rooms and Laboratory

    Medical Records Storage and Business Office
    Additional Areas Found in Many Offices
Medical Specialties
    Primary Care
    Osteopathy
    Podiatry
    Chiropractic
Practice Types
    Solo Practice
    Group Practice
    Clinic
Complementary and Alternative Medicine

CAAHEP CONTENT

Medical Law and Ethics
Legal Guidelines/Requirements for Health Care

Professional Components
Allied Health Professionals and Credentialing

ABHES CONTENT

Medical Terminology
Medical Specialties and Short Forms

Medical Law and Ethics
Ethical Decisions, Jurisprudence, and Confidentiality

KEY TERMS

ambulatory (AM-byoo-la-toe-ree) care
capitation (cap-ih-TAY-shun)
empirically (em-PEER-ih-clee)
fee-for-service
formulary (FORM-you-lay-ree)
health insurance

holistic (hole-IH-stick)
managed care
palliative (PAL-ee-a-tive) treatment
residency (RES-ih-dense-ee)
symptomatic (simp-toe-MA-tick) treatment
utilization review

Introduction to Health and the Health Care System

The World Health Organization (WHO) defines health as the absence of illness or disease and a state of being in which the individual feels well and is able to carry out the daily functions of life with no difficulties and no pain. In reality, no one reaches this optimum level of health. Everyone has aches and pains, psychological if not physical.

In our health care system, the physician's responsibility is to examine hundreds of people in the course of a week and try to focus on medical problems that meet the following criteria: The problem is causing or can cause severe difficulties in carrying out the daily functions of life. In addition, the problem can be treated either by reducing the effects of the symptoms or by eradicating the problem altogether.

Each individual the physician sees presents with a different group of physical symptoms, as well as a different set of social circumstances and emotional issues. The physician listens to the patient's description of his or her life, performs objective laboratory and diagnostic tests, identifies medical problems, and assesses the nature of each problem.

Physicians know that the vast majority of medical problems do not pose a long-term threat to health. Most medical conditions get better over time. Effective treatments are available to cure many conditions. In other cases the physician can reduce the symptoms even if the underlying medical condition is not significantly affected. This type of treatment is called **symptomatic treatment** (responding to symptoms) or **palliative treatment** (seeking to reduce the effects of a disease or condition without curing the underlying disease). For example, a patient who has diabetes mellitus receives palliative treatment. The patient is prescribed insulin, which alleviates the symptoms of the diabetes; however, the treatment does not cure the diabetes.

Most treatments are based on scientific study. In Western scientific medicine, as in no other medical tradition, approaches to diagnosis and treatment have been studied and tested over hundreds of years. As long ago as the fourth century BC, a physician named Hippocrates in Greece believed that disease was not a punishment for transgressions against the gods, but rather the result of physiologic

and environmental factors that could be studied. Since the time of Hippocrates, the practice of medicine has changed considerably, but this underlying belief has remained constant (Table 1-1).

SHIFT FROM HOSPITAL-BASED TO COMMUNITY-BASED HEALTH CARE

Three trends running in parallel through modern medicine have led to an increasingly important role for office-based health care, also known as *ambulatory health care.*

The first trend is the desire by those who pay the bills—employers, the federal and state governments, and insurance companies—to reduce the costs of health care whenever and wherever possible.

A second trend is the pressure for medical offices and clinics to provide a broad range of diagnostic and treatment services to avoid having to admit patients to the hospital. The increased cost of hospitalization has provided this pressure. Developments in diagnostic equipment, increased availability of home health care, and less invasive surgical procedures have facilitated the process.

The third trend is an increased understanding, through empiric evidence and research on outcomes, that people *feel better* the less they must be confined to a hospital or go to a hospital for treatment. Being able to be diagnosed and treated in an outpatient setting with follow-up at home allows people to feel more in control of their lives as medical patients. This is especially important for people who have frequent contact with the medical system, such as the parents of infants and children, the elderly, and those with chronic illnesses. Many people who would have been hospitalized for long periods or possibly even institutionalized 50, 25, or even 10 years ago are currently living independently in the community.

Today the hospital's role is primarily to provide acute care and diagnostic services. In order to be hospitalized, the patient's condition must be unstable or require constant regulation of therapy. If the patient does not meet these strict criteria, he or she either goes home to be followed as an outpatient; is transferred to a rehabilitation facility for intense, regular rehabilitative treatment; or is sent to a nursing home for long-term maintenance care.

Table 1-1 Milestones in the History of Medicine

3000 BC	Writings about the circulation of blood in China
c. 460 BC	Birth of Hippocrates (called the "Father of Medicine") in Greece—based medical care on observation and believed that illness was a natural biologic event
1514-1564	Andreas Vesalius—wrote the first relatively correct anatomy textbook
1578-1657	William Harvey—discovered circulation of blood (England)
1632-1723	Antony van Leeuwenhoek—discovered the microscope (Holland)
1728-1793	John Hunter—developed surgical techniques used in surgery
1749-1823	Edward Jenner—first vaccine for smallpox (England)
1818-1865	Ignaz Semmelweis—theorized that handwashing prevents childbirth fever (Austria); his theories were rejected during his lifetime and not accepted until the work of Pasteur and Lister
1820-1910	Florence Nightingale—began training for nurses; established first nursing school; before this time nurses received no training and the profession had little status (England)
1821-1912	Clara Barton—acted as a nurse on the battlefields of the Civil War; was a civil rights activist and suffragette; organized the American Red Cross
1821-1910	Elizabeth Blackwell—first woman to complete medical school in the United States; established a medical school in Europe for women only
1822-1895	Louis Pasteur—pasteurization of wine, beer, and milk to prevent growth of microorganisms; microbiology (France)
1827-1912	Joseph Lister—demonstrated that microorganisms cause illness; his experiments with phenol, carbolic acid, and other antiseptics laid the groundwork for modern surgery (England)
Mid-1800s	First large hospitals established in U.S. cities such as Bellevue, Johns Hopkins, and Massachusetts General. Discovery of anesthesia in the United States is credited to a Southern physician named Crawford Williamson Long
1843-1910	Robert Koch—isolated the bacteria that cause anthrax and cholera; established principles to determine that a specific bacteria causes a specific disease (German)
1845-1923	Wilhelm Roentgen—discovered x-rays (Germany) based on the discovery of radium and radioactivity by Marie (1867-1934) and Pierre Curie (1859-1906)
1851-1902	Walter Reed—a U.S. Army physician who proved that yellow fever is transmitted by mosquitoes, not direct contact. An aggressive spraying program made it possible to complete the Panama canal
1854-1915	Paul Ehrlich—coined the term *chemotherapy;* predicted autoimmunity; developed Salvarsan (arsphenamine), an effective treatment for syphilis in 1909. This led to the development of sulfa drugs and other antibiotics (Germany)
1881-1955	Alexander Fleming—discovered penicillin (England); identified it in 1929, but an efficient method of producing large amounts was not developed until needed in World War II. Other antibiotic medications such as sulfa were soon discovered
1891-1941	Frederick Banting—codiscoverer of insulin with Charles Best and John Macleod in 1922 (Canada)
1906-1993	Albert Sabin—developed oral polio vaccine
1914-1995	Jonas Salk—developed parenteral polio vaccine
1922-2001	Christian Neethling Barnard—South African surgeon who is remembered for succeeding at the first human-to-human heart transplant in 1967
1978	Birth of Louise Joy Brown, the first child born by in vitro fertilization, in Great Britain

Modified from Hunt SA: *Saunders fundamentals of medical assisting,* St. Louis, 2007, Saunders.

MANAGED CARE VERSUS PATIENT CARE: COMPETING FORCES FACING THE MEDICAL OFFICE IN THE TWENTY-FIRST CENTURY

Fee-for-Service Insurance Plans

Traditionally, medical care in the United States was paid for on a **fee-for-service** basis. Each service was billed and paid for as a separate charge: so much for the office visit, so much for the electrocardiogram, so much for the urinalysis, and so on. Fee-for-service payments can be thought of as ordering food at a restaurant à la carte: so much for the main course, so much for a salad, so much for coffee.

During the first part of the twentieth century, health insurance (if the patient had any) paid only for hospitalization and usually the patient completed most of the paperwork. **Health insurance** is a system by which a person or the person's employer pays an insurance company a yearly amount of money, and the insurance company pays some or most of the person's medical expenses for that year. The theory behind insurance is that, although a few people will have large medical bills over the course of the year, most people will have small bills. By setting the fee for everyone at a level above the actual cost of care for most people, the insurance company can pay for the care of the

Highlight on the History of Medical Treatment of Infectious Disease

Historians generally place the beginning of Western medicine with Hippocrates (c. 460-377 BC), a Greek physician who saw medicine as an independent discipline based on clinical practice rather than prayer and ritual. For several centuries there were few treatment methods other than rest, exercise, diet, and a few medications derived from plants. The intensive study of the human body in the 1500s fostered a better understanding of physiologic processes. For example, the English scientist William Harvey (1578-1657), who rejected the traditional belief that blood was made up of "spirits" and that body fluids were "humors," developed a theory, later proved true, that blood flows from the heart to the lungs, throughout the body via arteries, and back to the heart via veins.

Early microscope, about 1765. (Courtesy the Blocker History of Medicine Collections, Moody Medical Library, The University of Texas Medical Branch, Galveston, Tex.)

Physician in the Middle Ages taking a patient's pulse and holding a flask of urine. (Courtesy the Blocker History of Medicine Collections, Moody Medical Library, The University of Texas Medical Branch, Galveston, Tex.)

The first microscopic lens was invented in 1677 by Antony van Leeuwenhoek (1632-1723). Through his microscope van Leeuwenhoek saw yeasts, molds, and algae, adding evidence to the theory that diseases could be caused by particles too small to be seen with the eyes. He also identified red blood cells passing through capillaries.

Throughout the nineteenth century, other scientists and physicians advanced the understanding of the cause of disease. Some found ways to combat disease without understanding the mechanism by which the disease acted; others determined the actual cause of a particular disease.

In the 1840s the Viennese obstetric assistant Ignaz Semmelweis discovered that puerperal fever, or so-called childbed fever, a fatal illness of women who had just given birth, could be reduced if physicians washed their hands. He came to believe that physicians were infecting women by transferring bacteria from one woman to another.

Extracting blood for a transfusion, eighteenth century. (Courtesy the National Library of Medicine.)

Highlight on the History of Medical Treatment of Infectious Disease—cont'd

Semmelweis conducted what today would be called an *epidemiologic study*. He studied the records of women who had died and determined which physicians and medical students had attended which birth. His study of the records led him to conclude that most of the women who died had been attended to by physicians and medical students who had come into the birthing room directly from the anatomy laboratory, where they had worked with cadavers, without first washing their hands. Most of Semmelweis's colleagues dismissed his notion that simple handwashing could reduce childbirth deaths as nonsense, and during his lifetime, Semmelweis was ridiculed. It was not until decades later that physicians regularly began washing their hands.

The Scottish surgeon Joseph Lister (1827-1912) worked on similar ideas to develop the first practice of antisepsis (cleaning areas where germs may be) and later asepsis (creating a germ-free environment). Lister started by pouring carbolic acid on the wounds of those who had just had surgery. Over time, he found milder substances. Lister found that far fewer patients who were treated with these substances died from gangrene that developed in their open wounds.

Semmelweis, Lister, and others worked **empirically,** which means they determined a result through experimentation that proved the event could be repeated with the same results. They never completely understood what caused infectious diseases. Other scientists sought to determine that bacteria caused specific diseases.

The German physician Robert Koch (1843-1910) is called the "Father of Microbiology" because of his work with specific bacteria such as *Mycobacterium tuberculosis*, the bacterial agent that causes tuberculosis. Koch also isolated the bacterial agent that causes anthrax. Koch grew the anthrax bacterium in a number of different liquid media in his laboratory. He determined that all of them carried the same virulence, the potential for infection. Koch established that bacteria do not die out naturally. Today we know that it is possible to break the chain of illness by keeping those who are contagious away from those who are vulnerable to disease.

Koch's methods are used to prove that a particular infectious agent is causing a disease in more than one individual. He isolated a specific microorganism by identifying it microscopically, injected the organism into a healthy animal, waited for the animal to become sick, and then recovered the same organism from the sick animal.

The work of Louis Pasteur and Koch, among others, helped set the stage for the understanding of infectious disease and for worldwide vaccination programs to eradicate smallpox and to try to eradicate the "childhood illnesses" of mumps, measles, and rubella (German measles).

The first vaccination actually had occurred a century earlier. Edward Jenner (1749-1823), an English physician in the farming country of Gloucestershire, used the pus from one person's cowpox lesion to vaccinate another individual against smallpox in 1796.

Edward Jenner vaccinating an infant. (Courtesy the National Library of Medicine.)

Cowpox is a variant of smallpox. It is lethal to animals but relatively harmless to humans. For centuries, people had realized that people who had been infected with cowpox did not develop smallpox. Today, we understand what had happened—their immune systems had developed antibodies that prevented smallpox infection by attacking the smallpox virus.

Before Jenner, physicians had tried to immunize people against smallpox through a method known as *variolation,* deliberately infecting a person with a mild smallpox infection by taking the pus from a smallpox lesion. Variolation usually led to only mild cases of smallpox in those deliberately infected, but they remained contagious and unfortunately were able to pass on lethal cases to others.

Jenner used "humanized cowpox," taking pus from a lesion on a human and rubbing it into an open wound on another human. A couple of weeks later, he inoculated the second person with smallpox. Not only did the individual not become ill, but he also was not contagious. A century later Pasteur would discover fully the mechanism by which vaccination works. Vaccines were discovered for many diseases. By the beginning of the twentieth century, vaccines had been developed for diphtheria and tetanus, and most children received these vaccines as infants by the middle of the twentieth century. The development of the parenteral polio vaccine by Jonas Salk in 1952 led to a mass vaccination program of schoolchildren in the United States. This was repeated in the 1960s using the Sabin oral polio vaccine.

Medications to kill bacteria were another important tool in the fight against infectious disease. Paul Ehrlich is credited with the development of the first medication to kill bacteria. In 1909 he developed a drug called *Salvarsan* (arsphenamine), which could be used to effectively treat syphilis. Unfortunately the medication itself was extremely toxic. The first of the sulfanilamide drugs, Prontosil, was developed in 1932 in Germany. It was effective against infections caused by streptococci and some other types of bacteria. The

Continued

Highlight on the History of Medical Treatment of Infectious Disease—cont'd

sulfanilamides became popular before and during World War II because they were the only antiinfective agents widely available. Penicillin, a mold that kills bacteria, had been discovered in 1922 by Alexander Fleming in London after it attacked bacteria that he was growing on agar plates. Initially the scientific community did not believe that it would be effective inside the body, and little follow-up research was done. During World War II, two medical researchers, Howard Florey and Ernst Chain, took up the research on penicillin and managed to prove that the medication was effective. The first human was treated in 1941, and within a few years mass production had been established and penicillin was in widespread use.

Discovery of the first virus is credited to Dimitri Ivanowski, a Russian botanist, in 1892. He discovered that a substance could pass through a ceramic filter that trapped all known bacteria and still cause a disease of tobacco called *mosaic tobacco disease*. We now know that the culprit is the tobacco mosaic virus. Yellow fever was the first viral disease of humans to be identified. During construction of the Panama Canal, workers were devastated by this disease. Research done by Walter Reed (1851-1902) established that the disease was caused by a virus

transmitted by mosquitoes and not direct contact. Controlling mosquitoes facilitated the work on the canal. The development of the electron microscope in 1930 allowed viruses to be seen, but progress to control viral diseases was slow. For most viruses the body has adequate defenses to overcome the infection, but there are some significant exceptions. The retroviruses, such as human immunodeficiency virus (HIV), are notable because they are able to overcome the body's immune system. In the 1970s the first deaths from acquired immune deficiency syndrome (AIDS) were reported in the United States. Within the next 20 years, a worldwide epidemic occurred. By 1997 more than 6 million deaths worldwide had been caused by the AIDS virus. Treatments have been developed to slow the progression of the disease, but to date there is no effective immunization or cure for this disease. The World Health Organization currently takes a more proactive role to prevent the spread of highly contagious and serious viral diseases such as severe acute respiratory syndrome (SARS). Measures are also being taken to control avian influenza, a serious disease of birds that can be passed to humans from birds, although currently human-to-human contact has not been documented. ■

---

well, the occasionally ill, and the often ill and still make a profit.

This system encouraged health care providers to provide a high level of care for everyone with health insurance because the insurance paid for every test and every procedure. Physicians' incomes soared between the end of World War II and the early 1980s. With the increasing costs of laboratory and diagnostic testing, hospital services, and office visits, the cost of medical care increased far more rapidly than the cost of other goods and services in the U.S. economy. (In economic terms, health care inflation increased much more rapidly than the general rate of inflation.)

During this time, ever-better health insurance became a standard employee benefit at many companies. The first kind of health insurance offered, in the 1950s and 1960s, was coverage for hospital care. Coverage for office visits became standard in the 1970s.

Government Insurance Plans

Recognizing that there were large segments of the population without insurance because they are not employed, the federal government began to provide health insurance to large segments of the population starting in the 1960s. Medicaid began to provide health insurance for low-income children without parental support and later expanded to cover all low-income people. Medicare provides health insurance for the elderly, disabled, and those with end-stage kidney disease. CHAMPUS (now called TRICARE) provided health insurance for dependents of active-duty mili-

tary personnel. With these programs, the federal government has become the primary insurer for more than 50 million Americans. These plans, which included payments for office visits for illness, greatly increased the number of Americans who had medical insurance. There was little incentive for the consumer (the patient) to control costs because insurance was covering those costs and in most cases was "free" to the consumer.

Although most Americans who were insured did not feel that they were "paying" for their medical care, they were, indirectly. The huge increases in health care costs were one of the major sources of the generally high rates of inflation in the 1970s. Employers, who paid for the insurance, had to pay ever-rising premiums and offset these large premium increases with small increases in cash wages, which did not keep up with inflation. So American workers did, in fact, pay for health insurance and health care costs in lower purchasing power for the cash they received as salary.

Managed Care   *formulary*

The expansion of health care to cover office visits originally only covered visits for illness or injury and did not cover so-called routine care (well-child visits, immunizations, regular check-ups, or physical examinations).

Health maintenance organizations (HMOs) were originally formed with a belief that consistent, routine care would help prevent later expensive care. The theory was that increasing prevention and promoting early detection and diagnosis of chronic and life-threatening medical conditions would reduce costs. The HMO movement, which gained acceptance in the 1970s, pushed traditional health insurance companies to begin providing coverage for routine care.

In the late 1970s, insurance companies began to respond to escalating health care costs by reviewing care to find out if it was medically necessary. This process, called **utilization review,** identified patients who, according to the insurance companies, no longer needed to be hospitalized. Originally, utilization review was used by Medicare and Medicaid. Other insurance companies soon realized that shortening hospital stays was an important way of reducing overall health care costs. The combination of HMO insurance plans and strict utilization review for hospitalized patients is the basis of what we call **managed care.**

The original HMO model had two components: insurance and the provision of services including diagnostic tests and pharmacy. HMO plans set up full-service medical clinics. Physicians were employees. The HMO established a contractual relationship with a hospital for inpatient services, and patients had to go to the specific hospital with which the HMO had a contract.

In the later 1980s, a second type of HMO model based on networks of physicians who agreed to provide care for HMO patients came into being. Some of these networks operated under the old fee-for-service plans but agreed to discounted fees from the HMOs in exchange for access to the rapidly growing patient populations enrolled in HMOs. In an effort to reduce payments, HMOs tried to have physicians accept a flat monthly fee for each subscriber in their practice and agree to provide all necessary primary care for that fee. This type of payment is called **capitation.** This reduces the incentive to provide extra services because they will not be reimbursed separately.

The managed care movement in general, as well as the trend to decrease reimbursement for primary care in particular, put the burden on physicians to compete with each other to provide the most care for the least money. As a result, physicians feel pressure to limit diagnostic tests, reduce hospitalizations and the number of days patients stay in the hospital, and use generic instead of brand-name drugs. (Generics are identical in chemical formulation to brand-name drugs and can only be manufactured after the brand-name drug's patent protection has expired.)

Managed care also puts pressure on physicians to see more patients, spend less time with each patient, and justify all services including diagnostic tests and referrals. The expense of handling sicker patients is expected to be balanced by those patients who use less than the average amount of medical services.

In addition, insurance plans have tried to reduce their costs for prescription medications by restricting what drugs physicians can prescribe by devising lists of approved drugs. Such a list, called a **formulary,** usually limits physicians to one or two of the less expensive drugs for each possible medical condition. Exceptions are made if the physician can

show that the less expensive drugs have been ineffective for his or her patient and that a more expensive drug is necessary. In some plans the patient can receive a more expensive medication by paying more of the cost.

Despite these measures, however, in the late 1990s, insurance premiums began to increase at more than double and even triple the underlying rate of inflation. Managed care plans, even those that had instituted capitation in the early 1990s, saw their ability to limit costs severely hampered. In addition, prescription drug costs increased more than 15% per year in the late 1990s.

Consumers and physicians both became increasingly upset about the control of medical practice exacted by insurance companies. Physicians began banding together in larger groups to negotiate more rigorously with insurance companies. In many areas primary care practices were closed because they were losing money. It remains to be seen how managed care will evolve and respond to consumer and physician dissatisfaction.

Each form of providing health care services has advantages and disadvantages. A comparison of managed care and fee-for-service care is shown in Table 1-2.

AMBULATORY CARE

There is no such thing as a "typical" medical office. The style of any particular medical office depends on the personality of the physician or physicians who practice there, as well as the general population of patients who come there. Regardless of the physician's personality and the patients' personal background, the same kinds of activities occur in any physician's office setting.

Today, the trend in medical care is toward an increasing amount of **ambulatory care**—defined as the patient coming to the care rather than the patient receiving care in a home or hospital setting (Figure 1-1). To take advantage of ambulatory care, the patient must be able to walk into the physician's office or at least be brought to the office in a wheelchair. In addition to private physicians' offices, offices of physicians who make up a staff model HMO, community health centers, multispecialty clinics, and hospitals are increasingly making more space available for outpatient care.

Flow of Activity in Ambulatory Care

Regardless of the organizational setup of the physician's office, the flow of activities for each patient will be similar. The patient will do the following:
- Enter the office
- Approach the reception area, identify the physician and time of appointment, provide the office staff with personal and payment information, and make a copayment (if necessary)
- Be seen by a physician (or by a nurse practitioner or physician assistant if the practice uses such personnel)
- Undergo any necessary diagnostic or laboratory tests
- Receive a diagnosis, treatment, or a referral to another health care provider

Table 1-2 Comparison of Managed Care and Traditional Fee-for-Service Insurance Plans

Managed Care	Traditional Fee-for-Service
Physician Choice	**Physician Choice**
Patient must see a member physician	Patient can see any physician
Primary provider refers to specialists	Patient can choose to see a specialist
Patient may be seen by a provider other than own primary provider	Patient always sees physician of choice
Services	**Services**
Plan pays for routine and preventative care, as well as illness and injury	Plan covers illness or injury only
Each plan has own guidelines and schedules about how often routine procedures can be done	
Each plan has guidelines about what type of tests and treatment can be ordered for a specific diagnosis	Physician can order any tests or treatment
Plan pays part or all of medication, although the patient may be responsible for a greater portion if the medication is not on the list approved by the plan	Medications not covered
Plan pays part or all of other services such as eye examinations, glasses	Nonmedical services not covered
Patient Payments	**Patient Payments**
Patient pays a set fee (copayment) each visit or service	Patient pays an annual fee (deductible) and set percent of each service (coinsurance)
Insurance Payments	**Insurance Payments**
Physician may receive an annual payment for each patient (capitation) or may be paid by service at a significant discount from usual charge for the service	Physician paid by service; actual amount varies according to insurance; government plans may pay much less than the usual charge for the service

From Hunt SA: *Saunders fundamentals of medical assisting,* St. Louis, 2007, Saunders.

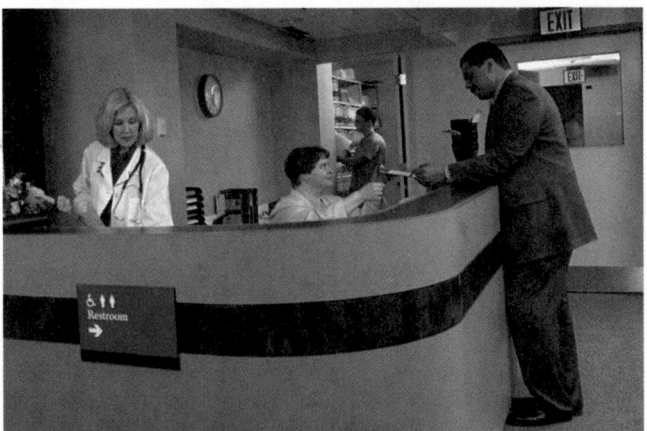

Figure 1-1. The patient check-in area in a clinic. (From Hunt SA: *Saunders fundamentals of medical assisting*, St. Louis, 2007, Saunders.)

- Receive instruction for follow-up care and any additional diagnostic tests before leaving the medical office; if seriously ill, the patient may be admitted to the hospital

Figure 1-2 is a flowchart of how a patient moves through the medical office.

Once a patient has been seen in the medical office, the office begins the process of obtaining payment for its services. The medical payment may come from a private insurance plan, a government-funded insurance program, and/or

from the patient. The patient may be responsible for a percentage of the charges or the entire bill if he or she does not have insurance.

After the examination, the patient receives instructions such as patient preparation for a test or procedure to be performed or information on medication that has been prescribed. Patients who are seen regularly because of a chronic illness may spend time with a physician or medical assistant reviewing the patient's individual treatment plan. A follow-up appointment is made if necessary.

Most medical offices provide health education materials in the waiting room. These materials may consist of pamphlets, article reprints, health education videos, or health news reports specially prepared for viewing in the medical office.

The Health Care Team

A medical assistant works as a member of a dedicated health care team. The physician or group of physicians expects each medical assistant to fill a slightly different role within the office team. This role will depend on the style of the practice, the region of the country where the practice is located, and what other types of medical professionals staff the team.

As the operations of a medical practice become more complex, physicians may employ individuals with more specialized medical business and medical management experience to run the business side of the office. In these offices, medical assistants play more of a clinical role. In

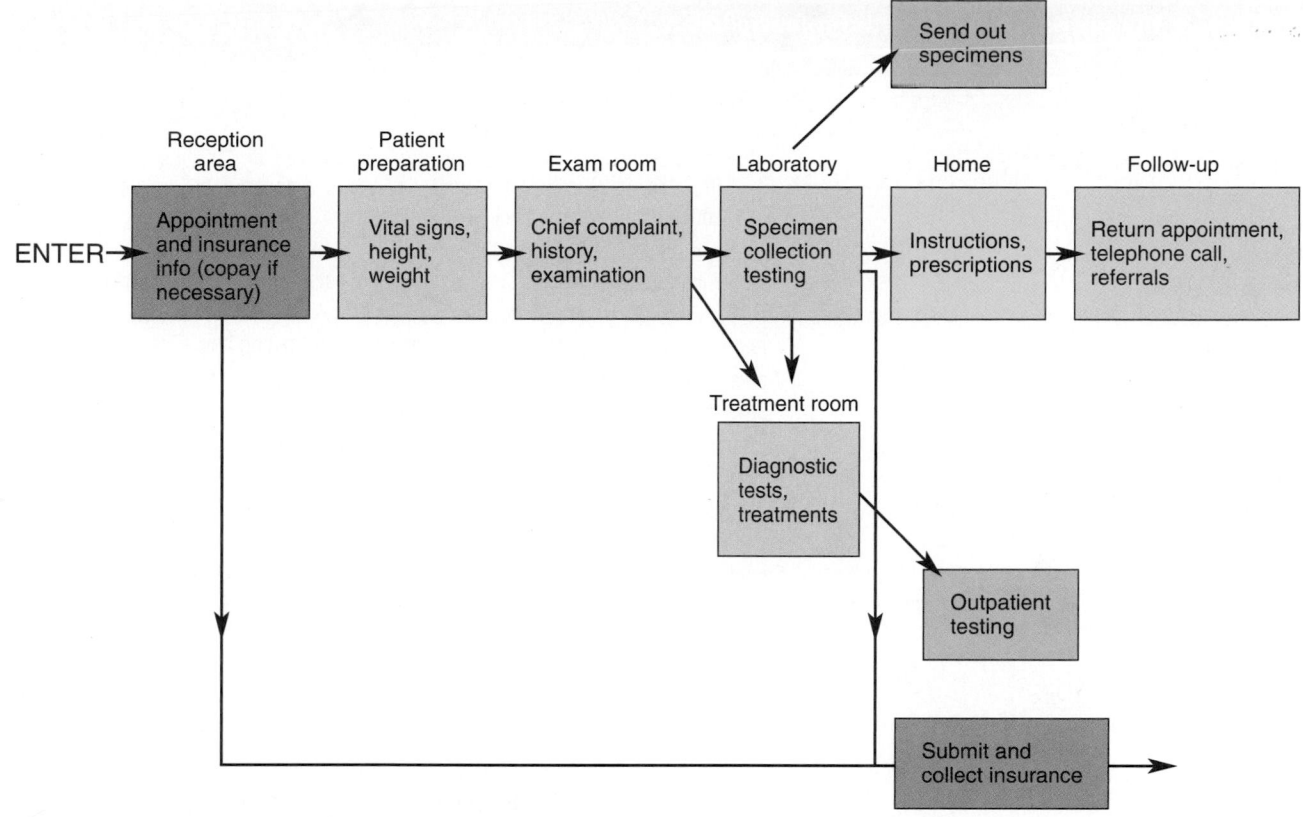

Figure 1-2. Patient progress through a medical office. (From Hunt SA: *Saunders fundamentals of medical assisting*, St. Louis, 2007, Saunders.)

Putting It All into Practice

My name is Aida Reyes, and I am the medical assistant for a primary care physician. I have been working here for 12 years, and in that time it seems to get busier and busier. We used to see about 15 patients in a typical morning or afternoon, and now we are seeing an average of 20 to 25. When I first took the job, I thought it would be a fairly relaxed environment. How busy could it be with only one physician? I didn't take into account all the different things I would have to do. I have to open the office, prepare for the day's patients, check patients in, assist the physician, check patients out, pull the charts for the next day's patients, restock the examination rooms, and close the office. Even though there is a receptionist and a file clerk working part time, I never catch up on the paperwork. I also have to do all the referrals myself because so many patients have some type of managed care insurance. We are fortunate to have a laboratory on the first floor of our building, but I still have to make sure that all laboratory requisitions are filled out completely for our patients. ∎

Prepare for Success

smaller offices, medical assistants usually perform both clinical and administrative activities.

Members of the Health Care Team

The members of the medical team who typically work in ambulatory care, be it a private practice, a community or public health clinic, or a hospital clinic, include physicians, nurse practitioners (NPs), physician assistants (PAs), medical assistants, registered nurses or licensed practical nurses, a business manager, a receptionist, a medical secretary, file clerks, and one or more insurance specialists. Medical transcription is occasionally done in the medical office, but increasingly it is outsourced or replaced by the electronic medical record. If the office performs moderate- or high-complexity laboratory tests, a certified medical technologist may also be on the staff or serve as a consultant.

Hospital or community-based clinics will possibly also have a staff of social workers, outreach workers, and case managers to provide social services to patients. Practices specializing in women's health (obstetrics/gynecology) may also have certified nurse-midwives.

Table 1-3 lists various nurses and allied health professionals and describes their roles.

Physicians and Other Health Care Providers

Physicians have either an MD (medical physician) or DO (doctor of osteopathy) degree, either of which is received

Table 1-3 Nurses and Allied Health Professionals

Occupation	Credentials	Responsibilities
Certified Coding Specialist–Physician-Based	CCS-P	Assigns codes to patient charges and diagnoses for insurance billing
Diagnostic Medical Sonographer	DMS	Performs ultrasound scans in hospitals and ambulatory care facilities. Ultrasound uses high-frequency sound waves to produce images. A sonographer may specialize in ultrasound of the heart (echocardiography)
Dietician Dietetic Technician	RD; DTR	Assists with nutrition of patients in hospitals and ambulatory care. Performs nutrition screening and counseling. Coordinates all aspects of food service in many settings
Emergency Medical Technician/ Paramedic	EMT; paramedic	Provides emergency services and life support in the community. Several levels of emergency service personnel exist, depending on training and experience
Health Information Specialist	RHIA; RHIT	Works with patient medical records; may provide assistance in planning, managing information, gathering data for medical research, and policy making
Medical Assistant	CMA (AAMA); RMA	Performs administrative and clinical tasks in ambulatory care
Medical Laboratory Technologist	MLT; MT	Performs laboratory tests in the clinical laboratory and may supervise laboratory operations or provide consulting services
Medical Secretary	CMS	Secretary who specializes in administrative procedures in a health care setting
Nuclear Medicine Technologist	CNMT	Operates cameras that detect and form images from radioactive isotopes in a patient's body
Nurse, Practical	LPN; LVN	Performs direct patient care and clinical procedures. May work in hospitals, nursing homes, and ambulatory care settings
Nurse Practitioner	NP	Specializes in a specific area such as internal medicine, pediatrics, and women's health and often manages routine patient care in ambulatory care settings
Nurse, Registered	RN	Plans and provides nursing care in inpatient settings. Provides supervision for caregivers in both inpatient and outpatient settings
Occupational Therapist Occupational Therapy Assistant	OT; OTA	Plans therapeutic activities for rehabilitation, especially for activities of daily living (ADLs). Implements treatment plans
Physical Therapist Physical Therapy Assistant	PT; PTA	Plans exercises for large muscle groups for rehabilitation and implements treatment plans
Physician Assistant	PA	Manages routine patient care under the supervision of a physician. Usually works in ambulatory care
Radiologic Technologist Nuclear Medicine Technologist	RT	Takes x-rays and assists with special radiographic examinations. After completing education, may specialize in nuclear medicine, computed tomography, mammography, or therapeutic radiation. A nuclear medicine technologist operates devices that detect and map absorption of radioactive substances given by injection to create diagnostic images
Respiratory Therapist	RRT	Provides respiratory treatments and manages patients on ventilators
Surgical Technologist	CST	Assists during surgery in hospital and day surgery centers by setting up operating rooms, preparing instruments and equipment, and passing instruments during surgery

after 4 years of college, then 4 years of medical or osteopathic school. In addition, they complete a hospital-based, intensive postgraduate training period, traditionally called a **residency,** which lasts from 2 to 7 years, depending on the specialty. To receive a medical license from the state where he or she will practice, the physician must pass Parts I, II, and III of the U.S. Medical Licensing Examination (USMLE). The first two parts of the examination are taken during medical school, but Part III cannot be taken until the physician has completed at least 1 year of residency (sometimes called an *internship*).

If a physician wants to be "board certified" in a specialty, he or she must pass another examination, administered by the certification board of the particular specialty. The physi-

cian does not need to be board certified to obtain a state license to practice medicine.

A physician assistant (PA) must have at least 2 years of college, plus 2 years of physician assistant school, although most PA programs award a master's degree. A physician assistant usually specializes (e.g., pediatrics, adult medicine) and manages a group of patients receiving routine care. He or she must practice with a physician. All states have laws regulating physician assistants, and students must pass the national certification examination.

A nurse practitioner (NP) is a registered nurse (RN) who studies in a program in advanced practice nursing, a program that usually grants a Master of Science in Nursing (MSN) or higher degree. Nurse practitioners can specialize in

What Would You Do? What Would You *Not* Do?

Case Study 1

In the examination room, Alicia Darwin, a new patient, tells Aida that she has switched physicians because she had often been seen by a nurse practitioner in the medical office where she used to go. "I don't think a nurse practitioner has as much experience as a doctor," she said, "and besides, the nurse practitioner can't give me medication if I need it." She asked Aida to confirm that she would always be seen by the physician in this office. She added, "I don't have anything against nurses like you; I just want to have a real doctor take care of me." ■

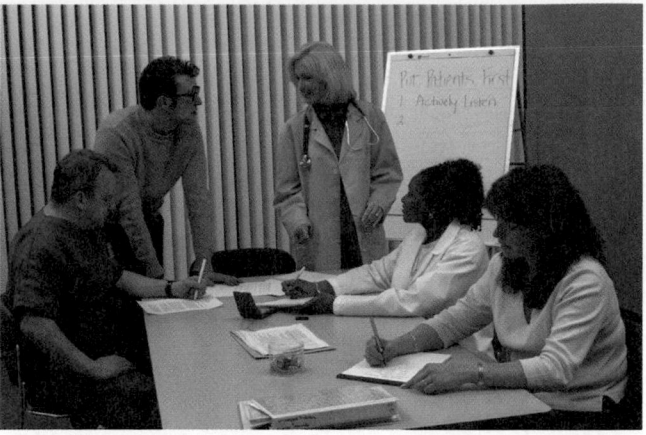

Figure 1-3. Team meetings can improve patient care. (From Hunt SA: *Saunders fundamentals of medical assisting*, St. Louis, 2007, Saunders.)

pediatrics, family practice, gerontology, or other specialty areas.

The scope of a nurse practitioner's ability to practice independently is determined by each state. In all states, nurse practitioners are allowed to carry a caseload and manage routine patient care. Some states allow nurse practitioners to write prescriptions; in other states a physician must cosign the order. In some states, nurse practitioners are allowed to practice independently, but in most they must practice in an office with supervision by a physician. In a few states, nurse practitioners are allowed to admit patients to hospitals.

Effective Teamwork

Working as an effective health care team does not just happen. To be effective, team members work together to provide appropriate care for each patient. The more people involved, the more crucial this teamwork is. Each member of the team must be committed to problem solving, communicating, and coordinating effective care.

Teamwork is reinforced at regular staff meetings, which can be directed by either the medical or business director of the office, depending on the particular topics of the meeting. But the true test of teamwork occurs on a daily basis as health care is provided (Figure 1-3).

Each health care team member has a certain responsibility and restrictions on activities and areas about which he or she is allowed to make decisions. Sometimes this scope is defined by federal or state law. For example, medical assistants are allowed to administer injections in some states, but in others they cannot.

The specific education and role of the medical assistant is discussed in Chapter 2. To function as an effective team member the medical assistant must learn what areas fall within the proper scope of decision-making responsibility. This may vary. Generally, on the clinical side, these areas will be limited to patient safety and comfort needs, as well as possibly to anticipating diagnostic tests that will be needed. In the administrative area, the medical assistant may have more freedom to make decisions.

In addition, the medical assistant must communicate well with other health team members. He or she cannot assume that the patient will repeat all information to the physician, so the medical assistant must communicate anything related to the patient's health verbally or through the medical record. At the same time, the medical assistant must be careful to avoid using diagnostic terminology in the medical record or giving medical advice to the patient (unless following specific guidelines established by the physician).

Teamwork is enhanced when each team member helps and supports other members and avoids blaming or criticizing others. Because the number of employees in a medical office is often small, it is important for everyone to do their best to get along and deal with conflict. When a problem arises, it is important to try to find solutions to the problem rather than focusing on who caused the problem or whose fault it is. It is also helpful to maintain perspective and accept that things do go wrong, and most problems can be dealt with. In any conflict situation, it is important to listen to the point of view of others and validate their feelings. Effective communication techniques are discussed in more detail in Chapter 4.

PARTS OF THE MEDICAL OFFICE

A physician's office has a number of different physical spaces in it. Each space has a particular purpose. Every physician's office has three basic areas: a reception area and waiting room, examination and treatment rooms, and an area for other activities. This may include medical records storage, if the office uses paper medical records; storage for supplies, and staff offices or cubicles.

In most offices, physicians also have their own offices, separate from examination rooms, but some physicians have examination tables in their offices, combining the two spaces in one room.

Larger offices may have several additional areas such as an office laboratory; separate treatment rooms or special procedure rooms; a business office, which is separate from the front office (reception, telephones, appointments); and a lunch or break room for the staff.

All physicians' offices must meet a number of specifications laid out by regulatory agencies. These include the federal Occupational Safety and Health Administration (OSHA), which regulates workplace health and safety. They also must meet the specifications of the Americans with Disabilities Act, which requires that doorways be at least 3 feet wide and hallways at least 5 feet wide. Restroom facilities must be available for both patients and staff. Office laboratories are regulated by the Clinical Laboratory Improvement Act (CLIA '88). Local boards of health also inspect and regulate hospitals and clinics.

Figure 1-4 shows the layout of a small physician office.

Reception Area and Waiting Room

The reception area and waiting room are the first place any new or prospective patient will see. First impressions are important. The waiting room should be clean and well lit. Furniture should be arranged and not haphazardly placed. Up-to-date, general-interest reading material should be available; many physicians also have patient education materials available in the waiting room. Waiting rooms in pediatric and family practice offices also have toys available for children. Large pediatric practices may have a separate waiting room for sick children or for adolescents.

The waiting room should have enough chairs for two people per patient visit, multiplied by the number of patients seen in 2 hours. It needs to present a calm atmosphere and look professional. Usually, the waiting area is carpeted. It should have comfortable chairs, grouped in blocks if possible rather than just lined up around the walls. Colors should be muted, and music should be soft. Red, yellow, and orange are typically avoided; today, physician's office decor often uses shades of green, dusty pink, or salmon. Music is usually a tape or radio station of the "easy listening" variety.

The reception area adjoins the waiting room. The medical assistant at the reception desk should greet each patient as he or she enters the waiting room. Most reception areas have a counter so that the patient can fill out or sign forms, and many have a sliding window so that patients cannot hear the conversations occurring behind the receptionist.

Patients check in here when they enter the office. New patient forms are received here, and health insurance cards are copied. Copayments are taken from patients whose insurance is provided through HMOs. Appointments may be made by the receptionist or in a separate area of the office.

Examination Rooms and Laboratory

Many offices have a small open area to take vital signs such as blood pressure, as well as height and weight, and to process simple laboratory tests, especially if there is no larger laboratory in the office (Figure 1-5). This allows the medical assistant to obtain preliminary data while the examination rooms are occupied. A telephone and small desk or computer may also be available so that clinical personnel can talk to patients about medical problems, take laboratory results, and make calls related to clinical care. If these areas are adjacent to corridors or walkways, it is important for the medical assistant to be sure to maintain patient privacy and avoid discussing any medical information when other patients might be passing near the area.

Examination rooms are designed for the convenience of the physician and assisting personnel who will work there. However, they also need to be as comfortable and calming to the patient as possible. Reading material should be available in each examination room. Although good scheduling will ensure that patients will not wait too long in these rooms for a physician, emergency phone calls, "corridor consults" with colleagues, and other short delays may occur.

Figure 1-4. Layout of a small medical office. (From Hunt SA: *Saunders fundamentals of medical assisting,* St. Louis, 2007, Saunders.)

Figure 1-5. Patient preparation area, with medical assistant measuring blood pressure.

Many physicians also perform treatments or diagnostic procedures in examination rooms, but complex procedures (such as suturing a laceration) are often performed in larger rooms with extra equipment and/or supplies. These are called *treatment rooms*.

If laboratory tests are performed in the medical office, there is a special room or area set aside for this. The 1988 amendments to the Clinical Laboratory Improvement Amendments (CLIA '88) regulate laboratory testing. Medical assistants are trained to perform low-complexity tests (CLIA-waived tests) and may also perform more complex texts with special training.

CLIA '88 specifies who can supervise laboratories and lays out the process for inspection and accreditation. It sets strict guidelines for quality control, quality assurance, handling of hazardous materials, documentation, and proficiency training. Offices that perform only CLIA-waived laboratory tests may perform laboratory testing in the patient preparation area. Ideally, the bathroom is adjacent to this area, with an opening in the wall so that urine samples can be passed directly into the laboratory area.

Medical Records Storage and Business Office

The medical records storage may be located near the reception area, in the business areas, adjacent to the patient preparation area, or in a separate room. Charts of active patients—those who have been seen within the past 2 to 3 years—are kept in the records storage area in the office. Inactive charts are removed regularly and stored in a less accessible location such as the basement of the building or off-site in a facility that maintains records in storage. Charts needed for patients who will be coming in during a specified period—morning, afternoon, or an entire day—are removed from the storage area and prepared for use.

What Would You Do? What Would You *Not* Do?

Case Study 2

The physician complains to Aida that there are always dishes in the sink in the break room and crumbs and used paper coffee cups on the table. Even though the area is not seen by patients, the physician is concerned that an insect or rodent problem could develop. Aida knows that the part-time file clerk and the part-time receptionist have a tendency to leave dirty dishes and trash after their afternoon break. She herself is so busy that she rarely has time to either clean or sit down in the break room. ■

Some practices are moving away from paper records to computerized medical records. In this case, patient records are stored on a computer's hard disk and are simply pulled up from the database as needed. The process of placing old records into the computerized record is lengthy, and many offices that use an electronic medical record also have the former paper record for established patients.

Posting of patient charges, billing, and computer operations may be performed in an area behind the reception desk or in a separate business office. If the practice has one or more satellite locations, the billing and insurance is usually done in the practice's main office for all locations. Some offices contract billing and insurance claim processing to an outside company, which may even be located in another state.

Additional Areas Found in Many Offices

Physicians' private offices are often a reflection of their personal tastes. This room is where a physician meets privately with patients, patients' families, and other visitors. He or she usually displays degrees and certificates of membership in professional organizations on the walls of the office. Even if the practice has a small library for the use of all staff, physicians will usually have at least a few important references in this office. Art and memorabilia that shows the physician's personal taste also helps to make the private office a pleasant place for the physician to do quiet work and hold meetings.

Recognizing the needs of staff for a quiet place to take their breaks and eat their lunch, newer offices often include a staff break/lunch room. This room may have a refrigerator and microwave for staff to prepare lunches they bring from home. There should be at least one table and chairs. The lunch or break room should not double as a storage area, and staff should avoid using the room for meetings that deprive others use of the room. Depending on the type of medical practice, particular rooms may be set aside for specific treatments or diagnostic procedures. Types of special rooms include the following:

1. A pediatrics examination/treatment room in a family practice group's office
2. Surgical procedure room in a general surgery group's office

3. A room for more complex testing such as colposcopy and pelvic ultrasounds in a group practice specializing in obstetrics/gynecology

4. A trauma room in a large clinic or community health center

Memories *from* Externship

Aida Reyes: The clinic where I did my externship was so large that at first I kept getting lost. Another thing that confused me was the doors that the staff used to get from one part of the clinic to another. It was arranged by department, but the layout of rooms in each department was different. I spent the majority of my time in internal medicine working with one medical assistant and one physician, but my preceptor arranged for me to spend time in other departments like medical records, billing, and pediatrics and with the referral coordinator. In addition to the full-time physicians, there were some specialists who came in once or twice a week, including a neurologist, an orthopedic surgeon, and an ophthalmologist. The clinic also employed a social worker and a dietician. In each department there was a nurse and at least two medical assistants in addition to the receptionist. The amazing thing was how quickly I adapted and became comfortable finding my way around. After only a few weeks, it felt like I belonged there. I was so proud when my preceptor said, "Aida, you have become one of the team. I don't know how we ever got along without you." ■

Prepare for Success

MEDICAL SPECIALTIES

Since the middle of the twentieth century, the practice of medicine has been broken down into fields of specialty and subspecialty. In 1950 most Americans received their medical care from a general practitioner, who took care of adults and children, often delivered babies, and performed many general surgical procedures.

Today, Americans may see two, three, or more physicians routinely. Box 1-1 describes the medical specialties recognized by the American Board of Medical Specialties. In many areas, there are several subspecialties. If the physician wants to work in a subspecialty, after the residency training he or she participates in additional training called a *fellowship* for 2 to 3 years. It is not possible to be board certified in any specialty or subspecialty without completing a residency.

Primary Care

Primary care physicians either specialize in internal medicine (treatment of the internal organs of adults by other than surgical means), pediatrics (general medical care of children and adolescents), or family medicine (general medical care of children, adolescents, and adults—today's equivalent of general practice).

Over the course of time, the activities of different types of physicians have shifted. For instance, fewer family practitioners deliver babies today than did general practitioners in the 1950s and 1960s, preferring to leave that task to obstetricians, due to the cost of malpractice insurance. Although some women continue to see a gynecologist for an annual pelvic examination and Pap test, the primary care

BOX 1-1 Medical Specialties

Allergy and Immunology (Allergist, Immunologist)
Treats adults and/or children with allergies and problems of the immune system. Many individuals experience allergies and/or asthma in the presence of allergens. The immune system can also malfunction through either inherited or acquired diseases. Allergists and immunologists diagnose, manage, and treat allergic diseases, immunodeficiency conditions, and autoimmune diseases.

Anesthesiology (Anesthesiologist)
Provides anesthesia during surgery and other procedures, as well as medical care to patients before, during, and after surgery. The anesthesiologist also supervises other anesthesia personnel in the operating room, such as nurse anesthetists and anesthesiology residents.

Colon and Rectal Surgery
Performs surgical treatment on the large intestine and rectum. These surgeons specialize in the diagnosis and treatment of diseases of the colon and rectum in addition to full training in general

surgery. They perform diagnostic and screening procedures and perform surgery when necessary.

Dermatology (Dermatologist)
Specializes in conditions of the skin. Dermatologists diagnose skin diseases and also perform surgery on the skin. Laser treatments are commonly used for skin conditions in addition to medication, cryotherapy, and surgery.

Emergency Medicine
Treats patients for emergency conditions, usually in the emergency department of a hospital. Emergency medicine focuses on treatment of acute illnesses and injuries that require immediate care. The physician is often an employee of a hospital emergency department or other urgent care center.

Family Medicine (Family Practitioner)
Treats adults and children for routine care and complaints; often the primary care physician for all family members. The family practitioner is concerned with the total health of the individual and the family. Specialized training is available for the subspecialties of geriatric medicine and sports medicine.

BOX 1-1 Medical Specialties—cont'd

Internal Medicine (Internist)

Provides medical treatment for conditions of various body systems. The internist may be the primary care provider for adults. Within the discipline of internal medicine are several subspecialties such as adolescent medicine, cardiovascular disease, critical care medicine, endocrinology, gastroenterology, geriatric medicine, hematology, medical oncology, nephrology, pulmonary disease, rheumatology, and sports medicine.

Medical Genetics

Provides diagnostic procedures and treatment for individuals with genetically linked diseases. Also provides genetic counseling and prenatal diagnosis. May specialize in laboratory testing or in research related to genetic diseases.

Neurologic Surgery (Neurosurgeon)

Performs prevention, diagnosis, surgical and nonsurgical treatment, and rehabilitation for conditions of the brain, spine, and nervous system. Also provides surgical and nonsurgical treatment of pain. Subspecialties include vascular neurosurgery and pediatric neurosurgery.

Nuclear Medicine

Specializes in diagnosis using radionuclides, atoms that give off electromagnetic radiation. Nuclear physicians are usually employed by a hospital or university (or both) and have little direct patient care. They are responsible for diagnosis and recommending treatment of abnormalities detected by the various imaging modalities used in the nuclear medicine department.

Obstetrics (Obstetrician) and Gynecology (Gynecologist)

Specializes in care during pregnancy and delivery (obstetrician); specializes in other care and surgery of the female reproductive system (gynecologist). The gynecologist is responsible for screening procedures, diagnostic procedures, and both medical and surgical treatments. He or she also frequently uses hormone-modulating treatments. Pep test, colposcopy

Ophthalmology (Ophthalmologist)

Specializes in the care of the eye. The ophthalmologist manages diseases and conditions of the eye with both medical and surgical treatment including laser treatments. May also manage errors of refraction and prescribe corrective lenses, although this is often delegated to an optometrist. Several subspecialties deal with specific eye diseases or parts of the eye.

Orthopedic Surgery (Orthopedic Surgeon)

Specializes in diagnosis and treatment of acute and traumatic injuries of the musculoskeletal system, as well as diseases of the muscular or skeletal system. Both surgical and nonsurgical treatments are used. Some orthopedic surgeons specialize in specific joints, specific age groups, orthopedic sports medicine, or orthopedic oncology.

Otolaryngology (Otolaryngologist or ENT)

Specializes in the care of the ear, nose, throat, head, and neck. The ENT is responsible for the diagnosis and surgical or nonsurgical treatment of a variety of disorders. Many physicians specialize in the care of only one organ or area and may focus on either reconstruction or diseases of that organ.

Pathology (Pathologist)

Examines cells, tissues, and other specimens to determine whether their structure is normal or abnormal; attempts to determine the nature or cause of disease. Pathologists examine tissue biopsies and other specimens to identify abnormal cells. They also perform autopsies. They may be trained within two primary specialty areas: clinical pathology and/or anatomic pathology.

Pediatrics (Pediatrician)

Specializes in the care of children from birth through adolescence. In the United States, pediatricians are considered to be primary care practitioners. However, many pediatricians specialize, and almost every specialty for adult medicine is represented as a pediatric subspecialty.

Physical Medicine and Rehabilitation (Physiatrist)

Specializes in the treatment and rehabilitation of patients with disabling conditions such as spinal cord injury and stroke. A physiatrist sees patients across several age groups and specialty areas and focuses on restoring maximal function to patients. He or she may specialize in specific age groups or types of injury such as spinal cord injury.

Plastic Surgery

Specializes in surgical and nonsurgical treatment of physical defects of various areas of the body. The plastic surgeon performs procedures for cosmetic enhancement or reconstruction of various parts of the body. Cosmetic surgery has become popular in the past 2 decades. Reconstructive surgery includes craniofacial surgery, hand surgery, and maxillofacial surgery to repair congenital defects and problems that result from injury or disease.

Preventative Medicine

Includes aerospace medicine, occupational medicine, and public health. In this medical specialty, physicians practice in one of the specialty areas or one of the subspecialties (medical toxicology or undersea and hyperbaric medicine).

Psychiatry (Psychiatrist) and Neurology (Neurologist)

Specializes in preventing, diagnosing, and treating mental illness and conditions of the nervous system. Psychiatrists have completed the same general training as any other physician, and they

Continued

BOX 1-1 Medical Specialties—cont'd

are able to prescribe medication for mental illness and monitor the effects of medication therapy. Like other mental health professionals, they usually also have training in psychotherapy, psychoanalysis, and/or cognitive behavioral therapy.

Radiology (Radiologist)

Specializes in the use of x-ray and other ionizing radiation for diagnosis (diagnostic radiology) and treatment (radiation oncology). A radiologist has the training to manage several types of diagnostic imaging including x-ray, computed tomography (CT) scan, and magnetic resonance imaging (MRI).

Surgery (General Surgeon or Vascular Surgeon)

Performs general surgical procedures or vascular surgical procedures. A general surgeon performs primarily abdominal surgery using traditional methods or laparoscopic methods. A vascular surgeon manages diseases or conditions of the arteries and veins, except for the blood vessels of the heart and brain. Cardiothoracic

surgeons manage conditions of the heart including the blood vessels, and neurosurgeons manage all conditions of the brain.

Thoracic Surgery (Thoracic Surgeon)

Performs surgery of the chest including cardiac surgery, although thoracic surgeons usually specialize in surgery of the chest or cardiac surgery. Because cardiac surgery requires a high degree of skill, preparation for this specialty requires long and intensive training. Thoracic surgeons may limit their practice by age group served or by type of condition (such as congenital heart disease or heart transplantation).

Urology (Urologist)

Specializes in the care of the urinary system in males and females and the reproductive tract in males; also specializes in surgery of the urinary tract and male reproductive tract. The urologist may provide medical conditions as for infections or surgical repair for abnormal growths or correction of congenital malformations.

---

provider performs these activities more often today than in the past.

Because of the requirements for a primary care provider in managed care plans, some specialists, especially obstetrician/gynecologists, also provide general care for some patients in their practice.

Osteopathy

Osteopathy is a mix of traditional scientific medicine and **holistic** medicine. This branch of medical practice seeks to balance the structure and function of the body through manipulation of muscles and joints. Osteopathy was started in the late 1800s by Andrew Taylor Still (1828-1917). Osteopaths see disease as the result of dysfunction in the skeletal and muscular systems. Pain, "asymmetry" (the difference in anatomy between one side of the body and the other or differences in joint movement), and tissue tenderness are used to gauge symptoms. Osteopaths, who hold DO degrees, today are given all the privileges of those with MD degrees. The majority of osteopaths practice as primary care doctors, where they believe their holistic and structural approach can be most effective.

Podiatry

Podiatrists use traditional medical and surgical techniques but are limited in their practice to treatment of disorders of the feet and ankles. Since the 1970s, podiatry has worked to enlarge its area of practice by focusing on surgery of the foot to alleviate such problems as bone spurs and bunions. This has put them into competition with orthopedic surgeons, who traditionally did this work. Podiatrists work closely with primary care doctors in the management of diabetic patients and the elderly, who tend to have many foot problems.

Chiropractic

Chiropractic is the technique of spinal manipulation. Chiropractors believe that vertebral subluxations (partially dislocated spinal joints) cause nerve blockages, which in turn lead to pain in the back, neck, shoulders, and legs. Begun in 1895 by Daniel David Palmer (1845-1913), chiropractic holds that the body has its own ability to heal and maintain balance. According to chiropractic theory, the nervous system is the center of all disease and healing. Some chiropractors believe that subluxation is the reason for all disease. Today's chiropractors, who are licensed by the state in which they practice, limit their treatment to discomfort clearly associated with the spine and integrate their practices into standard Western medical practice. Figure 1-6 demonstrates a chiropractic adjustment.

PRACTICE TYPES

Fifty years ago most physicians who were not on full-time hospital staffs worked by themselves in an office, either in their home or in an office building. They paid their office expenses, taxes, and liability insurance out of their income, and the difference was considered their "net income" from their practice. As their practice got busier, their income increased. Today many physicians work with other physicians. Some of them have an ownership position in the practice or facility they work for, but others are employees and receive a salary from their employer. The following categories refer to the way the office is structured, not the business arrangement or ownership.

Solo Practice

It is still possible for a physician to work in a solo practice. But to do so, he or she must make a number of trade-offs.

Figure 1-6. Spinal adjustment with patient in prone position. (Courtesy Gatterman MI: *Foundations of chiropractic: subluxation*, St. Louis, 1995, Mosby.)

Solo practices are limited in their size by the number of patients one physician can manage. When a physician practices alone, the medical assistant is usually responsible for aspects of both administrative and clinical support.

Even if a solo practitioner employs a nurse practitioner or physician's assistant to see additional patients, the physician still must factor into his or her workday some time to oversee the work of these nonphysician professionals. In addition, the physician, as the employer, is usually responsible for paying the malpractice insurance premiums for all of the licensed professionals in his or her office. Physicians in solo practice are also completely responsible for their patients. Usually they make arrangements with other physicians to share after-hours and weekend call and to cover for vacations.

Group Practice

Many physicians today participate in a group practice. The most common type of group practice includes three to four physicians of the same medical specialty who band together to share resources such as office space and personnel. In these groups, medical assistants usually specialize in either clinical or administrative work, although they expect to help out in other areas.

Depending on the business form used, patients are either the responsibility of one physician or "the group." In either case, if a patient's regular physician is not available, another physician in the office can see the patient. In addition, physicians who work in group practices usually share after-hours and weekend call responsibility. They usually split the cost of malpractice insurance, and the policy is written for the group rather than for each individual.

Large medical groups with physicians who provide primary care, as well as physicians with other medical specialties, are becoming increasingly common throughout the country. Their names often include the words "associates" or "medical associates." This organizational form allows a sharing of resources that, in turn, allows each physician in the group to provide a broader range of services. In the past, these groups have been more common in particular regions

and in rural areas, where a single group of physicians has the responsibility both as the physicians in town and the staff of small, rural hospitals. HMOs that provide all services in one building, so-called closed-panel HMOs, also operate as multispecialty groups.

These practices often have separate administrative departments for billing, appointment scheduling, and referrals and separate clinical departments for phlebotomy, electrocardiograms, laboratory work, and x-ray. In such practices, medical assisting jobs can be limited in scope, and specific responsibilities depend on the department where the medical assistant works.

Clinic

Traditionally a clinic was usually connected to a hospital and provided ambulatory care, often to patients with limited financial resources. Patients were either seen at no charge or billed by the clinic, and physicians were paid a salary for their services and/or saw patients as part of their residency program. Today a *clinic* usually refers to a public or non-profit facility that provides outpatient public health services, although multispecialty group practices may use the word "clinic" in their name. Community health centers, established by the federal government in the late 1960s, operate as clinics and have physicians, as well as nurse practitioners, physician's assistants, and nurse-midwives all on salary. In many states separate laws apply to clinics related to licensing and supervision by public health agencies.

COMPLEMENTARY AND ALTERNATIVE MEDICINE

Numerous other practices are used for the treatment of illness, some of which have a long tradition and some of which have developed more recently. Studies from the early 1990s found that Americans annually spend literally millions of dollars on therapies that are not part of their physician's standard approach. They often do not even tell their physicians about these other treatments. The term *complementary medicine* is usually used for medical treatments that patients use in addition to standard medical treatments. The term *alternative medicine* refers to practices that are used instead of standard medical treatment. For many patients, these may overlap. Acupuncture, for example, has been a definitive method of treatment in traditional Chinese medicine for centuries (Figure 1-7). In the United States it has become a popular treatment method used in addition to standard treatment. It has become so popular that there are many schools to train practitioners and the practice of acupuncture requires a license in about 40 states.

Since the early 1990s, scholars of medicine have begun to take an interest in studying complementary and alternative practices scientifically. The federal government has since established the National Center for Complementary and Alternative Medicine within the National Institutes of Health. This agency coordinates and funds scientific research to study the effectiveness of these health practices. The most well-respected medical journals such as the *New England*

Figure 1-7. Acupuncture involves the placement of several extremely thin needles in various parts of the body. (From Hunt SA: *Saunders fundamentals of medical assisting*, St. Louis, 2007, Saunders.)

What Would You Do? What Would You *Not* Do?

Case Study 3

While taking John Carter's medical history, he mentions that he has been getting acupuncture and taking several herbal preparations that he buys at a health food store. He also says that he wears shoe insoles with magnets in them because he has had heel pain for several months. He says, "You should try them. They have really helped my heel pain." ■

Journal of Medicine and the *Journal of the American Medical Association* have published a number of studies about the effectiveness of various nonstandard therapies, and numerous specialized journals have also been established to publish research about such therapies. When research demonstrates that practice is effective, physicians trained in the classical Western medical tradition are more accepting and may even incorporate some of these practices or refer patients to practitioners.

MEDICAL PRACTICE *and the* LAW

Although all states require a physician to have a license to practice medicine, it does not always have to be from the state in which the physician is working. Although individual state laws vary, in the following cases a physician is usually exempt.

1. A physician who is licensed in another state or country who is meeting with a physician of the state in question for the purposes of consultation
2. A physician who is licensed in another state or country who is visiting a medical school or teaching hospital to receive instruction or to provide instruction, as long as it is under the supervision of a licensed physician

3. A physician who is authorized by a foreign government may usually practice medicine in relation to that government's diplomatic, consular, or maritime staff
4. Any commissioned medical officer serving in the U.S. armed forces or public health service or any physician employed by the U.S. Veterans Administration

In addition, medical students and interns or residents in postgraduate programs who are under the supervision of a licensed physician may practice medicine in the institutions with which their training programs are affiliated. ■

What Would You Do? What Would You *Not* Do?   RESPONSES

Case Study 1
Page 11

What Did Aida Do?
❑ Accepted Alice Darwin's reason for changing medical offices without making a judgment.
❑ Stated that she hoped Alice would feel comfortable as a patient in their practice.
❑ Stated that she was a medical assistant, not a nurse, and explained the difference briefly.
❑ Clarified the legal position of a nurse practitioner in her state related to prescribing medications.

What Did Aida Not *Do?*
❑ Did not agree verbally or by implication that she is a nurse.
❑ Did not ask for additional information about Alice's previous physician or medical office.
❑ Did not make any critical remarks about nurse practitioners or Alice's previous physician.

❑ Did not make any statement that could be interpreted as a guarantee that Alice would like this physician better.

What Would You Do/What Would You *Not* Do? Review Aida's response and place a checkmark next to the information you included in your response. List the additional information you included in your response.

_____
_____
_____
_____

Case Study 2
Page 13

What Did Aida Do?
❑ Agreed that the condition of the break room could be improved.

What Would You Do? What Would You *Not* Do? RESPONSES—cont'd

❏ Promised to talk to all staff members about keeping the break room clean.

❏ Arranged time to speak to staff members either individually or as a group to discuss ways to keep the break room clean and make a plan.

❏ Encouraged all staff members to take an active part in developing a plan to keep the break room clean.

❏ Followed up to be sure that any plan made was implemented and was effective.

What Did Aida Not *Do?*

❏ Did not focus on identifying who was responsible either when talking to the physician or other staff members.

❏ Did not become defensive when talking to the physician or other staff members.

❏ Did not single out any staff member(s) as responsible for the problem.

❏ Did not complain about one staff member's behavior to any other staff member.

What Would You Do/What Would You *Not* Do? Review Aida's response and place a checkmark next to the information you included in your response. List the additional information you included in your response.

_____

_____

_____

_____

Case Study 3
Page 18

What Did Aida Do?

❏ Accepted John Carter's description of his complementary/alternative medical practices.

❏ Documented all practices in the medical record.

❏ Asked questions to explore the underlying problems such as heel pain or the reason for acupuncture.

What Did Aida Not *Do?*

❏ Tell John that he might be endangering his health because of his complementary/alternative medical practices.

❏ Tell John that acupuncture, magnets, or herbs would not help him.

❏ Ask John where to buy foot insoles with magnets.

❏ Dismiss John's practices as insignificant and fail to document them.

What Would You Do/What Would You *Not* Do? Review Aida's response and place a checkmark next to the information you included in your response. List the additional information you included in your response.

_____

_____

_____

_____

TERMINOLOGY REVIEW

Ambulatory care Medical care that is provided on an outpatient basis. The patient is able to come to the facility providing care and return home after receiving services.

Capitation A set payment provided by managed care insurance per patient per month regardless of the amount of service the patient receives.

Empirically Learned from observation or experiment.

Fee-for-service A means of payment for health care in which each service provided is reimbursed in full or in part.

Formulary A list of prescription drugs covered or preferred by a managed care insurance company.

Health insurance Purchase of protection for covered services related to health care.

Holistic Considering the whole; in medicine, considering the entire person when providing health care.

Managed care A system that manages the delivery of health care with the intention of controlling costs.

Palliative treatment Therapy that reduces the effects of disease or condition but does not remove the disease itself.

Residency A program to provide training in a medical specialty to a physician who has finished medical school.

Symptomatic treatment Therapy for symptoms of a disease or condition that does not remove the disease itself.

Utilization review Assessing medical services to determine whether they are appropriate, necessary, and high quality.

ON THE WEB

For Information on Health:

World Health Organization: www.who.int/en

National Institutes of Health: www.nih.gov

For Information on Physicians and Osteopathic Physicians:

American Medical Association: www.ama-assn.org

American Osteopathic Association: www.osteopathic.org

For Information on Medical Specialties:

American Board of Medical Specialties (ABMS): www.abms.org

For Information on Complementary and Alternative Medicine:

National Center for Complementary and Alternative Medicine (NCCAM), National Institutes of Health: nccam.nih.gov

PREPARE FOR CERTIFICATION   Visit the Evolve site at http://evolve.elsevier.com/Bonewit/today/ to actively Prepare for your Certification.

CD   *Check out the* **Companion CD** *bound with the book to access additional interactive activities.*

2

The Professional Medical Assistant

Professionalism
- Project a positive attitude.
- Maintain confidentiality at all times.
- Be a "team player."
- Be cognizant of ethical boundaries.
- Exhibit initiative.
- Adapt to change.
- Evidence a responsible attitude.
- Be courteous and diplomatic.
- Conduct work within scope of education, training, and ability.

Communication
- Professional components
- Allied health professions and credentialing

Legal Concepts
- Monitor legislation related to current health care issues and practices.
- Perform risk management procedures.

KEY TERMS

accreditation
continuing education units (CEUs)
externship

fee splitting
initiative
risk management

Introduction to Professional Medical Assisting

Medical assisting came into existence as a career during the second half of the twentieth century. As recently as 1950, most physicians established their own practice when they completed their medical education and hospital training. A physician (almost always a man) usually saw patients with no assistance, except possibly his wife who answered the telephone and often did the billing.

The physician spent a large portion of each day making house calls. During a house call the physician would examine a patient with only the equipment he could carry in his medical bag. The physician's office was often located in a room in his house or the first floor of a building, with the physician living in an apartment above. Patients who went to the physician's office may or may not have had an appointment. They expected to wait to be seen.

In the first 20 years following World War II (before the increasing use of technology caused medical costs to skyrocket), a physician usually charged $2 to $5, possibly $10, for an office visit, a sum that seems small today. For some patients, however, even this small charge was more than a day's pay. For physicians, the low fee was enough because the expenses of his practice were also low. In fact, physicians rarely pressed poor patients for full payment. They always had many patients who owed them money, and it was not uncommon for patients to pay small amounts on a weekly basis for many months or even years, especially the parents of young children. Sometimes physicians would even barter by exchanging medical care for goods or services provided by the patient. For example, a patient might pay for his medical care by bringing the physician fresh produce from his farm.

In the past 40 years, the practice of medicine has changed dramatically. This, in turn, changed the way in which physicians operated their medical practice. With the advent of government insurance programs, not only were office visits covered by insurance, but the medical office was also expected to complete and submit the insurance forms to receive payment. Physicians soon discovered that the cost of employing a person to complete these forms was offset by improved collections. Gradually almost all insurance billing shifted to the health care provider.

Advances in medical science made many more diagnostic tests, laboratory tests, and treatments available and even necessary for good medical care. It made sense to have an assistant in the office to perform these tests and allow the physician to concentrate on seeing patients.

Even as laboratory and diagnostic testing has increased in amount and in complexity, so too has the administrative equipment and technology used in a physician's office. Today there are computers, wireless electronic devices, printers, fax machines, photocopiers, intercoms, and voice-mail systems.

Physicians send claims to a number of different insurance companies. Many insurance plans require prior approval for certain medical procedures, referrals to specialists, or surgical procedures. Insurance companies and government programs prefer electronic claims filing and often make electronic payments directly into physicians' office accounts at banks. This creates a need not only for more staff, but also for more highly trained staff.

Physicians have also stopped or at least greatly reduced the number of house calls they make. Because of this, physicians need more office space. In addition, patients with more complex needs are seen in physician's offices, rather than the hospital emergency department or outpatient department. Sometimes patients must occupy an examination or treatment room for an extended period of time, such as when an individual with asthma is receiving an inhalation treatment.

Another change that has had an impact on the medical practice involves the increase in medical litigation. Since the 1970s physicians have practiced what has come to be called "defensive medicine." Because of the fear of a malpractice lawsuit and the high cost of malpractice insurance, physicians perform many laboratory and diagnostic tests to rule out even the most unlikely cause of an illness.

All of these factors—increased medical equipment, increased laboratory and diagnostic testing, increased clerical equipment, and increased space—push up the overhead costs of running a medical office. This forces physicians to see more patients, which in turn encourages the physician to transfer many procedures, once performed by the physician, to the medical staff.

As services expanded, physicians employed nurses to help them in their offices. This helped ease their burden of performing procedures and caring for patients, but nurses were often unable and unwilling to assist with the administrative aspects of the practice. As a result, many physicians found a willing candidate and trained that person to assist first with administrative duties and then with both patient care and administrative duties. This evolved over time into what today is a medical assistant.

In 1956 medical assistants from 15 states organized to form the American Association of Medical Assistants (AAMA). In 1978 the profession was recognized by the U.S. Department of Education. The AAMA and other organizations, especially the American Medical Technologists (AMT), have worked to define professional training for the medical assistant and to provide certification for medical assistants through national examinations. Figure 2-1 shows the logo of the AAMA. Figure 2-2 shows the logo of the AMT.

Figure 2-1. Logo of the American Association of Medical Assistants. (Courtesy the American Association of Medical Assistants.)

Figure 2-2. Logo of the American Medical Technologists. (Courtesy the American Medical Technologists.)

EDUCATIONAL PROGRAMS FOR MEDICAL ASSISTANTS

Initially medical assistants received on-the-job training, but as the profession grew, formal education programs were established. These programs vary in length from 6 months to 2 years. Medical assisting programs include theoretical and practical preparation in all aspects of the medical assisting profession. To maintain quality, many of these programs sought **accreditation,** credit, or recognition for maintaining certain standards by a regional or national organization. The two recognized accrediting agencies for medical assisting programs are the Commission on Accreditation of Allied Health Education Programs (CAAHEP) in collaboration with the AAMA and the Accrediting Bureau of Health Education Schools (ABHES).

A medical assisting program seeking accreditation from one of these agencies must prepare a written report showing how the educational standards of the agency are being met. After the report has been submitted, an accreditation visit is made to validate the information presented in the report. Once accreditation has been granted, graduates of the program are eligible to take either the CMA (AAMA) or RMA certification examination. Accredited programs must include at least 160 hours of practical work experience in a medical office or clinic, known as an **externship.**

CHARACTERISTICS OF MEDICAL ASSISTANTS

Medical assistants possess or develop a number of characteristics that make them effective in their work. Although a person's character and personality have been shaped by heredity and environment, a medical assisting student can work to enhance the traits that are important for health care delivery. Appearance and behavior are an important means of projecting competence in the medical field.

Character Traits

The most important character traits of a competent medical assistant are reliability, dependability, honesty, tolerance, and good organizational skills. The medical assistant is an integral part of the office practice and must arrive at work on time and not take days off, except when ill or if a family emergency arises. A medical assistant must be able to organize the day's work and be prepared for each patient interaction.

A medical assistant projects honesty by working within his or her "scope of practice"; that is, doing only what he or she is trained to do and being comfortable in saying "I don't know" or "I don't know how to" when appropriate. The medical assistant must always maintain confidentiality and behave ethically. The medical assistant must recognize that a high level of trust is an important component of quality patient care. Tolerance or a willingness to accept the beliefs and practices of others is an important character trait. Tolerance allows the medical assistant to work effectively with coworkers and patients from a variety of religious, ethnic, and cultural backgrounds.

Putting It All into Practice

My name is Beth Ann Wilson, and I am a certified medical assistant. I attended a medical assisting training program at the community college near my home. I was the first person in my family to go to college, and my family was very proud of me. After the first year (two semesters), I received a certificate in medical assisting, and I found a job in our town at a group practice specializing in obstetrics and gynecology. My instructor encouraged me to take the CMA (AAMA) examination, and I was glad when I found out that I had passed it. I continued to take night classes so that I could get my associate's degree. I also attend the state and local chapter meetings of the AAMA so that I can get the contact hours I need to renew my CMA (AAMA) certification.

When I started working, I spent most of my time at the front desk answering the telephone, checking patients in, and filing, but after about 8 months I began to escort patients back to the examination rooms, prepare them for examinations, perform laboratory tests, and assist during examinations. We do some specialized tests in our office, including colposcopy, and I was trained to set up for the test and assist the physicians. Janice, our office manager who is a CMA (AAMA), has asked me to be responsible for ordering all the supplies for the office and taking inventory. She has also encouraged me to take business courses and attend seminars related to changes in insurance billing. Not too long ago, Janice told me that she is planning to cut back her hours in the spring, and she hopes that I will be able to take over some of her duties in running the practice. That will be a big challenge, but I think I am ready for it. I have a few ideas of my own, and I will be glad for an opportunity to try them out. ■

Prepare for Success

Personality Traits

Certain personality traits are essential to being a successful medical assistant. A medical assistant needs to be genuinely interested in helping people. The medical assistant must be outgoing, warm and caring, and able to put the needs of others first. The ability to remain calm in challenging or difficult situations is also important.

The practice of medicine is one of the "caring professions." Each professional in the medical office needs to have a serious interest in helping people. Although the medical assistant must know how to perform the necessary administrative activities effectively and efficiently, the first priority is the care of patients who visit the office.

The concepts of warmth and caring are discussed in more detail in Chapter 4, in the section on communication. For now, it is important to say that caring is a key personality trait. Some aspects of caring can be learned and practiced. If an individual does not have a naturally caring personality, he or she will find it much harder to learn the necessary caring communication skills.

What Would You Do? What Would You *Not* Do?

Case Study 1

It is a busy Monday and Beth Ann is getting ready to leave the office for her lunch break at 1:30 PM when a male physician steps out of an examination room and asks her to assist him with a Pap test and pelvic examination. Beth Ann knows that it is office policy to always have a female staff member in the examination room when a pelvic examination is done. She tells the physician that she is about to go for lunch, but she will find someone to assist him. She goes to the front and finds one receptionist at the desk who is busy checking in patients, but neither of the two other medical assistants working that day is in sight. ■

The ability to put the needs of others first is important. The medical assistant must not allow personal circumstances to interfere with interactions with patients, colleagues, or physicians. Remaining objective and concentrating on the situation at hand is important. The patient's needs take precedence over the needs of the medical assistant.

The atmosphere in a medical office may change quickly from calm and orderly to rushed and somewhat disorganized. The medical assistant who can remain calm when things do not go as planned will be more successful than one who is thrown completely off balance by sudden changes in schedule or plans and becomes emotionally unable to respond effectively.

Appearance and Behavior

Personal appearance influences both the feelings and behavior of the medical assistant. It also influences the way in which the patients respond to the medical assistant. Psychologists have long recognized the importance of physical appearance. Important judgments are made within seconds of meeting a stranger on the basis of appearance and body language.

When the medical assistant calls a patient to come from the waiting room to the examination or treatment room, the patient immediately forms an impression of the quality of care the medical assistant—and the physician—are going to provide (Figure 2-3). A medical assistant who is neat, clean, and well groomed projects a sense of professionalism, authority, and competence. When medical assistants are courteous, they project respect for a person's dignity. This is important because many patients feel awkward, especially when dressed in underwear and an examination gown.

Most medical offices require that medical assistants wear a uniform when performing clinical tasks. The uniform worn by most medical assistants consists of scrub pants with either a scrub top or short-sleeve shirt, white soft-soled shoes, and a laboratory coat or jacket. The top and jacket may be patterned, especially in a pediatric practice (Figure 2-4). In some practices all staff wear coordinated uniforms. When performing administrative tasks, the medical assistant wears scrubs or street clothes. If street clothes are worn, they should project a business-like appearance (Figure 2-5).

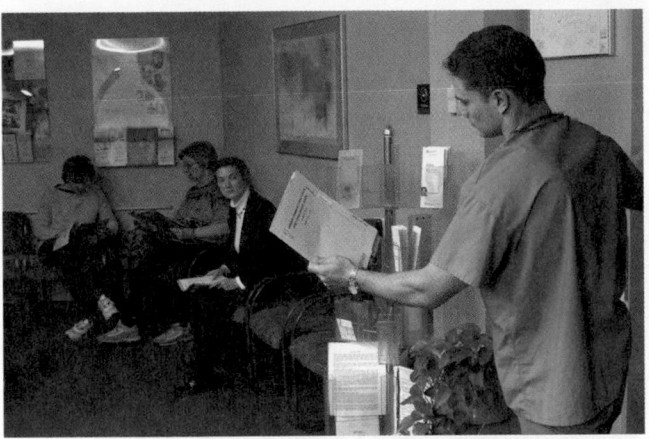

Figure 2-3. The patient judges the medical assistant's professionalism when called from the waiting room. (From Hunt SA: *Saunders fundamentals of medical assisting*, St. Louis, 2007, Saunders.)

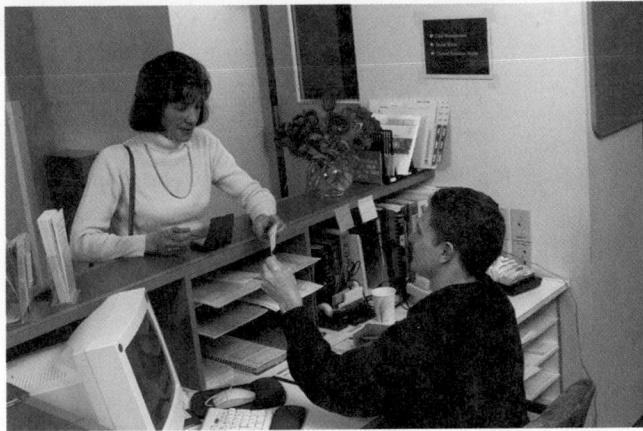

Figure 2-5. Street clothes may be worn for administrative tasks in some offices. (From Hunt SA: *Saunders fundamentals of medical assisting*, St. Louis, 2007, Saunders.)

Figure 2-4. A professional appearance increases the patient's confidence in the medical assistant.

Jeans, for example, are unacceptable attire in the medical office.

Neatness and good grooming are also important for health and safety reasons. Hair carries bacteria, even if regularly washed. Medical assistants who perform clinical activities should pull their hair back and tie it, usually in a ponytail. A little bit of makeup can enhance a professional image, but too much is not appropriate for a work environment. Dress, hair, and makeup should present a business-like appearance.

Nails should be kept relatively short and should not be polished. Long nails are not functional for keyboard work, patient care, or laboratory procedures. The Centers for Disease Control and Prevention (CDC) recommend that artificial nails not be worn and fingernails be kept ¼ inch or shorter when caring for patients at high risk of acquiring infections.

Traditionally, health professionals were only allowed to wear "functional" jewelry—a wristwatch and a plain wedding band—because jewelry is not regularly washed and can become tangled in equipment. Today, most medical offices allow staff to wear small earrings that do not dangle below the earlobe and necklaces that can be tucked into the shirtfront. Wearing rings other than a wedding band is not a good idea. Rings can cut through protective gloves or scrape a patient. Also, they need to be taken off frequently for handwashing. Most medical offices do not allow visible piercings, except for the ears. Many patients have a negative response when medical assistants or other health professionals have visible tattoos, and it may also be a policy of the medical office that visible tattoos must be covered.

Initiative is the ability to begin or follow through on a plan without being supervised. Initiative is an important quality for a medical assistant. The willingness to take initiative and perform tasks that need to be done without being specifically instructed to do so improves the functioning of the office as a whole.

Initiative, however, does not mean taking over. The office is the physician's place of business, and the physician expects to run it. Initiative does not mean redecorating the waiting room without asking the physician. It does mean doing things that need to be done without being asked, keeping up with current issues in practice without being told, and identifying helpful educational opportunities and asking permission to attend. It also means finding useful things to do when the office is slow, such as restocking supplies, ordering supplies, and cleaning out cabinets and cupboards.

Office managers who supervise medical assisting students during externships relay that some medical assisting students do not take enough initiative. Taking appropriate initiative is an important skill to develop. While in school, students learn to wait for someone to tell them exactly what to do and how to do it. In the workplace the opposite quality is valued. A medical assistant is expected to figure out what needs to be done and how to help out—even on an externship.

When a medical assistant begins an externship experience or a new position, he or she must learn when to jump in and perform a task without being asked. The task that is most comfortable for the medical assistant to perform may not be the one that shows the most initiative. Medical assisting students often work on filing during slack periods because they are comfortable with the task, but it might be more important to restock examination rooms or make telephone calls to remind patients about appointments.

Initiative is a quality that employers look for in new medical assistants. An employer may even test a new employee's initiative by showing them how to do something, such as restocking an examination room at the end of the day, and then watching to see if the new medical assistant restocks the examination room without being told.

The willingness to adapt to change is important for medical assistants, as well as all health care workers. The pace of change within ambulatory care is fairly rapid, so it is imprudent to become attached to one way of doing things. Changes in equipment, procedure, staff, and setting can occur quite frequently, but patient care needs to remain excellent. When the medical assistant approaches changes with tolerance and even enthusiasm, the office runs more smoothly. The medical assistant needs to adapt to the office setting rather than expecting the office to adapt to his or her preferences.

Finally, it is important for the medical assistant to work well with others and be a team player. Behavior that enhances patient care includes helping others, maintaining a positive attitude and not complaining, avoiding gossip, working within the established chain of command, and handling stress without losing emotional control or creating emotional scenes. Keeping perspective, accepting corrections or criticism without becoming defensive, and learning from mistakes are important. This facilitates working with others over the long term with a minimum of discord.

What Would You Do? What Would You *Not* Do?

Case Study 2

Dawn Elliot, a 48-year-old woman, brings her mother, Ruth Mitchell, who is 70 years old, to the office for complaints of vaginal bleeding. The physician asks for blood to be drawn in the office to determine if Mrs. Mitchell has anemia due to blood loss. Diane, a medical assisting externship student who has been working with Mrs. Mitchell, comes to Beth Ann and says, "Can you draw the blood from my patient? She says she doesn't want a student to draw her blood." Dawn notices that Diane is dressed in a professional manner. ∎

PROFESSIONALISM

Professionalism is behavior based on a body of knowledge and ethical standards to serve the public. The particular body of knowledge is different for each profession, but ethical standards for professionals are similar.

Professionalism for Physicians

For physicians, *professionalism* means treating patients based on the body of scientific knowledge they have accumulated, and continue to accumulate, over their working lifetime. In addition, physicians are bound by both ethical standards and legal regulations.

Most physicians rely on the American Medical Association's (AMA's) *Principles of Medical Ethics* for guidance. The AMA code of ethics is reviewed and updated periodically by that organization.

Other sources of professional guidance to physicians include the following:
- State and federal regulations
- Regulations of the hospital(s) to which the physicians admit patients
- Any open-panel health maintenance organizations or preferred provider organizations in which the physicians participate
- The national medical board of their specialty or subspecialty

Physicians may also take guidance from Hippocrates (c. 460-377 BC). Hippocrates was an ancient Greek physician who wrote the Hippocratic Oath. The Hippocratic Oath served as a guide to good conduct for ancient physicians, and parts of it are still applicable today. Few of today's physicians actually repeat the Hippocratic Oath when they graduate from medical school. Its philosophic underpinnings are still taught in medical school and adhered to by physicians, especially the key concept: "First, do no harm."

For more information on unprofessional activities of physicians, and by extension all office staff, see *Highlight on Unprofessional Conduct for a Physician.*

Professionalism for Medical Assistants

The AAMA maintains a code of ethics that is similar to the AMA principles for physicians. The AMT also maintains a set of standards that define professional practice. These codes of ethics can be viewed at the websites of each organization.

The medical assistant's ethical responsibilities are to admit mistakes, stay within the personal limits of his or her training, maintain confidentiality, stay current, and uphold the honor of the profession. This may mean having to confront a coworker who is not adhering to such principles.

Dealing with a coworker's inappropriate conduct is difficult, especially for a new employee or if the coworker is higher in the organizational hierarchy. We live in a society that does not like "tattletales." On the other hand, unprofessional behavior in a medical office is disruptive to the

Highlight on Unprofessional Conduct for a Physician

Even if they are not illegal, many activities are considered unprofessional for physicians, and by extension for their employees:

- Receiving payment for referrals to other physicians, laboratories, treatment centers, or pharmacies. Although physicians often make specific referrals, it is unethical for them to have arrangements to receive payments for those referrals, and especially to refuse to refer a patient unless a payment is made. This practice is sometimes called **fee splitting.** It is also unethical to charge a patient simply for being admitted to a hospital, without any other service being provided.

- Prescribing medication or diagnostic tests for financial gain rather than because of the patient's need for the test.

- Pressuring patients to use pharmacies or laboratories in which the physician has a financial interest. It is also unethical to prescribe medication, tests, or procedures that are not medically necessary. Billing an insurance company for unnecessary procedures is illegal.

- Accepting gifts from pharmaceutical companies or medical equipment manufacturers or suppliers in return for promoting the company's product or prescribing only the company's drug. Physicians may accept inexpensive or educational gifts with the understanding that they have no obligation to promote the product.

- Allowing another physician or surgeon to perform surgery without informing the patient. The patient has the right to know who is performing a procedure.

- Failing to disclose the source of sperm used for artificial insemination (e.g., husband, sperm bank, paid donor). The physician may not substitute sperm without informing the patient.

- Failing to practice medicine appropriately.

- Practicing medicine under the influence of mind-altering drugs, alcohol, or any prescription medication that may impair mental function, alertness, or physical performance.

- Allowing an unlicensed person to practice medicine.

- Failing to order a consultation for any medical problem that is beyond a physician's personal experience and expertise. For example, a gynecologist should not treat a patient for renal failure.

- Charging for missed appointments, or charging interest on unpaid bills, without informing patients that such a procedure is in effect.

- Failing to notify patients about any policy related to charges for missed appointments or appointments canceled without 24 hours' notice.

- Failing to notify patients about interest charges on past-due accounts, in accordance with state laws.

- Withholding information about a patient's medical care from another medical facility just because the patient has an outstanding bill.

- Putting a patient at risk of HIV infection, or refusing to treat a patient who is HIV positive. It is considered ethical for physicians to limit their practice to certain medical specialties and to refuse to accept specific types of insurance.

- Performing a procedure that might transmit the HIV virus to a patient if a physician or any other health care worker is HIV positive.

- Engaging in a sexual relationship with a patient. Something inherent in the relationship between two individuals in which one is perceived to be more influential than the other puts pressure on the "weaker" party to please the more powerful party. Because this makes it difficult to determine if consent is freely given, such a relationship should never be sexual in nature. Sexual relationships between professionals and the people they serve (e.g., physician-patient, attorney-client, teacher-student) are thus considered unethical and unprofessional. ■

concept of teamwork. Even if the unprofessional behavior does not pose an immediate threat to a patient, any behavior that results in people not working well together can lead to an uncomfortable or dangerous situation.

The medical assistant should first discuss the situation with the coworker by calmly and objectively describing the actions or behavior that he or she considers inappropriate. If the person does not correct the situation, it is appropriate to report the behavior to the office manager.

If the unprofessional behavior is being exhibited by a physician, the medical assistant should discuss the situation with the office manager. Serious infractions can be reported to the state authority that licenses that individual. These agencies have different names in different states; for example, Board of Registration (Massachusetts), Board of Medical Practice (Minnesota, Delaware, and Vermont), or Board of Medical Examiners (Oregon, Louisiana, New Jersey, Nevada, etc.). Any type of report must be based on firsthand evidence. In most states, reports can be made on-line. Information about professionals whose licenses have been revoked or suspended is also available on-line in many states. In most states these reports can be made anonymously.

What Would You Do? What Would You *Not* Do?

Case Study 3

Before examining Ruth Mitchell, the physician asked Beth Ann to recheck her blood pressure. It was 190/100 in the right arm and 186/98 in the right arm. Beth Ann noticed that the blood pressure had been taken that day by Diane, a medical assisting externship student, who had recorded it as 130/80. Beth Ann asked Diane if she was confident about the blood pressure she obtained on Mrs. Mitchell. Diane said, "It was really faint, and I didn't hear it that well, so I wrote down the same blood pressure as she had the last time she was here. I didn't want to look incompetent. Besides, I was afraid it might affect my grade if you thought I was having trouble hearing the blood pressure." ■

CREDENTIALS OF MEDICAL ASSISTANTS

Medical assistants usually graduate from an educational program that may vary in length from 6 months to 2 years. If the medical assistant graduates from a program accredited by CAAHEP or ABHES, he or she is eligible to take a national certification examination. Certification is a process by which an organization, often a national body, validates the credentials of an individual or a program. Certification is important for health care professionals. Certification is also important for medical assistants who live in a state that does not regulate unlicensed health professionals. When an unbiased national organization validates knowledge and skills, the employer can be sure that the medical assistant has excellent qualifications.

Two organizations provide nationally accepted certification for medical assistants: the AAMA and the AMT. In many areas, employers hire only medical assistants who have passed a certification examination. As medical assistants perform more specialized clinical tasks, employers have become increasingly concerned about validating skills and knowledge before hiring them.

Certified Medical Assistant

A certified medical assistant (CMA [AAMA]) has passed the certification examination administered by the AAMA. In order to take the examination, the individual must have graduated from a medical assisting program accredited by CAAHEP or ABHES.

The examination is computer-based (as of January 2009) and is administered at online testing centers. Most states have several testing locations.

Application material can be obtained from the AAMA Certification Department, 20 North Wacker Dr., Suite 1565, Chicago IL 60606-2903; from the director of accreditation at the medical assisting program attended; or from the AAMA website (www.aama-ntl.org).

Passing this examination allows a medical assistant to use the title CMA (AAMA) after his or her name on all official documents, including patient records and business cards.

Registered Medical Assistant

A registered medical assistant (RMA) has passed the examination administered by the AMT. The AMT is an organization that certifies medical assistants, medical technologists, medical laboratory technicians, phlebotomists, and other health professionals.

In order to take the RMA examination, an individual must have (1) graduated from a medical assisting program accredited by the ABHES or an organization approved by the U.S. Department of Education; (2) graduated from a formal medical services program of the U.S. armed forces; or (3) been employed in the profession of medical assisting for 5 years.

Applications for the RMA examination can be obtained from the Registrar's Office, American Medical Technologists, 710 Higgins Rd., Park Ridge IL 60068-5765. Information about the examination can be obtained from the AMT website. The RMA examination is given at Cogent testing center locations throughout the country on specific dates, or in many centers every week.

Passing this examination entitles the medical assistant to use the initials RMA after his or her name on all official documents.

Obtaining Additional Credentials

A medical assistant may need to validate other skills as a condition of employment.

Training in cardiopulmonary resuscitation (CPR) is offered directly through the American Red Cross (ARC) and the American Heart Association (AHA) and by hospitals and other health care agencies. Like other health professionals, medical assistants recertify every 1 to 2 years to be sure their skills are current as required by their professional organization and/or employer. Most health care facilities require current CPR credentials.

Medical assistants may also take courses in first aid, hearing tests, performing x-rays, or other specialized tests, depending on state law and the needs of the medical practice. In many areas, medical assisting certification or registration is a valid qualification to perform phlebotomy, but some states and/or institutions require separate certification in phlebotomy. This can be obtained through the AMT, the American Society of Clinical Pathologists (ASCP), or the American Society of Phlebotomy Technicians, Inc. The websites of these organizations are listed at the end of the chapter.

A medical assistant who obtains experience working for a podiatrist or ophthalmologist may obtain certification as a podiatric medical assistant, certified (PMAC) or a certified ophthalmic assistant (COA).

If the medical assistant specialized in the administrative area, additional credentials can be obtained, such as the Certified Medical Administrative Specialist (CMAS) from the AMT, or one of the various certifications in medical coding, such as a certified coding associate (CCA) or certified coding specialist–physician-based (CCS-P) from the American Health Information Management Association (AHIMA). The CCS-P is a coding practitioner who specializes in coding for physicians in settings, such as physician offices, group practices, multispecialty clinics, or specialty centers. Additional education may be required to obtain these credentials.

PROFESSIONAL ORGANIZATIONS

The AAMA and the AMT maintain professional organizations of medical assistants. For an annual membership fee, many benefits are available. Medical assisting students can join either the AAMA or the AMT for a reduced annual rate and receive member services. Membership information is available at the website for each organization.

Peer Support

Through local and national meetings and workshops, medical assistants are able to enter a network of peers with whom they can share and from whom they can learn. They can also obtain insurance at reasonable cost, professional journals, and other sources of information important to the profession.

Continuing Education

With the constant change in the medical field, it is not merely important but necessary to keep skills up to date, attain new skills, and obtain new information about professional practices. Most health professions require a certain amount of continuing education for licensure or certification renewal. These are designed either as contact hours or **continuing education units (CEUs).**

Medical assisting contact hours and CEUs can be obtained from educational programs that have been approved by the particular certifying agency. The AAMA validates continuing education programs given through the state and national organization. Attending meetings of professional organizations is the best way to find educational programs specifically for the needs of professional medical assistants. Home study programs are also available to obtain continuing education credit.

An individual must be recertified as a CMA (AAMA) every 5 years. This can be accomplished by retaking the certification examination or by successfully completing the required continuing education programs. Sixty contact hours must be accumulated during the 5-year period, 10 in the administrative area, 10 in the clinical area, and 10 in the general area, with 30 additional hours in any of the three categories. In addition, 30 of the contact hours must be from AAMA-approved programs.

If certified after January 2006, RMAs must accumulate 30 contact hours of continuing education every 3 years. Those who were certified before this date are expected to keep up to date with current practice, but there are no specific continuing education requirements.

Legislative Advocacy

One of the tasks of professional organizations is to monitor legislative initiatives at the state and national level that may affect the profession. In many states the profession of medical assisting is defined in state law, whereas in other states it is not. The state professional organization provides a forum to push for legislation that will advance the medical assisting profession.

Publications, Newsletters, and Websites

Both the national and state organizations provide a means for communication among professional medical assistants, including *CMA Today,* published by the AAMA, and the *Journal of Continuing Education Topics and Issues,* published by the AMT. The national organizations have state associations, often with several chapters within the state. The state organizations may produce newsletters and maintain websites. Conferences are held annually both nationally and at the state level to enhance communication and contact among members of the profession.

ROLE OF THE MEDICAL ASSISTANT
Administrative Responsibilities

Various administrative responsibilities must be performed on a daily basis in a medical office. We like to think of a physician's office as a place where patients receive medical treatment, but in reality much of the activity in a physician's office involves moving paperwork through specified processes. The medical assistant may be responsible for a number of these activities, although larger offices may employ specialists to perform these tasks.

1. Scheduling appointments, both over the telephone and in person, is a primary responsibility of the medical assistant. A patient may also need to have appointments made with other medical facilities; examples include a consultation with a specialist, a diagnostic procedure, outpatient surgery, continuing therapy or rehabilitation, and a hospital admission. Some patients may need to schedule multiple appointments with other facilities as the result of a single office visit. The medical assistant must learn the procedure for making and documenting each type of appointment (Figure 2-6).

2. Maintaining the medical record and filing records and reports has traditionally been one of the medical assistant's roles. With the increasing use of electronic medical records, there is less actual filing in many offices, but it still may be necessary to scan paper reports and keep track of laboratory and diagnostic test results. Each

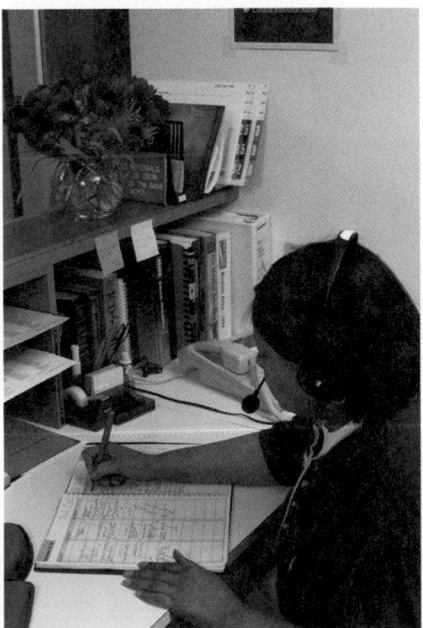

Figure 2-6. Medical assistant making an appointment. (From Hunt SA: *Saunders fundamentals of medical assisting,* St. Louis, 2007, Saunders.)

patient encounter with a clinician—physician, nurse practitioner (NP), or physician's assistant (PA)—is followed by documentation of the patient's visit. Clinicians create handwritten or dictated patient notes, or they may enter information directly into an electronic medical record. A medical assistant may be asked to perform medical transcription on these dictations, typing the notes and placing them into the chart. If the dictation method is used, it is currently more common to send the dictation to an outside service electronically. In this case the medical assistant prints the reports after they have been returned and files them in the correct medical record. Additionally, the medical assistant may write letters and prepare other documents for the physician.

3. Every patient visit generates a paper trail that is necessary for the physician to be paid for the services provided. The medical assistant must know how to accept and document payments (Figure 2-7), total and enter charges, code the procedures and/or diagnostic tests performed, and enter payments received. These charges and payments are entered either into the office computer and/or into various paper records, such as the day sheet, to keep track of money owed to the practice. In turn, the charges are used to generate insurance claims and patient bills. In larger offices and clinics, a separate business office usually handles financial matters. Small offices often send billing information to an outside billing service. If billing is performed in the office, the medical assistant must be able to create patient bills and submit insurance claims.

4. On a regular basis, checks and cash need to be deposited in the office's bank account. Preparing bank deposits and recording the deposits into the office's checkbook is an activity that medical assistants often perform.

5. Every business has bills to pay. These include rent (or mortgage, if the office is owned), electricity, lease payments on equipment, staff salaries, and a number of other regular payments, such as liability and malpractice insurance. Medical assistants, or business office personnel, usually write these checks and maintain records of these and other bills owed by the office. (Some offices have an outside bookkeeping service perform these tasks. Even in many offices that pay their own regular bills, salary is handled by an outside payroll service.)

Clinical Responsibilities

Depending on the type of medical office, clinical activities may provide the bulk of the medical assistant's responsibilities. The medical assistant prepares patients for examination, performs diagnostic tests, performs treatments, and assists the physician with examination and treatment.

1. Medical assistants are often asked to collect and process specimens. Some specimens are tested in the office, and others are sent to an outside laboratory.

2. Medical assistants perform several diagnostic tests, such as electrocardiograms and respiratory testing.

3. Medical assistants prepare patients for examination, including taking medical histories, weighing the patient, measuring vital signs, and obtaining the chief complaint. Having this done by a medical assistant may allow the physician to see at least one extra patient per hour.

4. Between each patient, the medical assistant prepares the examination and/or treatment room (Figure 2-8). This involves making sure there is fresh paper on the table, that the proper instruments and supplies are available for the next examination or procedure, and that the necessary equipment is available and in working order.

5. Medical assistants help the physician with examinations and procedures. The medical assistant settles a patient into an examination room and positions and drapes the patient for portions of the examination. Another duty is to pass instruments and supplies to the physician during procedures. The medical assistant may also remove

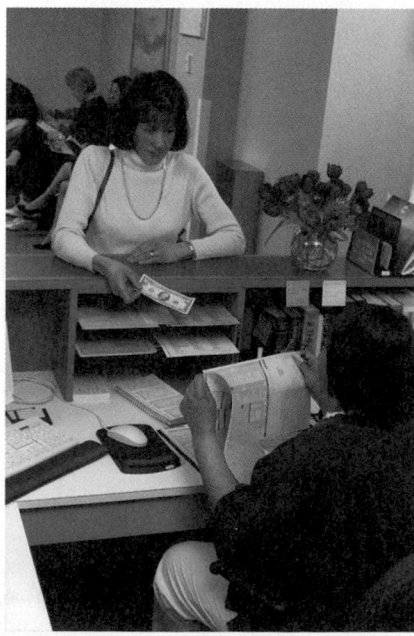

Figure 2-7. Medical assistant taking a payment. (From Hunt SA: *Saunders fundamentals of medical assisting*, St. Louis, 2007, Saunders.)

Figure 2-8. Medical assistant preparing an examination room. (From Hunt SA: *Saunders fundamentals of medical assisting*, St. Louis, 2007, Saunders.)

sutures and change sterile dressings. If minor surgery or sterile procedures are performed in the office, the medical assistant sets up the equipment and supplies and then assists the physician as needed.

6. Medical assistants perform treatments, including nebulizer and IPPB (intermittent positive-pressure breathing) treatments or application of hot and cold packs or compresses.

7. Medical assistants prepare and administer medications and immunizations. The administration of medication requires concentration and precision. All medications must be documented according to office procedure.

8. Sometimes a medical assistant also has to perform emergency care and administer first aid or assist with an office emergency. This does not happen often, but every medical assistant must be prepared.

Managing the Medical Office

The medical assistant may have many responsibilities to keep the medical office running smoothly.

1. Operational activities involve maintaining the inventory of supplies. This can include everything from purchasing tongue blades and gauze to contracting with a uniform service to launder the staff's laboratory coats or patient gowns. It may also involve evaluating and recommending changes in the supplies purchased and evaluating new equipment for potential purchase or lease.

2. A second group of activities involves personnel policy and procedures. Businesses are always reviewing their policies and procedures and updating and revising them as needed. As offices move from one or two physicians and a small staff to a larger organization, policies and procedures become more important to standardize the way all employees are dealt with.

3. **Risk management** is the development of policies and procedures that minimize the chances of the practice being sued by a patient or disciplined by a regulatory agency. Every physician's office needs to have one person responsible for risk management, which involves, among other areas, the promotion of health and safety for office personnel and patients, implementation of a quality control program, maintenance of proper infection control measures, fire prevention, and the proper disposal of hazardous waste and controlled substances.

4. Record-keeping is an important activity for the individual who manages a medical office. In addition to patient records, many other kinds of records must be kept, including office insurance records, quality control records, maintenance contracts, personnel records, and financial records.

Patient Education

Instructing patients is an important role for medical assistants because the medical assistant actually conveys information to the patient from the physician.

1. The medical assistant is often responsible for educating the patient about office procedures, including giving information to a new patient who is making the first appointment, as well as instructing an established patient whose circumstances have changed.

2. The medical assistant may provide information about maintaining health to patients directly as directed by the physician or by making educational materials available in the office. These are always reviewed by the physician before being given to patients (Figure 2-9).

3. The medical assistant may locate community resources for a patient or provide brochures from community agencies in order to improve follow-up care for a patient.

Memories *from* Externship

Beth Ann Wilson: I could not believe how nervous I was before I went to my externship the first day. I had worked at several jobs and even done filing at a medical office during the summer when I was in high school, but it felt totally different to know that I would be responsible to act like a "real" medical assistant. Fortunately, the staff members at my placement were wonderful. They let me shadow one of the medical assistants until I felt comfortable to work with patients on my own. They were also careful to expose me gradually to each part of the medical office, so it didn't get overwhelming. The person who helped me the most was Cheryl, the office manager. Every day she sought me out and asked how it was going. There was one time when a physician asked me to take out a patient's sutures, and I hadn't even seen someone perform that procedure. I didn't know what to say, but I told him I would find another medical assistant to help him. Then I went to Cheryl. She found someone else to perform the procedure and made sure that I had an opportunity to observe. I never could decide whether I liked checking patients in up front or assisting the physicians better, as long as I had a chance to interact with patients. It has always made me feel good to know that I am helping others. ∎

Prepare for Success

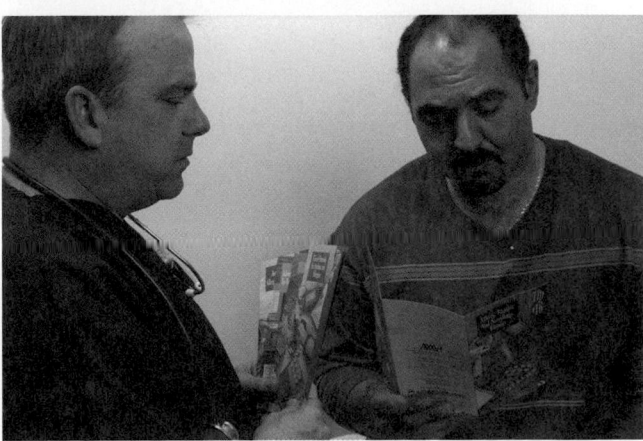

Figure 2-9. The medical assistant uses brochures to teach a patient. (From Hunt SA: *Saunders fundamentals of medical assisting*, St. Louis, 2007, Saunders.)

EMPLOYMENT OPPORTUNITIES

According to the U.S. Department of Labor Bureau of Labor Statistics, medical assisting is projected to be one of the fastest growing occupations in the period between 2006 and 2016. Job prospects are expected to be better for medical assistants who have completed a formal educational program.

In 2006 the majority of medical assistants worked in physician's offices. About 12% worked in public and private hospitals in either inpatient or outpatient areas. About 11% worked in offices of other health practitioners, such as chiropractors, podiatrists, or optometrists. Other employment opportunities included outpatient care centers, schools or other education facilities, medical laboratories, government agencies, employment services, and nursing care facilities.

The median annual income reported by medical assistants in May 2006 was $26,290, but salaries varied greatly depending on geographic location, skill level, and type of facility in which the medical assistant was employed.

The Bureau of Labor Statistics reported median annual income for medical assistants in May 2006 as follows:

General medical and surgical hospitals	$27,340
Outpatient care centers	$26,840
Offices of physicians	$26,620
Offices of chiropractors	$22,920
Offices of optometrists	$22,850

The most direct route for career advancement is probably to become an office, practice, or department manager. This may require additional education, especially in business administration, but often management skills can be learned mainly on the job. In order to become a medical assisting instructor, it is necessary to have an Associate in Science Degree or a higher degree in a related field and to be either a CMA (AAMA) or an RMA (for an accredited medical assisting program). Clinical advancement usually requires additional training in a formal education program preparing for a health career, such as dental hygiene, laboratory technology, nursing, radiologic technology, or respiratory therapy.

MEDICAL PRACTICE and the LAW

Medical assistants are not licensed, and in most states their role is not clearly defined in the law. State medical practice laws usually allow physicians to delegate clinical tasks to qualified medical assistants under their supervision, provided that the task is not prohibited by another law. Some states do define the role of a medical assistant, sometimes related to general duties and sometimes related to specific tasks that the medical assistant is allowed to perform. In some states, medical assistants are required to register with the state before practicing as a medical assistant. Because state laws vary so greatly, a medical assisting student should always find out the legal status of a medical assistant in his or her own state or the state in which he or she intends to work after graduation. ■

What Would You Do? What Would You Not Do? RESPONSES

Case Study 1
Page 24

What Did Beth Ann Do?
❑ Looked in the back part of the office for an available staff member.
❑ Asked the receptionist if she knew where one of the other medical assistants was.
❑ Used the intercom to locate a medical assistant.
❑ Checked the examination rooms with open doors to see if a medical assistant might be almost finished checking in a patient.
❑ Assisted the physician if she was unable to find another medical assistant to do it.

What Did Beth Ann Not Do?
❑ Leave for lunch without finding someone to assist the physician.
❑ Tell the physician that she was sorry she could not assist him at this time.
❑ Knock on closed examination room doors.

What Would You Do/What Would You Not Do? Review Beth Ann's response and place a checkmark next to the information you included in your response. List the additional information you included in your response.

_____
_____
_____
_____

Case Study 2
Page 26

What Did Beth Ann Do?
❑ Agreed to draw the blood without complaining.
❑ Tried to make the patient feel comfortable and confident.
❑ Explained to Diane later that some patients do not want students to perform certain procedures.
❑ Told Diane that she was glad she had called her to help.
❑ Reinforced that even if Diane's pride was slightly hurt, Diane did the correct thing by not showing this to the patient.

What Did Beth Ann Not Do?
❑ Did not make the patient feel as if she were asking for special treatment.
❑ Did not tell Diane that she looked very young or unprofessional.

❏ Did not talk about the incident as a funny story in the break room to other staff.

What Would You Do/What Would You *Not* Do? Review Beth Ann's response and place a checkmark next to the information you included in your response. List the additional information you included in your response.

_____

_____

_____

_____

Case Study 3
Page 27

What Did Beth Ann Do?
❏ Told the patient that the physician asked her to recheck the blood pressure because it sometimes changes when patients sit in a quiet examination room.
❏ Found a private place to speak to Diane and agreed with her that sometimes it is really hard to hear the blood pressure.
❏ Explained to Diane that it is important to take and record the blood pressure correctly even if she has to ask for assistance.

❏ Reminded Diane that the staff understands she is a student and will not be able to perform every procedure perfectly.
❏ Offered to work with Diane to improve her technique.
❏ Only discussed the incident with the office manager, if anyone.

What Did Beth Ann Not *Do?*
❏ Did not talk down to Diane or try to make her feel bad.
❏ Did not tell others in the office not to rely on Diane's blood pressure measurements.
❏ Did not tell the patient that Diane had not been sure of her measurement.

What Would You Do/What Would You *Not* Do? Review Beth Ann's responses and place a checkmark next to the information you included in your response. List the additional information you included in your response.

_____

_____

_____

_____

TERMINOLOGY REVIEW

Accreditation Credit or recognition for maintaining certain standards by a regional or national organization.

Continuing education unit (CEU) A standard unit of measure on continuing education for professionals, defined as 10 contact hours of participation.

Externship A work experience that is required in an educational program and usually unpaid.

Fee splitting The practice of sharing fees with colleagues, especially for making referrals.

Initiative The ability to begin or carry through on a plan of action independently.

Risk management Processes to protect a health care facility from the risk of legal action.

ON THE WEB

For Information on Professional Organizations:

Accrediting Bureau of Health Education Schools: www.abhes.org

American Association of Medical Assistants: www.aama-ntl.org

American Health Information Management Association: www.ahima.org

American Medical Association: www.ama-assn.org

American Medical Technologists: www.amt1.com

American Society for Clinical Pathology: www.ascp.org

American Society of Phlebotomy Technicians: www.aspt.org

American Society of Podiatric Medical Assistants: www.aspma.org

Commission on Accreditation of Allied Health Education Programs: www.caahep.org

Joint Commission on Allied Health Personnel in Ophthalmology: www.jcahpo.org/newsite/index.htm

For Information on Occupational Outlook for Medical Assistants:

U.S. Department of Labor Bureau of Labor Statistics: www.bls.gov

PREPARE FOR CERTIFICATION Visit the Evolve site at http://evolve.elsevier.com/Bonewit/today/ to actively Prepare for your Certification.

Check out the Companion CD bound with the book to access additional interactive activities.

3

Ethics and Law for the Medical Office

LEARNING OBJECTIVES

Ethics and Health Care

1. Identify key differences between law and ethics.
2. List reasons for medical assistants to study ethics.
3. Identify specific rights that patients have in relation to health care.
4. Correlate the concept of duties to the actions expected of health professionals.
5. Describe how certain ethical issues generate ethical conflict in society.
6. Describe six steps that may be used to make ethical decisions.
7. Discuss several ways that ethical decisions may be made by individuals, groups, and/or society.

Law and Professional Liability

1. Identify similarities and differences between public law and private law.
2. Identify the process through which laws are created on the federal and state level.
3. Differentiate between types of crimes, such as felonies and misdemeanors, as well as between violent and nonviolent crimes.
4. Differentiate between criminal law and civil law.
5. List and explain the elements of a valid contract.
6. State the rights and duties of each party in the physician-patient relationship.
7. Define "standard of care," and describe how this concept affects the behavior of health professionals.
8. Describe the medical assistant's role in obtaining informed consent.
9. Explain the principles of negligence and professional negligence as they apply to the behavior of health professionals.
10. Explain the purpose and need for professional liability insurance.
11. Describe the process of malpractice litigation.
12. List and explain specific defenses to intentional and unintentional torts.

Federal and State Laws Regulating the Medical Office

1. Describe and explain the laws regulating controlled substances and prescription medications.
2. List and explain several laws that protect employees of medical offices.
3. Describe how the provisions of the Health Insurance Portability and Accountability Act (HIPAA) affect the medical office.
4. List and explain the situations where mandatory reporting is required by the medical office.
5. Describe how states regulate the practice of medicine and health occupations.
6. Differentiate between licensing and voluntary accreditation for health care facilities.

CHAPTER OUTLINE

Introduction to Medical Ethics
Reasons to Study Ethics
Ethics and Health Care
    Ethical Concepts
    Ethical Conflict
    Process Used to Make Ethical Decisions
    Ethical Decisions

Introduction to Law
    Difference between Public Law and Private Law
    Lawsuits
    Specialized Areas of Public Law
    Creation of Laws
    Criminal Law
    Civil Law

Law and Professional Liability
  Physician-Patient Relationship
  Personal and Professional Liability
  Malpractice Litigation
  Tort Defenses
Federal and State Laws Affecting the Medical Office
  Controlled Substances and Prescriptions

Federal and State Law Protecting Employees
Health Insurance Portability and Accountability Act of 1996
Mandatory Reporting
State Regulation of Health Occupations
Facility Licensing and Accreditation

CAAHEP COMPETENCIES

General Competencies
Legal Concepts
- Identify and respond to issues of confidentiality.

- Perform within legal and ethical boundaries.
- Demonstrate knowledge of federal and state health care legislation and regulations.

ABHES COMPETENCIES

Legal Concepts
- Follow established policy in initiating or terminating medical treatment.

- Maintain licenses and accreditation.
- Monitor legislation related to current health care issues and practices.

KEY TERMS

abandonment
act
arbitration
assumption of risk
autonomy (ah-TAW-noe-mee)
beneficence (ben-IH-fih-sens)
bill
case law
certificate of need
civil law
cloning (KLOW-ning)
common law
comparative negligence (NEG-lih-jhens)
contingency (kon-TIN-jhen-see)
contributory negligence
controlled substance
crime
criminal law
defendant
do-not-resuscitate (DNR)
Drug Enforcement Administration (DEA)
duty
emancipated minor
embezzlement (em-BEZ-el-ment)
etiquette
felony
fidelity
fraud
gene therapy
genetic engineering
health care proxy (PROX-ee)

informed consent
larceny
liability
license
licensure (LI-sen-sur)
litigation (lih-tih-GAY-shun)
living will
malfeasance (mal-FEE-suns)
malpractice
mediation
misdemeanor (mis-de-MEAN-or)
misfeasance (mis-FEE-suns)
negligence (NEG-lih-jhens)
nonfeasance (non-FEE-suns)
nonmalfeasance (non-mal-FEE-suns)
plaintiff (PLANE-tiff)
prescription
privilege
prudent
reciprocity (re-sip-RAW-city)
respondeat superior (ray-SPON-day-at sue-peer-ee-or)
right
standard of care
statute of limitations (STA-chewt)
statutory law (STA-chew-toe-ree)
stem cells
subpoena (su-PEE-na)
subpoena *duces tecum* (su-PEE-na DEW-chess TAY-come)
tort
veracity (ver-ASS-ih-tee)

Introduction to Medical Ethics

Within a democracy, society tolerates a wide range of beliefs about what is moral or right and uses the democratic process to create rules and laws that regulate public behavior. This process allows for change and flexibility because laws are continually reviewed through the judiciary process.

It is important to remember that society's beliefs about right and wrong precede laws and also influence their interpretation. Currently, the rapid pace of technologic innovation and changing beliefs place considerable stress on the social structure.

There is also a wide diversity of expectations about normal, acceptable behavior, sometimes called **etiquette,** or manners. Breaches of etiquette are far less important than failure to adhere to high ethical standards, and they pose no true threat to the integrity of an individual or society. However, individuals may have just as strong an emotional reaction to what they see as bad manners as they would to a true ethical breach.

In the context of the medical office, a patient may feel that being rushed by the physician and treated "as a number, not a name" by the front-office staff is being treated without dignity. The patient's emotional response to how he or she is treated may seem more important than the actual quality of care.

REASONS TO STUDY ETHICS

Although ethics is an abstract discipline and medical assisting is firmly grounded in practice and procedure, medical assistants should study ethics for a number of reasons.

First, it is an important part of an individual's education to develop the intellectual skills to analyze complex problems and justify the choices made in particular situations. In the case of ethics, the choice is between alternative courses of action that have moral and social consequences.

Second, as society has become increasingly complex, average citizens are more aware that choices affect not only people living now, but those who will live in the future. People hesitate to allow only elected and appointed officials to deal with these choices. Learning about ethics and social issues encourages ordinary people to have input into social beliefs and expectations. There is also a greater sense of interconnections involving the whole word, sometimes called *globalism.* Many individuals feel some level of responsibility for all human beings, and indeed for all living beings on the earth.

Third, in the specific realm of medicine and science, more sophisticated medical treatment and new technologies are constantly becoming available. However, society does not have unlimited resources to provide everything to everyone, even in the developed world. There is a need to make informed choices about what care will be provided to whom, and when, rather than simply responding to special interests.

Fourth, every year new biomedical research makes it possible to do more things with which the world has no previous experience. Society must have informed citizens who can analyze issues and guide the future. Within the health care system, health professionals, including medical assistants, need skills in considering ethical questions in order to improve health care for individuals and society.

ETHICS AND HEALTH CARE
Ethical Concepts

Current thinking about biomedical ethics identifies several rights (very strong claims) for patients and duties (requirements) for the institutions and individuals who provide health care. Sources for these ideas include religious traditions, social belief systems, political documents such as the Declaration of Independence and the U.S. Constitution and the Bill of Rights, as well as ethical theories developed by individual philosophers.

Rights

A **right** is a claim that is expected to be honored. It is stronger than a wish or a need.

The early leaders of the American government believed in natural rights and the duty of any government to preserve them. Natural rights exist through the natural order or are granted by God. These include the following:
1. Right to life
2. Right to privacy
3. Right to autonomy
4. Right to the means to sustain life

Right to Life

One of the rights mentioned in the Declaration of Independence is the right to life.

Since the 1970s, the term "right to life" has come to be associated with the movement against abortion. But in a broader context, it reflects the belief that human beings may not kill others. The belief in the right to life is found in all major religions and traditions.

The right to life has many implications for medicine. Historically, physicians and other health care workers may not harm patients because this may threaten their lives. They may not assist with suicide; this is expressly stated in the Hippocratic Oath. In the United States today, however, many individuals want some control over death, including the choice of suicide assisted by their physician.

Two important areas of conflict appeared in the middle of the twentieth century. First, advances in medical care made it possible to keep people alive who could not recover their health. Sometimes, this sustaining of life came at the cost of prolonged suffering.

Second, the absolute right to life of an unborn fetus conflicts with the right of a woman to control her own reproductive capacity. Birth-control methods, artificial conception methods and abortion, if necessary, are measures to control the size of a woman's family. Many women and their physicians have come to believe they have a right to make decisions related to reproduction, including using available technology, as they see fit.

Right to Privacy

The Supreme Court has ruled that there is an implicit right to privacy in the Bill of Rights, specifically in the Fourth Amendment. A series of court decisions affirming a woman's right to use mechanical birth control and to have an abortion hinged on justices' perceiving this right to privacy.

Patient confidentiality, which has been upheld by courts, is another manifestation of the right to privacy. Patient confidentiality is discussed in detail later in this chapter.

Right to Autonomy

Currently, medical ethics takes the position that an individual has the right to **autonomy,** which means the right to make independent decisions about his or her health care according to individual values and concerns, without constraint or coercion from others. This right is preserved even when the individual's decisions do not match the values of the medical community or the individual physician. The right of autonomy is the basis for **informed consent.** Informed consent is consent based on understanding of a medical procedure and its possible outcomes. Health care professionals must provide complete information in order for patients to make informed decisions. The patient must have the mental capacity to reason and consider alternatives. Because of this, the law limits the autonomy of children or individuals with decreased mental capacity such as the mentally retarded or individuals whose mental capacity has been impaired by illness, those acting under the influence of drugs or alcohol, and those experiencing mental illness.

Respect for autonomy does not derive from the Hippocratic Oath. Rather, it comes from the thinking of European philosophers such as Immanuel Kant and John Locke.

Right to the Means to Sustain Life

Every society must grapple with the problem of equitable distribution of goods and services to its citizens and how to regulate that distribution over time.

This is not a problem when the supply is adequate, or when supply is greater than demand. For instance, in ordinary circumstances the supply of oxygen is more than adequate to meet the needs of the entire population.

It is when the amount of a particular resource is less than the desire for that resource that problems develop. In this case, resources are said to be scarce, and the society's government must determine who will have access to the scarce resources.

At a minimum, every individual should have access to what is necessary to sustain life and preserve human dignity. Consideration of justice in distribution and access is especially important in social and political movements. Any society must find ways to respond to need while also rewarding contribution and providing for stability within the social system.

Currently, in the allocation of health care resources in the United States, it is increasingly difficult to determine what is necessary for everyone. Many expensive procedures are available, some of which have limited expectations for success and some of which relate more to happiness than health.

Health care economists and nongovernmental organizations such as the World Health Organization are constantly engaging in this discussion, along with experts in biomedical ethics. For instance, for the same financial cost as one bone marrow transplant, with its attendant postsurgical care, many adolescent females could receive an immunization against cervical cancer.

Duties

A **duty** is a commitment to act in a certain way on the basis of religious beliefs, moral principles, or a particular professional code of conduct. Traditionally five main duties of a health care professional have been identified.

Putting It All into Practice

My name is Vicki Edmonds, and I have worked in a family practice for about 6 years. There are two physicians and two nurse practitioners in my practice, and I usually assist one of the physicians. Of course, if it is busy, or one of the other medical assistants is ill, we all pitch in and help out. Neither of the physicians in my practice has ever been sued, and we all work together to be sure it stays that way. We do everything we can so that our patients not only receive great care but are also satisfied with their treatment. We also document everything carefully because our physicians are aware that it is hard to prove that you gave good care if you don't write it down. Every once in a while we have a patient who constantly breaks appointments or doesn't take his or her medication, and if the physician thinks that it is harmful to the patient's health, sometimes he will instruct the patient to find another practitioner to care for him or her. I remember one time when the patient lived far away, and she said that it was difficult for her to make the trip to our office. After she missed three appointments in a row, the physician had me write a letter suggesting that she find another physician nearer to her home. He explained that he couldn't be responsible for her if she was unable to keep appointments. In the letter he gave her a month to find another physician, and he offered to help her if she was having difficulty. We sent that letter by certified mail and obtained a return receipt. Then we documented everything in the patient's medical record. The patient sent a letter back saying that she was going to an office much closer to home, and she thought that would work out better for her. ■

Prepare for Success

Do No Harm

The concept of **nonmalfeasance** means, first of all, doing no harm in any treatment given. This duty is found in the Hippocratic Oath. It is not taken in a literal sense because many treatments can have adverse effects. Rather, it is taken to mean that medical benefits should outweigh adverse effects.

This concept applies especially to scientific research. Guidelines for ethical research not only require informed consent but also restrict research with possible harmful effects to those patients whose conditions are so serious that doing nothing is likely to be as dangerous as the treatment or procedure being studied.

Do the Best Possible

The concept of **beneficence,** doing the best possible, is seen in some systems of ethics as a separate duty, whereas in others it is considered an extension of doing no harm. It is often difficult to pinpoint exactly what harm and good are; this may vary with a particular individual's viewpoint.

Be Faithful to Reasonable Expectations

The concept of **fidelity,** being faithful, comes from the Latin term *fides,* which means faithful. In the case of medical practice, fidelity is usually interpreted as meaning faithful to reasonable expectations. Although patient expectations vary, there is general agreement that a patient can reasonably expect to be treated with dignity, treated by individuals who honor their agreements, and treated by competent providers. Patients can also expect that they will be cared for by individuals who adhere to the ethical standards of their profession, to statutory law, and to accepted medical and scientific practice.

Tell the Truth

The concept of **veracity** has increased in importance since the nineteenth century. Veracity is not found in the Hippocratic Oath. It has developed with the evolution of the scientific tradition. Today it is seen as a proactive duty—physicians and other health care professionals must provide truthful information without having to be asked. It is a tenet of modern science that scientific knowledge belongs to all. Results of experiments must be accurate and reviewed by other scientists to see if the results can be replicated, then published for the benefit of all.

Give Each Person a Fair Share

The concept of justice requires that each individual is given his or her due and deserves a fair share of resources. However, there is often an underlying belief that an individual must contribute or bear a portion of the burden before being allowed to get certain resources. Justice in the context of medical practice appears not only in terms of distribution of medical resources, but also in the belief in the right to compensation if a mistake is made.

Many Americans believe that everyone is entitled to the benefit of health insurance. As a nation, we have not been able to agree on a means to provide universal health insurance, although we try to provide emergency care to all. Individuals without insurance often need to wait until their health status deteriorates to the level of an "emergency" before they can receive care. To many, this seems not only unfair, but a poor way to manage health care resources as well.

Deciding what is "fair" is often a matter of the situation. In the United States, the tendency is to believe in "first come, first served." But in an emergency department, serious conditions must take precedence.

Ethical Conflict

Many issues become controversial when there is a disagreement within society about the relative hierarchy of certain rights and duties.

Reproductive Issues

Conflict surrounds the issues of contraception, abortion, and other issues related to reproduction. In regard to pregnancy, some people feel that the duty to follow divine law or natural measures take precedence over an individual's right to autonomy. This results in differing beliefs about how appropriate it is to use contraception and artificial measures to become pregnant. There has been controversy about the "morning-after pill" (marketed under the name Plan B). Because it has been found to be relatively safe, it was finally approved as an over-the-counter medication for women older than age 18 by the Food and Drug Administration (FDA) in 2006.

Another controversial issue is abortion. Some argue that the fetus's right to life outweighs the woman's right to privacy in determining—with her physician—the proper course of her medical care. Since the original U.S. Supreme Court decision in 1973 upholding a woman's right to obtain an abortion in any state (Roe vs. Wade), the Court has been called on to rule many times on various state laws that seek to limit this right. The Partial-Birth Abortion Ban Act of 2003, which prohibits a specific abortion procedure that can done in the second trimester of pregnancy, is an example of a federal law that restricts a woman's right to abortion in some cases.

What Would You Do? What Would You *Not* Do?

Case Study 1

Denise Fitzgerald is a 16-year-old female who has come to the office for complaints of a sore throat and fever. While Vicki is doing vital signs, she notices a circular wound on Denise's arms that looks like a cigarette burn. It is red and has some crusted areas. When she asks Denise about it, the patient blushes and says in a low voice that her boyfriend burned her a few days ago to teach her a lesson. Then Denise says, "Please don't tell the doctor because he will tell my mother, and I'm afraid she will make me break up with my boyfriend." ■

Stem Cell Research

A promising area of research for medical treatment involves the use of embryonic **stem cells.** These cells, taken from fetal tissue, are able to mature into different types of tissue. Embryonic cells may be found to be able to reduce, or possibly even reverse, the symptoms of Parkinson's disease and other diseases.

The ethical conflict arises because a possible source of embryonic cells tissue is from aborted fetuses or fertilized ova not used for in vitro fertilization. Researchers who use fetal tissue stress that they use only tissue from spontaneous abortions (miscarriages). Antiabortion advocates argue that if there is an increased need for fetal tissue, a time may come when women might be influenced in their decision whether or not to have an abortion if they could sell their fetus's tissue for research and/or treatment. In 2001 the federal government introduced a policy that federal funding would only be available for the 64 then-existing stem cell lines. Since then there are been several unsuccessful efforts to introduce federal legislation to loosen restrictions. Some states have passed laws to promote funding for research from private and/or state sources.

Genetic Engineering and Cloning

A number of ethical issues surround the practices of **genetic engineering** (making, altering, or repairing genetic material) and **cloning** (reproducing genetically identical cells or individuals).

One is the issue of genetically engineered crops and other food products. This encompasses practices as diverse as injecting milk cows with growth hormones in order to get them to produce more milk to incorporating material from bacteria into plant seeds. Opponents argue that we cannot predict all of the possible effects of manipulating genetic material and are likely to see unexpected and unwanted consequences to ourselves or other species.

Gene therapy is a term used for experimental treatments that attempt to treat or cure disease by giving patients new genes or parts of genes that may have been synthesized in the laboratory, taken from human tissue, or engineered from genetic material of animals or other species. Research efforts are overseen by the Recombinant DNA Advisory Committee of the National Institutes of Health (NIH). A clinical study of a gene therapy treatment for arthritis was suspended in July 2007 after the death of a patient.

Human cloning is prohibited by several states, but efforts to pass legislation on the federal level have not succeeded to date. Experiments in animal cloning continue although critics claim that it results in unhealthy animals and needless suffering. There are serious concerns about safety and health if cloned animals were introduced into the food supply chain.

Refusing or Withholding Treatment and Physician-Assisted Suicide

The right to refuse treatment is well established for adults. The 1990 Patient Self-Determination Act establishes the duty of hospitals, nursing homes, and health maintenance organizations (HMOs) to inform patients or new subscribers of their right to express their wishes related to health care and to refuse treatment. The act also establishes the right of an individual to prepare an advance directive that specifies what treatments he or she would like to receive, and which he or she would not wish to receive, if the individual becomes incapable of making those decisions at a later time. Courts have held an individual's right to refuse treatment in such high regard that they have allowed mentally ill patients to refuse treatments for their mental illness.

When an individual requires resuscitation or life support to stay alive, there may come a point where it seems that the treatment is resulting in more suffering (harm) than benefit. This is especially true if it is unlikely that the person can recover his or her health or normal function. If there is a written document expressing the person's wishes, life support may be removed or discontinued. In the absence of an advance directive, an individual's family may bring to court a petition to remove life support. Such a petition must be supported by witnesses other than those who file the petition, stating that the incompetent individual expressed a desire to avoid being kept alive by artificial means. Life support has been interpreted to include ventilators, antibiotics, and even tube feedings.

Physician-assisted suicide and euthanasia (literally, "good death"), sometimes called *mercy killing,* evoke fears that the power to take life will be abused—that it will be used more for the convenience of others than for the well-being of those who are dying. Advocates for the disabled have argued that allowing physician-assisted suicide or euthanasia could be the first step in society's determining that the severely disabled are too much of a financial and physical burden, and having them euthanized.

Throughout the 1990s, an individual physician named Jack Kevorkian provided patients with degenerative, terminal illness a machine that provided an injection of lethal drugs. He was sentenced to 10 to 25 years in prison in 1999 and released after 8 years in 2007 after he promised not to assist in any additional deaths.

In 1997, Oregon became the first state to legalize physician-assisted suicide, allowing physicians to write a prescription for a patient of a lethal dose of pain killer or other medication. The physician is not allowed to administer the medication themselves. The U.S. Supreme Court upheld a challenge to the Oregon law in 2006. The discussion about physician-assisted suicide occurs in every state, but to date similar legislation has failed to pass in any other state.

Terminally ill patients and their families are often looking for a trusted advisor with whom they can discuss their fears and concerns. Even when a physician is not morally willing or legally able to provide a means for a patient to end his or her life, there is increasing recognition of the value of frank discussion and reassurance that patients will not be left to cope alone.

Process Used to Make Ethical Decisions

Making ethical decisions involves measures to respond to conflict between different values and their relative importance. In order to decide on a course of action, it is helpful to clarify the conflict and make a thoughtful choice. A six-step process can be used to make sure that actions are well considered and in accordance with beliefs about what is right and wrong, rather than simply impulse reactions.

Gathering Information

Information that needs to be gathered includes (1) background about the situation; (2) facts related to the specific problem; (3) information about the people involved, such as their knowledge of the situation or their mental capacity; and (4) the laws or institutional policies that relate to the situation.

Identifying Conflicting Values

A conflict does not always involve lofty values. It may be as simple as one person's wish not to cause problems, to save time, or to avoid a hassle. However, this desire may conflict with professional duties or with another individual's right.

If a medical assistant is working in a facility that does not always follow established procedures (e.g., does not always run controls for laboratory tests), the desire to go along with coworkers and avoid conflict may be strong; however, the duty to act with fidelity is not being met. The medical assistant may be personally performing the needed controls, but the knowledge that others are not doing so creates a conflict between reluctance to violate the autonomy of a coworker and the duty of fidelity to patients.

Determining Relative Importance of Conflicting Claims

To determine the relative importance of conflicting claims, an individual needs to clarify his or her goals and weigh the conflicting values. It is important to remember that when values conflict, an individual or group makes a decision about importance that is valid within its own context, but may not conform with the values of other individuals or groups.

For example, in the case of abortion, some people believe that the right of a fetus to life outweighs all other rights. Others believe that a woman's right to autonomy in medical decisions about her body, and the consequences to a child of being unwanted, diminish or outweigh the absolute right to life in the early stages of a pregnancy.

Exploring Alternatives

Once it has been established which values are more important, it is important to consider the possible outcomes of actions that may be taken. It is helpful to identify as many courses of action as possible, predict the consequences of each action, and project how different goals would be met or not met by following each possible course of action.

Choosing and Justifying One Alternative

Conflicting claims require choices. By analyzing hypothetic situations in detail, a person can construct some sort of personal framework for ethical decisions; once on the job, there is often little time to analyze each situation individually.

In the end, there are four ways to justify a decision:
1. By presenting logical arguments—deductions based on facts
2. By social justification—consideration of the larger consequences to society
3. By projection of consequences—imagining what might happen if a given alternative is chosen
4. By refuting alternative claims—stating explicitly why alternative choices have less merit than the one chosen

If it is impossible to select any alternative that seems comfortable, or "right," the choice to do nothing becomes a chosen alternative rather than simply the avoidance of a decision.

Implementing the Decision

The final step in this process is to put the ethical decision into action. The decision can be reconsidered and another solution can be tried.

Ethical Decisions

Individual

Often, the person who is responsible for the consequences makes the decision. In a medical office, the medical assistant refers decisions related to patient care to the physician.

This means that the medical assistant cannot ethically withhold from the physician information given by the patient related to medical condition. Even if the medical assistant does not agree with how the physician is managing a patient's care, the medical assistant cannot ethically (or legally) suggest another treatment plan for the patient.

On the other hand, the medical assistant makes decisions related to his or her own actions. For example, a medical assistant may refuse a request to reveal personal information about a patient to another staff member who is not directly involved in patient care.

Advance Directives

On the basis of personal beliefs, patients can formalize their decisions about treatment in terminal or end-of-life situations in a number of ways. These include **do-not-resuscitate (DNR)** orders, living wills, health care proxies, and organ donor cards, all of which fall under the heading of "advance directives" (Box 3-1). An advance directive may specify care to be given or avoided and name a person to make medical decisions for the individual should he or she become incompetent. This is usually a spouse, child older than age 18, member of the clergy, or close friend. Medical advance directives should always name a single individual to make decisions, with an alternate if possible. This is often a difficult choice, especially for an elderly person with several children.

BOX 3-1 Advance Directives

Do-Not-Resuscitate (DNR) Order

Requested by either patient or health care agent. A written order from the physician in the patient's medical record that allows medical staff to not resuscitate in the event of cardiac or respiratory arrest.

Living Will

Executed by an individual before or during illness. Identifies the patient's wishes about which life-prolonging actions should or should not be taken. In states that accept it, it provides instructions to health professionals about treatment to be provided and may include instructions to a health care agent as to which treatments he or she should authorize. Provisions for organ donation, autopsy, or donation of remains to a medical school are also usually included in a living will.

Health Care Proxy

Executed by an individual before or during illness. Names a health care agent who has the ability to make decisions about care, including signing a DNR. It may also outline the types of care that the individual does or does not wish to receive. It becomes effective only when the individual becomes incapable of making his or her own decisions.

Organ Donor Card

A card stating that an individual wishes to donate organs. Many states have done away with a separate organ donor card, preferring to place the organ-donor designation on an individual's driver's license.

Uniform Donor Card

I _____ hereby make this anatomical gift, if medically acceptable, to take effect upon my death. I give:

____ Any needed organs/tissues for any purpose

____ Only the following listed organs/tissues

_____

(Specify the organ[s] or tissue[s])

____ My body for anatomical study if needed

Limitations or special wishes: _____

_____

- -

This is a legal document under the Uniform Anatomical Gift or similar laws, signed by the donor and two witnesses in the presence of each other.

_____
Signature of Donor

_____   _____
Date Signed   *Donor's Date of Birth*

_____   _____
City   *City*

_____
Signature of Witness

_____
Signature of Witness

Figure 3-1. Organ donor card. (From Hunt SA: *Saunders fundamentals of medical assisting,* St. Louis, 2007, Saunders.)

In addition, the patient may want to provide for donation of any organs that are useful. If the patient does not make this decision ahead of time, the family can do it as part of their decision-making powers under an advance directive document. Signed originals rather than photocopies of the advance directives should be held by the named surrogate, and the patient should keep copies with his or her important papers. It should also be noted in the primary care physician's records with a copy if possible so that the surrogate can be contacted if necessary.

DNR orders should be in the medical record, and the staff should be informed of the patient's wishes. If the patient is at home, the family must have a copy of the DNR order to show emergency personnel, who otherwise will be legally obligated to resuscitate the patient.

Removal of life support means that no form of support, including mechanical breathing, feeding, or medications to prolong life, should be given. Pain medication and sedation are continued if necessary after removal of life support.

A **living will** is a document executed by an individual that gives medical professionals instructions about how that person wishes to be treated in the event he or she becomes incompetent. A living will may also give instructions regarding organ donation, autopsy, or donation of the remains to a medical school for anatomy dissection. Many states allow an individual's wishes to donate organs to be noted on his or her driver's license or on an organ donor card that can be carried in the wallet. In the event of a fatal auto accident, the police—who usually use the license or other documents to make identification—can notify ambulance personnel that the deceased is an organ donor. Figure 3-1 is an organ donor card.

A person usually names an agent to carry out his or her wishes if he or she is unable to do so. A **health care proxy** names the person who is charged with this responsibility and may also give specific instructions to the designated person concerning medical issues. Laws regulating living wills and health care proxies vary from state to state, and it is important for patients to use forms that will be valid where they live. This may require the assistance of an attorney.

Consensus

When a decision affects more than one person, there is often a need for discussion and agreement from all parties. For example, when an office or organization changes policy, each department affected must agree to the change.

A medical practice can look to a professional organization for guidance. Medical associations publish guidelines related to medical ethics. Professional associations for medical assistants can be a source of information and guidelines. For problems affecting the medical office, a discussion by all office staff may assist in decision making.

Ethics Committee

Hospitals and other health care institutions often form committees to review specific cases and decide on a course of action. These committees also establish institutional policies for situations that typically occur. The physicians in a medical office may be members of such ethics committees through hospitals or medical schools with which they are affiliated.

Law/Society/Organizations

Society attempts to regulate behavior by passing laws. But on many issues, society is divided as to the proper ethical course. There may be no specific law, or the law may not reflect the ethical beliefs of all members of the society, as in the case of abortion. Groups are often formed by those who support a specific position related to an ethical issue. They serve as sources of information, and they may raise funds to provide financial support for lobbying. The information provided by such groups, including publications and websites, usually favors only one point of view. Professional journals and professional organizations, however, usually provide more balanced information.

INTRODUCTION TO LAW
Difference between Public Law and Private Law

The legal system in the United States is primarily divided into two parts, public law and private law. Public law refers to laws that define the relationship between the individual and society as a whole. The term **criminal law** is used to refer to the set of laws that protect society. Examples include laws against robbery, rape, and operating a motor vehicle while under the influence of alcohol or a controlled drug. Private law, also called **civil law,** is the set of laws that deals with disputes between individuals and/or groups of people. This may involve two individuals or groups of people; individuals and corporations, government, or other organizations; or one corporate, government, or organizational entity and another such entity. Contracts are considered a part of civil law, and disputes about contracts that go to court are tried as part of the civil court system.

Lawsuits

Both civil and criminal action disputes can lead to lawsuits that are tried in the court system. In any court proceeding, there is a **plaintiff,** the person or entity that makes the complaint, and a **defendant,** the person or entity against whom a lawsuit is brought. In a criminal lawsuit, the plaintiff is the district or state's attorney, a representative of the government. In a civil lawsuit, the plaintiff is the injured party.

In criminal law the criminal activity itself is held to be harmful or potentially harmful to society or individual members of society. The act itself is punishable, regardless of whether anyone was actually harmed by the act. In civil law, an injury or damage must result because of someone's wrongful act for **liability** (legal responsibility) to arise. The same misdeed can provoke both a criminal charge and a civil lawsuit. The criminal suit will determine if the person is guilty of committing a crime punishable by an imprisonment or fine paid to the government. The civil suit will determine what liability the person has to the injured party, if any.

A well-known example of this dual legal picture is the O.J. Simpson case. Simpson was found not guilty by a jury of the murder of his ex-wife, Nicole, and her friend, Ronald Goldman. However, her estate filed a civil suit against him on the grounds of "wrongful death." In the civil case, he was found liable for their deaths, and more than 30 million dollars was awarded in damages. In a criminal case the charge must be proven "beyond a reasonable doubt," but in a civil case the burden of proof is only to a level where the supporting evidence is more convincing than the opposing evidence ("a preponderance of the evidence").

Specialized Areas of Public Law

Specialized areas of public law include constitutional law, international law, and administrative law. Constitutional law is the study of law of countries and other political organizations. International law concerns the relationships among countries and includes maritime law and regulations applying to ocean-going vessels. Administrative law refers to law arising from the actions of federal government agencies, such as the Social Security Administration and the Internal Revenue Service.

Creation of Laws

Law was created by tradition through accepted social practices and decisions of the courts. This type of law is called **common law** or **case law.** Today most laws are created through a vote by a legislative body. The term for this is **statutory law.** Legislators are elected by popular vote to serve either in the state or federal legislature. One of their important duties is to draft new legislation, which is called a **bill** while it is under consideration. Once passed by either the House of Representatives or the Senate, a bill that contains several parts becomes an **act.** Once passed by both houses, the act is signed into law by the President (for a federal law) or a state governor (for law applicable to one state). Cities and towns can also enact laws, called *ordinances;* these usually have to do with local issues, such as smoking in public places, parking, leash laws for pets, and curfews at parks.

All employees of the medical office must be aware of the federal and state laws that regulate the provision of health care and insurance reimbursement, as well as those related to the operation of a business.

Criminal Law

The branch of law that describes offenses against the public welfare is called *criminal law.* A **crime** is an offense in violation of a law that prohibits or requires certain behavior. When a person is convicted of a crime (or pleads guilty to a crime), punishment is imposed. A **felony** is a serious crime, punishable by death or imprisonment in a state or federal penal institution for more than 1 year. A **misdemeanor** is a less serious crime, punishable by a fine or imprisonment for less than 1 year, often in a local or county penal institution. Another term sometimes used to describe a criminal act is **malfeasance**—a wrongdoing that is illegal or contrary to official obligation.

Nonviolent Crimes

Occasionally a physician is charged with manslaughter or criminal negligence if a patient dies or suffers serious injury as a result of incorrect or negligent treatment. This is usually in addition to a civil lawsuit brought by the patient or family for wrongful death (see the discussion of professional malpractice later in this chapter). Euthanasia and assisted suicide (except for physician-assisted suicide in Oregon) are usually considered murder whether performed by a health professional or family member.

Two or more people who have joined together to commit an unlawful act may be accused of conspiracy; this may be applied to actions that are illegal in and of themselves, or actions to prevent detection of a prior crime.

Stealing another person's property (without violence) is called **larceny.** In the medical office, this may take the form of **embezzlement**—appropriating funds from a client, customer, or employer.

A growing problem in the health care industry is **fraud**—deliberate deception carried out to secure unfair or unlawful gain. Billing for services not provided, billing for services provided to imaginary patients, performing unneeded services, and even deliberately using codes from a higher level of service than that provided are all forms of insurance fraud. Every instance of such a billing can be considered a separate act. If the fraud involves the use of mail (mail fraud) or electronic resources (wire fraud), it becomes a federal offense.

In the mind of an office employee, there may be a difference between billing an insurance company using a code for more complex service than was actually provided, "because they pay us so little anyway," and billing for procedures that were never performed. But from a legal perspective, both are considered fraud and, if proved, both carry serious penalties.

Insurance companies and agencies of the federal and state government are victims of billions of dollars in fraudulent claims each year. They have increasing incentives to investigate health care facilities they suspect of fraudulent billing.

Civil Law

The branch of law that regulates interactions among individuals, groups, organizations, and the government is civil law. Disputes arise when one individual or group believes that the actions of another individual or group have caused personal injury or damage to property. In medical offices these usually relate to the actual care received by the patient and/or the relationship between the patient and the physician or office staff. Two types of obligations that may give rise to civil lawsuits are contracts and torts. In order for there to be a contract, there must be a mutual agreement and intent to do (or not do) something that is legal in exchange for service (called *consideration*) or for payment. A **tort** is an injury or wrong against a person or property that does not involve breach of contract. If a person knows, or should know, the consequences of their action, it is called an *intentional tort.* If the action is a mistake or has unintended consequences, it is called an *unintentional tort.* See Box 3-2 for a list of torts. Keep in mind that intentional torts may also be prosecuted as criminal acts if they are performed with specific intent to cause injury.

Two other terms may be used for acts that can result in civil lawsuits. The term **misfeasance** refers to a legal act performed in an improper way, especially if it causes injury or damage. The term **nonfeasance** means failing to perform an act that should have been performed if injury or damage results.

LAW AND PROFESSIONAL LIABILITY
Physician-Patient Relationship

The physician-patient relationship is a contractual relationship. Each party has certain rights and responsibilities under the relationship.

A contract does not have to be written or sometimes even discussed in detail. When clothes are left for dry cleaning, it is assumed that there will be an obligation to pay for the service. The same is true if a patient makes a visit to a medical office. Written contracts are used when there is a considerable amount of money at stake (such as a car loan or mortgage), but even in the medical office a patient may be asked to sign a statement confirming that payment will be made for any charges not covered by insurance.

Certain groups of people are not legally able to be a party to contracts, including most medical care contracts. These people are also not able to give informed consent. This includes the following:
1. Children younger than the age of 18
2. Mentally ill or retarded adults

BOX 3-2 Intentional and Unintentional Torts

Intentional Torts

Abandonment Failure to continue to provide medical care to a patient without proper notification.

Assault Threat to touch another person or his or her property without permission in a way that will cause pain, injury, or damage or is offensive.

Battery Touching of another person or his or her property without permission in a way that will cause pain, injury, or damage or is offensive.

Defamation Making a false claim that may harm a person's reputation, business, or group. If the claim is made verbally, it is called *slander.* If the claim is made in writing, it is called *libel.*

False imprisonment Confining a person without legal authority, such as using restraints without a proper physician order.

Invasion of privacy Public disclosure of private information, such as releasing medical information or photographs without consent of the patient.

Misrepresentation Providing information with knowledge that it is incorrect or reckless disregard for the truth.

Unintentional Torts

Negligence Failure to act with reasonable prudence in a situation. Negligence by a professional is also called *malpractice.*

Strict liability Responsibility for injury, even if there was no negligence. This is often applied when individuals are injured by products or equipment.

3. Individuals who are temporarily mentally incapacitated (including those who have received narcotic analgesics or other mind-altering medications)
4. Individuals who are under threat or duress (fear of a threat)
5. Individuals who have been found incompetent to handle their affairs

All consent forms should be signed and all implied contracts made with a competent party acting as a willing health care decision maker for the child or incompetent person. In some circumstances, adult rights, including the right to consent for medical treatment, are given to individuals younger than the age of 18. Such an individual is called an **emancipated minor.** In most states, one of the following three circumstances will allow a minor to become free of control of a parent or guardian:

1. Entry into the armed services
2. Marriage
3. Obtaining a court order from a judge after proving the ability to be financially independent

The Physician

Within the physician-patient relationship, the physician provides skillful care to the patient and continues to treat the patient unless he or she informs the patient that the relationship will be terminated. In this case the physician must give the patient time to make other arrangements for care. The physician arranges for someone else to treat the patient if the physician is unavailable (such as on nights, weekends, and vacations). The physician informs the patient about treatments or procedures and carries out only those treatments and procedures to which the patient consents. The physician informs the patient of test results, diagnoses, and medical conditions and gives the patient instructions for follow-up care and procedures to follow at home.

A physician has the following rights:
- To accept or decline to treat a patient
- To choose to limit the medical practice to a particular size or certain specialty
- To decide where to practice

Decisions not to treat particular patients must be based on general principles (such as limiting a practice to urology) rather than arbitrary decisions (based on a whim or subjective judgment).

The Patient

The patient agrees to keep appointments, give accurate information about his or her medical condition, provide an accurate medical history, follow directions, and pay for service.

The patient has the following rights:
- To refuse treatment
- To receive complete information about procedures
- To select a physician
- To continuity of care
- To confidentiality of verbal and written communication with the physician and the physician's agents
- To be treated with respect and dignity
- To receive complete information about the treatment suggested, alternatives, and possible consequences of alternatives or no treatment

Terminating the Physician-Patient Relationship

To end a relationship with a patient, a physician must notify the patient in writing. It is recommended that such a letter be sent using certified mail with return receipt requested. The letter needs to be dated, must state the reasons for termination of care, and should describe how medical records will be made available. Copies of any correspondence regarding termination and receipts should be kept in the medical record. Physicians also send written notification of termination of the physician-patient relationship to confirm a telephone conversation with the patient in which the patient has notified that physician that he or she wishes to terminate the relationship.

Common reasons for a physician terminating care of a patient include the following:

1. The physician moves
2. The physician retires
3. The physician dies
4. The physician closes the practice for other reasons
5. The patient regularly and continually breaks appointments
6. The patient regularly and continually refuses to follow medical advice

If a patient can convince a court that he or she was under the belief that a physician-patient relationship still existed and because of such belief did not seek out another practitioner, and suffered injury, a successful case can be made for **abandonment.** This is rare and should never happen if the physician keeps good written records about any termination notification. Figure 3-2 is a sample letter of termination.

Personal and Professional Liability

A person is responsible for his or her actions and may be held liable if those actions injure another person. In daily life we are required to act as a reasonable person would act in the same circumstances. The failure to act—or refrain from acting—as a reasonable person would act in similar circumstances is called **negligence.**

A common example of negligence relates to a wet floor. If someone washes the floor or spills water on the floor and does not wipe it up, the floor becomes slippery. When an unsuspecting person comes along and is not aware that the floor is wet, that person could slip and be injured. The person responsible for making the floor wet will be expected to know that the wet floor is slippery and could cause

someone to fall. A person who notices the spill is also expected to know that the wet floor could cause a fall.

If a person falls, is injured, and files a lawsuit, the person who washed the floor, or another person with responsibility for public safety who noticed the spill, could be found to be negligent and be responsible (liable) to pay for the injured person's medical care, lost wages, and any other costs caused by the fall on the wet floor.

Standard of Care

A person without any special training is held only to a standard of a "reasonably prudent person." The term **prudent** means careful or using common sense. For instance, any reasonably prudent person is expected to realize that an infant or unconscious person will not be able to remove a heating pad that is too hot. If an infant or unconscious person is burned by a heating pad, the person who placed it will be considered liable and will be responsible for medical bills, as well as pain and suffering.

A medical assistant is generally held to a professional standard, especially when performing procedures that are often done by a licensed health professional. The medical assistant must be especially careful to avoid offering advice or making decisions that may be interpreted as diagnosing illness or prescribing treatment.

If the medical assistant administers medication, he or she must do so correctly and must follow proper procedures and precautions to protect the patient from injury. A physician must be on the premises (not necessarily in the room) any time medication is given by a medical assistant, because in

---

October 28, 20XX

James Winston
824 Acacia Road
Blackburn, WI 54937

Dear Mr. Winston:

This letter is to inform you that our practice can no longer provide medical service to you. In order to maintain your health, your condition requires frequent monitoring and adherence to prescribed regimens. Since you have failed to keep your last three appointments, it has been impossible to provide adequate medical supervision. We do agree to provide care to you, if you wish, until December 31, 20XX. This should give you adequate time to arrange for care from another primary care provider.

We encourage you to find another physician promptly. We hope that you can establish an effective working relationship with another physician. Please feel free to call our office or the state medical society to obtain a referral to another physician.

Please notify us in writing when you have selected a new physician, and we will be happy to forward a copy of your medical record and a summary of your treatment.

Very truly yours,

Figure 3-2. Sample letter notifying a patient of the physician's withdrawal as primary care provider.

most states the medical assistant can only perform the procedure under the authority and supervision of a physician. Importantly, medical assistants must find out what they are legally allowed to do in the state where they work.

In emergency situations, when no qualified professional is available, health care practitioners are allowed to give care for which they have been trained but at which they may not be proficient. For instance, a psychiatrist who performs a tracheotomy, an incision through the neck and into the windpipe to allow a patient to breathe, in his office would have to meet the same standard as a surgeon. But if that same psychiatrist performed an emergency tracheotomy at the scene of an accident where a trauma victim's airway is blocked, he or she will be held to a lower standard. This allows a physician to extend himself or herself into an area in which he or she is less competent in order to save a patient's life without fear of a losing a malpractice lawsuit.

Patients make an assumption that in a medical office they will receive medical treatment, even in the event of an emergency. All medical office personnel are expected to be able to give advice in an emergency or to activate the local emergency medical system if they cannot handle the situation.

Many, if not most, medical offices, train all of their personnel in CPR and first aid. If a medical assistant, secretary, or receptionist tells any patient that a problem is not serious, and it is, he or she may be liable if there is injury to the patient due to delay of treatment. Failure to respond correctly to an emergency can be considered a "breach of contract" because there is an implied contract between a patient and a medical office that any emergency will be handled by competent staff.

Health professionals are generally held to a high standard of care. The physician's key legal obligation is to provide care to patients that meets an acceptable standard. For physicians and other health professionals, the term **standard of care** defines the level of appropriate care legally required of any other practitioner with the same education and training providing the same care in the same geographic region. In general, if a legal question arises, a medical assistant will be held to the standard of care of the professional who would normally perform the care in question.

For example, if a family practice physician prescribes blood pressure medication, he or she has to do it as competently as another family practice physician in the same area. If a nurse practitioner prescribes blood pressure medication, he or she has to meet the same standard as the family practice physician. If a patient suffers injury from taking the medication, in either case, the court would look at the appropriateness of the medication for the particular patient, the dose, and the follow-up to see whether either practitioner has acted at an acceptable level.

Informed Consent

Like a contract, consent is either implied or expressed. If a medical assistant says, "Roll up your sleeve so that I can give you an injection" and the patient does so, the patient has given implied consent to the medical assistant to administer the injection. Even though the patient has not verbally agreed, the act of preparing for the injection suggests that the patient is willing to undergo the procedure.

Again, as with a contract, expressed consent can be verbal or written. We know, however, that simply expressing consent does not always represent understanding. Patients today have the legal right to completely understand what will be done to them or for them. For this reason, many medical offices now use written consent forms to obtain informed consent.

Written consent forms are now always used for surgery; for procedures involving entry into a sterile body cavity, for procedures that carry a risk to the patient's health, and for testing for human immunodeficiency virus (HIV), the virus that causes AIDS. Written consent forms are increasingly being used as well for immunizations; treatment with birth control pills; transfusions of blood or blood products, such as plasma; and other treatments and procedures.

Legally, it is not the form, but the understanding by the person on whom the treatment or procedure will be performed, that truly represents consent. It is the responsibility of the person performing the procedure, prescribing the medication, or performing the test or examination to inform the patient about the potential risks of the action, the discomfort it may cause, the common side effects, and why it is important to do and the probable results if the test or procedure is not done.

Often the medical assistant is asked to obtain the signature on the consent form and witness that signature. If the medical assistant believes that the patient does not fully understand what he or she is consenting to, the matter should be referred back to the physician. This is a good example of the medical assistant acting as a liaison between the patient and the physician and being an advocate for the patient.

Depending on state law, there may be special consent forms for the release of information about HIV test results and/or treatment, drug and alcohol rehabilitation, services for mental health, or other health-related information.

A patient can rescind (withdraw) the authorization to release information at any time by notifying the medical office in writing.

What Would You Do? What Would You *Not* Do?

Case Study 2

Howard Morton is a 72-year-old patient who has come to the office for an office visit for severe back pain. After examining him, the physician referred him to an orthopedic surgeon for evaluation. While Vicki is preparing the referral form for Mr. Morton, he says, "If I see an orthopedic surgeon, he is probably going to want to do surgery. Do you think surgery is the best treatment for my kind of problem? What else could I try? Should I see a chiropractor? Or do you think acupuncture might help?" ■

Professional Negligence

Professional negligence is often called **malpractice.** To avoid lawsuits for malpractice, a health professional must be sure that he or she is acting within the limits of his or her profession and must act (or refrain from acting) in a given situation as a reasonable and prudent person of the same profession would. When the medical assistant performs procedures that are usually performed by other professionals, such as nurses, the medical assistant will be held to the same standard as the professional who usually performs the procedure. No one always does everything perfectly, and both negligence and malpractice are assumed to be mistakes and unintentional.

Requirements to Prove Professional Negligence

To prove that a professional is guilty of professional negligence and liable for the outcome, four things must be proved by a preponderance of the evidence. This means that it is more likely than not. Sometimes these things are called the *4 Ds of malpractice:*

1. The person who caused the injury has a *duty* to the person who was injured.
2. The person was *derelict* (neglectful) in performing that duty.
3. The failure to perform the duty was the *direct cause* of the injury and nothing could have intervened.
4. The failure to perform the duty caused *damage* or injury.

In some instances the plaintiff has no direct knowledge of the incident (e.g., if the plaintiff is under general anesthetic). In such a case a lawsuit may be allowed under the doctrine of *res ipsa loquitur,* where the court assumes that negligence must have occurred because of the type of injury. An example would be if the gallbladder was removed when the patient was scheduled for a hysterectomy.

A physician who gives casual medical advice at a party may not consider the person a patient he or she has a duty to take care of. But if the person fails to seek medical treatment on the basis of the physician's casual words, a court may have to decide if the physician owed a duty to the person.

If a professional does exactly what any other professional would have done, and the patient has a poor outcome, the physician is not necessarily negligent. For example, even with the best sterile technique it is possible to get a wound infection. A person with a wound infection must show that proper technique was not used. If the injured person does not follow directions to keep the wound dry and the wound gets infected, maybe the infection was not directly caused by the surgery, but because the patient did not follow directions.

If someone makes a mistake but there is no injury, the person who makes the mistake will not be liable and will not have to pay any damages. Many mistakes can be corrected if they are reported promptly.

Professional Liability Insurance

To protect against financial loss if the patient sues, physicians usually have professional liability insurance (also called *malpractice insurance*). This is for two reasons. One is to protect physicians for their own negligent actions. The second is to protect physicians if they are sued for the negligent actions of their employees while on the job.

If an injury occurs, the law allows the injured person to sue both the person responsible for causing the injury *and that person's employer,* provided that the incident occurred at work. This occurs under what is known as the doctrine of ***respondeat superior.*** The English translation of this Latin term is literally "let the master answer," meaning let the person at the head of the organization answer for the injuries caused by his or her employees.

This legal doctrine provides an incentive for employers to be sure that their employees are careful and gives the injured person a better chance of collecting actual money for any injury. Even if the employee does not have insurance to cover such an incident or enough money to pay the amount received in judgment, the employer ought to have liability insurance. Medical assistants who are members of the American Association of Medical Assistants have the opportunity to purchase their own inexpensive malpractice insurance through the professional organization.

Laws that protect health professionals from being sued for giving emergency care are called *Good Samaritan Acts.* They vary from state to state and may cover physicians, nurses, emergency medical technicians, anyone certified to perform CPR, and other professionals.

Malpractice Litigation

Litigation (the process of taking a lawsuit or criminal case through the courts) is complex. Having a general understanding of the process is important, even though less than 5% of all lawsuits brought against medical professionals or medical institutions ever reach the stage of going to trial.

Initiating a Lawsuit

A person who believes he or she has received inappropriate medical care consults an attorney, who obtains information from the patient and usually tries to obtain copies of the relevant medical records. A letter containing a patient's authorization to send a copy of medical records to a lawyer may be the first indication to the medical office that the patient is actively contemplating a lawsuit.

After receiving written authorization from the patient, the medical office provides a copy of the record to a lawyer. In most states, health care facilities, including physicians' offices, are allowed to charge a copying fee for records sent to an attorney. This contrasts with the policy of sending copies of records without charge to another physician or health care facility to provide continuity of care.

At the time a lawsuit is actually filed, the patient signs a document releasing the physician from the requirements of patient confidentiality. This is necessary because information about the patient's medical record becomes part of the public record in the litigation process.

When he or she obtains the patient's medical records, the attorney has them reviewed by physicians or other health professionals uninvolved in the patient's treatment to determine if a case can clearly be made for malpractice. Appropriateness of care is clearly the major issue in a suit for malpractice. However, incomplete, illegible, or altered records decrease the medical record's credibility, even if the care actually given was appropriate.

Most malpractice suits are accepted by attorneys on a **contingency** basis. In such a case the individual filing the lawsuit only pays for the attorney's time and effort if he or she collects an award from the party being sued. This is usually a percentage of the settlement or judgment amount. Contingency payments to the attorney are usually from 20% to 40% of the amount collected. The amounts are higher if the case goes to trial and lower if the case is settled out of court.

Response to a Possible Lawsuit

The first thing a physician should do on receiving a request for patient records by an attorney or on being served with notice of a lawsuit is to inform the company that provides his or her professional liability insurance. If a suit is filed, the malpractice insurance provider will appoint an attorney to represent the physician as a policyholder. The physician may also wish to hire an independent attorney because the physician's interests are not always the same as the malpractice insurance carrier's. If other staff members are named in the lawsuit, it may be in their best interest to hire their own attorneys as well.

As the legal process continues, the attorneys usually negotiate a settlement in order to avoid the time and expense of going to court, as well as the possibility of a large damage award. Because juries are unpredictable, the attorneys appointed by the insurance provider will hesitate to risk a jury trial, even if there does not appear to be any negligence in the care provided to the plaintiff. If there is a lawsuit, the court may issue a **subpoena,** a court order that requires an individual to be present to testify during some part of the trial process. In order to require that the original medical record is present, the court will issue a **subpoena** *duces tecum,* a court order requiring that documents (or other material evidence) be made available. An employee of the health care facility should bring the original medical record to court each day that it is required and be present wherever the medical record is at all times.

Alternative Dispute Resolution

Instead of a trial, both parties may agree to have their dispute decided by a neutral third party. This process can reduce time, expense, and publicity of a dispute. Such a process may take the form of mediation or arbitration.

Mediation uses a facilitator to help two parties in conflict settle their differences. This can be done in different ways, and if no settlement is reached, either party may find recourse in the court system.

Arbitration is a process whereby a neutral party settles the dispute. The arbitration can be either binding or nonbinding.

In nonbinding arbitration, the parties do not have to accept the decision and one party can proceed with a court case. In binding arbitration, the parties agree at the beginning to be bound by the decision of the arbitrator(s).

Various organizations provide lists of arbitrators, and depending on the circumstances and applicable state law, the parties in arbitration either select a mutually acceptable arbitrator or are assigned one from a list prepared during the arbitration process.

Arbitration is not common in malpractice cases; it is far more common in commercial contract and labor contract disputes.

Tort Defenses

Privilege

Privilege is a special right or permission granted to a certain group of individuals. For example, a health care facility's policy and procedure manual may give physicians the power to order soft restraints or leather restraints for a patient in certain circumstances. With such an order, other health professionals may legally apply the restraints. A patient who is placed in restraints according to established procedures could not make a case for false imprisonment, an intentional tort.

Consent

Consent has been already been discussed in detail. A patient may be asked to sign a consent form allowing photographs to be taken and published in a medical journal or textbook, or used as a slide in a lecture (without personal identifying information) for the purpose of providing education. If informed consent was obtained, especially if it is in writing, the patient cannot make a case for invasion of privacy.

Self-Defense or the Defense of Others

Self-defense or the defense of others is another defense against intentional tort. When physical contact occurs, a person accused of assault and/or battery may assert that he or she was defending against contact initiated by another person.

Expiration of the Statute of Limitations

Several defenses can be used against a charge of negligence or malpractice. The **statute of limitations** is the law that limits the time period during which a person can sue. The period varies from 1 to 3 years, depending on the laws of the particular state and whether the suit is for negligence or malpractice (negligence usually has a shorter statute of limitations than malpractice).

Although state law can vary slightly, the statute of limitations usually begins at one of three points:
1. When the injury occurs
2. When the individual first realizes that an injury has occurred; for instance, if a hemostat is left in the body during surgery, the statute of limitations begins to run when the instrument is discovered by an x-ray taken at a later date for another reason

3. When a minor reaches the age of majority or some other specific age (such as 21)

Contributory or Comparative Negligence

If the injured person has played a part in causing the injury, some states regard this as a complete defense (**contributory negligence**). Other states determine **comparative negligence**—how much of the negligence was caused by the professional and how much was caused by the injured individual. Judges and juries are asked to assess damages to the injured party depending on the percentage of the injury caused by the health care professional.

For example, following minor surgery a patient developed a wound infection that required additional surgery and resulted in an unsightly scar. The physician's attorney brought out that the patient had failed to seek medical attention for several days after noting swelling, drainage from the wound, and a fever of 102°F. Prompt medical attention, the attorney argued, would have prevented the second surgery and minimized scarring.

In a state using contributory negligence, establishing that the patient contributed to the injury would be a complete defense and the patient would not collect any damages. In a state using comparative negligence, the judge or jury would determine a percentage for the amount of negligence on the part of the physician and award the patient that percentage of the total damages established by the court.

Assumption of Risk

A patient who does not follow medical advice becomes responsible for any problems that occur as a result of his or her decision. This is called **assumption of risk.** This is easier to establish if the patient has signed a waiver, such as a form acknowledging that a patient is leaving the hospital against medical advice. In the medical office, there is usually no form for the patient to sign, so a complete note should be written in the patient's medical record if he or she refuses to follow medical advice. This note should include the patient's exact words if possible, and the name of any staff or family member who was present during the discussion. If a patient frequently misses appointments, it is also an example of disregarding medical advice. By documenting all missed appointments, the medical assistant can provide evidence that the patient, not the physician, is responsible for any problem that may arise.

What Would You Do? What Would You *Not* Do?

Case Study 3

While walking down the hall to call the next patient, Vicki notices a large wet area on the linoleum floor of the hall. She gets several dry paper towels and goes to clean up the spill. Just as she bends over to wipe up the water, the physician comes out of examination room #4. He looks at the open door of his other examination room, and noticing that it is empty, he says, "Where's my next patient? And can you take an ECG on the patient in room #4 right away?" ■

FEDERAL AND STATE LAWS AFFECTING THE MEDICAL OFFICE

Controlled Substances and Prescriptions

Controlled Substances

The **Drug Enforcement Administration (DEA)** enforces the Controlled Substances Act of 1970. A **controlled substance** is a drug that has a potential for addiction and/or abuse. Physicians who prescribe controlled substances must register with the DEA and renew their registration every year. The DEA updates the five schedules of controlled substances annually. Schedule I controlled substances have the highest potential for abuse and currently have no accepted medical use in the United States, whereas Schedule V controlled substances have the lowest potential for abuse. The specific medications are discussed in more detail in Chapter 26.

Federal law requires that controlled substances be stored away from other medications, in a sturdy, locked cabinet. It is recommended to use a double-locked box or drawer—a box or drawer with an outer lock or key and an inner compartment that also has a lock or key. A physician may not legally obtain Schedule I controlled substances, unless participating in an authorized experiment. Schedule II controlled substances are ordered from a manufacturer or a distributor using the Federal Triplicate Order Form DEA 222. Schedule III through V controlled substances do not require the special triplicate form; however, they do require that invoices and packing slips be kept for 2 years.

If controlled substances are kept in a medical office, an inventory sheet must be maintained. The controlled substance stock should be counted daily and verified by a second person. The two people must sign the inventory sheet. Every 2 years, a record of daily inventory of controlled substances must be submitted to the DEA. If controlled substances need to be wasted or destroyed, two witnesses must sign the inventory sheet. If any controlled substances are stolen, local police must be alerted immediately.

Prescribing, dispensing, and/or administering controlled substances also requires documentation. States vary on what paperwork is necessary; some require a special narcotic prescription form for Schedule II prescriptions. Any physician copies of controlled substance prescription forms should be kept in a secure, fireproof safe or other storage. If controlled substances are administered or dispensed only rarely, records can be kept in the patients' records and made available to DEA investigation.

The physician's DEA registration number should not be preprinted on prescription forms. The physician usually writes the DEA number on a prescription for a controlled substance. If a prescription does not have the DEA number, the pharmacy calls the physician's office to obtain it after the prescription has been delivered by the patient.

A medical assistant must know the legal requirements regarding controlled substances that have been set by the DEA and the state in which he or she works. A medical assistant will often be responsible for flagging the physician's DEA registration renewal date, as well as for providing security and inventory record keeping of all controlled substances. A medical assistant may also be responsible for properly disposing of expired controlled substances and keeping records. In some states medical assistants are not permitted to administer controlled substances, although they are allowed to administer other medications.

Prescriptions

Federal law also identifies drugs that require a prescription. A **prescription** is an order from a physician or other licensed health care provider to a pharmacist to dispense a supply of medication. Individual states have different regulations within a set of federal guidelines. The medical assistant must know the laws of the state in which he or she works.

In order to prevent theft or alteration of prescriptions, it is recommended that physicians adhere to the following recommendations:

1. Store all prescription blanks in a safe place where they cannot be stolen and keep the number of prescription pads in use to a minimum.
2. Write out the actual amount prescribed in words in addition to the number. This makes it more difficult to alter the amount.
3. Use prescription blanks only for writing prescriptions and not for notes.
4. Do not sign prescription blanks in advance.
5. Use tamper-resistant prescription pads.

The physician may also write on the prescription whether a generic substitute may be provided. Different states have different laws regarding substitution of a generic preparation for a brand-name drug.

Federal and State Laws Protecting Employees

Hiring and Firing

A person who works for an organization that has more than 15 employees is protected by federal Equal Opportunity Employment laws (Title VII of the Civil Rights Act of 1964) and the Federal Age Discrimination Act of 1967. These laws make it illegal for a company to discriminate in hiring practices on the basis of race, sex, religion, national origin, or age. Some states also have legislation making it illegal to discriminate on the basis of sexual orientation. Complaints about discrimination in hiring are submitted to the federal Equal Employment Opportunity Commission (EEOC).

Employment policies must treat employees equally and cannot discriminate against any category of employees by paying one group (such as men) more than another group for the same duties.

Preemployment Testing

Preemployment testing is only allowed to determine if the potential employee has the skills and abilities to perform a

Memories *from* Externship

Vicki Edmonds: When I was at my externship at a clinic affiliated with a community hospital, the employees were implementing a plan for the physicians to discuss advance directives with all patients. They hoped to have each patient prepare a written health care proxy and provide the office with a copy. When we pulled each patient's medical record for the visit, we checked the record to see if there was already a complete form. If not, we placed a blank health care proxy form loosely in the front of the folder for the physician to give to the patient. Then when patients checked out, we would remind them to return the completed form. At first I found this embarrassing because it seemed like such a private thing. Then one of our elderly patients told me that she was so grateful that her husband had signed a health care proxy before he had a stroke, which left him completely paralyzed and unable to speak. She said that the discussions they had had when he was preparing the form had helped her understand exactly what his wishes were. On the basis of those discussions, she had asked the hospital staff not to resuscitate him if he stopped breathing or his heart stopped. She told me that before they talked about it, she would not have been comfortable making that decision. I was impressed by this patient's ability to talk frankly about her family's preparations to face serious illness, and I was grateful because it helped me become more comfortable with the subject. ■

Prepare for Success

specific job. If keyboarding is included in the job description, the employer may administer a keyboarding test to test a candidate's qualifications for the position. This also applies to any testing done before an individual with a disability is hired.

The Americans with Disabilities Act (ADA) discusses the need for employers to make "reasonable accommodations" to any individual with a physical or mental disability who is otherwise qualified to perform the tasks necessary in the job. The law also deals with the necessity of making public accommodations accessible to disabled individuals. The EEOC also hears complaints about possible failure to comply with the workplace portions of the ADA.

Preemployment drug tests have been ruled legal for any position. However, random drug tests while on the job are usually legal only if the demands of public safety outweigh the employee's right to privacy. Some health care facilities perform drug tests on all new employees.

Health and Safety Act of 1970

The Occupational Safety and Health Administration (OSHA) was created in 1970 to be the federal agency responsible for the physical protection of employees in the workplace. OSHA regulates all workplace environments but has two specific functions related to the medical office.

Bloodborne Pathogen Standard

One OSHA regulation relates to preventing exposure to pathogens that cause disease. Effective March 1992, the Occupational Exposure to Bloodborne Pathogen Standard requires employers to have an exposure control plan, which identifies all employees who might come into contact with blood and other potentially hazardous materials. The plan must include safe handling procedures for specimens; contaminated needles, glass slides, and scalpel blades; contaminated laundry; and hazardous disposable waste.

Employers are required to provide employees with several safeguards:

1. Immunization against the hepatitis B virus (HBV)
2. Personal protective equipment
3. Labeling for biohazard waste containers and other hazards
4. Medical care if an employee is exposed to bloodborne pathogens or other hazardous material

Employees must receive initial training and have this training updated annually. A plan for follow-up after an exposure also must be in place.

Standard for Occupational Exposure to Hazardous Chemicals in the Laboratory

The second area of medical office practice that is of specific concern to OSHA relates to hazardous chemicals. OSHA maintains the Standard for Occupational Exposure to Hazardous Chemicals in the Laboratory.

Each employer must have a written plan and must designate a chemical safety officer. If potentially hazardous chemicals are in use, including stains, bleach, acetone, and isopropyl alcohol, any work site with employees is subject to regulation.

All potentially hazardous chemicals must be inventoried. Employees must be trained before handling any hazardous chemicals. Employees have a right to know of any hazardous chemicals in their environment. A manual containing safety information about all chemicals used must be created for each laboratory. This data is contained on Material Safety Data Sheets (MSDS), which are provided by the manufacturer. Information about these sheets is discussed in Chapter 18. The 1988 Clinical Laboratory Improvement Amendments, which regulate office laboratories, are discussed in detail in Chapter 29.

Family and Medical Leave Act

The Family and Medical Leave Act of 1993 (FMLA) applies to employers with 50 or more employees. Under FMLA, employees are entitled to up to 12 weeks of unpaid leave to accommodate a serious health crisis of any family member or the birth or adoption of a child. The employee must notify the employer before the beginning of the leave how much of the leave he or she intends to take. After the employee returns, he or she must be given former job and seniority status.

Sexual Harassment

Sexual harassment is defined as any unwanted physical or verbal sexual attention from anyone an individual interacts with on the job that causes that individual to fear reprisal if the attention is refused. Sexual harassment is not flirting. Flirting occurs when both parties engage in actions or verbal exchanges intended to attract or compliment the other. Harassment occurs when one party (most often a man) engages another party (most often a woman) in unwanted comments or physical contact of a sexual nature. If a comment or attention is unwanted, it should be clearly stated to the offending party. Sometimes individuals hesitate to "hurt the other person's feelings" or are uncomfortable speaking out, and communication is unclear.

Minimum Wage and Overtime

The federal Fair Labor Standards Act regulates the minimum wage, although some states have a higher minimum wage than that set under federal law. The Fair Labor Standards Act also requires overtime pay of one-and-one-half the employee's regular rate of pay for time worked beyond 40 hours in 1 week. Professional and supervisory employees are exempt from the law. Registered nurses and office managers are considered professional employees, but medical assistants are not and are covered by the overtime rules.

Employee Retirement Income Security Act

The Employment Retirement Income Security Act of 1974 (ERISA) regulates employee benefit plans, including managed care health plans, pension plans, and other employee benefits. ERISA sets minimum standards for pension plans to prevent unfair denial of pension rights. Under ERISA, employee health plans cannot use health status or medical condition to deny certain employees the right to insurance.

Health Insurance Portability and Accountability Act of 1996

The Health Insurance Portability and Accountability Act of 1996 (HIPAA) provides legislation related to several aspects of health insurance, privacy of patient information, and standards for filing health insurance claims electronically. This act has several sections.

Health Insurance Availability and Coverage

The first part deals with health insurance availability and coverage. It provides specific regulations for group health insurance plans to prevent eligibility rules that exclude patients with certain diagnoses or genetic conditions or require them to pay higher premiums. It also regulates the length of time that group health plans can refuse to pay for preexisting conditions, especially if the new subscriber had other health insurance before enrolling in the group insurance plan.

Privacy Rule

The HIPAA Privacy Rule (one part of the law) went into effect in 2003. This rule provides patients with control over the use and disclosure of their health information. The Privacy Rule contains provisions that describe how personal health information may be used, stored, maintained, or transmitted electronically. In addition, it describes how patients must be informed of their right to control their health information.

1. The medical office must inform patients in writing how their protected health information (PHI) will be used by the medical office. This document is called a *Notice of Privacy Practices* (NPP). Protected health information includes written, oral, and electronic health information that contains data through which the patient can be identified such as the Social Security number, name, and telephone number. Patients must sign a document indicating that they have received a notice of privacy protection.

2. A patient's written consent is not required for the use of or disclosure of PHI if the purpose of disclosure is medical treatment, payment, or health care operations. Therefore individuals who are involved in caring for the patient (including medical assistants and medical assisting students) may have access to protected health information.

3. Patients have the right to access their medical records and to request changes to the records if they believe they are inaccurate.

4. The medical office must have procedures in place to prevent unnecessary or inappropriate access to PHI, including request forms for information; procedures to prevent unauthorized individuals from viewing records, appointment books, computer screens, or other material that might contain PHI; and procedures for storing and destroying records containing PHI so that no unauthorized access occurs.

5. Patients have a right to request an accounting of the transfer of their information for purposes other than treatment, payment, or health care operations.

6. The medical office must have written agreements with each outside agency that handles PHI, such as medical laboratories, transcription services, law and accounting forms, software and hardware consultants, or billing services to ensure that these other agencies handle PHI in accordance with the HIPAA Privacy Rule.

7. All employees must be trained in privacy and security of PHI.

Transaction and Code Set Rule

The Transaction and Code Set Rule prescribes electronic data interchange standards for structuring information that must be used for Medicare and Medicaid insurance claims. As of July 1, 2005, almost all providers that file Medicare claims electronically must adhere to these electronic data interchange standards.

Security Rule

The Security Rule complements the Privacy Rule by setting standards to maintain security of personal health information that is transmitted electronically. It identifies adminis-trative, physical, and technical security safeguards for electronic protected health information (EPHI). The final compliance date was April 21, 2006.

Other Provisions

The Unique Identifiers Rule established a new provider identification number called the *National Provider Identifier* (NPI), a 10-digit identification number issued to each provider by the Centers for Medicare and Medicaid Services (CMS). As of May 23, 2007, this number was supposed to be required for all claims to Medicare, but the implementation was somewhat delayed. The NPI replaces other physician insurance identification numbers but not the DEA number or state physician license number.

The final part of HIPAA is the Enforcement Rule, which describes penalties for violating HIPAA rules.

Mandatory Reporting

For public health reasons and the good of society as a whole, physicians are required to make certain reports, usually to a state or local agency. Some are required by law and cannot be refused because the patient does not want the information released.

1. Records of births, stillbirths, and deaths.

2. Reports must be made to the medical examiner or coroner (the name depends on the state) for certain types of deaths, which may indicate suspicious circumstances or may be a result of a crime. The medical examiner then decides whether to investigate.

3. Reports of infectious disease cases have to be reported to the local board of health. Each state has a list of reportable diseases, which include diseases that pose a public health risk, such as rabies, measles, and AIDS. Dog bites and human bites must usually also be reported.

4. Injuries that may have occurred as a result of violence must be reported to the police. Sometimes a patient asks that the report not be made. Even if the injured person does not intend to press charges, the injury still must be reported. If there is a likely need for evidence to be collected from the injured person (e.g., in the case of a rape), the person should be directed to an emergency department, which has personnel trained in the procedure. If this kind of case seems likely when patients call to ask for an appointment, they should be referred to the emergency department with an explanation that staff there have been trained to collect evidence.

5. Possible abuse or neglect must be reported to the police or a particular state agency, depending on state law. Suspicion does not have to be backed up with evidence. Certain professions are mandated (legally required) to report, especially child abuse or elder abuse. Physicians and nurses are always required to make such reports, and in some states medical assistants, as allied health care professionals, are also included in the list of those required to make reports.

6. Various other reports are mandated by the states. Some states require reports of seizures (a symptom of epilepsy)

to the department of motor vehicles, and some states require that all cancer cases treated by health professionals be reported to a state cancer registry.

Failure to make a mandated report is a crime. When a report is required by law, the patient should be informed why the report is required and to whom the report will be made.

State Regulation of Health Occupations

The laws that regulate the practice of medicine are called *medical practice acts,* and they generally contain the following two elements:

1. Definition of the practice of medicine.
2. Limitation to qualified practitioners by **licensure**—the process by which the state examines a person's qualifications and issues a **license** to practice medicine. All states require a license to practice medicine, although a physician may practice in certain federal facilities and agencies with a license from a different state than the one in which the facility is located. Practicing medicine without a license is a criminal act.

In most states a physician can be licensed after he or she has met the following requirements:

1. Graduated from an accredited school including a 4-year postgraduate school of medicine with an MD degree, an accredited 4-year postgraduate school of osteopathy with a DO degree, or a recognized foreign medical school with an MD degree
2. Passed parts I, II, and III of the U.S. Medical Licensing Examination (USMLE), as well as an English language competence examination if foreign born and foreign educated
3. Received 1 to 2 years of hospital-based training in an approved program after graduation from medical school (Graduates from foreign medical schools must have 2-3 years of postgraduate hospital-based training depending on the state.)
4. Is found by the board of medical examiners to be of good moral character

Physicians can also be licensed in most states if they have held a medical license in another state for more than 5 to 10 years. This is called **reciprocity** or reciprocal licensing. Usually this is simply a matter of requesting a license if a physician is moving from one state to another. In states with many physicians, reciprocal licensing is more difficult to obtain. Florida severely limits reciprocal licensing in an effort to keep older physicians from "retiring" to Florida and then opening practices or taking hospital or clinic jobs.

The physician licensing board approves the original application for a license, then renews the license yearly or biannually—every 2 years.

Revoking or Suspending a Physician's License

A physician licensing board can revoke or suspend a physician's license for conviction of a crime, unprofessional activity, and physical or mental incapacity, including alcoholism, drug abuse, and senility. If convicted of a crime, the seriousness and nature of the crime will influence the physician licensing board's decision about the length of time a person's license may be suspended.

Similar laws govern the licensure and revocation of licenses for such professions as registered nurses, nurse practitioners, and physician assistants. These laws clarify what the member of the profession can and cannot do.

Facility Licensing and Accreditation

State Requirements

Each state requires certain types of health care facilities to obtain a license. This gives the state oversight into the activities of the facility and allows for on-site surveys to maintain quality standards. A list of these types of facilities can be found in Box 3-3. Physician offices are usually not included, but if laboratory testing is done in the office, it may be necessary to get a license or certificate of waiver for the laboratory depending on the type of testing being done. Health insurance companies and HMOs are also licensed by the state, which sets certain requirements for their business operations.

Many states also manage health care expansion through **certificate of need** programs. This type of program requires a health care facility to apply to the state for permission to construct new buildings, offer new services, or purchase new equipment costing more than a certain amount. The goal of these programs is to control health care costs and be sure that new health care services are provided where they are most needed.

Federal Requirements

In addition to state licensure, ambulatory surgical centers that bill Medicare and Medicaid for services must be certified by the CMS and meet physical plant, staffing, safety, and governance standards. These centers must enter into a written agreement with the CMS.

BOX 3-3 List of Health Care Facilities That May Be Licensed by the State

- Ambulatory surgical centers
- Blood banks
- Clinics or community clinics
- Commercial independent laboratories
- Drug treatment centers
- End-stage renal disease centers
- Health departments
- Home health agencies
- Hospitals
- Intermediate care facilities
- Nursing homes
- Physician office laboratories
- Pregnancy counseling centers

The CMS also participates with state and private agencies to regulate clinical laboratories and determine compliance with regulations to ensure the quality assurance. This is discussed in more detail in Chapter 29.

Voluntary Accreditation

Many health care facilities, including hospitals, ambulatory surgical centers, clinical laboratories, health clinics, and physician offices, seek voluntary accreditation by independent accrediting agencies as a means to improve health care and maintain high standards.

The Joint Commission (formerly known as *JCAHO*), was originally established in 1951 to accredit hospitals, rehabilitation centers, and nursing homes. In recent years it has expanded its activities to accredit almost all kinds of health care facilities, including clinics and physician offices. In order to become accredited, the health care facility must prepare a report demonstrating compliance with all standards of the Joint Commission. This is followed by a survey visit with follow-up to improve in any areas of weakness that might be found during that visit.

The Accreditation Association for Ambulatory Health Care (AAAHC) performs a similar type of accreditation for most types of ambulatory health care facilities.

MEDICAL PRACTICE and the LAW

Two elements are important to avoid malpractice suits. The first is to implement proper procedures to prevent mistakes. These procedures are part of the overall process of *risk management,* a term that is usually applied to measures taken to reduce risk of injury and lawsuits within the medical office.

Safety plans, chemical hygiene plans, evacuation plans, and standard precautions are all part of risk management, as are measures to avoid theft by patients or staff or fraud by financial staff. In addition, education and training of all staff help each staff member provide proper care to patients.

A second element of risk management is to prevent patients from becoming angry about the care (or lack of care) they receive. This requires all staff who interact with patients to be courteous, give complete explanations, and treat patients and their families with respect and dignity. If the office maintains good relations with patients, patients will be more likely to understand when there is a poor outcome or a mistake is made. Demonstrating respect and concern for patients at all times is one of the most important ways to prevent malpractice lawsuits.

Although the owners of the practice are ultimately responsible, the job of developing and implementing risk management plans usually falls to the office manager and, in a small office, to the head medical assistant. The best way to protect against malpractice lawsuits is to use the following procedures to prevent mistakes:

1. Make sure all equipment is in good working order and that staff have been properly trained to use it.
2. Make sure all staff members know how to do procedures and can review them in an up-to-date procedure manual.
3. Be sure that patients understand the nature of procedures and surgery and sign written consent forms for surgery and invasive procedures.
4. Always document accurately and completely. Promptly report any problems, and document your report.
5. Protect patients from injury by the proper use of equipment and safe transfers to and from wheelchairs.
6. Be sure that patients are not left alone if there is any question of their balance or mental status. Children should never be left unattended in an examination room or the waiting room.
7. Patients should be identified using two identifiers before administering medications or obtaining laboratory specimens.
8. All specimens should be labeled correctly. All results should be logged and tracked so that none slip through the cracks.
9. Patients should not be left unattended with hot packs or where hot water or hot pipes are present.
10. All liquid spills should be wiped up promptly and signs should be used if floors are wet.
11. Staff should not make promises about outcomes.
12. The physician should be notified of any patient complaints and/or requests for patient records from an attorney.
13. All patients should be followed up after surgery. ■

What Would You Do? What Would You *Not* Do? RESPONSES

Case Study 1
Page 38

What Did Vicki Do?
- ❑ Told Denise that she would have to point out the burn to the physician because he needed to be sure it was healing properly.
- ❑ Told Denise that she would have to tell the physician what Denise had said about the burn.
- ❑ Explained that burning someone with a cigarette is not acceptable behavior and encouraged Denise to discuss the incident with the physician or another adult.
- ❑ Asked Denise if her boyfriend had hurt her any other time.

What Did Vicki Not *Do?*
- ❑ Did not tell Denise that she needed to break up with her boyfriend immediately.
- ❑ Did not agree to hide the information about the burn from the physician.
- ❑ Did not promise that the physician would not tell her parents.
- ❑ Did not discuss Denise's burn or explanation for it with anyone other than the physician.

What Would You Do/What Would You *Not* Do? Review Vicki's response and place a checkmark next to the information you included in your response. List the additional information you included in your response.

_____

_____

_____

_____

Case Study 2
Page 46

What Did Vicki Do?
- ❑ Told Mr. Morton that the orthopedic surgeon specialized in musculoskeletal conditions and would not always recommend surgery.
- ❑ Asked Mr. Morton if he had asked the physician about other kinds of treatments.
- ❑ Asked Mr. Morton if he wanted her to complete the referral and make a new appointment.
- ❑ Asked Mr. Morton if he needed more time to speak to the physician.

What Did Vicki Not *Do?*
- ❑ Did not make recommendations about other types of treatment for back pain.

- ❑ Did not give an opinion about the benefits of one type of procedure compared with another.
- ❑ Did not promise that the orthopedic surgeon would not want to do surgery.
- ❑ Did not tell Mr. Morton that the physician should have done a better job explaining possible treatments.

What Would You Do/What Would You *Not* Do? Review Vicki's response and place a checkmark next to the information you included in your response. List the additional information you included in your response.

_____

_____

_____

_____

Case Study 3
Page 49

What Did Vicki Do?
- ❑ Told the physician politely that she has to finish cleaning up the spill in the hall because someone might slip and fall.
- ❑ Worked as quickly as possible to dry the floor of the hall and then called the next patient.
- ❑ Asked the physician if he wanted to talk to the next patient before she did the vital signs.
- ❑ Did the electrocardiogram (ECG) on the patient in room #4 after calling and preparing the physician's next patient.

What Did Vicki Not *Do?*
- ❑ Did not leave the spilled water on the floor while she called the next patient and took the ECG.
- ❑ Did not ask if the physician thought she could do two things at once.
- ❑ Did not go around the office later trying to find out who had spilled water without cleaning it up.

What Would You Do/What Would You *Not* Do? Review Vicki's response and place a checkmark next to the information you included in your response. List the additional information you included in your response.

_____

_____

_____

_____

↻ TERMINOLOGY REVIEW

Abandonment Failure to continue to provide medical care to a patient without proper notification.

Act A bill or measure that has become law. Often refers to legislation with several parts.

Arbitration A formal process where the parties to a dispute agree to submit to the decision of a neutral party.

Assumption of risk A defense to a lawsuit that establishes the plaintiff assumed the risk of whatever caused the injury.

Autonomy Ability to make independent decisions without constraint or coercion from others.

Beneficence Acting in the best possible way; performing good deeds.

Bill A law proposed by a legislative body.

Case law Law established by decisions of previous court cases.

Certificate of need A regulatory mechanism to ensure that new or expanded health care services will meet the needs of the community.

Civil law Law that regulates relationships and interactions between individuals and groups.

Cloning Producing genetically identical cells or individuals artificially.

Common law Unwritten body of law based on general custom.

Comparative negligence A defense to a lawsuit that establishes a percentage of responsibility for injury by the plaintiff.

Contingency A condition that must be met before a contract is binding.

Contributory negligence A defense to a lawsuit that establishes any responsibility for injury by the plaintiff.

Controlled substance A drug that has the potential for addiction or abuse.

Crime An offense in violation of a law that prohibits or requires certain behavior.

Criminal law Law that regulates offenses against the public welfare.

Defendant The person or group against whom an action is brought in a court of law.

Do-not-resuscitate (DNR) A medical order signed by a physician that relieves health care personnel from the obligation to resuscitate a patient who stops breathing or whose heart stops.

Drug Enforcement Administration (DEA) The federal agency that enforces the Controlled Substances Act of 1970.

Duty Commitment to act in a certain way.

Emancipated minor A person younger than the age of 18 with the rights of an adult including the ability to consent to medical care.

Embezzlement Fraudulent appropriation of funds or property of an employer or client.

Etiquette Rules of socially acceptable behavior; manners.

Felony A serious crime punishable by death or imprisonment.

Fidelity Faithfulness.

Fraud Intentional deception resulting in injury or loss.

Gene therapy Giving patients new genes or parts of genes to treat a disease or condition.

Genetic engineering Making, altering, or repairing genetic material.

Health care proxy A legal document that names an agent to make decisions about a person's medical care if he or she becomes unable to make wishes known.

Informed consent Agreement to a medical procedure based on understanding of the procedure and its possible consequences and effects.

Larceny Stealing another person's property or money without violence.

Liability Legal responsibility.

License Official permission to perform an activity or practice a profession.

Licensure The process by which the state examines qualifications and gives permission to an individual or organization to engage in a profession or business.

Litigation The process of taking a lawsuit through the courts.

Living will A legal document that specifies the kind of medical treatment a patient wants or does not want if he or she becomes incapacitated.

Malfeasance A crime or wrongdoing that is illegal or contrary to official obligation.

Malpractice Negligence by a professional.

Mediation Negotiation by a third party to help two parties resolve a dispute.

Misdemeanor A less serious crime, punishable by a fine or imprisonment for less than 1 year.

Misfeasance Performing a legal act in an improper way.

Negligence Failure to act (or refrain from acting) as a reasonably prudent person would in similar circumstances.

Nonfeasance Failing to perform an act that should have been performed, resulting in injury.

Nonmalfeasance Ethical concept requiring that an action do no harm, or do less harm than good.

Plaintiff The person or group that makes the complaint in a lawsuit.

Prescription An order to a pharmacist to dispense a supply of a medication.

Privilege A special immunity that protects against legal liability.

Prudent Using care or common sense.

Reciprocity Automatic issuing of a license in one state to the holder of a license in another state.

Respondeat superior A legal doctrine making an employer liable for the negligent acts of employees.

TERMINOLOGY REVIEW—cont'd

Right A claim that is expected to be honored.

Standard of care Level of appropriate care required of a health professional.

Statute of limitations A law limiting the time period for beginning a lawsuit.

Statutory law Law enacted by a legislative body.

Stem cells Cells that have the capacity to develop into various types of body tissue.

Subpoena A court order for a witness to appear and give testimony.

Subpoena *duces tecum* A court order to produce documents or records.

Tort An injury or wrong against a person or property that does not involve breach of contract.

Veracity Truthfulness.

ON THE WEB

For Information on Accreditation of Ambulatory Care Facilities:

Accreditation Association for Ambulatory Health Care (AAAHC): www.aaahc.org/eweb/StartPage.aspx

The Joint Commission: www.jointcommission.org

For Information on Federal Supervision of Laboratories and Ambulatory Surgery Centers:

U.S. Department of Health and Human Services: Centers for Medicare and Medicaid Services: www.cms.hhs.gov

For Information on Genetic Engineering:

Recombinant DNA Advisory Committee, National Institutes of Health: www.nih.gov

For Information on Organ and Tissue Donation:

U.S. Department of Health and Human Services: Information on Organ and Tissue Donation and Transplantation: www.organdonor.gov

For Information on Patient Rights and Duties of Health Care Providers:

Consumer Bill of Rights and Responsibilities from the *Report of the President's Advisory Commission on Consumer Protection and Quality in the Health Care Industry* (1997): www.hcqualitycommission.gov/cborr/

PREPARE FOR CERTIFICATION   Visit the Evolve site at http://evolve.elsevier.com/Bonewit/today/ to actively Prepare for your Certification.

CD *Check out the **Companion CD** bound with the book to access additional interactive activities.*

4

Interacting with Patients

ABHES COMPETENCIES

Communication

- Be attentive, listen, and learn.
- Be impartial and show empathy when dealing with patients.
- Adapt what is said to the recipient's level of comprehension.
- Serve as liaison between physician and others.
- Receive, organize, prioritize, and transmit information expediently.
- Recognize and respond to verbal and nonverbal communication.
- Principles of verbal and nonverbal communication
- Adaptation for individualized needs

Content

Psychology of Human Relations

- Dealing with difficult patients with normal/abnormal behavior
- Caring for patients with special and specific needs
- Emotional crises/patients and/or family
- Basic principles
- Hereditary, cultural, and environmental influences on behavior standards

KEY TERMS

acting out
active listening
anxiety
body language
chronic
closed questions
denial
ego defense mechanism
empathy
hierarchy (HIGH-er-ark-ee)
judgmental
nonverbal

open questions
oral
paraphrasing
physiologic
projection
reflecting
self-actualization
summarizing
sympathy
verbal
webcam

Introduction to Communication

In order to respond to a patient effectively, the medical assistant must be able to communicate effectively. A major component of health care includes reducing a patient's fear and anxiety, as well as helping the patient understand how to promote health and manage illness. To assess a patient's perception of his or her health status, the medical assistant must be effective at both sending and receiving messages.

COMMUNICATING WITH PATIENTS

Figure 4-1 outlines the basic model of communication. A sender sends a message to a receiver. The message can be **verbal,** meaning that spoken or written words are used to send the message. It can also be **nonverbal,** meaning the message is expressed without words through body language, facial expression, and other means. Most messages are sent using a combination of verbal and nonverbal communication.

Verbal and Nonverbal Communication

Verbal communication is either **oral** (spoken) or written. Written communication has traditionally been thought of as more formal than oral conversation—a formal letter rather than a phone call. Today, however, with the increasing use of e-mail, written communication may be as informal as oral communication.

Nonverbal communication refers to information that is received from body language. **Body language** is the way a person's body signals feelings or emotions. For example, hands folded across the chest and a rigid posture may signal anger. Nonverbal communication also includes the secondary communication that occurs during oral conversation. Secondary communication consists of the following: tone of voice, voice pitch, voice volume, and voice quality. Nonverbal communication often provides more information than the words themselves (Figure 4-2).

The response to a simple question such as, "How are you feeling today, Mr. Jackson?" may consist only of the words "All right." The quality of the voice—pinched, pained, flat, excited, spoken with a deep sigh—gives more information than the words about Mr. Jackson's physical condition and his state of mind.

Other types of nonverbal communication include facial expression, body position, and gestures used while speaking. These are known as *nonverbal cues.*

Interference with Communication

Numerous elements can interfere with communication between the sender and receiver. An analogy for interference is listening to the radio. The radio station can be thought of as the sender of a message. The message is sent through radio signals. Any number of outside elements can interfere with the radio station's signal to the receiver, such as a storm that causes electrical interference in the atmosphere, air traffic controllers switching to a radio frequency that interferes with the broadcast frequency, or the receiver

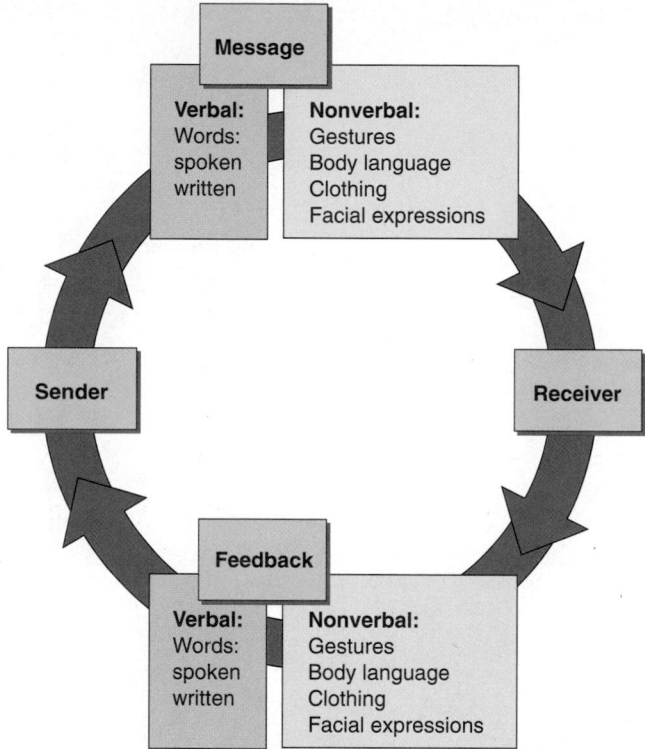

Figure 4-1. Model of communication. (From Hunt SA: *Saunders fundamentals of medical assisting,* St. Louis, 2007, Saunders.)

driving through a tunnel or over a bridge with steel suspension. In addition, interference can be caused by elements inside the receiver, such as strong emotions, thinking about something else or needing to concentrate on driving carefully.

Similarly, when communicating with a patient, interference can come from the outside or inside. Examples of outside interference include a distracting environment, noise, and lack of privacy during communication. Examples of inside interference include fatigue, fear, anxiety, anger, or being preoccupied with something else. All of these factors can cause the message to be diluted, changed, or not completely understood by the receiver. Other barriers arise because understanding or senses are impaired.

The ability to identify a patient's strong emotions or feelings from the nonverbal cues exhibited by the patient may cross cultural boundaries. For example, infants and children from all cultures cry when they receive immunizations. The ability for the medical assistant or a patient to interpret subtle feelings or gestures, however, does not typically cross cultural boundaries. For example, shaking the head from side to side does not always mean "no." In some cultures it may mean "yes," or it may be used to express other meanings such as an acknowledgement that the listener has heard what was said.

Individuals who come from different cultures also have a different idea of personal space and may interpret physical touch in a different way. Cultural sensitivity is especially important for communication to be effective. Nonverbal communication that is accepted in the sender's culture, such as smiling, looking straight into the speaker's eye, or lightly touching someone's shoulder to show concern, may create interference if the gesture has a different significance in the listener's culture.

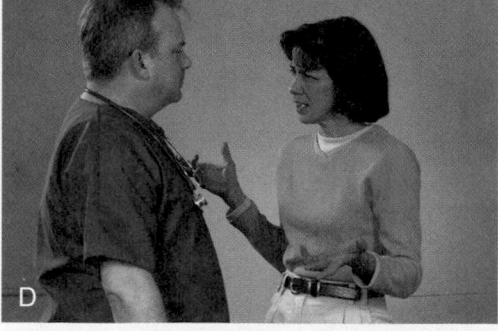

Figure 4-2. Most adults can easily identify the people in these photographs as expressing **A,** pleasure, **B,** uncertainty or lack of confidence, **C,** aggression, and **D,** confusion. (From Hunt SA: *Saunders fundamentals of medical assisting,* St. Louis, 2007, Saunders.)

Listening Skills

Good listening skills are major components of good communication. Some health professionals are naturally better listeners than others, but listening skills can be learned and practiced.

The most important listening skill is known as *active listening*. **Active listening** means being "in the moment" and paying close attention to what is being said without thinking about anything else. Focusing all the attention on the sender of the message is important. To receive a message clearly, the listener cannot allow emotions or thoughts to interfere with the sender's message.

What a sender says will naturally trigger a response. Letting go of the urge to respond verbally, take over the conversation, and air one's own views is important. By focusing on the sender, the medical assistant will not be tempted to let his or her own mental responses become spoken responses. It will also prevent the medical assistant from focusing on his or her mental responses, thereby preventing messages from the sender from being received clearly.

Additional guidelines for the medical assistant to demonstrate good listening techniques include the following:

1. Checking to make sure the patient's interpretation of a message is correct. This may involve asking the patient to repeat what has been said by rephrasing a question.
2. Listening for feelings. Medical assistants should be alert for key words or themes the patient uses frequently to describe his or her medical condition. These can be important clues as to the patient's emotional state. The medical assistant should also be aware of changes in his or her own feelings. The medical assistant's emotions may mirror the emotions of patients. For example, if the medical assistant begins to get impatient or aggravated with a patient, it may be a clue that the patient is upset or angry.
3. Being observant while listening. The patient's facial expressions, body language, tone of voice, and other nonverbal cues can tell a lot about what the patient is feeling.
4. Being patient and listening completely. Patients should be allowed to "tell their story" in their own time and in their own way. Interruption interferes with this process. Although there are questions that need to be asked, the medical assistant should introduce questions in a way that interferes as little as possible with the patient's natural storytelling flow.

Nonverbal Measures to Facilitate Communication

In the United States, eye contact is important (Figure 4-3). Maintaining eye contact is a sign of interest and involvement. However, being aware that in many cultures it is not respectful to look directly at older people is important. This is especially true in Asian and Native American cultures. Many Latinos also do not look directly at a person they respect, such as a teacher or a physician.

If the patient looks away and the medical assistant continues to seek eye contact, the patient may perceive this as

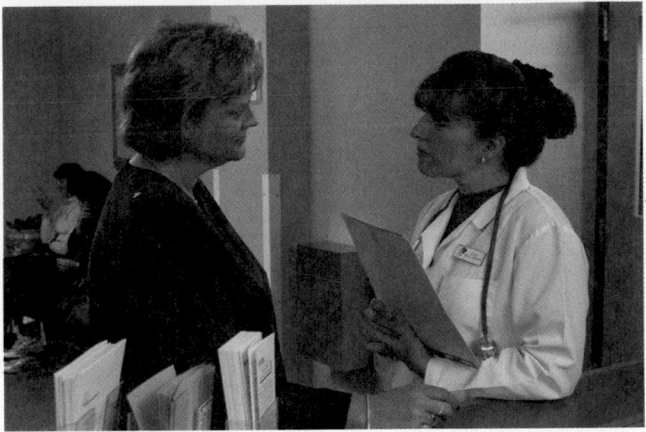

Figure 4-3. Photograph showing a comfortable talking distance and eye contact that is typical for the United States. (From Hunt SA: *Saunders fundamentals of medical assisting*, St. Louis, 2007, Saunders.)

aggression. Maintaining eye contact with someone who is culturally uncomfortable with that nonverbal communication creates a barrier between the two individuals.

For the most part, control of body language is unconscious. Therefore it is important for the medical assistant to be aware of the patient's nonverbal messages. Being alert to the patient's body language allows the medical assistant to notice when a patient feels uncomfortable or anxious. When a patient's words and body language do not match, the body language is usually a more genuine reflection of the patient's feelings.

Touching a person, even gently, can also be interpreted in many different ways. Moving closer can indicate interest, but it may also be viewed as aggressive. Many adults do not like to be touched by people they do not know well.

Cultural sensitivity is extremely important. For example, some Asians do not like to have their heads or their children's heads touched. This may present a problem when the medical assistant must measure the head circumference of an Asian infant. If this occurs, the medical assistant should stress to the infant's parent in a reassuring tone of voice that measuring head circumference is an important health assessment procedure and that there is no disrespect intended in the action.

A gentle pat on the shoulder can be reassuring to a patient, but it is important to notice if the patient becomes tense or appears uncomfortable when touched. If the medical assistant steps back, the patient will usually relax. In the United States, people normally maintain a distance of about 3 to 4 feet for conversation with others, but in other cultures this comfort zone varies.

If the medical assistant must penetrate the patient's personal comfort zone for a procedure, it may help to make a statement that prepares the patient for movement into the patient's personal space. For example, when applying a sterile dressing to a wound, the medical assistant might say, "I'm going to have to move in now so I have a better view of the area."

What Would You Do? What Would You *Not* Do?

Case Study 1

Nancy Walker, CMA (AAMA), has called Jennifer Boland, a 32-year-old married mother of three, from the waiting room. Nancy notices that Jennifer is not looking at her, but the patient cooperates with getting her weight and vital signs. When Nancy asks the reason for today's visit, it seems to take Jennifer a long time to answer. She picks at the sleeve of her jersey and finally says in a low voice that she is afraid she might be pregnant. Her voice cracks a little, and then she wipes one of her eyes. ∎

Interviewing Techniques

Closed Questions

Two types of questions can be used when conducting a patient interview. These include closed questions and open questions. **Closed questions** are questions that can be answered with one word (e.g., yes or no) or a short answer (e.g., I was born on 1/16/85). Closed questions are especially effective when the medical assistant needs to obtain specific information.

Examples of closed questions include the following:
- What is your date of birth?
- Who referred you to our office?
- Have you taken any medication for your pain?
- What medications are you currently taking?

Open Questions

Open questions consist of questions that encourage the patient to open up and talk. Examples of open questions include the following:
- What brings you to see the doctor today?
- What is your pain like?
- What has been going on with you since you were last here?
- How has your appetite changed over the past few months?

Open questions help the patient do the following:
- Identify what is important
- Express feelings
- Relay perceptions

Open questions are particularly effective in allowing the patient to describe a problem in his or her own words and explain how the patient feels about the problem. Because of this, open questions should be used to obtain a patient's chief complaint and conduct a patient interview. When using open questions, it is important for the medical assistant to employ active listening techniques.

If the medical assistant asks primarily closed questions, the patient may fail to give important details or mention other problems. If the medical assistant asks directly if the patient has been following a special diet or taking prescribed medication, the patient may feel pressure to agree, even if this has not always been the case. When a patient is encouraged to talk freely, a more realistic picture may emerge.

Keeping the Conversation Going

On occasion the medical assistant will need to employ techniques to keep a conversation going with a patient. For example, the medical assistant may need additional information from a patient, but the patient stops talking. When this occurs, the medical assistant should employ techniques that encourage the patient to continue speaking without steering the conversation in a particular direction. A useful technique in such a situation is to ask the patient an open question; however, "why" questions should not be used. Examples of "why" questions include the following:
- Why aren't you taking your medication?
- Why aren't you following your diet?

"Why" questions tend to make people defensive. Rather than having the patient justify his or her actions, it is important to identify the underlying reasons as to why the patient did not take the medication or stay on the diet. Effective questions that keep the conversation flowing without making a patient defensive include the following:
- How do you set up your meals and snacks?
- What problems are you having taking your medication?
- What do you think about having to take medication at school?

In answering these questions, the patient may provide clues as to the underlying reasons for not staying with the prescribed treatment plan.

Drawing Out Patients

Active listening includes techniques to draw a patient out and/or clarify what a patient is saying. This is especially important when the patient is trying to cope with strong feelings about his or her medical problems. Refer to Table 4-1 for a full listing of communication techniques that demonstrate active listening.

Avoiding Responses That Inhibit Communication

The medical assistant should avoid communication techniques that exhibit disapproval or blame as well as statements that are challenging or not genuine. If a patient feels that the medical assistant is not really listening, does not understand his or her point of view or does not validate emotions, the patient may become defensive or stop speaking altogether. The medical assistant's ability to demonstrate acceptance of strong emotions experienced by the patient is especially important.

When a patient expresses concerns, it is tempting to try to reassure the patient. For example, a patient might express anxiety about the results of a diagnostic test. If the medical assistant reassures the patient that the results will probably be normal, the fact that the patient is worried is not validated and the reassurance implies that the patient's worry is unreasonable or unacceptable. If the medical assistant confirms that it is difficult to wait for test results, the patient is more likely to feel that his or her feelings have been accepted.

Because the medical assistant's job is to make the person feel comfortable, it is important to avoid being too casual

Table 4-1 Communication Techniques That Demonstrate Active Listening

Technique	Description	Example
Using open questions	Asking questions that do not expect a particular answer, especially a yes or no answer	"What's been going on lately?" "How would you describe your stomach pain?"
Repeating or rephrasing	Saying the same thing as the patient either as a statement or a question to encourage agreement, disagreement, or clarification	*Patient:* " It feels like someone is stabbing me in the side." *Medical assistant:* "Like a knife in your side . . ."
Translating a nonverbal message into words	Translating the patient's nonverbal expression of emotion into a verbal expression	*Patient:* "All the doctor visits, the medication, the pain—it's really too much." *Medical assistant:* "You sound like you feel overwhelmed."
Reflecting	Turning a question or statement around to reflect back to the patient; this gives the patient confidence to continue	*Patient:* "Would you have this surgery if you were me?" *Medical assistant:* "What do you think about having the surgery?"
Paraphrasing and summarizing	Paraphrasing puts the patient's statement into the medical assistant's own words; summarizing restates the meaning but may leave out some of the details. The purposes are to validate that the medical assistant has understood and encourage clarification	*Medical assistant:* "So for the past week the pain has been getting steadily more intense and more frequent, and since this morning it hasn't let up at all."
Providing silence	Simply waiting for the patient to continue; allows the patient to choose whether to continue or choose a new topic	(Silence)
Verbalizing the implied	Saying what the patient seems to mean but has not expressed	*Patient:* "Usually I don't mind coming to see Dr. Hughes." *Medical assistant:* "But you didn't want to come today . . ."
Asking for clarification	Asking for more detail or a clearer statement; lets the patient know that the medical assistant has not understood and may show the patient how to make the message clearer	*Medical assistant:* "It's not clear to me how often you have been taking this medication. Do you take it before every meal, or just when you are at home?"

From Hunt SA: *Saunders fundamentals of medical assisting,* St. Louis, 2007, Saunders.

or familiar with a patient. If a subject is sensitive, but it is important to ask about it, the medical assistant can do so in a somewhat tentative way to make it easier for the patient to reply. The medical assistant can identify what the patient might be feeling, but the patient will not always agree. Many people are not always aware of their feelings and may deny feelings that they are communicating nonverbally. This should be respected. Others are only too glad to have their feelings recognized.

Medical assistants should express themselves honestly, without being **judgmental,** which means critical or negative. They can disagree with what a patient is saying, especially if that disagreement will get the patient to elaborate on what is being said. But they should not argue because arguing sets up a competitive situation. Because the medical assistant represents medical authority, the patient can easily feel threatened and unworthy.

The responses that should be avoided are summarized in Table 4-2.

Barriers to Effective Communication

Impaired Level of Understanding

Occasionally, a patient with an impaired level of understanding visits the medical office. When this occurs, the

Putting It All into Practice

My name is Nancy Walker, and I have been working for an oncologist for the past 5 years. Our patients have many different types of cancer and are at many different stages of their diseases. One thing that they all have in common is that they need a lot of emotional support. We provide this primarily by keeping the lines of communication open. We try to create an atmosphere where patients feel able to discuss whatever is on their minds. Some patients never say the word "cancer," and they talk about future plans as if they will be in the peak of health. Other patients are amazingly open and frank, even if they have not responded well to treatment. One patient told me that this is the only place she can talk about dying because her husband and her daughter become so emotional that she feels she has to spare them. We do not push patients to talk about anything they are uncomfortable with, but we do make time if patients want to talk about their feelings. The physicians also refer our patients to support groups or counselors because they believe that it is equally important to manage a patient's emotions and physical symptoms. ∎

Prepare for Success

Table 4-2 Responses That Inhibit Communication

Technique	Description	Example
Offering false reassurance	Telling the patient that everything will be all right; implies that the patient should not feel anxiety or concern. Especially inappropriate when the medical assistant does not know what will happen	"Don't worry, your husband will come through this with flying colors."
Disapproving, blaming	Making a negative value judgment about the patient's thinking or behavior; by implying or stating that a patient is responsible for his or her health problem, the medical assistant encourages the patient to defend against attack rather than establishing trust	"You shouldn't be smoking, you know. No wonder you have trouble breathing."
Challenging	Insisting that the patient prove a statement or belief	"Just show me something in writing that says people should never take a bath."
Defending	Protecting oneself or someone else from criticism, which implies that the patient does not have a right to have a different opinion	"Dr. Lawler's patients never have to wait very long."
Asking for explanations of feelings or behavior	Because patients often don't know why they feel or act as they do, asking why may be frustrating and cause them to become defensive	"Why don't you stick to your diet?" "Why are you angry?"
Belittling or negating feelings	Acting as if feelings are less intense than they are or not even present; this implies that the patient's feelings are not real or not justified	"You are really making a big deal out of a little cut."

Modified from Hunt SA: *Saunders fundamentals of medical assisting,* St. Louis, 2007, Saunders.

medical assistant needs to simplify his or her method of speaking. The medical assistant should use short sentences and simple words. Speaking slowly in a normal speaking tone is important. Raising one's voice does not help in this situation. The tone of voice should express concern and empathy without being condescending or implying that the patient is not intelligent. Strong and constant eye contact also helps the patient to focus.

It may be necessary to say the same thing more than once, either by repeating it or saying the same thing in a different way. In addition, gestures and demonstration help to reinforce the information.

Those with limited understanding of medical information—children, the elderly (especially those who suffer from some degree of dementia), and those who are mentally disabled—need constant reassurance. Giving a direct and complete explanation at the patient's level of understanding is important. Even young children need to be informed about what is going to be done to them. For instance, if the medical assistant is going to draw blood, it is not enough to say, "I'm going to draw your blood. It's going to hurt for just a moment."

It may be necessary to say something like, "I'm going to use this needle to take some blood from your arm. I'm going to put it through the skin, into where your blood is. It will feel kind of like someone is pinching you, but only for a second. Then I'll put a Band-Aid on it, and it will stop bleeding."

After an explanation to an individual with impaired understanding, the medical assistant should ask the patient to repeat the explanation back in his or her own words. If the patient simply repeats some of the explanation, communication may have been ineffective. If the medical assis-

tant explains a procedure like a colonoscopy, for example, he or she should then ask the patient, "Can you tell me what a colonoscopy is?" An answer that may indicate lack of understanding is, "It's when they do a colonoscopy." The medical assistant can then make another attempt to provide a simple explanation.

A young child or an individual with an impaired level of understanding cannot give informed consent. This must be obtained from an individual who can legally give informed consent for the impaired patient before the medical assistant can proceed.

Sight Impaired

Many degrees of vision loss exist. Total blindness is the complete inability to perceive light and form. Legally blind is a term used to describe individuals whose vision cannot be corrected beyond 20/200 in the better eye. This means that with glasses, the person sees the same or less at 20 feet than a person with normal vision sees at 200 feet. A person may be called *sight impaired* if his or her vision is better than 20/200 but they still have low vision or a decreased field of vision.

Importantly, the medical assistant should be verbally descriptive when working with a patient with impaired vision. The medical assistant should use touch and guidance when escorting patients who cannot see to walk safely from the waiting room to the examination room and also when helping them around the examination room. Patients with impaired vision usually prefer to take the medical assistant's arm and follow his or her movements rather than vice versa. To explain exactly where things are, a clock image sometimes helps. Saying that the examination table is at three o'clock tells a blind patient that the examination table is on the right directly to the side.

Hearing Impaired

The term *deaf* is usually used when individuals cannot hear well enough to use the sense of hearing to process information. However, there are many more individuals whose hearing is impaired than those who are deaf, especially in certain tone ranges or when sound is not loud enough.

Special techniques should be used with patients who are hearing impaired. The medical assistant should speak clearly, slowly, and in short sentences. The medical assistant's voice should be slightly louder than normal but not so loud that it loses clarity or sounds like shouting. Eye contact is also important when communicating with a hearing-impaired patient. Even if the hearing-impaired patient does not lip-read, most people who lose their hearing learn how to associate facial expression and mouth shape with words they know and recognize.

When beginning a conversation with a hearing-impaired patient, it may be necessary to touch the person gently to get his or her attention. If the patient is wearing a hearing aid, it may be helpful to ask if the hearing aid has been working well for him or her.

Sign language is often used to communicate with the deaf. Hand and finger positions represent letters or words. Several different systems exist, but American Sign Language is the recognized language in the United States.

Because each sign can represent an entire word, a person who uses sign language may be able to communicate as fast as, or faster than, a person who is speaking. Sign language has its own structure and grammar system, so it takes considerable practice to become fluent. A patient who uses sign language to communicate is usually accompanied by an interpreter. If the patient does not have an interpreter, the law requires the office to provide one. Sign language interpretation can be provided by an interpreter. It can also be provided by setting up a video relay service account. Video service links the deaf patient with a sign language interpreter. When using a sign language interpreter, it is important that the medical assistant maintain eye contact with the patient. Hearing-impaired and deaf patients are able to obtain information from facial expressions and body language. They may also be able to read lips.

Language Barriers

A language barrier interferes with communication as a result of speaking different languages. Depending on the patient's facility with English, this interference may vary from slight to severe.

The best way to work around language barriers is with translation assistance. Translators can be office staff, community volunteers, or patient family members. When scheduling an appointment for a patient with a language barrier, the medical assistant should inquire whether or not a family member will be accompanying the patient to provide translation assistance. If not, translation assistance must be provided by the medical office. Sometimes a patient with a language barrier brings a child to translate. The medical assistant should be aware that children are the least reliable translators because they have a tendency to skip over medical words they do not understand or cannot translate without realizing that important information may be lost. It may also be embarrassing for a patient to discuss certain medical problems if a child is translating for them.

When conversing with a patient through a translator, the medical assistant should speak to the patient and not to the translator. The medical assistant should allow the translator to translate a sentence before going on to the next sentence. The medical assistant should speak slowly and carefully, using simple terms and short sentences. Many people who do not feel comfortable speaking English can still understand much of what is said to them in English.

At times the medical assistant may need to improvise when working with a patient with a language barrier. This may be required during the following circumstances: the office does not have translation services, the translator is busy, or the patient's family member is translating but the patient wants to converse with the medical assistant in private. In these situations the medical assistant should use gestures and pantomime to convey his or her ideas.

Translation assistance is required before a patient with a language barrier gives written consent to an invasive procedure or minor office surgery. The law states that a patient must be fully informed as to the nature of his or her surgery or procedure. Consent forms are usually written in English, but the verbal explanation of the procedure needs to be in a language the patient understands well. If a practice has a large number of non–English-speaking patients, it is a good idea to have routine consent forms and instructional materials translated and available.

Telephone and video translation services can be purchased from several companies. Telephone translation assistance allows the patient, medical assistant, and/or physician to speak to the translator using a speakerphone. A video translation service requires a computer, a **webcam** (small video camera attached to the computer), and speakerphone and allows all parties to see each other during the conversation.

What Would You Do? What Would You *Not* Do?

Case Study 2

When Nancy calls Harold Underwood, a 67-year-old male, from the waiting room, he does not answer until she has repeated his name three times. Because he is a new patient, Nancy introduces herself. He says that he has moved into senior housing nearby so that he can be close to his daughter. Nancy finds that she has to repeat all instructions, and she notices that Harold is wearing a hearing aid in his left ear. When she asks him if he needs help to step up to sit on the examination table, he looks at her blankly. ■

UNDERSTANDING AND MEETING THE NEEDS OF PATIENTS

Patient Expectations of Health Care

Patient expectations depend on many factors including unmet needs and experiences the person has had in the past. Previous interactions with health care facilities also shape a patient's expectations. For example, if there is a long waiting time, a patient who has always had to spend 30 to 40 minutes in the waiting room will be less upset than a patient who is used to being seen within 10 minutes.

Patients usually want to be seen by a physician in a reasonable amount of time, and they hope that the physician will "fix" whatever is wrong. Patients do not expect to have long-term problems. They want to be treated as if they were cars and physicians were mechanics—"fix what's broken and get me back on the road of life!"

In addition, people expect physicians to take care of them when they are really sick and not fuss too much over them when they are generally well. People certainly do not want physicians to nag them about changing their lifestyle to improve their health. But physicians are much more likely today to bring up lifestyle issues, such as eating healthy foods in reasonable portions, not smoking, reducing alcohol intake, exercising, and using seat belts. Physicians are well aware that a healthy lifestyle can reduce the amount and intensity of medical care a person needs in the future.

Patients are sometimes so wrapped up in their primary concern—to get relief from pain or other symptoms—that they have difficulty accepting that physicians are often looking for the cause of their illness, not just to alleviate symptoms. This can cause a lot of frustration for patients, especially if no significant relief can be given or if the physician does not seem to think that alleviating the symptoms would be appropriate.

A common example of this is a viral illness such as the common cold. A patient may have a fever, muscle aches, weakness, vomiting, and diarrhea. Once the physician establishes that the patient is not suffering from a more serious condition, the physician may recommend only rest, fluids, and over-the-counter medications (e.g., acetaminophen or ibuprofen for fever reduction and relief of soreness). This plan of treatment can be frustrating for a patient, who wants to feel better and have a speedy recovery.

How Basic Needs Affect the Behavior of Patients

Maslow's Hierarchy of Needs

Abraham Maslow was an American psychiatrist. In his book titled *Motivation and Personality,* he defined what has come to be known as "Maslow's hierarchy of needs." A **hierarchy** is an arrangement in order of importance. Maslow describes human needs as a hierarchy with the most important needs at the lowest level. The image of a pyramid is often used to depict this visually, as shown in Figure 4-4. On the bottom of the pyramid (Level 1) are the **physiologic** needs. These are the basic biologic needs for survival, which include oxygen, water, food, excretion, sleep, shelter, and sexual expression.

Figure 4-4. Maslow's hierarchy of needs. (From Hunt SA: *Saunders fundamentals of medical assisting,* St. Louis, 2007, Saunders.)

On the next level of the pyramid (Level 2) are the needs for safety and security. Level 2 needs include avoiding harm, attaining physical safety, and the emotional security that comes with freedom from fear and anxiety.

On the middle level of the pyramid (Level 3) are the needs for love and belonging. Level 3 needs include both receiving and giving personal affection, companionship with another individual, and identification with a group.

On the fourth level of the pyramid (Level 4) are the needs for esteem and recognition. Level 4 needs include self-esteem, the respect of others in one's peer group, success in work, and prestige in the community.

Finally, at the pyramid's pinnacle (Level 5) is the need for **self-actualization.** This is the fulfillment of each individual's potential.

Effects of Unmet Needs during Illness

Understanding that an individual cannot step up to the next level on Maslow's pyramid until his or her needs have been fully met at the current level is important. An individual's current level may shift several times, even in the course of a day, as different needs are experienced. An individual moves up or down the pyramid depending on what needs are currently unmet. Only when lower-level needs are met will the person be able to devote a significant amount of energy or concern for needs that are higher on the pyramid. In fact, a person has all the needs (outlined on the pyramid) all the time but only becomes aware of higher-level needs once the lower-level needs are met.

This has a number of implications for how patients relate to the medical care they receive.

Many patients who come to the medical office are struggling to meet basic needs because they are ill. Health care professionals must recognize any difficulties in that area.

Health and happiness require more than just meeting basic needs, however. Part of the role of health professionals is to foster the meeting of needs beyond physiologic needs. For example, intervening for an abused child or battered woman helps meet needs for safety and security, as well as some sense of love and belonging, by knowing someone cares. Teaching patients how to manage a **chronic** disease—one that continues to exist over time—helps a person's self-esteem by making the person feel competent in self-care.

Another area where understanding the hierarchy of need helps in the health care setting includes learning to recognize situations when attention-getting behavior by patients might be an attempt to satisfy needs for love and belonging, or for esteem and recognition. When people are ill, their usual means for meeting their attention needs (both for love and belonging, as well as esteem and recognition) may be interrupted.

Medical assistants must be able to recognize that they cannot meet all of a patient's needs. For example, the medical assistant is not a close friend and should not attempt to be one, but recognizing when a patient feels a loss in this area, the medical assistant helps the person to identify his or her feelings and to cope with whatever need is not being met.

Establishing Caring Relationships

A patient who visits the medical office is often fragile, emotionally as well as physically. Illness interrupts an individual's daily routine and threatens self-concept and self-esteem. A patient who is ill often has a difficult time meeting his or her physiologic needs. One of the primary roles of a medical assistant is to create and maintain a caring relationship with the patient. The medical assistant is often the patient's earliest, most frequent, and most consistent point of contact with the medical office.

Empathy

In order to meet a patient's needs, the medical assistant must first be able to identify the patient's feelings. In addition, the medical assistant must be able to understand those feelings, not in an intellectual way but in an emotional way. This understanding is called *empathy*. **Empathy** is the capacity to make an emotional connection with another person's feelings without allowing the emotional connection to become overpowering. Empathy is often contrasted with sympathy. **Sympathy** is defined as experiencing the same emotions as another. Sympathy is often accompanied by a feeling of pity.

Empathy is more objective than sympathy. Experiencing empathy requires a person to retain perspective and have confidence that strong emotions are not dangerous. The medical assistant must be sensitive to the feelings patients have when they go through the medical office routine. Importantly, the medical assistant must be constantly aware that strong emotions may arise when individuals experience a threat such as an illness. By showing empathy to a patient, a medical assistant can support patients more effectively.

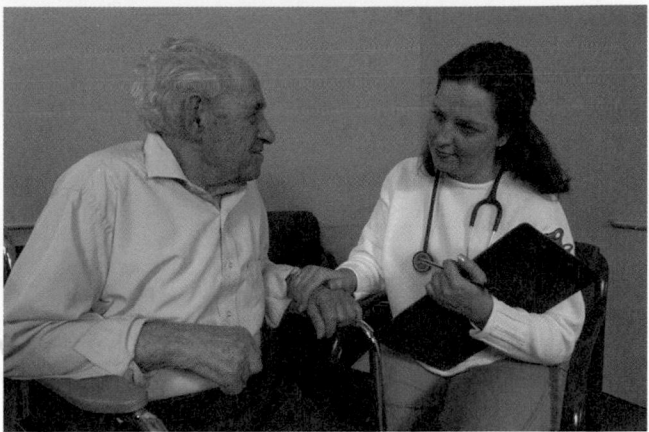

Figure 4-5. A medical assistant expresses caring through body position, eye contact, and touching the patient's hand. (From Hunt SA: *Saunders fundamentals of medical assisting,* St. Louis, 2007, Saunders.)

Expression of Caring

Caring can be expressed through words and body language. The medical assistant expresses caring through words, by drawing patients out and letting them tell their story in their own way, in their own time. This was described earlier in this chapter in the section on interviewing techniques. The medical assistant should accept and validate a patient's feelings. Patients benefit by being acknowledged and having someone else accept them.

Caring can also be expressed nonverbally through body language and through the way a medical assistant positions himself or herself during conversations with patients (Figure 4-5). The medical assistant should be positioned at the patient's eye level and at a distance of no more than 3 to 4 feet. If the medical assistant stands while the patient sits at a lower level, the patient may feel intimidated or inferior. Typically, the patient sits on the examining table while the medical assistant stands, which has both at almost equal height. If the patient is more comfortable sitting in the examining room chair, the medical assistant can sit on the physician's stool, which again puts both at about equal height. This is much more friendly than if the medical assistant stands while the patient sits in the chair.

Maintaining eye contact and lightly touching the patient, if it seems appropriate, also communicate interest and caring.

Value of Effective Relationships with Patients

The medical assistant is often the patient's most frequent, and long-term, point of contact with the medical office. A medical assistant who gets to know a patient well can be of invaluable assistance to both the patient and the physician, through trust established over time.

The experience of being understood and cared for is one of the most important steps in beginning to heal or cope effectively with illness, especially if the patient has a chronic illness. Ideally, each professional the patient comes in contact with at the office will convey this sense, but it is most important for those who are performing procedures. If the patient feels understood, he or she will also develop trust and be able to relax during procedures. This makes the procedure easier and less painful for the patient. It also makes it easier for the medical assistant to perform the procedure.

Emotional Responses to Illness
Guilt

Patients may feel guilt about their illness. The amount of guilt they feel varies from one patient to another. The amount of guilt that a patient is willing to express, as opposed to the amount that is repressed, varies from one patient to the next.

Some individuals engage in behaviors that are known to be risky to health, such as cigarette smoking, drinking, and drug abuse. These patients sometimes feel guilty about a respiratory disease, but others may display a devil-may-care attitude about their disease. People often know intellectually that their high-calorie, high-fat diet or sedentary lifestyle predisposes them to certain illnesses or conditions. Smokers, for example, have been bombarded with scientifically valid information for almost 40 years about the link between smoking and heart disease, lung cancer, and chronic obstructive pulmonary disease. Yet many of these individuals continue established habits without an outward sense of guilt. It seems as though they have convinced themselves that their risky behavior is not the cause of their disease or that they are somehow immune to the consequences of their behavior.

On the other hand, patients with conditions totally out of their control may experience guilt. For example, someone with pancreatic cancer might say that he could have avoided the disease if he had taken better care of himself, eaten a healthy diet, or gotten more exercise.

As with other emotions, the medical assistant should accept and validate a patient's description of his or her feelings. If the patient's previous behavior is partially responsible for current medical problems, the patient requires support and acceptance. If it is unlikely that previous behavior is related to the medical problem, the medical assistant can encourage the patient to discuss the causes of his or her condition with the physician.

Loss of Control

When people are ill, they often have a feeling of a loss of control. This is especially true if they have sought medical care for their condition. In addition to physiologic changes that may be unwelcome, they feel unable to control their schedule and/or environment. Some decisions are made for them. They have to take off their clothes. People get physically close to them and sometimes even touch them. People tell them to do things they do not want to do. They are anxious and become defensive. The medical assistant should respond to the patient's irritation with patience and kindness. It is important to give the patient choices and make every effort to accommodate the patient's wishes.

Anxiety

Anxiety is a response to a perceived threat. A person who is moderately to severely anxious is not able to converse coherently and will not pick up nonverbal cues that he or she would normally notice. When working with a patient who is anxious, the medical assistant must first get the person's attention, slow down the conversation, and then help the person to focus on the conversation. It is important to validate the patient's concern, which reduces his or her anxiety level. This allows the patient's energy to be channeled in a more productive way. When patients are anxious, they may not remember what they are told. The medical assistant can help the patient by creating memory aids. For example, the medical assistant can prompt the patient to record a follow-up appointment in his or her appointment calendar. It is also a good idea to write the instructions down or provide the patient with a preprinted instruction sheet.

Severe anxiety can be medically problematic. Physical symptoms occur with a full-blown anxiety attack, often termed a *panic attack*. An overly anxious person hyperventilates, has an extremely rapid heart rate, and becomes unresponsive. Some people experience numbness in their fingers and toes; others feel a sensation of fluid in their ears. Some people become intensely fearful and have an overpowering sense of dread.

An anxiety attack must be dealt with as a medical issue first. Helping the patient acknowledge the anxiety is important. Acknowledging the anxiety helps a person gain control. In addition, having strong emotions accepted by another person decreases the sense of fear that many people have about their emotions.

If the patient is breathing rapidly, the medical assistant should encourage the patient to take slow, deep breaths. Experts no longer recommend having a patient breathe into a brown paper bag because this may cause blood oxygen levels to fall dangerously low.

If possible, the medical assistant should encourage the patient to validate that anxiety is present without minimizing its significance. If the patient has not experienced severe anxiety before, he or she may not realize the effects it can cause. The medical assistant can explain that any physical symptoms are the result of anxiety and stay with the patient until the symptoms begin to subside. With most patients, the symptoms begin to diminish after 1 or 2 minutes. After the person has returned to a level of relative calm, it may be possible to discuss how the person handles anxiety. The physician may also refer the patient to a counselor to work on strategies to manage it.

Anger

Anger is a natural response to a perceived threat. Anger is often a subconscious response, which means that the patient is unaware of its cause, its intensity, or even its presence. A patient may express anger at a target that did not actually cause the angry feeling. Anger can also escalate quickly if it triggers an angry response from another individual. When dealing with an angry patient, the medical assistant needs to identify the emotion without feeling attacked. If possible, the medical assistant should help the angry person identify the true source of the anger.

Anger is one of the more difficult of the incapacitating emotions to deal with. Anger tests a medical assistant's empathy and ability to put aside private issues to help patients. The first instinct is to fight back at the angry patient, but this is counterproductive. It is more effective to respond with calmness and control using a quiet voice. Accepting that a patient is angry is not the same as allowing the patient to threaten office staff or other patients. It is perfectly acceptable to tell the patient that he or she is acting inappropriately, that he or she is making it difficult for other patients, or that shouting will not be tolerated. To protect the confidentiality of the patient who is temporarily out of control, the medical assistant should escort the patient to a private area. It is also appropriate for the medical assistant to request assistance from the office manager in dealing with an angry patient. Sometimes anger, like electricity, loses intensity when the connection is broken.

Ego Defense Mechanisms

When a threat seems unmanageable, the human psyche has several ways to avoid becoming overwhelmed. These are called *ego defense mechanisms*. **Ego defense mechanisms** are unconscious mental processes and behavioral strategies that offer psychological protection. Instead of experiencing a feeling directly, an individual may respond in one of the following ways: saying it is a feeling of someone else **(projection)**, failing to acknowledge the reality of the situation **(denial)**, or translating emotions into an inappropriate activity **(acting out)**.

Through empathy, the health care professional should have some idea of what the underlying emotion is; by accepting it he or she can help the patient to become more aware that such feelings are normal and can be worked with.

What Would You Do? What Would You *Not* Do?

Case Study 3

Julie Ann Reynolds is a 20-year-old patient who comes to the office and describes four or five recent episodes of shortness of breath, palpitations, feeling faint, sweating, and nausea. She states that she has just started taking classes at a local university after transferring from a community college. The episodes have mainly occurred either in the car on the way to school or shortly after she arrives. She says that on one occasion, her heart was beating so fast that she had to pull her car over and wait for about 10 minutes before she felt well enough to drive. She says that she has never had a heart problem, but she is afraid that now there is something wrong with her heart. She also says that her mother is worried about her and has suggested that she get an electrocardiogram and other tests because she might have a serious medical condition. ■

Medical assistants are often in a good position to do this, especially if they have established a good working relationship with the patient. Patients may need support to adopt unfamiliar coping strategies in response to stress, including illness.

If a patient seems angry, the medical assistant can say so and attempt to identify the reason. The patient often responds in an angry tone and may disagree with the medical assistant's guess about the cause of the anger. Then the medical assistant can allow the patient to vent and express his or her strong feelings. The medical assistant must avoid feeling personally attacked. This is easier if the medical assistant remembers that anger is often displaced (i.e., expressed toward a different person or event than the one who is really triggering the feeling).

If a patient is using denial, the medical assistant should remember that this is a defense against unmanageable anxiety. When patients appear to be avoiding reality, it is important not to agree with untrue statements or "feed into" the patients' denial. Equally important is not challenging patients who are in denial. They will start to accept reality when they are ready to handle the strong emotions.

Cultural Influences Affecting Health Care

Patients often come from cultures that have some level of distrust of Western scientific medicine and/or strong belief in their own medical traditions. In addition to seeking care from a physician, these patients may complement their care by visiting traditional practitioners. In many traditional practices, religion and medicine are tightly interwoven. Both patients and practitioners hope to affect health by

Memories *from* Externship

Nancy Walker: I did my externship in the adult medicine area of a clinic in a large metropolitan area. We had several African patients who came to our area as refugees from Somalia. If they were recent immigrants, we had to explain many things about our clinic to them because they were not familiar with preventative care from their own country. The female patients were modest; they did not shake hands with male physicians and avoided undressing for examinations. We tried to assign them to female practitioners, if possible, and everyone in the office learned to adapt procedures by having the patient remove the minimum possible amount of clothing. For example, the physicians usually listened to a female patient's heart and respirations just by placing the stethoscope under her clothing. One of these patients told me that some offices were not as accepting of their customs as we were. She said that it is considered immodest for a woman to remove clothing in front of any male, even a physician. She told me that if she had to do it, she would just stay sick. ■

Prepare for Success

Highlight on Ego Defense Mechanisms

Everyone uses defense mechanisms at some time or another to protect against being overwhelmed by painful feelings. Although people are sometimes aware of using these mechanisms, usually they operate on an unconscious level—that is, people are not aware that they are disguising or blocking emotions or impulses.

Everyone tends to use defense mechanisms that have been effective in the past to reduce stress or anxiety. When a person first encounters a situation that would provoke strong feelings, such as a diagnosis of serious illness, a defense mechanism like denial helps him or her avoid feeling overwhelmed and unable to cope. (Denial is unconsciously refusing to acknowledge something that is difficult to accept.) People say things like, "It doesn't seem real to me" or "This must be a mistake."

Denial allows the truth to penetrate gradually, so the person has a chance to get used to the threat, to seek privacy to experience intense emotion, and to avoid total disorientation. However, if a person continues to use denial without attempting to accept the situation, negative consequences may occur.

The person may not take appropriate actions to respond to illness. Friends and family may respond negatively to the person's perceived lack of responsibility. And the person may miss the opportunity to grow and strengthen his or her sense of self-worth and ability to cope with adversity.

If a medical assistant can identify a patient's defense mechanisms and coping patterns, he or she can gain a better understanding of the patient's underlying fears and concerns. The medical assistant can try to respond to these concerns but should not directly challenge the defenses or label them.

When defense mechanisms are attacked, it takes more energy to defend against threatening emotions. On the other hand, accepting defenses tends to promote a feeling of being understood and may decrease the need for rigidity in the defenses.

Example

Mr. Sykes has had to wait for about 45 minutes past his appointment time to see Dr. Lopez. When Kathy, the medical assistant, takes him back to the examination room, he says, "I think you should know that some of the people in the waiting room are really upset about how long they have been waiting."

Kathy may suspect that this is an example of projection—unconsciously identifying thoughts or feelings as originating in someone else when they really are one's own thoughts and feelings. She can be helpful to Mr. Sykes by responding in a way that reassures him that it is understandable for a person to be upset when there is an unusually long wait. Responses that are not helpful (because they reinforce Mr. Sykes' fear that it would be dangerous to express a negative emotion directly) are as follows:

1. Making it seem as though Mr. Sykes is overreacting and should not feel upset ("Oh, it hasn't been that long.")
2. Labeling or challenging the defense mechanism ("Do you always project your own feelings on people around you?")
3. Defending the physician or office staff ("Dr. Lopez has been very busy with several sick patients.")
4. Talking negatively about the patients in the waiting room ("Some people are never happy, no matter how quickly they are seen.")

Following is a list of several other ego defense mechanisms, with examples that might occur in a medical office. Remember that using defense mechanisms usually helps people adapt to stressful situations. ■

Other Ego Defense Mechanisms		
Selective inattention	Failing to hear or pay attention to information that may provoke anxiety	A patient expresses the belief that his cancer will definitely be cured if he has the primary tumor removed
Regression	Returning to the emotional adjustment of an earlier stage of growth and development	An ill person who could be independent asks for assistance with personal hygiene
Depersonalization	Removing feeling from something that is perceived as stressful	A medical assistant who is assisting with a lumbar puncture on a young child experiences the child as looking like a toy or doll
Rationalization	Assigning logical reasons or excuses for actions that may have been motivated by self-interest or other emotions the person does not wish to acknowledge	A patient might justify not telling the physician that he smokes by saying to himself, "The doctor isn't interested because he didn't ask about it"
Repression	Unconsciously excluding unacceptable ideas, impulses or emotions from awareness	A diabetic patient who hates finger sticks continuously forgets to test her blood sugar
Suppression	Deciding to put uncomfortable or painful thought out of awareness	A patient says, "I don't want to think about my surgery until the day before"
Displacement	Shifting an emotion or behavior from the original object to a more acceptable substitute	A medical assistant who has just been given a poor evaluation is extremely rude to the next person she talks to on the telephone
Undoing	An attempt to make amends for a feeling or behavior that makes a person feel guilty	A patient notices that she hates the medical assistant's hair style and hair color. Immediately she tells the medical assistant that she has beautiful eyes
Compensation	Attempting to overcome a real or perceived handicap by developing some other ability or trait	A person who thinks that she isn't very intelligent in school always offers to help the teacher

From Hunt SA: *Saunders fundamentals of medical assisting*, St. Louis, 2007, Saunders.

influencing spirits or gods in the unseen world. People from many cultures believe in the effectiveness of sacred words, tattoos, or amulets (objects worn to prevent injury or evil), as well as specific rituals that may involve chanting, fire, or even animal sacrifice.

Causes of Illness

Many cultures distinguish between illness caused by bad spirits or evil people and illness with physiologic origins. Importantly, one should not ridicule these theories if patients believe them. When patients feel that health professionals do not respect their beliefs, they may not follow recommendations or return for follow-up care. An open attitude and the willingness to listen to the patient's beliefs are required in order to establish a relationship of trust with the patient.

Fundamentals of scientific medical practice may be foreign to certain traditional practices, such as frequent handwashing to remove invisible organisms, taking medicine when one does not feel ill, and causing pain to healthy children by giving them immunizations.

Treatments and Traditional Practices

When patients have different beliefs, it is important for all members of the health care team to keep the lines of communication open. Patients need to be able to discuss other treatments that are being used. They also need to understand the importance of the treatments being offered by scientific medicine so that they can comply with standard medical treatment regimens in addition to their traditional practices.

As a general rule, the medical assistant should accept any traditional practice that is not dangerous. For example,

patients from Cambodia and other parts of Southeast Asia believe that rubbing the skin with the side of a coin dipped in a camphor preparation is a treatment for colds and headaches. This treatment, which is performed bilaterally on the upper chest or back, leaves bruises on the skin, but does not cause breaks in the skin. A child with bruises from this type of treatment is not a victim of child abuse, but the bruises might look like abuse. The medical assistant should learn about traditional treatments used by patients in the practice where he or she works.

One area in which family and cultural traditions may be strong relates to diet and herbal preparations. In many traditions, certain diseases and conditions are considered "hot" and others are considered "cold." The patient may be advised to either eat or avoid certain foods or to take certain herbal preparations in order to restore balance. If the patient can describe traditional treatments, it will be easier for the physician to identify any practices that might be harmful or that might interfere with prescribed medical treatments.

Behavioral Requirements

In some cultures there are specific behavioral requirements for women and men. There may be cultural norms requiring women to have a male escort when they leave their homes. In some cultures the oldest male in the family must make important decisions. For some individuals there are also cultural requirements prohibiting the removal of clothing, jewelry, and head coverings, even for medical examinations. Medical assistants must learn about cultural norms and respond with acceptance and sensitivity. If necessary, adaptations must be made so that the patient is not forced to violate personal standards.

MEDICAL PRACTICE and the LAW

The Civil Rights Act of 1964 and its amendments require access to federally funded health programs and services for individuals with limited English proficiency (LEP). State laws require similar access for state programs and services. This has been interpreted as a requirement for translation services to be provided by all government-funded health care providers. These services include consent forms in the languages of the service population and qualified medical interpreters either in person or by telephone. Health care providers are also required to provide sign language

interpreters if necessary under the provisions of the Americans with Disabilities Act.

The U.S. Department of Health and Human Services also requires translation services before informed consent can be given for medical research. Before enrolling a subject in a medical research program, it is necessary to provide written consent forms in the language that the subject understands and a translator fluent in English. ∎

What Would You Do? What Would You *Not* Do?   **RESPONSES**

Case Study 1
Page 62

What Did Nancy Do?
- ❑ Maintained a warm and accepting posture and a friendly tone of voice.
- ❑ Used an open response to encourage Jennifer to say more about how she felt about possibly being pregnant.
- ❑ Identified verbally that Jennifer seemed a little upset.

What Did Nancy Not *Do?*
- ❑ Did not immediately congratulate Jennifer or respond as if this was good news.
- ❑ Did not immediately assume a business-like tone of voice and ask closed questions to obtain information.
- ❑ Did not imply that Jennifer was experiencing a different emotion.
- ❑ Did not act as if the patient had nothing on her mind.
- ❑ Did appear to be in a hurry to finish the interview.

What Would You Do/What Would You *Not* Do? Review Nancy's responses and place a checkmark next to the information you included in your response. List the additional information you included in your response.

_____

_____

_____

_____

Case Study 2
Page 65

What Did Nancy Do?
- ❑ Made sure that Harold was looking at her when she spoke to him.
- ❑ Spoke clearly and a little slower than usual using a strong voice.
- ❑ Asked Harold if his hearing aid was working well for him.
- ❑ Used gestures to reinforce her directions.
- ❑ Used short sentences.
- ❑ Repeated instructions or questions as needed.

What Did Nancy Not *Do?*
- ❑ Did not speak so loudly that she was shouting.
- ❑ Did not express impatience in her tone of voice or body language.
- ❑ Did not speak in long, complicated sentences.
- ❑ Did not turn away from the patient and keep talking.
- ❑ Did not drop her voice at the end of sentences.

What Would You Do/What Would You *Not* Do? Review Nancy's responses and place a checkmark next to the information you included in your response. List the additional information you included in your response.

_____

_____

_____

_____

Case Study 3
Page 69

What Did Nancy Do?
- ❑ Expressed to Julie Ann that these symptoms are upsetting.
- ❑ Agreed that it is a good decision to see the doctor.
- ❑ Asked Julie Ann to describe the emotions she was experiencing during these episodes.
- ❑ Maintained an open, friendly, and calm demeanor during the interview.

What Did Nancy Not *Do?*
- ❑ Did not try to identify the cause of the episodes for Julie Ann.
- ❑ Did not rush through the interview so that the patient would be ready for the physician quickly.
- ❑ Did not say, "It's probably just anxiety."
- ❑ Did not say that there was probably nothing seriously the matter with Julie Ann.

What Would You Do/What Would You *Not* Do? Review Nancy's responses and place a checkmark next to the information you included in your response. List the additional information you included in your response.

_____

_____

_____

_____

TERMINOLOGY REVIEW

Acting out Translating unconscious emotions into inappropriate behavior.

Active listening Paying close attention to a speaker without thinking of anything else.

Anxiety A vague, unpleasant emotion of fear or dread often accompanied by restlessness or nervousness.

Body language Communication that is expressed through facial expressions, body position, muscle activity, and other nonverbal means.

Chronic Existing over a long period of time.

Closed questions Questions that anticipate a yes/no or short answer.

Denial Failure to acknowledge the reality of a situation.

Ego defense mechanism Unconscious mental process that offers psychological protection.

Empathy Objective awareness and sensitivity to the feelings and emotions of others.

Hierarchy Classified according to rank or importance.

Judgmental Making judgments about what is good or bad based on personal opinion.

Nonverbal Communication that occurs without words, such as through body posture or facial expression.

Open questions Questions that could have a variety of answers and encourage a personal response.

Oral Spoken; pertaining to the mouth.

Paraphrasing A restatement of the words of another, often to clarify meaning.

Physiologic Pertaining to body processes.

Projection Experiencing one's own emotions as those of another.

Reflecting Expressing the meaning and emotion of another's words back to the person.

Self-actualization The fulfillment of each individual's potential.

Summarizing Expressing the most important points of a conversation or written document.

Sympathy Feeling the same emotions as another.

Verbal Using words to communicate.

Webcam Small video camera attached to a computer that allows video to be transmitted on the Internet.

ON THE WEB

For Information on Multi-Cultural Resources:

U.S. National Library of Medicine—Multi-Cultural Resources for Health Information: sis.nlm.nih.gov/outreach/multicultural.html

For Information on Hearing Impairment:

National Association of the Deaf: www.nad.org

For Information on Limited English Proficiency:

Department of Health and Human Services Office for Civil Rights: Limited English Proficiency (LEP): www.hhs.gov/ocr/lep

For Information on Psychology:

American Psychological Association: www.apa.org

Social Psychology Network: www.socialpsychology.org

For Information on Vision Impairment:

American Foundation for the Blind: www.afb.org

National Association for Visually Handicapped: www.navh.org

 PREPARE FOR CERTIFICATION Visit the Evolve site at http://evolve.elsevier.com/Bonewit/today/ to actively Prepare for your Certification.

 *Check out the **Companion CD** bound with the book to access additional interactive activities.*

Introduction to Anatomy and Physiology

LEARNING OBJECTIVES

The Human Body
1. Explain why it is important for the medical assistant to be knowledgeable about anatomy and physiology.
2. Explain the relationship between anatomy and physiology.
3. State the six levels of organization within the human body.
4. List the 11 organ systems of the body, and describe the function of each.
5. Describe homeostasis and its importance to the human body.
6. Explain how the body maintains homeostasis using a negative feedback system.
7. List the four criteria used to describe the anatomic position.
8. Identify body planes, body regions, and relative positions using anatomic terms.
9. Distinguish between the dorsal body cavity and the ventral body cavity, and list the subdivisions of each cavity.

Cell Structure and Function
1. Describe the cell membrane.
2. Describe the composition of the cytoplasm.
3. Describe the components of the nucleus, and state the function of each component.
4. Identify and describe each of the cytoplasmic organelles, and state the function of each organelle.
5. Explain how the cell membrane regulates the composition of the cytoplasm.
6. Describe the various mechanisms that result in the transport of substances across the cell membrane.
7. List the phases of a cell cycle, and describe the events that occur in each phase.
8. Explain the difference between mitosis and meiosis.

Tissues and Membranes
1. List the four main types of tissues found in the body.
2. Describe the various types of epithelial tissues in terms of structure, location, and function.
3. Describe the general characteristics of connective tissue.
4. List three types of connective tissue cells, and state the function of each.
5. Describe the features and location of the various types of connective tissue.
6. Explain the differences among skeletal muscle, smooth muscle, and cardiac muscle in terms of structure, location, and control.
7. State the two categories of cells in nerve tissue, and explain their function.

CHAPTER OUTLINE

The Human Body
    Anatomy and Physiology
    Levels of Organization
    Organ Systems
    Homeostasis
    Anatomic Terms

Cell Structure and Function
    Structure of the Generalized Cell
    Cell Functions
Tissues and Membranes
    Body Tissues
    Body Membranes

CAAHEP COMPETENCIES

Content Competencies
Anatomy and Physiology
- Anatomy and physiology of all body systems

- Common pathology/diseases
- Diagnostic/treatment modalities

ABHES COMPETENCIES

Content Competencies
Anatomy and Physiology
- Anatomy and physiology

- Study of diseases and etiology
- All body systems
- Diagnostic/treatment modalities

KEY TERMS

active transport (AK-tiv TRANS-port)
anatomic position (an-ah-TOM-ih-kul poh-ZIH-shun)
chondrocyte (KON-droh-syte)
collagenous fibers (koh-LAJ-eh-nuss FYE-burs)
cytokinesis (sye-toh-kih-NEE-sis)
diffusion (dif-YOO-zhun)
elastic fibers (ee-LAS-tick FYE-burs)
fibroblast (FYE-broh-blast)
histology (hiss-TAHL-oh-jee)
homeostasis (hoh-mee-oh-STAY-sis)
human anatomy (ah-NAT-o-mee)
human physiology (fiz-ee-AHL-oh-jee)
macrophage (MAK-roh-fahj)

mast cell (MAST SELL)
meiosis (mye-OH-sis)
metabolism (meh-TAB-oh-lizm)
mitosis (mye-TOH-sis)
negative feedback (NEG-ah-tiv FEED-bak)
neuroglia (noo-ROG-lee-ah)
neuron (NOO-ron)
osmosis (os-MOH-sis)
osteocyte (AH-stee-oh-syte)
passive transport (PASS-iv TRANS-port)
phagocytosis (fag-oh-sye-TOH-sis)
pinocytosis (pin-oh-sye-TOH-sis)
tissue (TISH-yoo)

THE HUMAN BODY

The human body is an awesome masterpiece. Imagine billions of microscopic parts, each with its own identity, working together in an organized manner for the benefit of the total being. The human body is more complex than the greatest computer, yet it is personal. The study of the human body is as old as history itself because people have always had an interest in how the body is put together, how it works, why it becomes defective (illness), and why it wears out (aging).

The study of the human body is essential for those planning a career in health sciences, just as knowledge about automobiles is necessary for those planning to repair them. How can you fix an automobile if you do not know how it is put together or how it works? How can you help fix a human body if you do not know how it is put together or how it works?

Anatomy and Physiology

Human anatomy is the study of the shape and structure of the human body and its parts. It encompasses a wide range of study, including the development and microscopic organization of structures, the relationship between structures, and the interrelationship between structure and function. **Gross human anatomy** deals with the large structures of the human body that can be seen through normal dissection. **Microscopic anatomy** deals with the smaller structures and fine detail that can be seen only with the aid of a microscope.

Human physiology (fiz-ee-AHL-oh-jee) is the scientific study of the functions or processes of the human body. It answers how, what, and why anatomic parts work. Anatomy and physiology are interrelated because structure and function are always closely associated. The function of an organ, or how it works, depends on how it is put together. Conversely, the anatomy or structure provides clues to understanding how it works. The structure of the hand, with its long, jointed fingers, is related to its function of grasping things. The heart is designed as a muscular pump that can contract to force blood into the blood vessels. By contrast, lungs are made of a thin tissue and function to exchange oxygen and carbon dioxide between the outside environment and the blood. Imagine what would happen if the heart were made of thin tissue and the lungs were made of thick muscle. Structure and function are always related.

Levels of Organization

One of the most outstanding features of the complex human body is its order and organization—how all the parts, from tiny cells to visible organs, work together to make a functioning whole. The organizational scheme of the body has six levels (Figure 5-1).

Starting with the simplest and proceeding to the most complex, the six levels of organization are chemical, cellular, tissue, organ, body system, and total organism. The structural and functional characteristics of all organisms are determined by their chemical makeup.

Chemical Level   The **chemical level** deals with the interactions of atoms, such as hydrogen and oxygen, and their combinations into molecules, such as water. Molecules contribute to the makeup of a cell, which is the basic unit of life.

Cells   **Cells,** discussed later in this chapter, are the basic living units of all organisms. Estimates indicate that there are about 100 trillion dynamic, living cells in the human body. These cells represent a variety of sizes, shapes, and structures and provide a vast array of functions.

Tissues   Cells with similar structure and function are grouped together as **tissues.** All of the tissues of the body are grouped into four main types: epithelial, connective, muscle, and nervous. The tissue level of organization is also discussed in this chapter.

Organs   Two or more tissue types that together form a more complex structure and work together to perform one or more functions make up **organs,** the next higher level of organization. Examples of organs include the skin, heart, ear, stomach, and liver.

Body Systems   A **body system** consists of several organs that work together to accomplish a set of functions. Some examples of body systems include the nervous system, the digestive system, and the respiratory system.

Total Organism   Finally, the most complex of all the levels is the **total organism,** which is made up of several systems that work together to maintain life.

Organ level

Body system level

Tissue level

Photoreceptor cells in retina

Total organism level

Photoreceptor cell

Cellular level

Chemical level

Figure 5-1. Organizational scheme of the body. (From Applegate E: *The anatomy and physiology learning system,* ed 3, St. Louis, 2006, Saunders.)

Organ Systems

The human body has 11 major organ systems, each with specific functions, yet all are interrelated and work together to sustain life. Each system is described briefly here and then in more detail in later chapters. The organ systems are illustrated and summarized in Table 5-1.

Integumentary System *Integument* means skin. The integumentary (in-teg-yoo-MEN-tar-ee) system consists of the skin and the various accessory organs associated

Table 5-1 Organ Systems of the Body

Integumentary System	Skeletal System	Muscular System
COMPONENTS: Skin, hair, nails, sweat, sebaceous glands	COMPONENTS: Bones, cartilage, ligaments	COMPONENTS: Muscles
FUNCTIONS: Covers and protects body; regulates temperature	FUNCTIONS: Provides body framework and support; protects; attaches muscles to bones; provides calcium storage	FUNCTIONS: Produces movement; maintains posture; provides heat

Nervous System	Endocrine System	Cardiovascular System
COMPONENTS: Brain, spinal cord, nerves, sense receptors	COMPONENTS: Pituitary, adrenal, thyroid, other ductless glands	COMPONENTS: Heart, blood vessels, blood
FUNCTIONS: Coordinates body activities; receives and transmits stimuli	FUNCTIONS: Regulates metabolic activities and body chemistry	FUNCTIONS: Transports material from one part of the body to another; defends against disease

Continued

Table 5-1 Organ Systems of the Body—cont'd

Lymphatic System	Digestive System	Respiratory System
COMPONENTS: Lymph, lymph vessels, lymphoid organs	COMPONENTS: Mouth, esophagus, stomach, intestines, liver, pancreas	COMPONENTS: Air passageways, lungs
FUNCTIONS: Returns tissue fluid to the blood; defends against disease	FUNCTIONS: Ingests and digests food; absorbs nutrients into blood	FUNCTIONS: Exchanges gases between blood and external environment

Urinary System	Reproductive System	
	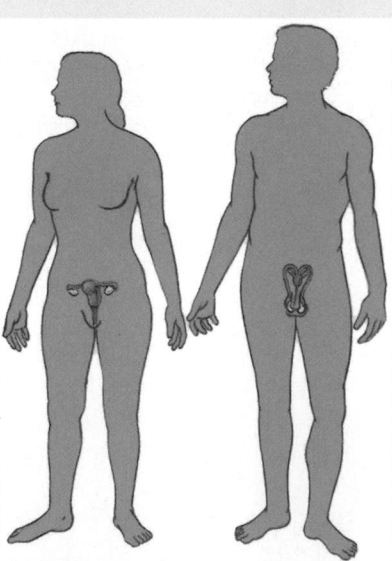	
COMPONENTS: Kidneys, ureters, urinary bladder, urethra	COMPONENTS: Testes, ovaries, accessory structures	
FUNCTIONS: Excretes metabolic wastes; regulates fluid balance and acid-base balance	FUNCTIONS: Forms new individuals to provide continuation of the human species	

From Applegate E: *The anatomy and physiology learning system,* ed 3, St. Louis, 2006, Saunders.

with it. These accessories include hair, nails, sweat glands, and sebaceous (oil) glands. The components of the integumentary system protect the underlying tissues from injury, protect against water loss, contain sense receptors, help in temperature regulation, and synthesize chemicals to be used in other parts of the body.

Skeletal System The skeletal (SKEL-eh-tull) system forms the framework of the body and protects underlying organs, such as the brain, lungs, and heart. It consists of the bones and joints along with ligaments and cartilage that bind the bones together. Bones serve as attachments for muscles and act with the muscles to produce movement. Tissues within bones produce blood cells and store inorganic salts containing calcium and phosphorus.

Muscular System Muscles are the organs of the muscular (MUS-kyoo-lar) system. As muscles contract, they create the forces that produce movement and maintain posture. Muscles can store energy in the form of glycogen and are the primary source of heat within the body.

Nervous System The nervous (NER-vus) system consists of the brain, spinal cord, and associated nerves. These organs work together to coordinate body activities. Nerve cells, or neurons, are specialized to transmit impulses from one point to another. In this way, body parts can communicate with each other and with the outside environment. Some nerve cells have special endings called *sense receptors* that detect changes in the environment.

Endocrine System The endocrine (EN-doh-krin) system includes all the glands that secrete chemicals called *hormones*. These hormones travel through the blood and act as messengers to regulate cellular activities. The endocrine and nervous systems work together to coordinate and regulate body activities to maintain a proper balance. The nervous system typically acts quickly, whereas the endocrine system acts slowly but with a more sustained effect. The endocrine system also regulates reproductive functions in both males and females.

Cardiovascular System The cardiovascular (kar-dee-oh-VAS-kyoo-lar) system consists of the blood, heart, and blood vessels. The blood transports nutrients, hormones, and oxygen to tissue cells and removes waste products such as carbon dioxide. Certain cells within the blood known as *white blood cells* defend the body against disease. The heart acts as a pump to create the forces necessary to maintain blood pressure and to circulate the blood. The blood vessels serve as pipes or channels for the flow of blood.

Lymphatic System The lymphatic (lim-FAT-ik) system consists of a series of vessels that transport fluid (lymph) from the tissues back into the blood. The system includes lymph nodes and lymphoid organs, such as the tonsils, spleen, and thymus, that filter the lymph to remove foreign particles as a protection against disease. Lymphoid organs also function in the body's defense mechanism by enhancing the activities of certain blood cells that produce immunity by inactivating specific pathogenic agents. The lymphatic system is sometimes considered to be a part of the cardiovascular system.

Digestive System The organs of the digestive (dye-JES-tiv) system include the mouth, pharynx, esophagus, stomach, small intestine, and large intestine (colon), which make up the digestive tract. Accessory organs of this system include the teeth, tongue, salivary glands, liver, gallbladder, and pancreas. The functions of this system are to ingest food, process it into molecules that can be used by the body, and then eliminate the residue.

Respiratory System The respiratory (reh-SPY-rah-tor-ee or res-per-ah-TOR-ee) system brings oxygen, in the form of air, into the lungs; removes the carbon dioxide; and provides a membrane for the exchange of these gases between the blood and lungs. The system consists of the nasal cavities, pharynx, larynx, trachea, bronchi, and lungs.

Urinary System The kidneys, ureters, urinary bladder, and urethra make up the urinary (YOO-rin-air-ee) system. The kidneys remove various waste materials, especially nitrogenous wastes, from the blood and help to regulate the fluid level and chemical content of the body. The product of kidney function is urine, which is transported through the ureters and urethra. The urinary bladder serves as a reservoir or storage area for the urine.

Reproductive System The reproductive (ree-pro-DUK-tiv) system is concerned with the production of new individuals. The system consists of the primary organs or gonads—ovaries in the female and testes in the male—that produce the reproductive cells, duct systems for transport, accessory glands, and supporting structures. In the female the reproductive system produces ova or eggs, receives sperm from the male, and provides for the support and development of the embryo and fetus. The male reproductive system is concerned with the production and maintenance of sperm and the transfer of these cells to the female.

Homeostasis

Homeostasis (hoh-mee-oh-STAY-sis) refers to the constant internal environment that must be maintained for the cells of the body. During homeostasis, the body systems are functioning normally and the internal environment of the body is in equilibrium; the body is in a healthy state. The word is derived from two Greek words: *homeo,* which means "alike" or "the same," and *stasis,* which means "always" or "staying." Putting these together, the word *homeostasis* means "staying the same." When the body is healthy, the internal environment always stays the same. It remains stable within limited normal ranges.

Everyone is familiar with aspects of the external environment—whether it is cold or hot, humid or dry, smoggy or clear. The internal environment is not quite as obvious. It refers to the tissue fluid that surrounds and bathes every cell of the body. Normal functional activities of the cell depend on the internal environment being maintained within limited normal ranges. The chemical content, volume, temperature, and pressure of the fluid must stay the same (homeostasis), regardless of external conditions, so that the cell can function properly. If the conditions in the tissue fluid deviate from normal, mechanisms respond that try to restore conditions to normal. If the mechanisms are unsuccessful, the cell malfunctions and dies. This leads to illness, disease, or, if homeostasis is not restored, eventually to death of the individual.

Negative and Positive Feedback

Any condition or stimulus that disrupts the homeostatic balance in the body is a **stressor.** When a stressor causes internal conditions to deviate from normal, all the body systems work to bring conditions back to the normal range. This is usually accomplished by a **negative feedback** mechanism. Negative feedback is a response mechanism of the body in which a stimulus initiates a reaction to reduce the stimulus. This mechanism works similar to a thermostat connected to a furnace and an air conditioner. When the temperature in the room decreases (stressor) below the thermostat setting (normal), the sensing device in the thermostat detects the change and causes the furnace to add heat to the room. When the room becomes too warm, the furnace stops and the air conditioner begins to cool the room. Negative feedback mechanisms do not prevent variation, but they keep variation within a normal range.

An example of a physiologic negative feedback mechanism in the human body involves blood pressure. When blood pressure decreases below normal, body sensors detect the deviation and initiate changes that bring the pressure back within the normal range. When the pressure increases above normal, changes occur to decrease the pressure to normal. Variations in blood pressure occur, but homeostatic mechanisms keep them within the limits of a normal range.

The nervous and endocrine systems work together to control homeostasis, but all the organ systems in the body help maintain the normal conditions of the internal environment. The brain contains centers that monitor temperature, pressure, volume, and the chemical conditions of body fluids. Endocrine glands secrete hormones in response to deviations from normal conditions, and these hormones affect other organs. The changes required to bring conditions back to the normal range are mediated by various organ systems. Good health depends on homeostasis. Illness results when the negative feedback mechanisms that maintain homeostasis are disrupted. Medical therapy attempts to assist the negative feedback process to restore balance, or homeostasis.

Anatomic Terms

Certain basic terms need to be understood to communicate effectively in the health care profession. In other words, you have to speak the language. This section explains some basic terms that relate to the anatomy of the body. They are used to describe directions and regions of the body.

Anatomic Position

If directional terms are to be meaningful, there must be some knowledge of the beginning position. If you give a person directions to go somewhere, you must have a starting reference point. When using directions in anatomy and physiology, it is assumed that the body is in **anatomic position.** In this position, the body is standing erect, the face is forward, and the arms are at the sides with the palms and toes directed forward. Figure 5-2 illustrates the body in anatomic position.

Directions in the Body

Directional terms are used to describe the relative position of one part to another. Note that in the following list of directional terms, the two items in each pair of terms are opposites.

Superior (soo-PEER-ee-or) means that a part is above another part, or closer to the head. The nose is superior to the mouth. **Inferior** (in-FEER-ee-or) means that a part is below another part, or closer to the feet. The heart is inferior to the neck.

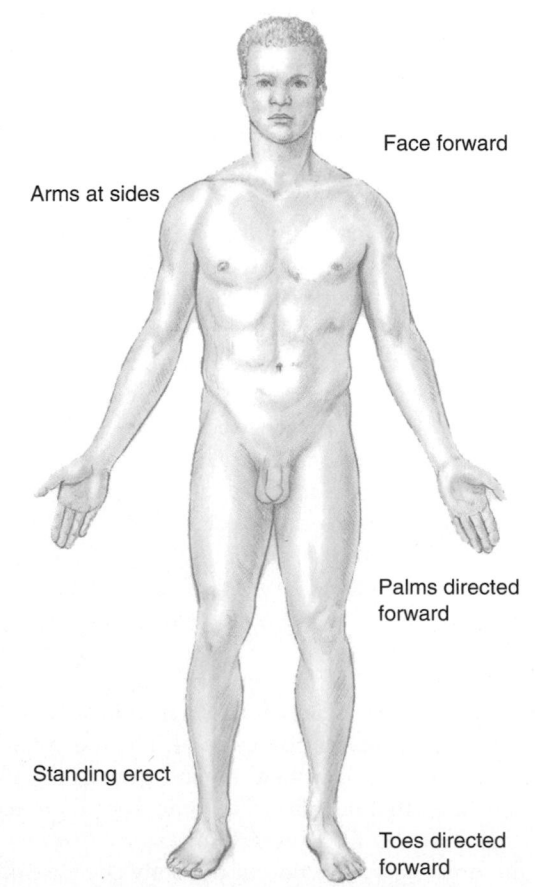

Face forward

Arms at sides

Palms directed forward

Standing erect

Toes directed forward

Figure 5-2. Anatomic position. (From Applegate E: *The anatomy and physiology learning system,* ed 3, St. Louis, 2006, Saunders.)

Anterior (an-TEER-ee-or) (or ventral) means toward the front surface. The heart is anterior to the vertebral column. **Posterior** (pos-TEER-ee-or) means that a part is toward the back. The heart is posterior to the sternum.

Medial (MEE-dee-al) means toward, or nearer, the midline of the body. The nose is medial to the ears. **Lateral** (LAT-er-al) means toward, or nearer, the side, away from the midline. The ears are lateral to the eyes.

Proximal (PRAHK-sih-mal) means that a part is closer to a point of attachment, or closer to the trunk of the body, than another part. The elbow is proximal to the wrist. The opposite of proximal is **distal** (DIS-tal), which means that a part is farther away from a point of attachment than is another part. The fingers are distal to the wrist.

Superficial (soo-per-FISH-al) means that a part is located on or near the surface. The superficial (or outermost) layer of the skin is the epidermis. The opposite of superficial is **deep,** which means that a part is away from the surface. Muscles are deep to the skin.

Visceral (VIS-er-al) pertains to internal organs or the covering of the organs. The visceral pericardium covers the heart. **Parietal** (pah-RYE-ih-tal) refers to the wall of a body cavity. The parietal peritoneum lines the wall of the abdominal cavity.

Planes and Sections of the Body

To aid in visualizing the spatial relationships of internal body parts, anatomists use three imaginary planes, each of which is cut through the body in a different direction. Figure 5-3 illustrates these three planes.

A **sagittal** (SAJ-ih-tal) **plane** refers to a lengthwise cut that divides the body into right and left portions. This is sometimes called a *longitudinal section.* If the cut passes through the midline of the body, it is called a **midsagittal plane,** and it divides the body into right and left halves.

A **transverse plane** or horizontal plane is perpendicular to the sagittal plane and cuts across the body horizontally to divide it into superior and inferior portions. Sections cut this way are sometimes called *cross sections.*

A **frontal plane** divides the body into anterior and posterior portions. It is perpendicular to both the sagittal plane and the transverse plane. This is sometimes called a **coronal** (ko-ROH-nal) **plane.**

Body Cavities

Spaces within the body that contain the internal organs or viscera are called *body cavities.* The two main cavities are the **dorsal cavity** and the larger **ventral cavity,** which are illustrated in Figure 5-4. The dorsal cavity is divided into the **cranial** (KRAY-nee-al) **cavity,** which contains the brain, and the **spinal** (SPY-nal) **cavity,** which contains the spinal cord. The cranial and spinal cavities join with each other to form a continuous space.

The ventral cavity is much larger than the dorsal cavity and is subdivided into the **thoracic** (tho-RAS-ik) **cavity** and the **abdominopelvic** (ab-dahm-ih-noh-PEL-vik) **cavity.** The thoracic cavity is superior to the abdominopelvic cavity and contains the heart, lungs, esophagus, and trachea. It is separated from the abdominopelvic cavity by the muscular diaphragm. Although there is no clear-cut partition to divide it, the abdominopelvic cavity is separated into the superior **abdominal** (ab-DAHM-ih-nal) **cavity** and the

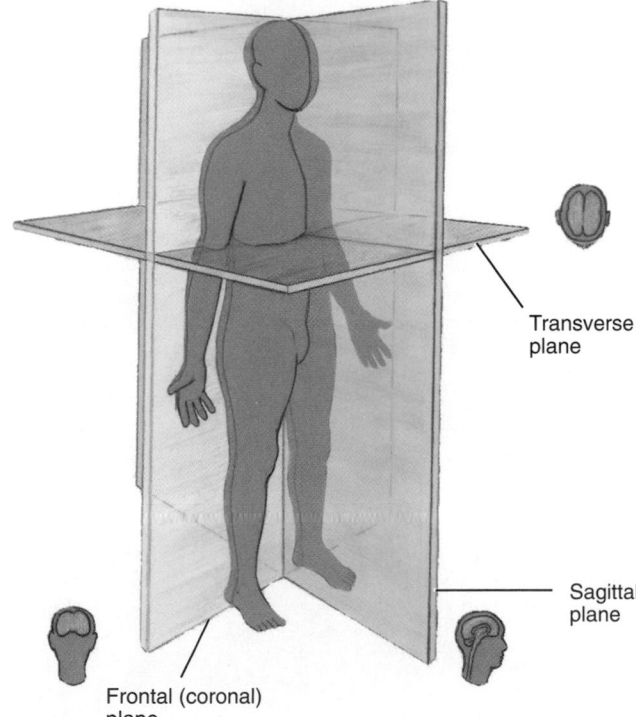

Figure 5-3. Transverse, sagittal, and frontal planes of the body. (From Applegate E: *The anatomy and physiology learning system,* ed 3, St. Louis, 2006, Saunders.)

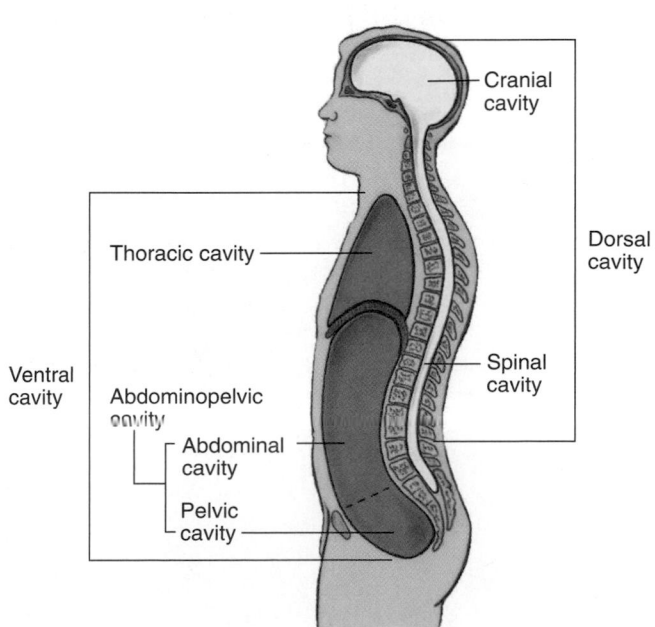

Figure 5-4. The two major cavities in the body. (From Applegate E: *The anatomy and physiology learning system,* ed 3, St. Louis, 2006, Saunders.)

inferior **pelvic** (PEL-vik) **cavity.** The stomach, liver, gallbladder, spleen, and most of the intestines are in the abdominal cavity. The pelvic cavity contains portions of the small and large intestines, the rectum, the urinary bladder, and the internal reproductive organs.

To help describe the location of body organs or pain, health care professionals frequently divide the abdominopelvic cavity into regions using imaginary lines. One such method uses the midsagittal plane and a transverse plane that passes through the umbilicus. This divides the abdominopelvic area into four quadrants, illustrated in Figure 5-5. Another system uses two sagittal planes and two transverse planes to divide the abdominopelvic area into the nine regions illustrated in Figure 5-6. The three central regions are, from superior to inferior, the **epigastric** (ep-ih-GAS-trik), **umbilical** (um-BIL-ih-kal), and **hypogastric** (hye-poh-GAS-trik) regions. Lateral to these, from superior to inferior, are the right and left **hypochondriac** (hye-poh-KAHN-dree-ak), right and left **lumbar,** and right and left **iliac** (ILL-ee-ak) or **inguinal** (IN-gwih-nal) regions.

Regions of the Body

The body may be divided into the **axial** (AK-see-al) portion, which consists of the head, neck, and trunk, and the **appendicular** (ap-pen-DIK-yoo-lar) portion, which consists of the limbs. The trunk, or **torso,** includes the thorax, abdomen, and pelvis. In addition to these terms and the nine abdominopelvic regions identified in the previous section, there are numerous other terms that apply to specific body areas. Some of these are listed in Table 5-2 and are identified in Figure 5-7.

CELL STRUCTURE AND FUNCTION
Structure of the Generalized Cell

Every individual begins life as a single cell, a fertilized egg. This single cell divides into 2 cells, then 4, 8, 16, and on and on, until the adult human body has an estimated 75 trillion cells. Cells are the structural and functional units of the human body. Homeostasis depends on the interaction between the cell and its environment.

Highlight on Anatomy and Physiology Pioneers: Anton van Leeuwenhoek

Anton van Leeuwenhoek was born on October 24, 1632, in Delft, Holland. He received little or no scientific education but was a cloth merchant and used hand-made lenses to study the fibers in fabrics. As a hobby, he taught himself new methods for grinding and polishing tiny lenses that gave magnifications up to 270 diameters. The lenses made by van Leeuwenhoek were unsurpassed for 200 years. The lenses he made led to the building of his microscopes. He was not the first to construct a microscope, but his microscopes are considered to be the first practical microscopes and for this he is called the **father of microscopy.** Using his own microscopes, van Leeuwenhoek made many pioneering biologic discoveries. He was the first to see free and independent cells, although he did not call them cells. The "cells" that he observed and described were red blood corpuscles, three types of bacteria, yeast cells, spermatozoa, and one-celled animals that we now call protozoa. van Leeuwenhoek made many other microscopic observations, reporting them to the Royal Society of England and the French Academy, until he died in Delft in 1723. ■

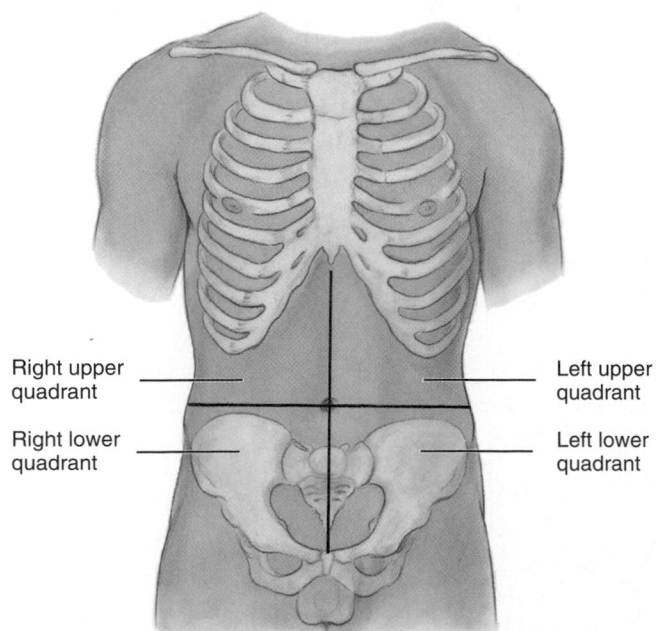

Figure 5-5. Abdominopelvic quadrants. (From Applegate E: *The anatomy and physiology learning system,* ed 3, St. Louis, 2006, Saunders.)

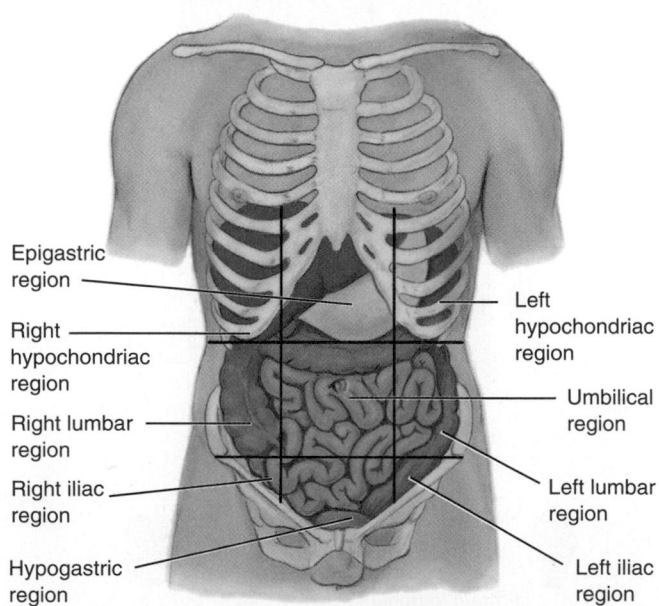

Figure 5-6. Nine abdominopelvic regions. (From Applegate E: *The anatomy and physiology learning system,* ed 3, St. Louis, 2006, Saunders.)

Table 5-2 Body Area Terms

Term	Meaning
Antecubital (an-te-KYOO-bih-tal)	Space in front of elbow
Axillary (AK-sih-lair-ee)	Armpit area
Brachial (BRAY-kee-al)	Arm; proximal portion of upper limb
Buccal (BUK-al)	Region of cheek
Carpal (KAR-pal)	Wrist
Celiac (SEE-lee-ak)	Abdomen
Cephalic (seh-FAL-ik)	Head
Cervical (SER-vih-kal)	Neck region
Costal (KAHS-tal)	Ribs
Cranial (KRAY-nee-al)	Skull
Cubital (KYOO-bih-tal)	Forearm; region between elbow and wrist; antebrachial
Cutaneous (kyoo-TAY-nee-us)	Skin
Femoral (FEM-or-al)	Thigh; part of lower extremity between hip and knee
Frontal (FRUN-tal)	Forehead
Gluteal (GLOO-tee-al)	Buttock region
Inguinal (IN-gwih-nal)	Depressed region between abdomen and thigh; groin
Leg (LEG)	Portion of lower extremity between knee and foot; also called *crural region*
Lumbar (LUM-bar)	Region of lower back and side between lowest rib and pelvis
Otic (OH-tik)	Ears
Palmar (PAWL-mar)	Palm of hand
Pectoral (PEK-toh-ral)	Chest region
Pedal (PED-al)	Foot
Pelvic (PEL-vik)	Inferior region of abdominopelvic cavity
Perineal (pair-ih-NEE-al)	Region between anus and pubic symphysis; includes region of external reproductive organs
Plantar (PLAN-tar)	Sole of foot
Popliteal (pop-LIT-ee-al or pop-lih-TEE-al)	Area behind knee
Sacral (SAY-kral)	Posterior region between hip bones
Sternal (STIR-nal)	Anterior midline of the thorax
Tarsal (TAHR-sal)	Ankle and instep of foot
Thoracic (tho-RAS-ik)	Chest; part of trunk inferior to neck and superior to diaphragm
Umbilical (um-BIL-ih-kal)	Navel; middle region of abdomen
Vertebral (ver-TEE-bral or VER-teh-bral)	Pertaining to spinal column; backbone

From Applegate E: *The anatomy and physiology learning system,* ed 3, St. Louis, 2006, Saunders.

During development, cells become specialized in size, shape, characteristics, and function, resulting in a large variety of cells in the body. For descriptive purposes it is convenient to imagine a typical, generalized cell that contains the components of all the different cell types. Not all the components of a "generalized" cell are present in every cell type, but each component is present in some cells and has its particular function to maintain life. A generalized cell is illustrated in Figure 5-8, and the structure and functions of the cellular components are summarized in Table 5-3.

Plasma Membrane

Every cell in the body is enclosed by a **plasma (cell) membrane.** The plasma membrane separates the material outside the cell (extracellular) from the material inside the cell (intracellular). It maintains the integrity of the cell. If the membrane ruptures, or is broken, the cell dies. The plasma membrane determines what can go into, or out of, the cell. It is **selectively permeable,** which means that some substances can pass through the membrane but others cannot. The main structural components of the plasma membrane are **phospholipids** and **proteins.**

Cytoplasm

The **cytoplasm** (SYE-toh-plazm) is the gel-like fluid inside the cell. The cytoplasm has numerous small structures, called **organelles,** suspended in it. These organelles (or-guh-NELZ), or "little organs," are the functional machinery of the cell, and each organelle type has a specific role in the metabolic reactions that take place in the cytoplasm.

The cytoplasm is primarily water known as the **intracellular fluid.** About two thirds of the water in the body is in the cytoplasm of cells. The intracellular fluid contains dissolved electrolytes, metabolic waste products, and nutrients such as amino acids and simple sugars.

Nucleus

The **nucleus** (NOO-klee-us) is the control center that directs the activities of the cell. All cells have at least one nucleus at some time during their existence; some, however, such as red blood cells, lose their nucleus as they mature. Other cells, such as skeletal muscle cells, have multiple nuclei.

The nucleus is a relatively large, spheric body that is usually located near the center of the cell (see Figure 5-8). It is enclosed by a double-layered **nuclear membrane** that separates the cytoplasm of the cell from the **nucleoplasm,** the fluid portion inside the nucleus.

The nucleus contains the genetic material of the cell. In the nondividing cell, the genetic material, deoxyribonucleic acid (DNA), is present as long, slender, filamentous threads called **chromatin** (see Figure 5-8). When the cell starts to divide or replicate, the chromatin condenses and becomes tightly coiled to form short, rodlike **chromosomes.** Each chromosome, composed of DNA with some protein, contains several hundred genes arranged in a specific linear

Figure 5-7. Terms for regions of the body. (From Applegate E: *The anatomy and physiology learning system,* ed 3, St. Louis, 2006, Saunders.)

Figure 5-8. Generalized cell. (From Applegate E: *The anatomy and physiology learning system,* ed 3, St. Louis, 2006, Saunders.)

Table 5-3 Structure and Function of Cellular Components

Component	Structure	Function
Plasma membrane	Bilayer of phospholipid and protein molecules	Maintains integrity of cell; controls passage of materials into and out of cell
Cytoplasm	Water; dissolved ions and nutrients; suspended colloids	Medium for chemical reactions; suspending medium for organelles
Nucleus	Spheric body near center of cell; enclosed in a membrane	Contains genetic material; regulates activities of cell
Nuclear membrane	Double-layered membrane around nucleus; has pores	Separates cytoplasm from nucleoplasm; pores allow passage of material as needed
Chromatin	Strands of DNA in nucleus	Genetic material of cell; becomes chromosomes during cell division
Nucleolus	Dense, nonmembranous body in nucleus; composed of RNA and protein molecules	Forms ribosomes
Mitochondria	Rod-shaped bodies enclosed by a double-layered membrane in cytoplasm; folds of inner membrane form cristae	Major site of adenosine triphosphate synthesis; converts energy from nutrients into a form that is usable by body
Ribosomes	Granules of RNA in cytoplasm	Protein synthesis
Endoplasmic reticulum	Interconnected membranous channels and sacs in cytoplasm	Transports material through cytoplasm; rough endoplasmic reticulum aids in synthesis of protein; smooth endoplasmic reticulum involved in lipid synthesis
Golgi apparatus	Group of flattened membranous sacs usually near nucleus	Packages products for secretion; forms lysosomes
Lysosomes	Membranous sacs of digestive enzymes in cytoplasm	Digest material taken into cell, debris from damaged cells, worn-out cell components
Cytoskeleton	Protein microfilaments and microtubules in cytoplasm	Provides support for cytoplasm; helps in movement of organelles
Centrioles	Pair of rod-shaped bodies composed of microtubules; located near nucleus at right angles to each other	Distribute chromosomes to daughter cells during cell division
Cilia	Membrane-enclosed bundles of microtubules that extend outward from cell membrane; short and numerous	Move substances across surface of cell
Flagella	Similar to cilia, except usually long and single	Cell locomotion

From Applegate E: *The anatomy and physiology learning system,* ed 3, St. Louis, 2006, Saunders.

order. Human cells have 23 pairs of chromosomes that together contain all the information necessary to direct the synthesis of more than 100,000 different proteins.

The **nucleolus** (noo-KLEE-oh-lus) ("little nucleus") appears as a dark-staining, discrete, dense body within the nucleus (see Figure 5-1). It has no enclosing membrane, and the number of nucleoli may vary from one to four in any given cell. The function of the nucleolus is to produce RNA and combine it with protein to form ribosomes. Ribosomes function in protein synthesis, as described later in this section. In growing cells and other cells that are making large amounts of protein, the nucleoli are large and distinct.

Cytoplasmic Organelles

Cytoplasmic organelles are "little organs" that are suspended in the cytoplasm of the cell. Each type of organelle has a definite structure and a specific role in the function of the cell.

Mitochondria

Mitochondria (mye-toh-KON-dree-ah) are elongated, oval, fluid-filled sacs in the cytoplasm that contain their own DNA and can reproduce themselves (see Figure 5-8). The membrane around a mitochondrion consists of two layers with a small space between the layers. The outer layer is smooth, but the inner layer has many invaginations that project like partitions into the interior matrix of the mitochondrion. These invaginations are called **cristae** (KRIS-tee) (Figure 5-9). Enzymes necessary for the production of adenosine triphosphate (ATP) are located along the cristae. ATP is a chemical that stores chemical energy within the cell and provides energy for use by the body cells. Mitochondria could be called the "power plant" of the cell because they convert energy from nutrients into ATP, which provides the energy needed by body cells.

Ribosomes

Ribosomes (RYE-boh-sohmz) consist of small granules of RNA located in the cytoplasm. The RNA in the ribosomes

Figure 5-9. Mitochondrion. (From Applegate E: *The anatomy and physiology learning system,* ed 3, St. Louis, 2006, Saunders.)

Figure 5-10. Golgi apparatus. (From Applegate E: *The anatomy and physiology learning system,* ed 3, St. Louis, 2006, Saunders.)

is from the nucleolus, and when fully assembled, ribosomes function in protein synthesis. Some ribosomes are found free in the cytoplasm. These ribosomes function in the synthesis of proteins for use within that same cell. Other ribosomes are attached to the membranes of the endoplasmic reticulum and function in the synthesis of proteins that are exported from the cell and used elsewhere.

Endoplasmic Reticulum

The **endoplasmic reticulum** (ER) (end-oh-PLAZ-mik reh-TICK-yoo-lum) is a complex series of membranous channels extending throughout the cytoplasm. The interconnected membranes form fluid-filled flattened sacs and tubular canals. The membranes are connected to the outer layer of the nuclear membrane, to the inner layer of the cell membrane, and to certain other organelles. The endoplasmic reticulum provides a path to transport materials from one part of the cell to another.

Some of the membranes of the endoplasmic reticulum have granular ribosomes attached to the outer surface (see Figure 5-8). This is called **rough endoplasmic reticulum** (RER) and, because of the ribosomes, it functions in the synthesis and transport of protein molecules. Other portions of the endoplasmic reticulum lack the ribosomes and appear smooth. This is the **smooth endoplasmic reticulum** (SER), which functions in the synthesis of certain lipid molecules, such as steroids.

Golgi Apparatus

The **Golgi apparatus** (GOL-jee ap-ah-RAT-us) is a series of four to six flattened membranous sacs, usually located near the nucleus, and connected to the endoplasmic reticulum (see Figure 5-8). It is the "packaging and shipping plant" of the cell.

Proteins from the RER and lipids from the SER are carried through the channels of the endoplasmic reticulum to the Golgi apparatus. Within the Golgi apparatus, the proteins may be modified or concentrated or have a carbohydrate component added. Then they are surrounded by a piece of the Golgi membrane and are pinched off the end of the apparatus to become a **secretory vesicle,** a temporary inclusion in the cytoplasm (Figure 5-10). The secretory

vesicles move to the cell membrane and release their contents to the exterior of the cell.

The Golgi apparatus is especially abundant and well developed in glandular cells that secrete a product, but they also function in nonsecretory cells. In these cells they appear to package intracellular enzymes in the form of lysosomes. Because of the secretory vesicles pinching off the ends of the flattened membranous sacs, the Golgi apparatus is sometimes described as looking like a stack of pancakes with syrup dripping off the edge.

Lysosomes

Lysosomes (LYE-soh-sohmz) are membrane-enclosed sacs of various enzymes that have been packaged by the Golgi apparatus. When cells are damaged, these enzymes destroy the cellular debris. They also function in the destruction of worn-out cell parts. The enzymes break down particles, such as bacteria, that have been taken into the cell. When a white blood cell phagocytizes or engulfs bacteria, the enzymes from the lysosomes destroy the bacteria. Lysosomal activity also seems to be responsible for decreasing the size of some body organs at certain periods. Atrophy of muscle because of lack of use, reduction in breast size after breastfeeding, and decrease in the size of the uterus after parturition all seem to be caused by lysosomal function.

Filamentous Protein Organelles

Several types of protein filaments are considered to be cellular organelles. The cytoskeleton and centrioles are in the cytoplasm, but the cilia and flagella project outward, away from the cell surface.

Cytoskeleton

The **cytoskeleton** helps to maintain the shape of the cell. At times it anchors certain organelles in position, but it may also move organelles from one position to another. Some parts of the cytoskeleton may move a portion of the cell membrane, whereas others may move the entire cell. The cytoskeleton also plays a role in muscle contraction.

The cytoskeleton is made up of protein **microfilaments** and **microtubules.** Microfilaments are long, slender rods of protein that support small projections of the cell membrane called **microvilli.** Microtubules are thin cylinders, larger than the microfilaments, and are composed of the protein **tubulin.** In addition to their role as part of the cytoskeleton, microtubules are also found in centrioles, cilia, and flagella.

Centrioles

A dense area called the **centrosome** (SEN-troh-sohm), located near the nucleus, contains a pair of **centrioles** (SEN-tree-ohlz) (see Figure 5-8). Each centriole is a nonmembranous rod-shaped structure composed of microtubules. The two members of the pair are at right angles to each other. Centrioles function in cell reproduction by aiding in the distribution of chromosomes to the new daughter cells.

Cilia

Cilia (SIL-ee-ah) are short, cylindric, hairlike processes that project outward from the cell membrane. Each cilium consists of specialized microtubules surrounded by a membrane and anchored under the cell membrane. Cilia have an organized pattern of movement that creates a wavelike motion to move substances across the surface of the cell. They are found in large quantities on the surfaces of cells that line the respiratory tract, where their motion moves mucus, in which particles of dust are embedded, upward and away from the lungs.

Flagella

Similar in structure to cilia, **flagella** (fluh-JELL-ah) are much longer and fewer. In contrast to cilia, which move substances across the surface of the cell, flagella beat with a whiplike motion to move the cell itself. In the human, the tail of the spermatozoon, or sperm cell, is a single flagellum that causes the swimming motion of the cell.

Cell Functions

The structural and functional characteristics of different types of cells are determined by the nature of the proteins present. Cells of various types have different functions because cell structure and function are closely related. A very thin cell is apparently not well suited for a protective function. Bone cells do not have an appropriate structure for nerve impulse conduction. Just as there are many cell types, there are varied cell functions. The specific functions of cells will become more apparent as the tissues, organs, and systems are studied. This section deals with the more generalized cell functions—the functions that relate to the sustained viability and continuation of the cell itself. These functions include movement of substances across the cell membrane, cell division to make new cells, and protein synthesis.

Movement of Substances across the Cell Membrane

The cell membrane provides a surface through which substances enter and leave the cell. The cell membrane controls the composition of the cell's cytoplasm by regulating the passage of substances through the membrane. If the membrane breaks, this control is removed and the cell dies. The survival of the cell depends on maintaining the difference between extracellular and intracellular material. Mechanisms of movement across the cell membrane include diffusion, osmosis, filtration, active transport, endocytosis, and exocytosis. These are summarized in Table 5-4.

Diffusion

Simple diffusion (dif-YOO-zhun) is the movement of substances from a region of high concentration to a region of low concentration. Odors permeate a room because the aromatic molecules diffuse through the air. A crystal of dye will color a whole beaker of water because the dye particles diffuse from the region of high concentration in the dye crystal to regions of low concentration in the water (Figure 5-11).

In the examples of diffusion cited, there has been no membrane involved. Diffusion can also occur across a membrane as long as the membrane is permeable to the substances involved. For example, oxygen and carbon dioxide are able to diffuse through the cell membrane. When carbon dioxide builds up in the capillaries to a concentration that is higher than in the lungs, the carbon dioxide diffuses into the lungs to be exhaled. Similarly, when the level of oxygen in the capillaries is lower than the

Table 5-4	Summary of Membrane Transport Mechanisms
Mechanism	**Description**
Passive	
Simple diffusion	Molecular movement down a concentration gradient
Osmosis	Movement of solvent toward high solute (low solvent) concentration; requires membrane
Filtration	Movement of solvent using hydrostatic pressure; requires membrane filter
Active	
Active transport	Movement of ions/molecules against a concentration gradient; requires carrier molecule and ATP
Phagocytosis	Ingestion of solid particles by creating vesicles; requires ATP
Pinocytosis	Ingestion of fluid by creating vesicles; requires ATP
Exocytosis	Secretion of cellular products by creating vesicles, then liberating contents to outside of cell; requires ATP

From Applegate E: *The anatomy and physiology learning system,* ed 3, St. Louis, 2006, Saunders.
ATP, Adenosine triphosphate.

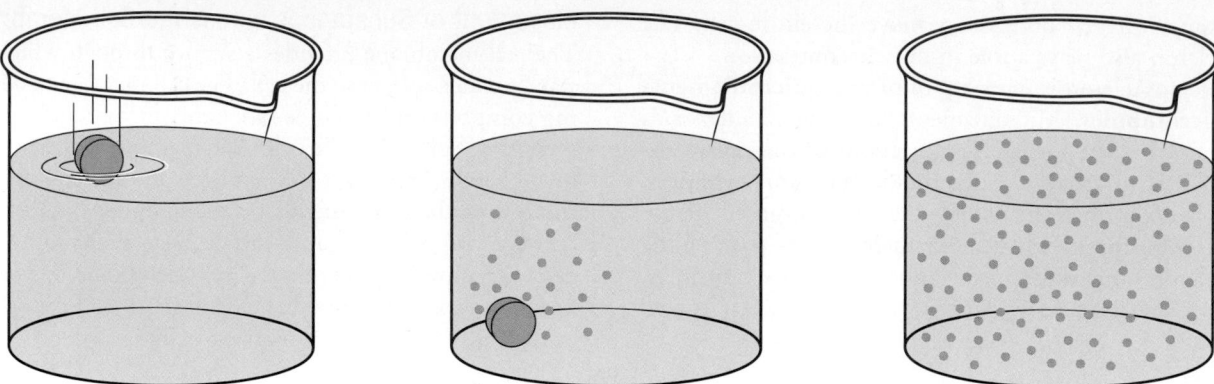

Figure 5-11. Simple diffusion. (From Applegate E: *The anatomy and physiology learning system,* ed 3, St. Louis, 2006, Saunders.)

Capillary with a high concentration of carbon dioxide molecules and a low concentration of oxygen

CO_2

Lung chamber with a high concentration of oxygen molecules and a low concentration of carbon dioxide

O_2

Figure 5-12. Diffusion of oxygen and carbon dioxide in the lungs. (From Applegate E: *The anatomy and physiology learning system,* ed 3, St. Louis, 2006, Saunders.)

level of oxygen in the lungs, oxygen diffuses into the capillaries for distribution to the body cells. In this way, the gases are exchanged between the air and the blood in the lungs, and between the blood and the cells of the various tissues (Figure 5-12).

Osmosis

Osmosis (os-MOH-sis) involves the movement of **solvent** (water) molecules through a **selectively permeable** membrane from a region of higher concentration of water molecules (where the **solute** concentration is lower) to a region of lower concentration of water molecules (where the solute concentration is higher). Figure 5-13 illustrates osmosis. When equilibrium is reached, the solutions on both sides of the membrane have the same concentration but the solution that was more concentrated at the start (had more solute) will now have a greater volume. Water molecules continue to pass through the membrane after equilibrium,

but because they move in both directions at the same rate there is no change in concentration or volume.

If a red blood cell, which contains 5% glucose, is placed in a container of 5% glucose solution, water will move in both directions at the same rate because the glucose concentrations inside and outside the cell are the same. Solutions that have the same solute concentration are **isotonic** (Figure 5-14A).

When a red blood cell is placed in a 10% glucose solution, water will leave the cell (where there are more water molecules) and enter the surrounding fluid (where there are fewer water molecules). When fluid leaves the cells, they will shrink or **crenate.** The 10% glucose solution is **hypertonic** (greater solute concentration) to the cell (Figure 5-14B).

When a red blood cell is placed in distilled water, water will enter the cell because there are more water molecules outside the cell than inside. The distilled water is **hypotonic** (lower solute concentration) to the cell. As water enters the cell, it will swell because of the increased volume. If enough water goes into the cell, it may rupture. This is called **lysis.** When this happens to a red blood cell, it is called **hemolysis** (hee-MAHL-ih-sis) (Figure 5-14C).

The terms *isotonic, hypotonic,* and *hypertonic* are relative. They are used to compare two solutions. A 5% glucose solution is hypertonic to distilled water but hypotonic to a 10% glucose solution.

Filtration

In diffusion and osmosis, particles (whether solute, solvent, or both) pass through a membrane by virtue of their own random movement, which is directed by a difference in concentration. In **filtration,** however, pressure pushes the particles through a membrane. Drip coffee makers, for example, use this principle. Water drips first through the coffee and then through the water, and small particles pass through a filter. The large granules of coffee are too big to go through the pores in the filter. The size of the pores determines the size of the particles that can pass through

Side A diluted
Side B concentrated

Water diffuses from A to B

Volume of A decreases
Volume of B increases

- Solvent (water molecules)
- Solute

Figure 5-13. Osmosis. (From Applegate E: *The anatomy and physiology learning system,* ed 3, St. Louis, 2006, Saunders.)

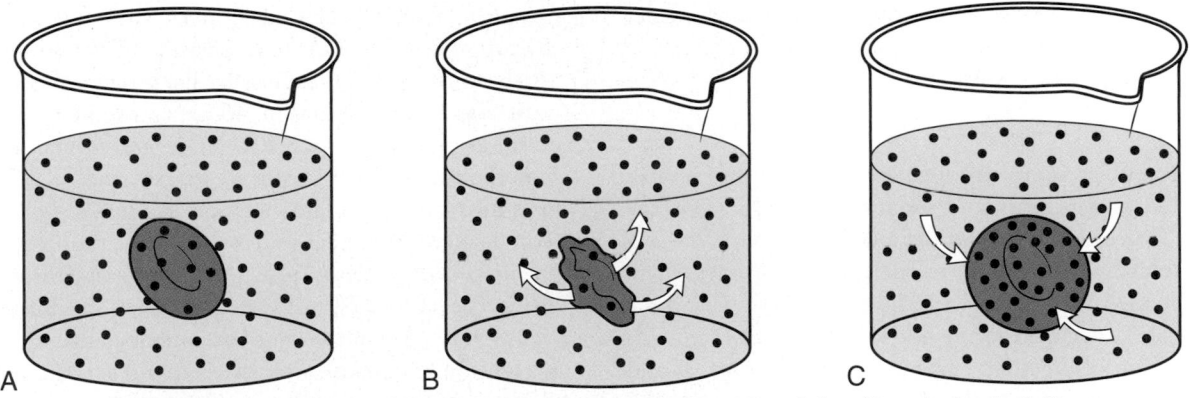

Figure 5-14. A, Isotonic solution. **B,** Hypertonic solution. **C,** Hypotonic solution. (From Applegate E: *The anatomy and physiology learning system,* ed 3, St. Louis, 2006, Saunders.)

the filter. The pressure is created by the weight of the water on the paper filter.

Contraction of the heart creates pressure in the blood. This fluid pressure or **hydrostatic pressure,** which is greater inside the blood vessels, pushes fluid, dissolved nutrients, and small ions through the capillary walls to form tissue fluid. The large protein molecules and blood cells are unable to pass through the pores in the capillary membrane. Blood is filtered through specialized membranes in the kidney as the initial step in urine formation. Water and small molecules and ions pass through the filtration membrane while blood cells and protein molecules remain in the blood.

Active Transport

In the transport mechanisms discussed thus far, no cellular energy has been involved and the molecules and/or ions moved from a region of high concentration to one of low concentration. **Active transport** differs from these processes in that it moves molecules and ions "uphill" from an area of lower concentration to an area of higher concentration. To accomplish this, cellular energy is required in the form of ATP. If ATP is not available, active transport ceases immediately. Active transport also uses a carrier molecule. Amino acids and glucose are transported from the small intestine into the blood by active transport.

As a result of active transport, substances such as electrolytes are present in significantly higher concentrations on one side of the cell membrane than on the other. For example, sodium ions are more concentrated outside the plasma membrane than inside the cell. Potassium is just the opposite; its concentration is higher inside the cell. Normal **passive transport,** such as diffusion and osmosis, tends to equalize the concentrations on the two sides of the membrane. Active transport, in this case known as the *sodium/potassium pump,* moves sodium and potassium against concentration gradients so that sodium is pumped out of the cell and potassium is pumped into the cell. This keeps a high sodium concentration outside the cell and a high potassium concentration inside the cell. The process requires ATP and a protein carrier molecule.

Endocytosis

Endocytosis (en-doh-sye-TOH-sis) refers to the formation of vesicles to transfer particles and droplets from outside to inside the cell. In this case, the material is too large to enter the cell by diffusion or active transport. The cell membrane surrounds the particle or droplet, and then that portion of the membrane pinches off to form a vesicle in the cytoplasm. The process requires energy in the form of ATP. **Phagocytosis** (fag-oh-sye-TOH-sis), which means "cell eating," involves solid material (Figure 5-15). The cell membrane engulfs a particle to form a vesicle in the cytoplasm. Lysosomes fuse with the vesicle and the enzymes digest the particle. Certain white blood cells are called *phagocytes* because they engulf and destroy bacteria in this manner. Another form of endocytosis is **pinocytosis** (pin-oh-sye-TOH-sis) or "cell drinking." It differs from phagocytosis in that the vesicles that are formed are much smaller and their contents are fluids. Pinocytosis is important in cells that function in absorption.

Exocytosis

In certain cells, secretory products are packaged into vesicles by the Golgi apparatus and are then released from the cell by a process called **exocytosis** (eck-soh-sye-TOH-sis). The secretory vesicle moves to the cell membrane, where the vesicle membrane fuses with the cell membrane and the contents are discharged to the outside of the cell (Figure 5-16). Secretion of digestive enzymes from the pancreas and secretion of milk from the mammary glands are examples of exocytosis. Exocytosis and endocytosis are similar except for working in opposite directions. They are both active processes that require cellular energy (ATP). Exocytosis

releases substances to the outside of the cell, and endocytosis transports substances to the inside of the cell.

Cell Division

Cell division is the process by which new cells are formed for growth, repair, and replacement in the body. This process includes division of the nuclear material and division of the cytoplasm. Periods of growth and repair are special periods in the life of an individual when it is obvious that new cells are needed either to increase the number of cells or to repair tissues after an injury. General maintenance and replacement needs of the body may not be quite as obvious. More than 2 million red blood cells are worn out and replaced in the body every second of every day. Skin cells are continually sloughed off the body's surface and must be replaced. The lining of the stomach is replaced every few days. All cells in the body (somatic cells), except those that give rise to the eggs and sperm (gametes), reproduce by **mitosis** (mye-TOH-sis). Egg and sperm cells are produced by a special type of nuclear division called **meiosis** (mye-OH-sis) in which the number of chromosomes is halved. Division of the cytoplasm is called **cytokinesis.**

Mitosis

All somatic cells reproduce by mitosis, in which a single cell divides to form two new "daughter cells," each identical to the parent cell. Humans have 23 pairs of chromosomes (or 46 chromosomes) in their cells. Each new cell that forms must also have 23 pairs or 46 chromosomes. For this to occur, events must proceed in an organized manner, chromosome material must replicate exactly, and then the chromosomes must separate precisely so that each new cell receives a set of chromosomes that is a carbon copy of the parent cells. For descriptive purposes, it is convenient to divide the events of mitosis into stages, as illustrated in Figure 5-17. It is important to remember that the process is a continual one and that there are no starting and stopping points along the way.

Interphase

The period between active cell divisions is called **interphase.** This is a time of growth and **metabolism** and is

Solid particle

Cell membrane wraps around particle

Vesicle

Figure 5-15. Phagocytosis. (From Applegate E: *The anatomy and physiology learning system,* ed 3, St. Louis, 2006, Saunders.)

Golgi apparatus

Secretory vesicle

Secretion

Figure 5-16. Exocytosis. (From Applegate E: *The anatomy and physiology learning system,* ed 3, St. Louis, 2006, Saunders.)

Figure 5-17. Mitosis. (From Applegate E: *The anatomy and physiology learning system,* ed 3, St. Louis, 2006, Saunders.)

usually the longest period of the cell cycle. In cells that are rapidly dividing it may last for as little as a few hours, but in other cells it may take days, weeks, or even months. Some highly specialized cells, such as nerve and muscle cells, may never divide and spend their whole life in interphase.

During interphase, the cell increases in size and synthesizes an exact copy of the DNA in its nucleus so that when the cell begins to divide it has identical sets of genetic information. Also just before division, the cell synthesizes an additional pair of centrioles and some new mitochondria. In addition to these synthetic activities that are a preparation for division, normal cellular function takes place during interphase.

Prophase

After interphase, the cell begins mitosis. The first stage of mitosis is **prophase.** During prophase, the chromatin shortens, thickens, and becomes tightly coiled to form chromosomes. As a result of the replication in interphase, each chromosome has two identical parts, called **chromatids,** that are joined by a special region on each called the **centromere.** The two pairs of centrioles separate and go to opposite ends of the cytoplasm. Microtubules called **spindle fibers** form and extend from the centromeres to the centrioles. The nucleolus and nuclear membrane disappear during the latter part of prophase.

Metaphase

Prophase ends when the nuclear membrane disintegrates, and this signals the beginning of the next stage, **metaphase.** The chromosomes align themselves along the center of the cell during metaphase. This is the time when the chromosomes are most clearly visible and distinguishable.

Anaphase

The third stage of mitosis is **anaphase.** After the chromosomes are aligned along the center of the cell, the centromeres separate so that each chromatid now becomes a chromosome. At this time, there are actually two sets of chromosomes in the cell. The two chromatids (now chromosomes) from each pair migrate to the centrioles at opposite ends of the cell. The microtubules that are attached to the centrioles and centromeres shorten and pull the chromosomes toward the centrioles. At the end of anaphase, the cytoplasm begins to divide.

Telophase

The final stage of mitosis is **telophase.** This stage is almost the reverse of prophase. After the chromosomes reach the centrioles at the ends of the cell, a new nuclear membrane forms around them. The spindle fibers disappear. The chromosomes start to uncoil to become long, slender strands of chromatin, and nucleoli appear in the newly formed nucleus. During this time, the cell membrane constricts in the middle to divide the cytoplasm and organelles into two parts that are approximately equal. Division of the cytoplasm is called **cytokinesis** (sye toh kih NEE-sis). Except for size, the two newly formed daughter cells are exact copies of the parent cell. The two daughter cells now become interphase cells to carry out designated cellular functions and to undergo mitosis as needed. The events of mitosis are summarized in Table 5-5.

Normally, body cells divide at a rate required to replace the dying ones. Normal cells are subject to control mechanisms that prevent overpopulation and competition for nutrients and space. Occasionally, a series of events occurs that alters some cells, so they lack the control mechanisms that tell them when to stop dividing. When the cells do not stop their mitotic activity, they form an abnormal growth called a *tumor,* or neoplasm.

Meiosis

Meiosis is a special type of cell division that occurs in the production of the gametes, or eggs and sperm. These cells have only 23 chromosomes, one half the number found in somatic cells, so that when fertilization takes place the resulting cell will again have 46 chromosomes, 23 from the egg and 23 from the sperm. Meiosis is discussed in greater detail in Chapter 16. In brief, meiosis consists of two divi-

sions, but DNA is replicated only once. The result is 4 cells, but each one has only 23 chromosomes. Table 5-6 and Figure 5-18 compare mitosis and meiosis.

DNA Replication and Protein Synthesis

Proteins that are synthesized in the cytoplasm function as structural materials, enzymes that regulate chemical reactions, hormones, and other vital substances. Because DNA in the nucleus directs the synthesis of the proteins in the cytoplasm, it ultimately determines the structural and functional characteristics of an individual. Whether a person has blue or brown eyes, brown or blond hair, or light or dark skin is determined by the types of proteins synthesized in response to the genetic information contained in the DNA in the nucleus. The portion of a DNA molecule that contains the genetic information for making one particular protein molecule is called a **gene.** If a cell produced for

Table 5-5 Summary of Mitotic Events	
Stage	**Events**
Interphase	DNA, mitochondria, and centrioles replicate
Prophase	Chromatin shortens and thickens to become chromosomes; centrioles move to opposite ends of cell; spindle fibers form; nucleolus and nuclear membrane disappear
Metaphase	Chromosomes align along center of cell
Anaphase	Centromeres separate and spindle fibers shorten to pull chromatids (chromosomes) toward centrioles at opposite ends of cell
Telophase	Chromosomes uncoil to become long filaments of chromatin; nuclear membrane and nucleolus reappear; cytokinesis occurs; daughter cells form and enter interphase

From Applegate E: *The anatomy and physiology learning system,* ed 3, St. Louis, 2006, Saunders.

Table 5-6 Comparison of Mitosis and Meiosis		
Feature	**Mitosis**	**Meiosis**
Type of cell where it occurs	Somatic cells	Reproductive cells
Chromosomes in parent cell	46 (23 pairs)	46 (23 pairs)
Chromosome replication	Yes—once	Yes—once
Number of cytoplasmic divisions	1	2
Number of cells formed	2	4
Number of chromosomes in each new cell formed	46 (23 pairs)	23

From Applegate E: *The anatomy and physiology learning system,* ed 3, St. Louis, 2006, Saunders.

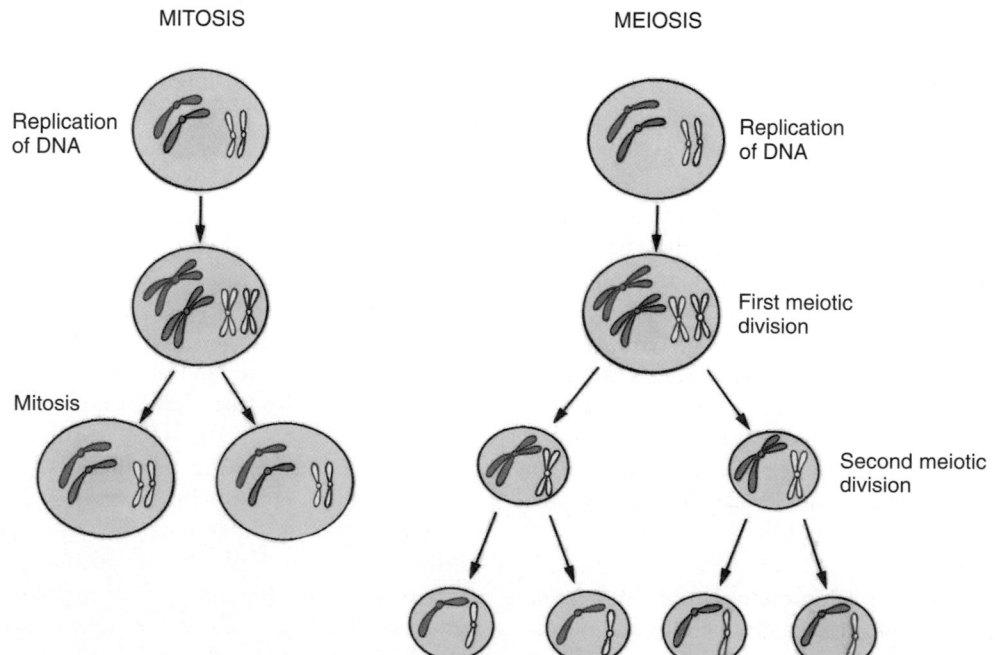

Figure 5-18. Comparison of mitosis and meiosis. (From Applegate E: *The anatomy and physiology learning system,* ed 3, St. Louis, 2006, Saunders.)

replacement or repair is to function exactly as its predecessor, then it must have the same genes, a carbon copy of the DNA. This is the purpose of DNA replication in cell division.

TISSUES AND MEMBRANES

A **tissue** is a group of cells that have similar structure and that function together as a unit. The microscopic study of tissues is called **histology** (hiss-TAHL-oh-jee). A nonliving material, called the **intercellular matrix,** fills the spaces between the cells. This may be abundant in some tissues and scarce in others. The intercellular matrix may contain special substances, such as salts and fibers, that are unique to a specific tissue and give that tissue distinctive characteristics.

Body Tissues

Four main tissue types are found in the body: epithelial, connective, muscle, and nervous. Each is designed for specific functions.

Epithelial Tissue

Epithelial (ep-ih-THEE-lee-al) **tissues** are widespread throughout the body. They form the covering of all body surfaces, line body cavities and hollow organs, and are the major tissue in glands. They perform a variety of functions that include protection, secretion, absorption, excretion, filtration, diffusion, and sensory reception.

The cells in epithelial tissue are tightly packed with little intercellular matrix. Because the tissues form coverings and linings, the cells have one free surface that is not in contact with other cells. Opposite the free surface, the cells are attached to underlying connective tissue by a noncellular **basement membrane.** This membrane is a mixture of carbohydrates and proteins secreted by the epithelial and connective tissue cells. Because epithelial tissues are typically **avascular** (without blood vessels), they must receive their nutrients and oxygen supply by diffusion from the blood vessels in the underlying tissues. Another characteristic of epithelial tissues is that they regenerate, or reproduce, quickly. For example, the cells of the skin and stomach are continually damaged and replaced, and skin abrasions heal quite rapidly.

Epithelia are classified according to cell shape and the number of layers in the tissue (Figure 5-19). Classified according to shape, the cells are squamous, cuboidal, or columnar, and the shape of the nucleus corresponds to the cell shape. **Squamous** cells are flat and the nuclei are usually broad and thin. **Cuboidal** cells are cubelike, as tall as they are wide, and the nuclei are spheric and centrally located. **Columnar** cells are tall and narrow, resembling columns, and the nuclei are usually in the lower portion of the cell near the basement membrane. According to the number of layers, epithelia are **simple** if they have only one layer of cells and **stratified** if they have multiple layers. Stratified epithelia are named according to the type of cells at the free

Highlight on Anatomy and Physiology

CONGENITAL ABNORMALITIES: Often congenital anatomic abnormalities must be surgically repaired so that disruptions in physiology are corrected. For example, a cleft palate (anatomy) is repaired so that food will enter (physiology) the pharynx instead of the nasal cavity. Broken bones (anatomy) are reset so that function (physiology) is restored.

CYSTIC FIBROSIS: Cystic fibrosis is an inherited disorder that afflicts 1 in every 2000 Caucasian live births. In cystic fibrosis the cell membrane proteins that function as channels for transporting chloride ions out of the cell are defective. Because chloride ion transport is altered, secretions such as mucus, sweat, and pancreatic juice are salty and thick. Thick mucus in the lungs leads to impaired breathing and increased infections. The ducts in the pancreas become plugged, which stops the flow of digestive enzymes. Life expectancy, with therapy, is about 27 years.

KIDNEY DIALYSIS: Normal-functioning kidneys remove waste products from the blood. When the kidneys do not function properly, waste molecules can be removed from the blood artificially by a process called *dialysis.* Dialysis is a form of diffusion in which the size of the pores in a selectively permeable membrane separates smaller solute particles from larger solutes. In kidney dialysis, small waste molecules pass through the membrane and are removed from the blood. The protein molecules, which are needed in the blood, are too large to pass through the pores and thus are retained.

NEOPLASMS: A benign neoplasm consists of highly organized cells that closely resemble normal tissue. In contrast, a malignant neoplasm, or cancer, consists of unorganized and immature cells that are incapable of normal function. These cells may detach from the tumor site and travel in the blood or lymph to another site and establish a new tumor. This is called *metastasis* and is probably the most devastating property of malignant cells. A benign tumor of glandular epithelial cells is called an *adenoma.* An adenocarcinoma is a cancerous tumor arising from glandular cells. Carcinomas are solid cancerous tumors that are derived from epithelial tissue. Approximately 85% of all malignant neoplasms are carcinomas. Sarcomas are cancerous tumors that are derived from connective tissue. These account for approximately 10% of all malignant neoplasms.

GENETIC DISORDERS: Genetic disorders are pathologic conditions caused by mistakes, or mutations, in a cell's genetic code. Mutations may occur naturally, or they may be induced by mutagens, such as radiation and certain chemicals. If the mutations occur in the gametes, the faulty code is passed from one generation to the next. Errors in the genes (DNA) cause the production of abnormal proteins, which result in abnormal cellular function. For example, in sickle cell anemia, a genetic blood disorder, red blood cells have abnormal hemoglobin because there is an "error" in the gene that directs hemoglobin synthesis.

PERITONITIS: An inflammation of the serous membranes in the abdominal cavity is called *peritonitis.* This is sometimes a serious complication of an infected appendix. ■

Squamous			Horizontal longer than vertical
Cuboidal			Horizontal and vertical equal
Columnar			Vertical greater than horizontal
Simple			One layer
Stratified			Many layers

Figure 5-19. Classification of epithelium. (From Applegate E: *The anatomy and physiology learning system,* ed 3, St. Louis, 2006, Saunders.)

Table 5-7 Summary of Epithelial Tissues

Type	Description	Location
Simple squamous	Single layer of thin, flat cells	Alveoli of lungs, capillary walls, kidneys
Simple cuboidal	Single layer of cuboidal cells	Ovary, thyroid gland, kidney tubules, pancreas, salivary glands
Simple columnar	Single layer of tall cells; often contains goblet cells	Stomach, intestines
Pseudostratified columnar	Single layer of uneven columnar cells; often contains cilia and goblet cells	Respiratory tract, tubes of reproductive system
Stratified squamous	Several layers with flat cells at the free surface	Skin, mouth, vagina, anus
Transitional	Specialized for stretching; several layers that decrease in number and cells that become thinner when distended	Urinary bladder

From Applegate E: *The anatomy and physiology learning system,* ed 3, St. Louis, 2006, Saunders.

Figure 5-20. Simple squamous epithelium. (From Applegate E: *The anatomy and physiology learning system,* ed 3, St. Louis, 2006, Saunders.)

surface of the tissue. Epithelial tissues are summarized in Table 5-7.

Simple Squamous Epithelium

Simple squamous epithelium (Figure 5-20) consists of a single layer of thin, flat cells that fit closely together with little intercellular matrix. Because it is so thin, simple squamous epithelium is well suited for areas in which diffusion and filtration take place. The alveoli or air sacs of the lungs, where diffusion of oxygen and carbon dioxide gases occurs, are made of simple squamous epithelium. This tissue is also found in the kidney, where the blood is filtered. Capillary walls, where oxygen and carbon dioxide diffuse between the blood and tissues, are made of simple squamous epithelium. Because it is so thin and delicate, this tissue is damaged easily and offers little protective function.

Simple Cuboidal Epithelium

Simple cuboidal epithelium (Figure 5-21) consists of a single layer of cube-shaped cells. These cells have more volume than squamous cells and also have more organelles. Simple cuboidal epithelium is found as a covering of the ovary, as a lining of kidney tubules, and in many glands, such as the thyroid, pancreas, and salivary glands. In the kidney tubules, the tissue functions in absorption and secretion. In glands, simple cuboidal cells form the secretory portions and the ducts that deliver the products to their destination.

Figure 5-21. Simple cuboidal epithelium. (From Applegate E: *The anatomy and physiology learning system,* ed 3, St. Louis, 2006, Saunders.)

Figure 5-22. Simple columnar epithelium. (From Applegate E: *The anatomy and physiology learning system,* ed 3, St. Louis, 2006, Saunders.)

Simple Columnar Epithelium

A single layer of cells that are taller than they are wide makes up **simple columnar epithelium** (Figure 5-22). The nuclei are in the bottom portion of the cell near the basement membrane. Simple columnar epithelium is found lining the stomach and intestines, where it secretes digestive enzymes and absorbs nutrients. Because the cells are taller (or thicker) than either squamous or cuboidal cells, this tissue offers some protection to underlying tissues.

In regions where absorption is of primary importance, such as in parts of the digestive tract, the cell membrane on the free surface has numerous small projections called **microvilli.** Microvilli increase the surface area that is available for absorption of nutrients. **Goblet cells** are frequently interspersed among the simple columnar cells. Goblet cells are flask- or goblet-shaped cells that secrete mucus onto the free surface of the tissue. **Cilia** may be present to move secretions along the surface.

Figure 5-23. Pseudostratified columnar epithelium. (From Applegate E: *The anatomy and physiology learning system,* ed 3, St. Louis, 2006, Saunders.)

Pseudostratified Columnar Epithelium

Pseudostratified columnar epithelium (Figure 5-23) appears to have multiple layers (stratified), but it really does not. This is because the cells are not all the same height. Some cells are short and some are tall, and the nuclei are at different levels. Close examination reveals that all the cells are attached to the basement membrane but that not all cells reach the free surface of the tissue. Cilia and goblet cells are often associated with pseudostratified columnar epithelium. This tissue lines portions of the respiratory tract in which the mucus, produced by the goblet cells, traps dust particles and is then moved upward by the cilia. Pseudostratified columnar epithelium also lines some of the tubes of the male reproductive system. Here the cilia help propel the sperm from one region to another.

Stratified Squamous Epithelium

Stratified squamous epithelium, the most widespread stratified epithelium, is thick because it consists of many layers of cells (Figure 5-24). Because stratified epithelia are named according to the shape of the surface cells, it follows that the cells on the surface are flat. The cells on the bottom layer, next to the basement membrane, are usually cuboidal or columnar, and these are the cells that undergo mitosis. As the cells are pushed toward the surface, they become thinner, so the surface cells are squamous. As the cells are pushed farther away from the basement membrane, it is more difficult for them to receive oxygen and nutrients from underlying connective tissue and the cells die. As cells on the surface are damaged and die, they are sloughed off and replaced by cells from the deeper layers. Because this tissue is thick, it is found in areas in which protection is a primary function. Stratified squamous epithelium forms the outer layer of the skin and extends a short distance into every body opening that is continuous with the skin.

Figure 5-24. Stratified squamous epithelium. (From Applegate E: *The anatomy and physiology learning system,* ed 3, St. Louis, 2006, Saunders.)

Figure 5-25. Transitional epithelium. (From Applegate E: *The anatomy and physiology learning system,* ed 3, St. Louis, 2006, Saunders.)

Transitional Epithelium

Transitional epithelium (Figure 5-25) is a specialized type of tissue that has several layers but can be stretched in response to tension. The lining of the urinary bladder is a good example of this type of tissue. When the bladder is empty and contracted, the epithelial lining has several layers of cuboidal cells. As the bladder fills and is distended or stretched, the cells become thinner and the number of layers decreases.

Glandular Epithelium

Glandular epithelium consists of cells that are specialized to produce and secrete substances. Glandular epithelium normally lies deep to the epithelia that cover and line parts of the body. If the gland secretes its product onto a free surface via a duct, it is called an **exocrine gland.** Examples of exocrine glands include sebaceous glands, mammary glands, and salivary glands. If the gland secretes its product directly into the blood, it is a ductless gland, or **endocrine gland.** Endocrine glands are discussed in Chapter 11.

Connective Tissue

Connective tissues bind structures together, form a framework and support for organs and the body as a whole, store fat, transport substances, protect against disease, and help repair tissue damage. They occur throughout the body. Connective tissues are characterized by an abundance of intercellular matrix with relatively few cells. Connective tissue cells are able to reproduce but not as rapidly as epithelial cells. Most connective tissues have a good blood supply, but some do not. Examples of connective tissue include adipose tissue, cartilage, and bone.

The intercellular matrix in connective tissue has a gel-like base of water, nonfibrous protein, and other molecules. Various mineral salts in the matrix of some connective tissues, such as bone, make them hard. Two types of fibers, collagenous (koh-LAJ-eh-nus) and elastic, are frequently embedded in the matrix. **Collagenous fibers,** composed of the protein collagen, are strong and flexible but are only slightly elastic. They are able to withstand considerable pulling force and are found in areas in which this is important, such as in tendons and ligaments. When collagenous fibers are grouped together in parallel bundles, the tissue appears white, so they are sometimes called *white fibers.* **Elastic fibers,** composed of the protein elastin, are not very strong, but they are elastic. They can be stretched and will return to their original shape and length when released. Elastic fibers, also called *yellow fibers,* are located where structures are stretched and released, such as the vocal cords.

Numerous cell types are found in connective tissue. Three of the most common are the **fibroblast, macrophage,** and **mast cell.** As the name implies, fibroblasts produce the fibers that are in the intercellular matrix. Macrophages are large phagocytic cells that are able to move about and clean up cellular debris and foreign particles from the tissues. Mast cells contain heparin, an anticoagulant, and histamine, a substance that promotes inflammation and that is active in allergies.

Loose Connective Tissue

Loose connective tissue, also called **areolar** (ah-REE-oh-lar) **connective tissue,** is one of the most widely distributed tissues in the body. It is the packing material in the body. It attaches the skin to the underlying tissues and fills the spaces between muscles. Most epithelial tissue is anchored to this tissue by the basement membrane, and the blood vessels in the loose connective tissue supply nutrients to the epithelium above. The matrix is characterized by a loose network of collagenous and elastic fibers. The predominant cell is the fibroblast, but other connective tissue cells are also present (Figure 5-26).

Figure 5-26. Loose (areolar) connective tissue. (From Applegate E: *The anatomy and physiology learning system,* ed 3, St. Louis, 2006, Saunders.)

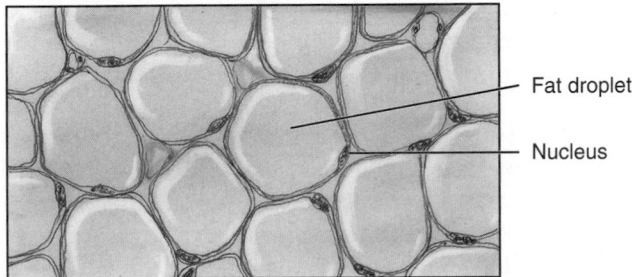

Figure 5-27. Adipose tissue. (From Applegate E: *The anatomy and physiology learning system,* ed 3, St. Louis, 2006, Saunders.)

Figure 5-28. Fibrous connective tissue. (From Applegate E: *The anatomy and physiology learning system,* ed 3, St. Louis, 2006, Saunders.)

Adipose Tissue

Commonly called *fat,* **adipose** (ADD-ih-pose) **tissue** is really a specialized form of loose connective tissue in which there is little intercellular matrix. Some of the cells accumulate liquid triglyceride, or fat, droplets. When this happens, the cytoplasm and nucleus are pushed off to one side, and the cells swell and become closely packed together (Figure 5-27). Fat cells have the ability to take up fat and then release it at a later time. Adipose tissue forms a protective cushion around the kidneys, heart, eyeballs, and various joints. It also accumulates under the skin, where it provides insulation for heat. Adipose tissue is an efficient energy storage material for excess calories.

Dense Fibrous Connective Tissue

Dense fibrous connective tissue is characterized by closely packed parallel bundles of collagenous fibers in the intercellular matrix (Figure 5-28). There are relatively few cells, and

Figure 5-29. Hyaline cartilage. (From Applegate E: *The anatomy and physiology learning system,* ed 3, St. Louis, 2006, Saunders.)

the ones that are present are fibroblasts to produce the collagenous fibers. This is the tissue that makes up **tendons,** which connect muscles to bones, and **ligaments,** which connect bones to bones. Dense fibrous connective tissue has a poor blood supply, and this, along with the relatively few cells, accounts for the slow healing of this tissue.

Elastic Connective Tissue

Elastic connective tissue has closely packed elastic fibers in the intercellular matrix. This type of tissue yields easily to a pulling force and then returns to its original length as soon as the force is released. The vocal cords and the ligaments that connect adjacent vertebrae are composed of elastic connective tissue.

Cartilage

Cartilage has an abundant matrix that is solid, yet flexible, with fibers embedded in it. The matrix contains the protein **chondrin** (KON-drihn). Cartilage cells, or **chondrocytes** (KON-droh-sytes), are located in spaces called **lacunae** (lah-KOO-nee) that are scattered throughout the matrix. Typically, cartilage is surrounded by a dense fibrous connective tissue covering called the **perichondrium.** The perichondrium has blood vessels, but they do not penetrate the cartilage itself, and the cells obtain their nutrients by diffusion through the solid matrix. Cartilage heals slowly because there is no direct blood supply, and this also contributes to slow cellular reproduction. Cartilage protects underlying tissues, supports other structures, and provides a framework for attachments.

Hyaline cartilage (Figure 5-29) is the most common type of cartilage. It has fine collagenous fibers in the matrix and a shiny, white, opaque appearance. It is found at the ends of long bones, in the costal cartilage that connect the ribs to the sternum, and in the supporting rings of the trachea. Most of the fetal skeleton is formed of hyaline cartilage before it is replaced by bone.

Fibrocartilage has an abundance of strong collagenous fibers embedded in the matrix. This allows it to withstand compression, act as a shock absorber, and resist pulling forces. It is found in the intervertebral discs, or pads between the vertebrae; in the symphysis pubis, or pad between the two pubic bones; and between the bones in the knee joint.

Elastic cartilage has numerous yellow elastic fibers embedded in the matrix, which makes it more flexible than hyaline cartilage or fibrocartilage. It is found in the framework of the external ear, the epiglottis, and the auditory tubes.

Bone

Osseous tissue or **bone** is the most rigid of all the connective tissues. Collagenous fibers in the matrix give strength to bone, and its hardness is derived from the mineral salts, particularly calcium, that are deposited around the fibers. Bones form the framework for the body and help protect underlying tissues. They serve as attachments for muscles and act as mechanical levers in producing movement. Bone also contributes to the formation of blood cells and functions as a storage area for mineral salts.

Cylindric structural units, called **osteons** or **haversian** (hah-VER-shun) **systems,** are packed together to form the substance of compact bone (Figure 5-30). The center or hub of the osteon is a tubular **osteonic** or **haversian** canal that contains a blood vessel. The matrix is deposited in concentric rings called **lamellae** (lah-MEL-ee) around the canal. **Osteocytes,** or bone cells, are located in lacunae between the lamellae so that they are also arranged in concentric rings. Slender processes from the bone cells extend, through tiny tubes in the matrix called **canaliculi** (kan-ah-LIK-yoo-lye), to other cells or to the osteonic canals. This provides a readily available blood supply for the bone cells,

which allows a faster repair process for bone than for cartilage.

Blood

Blood is a unique connective tissue because it is the only one that has a liquid matrix. It is a vehicle for transport of substances throughout the body. **Erythrocytes,** or red blood cells, and **leukocytes,** or white blood cells, are suspended in a liquid matrix called **plasma** (Figure 5-31). The red blood cells transport oxygen from the lungs to the tissues. White blood cells are important in fighting disease. Another formed element in the blood is the **platelet,** or **thrombocyte,** which is not actually a cell but a fragment of a giant cell in the bone marrow. Platelets are important in initiating the blood clotting process. Blood is discussed in more detail in Chapter 12.

Muscle Tissue

Muscle tissue is composed of cells that have the special ability to shorten or contract in order to produce movement of body parts. The tissue is highly cellular and is well supplied with blood vessels. The cells are long and slender, so they are sometimes called *muscle fibers,* and these are usually arranged in bundles or layers that are surrounded by connective tissue. The contractile proteins **actin** and **myosin** form microfilaments in the cytoplasm and are responsible for contraction. Muscle tissue is of three types: skeletal muscle, smooth muscle, and cardiac muscle. Features of muscle tissue are summarized in Table 5-8.

Figure 5-30. Compact bone (osseous tissue). (From Applegate E: *The anatomy and physiology learning system,* ed 3, St. Louis, 2006, Saunders.)

Labels: Canaliculi; Osteocyte in lacuna; Osteonic (haversian) canal; Lamellae

Figure 5-31. Blood. (From Applegate E: *The anatomy and physiology learning system,* ed 3, St. Louis, 2006, Saunders.)

Labels: Red blood cells; White blood cells; Platelets; Plasma

Table 5-8 Summary of Muscle Tissues			
Feature	Skeletal	Smooth	Cardiac
Location	Attached to bones	Walls of internal organs and blood vessels	Heart
Function	Produces body movement	Contracts viscera and blood vessels	Pumps blood through heart and blood vessels
Cell shape	Cylindric	Spindle shaped, tapered ends	Cylindric, branching, intercalated discs join cells together end to end
Number of nuclei	Many; peripherally located	One; centrally located	One; centrally located
Striations	Present	Absent	Present
Speed of contraction	Fastest	Slowest	Intermediate
Length of contraction	Least	Greatest	Intermediate
Type of control	Voluntary	Involuntary	Involuntary

From Applegate E: *The anatomy and physiology learning system,* ed 3, St. Louis, 2006, Saunders.

Skeletal Muscle

Skeletal muscle tissue (Figure 5-32) is what is commonly thought of as "muscle." It is the meat of animals, and it constitutes about 40% of an individual's body weight. Skeletal muscle cells (fibers) are long and cylindric with many nuclei (multinucleated) peripherally located next to the cell membrane. The cells have alternating light and dark bands that are perpendicular to the long axis of the cell. These bands are a result of the organized arrangement of the contractile proteins in the cytoplasm and give the cell a **striated** appearance. Skeletal muscle fibers are collected into bundles and wrapped in connective tissue to form the muscles, which are attached to the skeleton and which cause body movements when they contract in response to nerve stimulation. Skeletal muscle action is under conscious or voluntary control. Chapter 8 describes skeletal muscles in more detail.

Smooth Muscle

Smooth muscle tissue (Figure 5-33) is found in the walls of hollow body organs, such as the stomach, intestines, urinary bladder, uterus, and blood vessels. It normally acts to propel substances through the organ by contracting and relaxing. It is called *smooth muscle* because it lacks the striations evident in skeletal muscle. Because it is found in the viscera or body organs, it is sometimes called **visceral muscle.** Smooth muscle cells are shorter than skeletal muscle cells, are spindle shaped and tapered at the ends, and have a single, centrally located nucleus. Smooth muscle usually cannot be stimulated to contract by conscious or voluntary effort, so it is called *involuntary muscle.*

Cardiac Muscle

Cardiac muscle tissue (Figure 5-34) is found only in the wall of the heart. The cardiac muscle cells are cylindric and appear striated, similar to skeletal muscle cells. Cardiac muscle cells are shorter than skeletal muscle cells and have only one nucleus per cell. The cells branch and interconnect to form complex networks. At the point where one cell attaches to another, there is a specialized intercellular connection called an *intercalated* (in-TER-kuh-lay-ted) *disc.* Cardiac muscle appears striated like skeletal muscle, but its contraction is involuntary. It is responsible for pumping the blood through the heart and into the blood vessels.

Nervous Tissue

Nervous tissue is found in the brain, spinal cord, and nerves. It is responsible for coordinating and controlling many body activities. It stimulates muscle contraction, creates an awareness of the environment, and plays a major role in emotions, memory, and reasoning. To do all of these things, cells in nervous tissue need to be able to communicate with each other by way of electrical nerve impulses.

The cells in nervous tissue that generate and conduct impulses are called **neurons** (NOO-rons) or **nerve cells.** These cells have three principal parts: the dendrites, the cell body, and one axon (Figure 5-35). The main part of the cell, the part that carries on the general functions, is the **neuron cell body. Dendrites** are extensions, or processes, of the cytoplasm that carry impulses to the cell body. An extension or process called an **axon** carries impulses away from the cell body.

Figure 5-32. Skeletal muscle. (From Applegate E: *The anatomy and physiology learning system,* ed 3, St. Louis, 2006, Saunders.)

Figure 5-34. Cardiac muscle. (From Applegate E: *The anatomy and physiology learning system,* ed 3, St. Louis, 2006, Saunders.)

Figure 5-33. Smooth muscle. (From Applegate E: *The anatomy and physiology learning system,* ed 3, St. Louis, 2006, Saunders.)

Figure 5-35. Neuron (nervous tissue). (From Applegate E: *The anatomy and physiology learning system,* ed 3, St. Louis, 2006, Saunders.)

Highlight on Conditions Affecting Tissues

Adhesion (add-HEE-shun) Abnormal joining of tissues by fibrous scar tissue

Carcinoma (kar-sih-NOH-mah) A malignant growth derived from epithelial cells

Lipoma (lih-POH-mah) Benign tumor derived from fat cells

Marfan syndrome (mahr-FAHN SIN-drohm) A congenital disorder of connective tissue characterized by abnormal length of the extremities and cardiovascular abnormalities

Myoma (mye-OH-mah) Benign tumor formed of muscle tissue

Papilloma (pap-ih-LOH-mah) Benign epithelial tumor; may occur on any epithelial surface or lining

Sarcoma (sar-KOH-mah) A malignant growth derived from connective tissue cells

Scurvy (SKUR-vee) A condition caused by a deficiency of vitamin C in the diet, which results in abnormal collagen synthesis

Systemic lupus erythematosus (sih-STEM-ik LOO-pus air-ith-eh-mah-TOH-sis) Chronic autoimmune connective tissue disease characterized by injury to the skin, joints, kidneys, nervous system, and mucous membranes, but can affect any organ of the body ■

Figure 5-36. Body membranes. (From Applegate E: *The anatomy and physiology learning system,* ed 3, St. Louis, 2006, Saunders.)

Nervous tissue also includes cells that do not transmit impulses but instead support the activities of the neurons. These are the **glial** (GLEE-al) **cells** (or neuroglial cells), together termed the **neuroglia** (noo-ROG-lee-ah). Supporting, or glial, cells bind neurons together and insulate the neurons. Some are phagocytic and protect against bacterial invasion, whereas others provide nutrients by binding blood vessels to the neurons. Further detail on nerve tissue is presented in Chapter 9.

Body Membranes

Body membranes are thin sheets of tissue that cover the body, line body cavities, cover organs within the cavities, and line the cavities in hollow organs. By this definition, the skin is a membrane because it covers the body, and indeed, the skin, or integument, is sometimes called the **cutaneous membrane.** This membrane is discussed in Chapter 6. This section examines two epithelial membranes and two connective tissue membranes. Epithelial membranes consist of epithelial tissue and the connective tissue to which it is attached. The two main types of epithelial membranes are the mucous membranes and serous membranes. Connective tissue membranes contain only connective tissue. Synovial membranes and meninges belong to this category.

Mucous Membranes

Mucous membranes are epithelial membranes that consist of epithelial tissue attached to underlying loose connective tissue. These membranes (sometimes called **mucosae**) line the body cavities that open to the outside. The entire digestive tract is lined with mucous membranes. Other examples include the respiratory, urinary, and reproductive tracts. The type of epithelium varies depending on its function. In the mouth, the epithelium is stratified squamous for its protection function, but the stomach and intestines are lined with simple columnar epithelium for absorption and secretion. The mucosa of the urinary bladder is transitional epithelium so that it can expand. Mucous membranes get their name from the fact that the epithelial cells secrete mucus for lubrication and protection.

Serous Membranes

Serous membranes line body cavities that do not open directly to the outside, and they cover the organs located in those cavities. A serous membrane, or **serosa**, consists of a thin layer of loose connective tissue covered by a layer of simple squamous epithelium called **mesothelium.** These membranes always have two parts. The part that lines a cavity wall is the **parietal** layer, and the part that covers the organs in the cavity is the **visceral** layer (Figure 5-36). Serous membranes are covered by a thin layer of **serous fluid** that is secreted by the epithelium. Serous fluid lubricates the membrane and reduces friction and abrasion when organs in the thoracic or abdominopelvic cavity move against each other or the cavity wall.

Serous membranes have special names given according to their location. The serous membrane that lines the thoracic cavity and covers the lungs is the **pleura,** with the parietal pleura lining the cavity and the visceral pleura covering the lungs. The **pericardium** (pair-ih-KAR-deeum) lines the pericardial cavity and covers the heart. The serous membrane in the abdominopelvic cavity is the **peritoneum** (pair-ih-toh-NEE-um).

Synovial Membranes

Synovial (sih-NOH-vee-al) **membranes** are connective tissue membranes that line the cavities of the freely movable joints such as the shoulder, elbow, and knee. Similar to serous membranes, they line cavities that do not open to the outside. Unlike serous membranes, they do not have a layer of epithelium. Synovial membranes secrete **synovial fluid** into the joint cavity, and this lubricates the cartilage on the ends of the bones so that they can move freely and without friction. In certain types of arthritis, these membranes become inflamed and the fluid becomes viscous.

This reduces lubrication and increases friction, and movement becomes difficult and painful.

Meninges

The connective tissue coverings around the brain and spinal cord, within the dorsal cavity, are called **meninges** (meh-NIN-jeez). They provide protection for these vital structures. The outermost layer of the meninges is the toughest and is called the **dura mater** (DOO-rah MAY-ter). The middle layer, the **arachnoid** (ah-RAK-noyd), is quite fragile. The **pia mater** (PEE-ah MAY-ter), the innermost layer, is delicate and closely adherent to the surface of the brain and spinal cord. Inflammation of the meninges is **meningitis.** Further discussion of the meninges appears in Chapter 9.

⟲ TERMINOLOGY REVIEW

Active transport Membrane transport process that requires cellular energy.

Anatomic position Standard reference position for the body.

Chondrocyte Cartilage cell.

Collagenous fibers Strong and flexible connective tissue fibers that contain the protein collagen.

Cytokinesis Division of the cytoplasm at the end of mitosis to form two separate daughter cells.

Diffusion Movement of substances from a region of high concentration to a region of low concentration.

Elastic fibers Yellow connective tissue fibers that are not particularly strong, but can be stretched and will return to their normal shape when released.

Fibroblast Connective tissue cell that produces fibers.

Histology Branch of microscopic anatomy that studies tissues.

Homeostasis A normal stable condition in which the body's internal environment remains the same; constant internal environment.

Human anatomy Study of body shape and structure and the relationships of its parts.

Human physiology Study of the functions of living organisms and their parts.

Macrophage Large phagocytic connective tissue cell that functions in immune responses.

Mast cell A connective tissue cell that produces heparin and histamine.

Meiosis Type of nuclear division in which the number of chromosomes is reduced to one half the number found in a body cell; results in the formation of an egg or sperm.

Metabolism The total of all biochemical reactions that take place in the body; includes anabolism and catabolism.

Mitosis Process by which the nucleus of a body cell divides to form two new cells, each identical to the parent cell.

Negative feedback A mechanism of response in which a stimulus initiates reactions that reduce the stimulus.

Neuroglia Supporting cells of nervous tissue; cells in nervous tissue that do not conduct impulses.

Neuron Nerve cell, including its processes; conducting cell of nervous tissue.

Osmosis Diffusion of water through a selectively permeable membrane.

Osteocyte Mature bone cell.

Passive transport Membrane transport process that does not require cellular energy.

Phagocytosis Cell eating; a form of endocytosis in which solid particles are taken into the cell.

Pinocytosis Cell drinking; a form of endocytosis in which fluid droplets are taken into the cell.

Tissue Group of similar cells specialized to perform a certain function.

ON THE WEB

For Information on the Human Body:

American Medical Association: www.ama-assn.org

MadSci Network: www.madsci.org

Inner Body: Human Anatomy Online: www.innerbody.com

Medtropolis: The Virtual Body: www.medtropolis.com

University of Utah Health Sciences Center: library.med.utah.edu

Healthfinder: www.healthfinder.gov

Medscape: www.medscape.com

The Visible Human Project: www.nlm.nih.gov/research/visible

MedlinePlus Tutorials: www.nlm.nih.gov/medlineplus/tutorials

Cell Biology: www.cytochemistry.net/cell-biology

Cells Alive: www.cellsalive.com

The Virtual Cell Web Page: www.ibiblio.org/virtualcell

Loyola University Medical Education Network: www.lumen.luc.edu/lumen/meded/histo/frames/histo_frames.html

 PREPARE FOR CERTIFICATION   Visit the Evolve site at http://evolve.elsevier.com/Bonewit/today/ to actively Prepare for your Certification.

 Check out the Companion CD bound with the book to access additional interactive activities.

6

Integumentary System

LEARNING OBJECTIVES

1. Describe the structure of the two layers of the skin.
2. Name the supporting layer of the skin, and describe its structure.
3. List three factors that influence skin color.
4. Describe the structure of hair and nails and their relationship to the skin.
5. Discuss the characteristics and functions of the various glands associated with the skin.
6. List and describe four functions of the integumentary system.

CHAPTER OUTLINE

Introduction to the Integumentary System
Structure of the Skin
  Epidermis
  Dermis
  Subcutaneous Layer
Skin Color
Epidermal Derivatives
  Hair and Hair Follicles

Nails
Glands
Functions of the Skin
  Protection
  Sensory Reception
  Regulation of Body Temperature
  Synthesis of Vitamin D

CAAHEP COMPETENCIES

Content Competencies
Anatomy and Physiology
- Anatomy and physiology of all body systems

- Common pathology/diseases
- Diagnostic/treatment modalities

ABHES COMPETENCIES

Content Competencies
Anatomy and Physiology
- Anatomy and physiology

- Study of diseases and etiology
- All body systems
- Diagnostic/treatment modalities

KEY TERMS

arrector pili (ah-REK-tor PY-lee)
ceruminous gland (see-ROOM-in-us GLAND)
dermis (DER-mis)
epidermis (ep-ih-DER-mis)
keratinization (ker-ah-tin-ih-ZAY-shun)

melanin (MEL-ah-nin)
sebaceous gland (see-BAY-shus GLAND)
subcutaneous layer (sub-kyoo-TAY-nee-us LAY-ER)
sudoriferous gland (soo-door-IF-er-us GLAND)

Introduction to the Integumentary System

The skin and the glands, hair, nails, and other structures that are derived from it make up the **integumentary** (in-teg-yoo-MEN-tar-ee) **system.** Because it is on the outside of the body, this is the organ system with which we are most familiar. This is our contact with the external environment. It is the part that is, at least partially, exposed so that others can see it. Probably no other system receives as much personal attention. We spend millions of dollars each year in attempts to "beautify" the integumentary system through creams, lotions, oils, color, rinses, conditioners, permanents, manicures, pedicures, polishes, and more. The list goes on and on. Yet because it is on the outside of the body, this system is subjected to continual abuse in the form of bumps, abrasions, cuts, scrapes, toxic chemicals, pollutants, wind, and sun. However, the skin is resilient and versatile. Generally, it quickly repairs itself and continues to perform its many functions year after year.

STRUCTURE OF THE SKIN

The skin (sometimes called the **cutaneous** [kyoo-TAY-nee-us] **membrane)** consists of two distinct layers of tissues. The outer layer is the **epidermis,** and the inner layer is the **dermis.** These are anchored to underlying structures by a third layer, the **subcutaneous tissue.**

The structure of the skin is illustrated in Figures 6-1 and 6-2.

Epidermis

The outer layer of the skin is the **epidermis.** This layer consists of stratified squamous epithelium (see Figure 6-1). Because the epidermis is epithelium, there are no blood vessels present and the cells receive their nutrients, by diffusion, from vessels in the underlying tissue. The cells on the bottom, near the basement membrane, receive adequate nutrients and actively grow and divide. As cells are pushed upward toward the surface by the growing cells next to the basement membrane, they receive fewer nutrients. They also undergo a process called **keratinization** (ker-ah-tin-ih-ZAY-shun). During keratinization, a protein called *keratin* is deposited in the cell. This causes the chemical composition of the cell to change and the cell changes shape. By the time the cells reach the surface, they are flat or squamous and dead from lack of nutrients and are sloughed off. They are replaced by other cells that are pushed upward from below. As cells are pushed upward, away from the nutrient supply, and become keratinized, they take on different appearances and characteristics to form distinct regions. In thick skin, such as that on the soles of the feet and palms of the hand, the epidermis consists of five regions, or strata, of cells (see Figure 6-2). In the skin that covers the rest of the body, the regions are thinner and there are only four strata.

Highlight on the Integumentary System

SKIN: For an "average" person, the skin weighs about 5 kg, has a surface area of approximately 2 m², and varies in thickness from 0.05 to 0.4 cm.

NEOPLASMS: Cancerous neoplasms composed of melanocytes, called *malignant melanomas,* account for 3% of all cancers, and the incidence is rising at a rate of 4.5% annually. Exposure to sunlight is the major risk factor for the development of malignant melanoma, and individuals with fair skin and light hair are at greatest risk. Melanomas often metastasize to the lung, liver, and brain.

DERMIS: The dermis is the portion of an animal's skin that is used to make leather because the collagen in the dermis becomes tough when treated with tannic acid.

BLISTER: A blister is a fluid-filled pocket between the dermis and the epidermis. When the skin is burned or irritated, some plasma escapes from the blood vessels in the dermis and accumulates between the two layers, where it forms the blister.

DERMAL BLOOD VESSELS: In people with light skin, when dermal blood vessels dilate and blood flow increases (e.g., during blushing and increased temperature), the skin may be quite red. If the vessels constrict and blood flow decreases, the individual is pale or "white as a sheet."

HAIR TYPE: The shape of the hair shaft determines whether hair is straight or curly. If the shaft is round, the hair is straight. If it is oval, the hair is wavy. If it is flat, the hair is curly or kinky. A permanent flattens the hair to make it curly.

ACNE: Acne is a problem that plagues many teenagers. Increased hormone activity at puberty causes an increase in sebaceous gland activity. Sebum and dead cells may block the hair follicle and form blackheads. Bacteria infect the blocked follicle, and the sebum/dead cell mixture accumulates until the follicle ruptures. This initiates an inflammatory response that soon appears on the surface as a pus-filled pimple.

ADIPOSE TISSUE: People who lose weight rapidly may feel cold because they have reduced their adipose insulation. ■

Stratum basale   The bottom row of cells in the stratified squamous epithelium that makes up the epidermis consists of actively dividing (mitotic) columnar cells. This layer is the stratum basale (BAY-sah-lee), the layer next to the basement membrane and closest to the blood supply (see Figure 6-2). About one fourth of the cells in the stratum basale are melanocytes (meh-LAN-oh-sytes). Melanocytes consist of specialized epithelial cells that produce a dark pigment called *melanin* (MEL-ah-nin). All individuals have the same number of melanocytes. However, melanocyte activity (the amount of melanin produced) differs according to genetic and environmental factors.

Stratum spinosum   The stratum spinosum (spy-NOH-sum) consists of several layers of cells immediately above the stratum basale (see Figure 6-2). These cells have

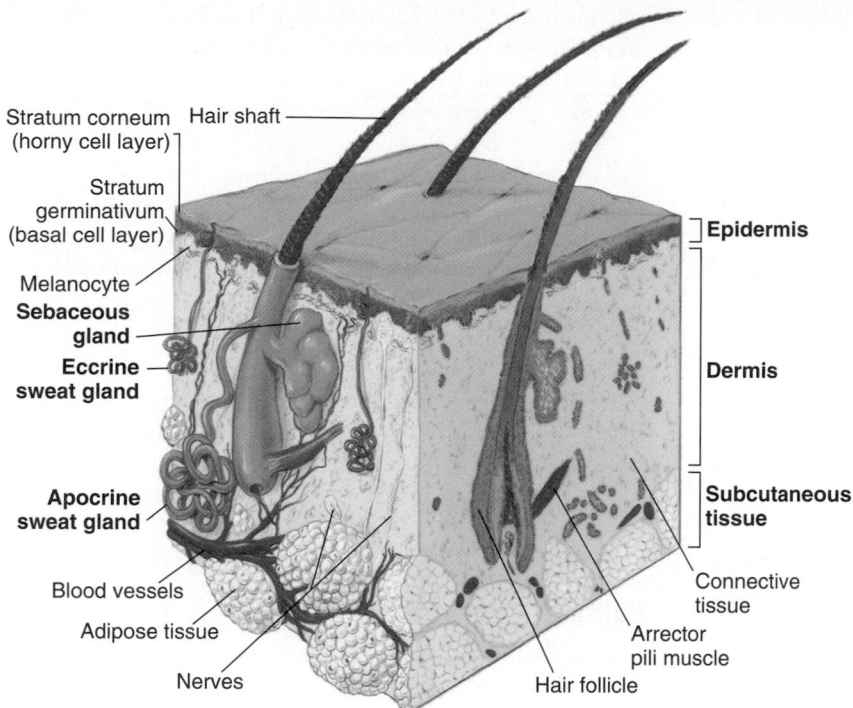

Stratum corneum
(horny cell layer)   Hair shaft

Stratum
germinativum
(basal cell layer)

Melanocyte

**Sebaceous
gland**

**Eccrine
sweat gland**

**Apocrine
sweat gland**

Blood vessels

Adipose tissue

Nerves

Epidermis

Dermis

**Subcutaneous
tissue**

Connective
tissue

Arrector
pili muscle

Hair follicle

Figure 6-1. Structure of the skin. (From Jarvis C: *Physical examination and health assessment,* ed 5, St. Louis, 2008, Saunders.)

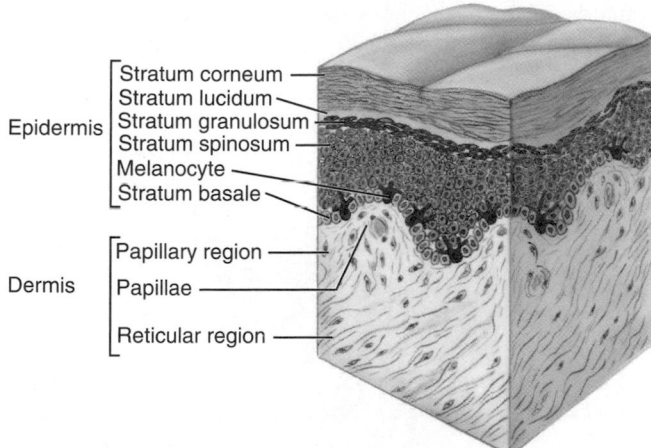

Epidermis

Stratum corneum
Stratum lucidum
Stratum granulosum
Stratum spinosum
Melanocyte
Stratum basale

Dermis

Papillary region
Papillae
Reticular region

Figure 6-2. Subdivisions of the epidermis and dermis. (From Applegate E: *The anatomy and physiology learning system,* ed 3, St. Louis, 2006, Saunders.)

slender projections, or spiny processes, that connect them with other cells. When a cell in the stratum basale undergoes mitosis and divides into two cells, one of the daughter cells remains in the stratum basale and the other one is pushed upward into the stratum spinosum. Because the cells in the stratum spinosum show limited mitotic ability, this layer combined with the stratum basale is called the *stratum germinativum* (JER-mih-nah-tiv-um).

Stratum granulosum   The stratum granulosum (gran-yoo-LOH-sum) is a thin region consisting of two or three layers of flattened cells (see Figure 6-2). Keratiniza-

tion begins in this layer. The cells appear granular, which gives this layer its name.

Stratum lucidum   The stratum lucidum (LOO-sih-dum) appears as a translucent band just above the stratum granulosum (see Figure 6-2). It consists of a few layers of flattened, anucleate cells. The stratum lucidum is present only in thick skin.

Stratum corneum   The stratum corneum (KOR-nee-um) is the outermost or surface region of the epidermis and constitutes about three fourths of the epidermal thickness. It consists of 20 to 30 layers of flattened, dead, completely keratinized cells (see Figure 6-2). The cells in the stratum corneum are continually shed and replaced. About 5 weeks after a cell has been produced in the stratum basale, it is sloughed off the surface of the stratum corneum. The keratin that is present is a tough, water-repellent protein, and its inclusion in the stratum corneum provides protection against water loss from the body.

Dermis

The **dermis,** or **stratum corium** (KOR-ee-um), is dense connective tissue that is deeper and usually thicker than the epidermis (see Figure 6-1). Hair, nails, and certain glands (although derived from the stratum basale of the epidermis) are embedded in the dermis. The dermis contains both collagenous and elastic fibers to give it strength and elasticity. If the skin is overstretched, the dermis may be damaged, leaving white scars called **striae** (STRY-ee), commonly called "stretch marks." Fibers also form a framework for the numerous blood vessels and nerves that are present in the dermis but generally absent in the epidermis. Many of the nerves in the dermis have specialized endings called **sensory receptors** that detect changes in the environment, such as heat, cold, pain, pressure, and touch. Because there are no nerves in the epidermis, these receptors are the body's contact with the environment.

The dermis is divided into two indistinct layers. The upper **papillary** (PAP-ih-lair-ee) **layer** derives its name from the numerous **papillae,** or projections, that extend into the epidermis (see Figure 6-2). Blood vessels, nerve endings, and sensory receptors extend into the papillae to bring them into closer proximity to the epidermis and the surface. On the palms, fingertips, and the soles of the feet, the papillae form distinct patterns or ridges that provide friction for grasping objects. The patterns are genetically determined and are unique for each individual. These are the basis of fingerprints and footprints.

The **reticular** (reh-TICK-yoo-lar) **layer** of the dermis is deeper and thicker than the papillary layer (see Figure 6-2). Bundles of connective tissue fibers run in many different directions to provide the strength and resilience needed to stretch in many planes. More bundles usually run in one direction than in the others, and this produces **cleavage lines.** Incisions across cleavage lines tend to gape more and produce more scar tissue than those that are parallel to the cleavage lines.

Subcutaneous Layer

The **subcutaneous layer** (see Figure 6-1) is not actually a part of the skin, but it loosely anchors the skin to underlying organs. Because it is beneath the dermis, it is sometimes called the **hypodermis.** It is also referred to as **superficial fascia.** The subcutaneous layer consists largely of loose connective tissue and adipose tissue. The fibers in the loose connective tissue are continuous with those in the dermis and, as a result, there is no distinct boundary between the dermis and the subcutaneous tissue.

The adipose tissue in the subcutaneous layer cushions the underlying organs from mechanical shock and acts as a heat insulator in temperature regulation. Fat in the adipose tissue can be mobilized and used for energy when necessary. The distribution of subcutaneous adipose tissue is largely responsible for the differences in body contours between men and women.

SKIN COLOR

Skin color is a result of many factors: some genetic, some physiologic, and some environmental. Basic skin color is caused by the dark pigment **melanin** produced by the melanocytes in the stratum basale of the epidermis. Melanocytes have long slender processes by which they transfer the melanin to surrounding cells in the skin and in hair. Everyone has about the same number of melanocytes. The activity of the melanocytes, however, is genetically controlled. A large number of melanin granules results in dark skin; fewer granules result in lighter skin. Although many genes are responsible for skin color, a single mutation can result in an inability to produce melanin. This results in a condition called **albinism** (AL-bih-nizm) in which individuals have light skin, white hair, and unpigmented irises in the eyes.

Some people have the yellowish pigment **carotene** (KAIR-oh-teen) in addition to melanin. This gives a yellow tint to the skin. A pinkish tint in the skin is attributable to the blood vessels in the dermis. Ultraviolet light increases melanocyte activity so that more melanin is produced and the skin becomes darker or tanned.

EPIDERMAL DERIVATIVES

Accessory structures of the skin include hair, nails, sweat glands, and sebaceous glands. They are derived from the stratum basale of the epidermis and are embedded in the reticular layer of the dermis. Figure 6-1 illustrates some of the accessory structures associated with the skin.

Hair and Hair Follicles

Hair is found on nearly all body surfaces. It is absent on the palms of the hands, soles of the feet, lips, nipples, certain external genitalia, and distal segments of the fingers and toes. All hair has essentially the same structure. It consists of a shaft and a root that are composed of dead, keratinized epithelial cells. The root is enclosed in a hair follicle that extends through the epidermis and is embedded in the dermis. The structure of hair and hair follicles is illustrated in Figure 6-3.

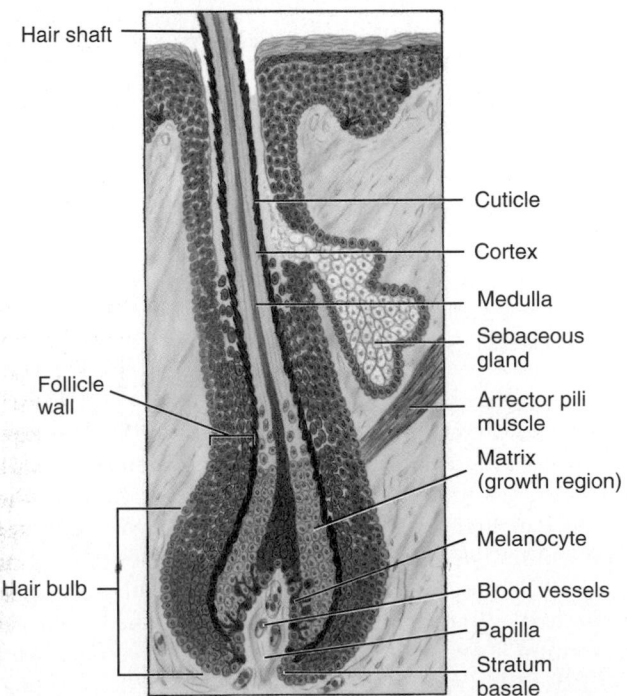

Figure 6-3. Structure of hair and hair follicles. (From Applegate E: *The anatomy and physiology learning system,* ed 3, St. Louis, 2006, Saunders.)

The **shaft** of a hair is that portion that extends beyond the surface of the epidermis. It is the part that you can see. Because it contains no nerves, it can be cut with no sensation of pain. The **root** is the portion of the hair that is below the surface of the skin. It is surrounded by a hair follicle. The shaft and root are continuous and together make up the hair, which is produced by the hair follicle. The central core of a hair is the **medulla.** This is surrounded by several layers of cells called the **cortex.** The outermost covering is a single layer of overlapping, keratinized cells called the **cuticle.** On the shaft of the hair, the cuticle is exposed to the environment and subjected to abrasion. It tends to wear away at the tip of the shaft. When this happens, the keratin fibers in the cells of the cortex and medulla project from the tip of the shaft, resulting in "split ends."

The root of a hair is enclosed in a tubular **hair follicle.** At the end deep in the dermis, the follicle expands to form a **hair bulb.** A **papilla** of dermis with a cluster of blood vessels projects into the center of the bulb. This provides the blood supply for the epithelial cells. As the follicle nears the hair bulb, the follicle becomes thinner so that only a single layer of stratum basale cells covers the papilla. The stratum basale cells, like those in the skin, provide the mitotic cells that divide and undergo keratinization to produce the hair.

Hair color is determined by the type of melanin produced by the melanocytes in the stratum basale. Yellow, brown, and black pigments are present in varying proportions to produce different hair colors. With age, the melanocytes become less active. Hair in which melanin is replaced with air bubbles is white.

A bundle of smooth muscle cells, called the **arrector pili** (ah-REK-tor PY-lee) muscle, is associated with each hair follicle. Most hair follicles are at a slight angle to the surface of the skin. The arrector pili muscles are attached to the hair follicles in such a way that contraction pulls the hair follicles into an upright position or causes the hair to "stand on end." Contraction of the arrector pili muscles also causes raised areas on the skin, or "goose bumps." Action of the arrector pili muscles is controlled by the nervous system in response to cold and fright.

Nails

Nails are thin plates of dead stratum corneum that contain a very hard type of keratin and cover the dorsal surfaces of the distal ends of the fingers and toes (Figure 6-4). Each nail has a **free edge;** a **nail body,** which is the visible portion; and a **nail root,** which is covered with skin. The **eponychium** (eh-poh-NICK-ee-um) or **cuticle** is a fold of stratum corneum that grows onto the proximal portion of the nail body. Stratum basale from the epidermis grows under the nail body to form the **nail bed.** This is thickened at the proximal end to form the **nail matrix,** which is responsible for nail growth. As cells are produced by the matrix, they become keratinized and slide over the nail bed. The portion of the body over the matrix appears as a whitish, crescent-shaped area called the **lunula** (LOO-nyoo-lah).

Figure 6-4. Structure of nails. (From Jarvis C: *Physical examination and health assessment,* ed 5, St. Louis, 2008, Saunders.)

Nails appear pink because of the rich supply of blood vessels in the underlying dermis.

Glands

The two major glands associated with the skin are the **sebaceous** (see-BAY-shus) **glands** and the **sweat glands.** A third type, the **ceruminous** (see-ROOM-ih-nus) **glands,** are modified sweat glands.

Sebaceous Glands

Generally, sebaceous glands are associated with hair follicles and are found in all areas of the body that have hair (see Figures 6-1 and 6-3). Those not associated with hair follicles open directly onto the surface of the skin. The oily secretion, called **sebum,** is transported by a duct into a hair follicle, and from there it reaches the surface of the skin. Sebum functions to keep hair and skin soft and pliable. It also inhibits growth of bacteria on the skin and helps to prevent water loss. Secretory activity of the sebaceous glands is stimulated by sex hormones; consequently, the glands are relatively inactive in childhood, become highly active during puberty, and decrease in activity during old age. Decreased sebum, in part, accounts for the dry skin and brittle hair that are common in older people.

Sweat (Sudoriferous) Glands

Sweat glands (also called **sudoriferous** [soo-door-IF-er-us] **glands**) are widely distributed over the body, except for the lips, nipples, and parts of the external genitalia. They are most numerous in the palms and soles. Estimates indicate that an individual has more than 2.5 million sweat glands.

Merocrine sweat glands are the more numerous and more widely distributed of the two types of sweat glands. The glandular portion is a coiled tube that is embedded in the dermis of the skin, and the duct opens onto the surface of the skin through a **sweat pore** (see Figure 6-1). The secretion of these glands is primarily water with a few salts. When the body's temperature increases, the glands are stimulated to produce sweat, which evaporates and has a cooling effect. Sweat, or **perspiration,** is also produced in response to nerve stimulation as a result of emotional stress.

Apocrine sweat glands are larger than the merocrine glands, and their distribution is limited to the axillae and external genitalia. Their ducts open into the hair follicles in these regions. Their secretion consists of water and salts and also contains organic compounds, such as fatty acids and proteins. These glands become active at puberty and are stimulated by the nervous system in response to pain, emotional stress, and sexual arousal. The secretion is odorless when released but is quickly broken down by bacteria to cause what is known as *body odor.*

Ceruminous Glands

Ceruminous glands are modified sweat glands that are found in the external auditory (ear) canal. They secrete an oily, sticky substance called **cerumen** (see-ROOM-men), or earwax, that is thought to repel insects and trap foreign material.

FUNCTIONS OF THE SKIN
Protection

The skin forms a protective covering over the entire body. The keratin in the cells waterproofs the cells and helps prevent fluid loss from the body. This waterproofing also prevents too much water from entering the body during swimming and bathing. Unbroken skin forms the first line of defense against bacteria and other invading organisms. The oily secretions of the sebaceous glands are acidic and inhibit bacterial growth on the skin. Melanin pigment absorbs light and helps protect underlying tissues from the damaging effects of ultraviolet light. Skin also protects underlying tissues from mechanical, chemical, and thermal injury.

Sensory Reception

The dermis contains numerous sensory receptors for heat, cold, pain, touch, and pressure. Even though hair itself has no sensory receptors, the movement of hair can be detected by receptors clustered around a hair follicle. The sensory receptors in the dermis relay information about the environment to the brain so that changes can be made to prevent or minimize injury. The sensory receptors are also a means of communication between individuals.

Regulation of Body Temperature

Normally, body temperature is maintained at 37°C (98.6°F). It is important that body temperature be regulated because changes in temperature alter the speed of chemical reactions in the body. About 40% of the energy in a glucose molecule is stored in the bonds of adenosine triphosphate (ATP) to be used by the cells. The remaining 60% of the energy is heat to maintain body temperature. Often this amount is more than is necessary to maintain body temperature, and

---

Highlight on Conditions Affecting the Integumentary System

Alopecia (al-oh-PEE-shee-ah) Absence of hair from skin areas where it normally grows; baldness; may be hereditary or due to disease, injury, or chemotherapy or may occur as part of aging

Basal cell carcinoma (BAY-sal SELL kar-sih-NOH-mah) Malignant tumor of the basal cell layer of the epidermis; most common form of skin cancer and usually grows slowly

Cellulitis (sell-yoo-LYE-tis) Infection of connective tissue with severe inflammation of the dermis and subcutaneous layers of the skin

Dermatitis (der-mah-TYE-tis) Inflammation of the skin

Eczema (ECK-zeh-mah) An inflammatory skin disease with red, itching, vesicular lesions that may crust over; common allergic reaction, but may occur without any obvious cause

Eschar (ESS-kar) A slough produced by a burn or gangrene

Impetigo (im-peh-TYE-go) Superficial skin infection caused by staphylococcal or streptococcal bacteria and characterized by vesicles, pustules, and crusted-over lesions; most common in children

Malignant melanoma (mah-LIG-nant mel-ah-NOH-mah) Cancerous growth composed of melanocytes; often arises in a preexisting mole; an alarming increase in the prevalence of malignant melanoma is attributed to excessive exposure to sunlight

Nevus (NEE-vus) An elevated, pigmented lesion on the skin; commonly called a *mole;* a dysplastic nevus is a mole that does not form properly and may progress to a type of skin cancer; plural, nevi

Pruritus (proo-RYE-tus) Severe itching; one of the most common problems in dermatology; arises as a result of stimulation of nerves in the skin by enzymes released in allergic reactions or by other irritating substances

Urticaria (ur-tih-KAIR-ee-ah) Allergic transient skin eruptions characterized by elevated lesions, called *wheals,* and often accompanied by severe itching and burning; also called *hives*

Wart (WORT) Epidermal growth on the skin caused by a virus; plantar warts occur on the soles of the feet, juvenile warts occur on the hands and face of children, and venereal warts occur in the genital area

Xeroderma pigmentosum (zee-roh-DER-mah pig-men-TOH-sum) A pigmentary and atrophic inherited disease of the skin and eyes that is characterized by vascular lesions, excessive freckling, keratinous growths, carcinoma, photophobia, ocular opacities, and tumors; involves defect in the enzymes active in the repair of DNA damaged by ultraviolet light ■

Highlight on Skin Aging

As the skin ages, the number of elastic fibers decreases and adipose tissue is lost from the dermis and subcutaneous layer. This causes the skin to wrinkle and sag. Loss of collagen fibers in the dermis makes the skin more fragile and makes it heal more slowly. Mitotic activity in the stratum basale slows so that the skin becomes thinner and appears more transparent. Reduced sebaceous gland activity causes dry, itchy skin. Loss of adipose tissue in the subcutaneous layer and reduced sweat gland activity lead to an intolerance of cold and susceptibility to heat. The ability of the skin to regulate temperature is reduced. There is a general reduction in melanocyte activity, which decreases protection from ultraviolet light, resulting in increased susceptibility to sunburn and skin cancer. Some melanocytes, however, may increase melanin production, resulting in "age spots."

Despite all the creams and "miracle" lotions, there is no known way to prevent skin from aging. Good nutrition and cleanliness may slow the aging process. Because skin that is exposed to sunlight ages more rapidly than unexposed skin, one of the best ways to slow the aging process is to avoid exposure by wearing protective clothing and by using sunblock whenever possible. ■

the excess heat must be removed from the body. The skin helps to regulate body temperature in two ways: by dilation and constriction of blood vessels, and by activity or inactivity of the sweat glands. Both of these mechanisms are examples of negative feedback in maintaining homeostasis. The adipose tissue in the subcutaneous layer also helps by acting as an insulator.

When there is excess heat in the body, and body temperature rises above normal, the small arteries in the dermis dilate to increase blood flow through the skin. This brings the heat from the deeper tissues to the surface so that it can escape into the surrounding air. Sweat glands become active in response to increased body temperature. Moisture, in the form of sweat, accumulates on the surface of the skin and then evaporates to provide cooling.

If body temperature falls below normal, the sweat glands are inactive and the blood vessels in the skin constrict to reduce blood flow. This constriction of the blood vessels reduces the amount of heat that is transferred from the deeper tissues to the surface. However, if the skin becomes too cold, below 15°C (59°F), cutaneous blood vessels will begin to dilate in order to bring warm blood to the region. This process ensures that the tissues are not damaged by the cold.

Synthesis of Vitamin D

Vitamin D is required for calcium and phosphorus absorption in the small intestine. The calcium and phosphorus are essential for normal bone metabolism and muscle function. Skin cells contain a precursor molecule that is converted to vitamin D when the precursor is exposed to ultraviolet rays in sunlight. It takes only a small amount of ultraviolet light to stimulate vitamin D production, so this should not be used as an excuse to expose the skin to sun unnecessarily and to risk the damage that may result.

↻ TERMINOLOGY REVIEW

Arrector pili Muscle associated with hair follicles.

Ceruminous gland A gland in the ear canal that produces cerumen or ear wax.

Dermis Inner layer of the skin that contains the blood vessels, nerves, glands, and hair follicles; also called *stratum corium.*

Epidermis Outermost layer of the skin.

Keratinization Process by which the cells of the epidermis become filled with keratin and move to the surface, where they are sloughed off.

Melanin A dark brown or black pigment found in parts of the body, especially skin and hair.

Sebaceous gland An oil gland of the skin that produces sebum or body oil.

Subcutaneous layer Below the skin; a sheet of areolar connective tissue and adipose tissue beneath the dermis of the skin; also called *hypodermis* or *superficial fascia.*

Sudoriferous gland A gland in the skin that produces perspiration; also called *sweat gland.*

ON THE WEB

For Information on the Integumentary System:

Merck Manual—Dermatologic Disorders: www.merck. com/mmpe *(Click on "Dermatologic Disorders")*

Loyola University Medication Education Network: Dermatology Atlas: www.meddean.luc.edu/lumen/ MedEd/medicine/dermatology/melton/title.htm

University of Delaware—Integumentary System: www. udel.edu/biology/Wags/histopage/colorpage/cin/cin. htm

Skin Cancer Risk Analyzer: www.telemedicine.org/mela-noma.htm

British Medical Journal: Dermatology: www.bmj.com/ cgi/collection/dermatology

 PREPARE FOR CERTIFICATION   Visit the Evolve site at http://evolve.elsevier.com/Bonewit/today/ to actively Prepare for your Certification.

 Check out the Companion CD bound with the book to access additional interactive activities.

7

Skeletal System

CAAHEP COMPETENCIES

Content Competencies
Anatomy and Physiology
- Anatomy and physiology of all body systems

- Common pathology/diseases
- Diagnostic/treatment modalities

ABHES COMPETENCIES

Content Competencies
Anatomy and Physiology
- Anatomy and physiology

- Study of diseases and etiology
- All body systems
- Diagnostic/treatment modalities

amphiarthrosis (am-fee-ahr-THROH-sis)
diaphysis (dye-AF-ih-sis)
diarthrosis (dye-ahr-THROH-sis)
epiphyseal plate (ep-ih-FIZ-ee-al PLATE)
epiphysis (ee-PIF-ih-sis)

osteoblast (AH-stee-oh-blast)
osteoclast (AH-stee-oh-clast)
osteocyte (AH-stee-oh-syte)
osteon (OH-stee-ahn)
synarthrosis (sin-ahr-THROH-sis)

Introduction to the Skeletal System

The skeletal system consists of the bones and the cartilage, ligaments, and tendons associated with the bones. It accounts for about 20% of the body weight. Bones are rigid structures that form the framework for the body. People often think of bones as dead, dry, inert pipes and plates because that is how they are seen in the laboratory. In reality, the living bones in our bodies contain active tissues that consume nutrients, require a blood supply, use oxygen and discharge waste products in metabolism, and change shape or remodel in response to variations in mechanical stress. The skeletal system is strong but lightweight. It is well adapted for the functions it must perform. It is a masterpiece of design.

OVERVIEW OF THE SKELETAL SYSTEM

Functions of the Skeletal System

The skeletal system gives form and shape to the body. Without the skeletal components, we would appear as big "blobs" inefficiently "oozing" around on the ground. Besides contributing to shape and form, our bones perform several other functions and play an important role in homeostasis.

Support

Bones provide a rigid framework that supports the soft organs of the body. Bones support the body against the pull of gravity, and the large bones of the lower limbs support the trunk when standing.

Protection

The skeleton protects the soft body parts. The fused bones of the cranium surround the brain to make it less vulnerable to injury. The vertebrae surround and protect the spinal cord. The bones of the rib cage help protect the heart and lungs in the thorax.

Movement

Bones provide sites for muscle attachment. Bones and muscles work together as simple mechanical lever systems to produce body movement. A mechanical lever system has four components: (1) a rigid bar, (2) a pivot or fulcrum, (3) an object or weight that is moved, and (4) a force that sup-

plies the mechanical energy for the movement. In the body, bones are the rigid bars, the joints between the bones are the pivots, the body or a part of it is the weight that is moved, and the muscles supply the force.

Storage

The intercellular matrix of bone contains large amounts of calcium salts, the most important being calcium phosphate. Calcium is necessary for vital metabolic processes. When blood calcium levels decrease below normal, calcium is released from the bones so that there will be an adequate supply for metabolic needs. When blood calcium levels are increased, the excess calcium is stored in the bone matrix. Storage and release are dynamic processes that go on almost continually.

Bone tissue contains lesser amounts of other inorganic ions, such as sodium, magnesium, potassium, and carbonate. Fat is stored in the yellow bone marrow.

Blood Cell Formation

Blood cell formation, called **hematopoiesis** (hee-mat-oh-poy-EE-sis), takes place mostly in the red marrow of bones. Red marrow is found in the cavities of most bones in an infant. With age, it is largely replaced by yellow marrow for fat storage. In the adult, red marrow is limited to the spongy bone in the skull, ribs, sternum, clavicles, vertebrae, and pelvis. Red marrow functions in the formation of red blood cells, white blood cells, and blood platelets.

Structure of Bone Tissue

There are two types of bone tissue: compact and spongy. As the names imply, the two types differ in density, or how tightly the tissue is packed together. Three types of cells contribute to bone homeostasis. Osteoblasts are bone-forming cells, osteoclasts resorb or break down bone, and osteocytes are mature bone cells. An equilibrium between osteoblasts and osteoclasts maintains bone tissue.

Compact Bone

The microscopic unit of compact bone is known as the **osteon** (haversian system) and was described in Chapter 5 The osteon consists of a central canal called the *osteonic* (haversian) *canal* that is surrounded by concentric rings (lamellae) of hard, calcified matrix. Between the rings of matrix, the bone cells (osteocytes) are located in spaces called *lacunae.* Small channels (canaliculi) radiate from the lacunae

Highlight on the Skeletal System

OSTEOPOROSIS: Osteoporosis is a bone disorder caused by decreased osteoblast activity. It is characterized by loss of the organic matrix, collagenous fibers, and minerals in the bone tissue. People with osteoporosis are susceptible to deformities of the vertebral column and fractures because the bones are too weak to support the weight of the body. Osteoporosis occurs most frequently in postmenopausal Caucasian women. Factors that influence its occurrence are aging, malnutrition, lack of exercise, and hormone imbalance. Supplemental estrogen after menopause may be of benefit, and exercise is always important in maintaining bone strength.

EPIPHYSEAL PLATE: The epiphyseal plates of specific long bones ossify at predictable times. Radiologists frequently can determine a young person's age by examining the epiphyseal plates to see whether they have ossified. A difference between bone age and chronologic age may indicate some type of metabolic dysfunction.

MASTOIDITIS: The mastoid air cells are separated from the cranial cavity by only a thin partition of bone. A middle ear infection that spreads to the mastoid air cells (mastoiditis) is serious because there is danger that the infection will spread from the air cells to the membranes around the brain.

SINUS PROBLEMS: The bones with paranasal sinuses are the frontal, sphenoid, ethmoid, and the two maxillae. The sinuses are lined with mucous membranes that are continuous with the nasal cavity. Allergies and infections cause inflammation of the membranes, which results in sinusitis. The swollen membranes may reduce drainage from the sinuses so that pressure within the cavities increases, resulting in sinus headaches.

SOFT SPOTS: The bones in the skull of a newborn are not completely joined together but are separated by fibrous membranes. The six large areas of membranes are called **fontanels,** or soft spots. The anterior fontanel is on the top of the head, at the junction of the frontal and parietal bones. The posterior fontanel is at the junction of the occipital and parietal bones. On each side of the head there is a mastoid (posterolateral) fontanel near the mastoid region of the temporal bone and a sphenoid (anterolateral) fontanel just superior to the sphenoid bone.

ABNORMAL SPINAL CURVATURES: An abnormally exaggerated lumbar curvature is called *lordosis,* or swayback. This is often seen in pregnant women as they adjust to their changing center of gravity. An increased roundness of the thoracic curvature is kyphosis, or hunchback. This is frequently seen in elderly people. Abnormal side-to-side curvature is scoliosis. Abnormal curvatures may interfere with breathing and other vital functions.

YES AND NO: The atlas holds up the skull and permits you to nod "yes." The axis allows you to rotate your head from side to side to indicate "no."

MARROW BIOPSY: The sternum is frequently used for a red marrow biopsy because it is accessible. The sample for biopsy is obtained by performing a sternal puncture, in which a large needle is inserted into the sternum to remove a sample of red bone marrow.

FRACTURED CLAVICLE: The clavicle is the most frequently fractured bone in the body because it transmits forces from the arm to the trunk. The force from falling on the shoulder or outstretched arm is often sufficient to fracture the clavicle.

TENNIS ELBOW: Tennis elbow is an inflammation of the tissues surrounding the lateral epicondyle of the humerus. Six muscles that control movement of the hand attach in this region, and repeated contraction of these muscles irritates the attachments. The medical term for tennis elbow is lateral epicondylitis.

PELVIC OUTLET AND CHILDBIRTH: The female pelvis is shaped to accommodate childbearing. Because the fetus must pass through the pelvic outlet, the physician carefully measures this opening to make sure there is enough room. The distance between the two ischial spines is a good indication of the size of the pelvic outlet. If the opening is too small, a cesarean delivery is indicated.

BROKEN HIP: Elderly people, particularly those with osteoporosis, are susceptible to "breaking a hip." The femur is a weight-bearing bone, and when it is weakened, it cannot support the weight of the body and the neck of the femur fractures under the stress. Instead of saying, "Grandma fell and broke her hip," often it is more appropriate to say, "Grandma broke her hip, then fell."

BUNION: Poorly fitted shoes may compress the toes so that there is a lateral deviation of the big toe toward the second toe. When this occurs, a bursa and callus form at the joint between the first metatarsal and proximal phalanx. This creates a bunion.

GOUT: Gout was commonly known as the disease of the kings because it was believed to be caused by a rich diet and fine wines. Gout is an equal-opportunity disease, however, and occurs across the entire population. A rich diet and fine wines may contribute to the disease, but they are not the definitive cause. Gout is caused by the excessive accumulation of uric acid that forms needle-like crystals within the joint, producing pain and inflammation. The great toe is the most commonly affected joint. The disorder is diagnosed by aspirating joint fluid and observing the crystals under the microscope. Although there is no cure for gout, it can be effectively controlled with antiinflammatory drugs and dietary measures.

KNEE PROBLEMS: The term *torn cartilage* refers to a damaged meniscus, usually the medial, in the knee. Frequently this can be repaired with relatively minor arthroscopic surgery. A torn ligament in the knee usually involves one of the cruciate ligaments. The surgical procedure to repair this damage is quite involved, and recovery of function may require months of rehabilitative therapy. ■

to the osteonic (haversian) canal to provide passageways through the hard matrix. In compact bone the haversian systems are packed tightly together to form what appears to be a solid mass. The osteonic canals contain blood vessels that are parallel to the long axis of the bone. These blood vessels interconnect, by way of perforating (Volkmann's) canals, with vessels on the surface of the bone. The microscopic structure of compact bone is illustrated in Figure 7-1.

Spongy (Cancellous) Bone

Spongy (cancellous) bone is lighter and less dense than compact bone (see Figure 7-1). Spongy bone consists of plates and bars of bone adjacent to small, irregular cavities that contain red bone marrow. The plates of bone are called **trabeculae** (trah-BEK-yoo-lee). The canaliculi, instead of connecting to a central haversian canal, connect to the adjacent cavities to receive their blood supply. It may appear that the trabeculae are arranged in a haphazard manner, but they are organized to provide maximum strength in the same way that braces are used to support a building. The trabeculae of spongy bone follow the lines of stress and can realign if the direction of stress changes.

Classification of Bones

Bones come in a variety of sizes and shapes. Bones that are longer than they are wide are called **long bones.** They consist of a long shaft with two bulky ends or extremities. They are primarily compact bone but may have a large amount of spongy bone at the ends. Examples of long bones are those in the thigh, leg, arm, and forearm.

Short bones are roughly cube shaped with vertical and horizontal dimensions approximately equal. They consist primarily of spongy bone, which is covered by a thin layer of compact bone. Examples of short bones include the bones of the wrist and ankle.

Flat bones are thin, flattened, and often curved. They are usually arranged similar to a sandwich with a middle layer of spongy bone called the **diploë** (DIP-loh-ee). The diploë is covered on each side by a layer of compact bone; these layers are called the **inner** and **outer tables.** Most of the bones of the cranium are flat bones.

Bones that are not in any of the previously mentioned three categories are classified as **irregular bones.** They are primarily spongy bone that is covered with a thin layer of compact bone. The vertebrae and some of the bones in the skull are irregular bones.

General Features of a Long Bone

Most long bones have the same general features, which are illustrated in Figure 7-2.

Diaphysis   The shaft of a long bone is called the *diaphysis* (dye-AF-ih-sis). It is formed from relatively thick compact bone that surrounds a hollow space called the *medullary* (MED-yoo-lair-ee) *cavity.*

Medullary cavity   In adults the medullary cavity contains yellow bone marrow, so it is sometimes called the *yellow marrow cavity.*

Epiphysis   At each end of the diaphysis, there is an expanded portion called the *epiphysis* (ee-PIF-ih-sis). The epiphysis is spongy bone covered by a thin layer of compact bone. The end of the epiphysis, where it meets another bone, is covered by hyaline cartilage, called the *articular cartilage.* This provides smooth surfaces for movement in the joints. In growing bones, there is an **epiphyseal** (ep-ih-FIZ-ee-al) **plate** of hyaline cartilage between the diaphysis and epiphysis. Bones grow in

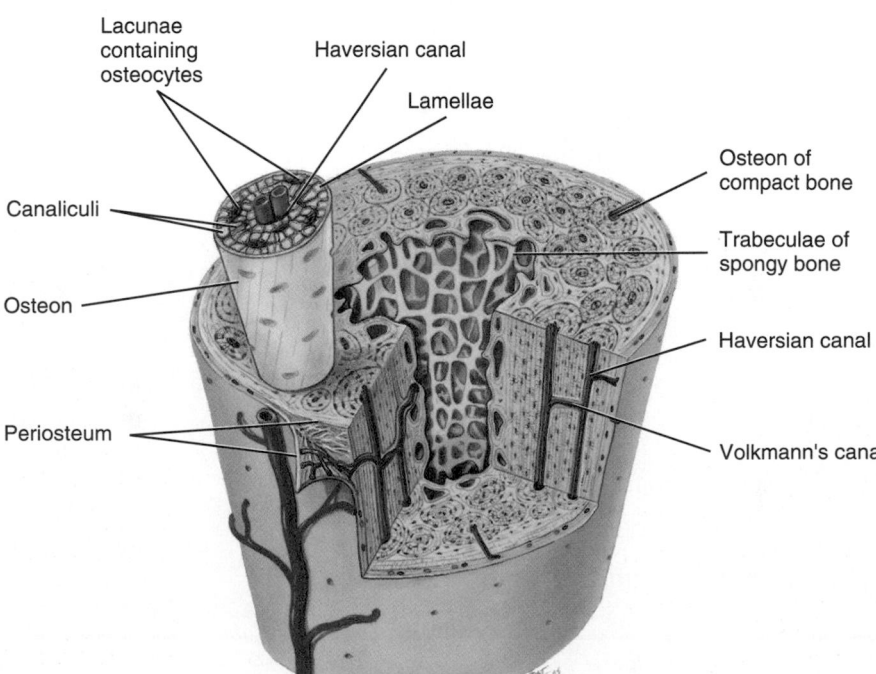

Figure 7-1. Structure of compact and spongy bone. (From Applegate E: *The anatomy and physiology learning system,* ed 3, St. Louis, 2006, Saunders.)

Lacunae containing osteocytes

Haversian canal

Lamellae

Canaliculi

Osteon of compact bone

Osteon

Trabeculae of spongy bone

Haversian canal

Periosteum

Volkmann's canal

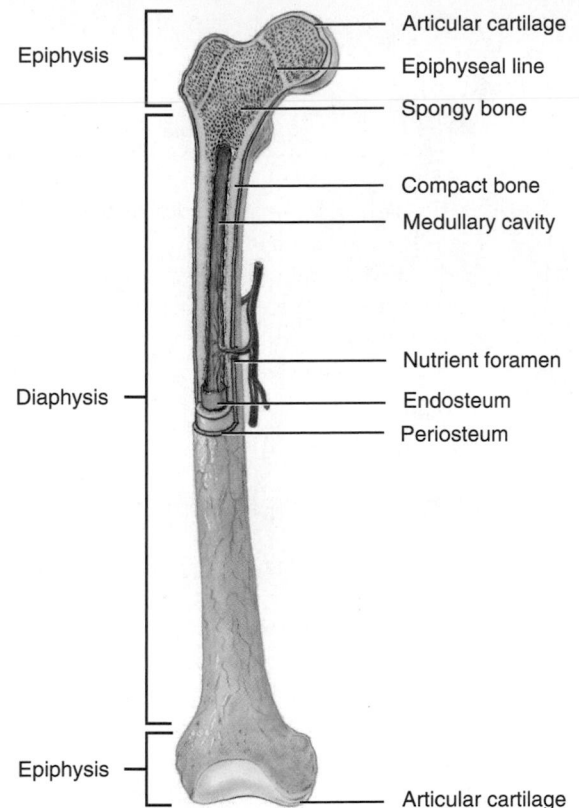

Epiphysis

Diaphysis

Epiphysis

- Articular cartilage
- Epiphyseal line
- Spongy bone
- Compact bone
- Medullary cavity
- Nutrient foramen
- Endosteum
- Periosteum
- Articular cartilage

Figure 7-2. General features of long bones. (From Applegate E: *The anatomy and physiology learning system,* ed 3, St. Louis, 2006, Saunders.)

length at the epiphyseal plate. Growth ceases when the cartilaginous epiphyseal plate is replaced by a bony epiphyseal line.

Periosteum   Except in the region of the articular cartilage, the outer surface of long bones is covered by a tough, fibrous connective tissue called the *periosteum.* The periosteum is richly supplied with nerve fibers, lymphatic vessels, blood vessels, and osteoblasts.

Nutrient foramina   Blood vessels enter the diaphysis of the bone through small openings called *nutrient foramina.*

Endosteum   The surface of the medullary cavity is lined with a thinner connective tissue membrane, the endosteum, which contains osteoclasts.

In addition to the general features that are present in most long bones, all bones have surface markings and characteristics that make a specific bone unique. Bones have holes, depressions, smooth facets, lines, projections, and other markings. These usually represent passageways for vessels and nerves, points of articulation with other bones, or points of attachment for tendons and ligaments.

Bone Development and Growth

The terms **osteogenesis** and **ossification** are often used synonymously to indicate the process of bone formation. Parts of the skeleton form during the first few weeks after conception. By the end of the eighth week after conception,

the skeletal pattern is formed in cartilage and connective tissue membranes and ossification begins. Bone development continues throughout adulthood. Even after adult stature is attained, bone development continues for repair of fractures and for remodeling to meet changing lifestyles. Three types of cells are involved in the development, growth, and remodeling of bones. **Osteoblasts** are bone-forming cells; **osteocytes** are mature bone cells; and **osteoclasts** break down and reabsorb bone.

Bone Growth in Length

Bones grow in length at the epiphyseal plate located between the diaphysis and epiphysis of a long bone. The hyaline cartilage in the region of the epiphyseal plate next to the epiphysis continues to grow by mitosis. The chondrocytes in the region next to the diaphysis age and degenerate. Osteoblasts move in and ossify the matrix to form bone. This process continues throughout childhood and adolescence until the cartilage growth slows and finally stops. When cartilage growth ceases, usually in the early 20s, the epiphyseal plate completely ossifies so that only a thin **epiphyseal line** remains and the bones can no longer grow in length. Bone growth is under the influence of growth hormone from the anterior pituitary gland and sex hormones from the ovaries and testes.

Even though bones stop growing in length in early adulthood, they can continue to increase in thickness or diameter throughout life in response to stress from increased muscle activity or to weight gain. The increase in diameter is called **appositional** (ap-poh-ZISH-un-al) **growth.** Osteoblasts in the periosteum form compact bone around the external bone surface. At the same time, osteoclasts in the endosteum break down bone on the internal bone surface, around the medullary cavity. These two processes together increase the diameter of the bone and, at the same time, keep the bone from becoming excessively heavy and bulky.

Divisions of the Skeleton

The typical adult human skeleton consists of 206 named bones. For convenience, the bones of the skeleton are grouped in two divisions, as illustrated in Figure 7-3. The 80 bones of the **axial skeleton** form the vertical axis of the body. They include the bones of the head, vertebral column, ribs, and breastbone or sternum. The **appendicular skeleton** consists of 126 bones and includes the free appendages and their attachments to the axial skeleton. The free appendages are the upper and lower extremities, or limbs, and their attachments are called *girdles.*

BONES OF THE AXIAL SKELETON

The axial skeleton, with 80 bones, is divided into the skull, hyoid, vertebral column, and rib cage.

Skull

The skull has 28 bones, as illustrated in Figures 7-4 through 7-6. Eight of these form the **cranium,** which houses the

Figure 7-3. Divisions of the skeleton with major bones identified. Yellow = axial skeleton. Blue = appendicular skeleton. (From Applegate E: *The anatomy and physiology learning system,* ed 3, St. Louis, 2006, Saunders.)

Highlight on Aging and the Skeletal System

The major age-related change in the skeletal system is the loss of calcium from the bones. Calcium loss occurs in both men and women, but it starts at an earlier age and is more severe in women. The exact reasons for the loss are unknown and possibly involve a combination of several factors. These may include an imbalance between osteoblast and osteoclast activity, imbalance between calcitonin and parathormone levels, reduced absorption of calcium and/or vitamin D from the digestive tract, poor diet, and lack of exercise. Whatever the cause, there is no sure way of preventing the loss, but adequate calcium and vitamin D in the diet may help reduce the effects.

Another change with age is a decrease in the rate of collagen synthesis. This means that the bones have less strength and are more brittle. Bones fracture more readily in elderly individuals and the healing process may be slow or incomplete. Tendons and ligaments become less flexible because of the changes in collagen.

The articular cartilage at the ends of bones tends to become thinner and deteriorates with age. This causes joint disorders that are commonly found in older individuals. People also appear to get shorter as they get older. This is partially due to loss of bone mass and partially due to compression of the intervertebral discs.

Age-related changes in the skeletal system cannot be prevented. An active and healthy lifestyle with appropriate exercise and an adequate diet help reduce the effect of the changes in the skeletal system. ■

brain. The anterior aspect of the skull, the face, consists of 14 bones. The remaining six bones are the auditory ossicles, tiny bones in the middle ear cavity. With the exception of the lower jaw, or mandible, and the auditory ossicles, the bones in the skull are tightly interlocked along irregular lines called **sutures.** Some of the bones in the skull contain **sinuses,** which are air-filled cavities lined with mucous membranes. The sinuses help to reduce the weight of the skull. The paranasal sinuses are arranged around the nasal cavity and drain into it.

Cranium

The eight bones of the cranium are interlocked to enclose the brain (see Figures 7-4 through 7-6).

Frontal Bone

The frontal bone forms the anterior portion of the skull above the eyes (forehead), a portion of the nose, and the superior portion of the orbit (eye socket). On either side of the midline, just above the eyes, there is a cavity in the frontal bone. These are the paranasal **frontal sinuses.**

Parietal Bones

The two parietal (pah-RYE-eh-tal) bones form most of the superolateral aspect of the skull. They are joined to each other in the midline by the **sagittal suture** and to the frontal bone by the **coronal suture.**

Occipital Bone

The single occipital (ahk-SIP-ih-tal) bone forms most of the dorsal part of the skull and the base of the cranium. It is joined to the parietal bones by the **lambdoid** (lamm-DOYD) **suture.** The **foramen magnum** is a large opening on the lower surface of the occipital bone. The spinal cord passes through this opening. **Occipital condyles** are rounded processes on each side of the foramen magnum. They articulate with the first cervical vertebra.

Temporal Bones

The two temporal bones, one on each side of the head, form parts of the sides and base of the cranium. On each side, a temporal bone meets the parietal bone at the **squamous** (SKWAY-mus) **suture.** Near the inferior margin of the temporal bone, there is an opening, the **external auditory meatus,** which is a canal that leads to the middle ear. Just anterior to the external auditory meatus, there is a shallow depression, the **mandibular** (man-DIB-yoo-lar) **fossa,** that articulates with the mandible. Posterior and inferior to each external auditory meatus, there is a rough protuberance, the **mastoid process.** The mastoid process contains air cells that drain into the middle ear cavity. The **styloid process** is a long, pointed projection inferior to the external auditory meatus. A **zygomatic** (zye-goh-MAT-ik) **process** projects anteriorly from the temporal bone and helps form the prominence of the cheek.

Sphenoid Bone

The sphenoid (SFEE-noyd) bone is an irregularly shaped bone that spans the entire width of the cranial floor. It is wedged between other bones in the anterior portion of the cranium. This bone helps form the sides of the skull, the base of the cranium, and the lateral and inferior

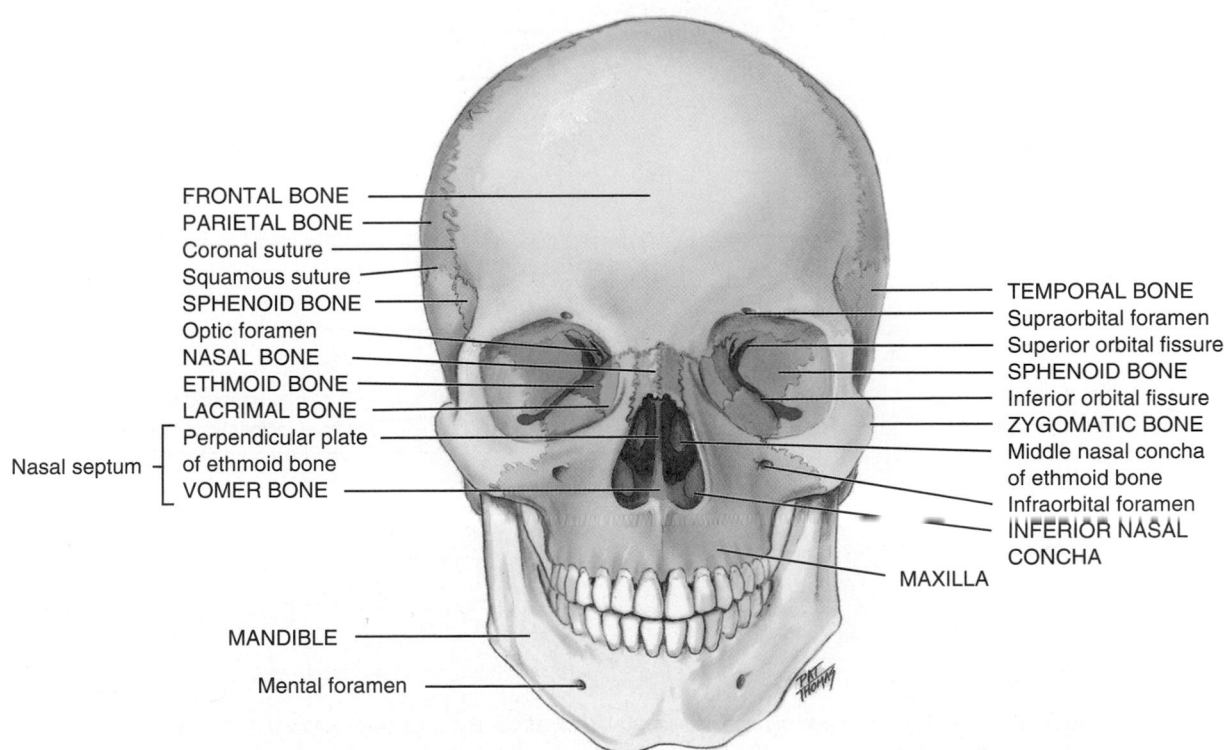

FRONTAL BONE
PARIETAL BONE
Coronal suture
Squamous suture
SPHENOID BONE
Optic foramen
NASAL BONE
ETHMOID BONE
LACRIMAL BONE
Perpendicular plate of ethmoid bone
VOMER BONE
Nasal septum

TEMPORAL BONE
Supraorbital foramen
Superior orbital fissure
SPHENOID BONE
Inferior orbital fissure
ZYGOMATIC BONE
Middle nasal concha of ethmoid bone
Infraorbital foramen
INFERIOR NASAL CONCHA
MAXILLA
MANDIBLE
Mental foramen

Figure 7-4. Skull, anterior view. (From Applegate E: *The anatomy and physiology learning system,* ed 3, St. Louis, 2006, Saunders.)

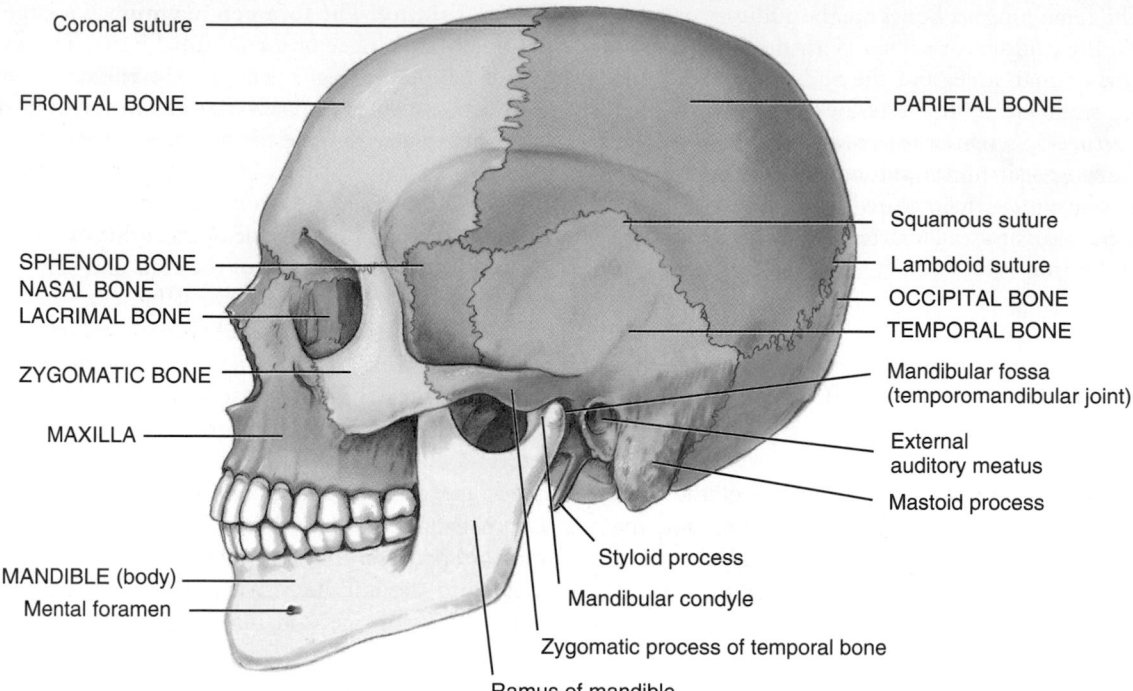

Coronal suture

FRONTAL BONE

PARIETAL BONE

Squamous suture

SPHENOID BONE
NASAL BONE
LACRIMAL BONE

Lambdoid suture
OCCIPITAL BONE
TEMPORAL BONE

ZYGOMATIC BONE

Mandibular fossa
(temporomandibular joint)

MAXILLA

External
auditory meatus

Mastoid process

MANDIBLE (body)
Mental foramen

Styloid process

Mandibular condyle

Zygomatic process of temporal bone

Ramus of mandible

Figure 7-5. Skull, lateral view. (From Applegate E: *The anatomy and physiology learning system*, ed 3, St. Louis, 2006, Saunders.)

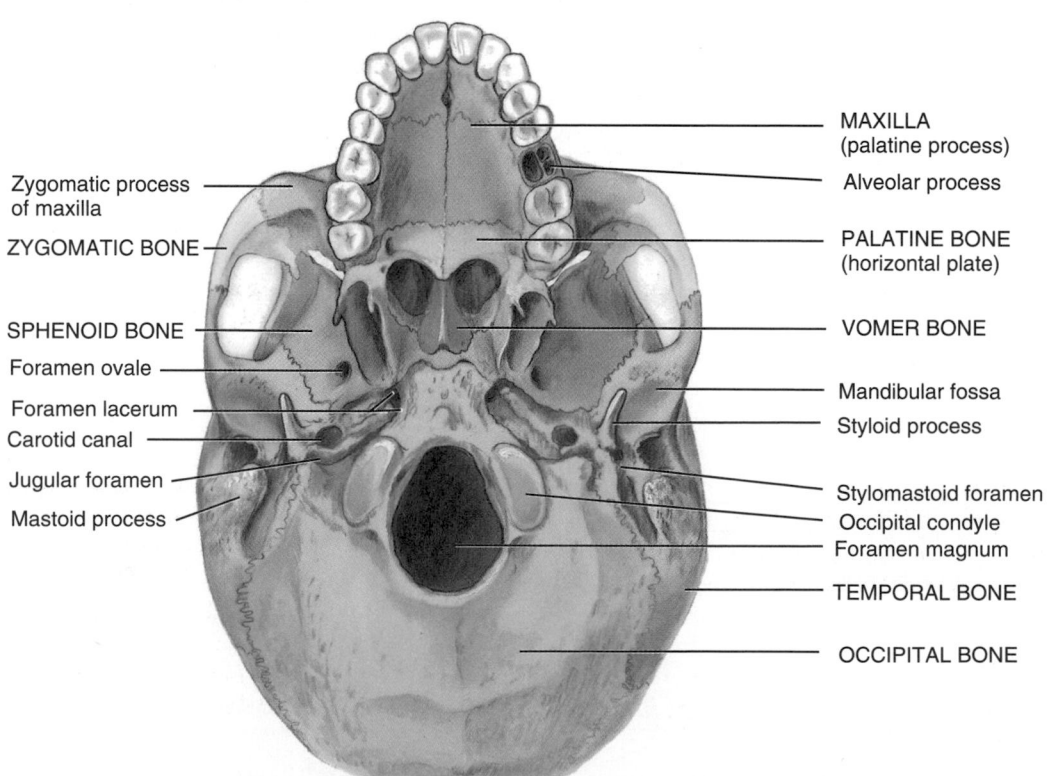

Zygomatic process
of maxilla

ZYGOMATIC BONE

MAXILLA
(palatine process)

Alveolar process

PALATINE BONE
(horizontal plate)

SPHENOID BONE
Foramen ovale
Foramen lacerum
Carotid canal
Jugular foramen
Mastoid process

VOMER BONE

Mandibular fossa
Styloid process

Stylomastoid foramen
Occipital condyle
Foramen magnum

TEMPORAL BONE

OCCIPITAL BONE

Figure 7-6. Skull, inferior view. (From Applegate E: *The anatomy and physiology learning system,* ed 3, St. Louis, 2006, Saunders.)

portions of each orbit. Within the cranial cavity, there is a saddle-shaped central portion, called the **sella turcica** (SELL-ah TUR-sih-kah), with a depression for the pituitary gland. Anterior to the sella turcica are two openings, one on each side, called the **optic foramina,** for the passage of the optic nerve. The **greater wings** extend laterally from the region of the sella turcica and are the portions of the sphenoid seen in the orbits and external wall of the skull. The sphenoid bone also contains paranasal **sphenoid sinuses.**

Ethmoid Bone

The ethmoid (ETH-moyd) bone is located anterior to the sphenoid bone and forms most of the bony area between the nasal cavity and the orbits. Delicate, scroll-like projections, called the **superior and middle nasal conchae** (KONG-kee) or **turbinates,** form ledges along the lateral walls of the nasal cavity. The conchae are lined with mucous membranes to warm and moisten inhaled air. The ethmoid bone contains many small, paranasal **ethmoidal sinuses.**

Facial Bones

The facial skeleton consists of 14 bones. Thirteen of these are interlocked, and there is one movable mandible, the lower jawbone. These bones form the basic framework and shape of the face. They also provide attachments for the muscles that control facial expression and move the jaw for chewing. All facial bones except the vomer and mandible are paired. Facial bones are illustrated in Figures 7-4 through 7-6.

Maxillary Bones

The maxillary bones, or **maxillae** (maks-ILL-ee), form the upper jaw. Additionally, they form the lateral walls of the nose, the floor of the orbits, and the anterior part of the roof of the mouth. The portion in the hard palate, or roof of the mouth, is the **palatine process.** The inferior border of each maxilla projects downward to form the **alveolar** (al-VEE-oh-lar) **process,** which contains the teeth. Each maxilla has a large paranasal **maxillary sinus.** These are the largest of all the paranasal sinuses.

Palatine Bones

The palatine (PAL-ah-tyne) bones are behind, or posterior to, the maxillae. Each one is roughly L-shaped. The **horizontal plates** form the posterior portion of the hard palate. The vertical portions help form the lateral walls of the nasal cavity.

Nasal Bones

The two nasal bones are small rectangular bones that form the bridge of the nose.

Lacrimal Bones

The small, thin lacrimal (LACK-rih-mal) bones are located in the medial walls of the orbits, between the ethmoid bone and the maxilla. Each one has a small **lacrimal groove** that is a pathway for a tube that carries tears from the eyes to the nasal cavity.

Zygomatic Bones

The zygomatic (zye-goh-MAT-ik) bones, also called **malar** bones, form the prominences of the cheeks and a portion of the lateral walls of the orbits. Each one has a **temporal process** that projects toward the zygomatic process of the temporal bone to form the **zygomatic arch.**

Inferior Nasal Conchae

The inferior nasal conchae (KONG-kee) are thin, curved bones that are attached to the lateral walls of the nasal cavity. They project into the nasal cavity just below the middle conchae of the ethmoid bone.

Vomer

The thin, flat vomer (VOH-mer) is in the inferior portion of the midline in the nasal cavity. It joins with the perpendicular plate of the ethmoid bone to form the **nasal septum.**

Mandible

The mandible (MAN-dih-bul) is the lower jaw. It has a horseshoe-shaped **body** that forms the chin and a flat portion, the **ramus,** that projects upward at each end. On the superior portion of the ramus, there is a knoblike process, the **mandibular condyle,** that fits into the mandibular fossa of the temporal bone to form the **temporomandibular** (tem-por-oh-man-DIB-yoo-lar) joint. The superior border of the mandible projects upward to form the **alveolar process** that contains the teeth.

Auditory Ossicles

Three tiny bones form a chain in each middle ear cavity in the temporal bone. These are the **malleus, incus,** and **stapes.** These bones transmit sound waves from the tympanic membrane, or eardrum, to the inner ear where the sound receptors are located.

Hyoid Bone

The hyoid bone is not really part of the skull, so it is listed separately. It is a U-shaped bone in the neck, between the mandible and the larynx, or voice box. Figure 7-7 illustrates the position and shape of the hyoid bone. It is unique because it is the only bone in the body that does not articulate directly with another bone. Instead, it is suspended under the mandible and anchored by ligaments to the styloid processes of the temporal bones. It functions as a base for the tongue and as an attachment for several muscles associated with swallowing.

Vertebral Column

The vertebral column extends from the skull to the pelvis and contains 26 bones called **vertebrae** (singular, vertebra). The bones are separated by pads of fibrocartilage called **intervertebral discs.** The discs act as shock absorbers and

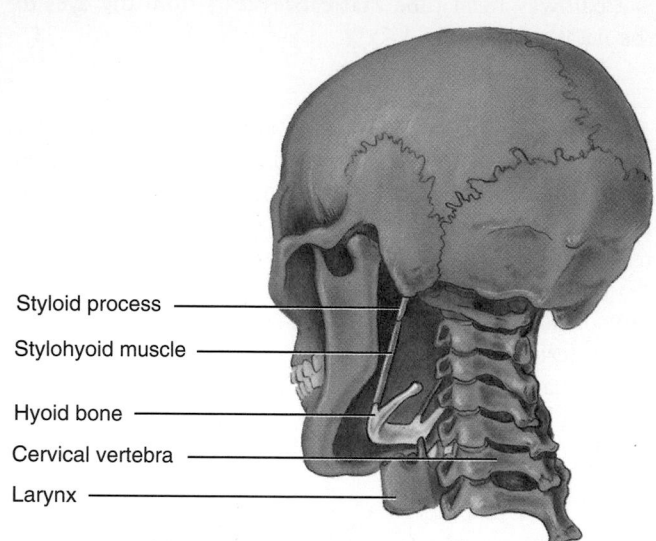

Figure 7-7. Hyoid bone. (From Applegate E: *The anatomy and physiology learning system,* ed 3, St. Louis, 2006, Saunders.)

allow the column to bend. Normally there are four curvatures, illustrated in Figure 7-8, that increase the strength and resilience of the column. They are named according to the region in which they are located. The **thoracic** and **sacral curvatures** are concave anteriorly and are present at birth. The **cervical curvature** develops when an infant begins to hold his or her head erect. The **lumbar curvature** develops when an infant begins to stand and walk. Both the cervical and lumbar curvatures are convex anteriorly.

General Structure of Vertebrae

All vertebrae have a common structural pattern, illustrated in Figure 7-9, although there are variations among them. The thick anterior, weight-bearing portion is the **body** or **centrum.** The posterior curved portion is the **vertebral arch.** The vertebral arch and body surround a central large opening, the **vertebral foramen.** When all the vertebrae are stacked together in a column, the vertebral foramina make a canal that contains the spinal cord. **Transverse processes** project laterally from the vertebral arch, and in the posterior midline there is a **spinous process.** These processes are places for muscle attachment. The spinous processes can be felt as bony projections along the midline of the back.

Composition of the Vertebral Column

The seven **cervical vertebrae** are designated C1 through C7. The 12 **thoracic vertebrae** are designated T1 through T12. Five **lumbar vertebrae,** designated L1 through L5, make up the part of the vertebral column in the small of the back. The lumbar vertebrae have large, heavy bodies because they support most of the body weight and have many back muscles attached to them.

The **sacrum** is a triangular bone just below the lumbar vertebrae. In the child there are five separate bones, but these fuse to form a single bone in the adult. The sacrum

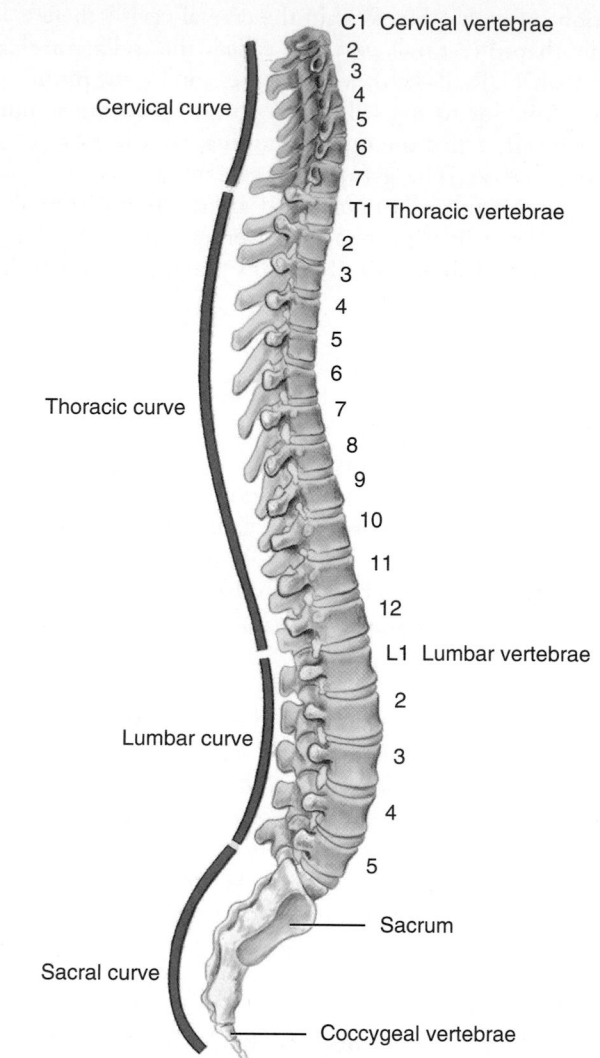

Figure 7-8. Curvatures of the vertebral column. (From Applegate E: *The anatomy and physiology learning system,* ed 3, St. Louis, 2006, Saunders.)

Figure 7-9. General features of vertebrae, viewed from above. (From Applegate E: *The anatomy and physiology learning system,* ed 3, St. Louis, 2006, Saunders.)

articulates with the pelvic girdle laterally, at the **sacroiliac** (say-kro-ILL-ee-ak) **joint,** and forms the posterior wall of the pelvic cavity.

The **coccyx** (KOK-siks), or tailbone, is the last part of the vertebral column (see Figure 7-8). A child has four (the number varies from three to five) separate small bones, but these fuse to form a single bone in the adult.

Thoracic Cage

The thoracic cage, or bony thorax, protects the heart, lungs, and great vessels. It also supports the bones of the shoulder girdle and plays a role in breathing. The components of the thoracic cage are the thoracic vertebrae dorsally, the ribs laterally, and the sternum and costal cartilage anteriorly.

Sternum

The **sternum,** or breastbone, is in the anterior midline (Figure 7-10). It consists of three parts: the superior, triangular **manubrium** (mah-NOO-bree-um); the middle, slender **body;** and the inferior, small **xiphoid** (ZYE-foyd) **process.** The xiphoid process, for muscle attachment, is composed of hyaline cartilage in the child, but it ossifies in the adult. An important anatomic landmark, the **jugular (suprasternal) notch** is an easily palpable, central indentation in the superior margin of the manubrium. The manubrium articulates with the clavicles and the first two pairs of ribs. The manubrium and body of the sternum meet at a slight angle that can be felt as a horizontal ridge below the jugular notch. This is the **sternal angle,** and it is a convenient way to locate the second rib (see Figure 7-10). The body of the sternum has notches along the sides where it attaches to the cartilage of the third through seventh ribs.

Ribs

Twelve pairs of **ribs,** illustrated in Figure 7-10, form the curved, lateral margins of the thoracic cage. One pair is attached to each of the 12 thoracic vertebrae. The upper seven pairs of ribs are called **true,** or **vertebrosternal** (ver-TEE-broh-stir-nal), **ribs** because they attach to the sternum directly by their individual **costal cartilage.** The lower five pairs of ribs are called **false ribs** because their costal cartilage does not reach the sternum directly. The first three pairs of false ribs reach the sternum indirectly by joining with the cartilage of the ribs above. These are called **vertebrochondral** (ver-TEE-broh-kahn-dral) **ribs.** The bottom two rib pairs have no anterior attachment and are called **vertebral ribs,** or **floating ribs.**

BONES OF THE APPENDICULAR SKELETON

The 126 bones of the appendicular skeleton are suspended from two yokes or girdles that are anchored to the axial skeleton. They are additions or appendages to the axis of the body. The appendicular skeleton is designed for movement. If a portion is immobilized for a period of time, life without appendicular movement can be awkward.

Pectoral Girdle

Each half of the **pectoral girdle,** or **shoulder girdle,** consists of two bones: an anterior **clavicle** (KLAV-ih-kul) and a posterior **scapula** (SKAP-yoo-lah). The term *girdle* implies something that encircles or makes a complete ring. The pectoral girdle, however, is an incomplete ring. Anteriorly, the bones are separated by the sternum. Posteriorly, there is a gap between the two scapulae because they do not articulate with each other or with the vertebral column. The bones of the pectoral girdle, illustrated in Figure 7-11, form the connection between the upper extremities and the axial skeleton. The clavicles and scapulae, with their associated muscles, also form the shoulder.

The **clavicle** is commonly called the **collarbone.** It is an elongated, S-shaped bone that articulates proximally with the manubrium of the sternum. The distal end articulates with the scapula.

1st thoracic vertebra (T1)

1
2
3
4
5
6
7
8
9
10
11
12

TRUE RIBS

FALSE RIBS

Jugular notch
Manubrium
Sternal angle
STERNUM
Body
Xiphoid process
Costal cartilage
12th thoracic vertebra (T12)
1st lumbar vertebra (L1)

Figure 7-10. Thoracic cage. (From Applegate E: *The anatomy and physiology learning system,* ed 3, St. Louis, 2000, Saunders.)

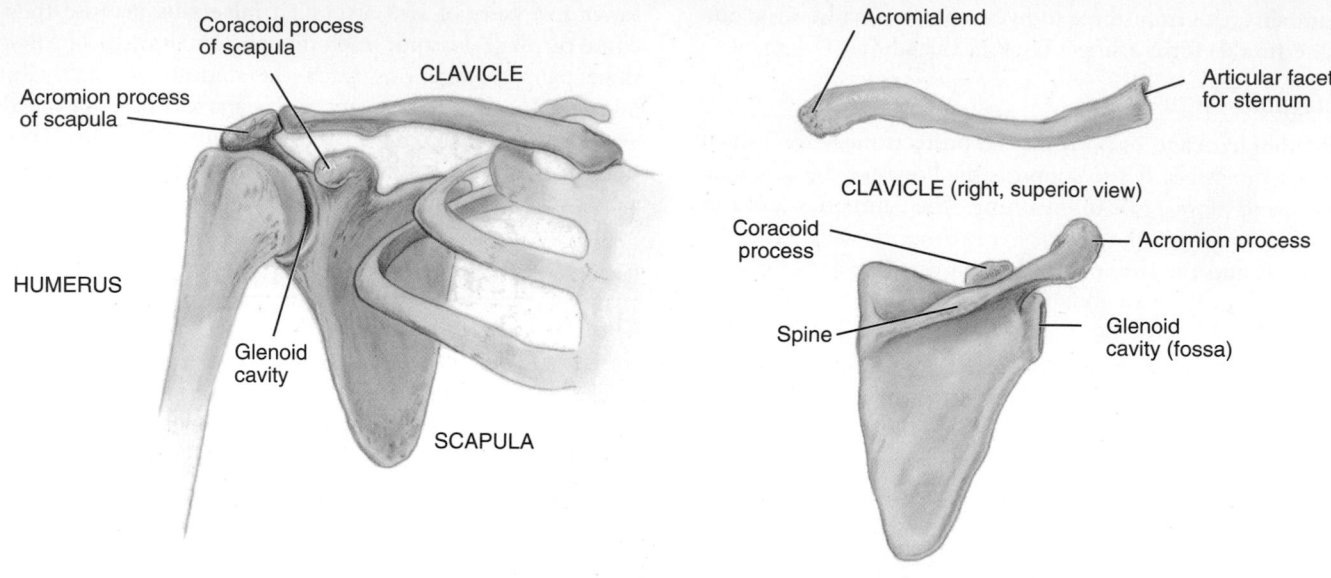

Figure 7-11. Components of the pectoral girdle. (From Applegate E: *The anatomy and physiology learning system,* ed 3, St. Louis, 2006, Saunders.)

The **scapula,** commonly called the **shoulder blade,** is a thin, flat triangular bone on the posterior surface of the thoracic wall. It articulates with the clavicle and the humerus. The scapula has points of attachment for numerous muscles that are involved in movement of the shoulder and arm. A bony ridge called the **spine** divides the dorsal surface into two unequal portions. The lateral end of the spine broadens to form the **acromion** (ah-KRO-mee-on) **process,** which articulates with the clavicle and is a site of muscle attachment. It forms the point of the shoulder. Another process, the **coracoid** (KOR-ah-koyd) **process,** forms a hook that projects forward, under the clavicle. It also serves as a place for muscle attachments. Between the two processes there is a shallow depression, the **glenoid cavity** (fossa), where the head of the humerus connects to the scapula.

Upper Extremity

The upper extremity (limb) consists of the bones of the arm, forearm, and hand.

Arm

The arm, or **brachium,** is the region between the shoulder and the elbow. It contains a single long bone, the **humerus,** illustrated in Figure 7-12. The **head** is the large, smooth, rounded end that fits into the scapula. Lateral to the head, there are two blunt projections for muscle attachment. These are the **greater** and **lesser tubercle.** The **deltoid tuberosity** is an elongated rough area along the shaft. The deltoid muscle attaches to the humerus along this region. The **lateral** and **medial epicondyles,** for the attachment of forearm muscles, project from the sides of the humerus at the distal end, near the elbow region. On the posterior surface, between the two epicondyles, there is a depression, the **olecranon**

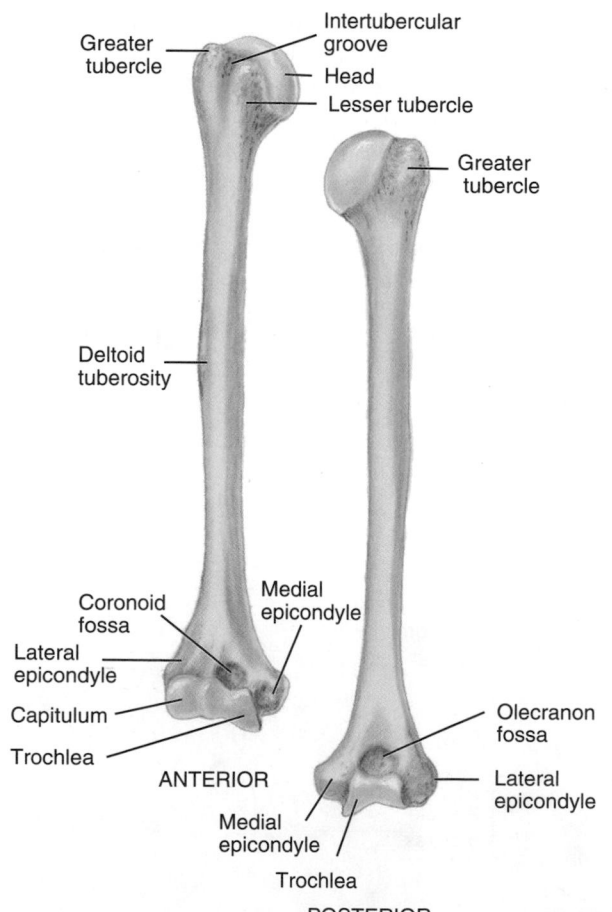

Figure 7-12. Humerus. (From Applegate E: *The anatomy and physiology learning system,* ed 3, St. Louis, 2006, Saunders.)

fossa, where the ulna fits with the humerus to form the hinged elbow joint. On the anterior surface is a shallow depression, the **coronoid fossa,** also for the ulna. Two smooth, rounded projections are evident on the distal end of the humerus. The **capitulum** is on the lateral side and articulates with the radius of the forearm. The **trochlea** is on the medial side and articulates with the ulna of the forearm.

Forearm

The forearm is the region between the elbow and wrist. It is formed by the **radius** on the lateral side and the **ulna** on the medial side when the forearm is in anatomic position. When the hand is turned so that the palm faces backward, the radius crosses over the ulna. The radius and ulna are illustrated in Figure 7-13.

The radius has a circular, disclike **head** on the proximal end. This articulates with the capitulum of the humerus. Just inferior to the head and on the medial side of the bone, there is a small, rough region called the **radial tuberosity,** which is an attachment for the biceps brachii muscle. On the distal end, the prominent markings of the radius are the **styloid process,** a pointed projection on the lateral side, and the **ulnar notch,** a smooth region on the medial side.

The proximal end of the ulna has a wrenchlike shape, with the opening of the wrench being the **trochlear notch,** or semilunar notch. The projection at the upper end of the notch is the **olecranon process,** which fits into the olecranon fossa of the humerus and forms the bony point of the elbow. The projection at the lower end of the notch is the

coronoid process, which fits into the coronoid fossa of the humerus. The **radial notch,** a smooth region on the lateral side of the coronoid process, is where the head of the radius fits. The **head** is at the distal end, and on the medial side of the head the pointed **styloid process** serves as an attachment point for ligaments of the wrist.

Hand

The hand, illustrated in Figure 7-14, is composed of the wrist, palm, and five fingers. The wrist, or **carpus,** contains eight small **carpal bones,** tightly bound by ligaments and arranged in two rows of four bones each. The carpal bones are identified in Figure 7-14. The palm of the hand, or **metacarpus,** contains five **metacarpal bones,** one in line with each finger. These bones are not named but are numbered 1 to 5 starting on the thumb side. The 14 bones of the fingers are called **phalanges** (fah-LAN-jeez). Some people refer to these as digits. Three phalanges are in each finger (a proximal, middle, and distal phalanx) except the thumb, or pollex, which has two. The thumb lacks a middle phalanx. The proximal phalanges articulate with the metacarpals.

Pelvic Girdle

The **pelvic girdle,** or **hip girdle,** attaches the lower extremities to the axial skeleton and provides a strong support for the weight of the body. It also provides support and protection for the urinary bladder, a portion of the large intestine, and the internal reproductive organs, which are located in the pelvic cavity.

Olecranon process

Trochlear notch

Head of radius

Coronoid process

Radial notch

Radial tuberosity

RADIUS   ULNA

Ulnar notch of radius

Head of ulna

Styloid process

Styloid process

Figure 7-13. Radius and ulna. (From Applegate E: *The anatomy and physiology learning system,* ed 3, St. Louis, 2006, Saunders.)

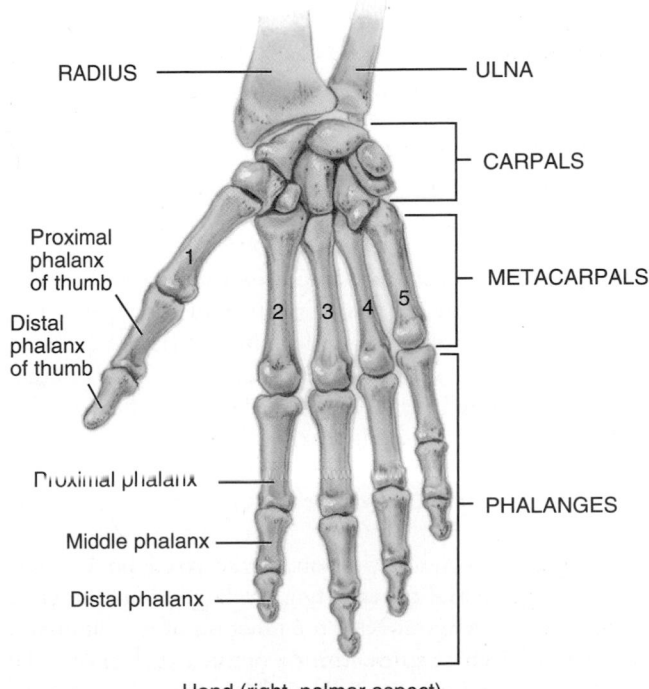

RADIUS   ULNA

CARPALS

Proximal phalanx of thumb

METACARPALS

Distal phalanx of thumb

1 2 3 4 5

Proximal phalanx

Middle phalanx

Distal phalanx

PHALANGES

Hand (right, palmar aspect)

Figure 7-14. Hand. (From Applegate E: *The anatomy and physiology learning system,* ed 3, St. Louis, 2006, Saunders.)

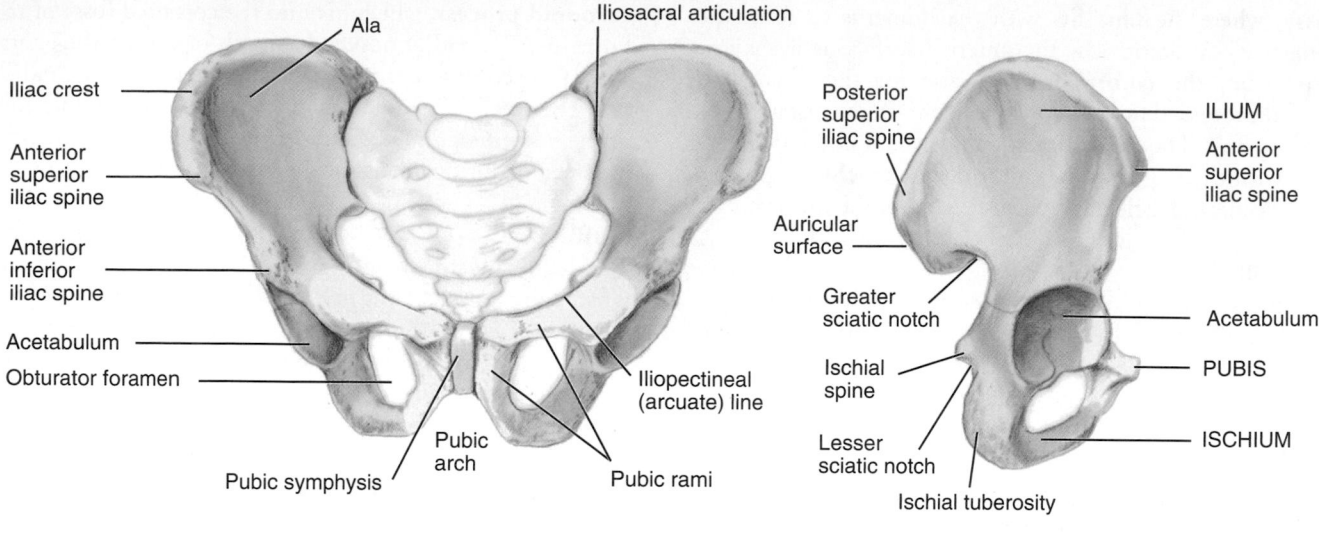

Iliac crest

Ala

Iliosacral articulation

Anterior superior iliac spine

Anterior inferior iliac spine

Acetabulum

Obturator foramen

Pubic symphysis

Pubic arch

Iliopectineal (arcuate) line

Pubic rami

Posterior superior iliac spine

ILIUM

Anterior superior iliac spine

Auricular surface

Greater sciatic notch

Ischial spine

Lesser sciatic notch

Ischial tuberosity

Acetabulum

PUBIS

ISCHIUM

PELVIC GIRDLE (anterior view)

OS COXAE (right, lateral view)

Figure 7-15. Bones of the pelvic girdle. (From Applegate E: *The anatomy and physiology learning system,* ed 3, St. Louis, 2006, Saunders.)

The pelvic girdle consists of two **coxal (hip) bones,** illustrated in Figure 7-15. The coxal bones are also called the **ossa coxae,** or **innominate bones.** Anteriorly, the two bones articulate with each other at the **symphysis pubis;** posteriorly, they articulate with the sacrum at the **iliosacral joints.** During childhood, each coxal bone consists of three separate parts: the **ilium, ischium,** and **pubis.** In the adult, these bones are firmly fused to form a single bone. Where the three bones meet, there is a large depression, the **acetabulum** (as-seh-TAB-yoo-lum), which holds the head of the femur. The **obturator foramen** is a large opening between the pubis and ischium that functions as a passageway for blood vessels, nerves, and muscle tendons.

The major portion of the coxal bone is formed by the ilium, which has a large, flared region called the **ala,** or wing. The concavity on the medial surface of the ala is the **iliac fossa.** The superior margin of the ala is the **iliac crest,** which ends anteriorly as a blunt projection, the **anterior superior iliac spine.** Just inferior to this is another blunt projection, the **anterior inferior iliac spine.** Posteriorly, the crest ends in the **posterior superior iliac spine** and just inferior to this there is a **posterior inferior iliac spine.** The **greater sciatic notch** forms a deep indentation in the posterior region. The sciatic nerve passes through this notch. The **auricular surface** is the rough region on the posterior part of the ilium, where it meets the sacrum to form the iliosacral (sacroiliac) joint. The **iliopectineal line,** a sharp line at the inferior margin of the iliac fossa, marks the pelvic brim.

The lower, posterior portion of the coxal bone is the ischium. The **ischial tuberosity** is the large, rough, inferior portion of the ischium. Near the junction of the ilium and ischium, the **ischial spine** forms a pointed projection. The indentation inferior to the spine is the **lesser sciatic notch.**

The most anterior portion of the coxal bone is the pubis. The two pubic bones meet at the pubic symphysis and

extend laterally and inferiorly from this point. The armlike extensions are the **pubic rami.** Inferiorly the pubic rami form a V-shaped arch called the **pubic arch.**

Together, the sacrum, coccyx, and pelvic girdle form the basin-shaped pelvis. The **false pelvis** (greater pelvis) is surrounded by the flared portions of the ilium bones and the lumbar vertebrae. The **true pelvis** (lesser pelvis) is smaller and inferior to the false pelvis. It is the region below the **pelvic brim,** or **pelvic inlet,** and it is encircled by bone. The large opening at the bottom of this region is the **pelvic outlet.** The dimensions of the true pelvis are especially important in childbirth.

Lower Extremity

The lower extremity (limb) consists of the bones of the thigh, leg, foot, and patella, or kneecap. The lower extremities support the entire weight of the body when we are erect and they are exposed to tremendous forces when we walk, run, and jump. With this in mind, it is not surprising that the bones of the lower extremity are larger and stronger than those in the upper extremity.

Thigh

The **thigh** is the region from the hip to the knee. It contains a single long bone, the **femur,** illustrated in Figure 7-16. It is the largest, longest, and strongest bone in the body.

The large, smooth, ball-like **head** of the femur has a small depression called the **fovea capitis.** A ligament attaches here. Prominent projections at the proximal end, the **greater** and **lesser trochanters,** are major sites for muscle attachment. The **intertrochanteric crest** on the posterior side and the **intertrochanteric line** on the anterior side are between the trochanters and are also for muscle attachment. The **neck** is between the head and the trochanters. On the posterior surface, a rough area, the **gluteal tuberosity,** continues inferiorly as the **linea aspera.** Both

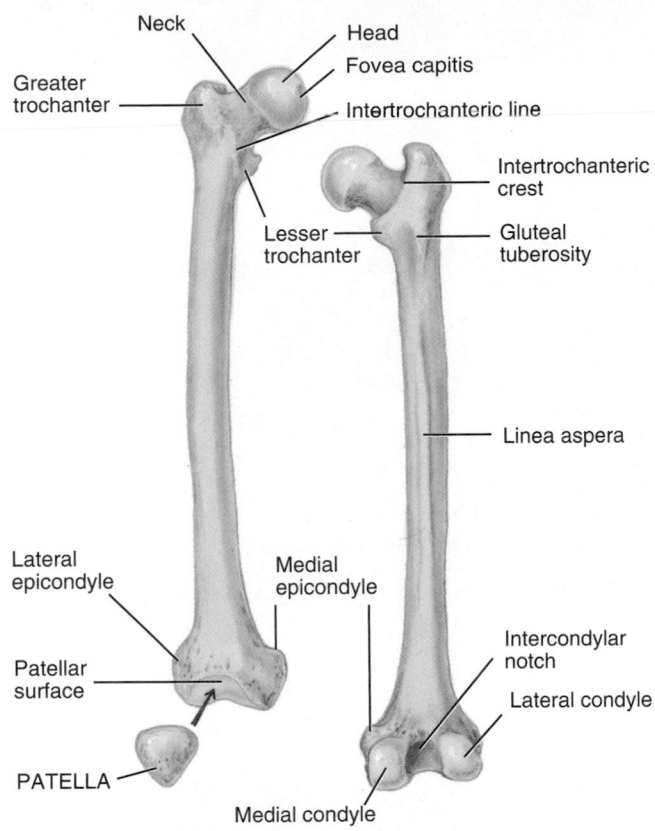

FEMUR and PATELLA (right)

Figure 7-16. Femur. (From Applegate E: *The anatomy and physiology learning system,* ed 3, St. Louis, 2006, Saunders.)

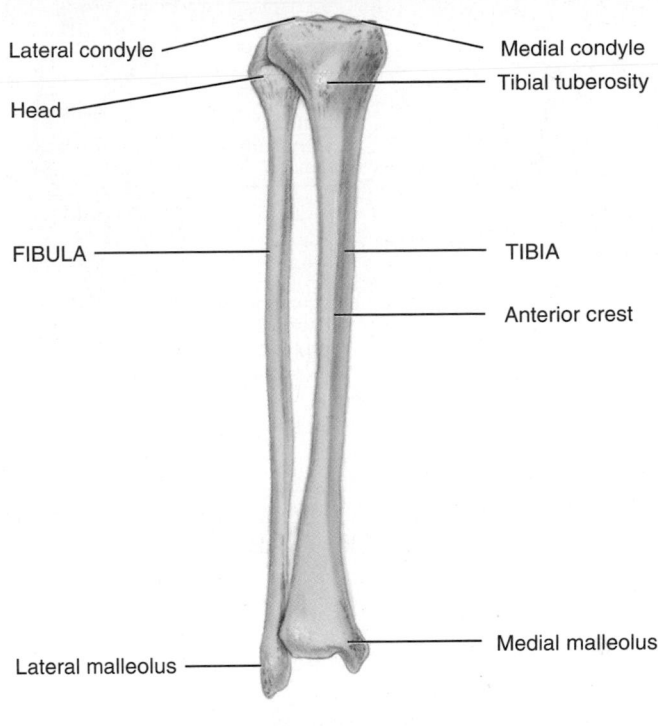

Anterior view (right)

Figure 7-17. Tibia and fibula. (From Applegate E: *The anatomy and physiology learning system,* ed 3, St. Louis, 2006, Saunders.)

of these are regions of muscle attachment. The distal end is marked by two large, rounded surfaces, the **lateral** and **medial condyles.** These form joints with the bones of the leg. The **intercondylar notch** is a depression between the condyles that contains ligaments associated with the knee joint. Two small projections superior to the condyles are the **epicondyles.** On the anterior surface, between the condyles, a smooth **patellar surface** marks the area for the kneecap.

Leg
The **leg** is the region between the knee and the ankle. It is formed by the slender **fibula** (FIB-yoo-lah) on the lateral side and the larger, weight-bearing **tibia** (TIB-ee-ah), or shin bone, on the medial side. The tibia articulates with the femur to form the knee joint and with the **talus** (one of the foot bones) to allow flexion and extension at the ankle.

The proximal end of the fibula is the **head** and the projection at the distal end is the **lateral malleolus,** which forms the lateral bulge of the ankle. The superior surface of the tibia is flattened and smooth, with two slightly concave regions called the **lateral** and **medial condyles.** The condyles of the femur fit into these regions. Just below the condyles, the **tibial tuberosity** forms a rough area for the attachment of ligaments associated with the knee. The

anterior crest is a sharp ridge on the anterior surface and forms the shin. On the medial side of the distal end, the **medial malleolus** forms the medial bulge of the ankle. Figure 7-17 illustrates the tibia and fibula.

Foot
The **foot,** illustrated in Figure 7-18, is composed of the ankle, instep, and five toes. The ankle, or **tarsus,** contains seven **tarsal bones.** These correspond to the carpals in the wrist. The largest tarsal bone is the **calcaneus** (kal-KAY-nee-us), or heel bone. The **talus,** another tarsal bone, rests on top of the calcaneus and articulates with the tibia. The tarsal bones are identified in Figure 7-18. The instep of the foot, or **metatarsus,** contains five **metatarsal bones,** one in line with each toe. The distal ends of these bones form the ball of the foot. These bones are not named but are numbered one through five starting on the medial side. The tarsals and metatarsals, together with strong tendons and ligaments, form the arches of the foot. The 14 bones of the toes are called **phalanges.** Three phalanges are in each toe (a proximal, middle, and distal phalanx), except in the great (or big) toe, or hallux, which has only two. The great toe lacks a middle phalanx. The proximal phalanges articulate with the metatarsals.

Patella
The **patella,** or **kneecap,** is a flat, triangular sesamoid bone enclosed within the major tendon that anchors the anterior

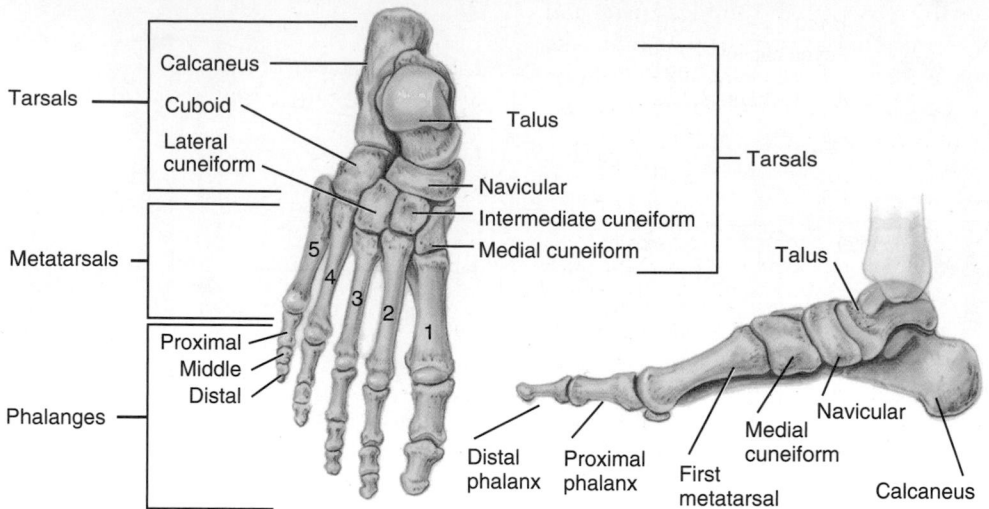

Figure 7-18. Bones of the foot. (From Applegate E: *The anatomy and physiology learning system,* ed 3, St. Louis, 2006, Saunders.)

thigh muscle to the tibia. It provides a smooth surface for the tendon as it turns the corner between the thigh and leg when the knee is flexed. It also protects the knee joint anteriorly.

ARTICULATIONS

An **articulation** (ahr-tik-yoo-LAY-shun), or joint, is where two bones come together. In terms of the amount of movement they allow, there are three types of joints: immovable, slightly movable, and freely movable.

Synarthroses

Synarthroses (sin-ahr-THROH-seez) are immovable joints. The singular form is synarthrosis. In these joints, the bones come in close contact and are separated only by a thin layer of fibrous connective tissue. The **sutures** in the skull are examples of immovable joints.

Amphiarthroses

Slightly movable joints are called **amphiarthroses** (am-fee-ahr-THROH-seez). The singular form is amphiarthrosis. In this type of joint, the bones are connected by hyaline cartilage or fibrocartilage. The ribs connected to the sternum by costal cartilage are slightly movable joints connected by hyaline cartilage. The symphysis pubis is a slightly movable joint in which there is a fibrocartilage pad between the two bones. The joints between the vertebrae, the intervertebral discs, are also of this type.

Diarthroses

Most joints in the adult body are **diarthroses** (dye-ahr-THROH-seez), or freely movable joints. The singular form is diarthrosis. In this type of joint, the ends of the opposing

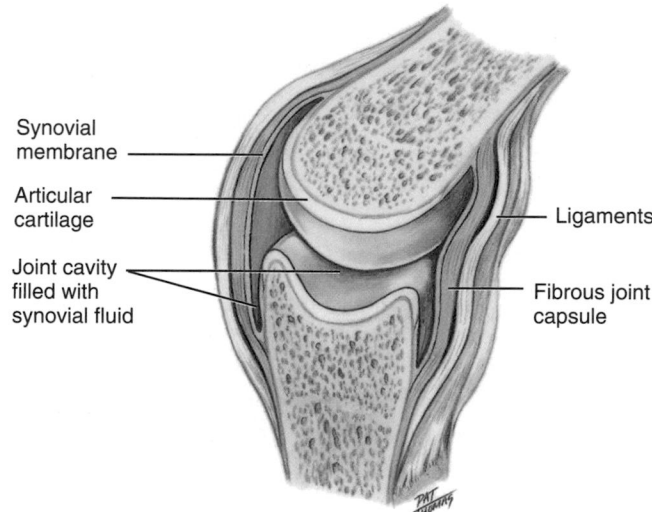

Figure 7-19. Generalized structure of a synovial joint. (From Applegate E: *The anatomy and physiology learning system,* ed 3, St. Louis, 2006, Saunders.)

bones are covered with hyaline cartilage, the **articular cartilage,** and they are separated by a space called the **joint cavity.** The components of the joints are enclosed in a dense fibrous **joint capsule** (Figure 7-19). The outer layer of the capsule consists of the ligaments that hold the bones together. The inner layer is the **synovial membrane** that secretes **synovial fluid** into the joint cavity for lubrication. Because all of these joints have a synovial membrane, they are sometimes called **synovial joints.**

Some diarthroses have pads and cushions associated with them. The knee has fibrocartilaginous pads, called **semilunar cartilages** or the **lateral meniscus** (meh-NISkus) and **medial meniscus,** which rest on the lateral and medial condyles of the tibia. The pads help stabilize the joint and act as shock absorbers. **Bursae** are fluid-filled sacs that act as cushions and help reduce friction. Bursae are lined with a synovial membrane that secretes synovial fluid into the sac. They are commonly located between the skin and underlying bone or between tendons and ligaments. Inflammation of a bursa is called **bursitis.** Figure 7-20 illustrates some menisci and bursae associated with the knee joint.

There are six types of diarthrotic or freely movable joints based on the shapes of their parts and the types of movement they allow. These are described in Table 7-1.

Figure 7-20. Sagittal section of the knee joint illustrating bursae and menisci. (From Applegate E: *The anatomy and physiology learning system,* ed 3, St. Louis, 2006, Saunders.)

Highlight on Conditions Affecting the Skeletal System

Ankylosing spondylitis (ANG-kih-loh-sing spahn-dih-LYE-tis) Inflammation of the spine that is characterized by stiffening of the spinal joints and ligaments so that movement becomes increasingly painful and difficult; also called *rheumatoid spondylitis*

Arthritis (ahr-THRYE-tis) Inflammation of a joint

Bunion (BUN-yun) Abnormal swelling of the joint between the big toe and the first metatarsal bone, resulting from a buildup of soft tissues and bone caused by chronic irritation from ill-fitting shoes

Carpal tunnel syndrome (KAHR-pull TUH-nul SIN-drohm) Condition characterized by pain and burning sensations in the fingers and hand, caused by compression of the median nerve as it passes between a wrist ligament and the bones and tendons of the wrist

Dislocation (dis-loh-KAY-shun) Displacement of a bone from its joint with tearing of ligaments, tendons, and articular capsule; also called *luxation*

Gout (GOWT) A form of acute arthritis in which uric acid crystals develop within a joint and irritate the cartilage, causing acute inflammation, swelling, and pain; most commonly occurs in middle-aged and older men

Lyme disease (LYME dih-ZEEZ) A bacterial disease transmitted to humans by deer ticks; characterized by joint stiffness, headache, fever and chills, nausea, and back pain; complications include severe arthritis and cardiac problems; early stages of the disease respond well to antibiotics

Osteoarthritis (ahs-tee-oh-ahr-THRYE-tis) A noninflammatory disease of the joints that is characterized by degeneration of the articular cartilage and changes in the synovial membrane; also called *degenerative joint disease* (DJD)

Osteomalacia (ahs-tee-oh-mah-LAY-shee-ah) Softening of bone because of inadequate amounts of calcium and phosphorus; bones bend easily and become deformed; in childhood this is called *rickets*

Osteomyelitis (ahs-tee-oh-my-eh-LYE-tis) Inflammation of the bone marrow caused by bacteria

Osteoporosis (ahs-tee-oh-por-OH-sis) Decrease in bone density and mass; commonly occurs in postmenopausal women as a result of increased osteoclast activity caused by diminished estrogen levels; bones fracture easily

Osteosarcoma (ahs-tee-oh-sahr-KOH-mah) Malignant tumor derived from bone; also called *osteogenic sarcoma;* osteoblasts multiply without control and form large tumors in bone

Rheumatoid arthritis (ROO-mah-toyd ahr-THRYE-tis) A chronic systemic disease with changes occurring in the connective tissues of the body, especially the joints; in contrast to osteoarthritis, the symptoms are usually more generalized and severe; evidence indicates it may be an autoimmune disease

Spina bifida (SPY-nah BIFF-ih-dah) A developmental anomaly in which the vertebral laminae do not close around the spinal cord, leaving an opening through which the cord and meninges may or may not protrude

Sprain (SPRAYN) Twisting of a joint with pain, swelling, and injury to ligaments, tendons, muscles, blood vessels, and nerves; most often occurs in the ankle; more serious than a strain, which is the overstretching of the muscles associated with a joint

Talipes (TAL-ih-peez) Congenital deformity of the foot in which the patient cannot stand with the sole of the foot flat on the ground; also called *clubfoot* ■

Table 7-1 Types of Freely Movable Joints

Type	Shape of Joint Surfaces	Range of Movement	Examples
Ball-and-socket	Ball-shaped end of one bone fits into cup-shaped socket of another	Permits widest range of movement in all planes including rotation	Shoulder, hip
Condyloid	Oval-shaped condyle fits into elliptical cavity of another	Angular motion but not rotation	Occipital condyles with atlas; metacarpals and metatarsals with phalanges
Saddle	Articulating surfaces of both bones have concave and convex regions; shapes of two bones complement each other	Permits wide range of movement	Carpometacarpal joint of thumb is only saddle joint in body
Pivot	Rounded or conical surface of one bone fits into ring of bone or tendon	Rotation	Joint between atlas and axis; proximal radioulnar joint
Hinge	Convex projection of one bone fits into concave depression in another	Permits flexion and extension only	Elbow and knee joints
Gliding	Flat or slightly curved surfaces moving against each other	Sliding or twisting without circular movement	Between carpals in wrist and between tarsals in ankle

From Applegate E: *The anatomy and physiology learning system*, ed 3, St. Louis, 2006, Saunders.

TERMINOLOGY REVIEW

Amphiarthrosis A slightly movable joint; plural, amphiarthroses.
Diaphysis The long straight shaft of a long bone.
Diarthrosis Freely movable joint characterized by a joint cavity; also called a *synovial joint;* plural, diarthroses.
Epiphyseal plate The cartilaginous plate between the epiphysis and diaphysis of a bone; responsible for the lengthwise growth of a long bone.

Epiphysis The end of a long bone.
Osteoblast Bone-forming cell.
Osteoclast Cell that destroys or resorbs bone tissue.
Osteocyte Mature bone cell.
Osteon Structural unit of bone; haversian system.
Synarthrosis An immovable joint; plural, synarthroses.

ON THE WEB

For Information on the Skeletal System:

Merck Manual: Bone, Joint, and Muscle Disorders: www. merck.com/mmhe *(Click on "Bone, Joint, and Muscle Disorders")*

Loyola University Medical Education Network: Pick a Bone: www.meddean.luc.edu/lumen/MedEd/Gross Anatomy/learnem/bones/main_bone.htm

National Osteoporosis Foundation: www.nof.org

PREPARE FOR CERTIFICATION
Visit the Evolve site at http://evolve.elsevier.com/Bonewit/today/ to actively Prepare for your Certification.

 *Check out the **Companion CD** bound with the book to access additional interactive activities.*

8

Muscular System

LEARNING OBJECTIVES

1. State the characteristics and functions of muscle tissue.
2. Describe the structure of a skeletal muscle.
3. List and describe the sequence of events involved in the contraction of a skeletal muscle fiber.
4. Explain how energy is provided for a muscle contraction.
5. Describe oxygen debt.
6. Describe and illustrate the movements accomplished by the contraction of skeletal muscle.
7. Identify and describe the major muscles making up the axial skeleton.
8. Identify and describe the major muscles making up the appendicular skeleton.

CHAPTER OUTLINE

Introduction to the Muscular System
Characteristics and Functions of the Muscular System
Structure of Skeletal Muscle
  Whole Skeletal Muscle
  Skeletal Muscle Attachments
  Skeletal Muscle Fibers
  Nerve and Blood Supply
Contraction of Skeletal Muscle
  Stimulus for Contraction

Energy Sources and Oxygen Debt
Movements
Skeletal Muscle Groups
  Naming Muscles
  Muscles of the Head and Neck
  Muscles of the Trunk
  Muscles of the Upper Extremity
  Muscles of the Lower Extremity

CAAHEP COMPETENCIES

Content Competencies
Anatomy and Physiology
- Anatomy and physiology of all body systems

- Common pathology/diseases
- Diagnostic/treatment modalities

ABHES COMPETENCIES

Content Competencies
Anatomy and Physiology
- Anatomy and physiology

- Study of diseases and etiology
- All body systems
- Diagnostic/treatment modalities

KEY TERMS

antagonist (an-TAG-oh-nist)
insertion (in-SIR-shun)
motor unit (MOH-toar YOO-nit)
neuromuscular junction (noo-roe-MUSK-yoo-lar JUNK-shun)

neurotransmitter (noo-roh-TRANS-mit-ter)
origin (OR-ih-jin)
prime mover (PRYM MOO-ver)
synergist (SIN-er-gist)

Introduction to the Muscular System

As described in Chapter 5, there are three types of muscle tissue: skeletal, visceral, and cardiac. These are reviewed in Table 8-1. This chapter takes a closer look at skeletal muscle, which makes up about 40% of an individual's body weight. It forms more than 600 muscles that are attached to the bones of the skeleton. Skeletal muscles are under conscious control and when they contract they move the bones. Skeletal muscles also allow us to smile, frown, pout, show surprise, and exhibit other forms of facial expression.

CHARACTERISTICS AND FUNCTIONS OF THE MUSCULAR SYSTEM

Skeletal muscle has four primary characteristics that relate to its functions:

Excitability Excitability (eks-eye-tah-BILL-ih-tee) is the ability to receive and respond to a stimulus. To function properly, muscles have to respond to a stimulus from the nervous system.

Contractility Contractility (kon-track-TILL-ih-tee) is the ability to shorten or contract. When a muscle responds to a stimulus, it shortens to produce movement.

Extensibility Extensibility (eks-ten-sih-BILL-ih-tee) means that a muscle can be stretched or extended. Skeletal muscles are often arranged in opposing pairs. When one muscle contracts, the other muscle is relaxed and stretched.

Elasticity Elasticity (ee-lass-TISS-ih-tee) is the capacity to recoil or return to the original shape and length after contraction or extension.

Muscle contraction fulfills four important functions in the body:

*   Movement
*   Posture
*   Joint stability
*   Heat production

Nearly all **movement** in the body is the result of muscle contraction. Some exceptions to this are the action of cilia, the motility of the flagellum on sperm cells, and the ameboid movement of some white blood cells. The integrated action of joints, bones, and skeletal muscles produces obvious movements such as walking and running. Skeletal muscles also produce more subtle movements that result in various facial expressions, eye movements, and respiration. **Posture,** such as sitting and standing, is maintained as a result of muscle contraction. The skeletal muscles are continually making fine adjustments that hold the body in stationary positions. Skeletal muscles contribute to **joint stability.** The tendons of many muscles extend over joints and in this way contribute to joint stability. This is particularly evident in the knee and shoulder joints, where muscle tendons are a major factor in stabilizing the joint. **Heat production,** to maintain body temperature, is an important by-product of muscle metabolism. Nearly 85% of the heat produced in the body is the result of muscle contraction.

STRUCTURE OF SKELETAL MUSCLE

A whole skeletal muscle is considered an organ of the muscular system. For example, the biceps muscle is an organ of the muscular system. Each organ or muscle consists of skeletal muscle tissue, connective tissue, nerve tissue, and blood or vascular tissue.

Whole Skeletal Muscle

An individual skeletal muscle such as the biceps muscle may consist of hundreds, or even thousands, of muscle fibers bundled together and wrapped in a connective tissue covering. Each muscle is surrounded by a connective tissue sheath called the **epimysium** (ep-ih-MYE-see-um). Fascia consists of connective tissue located outside the epimysium. Fascia surrounds and separates the muscles. Portions of the epimysium project inward to divide the muscle into compartments. Each compartment contains a bundle of muscle fibers. Each bundle of muscle fibers is called a **fasciculus** (fah-SIK-yoo-lus) and is surrounded by a layer of connective tissue called the **perimysium** (pair-ih-MYE-see-um). Within the fasciculus, each individual muscle cell, called a *muscle fiber,* is surrounded by connective tissue called the **endomysium** (end-oh-MYE-see-um). Connective tissue fibers of the endomysium are continuous with those in the perimysium, which, in turn, are continuous with the epimysium. Skeletal muscle cells (fibers), like other body cells, are soft and fragile. The connective tissue coverings furnish

Table 8-1 Summary of Muscle Tissue

Feature	Skeletal	Visceral	Cardiac
Location	Attached to bones	Walls of internal organs and blood vessels	Heart
Function	Produce body movement	Contraction of viscera and blood vessels	Pump blood through heart and blood vessels
Cell shape	Cylindric	Spindle shaped, tapered ends	Cylindric, branching
Number of nuclei	Many	One	One
Striations	Present	Absent	Present
Type of control	Voluntary	Involuntary	Involuntary

From Applegate E: *The anatomy and physiology learning system,* ed 3, St. Louis, 2006, Saunders.

Highlight on the Muscular System

RIGOR MORTIS: The term *rigor mortis* means the "stiffness of death." Within a short time of death, the adenosine triphosphate in muscles breaks down. This causes the myofilaments to remain locked in a contracted position and the body becomes rigid. A day or so later, muscle proteins begin to deteriorate and the rigor mortis disappears.

TETANUS: The word *tetanus* is often confusing because it means different things to different people. In reference to muscle contraction, the term denotes a steady contraction of a muscle fiber, without a relaxation phase. The word also refers to a disease, commonly called "lockjaw," that is caused by the bacterium *Clostridium tetani.* The toxin from the bacteria causes nerves to be highly excitable, which, in turn, causes uncontrollable muscle contractions, or spasms. A third use of the word is to denote a condition caused by a deficiency of calcium ions in the extracellular fluid. The lack of calcium increases nerve excitability with resulting muscle spasms, particularly of the extremities. The word *tetany* is also sometimes used to mean tetanus.

CRAMPS: Cramps are painful, spastic contractions of muscles. They are usually caused by an irritation within the muscles that results in reflex contractions. Local inflammation from the accumulation of lactic acid is one source of irritation.

WRYNECK: Injury to one of the sternocleidomastoid muscles may result in torticollis, or wryneck. This is characterized by a twisting of the neck and an unnatural position of the head.

DIAPHRAGM: Voluntary forceful contractions of the diaphragm increase intraabdominal pressure to assist in urination, defecation, and childbirth.

ELECTRICAL SHOCK: The muscles that flex the fingers and hand are stronger than the extensor muscles. In a normal relaxed position the fingers are slightly flexed because the normal muscle tone is greater in the flexors. Persons who receive a high-voltage electrical shock through the arms flex their hands tightly and "can't let go." All of the flexors and extensors receive the electrical stimulus, but because the flexor muscles are stronger, they contract more forcefully.

INTRAMUSCULAR INJECTIONS: The gluteus medius is a common site for intramuscular injections. Generally, the injection is given in the center of the upper outer quadrant of the buttock, or gluteal, area. The gluteus medius, rather than the gluteus maximus, is used to avoid damaging the sciatic nerve.

HORSEBACK RIDING: The adductor muscles in the medial compartment are the horse rider's muscles. These muscles adduct, or press, the thighs together to keep a person on a horse.

QUADS: The quadriceps femoris group is a powerful knee extensor that is used in climbing, running, and rising from a chair. ∎

---

support and protection for the delicate cells and allow them to withstand the forces of contraction. The coverings also provide pathways for the passage of blood vessels and nerves. The organization and connective tissue wrappings of skeletal muscle fibers are illustrated in Figure 8-1.

Skeletal Muscle Attachments

In some instances, fibers of the epimysium fuse directly with the periosteum of a bone to form a **direct** attachment. The fleshy part of the muscle is known as the **belly** or **gaster.** More commonly, the epimysium, perimysium, and endomysium extend beyond the belly of the muscle to form a thick, ropelike **tendon** or a broad, flat, sheetlike **aponeurosis** (ah-pah-noo-ROE-sis). The tendon or aponeurosis form **indirect** attachments from muscles to the periosteum of bones or to the connective tissue of other muscles. Typically, a muscle spans a joint and is attached to bones by tendons at both ends. One of the bones remains relatively fixed or stable while the other end moves as a result of muscle contraction. The fixed or stable end is called the **origin** of the muscle, and the more movable attachment is called the **insertion.**

Skeletal Muscle Fibers

Each individual skeletal muscle fiber consists of a single cylindric muscle cell. The cell membrane is called the **sar-**colemma (sar-koh-LEM-mah), the cytoplasm is the **sarcoplasm** (SAR-koh-plazm), and a specialized form of smooth endoplasmic reticulum that stores calcium ions is the **sarcoplasmic reticulum** (sar-koh-PLAZ-mik reh-TIK-yoo-lum). Multiple nuclei are next to the sarcolemma at the periphery of the cell. Because the muscle cell needs energy for contraction, there are numerous mitochondria. The sarcolemma has multiple inward extensions, or invaginations, called *transverse tubules* or **T tubules.**

Nerve and Blood Supply

Skeletal muscles have an abundant supply of blood vessels and nerves. This is directly related to the primary function of skeletal muscle-contraction. Before a skeletal muscle fiber can contract, it must receive an impulse from a nerve cell. Muscle contraction requires adenosine triphosphate (ATP), and blood vessels deliver the necessary nutrients and oxygen to produce it. Blood vessels also remove the waste products that are produced as a result of muscle contraction.

In general, an artery and at least one vein accompany each nerve that penetrates the epimysium of a skeletal muscle. Branches of the nerve and blood vessels follow the connective tissue components of the muscle so that each muscle fiber is in contact with a branch of a nerve cell and with one or more minute blood vessels called *capillaries.*

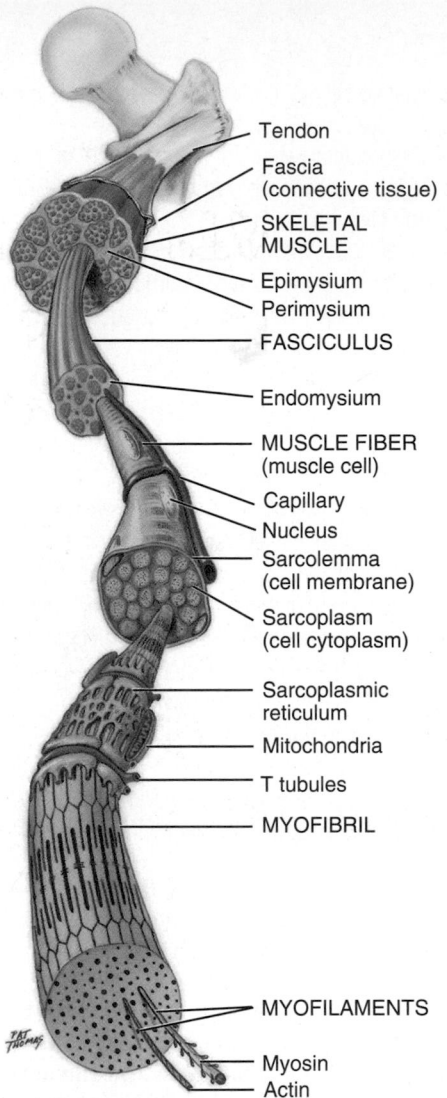

Figure 8-1. Organization and connective tissue components of skeletal muscle. (From Applegate E: *The anatomy and physiology learning system,* ed 3, St. Louis, 2006, Saunders.)

Labels:
- Tendon
- Fascia (connective tissue)
- SKELETAL MUSCLE
- Epimysium
- Perimysium
- FASCICULUS
- Endomysium
- MUSCLE FIBER (muscle cell)
- Capillary
- Nucleus
- Sarcolemma (cell membrane)
- Sarcoplasm (cell cytoplasm)
- Sarcoplasmic reticulum
- Mitochondria
- T tubules
- MYOFIBRIL
- MYOFILAMENTS
- Myosin
- Actin

CONTRACTION OF SKELETAL MUSCLE

Skeletal muscle contraction is the result of a complex series of events, based on chemical reactions, at the cellular (muscle fiber) level. This chain of reactions begins with stimulation by a nerve cell and ends when the muscle fiber is again relaxed. Contraction of a whole muscle is the result of the simultaneous contraction of many muscle fibers.

Stimulus for Contraction

Skeletal muscles are stimulated to contract by special nerve cells called **motor neurons.** As the axon of the motor neuron penetrates the muscle, the axon branches, so there is an axon terminal for each muscle fiber. A single motor neuron and all the muscle fibers it stimulates is called a **motor unit.** Some motor units include several hundred

individual fibers; others contain fewer than 10. Because all the muscle fibers in a motor unit receive a nerve impulse at the same time, all the fibers contract at the same time.

The region in which an axon terminal meets a muscle fiber is called a **neuromuscular,** or myoneural, **junction,** which is illustrated in Figure 8-2. The axon terminal does not actually touch the sarcolemma of the muscle cell but fits into a shallow depression in the cell membrane. The fluid-filled space between the axon terminal and sarcolemma is called a **synaptic cleft** (gap). **Acetylcholine (ACh)** (ah-see-till-KOH-leen), a **neurotransmitter,** is contained within synaptic vesicles in the axon terminal. Receptor sites for the acetylcholine are located on the sarcolemma.

Highlight on Conditions and Procedures Related to the Muscular System

Conditions

Cramp (KRAMP) Painful involuntary muscle spasm; often caused by myositis but can be a symptom of any irritation or ion imbalance

Muscular dystrophy (MUSS-kyoo-lar DIS-troh-fee) An inherited, chronic, progressive wasting and weakening of muscles without involvement of the nervous system

Myasthenia gravis (mye-as-THEE-nee-ah GRAY-vis) An autoimmune disease, more common in females, that is characterized by weakness of skeletal muscles caused by an abnormality at the neuromuscular junction

Myoparesis (mye-oh-pah-REE-sis) Weakness or slight paralysis of a muscle

Myopathy (mye-AHP-ah-thee) Muscle disease

Myorrhexis (mye-oh-REK-sis) Rupture of a muscle

Myositis (mye-oh-SYE-tis) Inflammation of muscle tissue

Repetitive stress disorder (ree-PET-ah-tiv STRESS dis-OAR-der) Condition with symptoms caused by repetitive motions that involve muscles, tendons, nerves, and joints; most commonly occur as work-related or sports injuries

Shin splint (SHIN SPLINT) Strain of the long flexor muscle of the toes resulting in pain along the tibia (shinbone); usually caused by repeated stress to the lower leg

Tic (TIK) A spasmodic involuntary twitching of a muscle that is normally under voluntary control

Procedures

Electromyography (ee-lek-troh-mye-AHG-rah-fee) The process of recording the strength of muscle contraction as a result of electrical stimulation

Muscle biopsy (MUSS-uhl BYE-ahp-see) Removal of muscle tissue for microscopic examination

Tenomyoplasty (ten-oh-MY-oh-plas-tee) Surgical repair of a tendon and muscle; applied especially to an operation for inguinal hernia

Tenoplasty (TEN-oh-plas-tee) Surgical repair of a tendon

Tenorraphy (ten-OAR-ah-fee) Suture of a tendon ∎

Figure 8-2. Neuromuscular junction. *ACh,* Acetylcholine. (From Applegate E: *The anatomy and physiology learning system,* ed 3, St. Louis, 2006, Saunders.)

When a nerve impulse reaches the axon terminal, acetylcholine is released. The acetylcholine diffuses across the synaptic cleft and binds with the receptor sites on the sarcolemma. This reaction is the stimulus for contraction. A **stimulus** is a change in the cellular environment that alters the cell membrane (i.e., the acetylcholine binding with the receptor sites). The stimulus causes a **response.** In this case, the response is a muscle impulse, similar to a nerve impulse, that travels in all directions on the sarcolemma. From the sarcolemma, it travels into the T tubules, where it initiates physiologic activity within the muscle cell that results in contraction.

Meanwhile, back at the synaptic cleft, the acetylcholine that was released is rapidly inactivated by the enzyme **acetylcholinesterase** (ah-see-till-koh-lin-ES-ter-ase). This ensures that one nerve impulse will result in only one muscle impulse and only one contraction of the muscle fiber. Anything that interferes with the production, release, or inactivation of acetylcholine, or its ability to bind with the receptor sites on the sarcolemma, will have an effect on muscle contraction. Muscle relaxant drugs work in this manner.

Energy Sources and Oxygen Debt

The immediate or initial source of energy for muscle contraction is **ATP** (Figure 8-3A). Surprisingly, muscles have limited storage facilities for ATP. In working muscles the stored ATP is depleted in about 6 seconds, and new ATP must be regenerated if muscle contraction is to continue.

Creatine phosphate (KREE-ah-tin FOS-fate) is a unique high-energy compound that is stored in muscles (Figure 8-3B). This compound provides an almost instantaneous transfer of its energy and a phosphate group to adenosine diphosphate (ADP) molecules to regenerate ATP:

Creatine phosphate + ADP → creatine + ATP

This reaction is so effective that there is little change in ATP levels during the initial stages of muscle contraction. When ATP levels are high, this reaction is reversed to form more creatine phosphate. Muscles store enough creatine phosphate to regenerate sufficient ATP to sustain contraction for about 10 seconds.

When muscles are actively contracting for extended periods of time, **fatty acids** and **glucose** become the primary energy sources. Glucose and fatty acids are present in the blood that circulates through the muscles, and glucose is stored in muscles as glycogen. As ATP and creatine phosphate stores are being used, more ATP is produced from the metabolism of glucose and fatty acids.

If adequate oxygen is available, fatty acids and glucose are broken down in the mitochondria by a process called **aerobic respiration** (Figure 8-3C). The products are carbon dioxide, water, and large amounts of ATP:

Fatty acids or glucose + oxyen → carbon dioxide + water + ATP

Limited amounts of oxygen can be stored in muscle fibers. Certain fibers, called *red fibers,* contain reddish protein pigment molecules called *myoglobin* (mye-oh-GLOH-bin). This pigment contains iron groups that attract and temporarily bind with oxygen. When the oxygen levels inside the muscle fiber diminish, the oxygen can be resupplied from myoglobin. Muscle fibers that contain little myoglobin are called *white fibers.*

When muscles are contracting vigorously for long periods of time, myoglobin and the circulatory system are unable to deliver oxygen fast enough to maintain the aerobic pathways. Processes that do not require oxygen are necessary. Under these conditions, glucose is the primary energy source. If adequate oxygen is not available, glucose is broken down by a process called **anaerobic respiration** (Figure

8-3D). The products of the anaerobic pathway are lactic acid and a small amount of ATP.

$$\text{Glucose} \rightarrow \text{lactic acid} + \text{ATP}$$

Some of the lactic acid accumulates in the muscle and causes a burning sensation. Most of it diffuses out of the muscle and into the bloodstream, which takes it to the liver. Later, when sufficient oxygen is available, the liver converts the lactic acid back to glycogen, the storage form of glucose.

The aerobic pathway produces about 20 times more ATP than the anaerobic pathway. However, the anaerobic pathway provides ATP about two and one-half times faster than the aerobic pathway. Most of the energy for vigorous activity over a moderate period of time comes from anaerobic respiration. Prolonged activities requiring endurance depend on aerobic mechanisms.

After periods of strenuous exercise that require anaerobic mechanisms to regenerate ATP, there is an accumulation of lactic acid in the muscle. This causes temporary muscular pain and cramping. The ATP and creatine phosphate in the muscle are depleted and need to be replenished. This creates an **oxygen debt** that must be repaid before equilibrium can be restored. Additional oxygen is necessary to convert the lactic acid into glycogen, a process that occurs in the liver. Oxygen is also necessary to replenish the ATP and the creatine phosphate in the muscle. Oxygen debt is defined as the additional oxygen that is required after physical activity to restore resting conditions. The debt is paid back by labored breathing that continues after the activity has stopped.

Movements

Most intact skeletal muscles are attached to bones by tendons that span joints. When the muscle contracts, one bone (the insertion) moves relative to the other bone (the origin). Frequently muscles work in groups to perform a particular movement. If one muscle has a primary role in providing a movement, it is called a **prime mover.** Muscles that work with, or assist, the prime mover to cause a movement are called **synergists** (SIN-er-jists). Often muscles span more than one joint, and a synergist will stabilize one joint while the prime mover acts on the other joint. For example, the

Figure 8-3. Energy sources for muscle contraction. **A,** Initial source is adenosine triphosphate *(ATP)*. **B,** ATP is replenished by creatine phosphate.

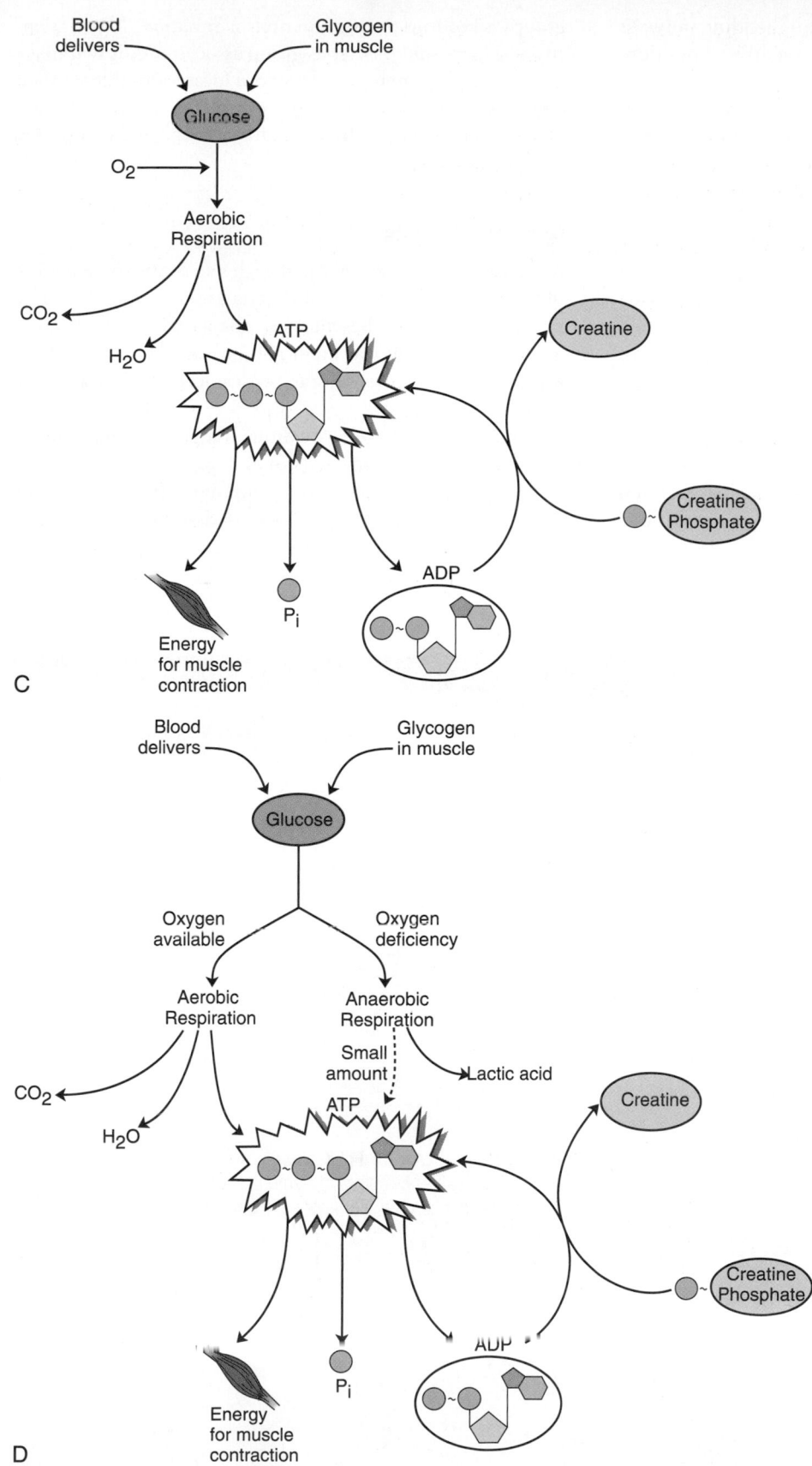

Figure 8-3, cont'd. C, Aerobic breakdown of glucose and fatty acids provides additional ATP. **D,** Vigorous activity may require the anaerobic breakdown of glucose, which produces lactic acid and ATP. *ADP,* Adenosine diphosphate. (From Applegate E: *The anatomy and physiology learning system,* ed 3, St. Louis, 2006, Saunders.)

fingers can be flexed to make a fist without bending the wrist because certain muscles fix the wrist in a stabilized position. **Antagonists** are muscles that oppose, or reverse, a particular movement. The biceps brachii muscle on the anterior arm flexes the forearm at the elbow. The triceps brachii muscle on the posterior arm extends the forearm at the elbow. The two muscles are on opposite sides of the humerus and have opposite functions. They are antagonists.

Bones and muscles work together to perform different types of movement at the various joints. When describing muscular action or movement at joints, you need a frame of reference and descriptive terminology with definite meaning. Some commonly used terms that are used to describe particular movements are defined in Table 8-2.

SKELETAL MUSCLE GROUPS

The body is composed of more than 600 skeletal muscles. A discussion of each muscle is certainly beyond the scope of this book. Only the more significant and obvious muscles are identified and described here. These are arranged in groups according to location and/or function. If you identify and learn the muscles as group associations, it will make them easier to remember. If you can locate a muscle on your own body, you will be able to contract the muscle and describe its action. Learning anatomy in this manner makes it more meaningful.

Naming Muscles

Most skeletal muscles have names that describe some feature of the muscle. Often several criteria are combined into one name. Associating the muscles' characteristics with their name will help you learn and remember them. The following are some terms relating to muscle features that are used in naming muscles:

- **Size:** vastus (huge); maximus (large); longus (long); minimus (small); brevis (short)
- **Shape:** deltoid (triangular); rhomboid (like a rhombus with equal and parallel sides); latissimus (wide); teres (round); trapezius (like a trapezoid, a four-sided figure with two sides parallel)

Table 8-2 Types of Body Movements	
Flexion (FLEK-shun)	**Dorsiflexion (dor-sih-FLEK-shun)**
Description: Means "to bend." Flexion usually brings two bones closer together and decreases the angle between them. Example: bending the elbow or the knee	*Description:* Flexion of the ankle in which the dorsum or top of the foot is lifted upward, decreasing the angle between the foot and leg. Example: standing on your heels
Extension (ek-STEN-shun)	**Plantar flexion (PLAN-tar FLEK-shun)**
Description: Means "to straighten." Extension is the opposite of flexion. It increases the angle between two bones. Example: straightening the elbow or the knee after it has been flexed	*Description:* Plantar flexion is movement at the ankle that increases the angle between the foot and leg. Example: standing on your toes

Table 8-2 Types of Body Movements—cont'd

Hyperextension (hye-per-ek-STEN-shun)
Description: Hyperextension occurs when a part of the body is extended beyond the anatomic position. The joint angle becomes greater than 180 degrees. Example: moving the head backward

Abduction (ab-DUCK-shun)
Description: Means "to take away." Abduction moves a bone or limb away from the midline or axis of the body. Examples: the outward movement of the legs in "jumping jacks," moving the arms away from the body, or spreading the fingers apart

Adduction (ad-DUCK-shun)
Description: Means "to bring together." Adduction is the opposite of abduction. It moves a bone or limb toward the midline of the body. Examples: bringing the arms back to the sides of the body after they have been abducted or moving the legs back to anatomic position after abduction

Circumduction (sir-kum-DUCK-shun)
Description: Circumduction is the conelike, circular movement of a body segment. The proximal end of the segment remains relatively stationary while the distal end outlines a large circle. Example: the movement of the arm at the shoulder joint, with the elbow extended, so that the tips of the fingers move in a large circle

Rotation (roh-TAY-shun)
Description: Rotation is the movement of a bone around its own axis in a pivot joint. Example: shaking your head "no"

Inversion (in-VER-zhun)
Description: Inversion is the movement of the sole of the foot inward or medially

Continued

Table 8-2 Types of Body Movements—cont'd

Supination (soo-pih-NAY-shun)
Description: Supination is a specialized rotation of the forearm that turns the palm of the hand forward or anteriorly. If the elbow is flexed, supination turns the palm of the hand upward or superiorly

Eversion (ee-VER-zhun)
Description: Eversion is the opposite of inversion. It is the movement of the sole of the foot outward or laterally

Pronation (proh-NAY-shun)
Description: Pronation is the opposite of supination. It is a specialized rotation of the forearm that turns the palm of the hand backward or posteriorly. If the elbow is flexed, pronation turns the palm of the hand downward or inferiorly

From Applegate E: *The anatomy and physiology learning system,* ed 3, St. Louis, 2006, Saunders.

- **Direction of fibers:** rectus (straight); transverse (across); oblique (diagonal); orbicularis (circular)
- **Location:** pectoralis (chest); gluteus (buttock or rump); brachii (arm); supra- (above); infra- (below); sub- (under or beneath); lateralis (lateral)
- **Number of origins:** biceps (two heads); triceps (three heads); quadriceps (four heads)
- **Origin and insertion:** sternocleidomastoid (origin on the sternum and clavicle, insertion on the mastoid process); brachioradialis (origin on the brachium or arm, insertion on the radius)
- **Action:** abductor (to abduct a structure); adductor (to adduct a structure); flexor (to flex a structure); extensor (to extend a structure); levator (to lift or elevate a structure); masseter (to chew)

Muscles of the Head and Neck

Muscles of Facial Expression

Humans have well-developed muscles in the face that permit a large variety of facial expressions. Because these muscles are used to show surprise, disgust, anger, fear, and other emotions, they are an important means of nonverbal communication. The following are some of the muscles used to produce facial expressions.

The **frontalis** (frun-TAL-is) is over the frontal bone of the forehead. It is attached to the soft tissue of the eyebrow; when it contracts, it raises the eyebrows and wrinkles the forehead. The **orbicularis oris** (oar-BIK-yoo-lair-is OAR-is) is a sphincter that encircles the mouth. This muscle is used to close the mouth, to form words, and to pucker the lips as in kissing. The **orbicularis oculi** (oar-BIK-yoo-lair-is OK-yoo-lye) is another sphincter but is around the eye (oculus). The actions of winking, blinking, and squinting use this muscle. The **buccinator** (BUCK-sin-ay-ter) is the principal muscle in the cheek area and is used to compress the cheek when whistling, sucking, or blowing air out. It is sometimes called the *trumpeter's muscle*. The **zygomaticus** (zye-goh-MAT-ih-kus) extends from the zygomatic arch to the corners of the mouth. It contracts to raise the corner of the mouth when we smile.

Muscles of Mastication

Four pairs of muscles are responsible for chewing movements or mastication. All of these muscles insert on the mandible, and they are some of the strongest muscles in the body. Two of the muscles, the **temporalis** (tem-poar-AL-is) and **masseter** (MASS-eh-ter), are superficial and are identified in Table 8-3 and Figure 8-4. The others, the lateral and medial pterygoids, are deep to the mandible and are not shown in the figure. The **temporalis** is the largest of the mastication muscles. As the name implies, it has its origin on the temporal bone. The **masseter** is located along the ramus of the mandible and is a synergist of the temporalis.

Table 8-3 Muscles of the Head and Neck

Muscle	Description	Origin	Insertion	Action
Muscles of Facial Expression				
Frontalis (frun-TAL-is)	Flat muscle that covers forehead	Galea aponeurotica	Skin of eyebrow and nose	Raises eyebrows
Orbicularis oris (oar-BIK-yoo-lair-is OAR-is)	Circular muscle around mouth	Maxilla and mandible	Skin around lips	Closes and purses lips
Orbicularis oculi (oar-BIK-yoo-lair-is OK-yoo-lye)	Circular muscle around eyes	Maxilla and frontal bones	Tissue of eyelid	Closes eye; winking, blinking, squinting
Buccinator (BUK-sin-ay-ter)	Horizontal cheek muscle; deep to masseter	Maxilla and mandible	Corner of mouth	Compresses cheek; trumpeter's muscle
Zygomaticus (zye-goh-MAT-ih-kus)	Extends diagonally from corner of mouth to cheekbone	Zygomatic bone	Skin and muscle at corner of mouth	Elevates corner of mouth as in smiling
Muscles of Mastication				
Temporalis (tem-por-AL-is)	Flat, fan-shaped muscle over temporal bone	Flat portion of temporal bone	Mandible	Closes jaw
Masseter (MASS-eh-ter)	Covers lateral aspect of jaw	Zygomatic arch	Mandible	Closes jaw
Neck Muscles				
Sternocleidomastoid (stir-noh-klye-doh MAS-toyd)	Straplike muscle that ascends obliquely over neck	Sternum and clavicle	Mastoid process	Flexes and rotates head
Trapezius (trah-PEEZ-ee-us)	Large, flat, triangular muscle on posterior neck and shoulder	Occipital bone and spines of thoracic vertebrae	Scapula	Extends head; also moves scapula

From Applegate E: *The anatomy and physiology learning system,* ed 3, St. Louis, 2006, Saunders.

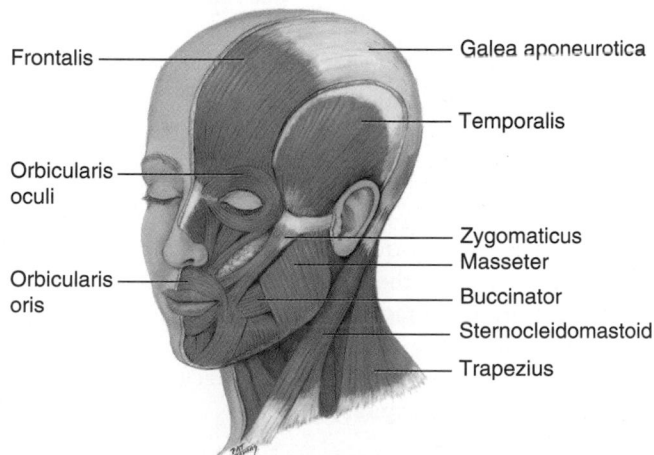

Frontalis

Galea aponeurotica

Temporalis

Orbicularis oculi

Orbicularis oris

Zygomaticus

Masseter

Buccinator

Sternocleidomastoid

Trapezius

Figure 8-4. Muscles of the head and neck. (From Applegate E: *The anatomy and physiology learning system,* ed 3, St. Louis, 2006, Saunders.)

Neck Muscles

Only two of the more obvious and superficial neck muscles are considered here. Numerous muscles are associated with the throat, hyoid bone, and vertebral column, a discussion of which is beyond the scope of this text.

Sternocleidomastoid (stir-no-klye-doh-MAS-toyd) muscles ascend obliquely across the anterior neck from the sternum and clavicle to the mastoid process. When both of

these muscles contract together, the neck is flexed and the head is bent toward the chest. When one of the muscles contracts, the head turns toward the direction opposite the side that is contracting. When the left muscle contracts, the head turns to the right. A portion of the **trapezius** (trah-PEEZ-ee-us) muscle is in the neck region and moves the head. Each trapezius muscle extends from the occipital bone at the base of the skull to the end of the thoracic vertebrae and also inserts on the scapula laterally. A portion of this muscle functions to extend the head and is antagonistic to the sternocleidomastoid.

Muscles of the Trunk

The muscles of the trunk (Table 8-4) include those that move the vertebral column, the muscles that form the thoracic and abdominal walls, and those that cover the pelvic outlet.

Vertebral Column Muscles

The **erector spinae** (ee-REK-ter SPY-nee) group of muscles on each side of the vertebral column is a large muscle mass that extends from the sacrum to the skull. These muscles are primarily responsible for extending the vertebral column to maintain erect posture. Muscle contraction on only one side bends the vertebral column to that side. The **deep back muscles** occupy the space between the spinous and transverse processes of adjacent vertebrae. Each individual muscle is short, but as a group the muscles extend the length

Table 8-4 Muscles of the Trunk

Muscle	Description	Origin	Insertion	Action
Muscles That Move the Vertebral Column				
Erector spinae (ee-REK-ter SPY-nee)	Intrinsic back muscles on each side of vertebral column	Vertebrae	Superior vertebrae and ribs	Extends vertebral column
Deep back muscles	Short, intrinsic muscles in space between spinous and transverse processes of vertebrae	Vertebrae	Vertebrae	Move vertebral column
Muscles of the Thoracic Wall				
External intercostals (inter-KOS-talz)	Short muscles in intercostal spaces between ribs	Ribs	Next rib below origin	Inspiration
Internal intercostals (inter-KOS-talz)	Short muscles in intercostal spaces between ribs	Ribs	Next rib above origin	Forced expiration
Diaphragm (DYE-ah-fram)	Dome-shaped muscle that forms partition between thorax and abdomen	Interior body wall	Central tendon of diaphragm	Inspiration
Abdominal Wall Muscles				
External oblique (ek-STIR-null oh-BLEEK)	Largest and most superficial of lateral abdominal wall muscles	Rib cage	Iliac crest and fascia	Compresses abdomen
Internal oblique (in-TER-null oh-BLEEK)	Underlies external oblique; fibers perpendicular to external oblique	Iliac crest and fascia	Lower ribs and fascia	Compresses abdomen
Transversus abdominis (trans-VER-sus ab-DOM-ih-nis)	Deepest muscles of abdominal wall; fibers run horizontally	Fascia and lower ribs	Linea alba and pubis	Compresses abdomen
Rectus abdominis (REK-tus ab-DOM-ih-nis)	Long, straight muscle on each side of linea alba	Pubic bone	Ribs and sternum	Flexes vertebral column and compresses abdomen
Muscles of the Pelvic Outlet				
Pelvic diaphragm; primarily levator ani muscle	Superior (deep) muscle hammock that forms floor of pelvic cavity	Pubis and ischium	Sacrum and coccyx	Supports and maintains position of pelvic viscera
Urogenital diaphragm	Superficial to pelvic diaphragm; between two sides of pubic arch	Ischium and genitalia	Genitalia and perineum	Supports pelvic viscera and assists in function of genitalia

From Applegate E: *The anatomy and physiology learning system*, ed 3, St. Louis, 2006, Saunders.

of the vertebral column. They are responsible for several movements of the vertebral column.

Thoracic Wall Muscles

The muscles of the thoracic wall (Figure 8-5) are involved primarily in the process of breathing. The intercostal muscles are located in spaces between the ribs. Fibers of the **external intercostal muscles** are directed forward and downward, whereas those of the **internal intercostals** are directed backward and downward. The internal intercostal fibers are at right angles to the external intercostal fibers. External intercostal muscles contract to elevate the ribs during the inspiration phase of breathing. The internal intercostals contract during forced expiration.

The **diaphragm** is a dome-shaped muscle that forms a partition between the thorax and the abdomen. It has three openings in it for structures that have to pass from the thorax to the abdomen. One opening is for the inferior vena cava, one is for the esophagus, and one is for the aorta. The diaphragm is responsible for the major movement in the

thoracic cavity during quiet, relaxed breathing. When the diaphragm contracts, the dome is flattened. This increases the volume of the thoracic cavity and results in inspiration. When the muscle relaxes, it again resumes its dome shape and decreases the volume of the thoracic cavity, which forces air out during expiration.

Abdominal Wall Muscles

The abdomen, unlike the thorax and pelvis, has no bony reinforcements or protection. The wall consists entirely of four muscle pairs, arranged in layers, and the fascia that envelops them (Figure 8-6). The aponeuroses of the muscles on opposite sides meet in the anterior midline to form the **linea alba** ("white line"), a band of connective tissue that extends from the sternum to the pubic symphysis. The outer muscle layer is the **external oblique** with fibers that run inferiorly and medially. With fibers oriented perpendicularly to the external oblique, the **internal oblique** lies just underneath it. The deepest layer of muscle is the **transversus abdominis** with its fibers running in a

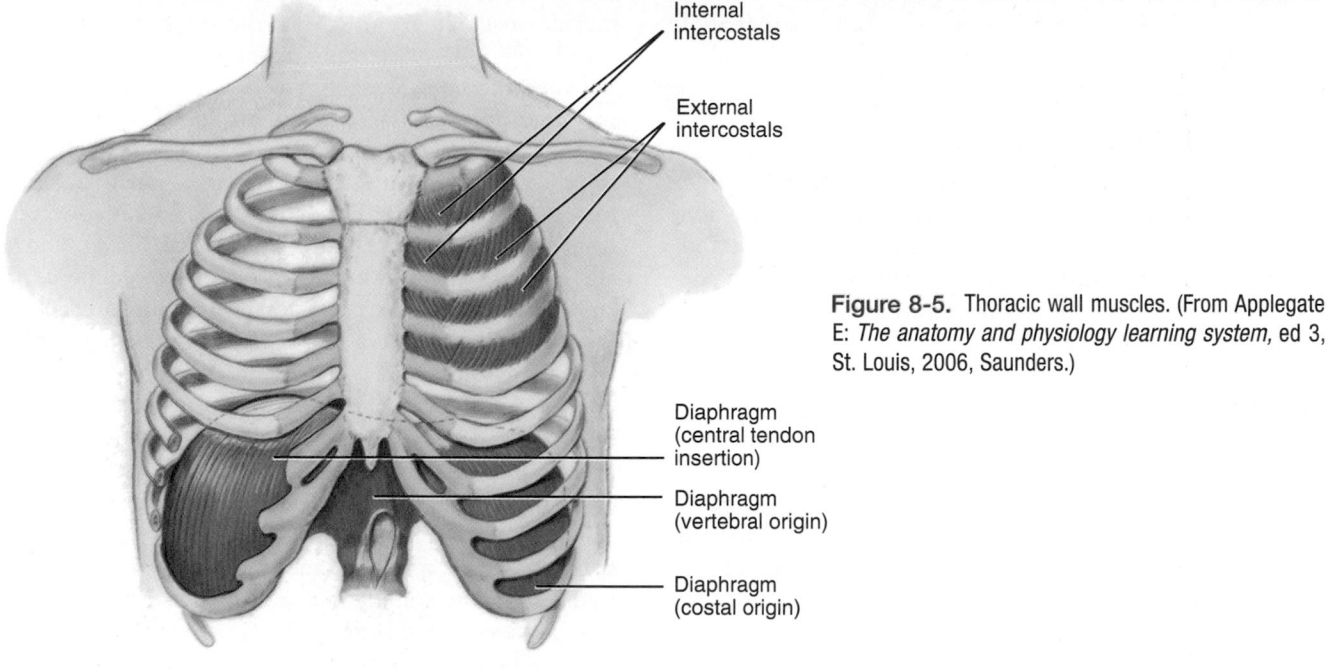

Figure 8-5. Thoracic wall muscles. (From Applegate E: *The anatomy and physiology learning system,* ed 3, St. Louis, 2006, Saunders.)

Internal intercostals

External intercostals

Diaphragm (central tendon insertion)

Diaphragm (vertebral origin)

Diaphragm (costal origin)

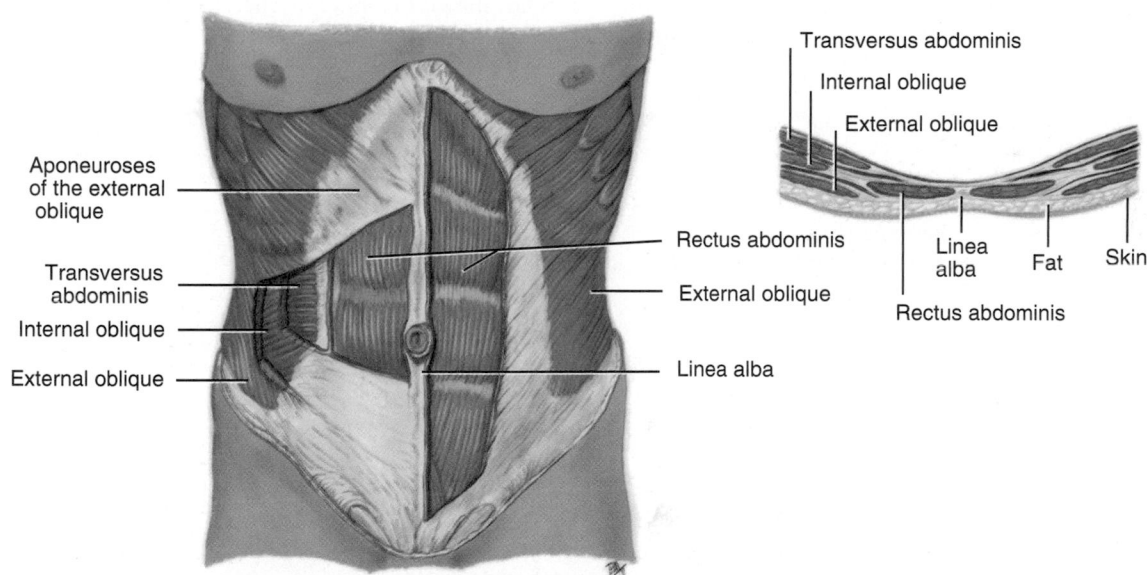

Aponeuroses of the external oblique

Transversus abdominis

Internal oblique

External oblique

Rectus abdominis

External oblique

Linea alba

Transversus abdominis

Internal oblique

External oblique

Linea alba   Fat   Skin

Rectus abdominis

Figure 8-6. Abdominal wall muscles. (From Applegate E: *The anatomy and physiology learning system,* ed 3, St. Louis, 2006, Saunders.)

horizontal direction. The arrangement of the muscle layers with the fibers in each layer going in different directions is similar to the type of construction found in plywood and adds strength to the anterolateral abdominal wall. The fascia of these muscles extends anteriorly to form a broad aponeurosis along much of the anterior aspect of the abdomen. The fascia also envelops the **rectus abdominis** muscle that runs vertically from the pubic bones to the ribs and the sternum on each side of the midline. All of these muscles compress the abdominal wall and increase intraabdominal pressure. The rectus abdominis also flexes the vertebral column.

Pelvic Floor Muscles

The pelvic outlet is formed by two muscular sheets and their associated fascia. The deeper or more superior muscular sheet is the **pelvic diaphragm,** which forms the floor of the pelvic cavity. Most of the pelvic diaphragm is formed by the two **levator ani** muscles that support the pelvic viscera. They resist increased pressure in the abdominopelvic cavity and thus play a role in the control of the urinary bladder and rectum. The superficial muscle group, the **urogenital diaphragm,** fills the space within the pubic arch and is associated with the genitalia.

Muscles of the Upper Extremity

The muscles of the upper extremity include those that attach the scapula to the thorax and generally move the scapula, those that attach the humerus to the scapula and generally move the arm, and those that are located in the arm or forearm and move the forearm, wrist, and hand (Table 8-5 and Figure 8-7).

Muscles That Move the Shoulder and Arm

The **trapezius** and **serratus anterior** (seh-RAY-tus anterior) are two of the muscles that attach the scapula to the axial skeleton. The trapezius is a large superficial triangular muscle of the back. It is attached to the thoracic vertebrae and the scapula. When the trapezius contracts, it adducts and elevates the scapula, as in shrugging the shoulders. The serratus anterior is located on the side of the chest where it runs from the ribs to the scapula. When the serratus anterior contracts, it pulls the shoulder downward and forward, as in pushing something.

Both the **pectoralis major** (pek-tor-AL-iss MAY-jer) and the **latissimus dorsi** (lah-TISS-ih-mus DOR-sye) muscles attach the humerus to the axial skeleton. The pectoralis major is a superficial muscle on the anterior chest. It has a broad origin on the sternum, costal cartilages, and clavicle, but then the fibers converge to insert on the humerus by way of a short tendon. The primary function of the pectoralis major is to adduct and rotate the arm medially across the chest. The latissimus dorsi is a large, superficial muscle located in the lower back region. It has an extensive origin from the spines of the thoracic vertebrae, ilium, and ribs and then extends upward to insert on the humerus. The latissimus dorsi adducts and rotates the arm medially and lowers the shoulder. It is an important muscle in swimming and rowing motions.

The **deltoid** is a large, fleshy muscle that covers the shoulder and attaches the humerus to the scapula. This muscle abducts the arm to a horizontal position. It is a common site for administering intramuscular injections. Another group of four muscles, the **infraspinatus, supraspinatus, subscapularis,** and **teres minor,** attaches the humerus to the scapula and moves the humerus in some way. These muscles, collectively, are called the **rotator cuff muscles** because they form a cuff or cap over the proximal humerus. A rotator cuff injury involves damage to one or more of these muscles or their tendons. The subscapularis is not shown in Figure 8-7 because it is on the costal surface of the scapula and not visible.

Table 8-5 Muscles of the Upper Extremity

Muscle	Description	Origin	Insertion	Action
Muscles That Move the Shoulder and Arm				
Trapezius (trah-PEEZ-ee-us)	Triangular muscle on posterior neck and shoulder; right and left trapezius together form trapezoid	Occipital bone and vertebrae	Scapula	Adducts, elevates, and rotates scapula; also extends head
Serratus anterior (seh-RAY-tus anterior)	Deep and inferior to pectoral muscles; forms medial wall of axilla; has serrated appearance	Ribs	Medial border of scapula	Pulls scapula anteriorly and downward
Pectoralis major (pek-tor-AL-iss MAY-jer)	Large, fan-shaped muscle that covers anterior chest	Sternum, clavicle, ribs	Humerus	Adducts and flexes arm across the chest
Latissimus dorsi (lah-TISS-ih-mus DOAR-sye)	Large, broad, flat muscle of lower back region; swimmer's muscle	Vertebrae	Humerus	Adducts and medially rotates arm
Deltoid (DELL-toyd)	Thick muscle that forms contour of shoulder	Clavicle and scapula	Humerus	Abducts arm
Rotator cuff	Group of four muscles that attach humerus to scapula and form cap or cuff over proximal humerus	Scapula	Humerus	Rotates arm
Muscles That Move the Forearm and Hand				
Triceps brachii (TRY-seps BRAY-kee-eye)	Only muscle in posterior compartment of arm; has three heads of origin	Humerus and scapula	Olecranon of ulna	Extends forearm
Biceps brachii (BY-seps BRAY-kee-eye)	Major muscle in anterior compartment of arm; has two heads of origin	Scapula	Radius	Flexes and supinates forearm
Brachialis (bray-kee-AL-is)	Strong muscle deep to biceps brachii in anterior compartment of arm	Humerus	Ulna	Flexes forearm
Brachioradialis (bray-kee-oh-ray-dee-AL-is)	Superficial muscle on lateral forearm	Distal humerus	Distal radius	Flexes forearm

From Applegate E: *The anatomy and physiology learning system,* ed 3, St. Louis, 2006, Saunders.

Muscles That Move the Forearm and Hand

The muscles that move the forearm are located along the humerus. The arm is divided into anterior and posterior muscle compartments. The **triceps brachii,** the primary extensor of the forearm, is the only muscle in the posterior compartment. As the name implies, it has three heads of origin. The anterior muscle compartment contains the **biceps brachii** and **brachialis** (bray-kee-AL-is). These muscles are the primary flexors of the forearm. In addition, the **brachioradialis** (bray-kee-oh-ray-dee-AL-is), a prominent muscle along the lateral side of the forearm, helps to flex the forearm. The brachioradialis extends from the lower part of the humerus to the radius and is generally considered to be a posterior forearm muscle.

The 20 or more muscles that cause most wrist, hand, and finger movements are located along the forearm. These muscles are divided into anterior and posterior compartments. Most of the anterior compartment muscles flex the wrist and fingers, whereas the posterior muscles cause extension.

Muscles of the Lower Extremity

The muscles of the lower extremity include those that are located in the hip region and generally move the thigh, those that are located in the thigh and move the leg, and those that are located in the leg and move the ankle and foot (Table 8-6).

Muscles That Move the Thigh

The muscles that move the thigh have their origins on some part of the pelvic girdle and their insertions on the femur. The largest muscle mass belongs to the posterior group, the

Deltoid

Biceps
brachii

Serratus
anterior

Brachioradialis

Tensor
fasciae latae

Sartorius

Gastrocnemius

Tibialis anterior

Soleus

Trapezius

Pectoralis major

Brachialis

Linea alba

External
abdominal
oblique

Iliopsoas

Adductor
longus

Adductor
magnus

Gracilis

Vastus medialis

Rectus femoris

Vastus lateralis

Figure 8-7. General overview of body musculature: **A,** Anterior view.

Continued

A

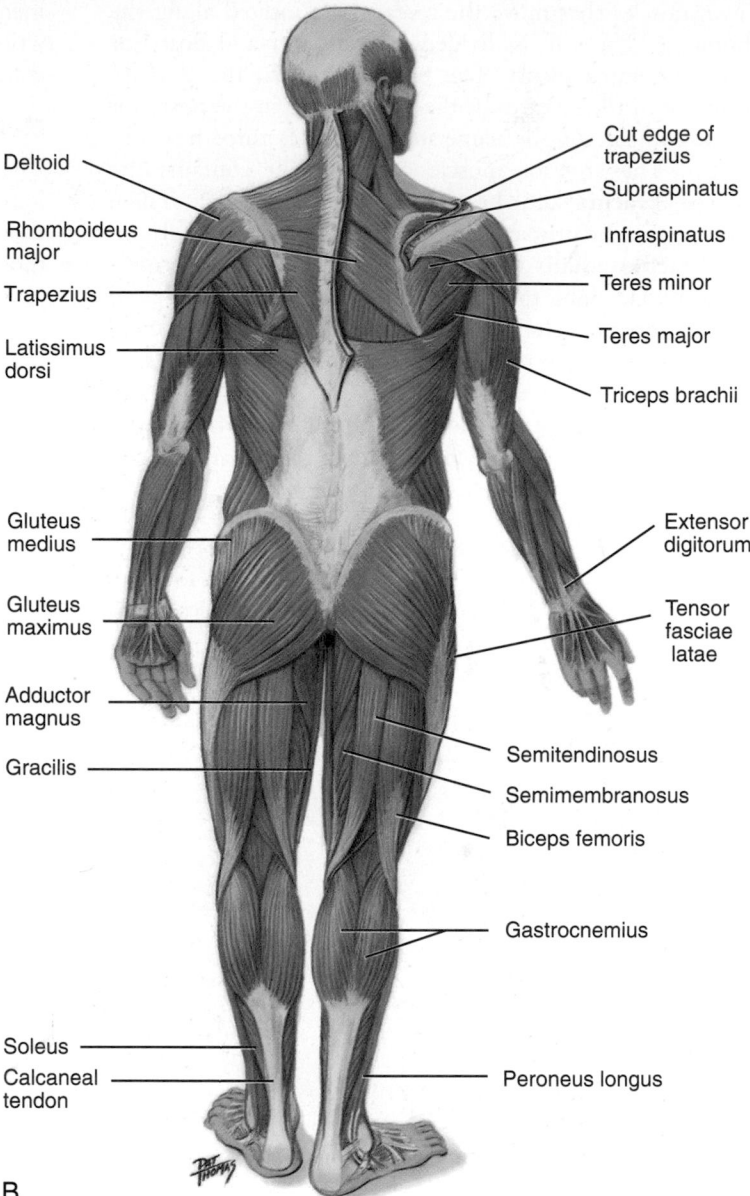

Figure 8-7, cont'd. **B,** Posterior view. (From Applegate E: *The anatomy and physiology learning system,* ed 3, St. Louis, 2006, Saunders.)

gluteal muscles. The **gluteus maximus** forms the area of the buttocks. The **gluteus medius,** a common site for intramuscular injections, is superior and deep to the gluteus maximus. The **gluteus minimus** is the smallest and deepest of the gluteal muscles. It is not illustrated in Figure 8-7. Although the **tensor fasciae latae** (TEN-soar FAH-she-ee LAY-tee) is a superficial muscle on the lateral side of the thigh, its function and innervation associate it with the gluteal muscles. These muscles abduct the thigh; that is, they raise the thigh sideways to a horizontal position. The gluteus maximus also extends or straightens the thigh at the hip for walking or climbing stairs.

The anterior muscle that moves the thigh is the **iliopsoas** (ill-ee-oh-SOH-as). This muscle is formed from the iliacus that originates on the iliac fossa and the psoas that originates on the lumbar vertebrae. The fibers converge into the ilio-

psoas and insert on the femur. The iliopsoas flexes the thigh, making it antagonistic to the gluteus maximus.

The medial muscles adduct the thigh; that is, they press the thighs together. This group includes the **adductor longus, adductor brevis, adductor magnus,** and **gracilis** (grah-SILL-is) muscles. The adductor brevis is not illustrated in Figure 8-7 because it is deep to the adductor longus.

Muscles That Move the Leg

Muscles that move the leg are located in the thigh region. The **quadriceps femoris** (KWAHD-rih-seps FEM-oar-is) includes four muscles that are on the anterior and lateral sides of the thigh, namely, the **vastus lateralis, vastus intermedius, vastus medialis,** and **rectus femoris.** As a group, these muscles are the primary extensors of the leg, straight-

Table 8-6 Muscles of the Lower Extremity

Muscle	Description	Origin	Insertion	Action
Muscles That Move the Thigh				
Iliopsoas (ill-ee-oh-SOH-as)	Composite of iliacus and psoas muscles; located in groin	Iliac fossa and vertebrae	Femur	Flexes and rotates thigh
Tensor fasciae latae (TEN-soar FAH-she-ee LAY-tee)	Most lateral muscle in hip region	Anterior ilium	Tibia by way of iliotibial tract	Flexes and abducts thigh; synergist of iliopsoas
Gluteus maximus (GLOO-tee-us MAK-sih-mus)	Largest and most superficial of gluteal muscles	Ilium, sacrum, and coccyx	Femur	Extends thigh; antagonist of iliopsoas
Gluteus medius (GLOO-tee-us MEE-dee-us)	Thick muscle deep to gluteus maximus; common site for intramuscular injections	Ilium	Femur	Abducts and rotates thigh
Gluteus minimus (GLOO-tee-us MIN-ih-mus)	Smallest and deepest of gluteal muscles	Ilium	Femur	Abducts and rotates thigh
Adductor longus (ad-DUCK-toar LONG-us)	Most anterior of adductor muscles in medial compartment of thigh	Pubis	Femur	Adducts thigh
Adductor brevis (ad-DUCK-toar BREH-vis)	Short adductor muscle deep to adductor longus	Pubis	Femur	Adducts thigh
Adductor magnus (ad-DUCK-toar MAG-nus)	Largest and deepest of adductor muscles	Pubis	Femur	Adducts thigh
Gracilis (grah-SILL-is)	Long, superficial, straplike muscle on medial aspect of thigh	Pubis	Tibia	Adducts thigh; flexes leg
Muscles That Move the Leg				
Sartorius (sar-TOAR-ee-us)	Long, straplike muscle that courses obliquely across thigh; longest muscle in body	Ilium	Tibia	Flexes thigh; flexes and rotates leg

Quadriceps femoris (KWAHD-rih-seps FEM-oar-is)
  Rectus femoris (REK-tus FEM-oar-is)
  Vastus lateralis (VASS-tus lat-er-AL-is)
  Vastus medialis (VASS-tus mee-dee-AL-is)
  Vastus intermedius (VASS-tus in-ter-MEE-dee-us)
	Group of four muscles that form fleshy mass of anterior thigh; form a common tendon that passes over patella	Femur; except for rectus femoris, which originates on ilium	Tibial tuberosity, by way of patellar tendon	Extends leg; rectus femoris also flexes thigh

Hamstrings
  Biceps femoris (BYE-seps FEM-oar-is)
  Semimembranosus (sem-ee-MEM-brah-noh-sus)
  Semitendinosus (sem-ee-TEN-dih-noh-sus)
	Large, fleshy muscle mass in posterior thigh	Ischium; one head of biceps femoris arises from femur	Biceps femoris inserts on fibula; others on tibia	Flexes leg and extends thigh; antagonist to quadriceps femoris

Muscles That Move the Ankle and Foot				
Tibialis anterior (tib-ee-AL-is an-TEAR-ee-or)	Superficial muscle of anterior leg	Tibia	Medial cuneiform and first metatarsal	Dorsiflexes foot
Gastrocnemius (gas-trok-NEE mee-us)	Superficial muscle on posterior surface of leg; forms curve of calf	Femur	Calcaneus by way of Achilles tendon	Plantar flexes foot
Soleus (SOH-lee-us)	Deep to gastrocnemius on posterior leg; has a common tendon for insertion with gastrocnemius	Tibia and fibula	Calcaneus by way of Achilles tendon	Plantar flexes foot
Peroneus (pear-oh-NEE-us)	Forms lateral compartment of leg	Tibia and fibula	Tarsals and metatarsals	Plantar flexes and everts foot

From Applegate E: *The anatomy and physiology learning system,* ed 3, St. Louis, 2006, Saunders.

ening the leg at the knee. The vastus intermedius is deep to the rectus femoris and is not illustrated. The other muscle on the anterior surface of the thigh is the long, straplike **sartorius** (sar-TOAR-ee-us) that passes obliquely over the quadriceps group. The sartorius, the longest muscle in the body, flexes and medially rotates the leg when you sit cross-legged.

The posterior thigh muscles are called the **hamstrings,** and they are used to flex the leg at the knee. All have origins on the ischium and insert on the tibia. Because these muscles extend over the hip joint, as well as over the knee joint, they also extend the thigh. The strong tendons of these muscles can be felt behind the knee. These same tendons are present in hogs, and butchers used them to hang the hams for smoking and curing, so they were called "ham strings." The hamstring muscles are the **biceps femoris, semimembranosus** (sem-ee-MEM-brah-noh-sus), and **semitendinosus** (sem-ee-TEN-dih-noh-sus). A "pulled hamstring" is a tear in one or more of these muscles or their tendons.

Muscles That Move the Ankle and Foot

The muscles located in the leg that move the ankle and foot are divided into anterior, posterior, and lateral compartments. The **tibialis anterior** is the primary muscle in the anterior group. Contraction of the muscles in the anterior group, including the tibialis anterior, causes dorsiflexion of the foot. **Peroneus** (pear-oh-NEE-us) muscles occupy the lateral compartment of the leg. Contraction of these muscles everts the foot and also helps in plantar flexion. The **gastrocnemius** (gas-trok-NEE-mee-us) and **soleus** (SOH-lee-us) are the major muscles in the posterior compartment. These two muscles form the fleshy mass in the calf of the leg. They have a common tendon called the **calcaneal tendon** or **Achilles tendon.** These muscles are strong plantar flexors of the foot. They are sometimes called the *toe dancer's muscles* because they allow you to stand on tiptoe. Numerous other deep muscles in the leg cause flexion and extension of the toes.

TERMINOLOGY REVIEW

Antagonist A muscle that has an action opposite to the prime mover.

Insertion The end of a muscle that is attached to a relatively movable part; the end opposite the origin.

Motor unit A single neuron and all the muscle fibers it stimulates.

Neuromuscular junction The area of communication between the axon terminal of a motor neuron and the sarcolemma of a muscle fiber; also called a *myoneural junction.*

Neurotransmitter A chemical substance that is released at the axon terminals to stimulate a muscle fiber contraction or an impulse in another neuron.

Origin The end of a muscle that is attached to a relatively immovable part; the end opposite the insertion.

Prime mover The muscle that is mainly responsible for a particular body movement; also called *agonist.*

Synergist A muscle that assists a prime mover but is not capable of producing the movement by itself.

ON THE WEB

For Information on Muscles and Joints:

Merck Manual: Musculoskeletal Disorders: www.merck.com/mmpe/sec04.html

University of Wisconsin Medical School: Anatomy Dissections: www.anatomy.wisc.edu/courses/gross/index.html

San Diego State University College of Sciences: Actin Myosin Crossbridges: www.sci.sdsu.edu/movies/actin_myosin_gif.html

Science Animations: science.nhmccd.edu/biol/animatio.htm

Skeletal Muscles of the Human Body: ptcentral.com/muscles

Loyola University Medical Education Network: Master Muscle List: www.meddean.luc.edu/lumen/meded/grossanatomy/dissector/mml/index.htm

Gateway Community College: Muscles Tutorial: www.gwc.maricopa.edu/class/bio201/muscle/mustut.htm

University of Washington: Upper Extremity Muscle Atlas: www.rad.washington.edu/atlas

University of Washington: Lower Extremity Muscle Atlas: www.rad.washington.edu/atlas2

Skeleton: The Joints: www.zoology.ubc.ca/%7Ebiomania/tutorial/bonejt/outline.htm

PREPARE FOR CERTIFICATION   Visit the Evolve site at http://evolve.elsevier.com/Bonewit/today/ to actively Prepare for your Certification.

*Check out the **Companion CD** bound with the book to access additional interactive activities.*

9

Nervous System

CAAHEP COMPETENCIES

Content Competencies
Anatomy and Physiology
- Anatomy and physiology of all body systems

- Common pathology/diseases
- Diagnostic/treatment modalities

ABHES COMPETENCIES

Content Competencies
Anatomy and Physiology
- Anatomy and physiology

- Study of diseases and etiology
- All body systems
- Diagnostic/treatment modalities

KEY TERMS

action potential (ACK-shun po-TEN-shall)
brain stem (BRAYN STEM)
cerebellum (sair-eh-BELL-um)
cerebrum (se-REE-brum)
diencephalon (dye-en-SEF-ah-lon)

myelin (MY-eh-lin)
neurilemma (noo-rih-LEM-mah)
saltatory conduction (SAL-tah-toar-ee kon-DUCK-shun)
synapse (SIN-aps)
threshold stimulus (THRESH-hold STIM-yoo-lus)

Introduction to the Nervous System

The nervous system is the major controlling, regulatory, and communicating system in the body. It is the center of all mental activity, including thought, learning, and memory. Together with the endocrine system, the nervous system is responsible for regulating and maintaining homeostasis. Through its receptors, the nervous system keeps us in touch with our environment, both external and internal.

Like other systems in the body, the nervous system is composed of organs, principally the brain, spinal cord, nerves, and ganglia. These, in turn, consist of various tissues, including nerve, blood, and connective tissues. Together these carry out the complex activities of the nervous system.

FUNCTIONS OF THE NERVOUS SYSTEM

The various activities of the nervous system can be grouped together as three general functions:
- Sensory functions
- Integrative functions
- Motor functions

Together these functions keep us in touch with our environments, maintain homeostasis, and account for thought, learning, and memory.

Millions of sensory receptors detect changes, called *stimuli,* that occur inside and outside the body. They monitor such things as temperature, light, and sound from the external environment. Inside the body, the internal environment, receptors detect variations in pressure, pH, carbon dioxide concentration, and the levels of various electrolytes. All of this gathered information is called **sensory input.**

Sensory input is converted into electrical signals called *nerve impulses* that are transmitted to the brain. In the brain the signals are brought together to create sensations, produce thoughts, or add to memory. Decisions are made each moment on the basis of sensory input. This is called **integration.**

Based on the sensory input and integration, the nervous system responds by sending signals to muscles, causing them to contract, or to glands, causing them to produce secretions. Muscles and glands are called **effectors** because they cause an effect in response to directions from the nervous system. This is the **motor output** or **motor function.**

ORGANIZATION OF THE NERVOUS SYSTEM

There is really only one nervous system in the body, although terminology seems to indicate otherwise. Although each subdivision of the system is also called a "nervous system," all of these smaller systems belong to the single, highly integrated nervous system. Each subdivision has structural and functional characteristics that distinguish it from the others. The nervous system as a whole is divided into two subdivisions: the **central nervous system** (CNS) and the **peripheral nervous system** (PNS) (Figure 9-1).

Central Nervous System

The **brain** and **spinal cord** are the organs of the **central nervous system.** Because they are so vitally important, the brain and spinal cord, located in the dorsal body cavity, are encased in bone for protection. The brain is in the cranial vault, and the spinal cord is in the vertebral canal of the vertebral column. Although considered to be two separate organs, the brain and spinal cord are continuous at the foramen magnum.

Peripheral Nervous System

The organs of the **peripheral nervous system** are the **nerves** and **ganglia.** Nerves are bundles of nerve fibers, much like muscles are bundles of muscle fibers. Cranial nerves (12 pairs) and spinal nerves (31 pairs) extend from the CNS to peripheral organs, such as muscles and glands. Ganglia are collections, or small knots, of nerve cell bodies outside the CNS.

The PNS is further subdivided into an **afferent (sensory) division** and an **efferent (motor) division.** The afferent or sensory division transmits impulses from peripheral organs to the CNS. The efferent or motor division transmits impulses from the CNS out to the peripheral organs to cause an effect or action.

Highlight on Conditions Affecting the Nervous System

Amyotrophic lateral sclerosis (a-my-oh-TROF-ick LAT-er-al sclair-OH-sis) A neurologic disease caused by degeneration of motor neurons of the spinal cord, medulla, and cortex; marked by progressive muscular weakness and atrophy with spasticity and exaggerated reflexes; mental capabilities are not impaired; also called *Lou Gehrig disease* or *motor neuron disease*

Bell's palsy (BELL'S PAUL-zee) Neuropathy of the seventh cranial nerve (facial) that causes paralysis of the muscles on one side of the face with sagging of the mouth on the affected side of the face

Cerebral concussion (seh-REE-brull kon-KUSH-un) Loss of consciousness as the result of a blow to the head; usually clears within 24 hours; no evidence of permanent structural damage to the brain tissue

Cerebral contusion (seh-REE-brull kon-TOO-shun) Bruising of brain tissue as a result of direct trauma to the head; neurologic problems persist longer than 24 hours

Cerebral palsy (seh-REE-brull PAWL-zee) Partial paralysis and lack of muscular coordination caused by damage to the cerebrum during fetal life, birth, or infancy

Cerebrovascular accident (CVA) (seh-ree-broh-VAS-kyoo-lar AK-sih-dent) Most common brain disorder; may be due to decreased blood supply to the brain or rupture of a blood vessel in the brain; commonly called a *stroke*

Multiple sclerosis (MS) (MULL-tih-pull skler-OH-sis) A disorder in which there is progressive destruction of the myelin sheaths of central nervous system neurons, interfering with their ability to transmit impulses; characterized by progressive loss of function interspersed with periods of remission; cause is unknown and there is no satisfactory treatment

Reye's syndrome (RS) (RIZ SIN-drohm) Brain dysfunction that occurs primarily in children and teenagers and is characterized by edema of the brain that leads to disorientation, lethargy, and personality changes and may progress to a coma; seems to occur after chickenpox and influenza, and taking aspirin is a risk factor

Shingles (SHING-gulls) Viral disease affecting peripheral nerves; characterized by blisters and pain spread over the skin in a bandlike pattern that follows the affected nerves; caused by the same herpesvirus that causes chickenpox

Tic douloureux (TICK doo-loo-ROO) A painful disorder of the fifth cranial nerve (trigeminal) that is characterized by sudden, intense, sharp pain in the face and forehead on the affected side; also known as *trigeminal neuralgia*

Transient ischemic attack (TIA) (TRANS-ee-ent iss-KEE-mik ah-TACK) An episode of temporary cerebral dysfunction caused by impaired blood flow to the brain; the onset is sudden, is of short duration, and leaves no long-lasting neurologic impairment; common causes are blood clots and atherosclerosis ∎

Finally, the efferent or motor division is again subdivided into the **somatic nervous system** and the **autonomic nervous system.** The somatic nervous system, also called *somatomotor* or *somatic efferent,* supplies motor impulses to the skeletal muscles. Because these nerves permit conscious control of the skeletal muscles, the somatic nervous system is sometimes called the **voluntary nervous system.** The autonomic nervous system, also called *visceral efferent,* supplies motor impulses to cardiac muscle, smooth muscle, and glandular epithelium. It is further subdivided into **sympathetic** and **parasympathetic** divisions. Because the autonomic nervous system regulates involuntary or automatic functions, it is sometimes called the **involuntary nervous system.**

NERVE TISSUE

Although the nervous system is complex, there are only two main types of cells in nerve tissue. The actual nerve cell is the **neuron.** It is the "conducting" cell that transmits impulses. It is the structural unit of the nervous system. The other type of cell is the **neuroglia,** or **glial,** cell. The word *neuroglia* means "nerve glue." These cells are nonconductive and provide a support system for the neurons. They are a special type of "connective tissue" for the nervous system.

Neurons

Neurons, or nerve cells, carry out the functions of the nervous system by conducting nerve impulses. They are highly specialized and amitotic. This means that if a neuron is destroyed, it cannot be replaced because neurons do not undergo mitosis.

Each neuron has three basic parts:
- Cell body
- One or more dendrites
- A single axon

Figure 9-2 illustrates a typical neuron. The main part of the neuron is the **cell body** or **soma.** In many ways, the cell body is similar to other types of cells. It has a nucleus with at least one nucleolus and contains many of the typical cytoplasmic organelles. It lacks centrioles, however. Because centrioles function in cell division, the fact that neurons lack these organelles is consistent with the amitotic nature of the cell.

Dendrites and **axons** are cytoplasmic extensions, or processes, that project from the cell body. They are sometimes referred to as **fibers.** Dendrites are usually, but not always, short and branching, which increases their surface area to receive signals from other neurons. The number of dendrites on a neuron varies. They are called *afferent processes* because they transmit impulses to the neuron cell body. Only one axon projects from each cell body. It is usually

Highlight on the Nervous System

BRAIN TUMORS: Because neurons are not capable of mitosis, primary malignant tumors of the brain are tumors of the glial cells, rather than of the neurons themselves. These tumors, called *gliomas,* have extensive roots, making them extremely difficult to remove.

BLOOD-BRAIN BARRIER: Neuroglia, particularly astrocytes, form a wall around the outside of the blood vessels in the nervous system. This astrocyte wall plus the blood vessel wall forms the blood-brain barrier. Water, oxygen, carbon dioxide, alcohol, and a few other substances are able to pass through this barrier and move between the blood and brain tissue. Other substances, such as toxins, pathogens, and certain drugs, cannot pass through this barrier. This is a protective mechanism to keep harmful substances out of the brain. It has clinical significance because drugs, such as penicillin, that may be used to treat disorders in other parts of the body have no effect on the brain because they do not cross the blood-brain barrier.

ANESTHETICS: Some anesthetics produce their effects by inhibiting the diffusion of sodium through the cell membrane and thus blocking the initiation and conduction of nerve impulses.

MENINGITIS: Meningitis is an acute inflammation of the pia mater and the arachnoid. It is most commonly caused by bacteria. However, viral infections, fungal infections, and tumors may also cause inflammation of the meninges. Depending on the primary cause, meningitis may be mild or it may progress to a severe and life-threatening condition.

LEFT AND RIGHT BRAIN: In most people (≈90%), the left cerebral hemisphere dominates for language and mathematic abilities. It is the reasoning and analytic side of the brain. The right cerebral hemisphere is involved with motor skills, intuition, emotion, art, and music appreciation. It is the poetic and creative side of the brain. These people are generally right-handed. In about 10% of the people, these sides are reversed. In some cases, neither hemisphere dominates. This may result in "confusion" and learning disabilities.

PARKINSON'S DISEASE: Parkinson's disease is a condition in which the basal ganglia do not produce enough of the inhibitory transmitter dopamine. Without dopamine, there is an excess of excitatory signals that affect certain voluntary muscles, producing rigidity and tremors.

EMOTIONS: The **limbic system** consists of scattered but interconnected regions of gray matter in the cerebral hemispheres and diencephalon. The limbic system is involved in memory and in emotions such as sadness, happiness, anger, and fear. It is our emotional brain.

HYDROCEPHALUS: In hydrocephalus, an obstruction in the normal flow of cerebrospinal fluid (CSF) causes the fluid to accumulate in the ventricles. The obstruction may be a congenital defect or an acquired lesion such as a tumor. As the fluid accumulates, it causes the ventricles to enlarge and CSF pressure to increase. When this happens in an infant, before the cranial bones ossify, the cranium enlarges. In an older child or adult, the pressure damages the soft brain tissue.

LUMBAR PUNCTURE: A lumbar puncture is the withdrawal of some CSF from the subarachnoid space in the lumbar region of the spinal cord. The extension of the meninges beyond the end of the cord makes it possible to do this without injury to the spinal cord. The needle is usually inserted just above or just below the fourth lumbar vertebra, and the spinal cord ends at the first lumbar vertebra. The CSF that is removed can be tested for abnormal characteristics that may indicate an injury or infection.

CARPAL TUNNEL SYNDROME: Carpal tunnel syndrome is a common occupational injury to the hand and wrist that is associated with repetitive hand motions. It is also associated with several diseases, including arthritis, diabetes, and gout. Symptoms, which include tingling of the thumb and fingers, result from the compression of the median nerve because of inflammation and swelling of the tendons within the carpal tunnel. ■

---

elongated, and because it carries impulses away from the cell body, it is called an *efferent process.*

An axon may have infrequent branches called **axon collaterals.** Axons and axon collaterals terminate in many short branches or **telodendria** (tell-oh-DEN-dree-ah). The distal ends of the telodendria are slightly enlarged to form **synaptic bulbs.** Many axons are surrounded by a segmented, white, fatty substance called **myelin** (MY-eh-lin) or the **myelin sheath.** Myelinated fibers make up the white matter in the CNS, whereas cell bodies and unmyelinated fibers make up the gray matter. The unmyelinated regions between the myelin segments are called the **nodes of Ranvier** (nodes of ron-vee-AY). In the PNS, the myelin is produced by Schwann cells. The cytoplasm, nucleus, and outer cell membrane of the Schwann cell form a tight covering around the myelin and around the axon itself at the

nodes of Ranvier. This covering is the **neurilemma** (noo-rih-LEM-mah), which plays an important role in the regeneration of nerve fibers. In the CNS, **oligodendrocytes** (ah-lee-go-DEN-droh-sites) produce myelin, but there is no neurilemma, which is why fibers within the CNS do not regenerate. The structure of an axon and its coverings is illustrated in Figure 9-2.

Functionally, neurons are classified as afferent, efferent, or interneurons (association neurons) according to the direction in which they transmit impulses relative to the CNS (Table 9-1). **Afferent,** or **sensory, neurons** carry impulses from peripheral sense receptors to the CNS. They usually have long dendrites and relatively short axons. **Efferent,** or **motor, neurons** transmit impulses from the CNS to effector organs, such as muscles and glands. Efferent neurons usually have short dendrites and long axons.

Central Nervous System (CNS)
— Brain
— Spinal cord

Peripheral Nervous System (PNS)
— Ganglia
— Nerves

From CNS

To CNS

Efferent Division (Motor)

Afferent Division (Sensory)

Somatic

Autonomic

Visceral

Somatic

Sympathetic uses energy   Parasympathetic conserves energy

Figure 9-1. Organization of the nervous system. (From Applegate E: *The anatomy and physiology learning system,* ed 3, St. Louis, 2006, Saunders.)

Dendrites

Cell body

Collateral branch

Nucleolus

Nucleus

Axon

Direction of impulse

Telodendria

Synaptic bulb

Node of Ranvier

Neurilemma

Myelin

Nucleus of Schwann cell

Axon

Figure 9-2. Structure of a typical neuron. (From Applegate E: *The anatomy and physiology learning system,* ed 3, St. Louis, 2006, Saunders.)

Table 9-1 Types of Neurons Classified According to Function

Type of Neuron	Structure	Function
Afferent (Sensory)	Long dendrites and short axon; cell body located in ganglia in PNS; dendrites in PNS; axon extends into CNS	Transmits impulses from peripheral sense receptors to CNS
Efferent (Motor)	Short dendrites and long axon; dendrites and cell body located within CNS; axons extend to PNS	Transmits impulses from CNS to effectors, such as muscles and glands in periphery
Association (Interneurons)	Short dendrites; axon may be short or long; located entirely within CNS	Transmits impulses from afferent neurons to efferent neurons

From Applegate E: *The anatomy and physiology learning system,* ed 3, St. Louis, 2006, Saunders.
PNS, Peripheral nervous system; *CNS,* central nervous system.

Table 9-2 Neuroglial Cell Types

Cell Type	Location	Description	Special Function
Astrocytes	CNS	Star shaped; numerous radiating processes with bulbous ends for attachment	Bind blood vessels to nerves; regulate composition of fluid around neurons
Ependymal cells	CNS (line ventricles of brain and central canal of spinal cord)	Columnar cells with cilia	Active role in formation and circulation of cerebrospinal fluid
Microglia	CNS	Small cells with long processes; modified macrophages	Protection; become mobile and phagocytic in response to inflammation
Oligodendrocytes	CNS	Small cells with few, but long, processes that wrap around axons	Form myelin sheaths around axons in CNS
Schwann cells*	PNS	Flat cells with long, flat process that wraps around axon in PNS	Form myelin sheaths around axons in PNS; active role in nerve fiber regeneration
Satellite cells*	PNS	Flat cells, similar to Schwann cells	Support nerve cell bodies within ganglia

From Applegate E: *The anatomy and physiology learning system,* ed 3, St. Louis, 2006, Saunders.
CNS, Central nervous system; *PNS,* peripheral nervous system.
*Some authorities do not consider these to be neuroglia because they are in the PNS.

Interneurons, or association neurons, are located entirely within the CNS, where they form the connecting link between the afferent and efferent neurons. They have short dendrites and may have either a short or long axon.

Neuroglia

Neuroglia cells do not conduct nerve impulses; instead, they support, nourish, and protect the neurons. They are far more numerous than neurons and, unlike neurons, are capable of mitosis. Table 9-2 describes the six types of neuroglia cells. Some authorities classify only the four supporting cell types found in the CNS as true neuroglia.

NERVE IMPULSES

The functional characteristics of neurons are **excitability** and **conductivity.** Excitability is the ability to respond to a stimulus; conductivity is the ability to transmit an impulse from one point to another. All the functions associated with the nervous system, including thought, learning, and memory, are based on these two characteristics. These functional characteristics are the result of structural features of the cell membrane.

Resting Membrane

A **resting membrane** is the cell membrane of a nonconducting, or resting, neuron. The membrane is impermeable to the passive diffusion of sodium (Na^+) and potassium (K^+) ions. An active transport mechanism, the sodium-potassium pump, maintains a difference in concentration of these ions on the two sides of the membrane. Sodium ions are concentrated in the extracellular fluid, whereas the potassium ions are inside the cell, as illustrated in Figure 9-3A. The intracellular fluid also contains proteins and other negatively charged ions. The result is a polarized membrane with more positive charges outside the cell and more negative charges inside the cell. This difference in charges on the two sides of the resting membrane is the **resting membrane potential.** Electrical measurements show the resting membrane potential to be about −70 millivolts (mV), which means that the inside of the membrane is 70 mV less positive (more negative) than the outside.

Stimulation of a Neuron

A stimulus is a physical, chemical, or electrical event that alters the neuron cell membrane and reduces its polarization for a brief time. The stimulus changes the membrane so

A Resting Membrane

The resting membrane is polarized with the inside negative to the outside. Sodium ions are concentrated on the outside and potassium ions on the inside.

B Depolarizing Membrane

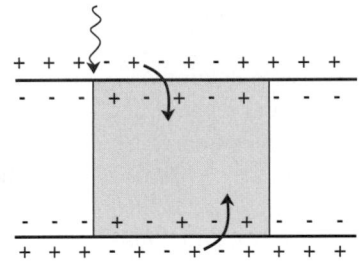

When stimulus is applied, membrane becomes permeable to sodium, which diffuses inward and makes the inside more positive.

C Reverse Polarization

The rapid inward movement of sodium makes the inside of the membrane positive to the outside.

D Repolarization

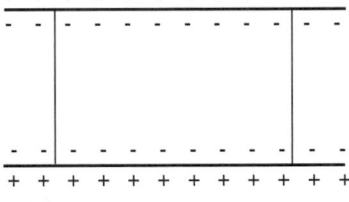

Sodium channels close and potassium channels open, which allows potassium to diffuse out of the cell. This restores the polarity of the membrane. Active transport mechanisms restore sodium and potassium to resting conditions.

Figure 9-3. Generation of an action potential (From Applegate E: *The anatomy and physiology learning system,* ed 3, St. Louis, 2006, Saunders.)

that it becomes permeable to sodium ions, which diffuse into the cell. If the stimulus is weak, the membrane is only slightly permeable and the inward movement of sodium is offset by an outward movement of potassium. In this case, the resting membrane potential is maintained and no response is initiated.

If the stimulus is strong enough, the membrane becomes highly permeable to sodium at the point of the stimulation. Positively charged sodium ions rapidly diffuse through the membrane to the inside of the cell. This movement is driven by the concentration gradient and the electrical gradient. (Remember, the inside is negatively charged, which attracts the positive sodium ions.) As the positive ions enter the cell, the inside of the membrane becomes more positively charged, reducing the polarization found in the resting membrane (Figure 9-3B). This is **depolarization.**

For just an instant, the influx of sodium ions reverses the membrane polarity with more positive charges inside the cell than outside. This is **reverse polarization** (Figure 9-3C).

Quickly, the membrane again becomes impermeable to sodium, with the sodium ions trapped inside the cell. Next the membrane becomes permeable to the intracellular potassium ions for a fraction of a millisecond, and they rapidly diffuse down the concentration gradient to the outside of the cell. Because these are positive ions, this action removes the intracellular positive charge and restores the resting membrane potential of −70 mV. This process is called **repolarization** (Figure 9-3D).

The rapid sequence of events in response to a stimulus, namely, depolarization, reverse polarization, and repolarization, is called the **action potential**. Electrical measurements show the action potential to peak at approximately +30 mV (Figure 9-4). At the conclusion of the action potential, the sodium-potassium pump actively transports sodium ions out of the cell and potassium ions into the cell to completely restore resting conditions.

The minimum stimulus necessary to initiate an action potential is called a **threshold (liminal) stimulus**. A weaker stimulus, called a **subthreshold (subliminal) stimulus,** does not cause sufficient depolarization to elicit an action potential.

Conduction along a Neuron

Once a threshold stimulus has been applied and an action potential generated, it must be conducted along the total length of the neuron either to an effector or to another neuron.

Figure 9-4. Recording of an action potential. (From Applegate E: *The anatomy and physiology learning system,* ed 3, St. Louis, 2006, Saunders.)

Propagated Action Potentials

The threshold stimulus causes a localized area of reverse polarization on the membrane. In that one area, the membrane is negative on the outside and positive on the inside. The rest of the membrane is in the resting condition. When a given area reverses its polarity, the difference in potential between that area and the adjacent area creates a current flow that depolarizes the second point (Figure 9-5A). When the second point reverses its polarity, current flow between the second point and the third point depolarizes the third point. This continues point by point, in domino fashion, along the entire length of the neuron, creating a **propagated action potential,** or **nerve impulse.** The following list summarizes the events that occur during nerve impulse conduction:

- Resting membrane has sodium ions on the outside and potassium ions on the inside. Intracellular negative ions produce a resting membrane potential of −70 mV.
- Receptors are stimulated by a physical, chemical, or electrical event.
- Stimulus alters permeability of neuron cell membrane; sodium channels open and sodium ions diffuse to the inside of the cell.
- Influx of sodium ions depolarizes the cell membrane.
- Sodium ions continue inward diffusion to reverse the membrane's polarity to +30 mV.
- Sodium channels close and potassium channels open.
- Potassium ions diffuse out of the cell.
- Outward diffusion of potassium ions restores resting membrane potential of −70 mV.
- Sodium-potassium pump transports sodium ions out of the cell and potassium ions back into the cell to restore resting conditions.
- Reverse polarity at one point is the stimulus that depolarizes an adjacent point to propagate the action potential.

Saltatory Conduction

The conduction described in the previous paragraphs is representative of an unmyelinated axon. Because myelin is an insulating substance, it inhibits the flow of current from one point to another. In myelinated fibers, depolarization occurs only at the places where there is no myelin, at the nodes of Ranvier (Figure 9-5B). The action potential "jumps" from node to node. This "jumping" is **saltatory** (SAL-tah-toar-ee) **conduction,** which is faster than conduction in unmyelinated fibers.

Refractory Period

The period of time during which a point on the cell membrane is "recovering" from depolarization is called the **refractory period.** Although the membrane is permeable to sodium ions, it cannot respond to a second stimulus, no matter how strong the stimulus. This is the **absolute refractory period.** For a brief period after the absolute refractory period, roughly comparable to the time of altered membrane permeability to potassium, it takes a stronger than

A

Unmyelinated fiber (continuous)

B

Myelinated fiber (saltatory)

Figure 9-5. Propagation of an action potential. (From Applegate E: *The anatomy and physiology learning system,* ed 3, St. Louis, 2006, Saunders.)

normal stimulus to reach threshold. This is the **relative refractory period.**

All-or-None Principle

Nerve fibers obey the **all-or-none principle.** If a threshold stimulus is applied, an action potential is generated and propagated along the entire length of the neuron at maximum strength and speed for the existing conditions. A stronger stimulus does not increase the strength of the action potential or change the rate of conduction. A weaker stimulus is subthreshold and does not evoke an action potential. If a stimulus is threshold or greater, an impulse is conducted. If the stimulus is subthreshold, there is no conduction.

Conduction across a Synapse

A nerve impulse, or propagated action potential, travels along a nerve fiber until it reaches the end of the axon; then it must be transmitted to the next neuron. The region of communication between two neurons is called a **synapse** (SIN-aps). A synapse has three parts (Figure 9-6):

• Synaptic knob
• Synaptic cleft
• Postsynaptic membrane

The first neuron, the one preceding the synapse, is called the **presynaptic neuron;** the second neuron, the one following the synapse, is called the **postsynaptic neuron.** Synaptic knobs are tiny bulges at the end of the telodendria on the presynaptic neuron. Small sacs within the synaptic knobs, called **synaptic vesicles,** contain chemicals known as **neurotransmitters** (noo-roh-TRANS-mitters).

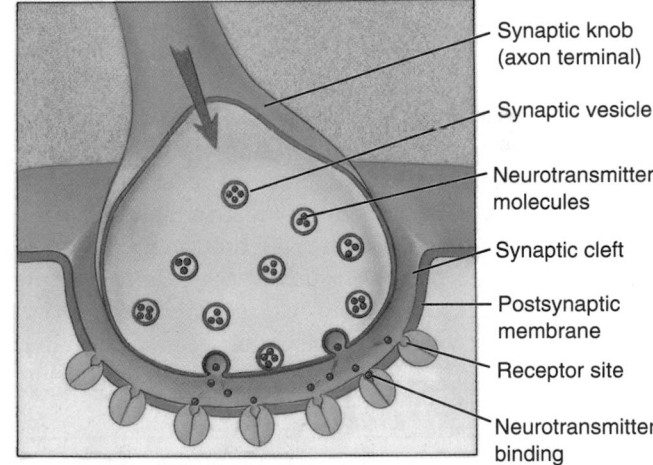

Figure 9-6. Components of a synapse. (From Applegate E: *The anatomy and physiology learning system,* ed 3, St. Louis, 2006, Saunders.)

When a nerve impulse reaches the synaptic knob, a series of reactions releases neurotransmitters into the synaptic cleft. The neurotransmitters diffuse across the synaptic cleft and react with receptors on the postsynaptic cell membrane. This is synaptic transmission. To prevent prolonged reactions with the postsynaptic receptors, the transmitters are quickly inactivated by enzymes. One of the best known neurotransmitters is **acetylcholine** (ah-see-till-KOH-leen), which is inactivated by the enzyme **cholinesterase** (koh-lin-ES-ter-ase). Table 9-3 lists some of the common neurotransmitters.

Table 9-3 Some Common Neurotransmitters

Neurotransmitter	Location	Function	Comments
Acetylcholine	CNS and PNS	Generally excitatory but inhibitory to some visceral effectors	Found in skeletal neuromuscular junctions and in many ANS synapses
Norepinephrine	CNS and PNS	May be excitatory or inhibitory depending on receptors	Found in visceral and cardiac muscle neuromuscular junctions; cocaine and amphetamines exaggerate effects
Epinephrine	CNS and PNS	May be excitatory or inhibitory depending on receptors	Found in pathways concerned with behavior and mood
Dopamine	CNS and PNS	Generally excitatory	Found in pathways that regulate emotional responses; decreased levels in Parkinson's disease
Serotonin	CNS	Generally inhibitory	Found in pathways that regulate temperature, sensory perception, mood, onset of sleep
Gamma-aminobutyric acid (GABA)	CNS	Generally inhibitory	Inhibits excessive discharge of neurons
Endorphins and enkephalins	CNS	Generally inhibitory	Inhibit release of sensory pain neurotransmitters; opiates mimic effects of these peptides

From Applegate E: *The anatomy and physiology learning system*, ed 3, St. Louis, 2006, Saunders.
CNS, Central nervous system; *PNS*, peripheral nervous system; *ANS*, autonomic nervous system.

In **excitatory transmission,** the neurotransmitter-receptor reaction on the postsynaptic membrane depolarizes the membrane and initiates an action potential. This is excitation or stimulation. Acetylcholine is typically an excitatory neurotransmitter. Some neurotransmitters result in **inhibitory transmission.** In this case, the reaction between the neurotransmitter and the receptor opens potassium channels in the membrane so that potassium diffuses out of the cell but has no effect on the sodium channels. This action makes the inside of the membrane even more negative than it is in the resting condition; it **hyperpolarizes** the membrane, which makes it more difficult to generate an action potential. This is inhibition. Gamma-aminobutyric acid (GABA) is an inhibitory neurotransmitter in the CNS.

The billions of neurons in the CNS are organized into functional groups called **neuronal pools.** The neuronal pools receive information, process and integrate that information, and then transmit it to some other destination. Neuronal pools are arranged in pathways, or circuits, over which the nerve impulses are transmitted. The simplest pathway is the **simple series circuit** in which a single neuron synapses with another neuron, which in turn synapses with another, and so on. Most pathways are more complex. In a **divergence circuit** (Figure 9-7A), a single neuron synapses with multiple neurons within the pool. This permits the same information to diverge or go along different pathways at the same time. This type of pathway is important in muscle contraction when many muscle fibers, or even several muscles, must contract at the same time. Another type of pathway is the **convergence circuit** (Figure 9-7B). In this case, several presynaptic neurons synapse with a single postsynaptic neuron. This accounts for the fact that many different stimuli may have the same ultimate effect. For example, thinking about food, smelling food, and seeing food all have the same effect—the flow of saliva.

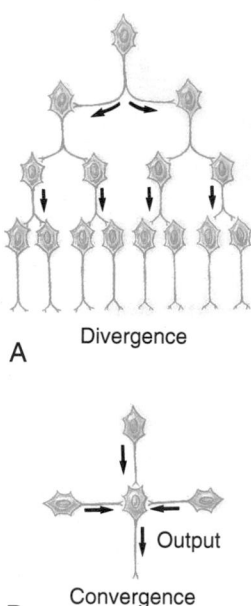

Figure 9-7. Divergence and convergence in neuronal pools. (From Applegate E: *The anatomy and physiology learning system,* ed 3, St. Louis, 2006, Saunders.)

Reflex Arcs

The neuron is the structural unit of the nervous system; the **reflex arc** is the functional unit. The reflex arc is a type of conduction pathway. It is similar to a one-way street because it allows impulses to travel in only one direction. The simplest reflex arc consists of two neurons, but most have three or more neurons in the conduction pathway. Figure 9-8 illustrates a three-neuron reflex arc. There are five basic components in a reflex arc (Table 9-4):

- Receptor
- Sensory neuron

Table 9-4 Components of a Reflex Arc

Component	Description	Function
Receptor	Site of stimulus action; receptor end of dendrite or special cell in receptor organ	Responds to some change in internal or external environment
Sensory neuron	Afferent neuron; cell body is in ganglion outside CNS; axon extends into CNS	Transmits nerve impulses from receptor to CNS
Integration center	Always within CNS; in simplest reflexes, it consists of synapse between sensory and motor neurons; more commonly one or more interneurons are involved	Processing center; region in CNS where incoming sensory impulses generate appropriate outgoing motor impulses
Motor neuron	Efferent neuron; dendrites and cell body are in CNS; axon extends to periphery	Transmits nerve impulses from integration center in CNS to effector organ
Effector	Muscle or gland outside CNS	Responds to impulses from motor neuron to produce an action, such as contraction or secretion

From Applegate E: *The anatomy and physiology learning system,* ed 3, St. Louis, 2006, Saunders.
CNS, Central nervous system.

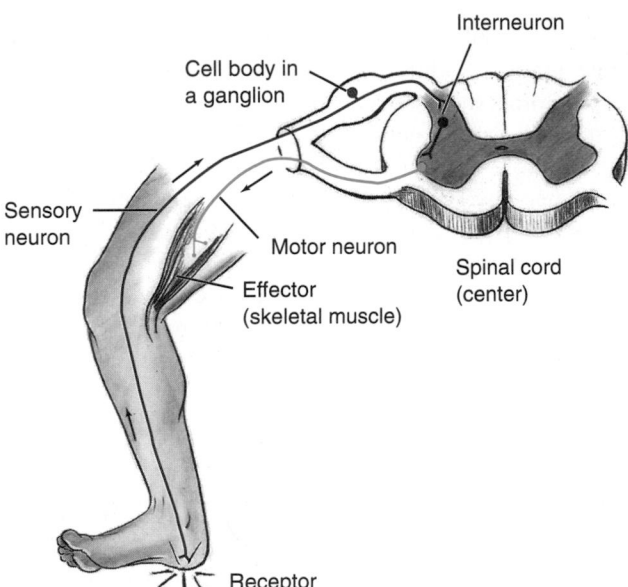

Figure 9-8. Components of a generalized reflex arc. (From Applegate E: *The anatomy and physiology learning system,* ed 3, St. Louis, 2006, Saunders.)

Figure 9-9. Meninges of the central nervous system. (From Applegate E: *The anatomy and physiology learning system,* ed 3, St. Louis, 2006, Saunders.)

- Center
- Motor neuron
- Effector

A **reflex** is an automatic, involuntary response to some change, either inside or outside the body. Reflexes are important in maintaining homeostasis by making adjustments to heart rate, breathing rate, and blood pressure. Reflexes are also involved in coughing, sneezing, and reactions to painful stimuli. Everyone is familiar with the withdrawal reflex. When you step on a tack or touch a hot iron, you immediately, without conscious thought, withdraw the injured foot or hand from the source of the irritation. Clinicians frequently test an individual's reflexes to determine if the nervous system is functioning properly.

CENTRAL NERVOUS SYSTEM

The CNS consists of the brain and spinal cord, which are located in the dorsal body cavity. These are vital to our well-being and are enclosed in bone for protection. The brain is surrounded by the cranium, and the spinal cord is protected by the vertebrae. The brain is continuous with the spinal cord at the foramen magnum. In addition to bone, the CNS is surrounded by connective tissue membranes, called **meninges,** and by **cerebrospinal fluid** (CSF).

Meninges

Three layers of meninges (men-IN-jeez) surround the brain and spinal cord (Figure 9-9). The outer layer, the **dura mater** (DOO-rah MAY-ter), is tough, white fibrous connective tissue. It is just inside the cranial bones and lines the vertebral canal. The dura mater contains channels, called **dural sinuses,** that collect venous blood to return it to the cardiovascular system. The **superior sagittal sinus,** located in the midsagittal line over the top of the brain, is the largest of the dural sinuses.

The middle layer of meninges is the **arachnoid** (ah-RAK-noyd). The arachnoid, which resembles a cobweb in appearance, is a thin layer with numerous threadlike strands that attach it to the innermost layer. The space under the arachnoid, the **subarachnoid space,** is filled with CSF and contains blood vessels.

The **pia mater** (PEE-ah MAY-ter) is the innermost layer of meninges. This thin, delicate membrane is tightly bound to the surface of the brain and spinal cord and cannot be dissected away without damaging the surface. It closely follows all surface contours.

Brain

The brain is divided into the cerebrum, diencephalon, brain stem, and cerebellum.

Cerebrum

The largest and most obvious portion of the brain is the **cerebrum** (seh-REE-brum), which is divided by a deep **longitudinal fissure** (FISH-ur) into two **cerebral hemispheres.** The two hemispheres are two separate entities but are connected by an arching band of white fibers, called the **corpus callosum** (KOR-pus kah-LOH-sum), that provides a communication pathway between the two halves. An extension of dura mater, the **falx cerebri** (FALKS SAYR-eh-brye), projects into the longitudinal fissure down to the corpus callosum. The superior sagittal sinus, a dural sinus mentioned earlier, is in the superior margin of the falx cerebri. The surface of the cerebrum is marked by convolutions, or **gyri** (JYE-rye), separated by grooves, or **sulci**

(SULL-see). The pia mater closely follows the convolutions and goes deep into the sulci, and then up and over the gyri.

Each cerebral hemisphere is divided into five lobes, as illustrated in Figure 9-10. Four of the lobes have the same name as the bone over them. The **frontal lobe,** under the frontal bone, is the most anterior portion of each hemisphere. The posterior boundary of the frontal lobe is the **central sulcus.** The **parietal lobe** is immediately posterior to the central sulcus, under the parietal bone. The **occipital lobe,** under the occipital bone, is the most posterior portion of the cerebral hemisphere. Laterally, the **temporal lobe** is inferior to the frontal and parietal lobes. The **lateral sulcus** (fissure) separates the temporal lobe from the two lobes that are superior to it. A fifth lobe, the **insula** (IN-sull-ah) or **island of Reil,** lies deep within the lateral sulcus. It is covered by parts of the frontal, parietal, and temporal lobes.

The cerebral hemispheres consist of gray matter and white matter. A thin layer of **gray matter,** the **cerebral cortex,** forms the outermost portion of the cerebrum. Gray matter consists of neuron cell bodies and unmyelinated fibers. Nearly three fourths of the neuron cell bodies in the entire nervous system are found in the cerebral cortex. Additional regions of gray matter, the **basal ganglia,** are scattered throughout the white matter. The **white matter,** which makes up the bulk of the cerebrum, is just beneath the cerebral cortex. White matter is myelinated nerve fibers that form three types of communication pathways in the cerebrum (Table 9-5).

Central sulcus

Longitudinal fissure

Precentral gyrus
Somatomotor cortex

Postcentral gyrus
Somatosensory cortex

PARIETAL LOBE
Sensation

FRONTAL LOBE
Personality
Behavior
Emotion
Intellectual functions

OCCIPITAL LOBE
Vision

Gnostic area
Stores complex
memory patterns

Sulcus

Gyrus

Gustatory area
Taste

RIGHT CEREBRAL
HEMISPHERE

Wernicke's area
Language
comprehension

LEFT CEREBRAL
HEMISPHERE

Lateral sulcus

Broca's area
Motor speech

TEMPORAL LOBE
Hearing, smell

INSULA
Visceral effects

Figure 9-10. Lobes and functional areas of the cerebrum. (From Applegate E: *The anatomy and physiology learning system,* ed 3, St. Louis, 2006, Saunders.)

Table 9-5	Pathways of White Matter in the Cerebrum
Type of Fibers	**Function**
Association	Transmit impulses from one gyrus to another within same hemisphere
Commissural	Transmit impulses from one cerebral hemisphere to another; allow one side to know what other side is doing; corpus callosum is large band of commissural fibers
Projection	Transmit impulses from cerebrum to other parts of central nervous system

From Applegate E: *The anatomy and physiology learning system,* ed 3, St. Louis, 2006, Saunders.

The cerebral cortex is the neural basis of what makes us "human." It is the center for sensory and motor functions. It is concerned with memory, language, reasoning, intelligence, personality, and all the other factors that we associate with human life. Even though the two cerebral hemispheres are nearly symmetric in structure, they are not always equal in function; instead, there are areas of specialization. However, there is considerable overlap in these regions and no area really works alone; all the areas are dependent on each other for mental "consciousness"—those abilities that involve higher mental processing, such as memory, reasoning, logic, and judgment.

It is possible to identify regions of the cerebral cortex that have specific functions. Some of these regions are illustrated in Figure 9-10. **Sensory areas** in the parietal, occipital, and temporal lobes receive information from the various sense organs and receptors throughout the body. The primary sensory area, the **somatosensory** (soh-mat-oh-SEN-soar-ee) **cortex,** is located in the **postcentral gyrus** of the parietal lobe, immediately posterior to the central sulcus. This region receives sensory input from sensory receptors in the skin and skeletal muscles. The right side of the somatosensory cortex receives input from the left side of the body and vice versa. The somatosensory cortex is highly organized with specific regions responsible for receiving sensory input from specific parts of the body. Larger areas of the cortex are devoted to the face and hands than to other parts of the body. Other areas of the cerebrum are responsible for vision, hearing, taste, and smell.

Motor areas responsible for muscle contraction are located in the frontal lobe. The primary motor area, the **somatomotor** (soh-mat-oh-MOH-ter) **cortex,** is in the **precentral gyrus,** immediately anterior to the central sulcus. Neurons in this area allow us to consciously control our skeletal muscles. The right primary motor gyrus controls muscles on the left side of the body and vice versa. The primary motor cortex is also highly organized in a manner similar to the primary sensory cortex, with neurons in a specific region responsible for controlling movement in a specific part of the body.

Association areas of the cerebral cortex are involved in the process of recognition. They analyze and interpret sensory information, and based on previous experiences they integrate appropriate responses through the motor areas. Table 9-6 describes some of the specific functional areas of the cerebral cortex.

The **basal ganglia** are functionally related regions of gray matter that are scattered throughout the white matter of the cerebral hemispheres. These regions function as relay stations, or areas of synapse, in pathways going to and from the cortex. The major effects of the basal ganglia are to decrease muscle tone and inhibit muscular activity. Because of these effects, they play an important role in posture and coordinating motor movements. Also, nearly all the inhibitory neurotransmitter dopamine is produced in the basal ganglia.

Diencephalon

The **diencephalon** (dye-en-SEF-ah-lon) is centrally located and is nearly surrounded by the cerebral hemispheres. It includes the **thalamus, hypothalamus,** and **epithalamus.** Regions of the diencephalon are illustrated in Figure 9-11.

The **thalamus** (THAL-ah-mus), about 80% of the diencephalon, consists of two oval masses of gray matter that serve as relay stations for sensory impulses, except for the sense of smell, going to the cerebral cortex. When the impulses reach the thalamus, there is a general awareness and crude recognition of sensation. The thalamus channels the impulses to the appropriate region of the cortex for discrimination, localization, and interpretation.

The **hypothalamus** (HYE-poh-thal-ah-mus) is a small region below the thalamus. It plays a key role in maintaining homeostasis because it regulates many visceral activities. The hypothalamus also serves as a link between the nervous and endocrine systems because it regulates secretion of hormones from the pituitary gland. A slender stalk, the **infundibulum,** extends from the floor of the hypothalamus to the pituitary gland and acts as a connector between the two structures. Two visible "bumps" on the posterior portion of the hypothalamus, the **mammillary bodies,** are involved in memory and emotional responses to different odors (Box 9-1).

The **epithalamus** (ep-ih-THAL-ah-mus) is the most dorsal, or superior, portion of the diencephalon. The **pineal** (PIE-nee-al) **gland,** or **body,** extends from its posterior margin. This small gland is involved with the onset of puberty and rhythmic cycles in the body. It is similar to a biologic clock.

Brain Stem

The **brain stem** is the region between the diencephalon and the spinal cord. It consists of three regions:
- Midbrain
- Pons
- Medulla oblongata

Regions of the brain stem are illustrated in Figure 9-11.

Table 9-6 Functional Regions of the Cerebral Cortex

Functional Region	Location	Description	Comments
Primary sensory cortex (somatosensory cortex)	Postcentral gyrus in parietal lobe	Receives sensory input from receptors in skin and skeletal muscles	Functions in sensations of temperature, touch, pressure, pain
Somatosensory association area	Parietal lobe, immediately posterior to primary sensory cortex	Integrates and analyzes input received by primary sensory cortex	Analyzes and interprets current sensory information and compares it with previous experience to form a basis for recognition
Primary visual cortex	Posterior region of occipital lobe	Receives sensory input from retina of eye	Perceives current visual image
Visual association area	Anterior to primary visual cortex in occipital lobe	Integrates and analyzes input received by primary visual cortex	Compares present visual information with previous experience as a basis for recognition; attaches significance to what you see
Auditory cortex	Superior margin of temporal lobe, along lateral sulcus	Receives auditory impulses related to pitch, rhythm, and loudness from inner ear	Allows you to hear "sounds"
Auditory association area	Adjacent to primary auditory area in temporal lobe	Integrates and analyzes input received by primary auditory area	Permits recognition of sounds (e.g., speech, music, noise); involved in memory of music
Olfactory cortex	Medial aspect of temporal lobe	Receives input from olfactory (smell) receptors in nasal cavity	Permits perception of different odors
Gustatory cortex	Parietal lobe where it is overlapped by temporal lobe	Receives input from taste buds on tongue	Permits perception of different tastes
Wernicke's area	Posterior aspect of temporal lobe of one hemisphere, usually the left	Receives input from auditory and visual association areas	Permits comprehension of spoken and written language
Primary motor cortex (somatomotor cortex)	Precentral gyrus in frontal lobe	Initiates efferent action potentials that control voluntary movements	Permits skeletal muscle contraction
Premotor cortex	Anterior to primary motor cortex in frontal lobe	Controls learned motor skills that involve skeletal muscles, either simultaneously or sequentially	Examples of learned motor skills are playing piano, typing, writing
Broca's area (motor speech area)	Inferior portion of frontal lobe in one hemisphere, usually the left	Programs and coordinates muscular movements necessary to articulate words	Person with injury in this area is able to understand words but is unable to speak because of inability to coordinate muscles necessary to form words
Prefrontal cortex	Anterior portion of frontal lobes	Involved with thought, reasoning, intelligence, judgment, planning, conscience	This area is well developed only in humans
Gnostic area (general interpretation area)	Region where parietal, temporal, and occipital lobes meet; found in one hemisphere (usually the left)	Integrates sensory interpretations from adjacent association areas to form thoughts; then transmits signals for appropriate responses	Stores complex memory patterns; allows person to recognize words and arrange them appropriately to express thoughts or to read and understand written ideas

From Applegate E: *The anatomy and physiology learning system,* ed 3, St. Louis, 2006, Saunders.

The **midbrain** is the most superior portion of the brain stem, the region next to the diencephalon. Two **cerebral peduncles** (seh-REE-brull pee-DUNK-als) form the ventral aspect of the midbrain. These bundles of myelinated fibers contain the voluntary motor tracts that descend from the cerebral cortex. On the dorsal aspect of the midbrain, four rounded protuberances form the **corpora quadrigemina** (KOR-poar-ah kwad-rih-JEM-ih-nah). The two superior bodies, the **superior colliculi** (soo-PEER-ee-or koh-LIK-yoo-lye), function as visual reflex centers. The other two, the **inferior colliculi,** contain auditory reflex centers. A narrow channel for CSF, the **cerebral aqueduct** (seh-REE-brull AH-kweh-dukt), descends through the center of the midbrain.

Figure 9-11. Midsagittal section of the brain showing the major portions of the diencephalon, brain stem, and cerebellum. (From Applegate E: *The anatomy and physiology learning system,* ed 3, St. Louis, 2006, Saunders.)

BOX 9-1 Functions of the Hypothalamus

- Regulates and integrates the autonomic nervous system

    The hypothalamus influences the autonomic centers in the brain stem and spinal cord. In this way it regulates many visceral activities, such as heart rate, blood pressure, respiratory rate, and motility of the digestive tract.

- Regulates emotional responses and behavior

    The hypothalamus acts through the autonomic nervous system to mediate the physical responses to emotion and mind-over-body phenomena. Nuclei involved in feelings of rage, aggression, fear, pleasure, and the sex drive are localized in the hypothalamus.

- Regulates body temperature

    Certain cells of the hypothalamus act as a body thermostat and activate appropriate responses.

- Regulates food intake

    The feeding or hunger center in the hypothalamus is responsible for hunger sensations. After food ingestion, the satiety center inhibits the hunger center.

- Regulates water balance and thirst

    Osmoreceptors in the hypothalamus monitor the volume and concentration of body fluids and then initiate appropriate responses from the thirst center and antidiuretic hormone.

- Regulates sleep-wake cycles

    Centers in the hypothalamus act with other brain centers to maintain alternating periods of sleep and wakefulness.

- Regulates endocrine system activity

    The hypothalamus produces releasing factors that control the release of hormones from the anterior pituitary gland. It also produces two hormones, antidiuretic hormone and oxytocin, that are stored in the posterior pituitary gland.

From Applegate E: *The anatomy and physiology learning system,* ed 3, St. Louis, 2006, Saunders.

The **pons** is the bulging middle portion of the brain stem. This region primarily consists of nerve fibers that form conduction tracts between the higher brain centers and the spinal cord. Four cranial nerves originate in the pons. It also contains the **pneumotaxic** (noo-moh-TACK-sik) and **apneustic** (ap-NOO-stick) **areas** that help regulate breathing movements.

The **medulla oblongata** (meh-DULL-ah ahb-long-GAH-tah), or simply **medulla,** extends inferiorly from the pons. It is continuous with the spinal cord at the foramen magnum. All the ascending (sensory) and descending (motor) nerve fibers connecting the brain and spinal cord pass through the medulla. Most of the descending fibers cross over from one side to the other. In other words, fibers descending on the left side cross over to the right and vice versa. This is called **decussation** (dee-kuh-SAY-shun). Because the fibers decussate, or cross over, the brain controls motor functions on the opposite side of the body. Five pairs of cranial nerves originate in the medulla. In addition, the medulla contains three vital centers that control visceral activities. The **cardiac center** adjusts the heart rate and contraction strength to meet body needs. The **vasomotor center** regulates blood pressure by effecting changes in blood vessel diameter. The **respiratory center** acts with the centers in the pons to regulate the rate, rhythm, and depth of breathing. Other centers are involved in coughing, sneezing, swallowing, and vomiting.

Cerebellum

The **cerebellum** (sair-eh-BELL-um), the second largest portion of the brain, is located below the occipital lobes of the cerebrum and is separated from them by the **transverse fissure.** It consists of two **cerebellar hemispheres** connected in the middle by a structure called the **vermis.** An extension of dura mater, the **falx cerebelli** (FALKS sair-eh-BELL-eye), forms a partial partition between the hemispheres. Another extension of dura mater, the **tentorium cerebelli** (ten-TOAR-ee-um sair-eh-BELL-eye), is found in the transverse fissure between the cerebellum and the occipital lobes of the cerebrum.

Like the cerebrum, the cerebellum consists of white matter surrounded by a thin layer of gray matter, the **cerebellar cortex.** Because the surface convolutions are less prominent in the cerebellum than in the cerebrum, the cerebellum has proportionately less gray matter. The branching arrangement of white matter is called **arbor vitae** (AR-bor VEE-tay).

Three paired bundles of myelinated nerve fibers, called **cerebellar peduncles,** form communication pathways between the cerebellum and other parts of the CNS. The **superior cerebellar peduncles** connect the cerebellum to the midbrain; the **middle cerebellar peduncles** communicate with the pons; and the **inferior cerebellar peduncles** consist of pathways between the cerebellum and the medulla oblongata and spinal cord.

The cerebellum functions as a motor area of the brain that mediates subconscious contractions of skeletal muscles necessary for **coordination, posture,** and **balance.** The cerebellum coordinates skeletal muscles to produce smooth muscle movement rather than jerky, trembling motion. When the cerebellum is damaged, movements such as running, walking, and writing become uncoordinated. Posture is dependent on muscle tone, which is mediated by the cerebellum. Impulses from the inner ear concerning position and equilibrium are directed to the cerebellum, which uses that information to maintain balance.

Ventricles and Cerebrospinal Fluid

A series of interconnected, fluid-filled cavities are found within the brain (Figure 9-12A). These cavities are the **ventricles** of the brain, and the fluid is **cerebrospinal** (seh-ree-broh-SPY-null) **fluid** (CSF). The **lateral ventricles** in the cerebrum are the largest of these cavities. One lateral ventricle exists in each cerebral hemisphere. A single, narrow, slitlike, midline **third ventricle** is enclosed by the diencephalon. The two lateral ventricles open into the third ventricle through the **interventricular foramina.** The

Figure 9-12. A, Ventricles of the brain. **B,** Circulation of cerebrospinal fluid. (From Applegate E: *The anatomy and physiology learning system,* ed 3, St. Louis, 2006, Saunders.)

fourth ventricle is at the level of the cerebellum and pons. A long, narrow channel, the **cerebral aqueduct,** passes through the midbrain to connect the third and fourth ventricles. The fourth ventricle is continuous with the central canal of the spinal cord. Openings in the wall of the fourth ventricle permit CSF to enter the subarachnoid space.

The CSF is a clear fluid that forms as a filtrate from the blood in specialized capillary networks, the **choroid plexus** (KOR-oyd PLEKS-us), within the ventricles. The circulation of the CSF is illustrated in Figure 9-12B. Ependymal cells, a type of neuroglia cell, aid in the circulation of CSF through the ventricles and central canal. CSF then enters the subarachnoid space through foramina in the fourth ventricle. From the subarachnoid space, CSF carrying waste products filters through **arachnoid granulations** (villi) into the dural sinuses and is returned to the blood. In addition to providing support and protection for the CNS, the CSF helps to nourish the brain and maintain constant ionic conditions for the brain and spinal cord and provides a pathway for removal of waste products.

Spinal Cord

The **spinal cord,** illustrated in Figure 9-13, extends from the foramen magnum at the base of the skull to the level of

the first lumbar vertebra, a distance of about 43 to 46 cm (17 or 18 inches). The cord is continuous with the medulla oblongata at the foramen magnum. Distally, it terminates in the **conus medullaris** (KOH-nus med-yoo-LAIR-is). Like the brain, the spinal cord is surrounded by bone, meninges, and CSF. Unlike the dura mater around the brain, the spinal dura is separated from the vertebral bones by an **epidural space** (Figure 9-14). This space is filled with loose connective tissue and adipose tissue. The meninges extend beyond the end of the spinal cord, down to the upper part of the sacrum. From there, a fibrous cord of pia mater, the **filum terminale** (FYE-lum term-ih-NAL-ee), extends down to the coccyx where it is anchored.

The spinal cord is divided into 31 segments with each segment giving rise to a pair of spinal nerves. At the distal end of the cord, many spinal nerves extend beyond the conus medullaris to form a collection that resembles a horse's tail. This is the **cauda equina** (KAW-dah ee-KWYNE-ah). There are two enlargements in the cord, one in the cervical region and one in the lumbar region. The **cervical enlargement** gives rise to the nerves that supply the upper extremity. Nerves from the **lumbar enlargement** supply the lower extremity.

In cross section, the spinal cord appears oval (see Figure 9-14). A narrow, deep, **dorsal (posterior) median sulcus** and a shallower, but wider, **ventral (anterior) median fissure** partially divide the cord into right and left halves. Peripheral white matter surrounds a core of gray matter that resembles a butterfly or the letter H. Each side of the gray matter is divided into **dorsal, lateral,** and **ventral horns.** These contain the terminal portions of sensory neuron axons, entire interneurons, and the dendrites and cell bodies of motor neurons. The central connecting bar between the two large areas of gray matter is the **gray commissure** (KOM-ih-shur). This surrounds the **central canal,** which contains CSF. The gray matter divides the surrounding white matter into three regions on each side. These regions are the **dorsal, lateral,** and **ventral funiculi** (fuh-NIK-yoo-lee) or **columns.** The white matter contains longitudinal bundles of myelinated nerve fibers, called **nerve tracts.**

The spinal cord has two main functions. It is a conduction pathway for impulses going to and from the brain, and it serves as a reflex center.

The conduction pathways that carry sensory impulses from body parts to the brain are called **ascending tracts.** Pathways that carry motor impulses from the brain to muscles and glands are **descending tracts.** Tracts are often named according to their points of origin and termination. For example, **spinothalamic** (spy-noh-tha-LAM-ik) **tracts** are ascending (sensory) tracts that begin in the spinal cord and conduct impulses to the thalamus. They function in the sensations of touch, pressure, pain, and temperature. **Corticospinal** (kor-tih-koh-SPY-null) **tracts,** also called **pyramidal** (pih-RAM-ih-dal) **tracts,** are descending (motor) tracts that begin in the cerebral cortex and end in the spinal cord. These tracts function in the control of skeletal muscle movement. All other descending tracts are grouped together

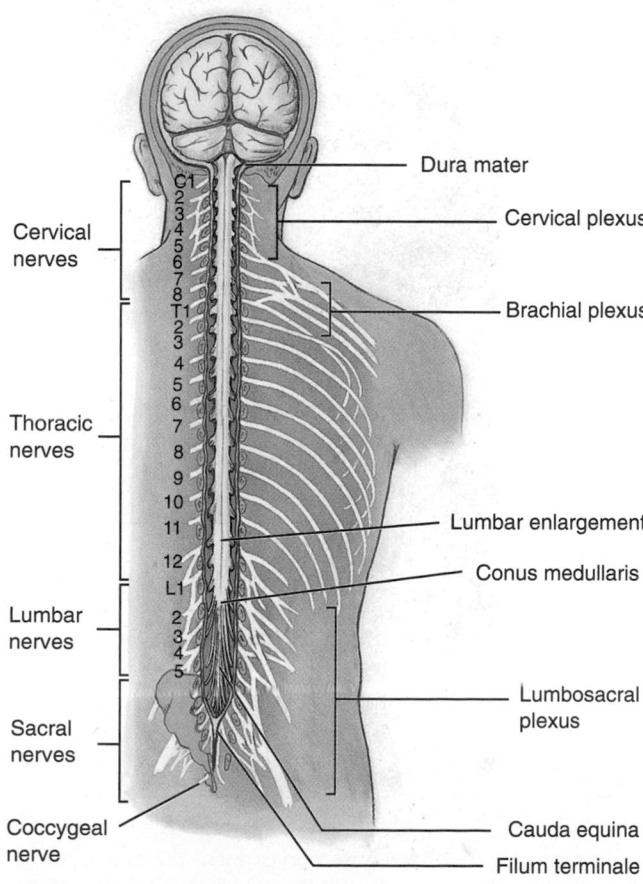

Figure 9-13. Gross anatomy of the spinal cord. (From Applegate E: *The anatomy and physiology learning system,* ed 3, St. Louis, 2006, Saunders.)

Cervical nerves

Thoracic nerves

Lumbar nerves

Sacral nerves

Coccygeal nerve

Dura mater

Cervical plexus

Brachial plexus

Lumbar enlargement

Conus medullaris

Lumbosacral plexus

Cauda equina

Filum terminale

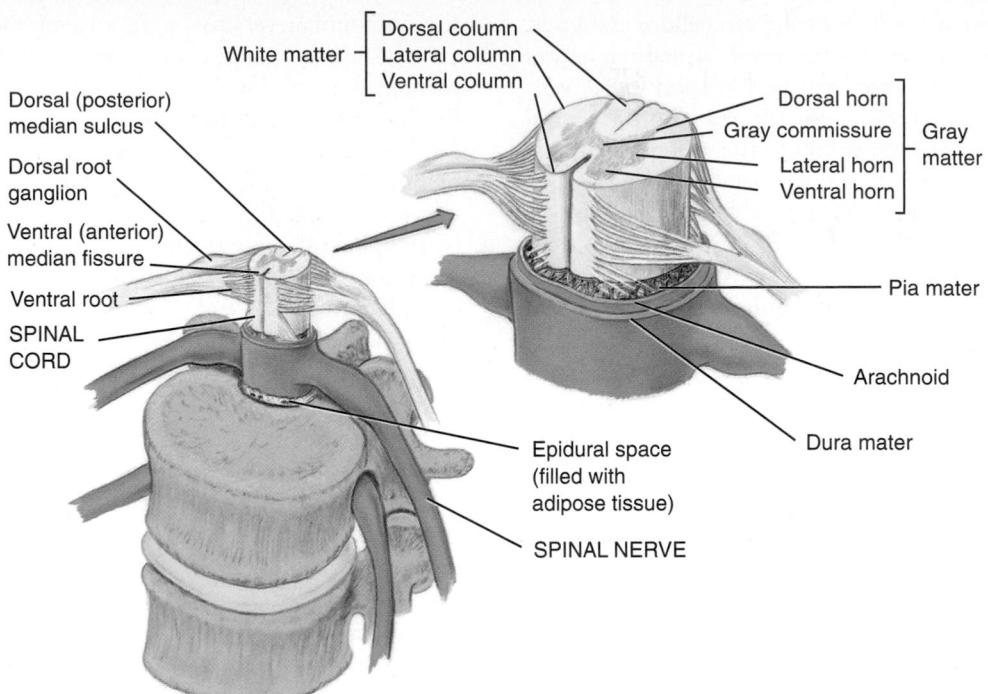

Figure 9-14. Cross section of the spinal cord. (From Applegate E: *The anatomy and physiology learning system,* ed 3, St. Louis, 2006, Saunders.)

Table 9-7 Some Clinically Significant Reflexes		
Reflex	**Description**	**Indications**
Patellar (knee-jerk reflex)	Stretch reflex; two-neuron path; reflex hammer strikes patellar tendon just below knee; receptors in quadriceps femoris muscle are stretched; reflex results in immediate "kick"	Reflex is blocked by damage to nerves involved and by damage to lumbar segments of spinal cord; also absent in people with chronic diabetes mellitus and neurosyphilis
Achilles tendon (ankle-jerk reflex)	Stretch reflex; two-neuron path; reflex hammer strikes Achilles tendon just above heel; gastrocnemius and soleus muscles contract to plantar flex foot	Weak or no reflex action indicates damage to nerves involved or to L5-S2 segments of spinal cord; also absent in chronic diabetes, neurosyphilis, and alcoholism
Abdominal	Stroking lateral abdominal wall produces reflex action that compresses abdominal wall and moves umbilicus toward stimulus	Absent in lesions of peripheral nerves, in lesions in thoracic segments of spinal cord, and in multiple sclerosis
Babinski's	Lateral sole of foot is stroked from heel to toe; positive sign results in dorsiflexion of big toe and spreading of other toes; negative sign results in toes curling under with a light inversion of foot	Positive Babinski's sign is normal in children younger than 18 months of age; negative sign is normal after 18 months of age; if motor tracts in spinal cord are damaged, positive Babinski's sign reappears

From Applegate E: *The anatomy and physiology learning system,* ed 3, St. Louis, 2006, Saunders.

as **extrapyramidal** (eks-trah-pih-RAM-ih-dal) **tracts,** and they function in muscle movements associated with posture and balance.

In addition to serving as a conduction pathway, the spinal cord functions as a center for spinal reflexes. The reflex arc, described earlier in this chapter and illustrated in Figure 9-9, is the functional unit of the nervous system. Reflexes are responses to stimuli that do not require conscious thought and, consequently, they occur more quickly than reactions that require thought processes. For example, with the withdrawal reflex, the reflex action withdraws the affected part

before you are aware of the pain. Many reflexes are mediated in the spinal cord without going to the higher brain centers. Table 9-7 describes some clinically significant reflexes.

PERIPHERAL NERVOUS SYSTEM

The PNS consists of the nerves that branch out from the brain and spinal cord. These nerves form the communication network between the CNS and the remainder of the body. The PNS is further subdivided into the **somatic nervous system** and the **autonomic nervous system.** The somatic nervous system consists of nerves that go to the skin and muscles and is involved in conscious activities. The autonomic nervous system consists of nerves that connect the CNS to the visceral organs such as the heart, stomach, and intestines. It mediates unconscious activities.

Structure of a Nerve

A nerve contains bundles of nerve fibers, either axons or dendrites, surrounded by connective tissue. **Sensory nerves** contain only afferent fibers—long dendrites of sensory neurons. **Motor nerves** have only efferent fibers—long axons of motor neurons. **Mixed nerves** contain both types of fibers.

Each nerve is surrounded by a connective tissue sheath called the **epineurium** (ep-ih-NOO-ree-um). Portions of the epineurium project inward to divide the nerve into compartments, each containing a bundle of nerve fibers. Each bundle of nerve fibers is called a **fasciculus** and is surrounded by a layer of connective tissue called the **perineurium** (pair-ih-NOO-ree-um). Within the fasciculus, each individual nerve fiber, with its myelin and neurilemma, is surrounded by connective tissue called the **endoneurium** (end-oh-NOO-ree-um). A nerve may also have blood vessels enclosed in its connective tissue wrappings (Figure 9-15).

Cranial Nerves

Twelve pairs of cranial nerves, illustrated in Figure 9-16, emerge from the inferior surface of the brain. All of these

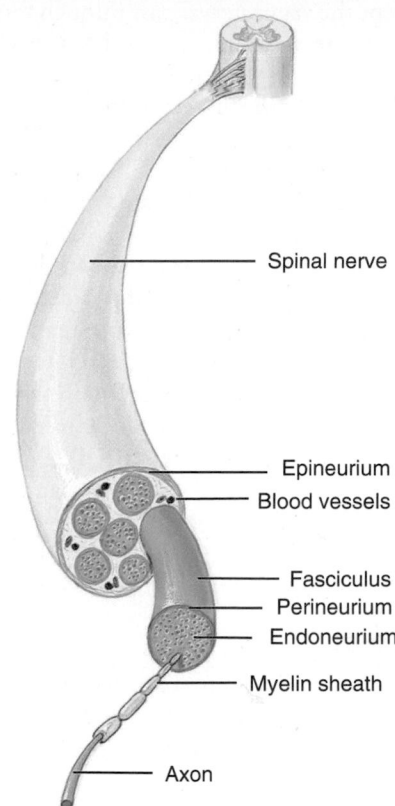

Figure 9-15. Structure of a nerve. (From Applegate E: *The anatomy and physiology learning system,* ed 3, St. Louis, 2006, Saunders.)

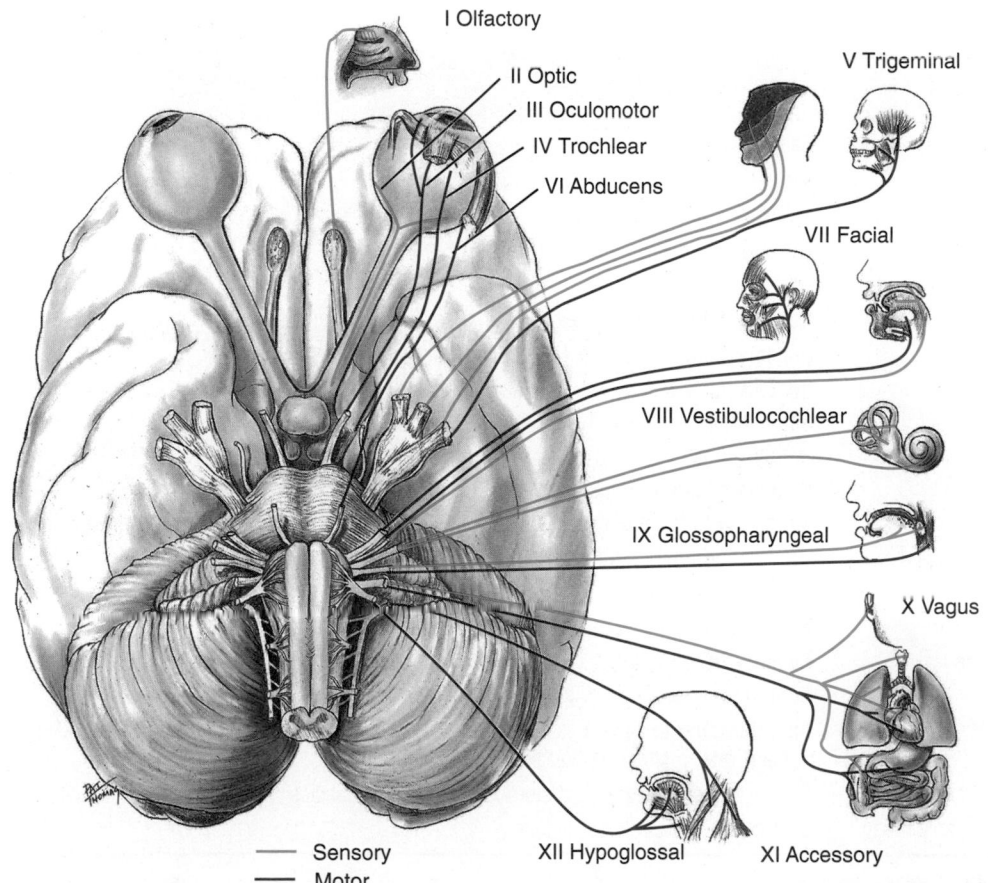

Figure 9-16. Cranial nerves. (From Applegate E: *The anatomy and physiology learning system,* ed 3, St. Louis, 2006, Saunders.)

nerves, except the vagus nerve, pass through foramina of the skull to innervate structures in the head, neck, and facial region. The vagus nerve, cranial nerve X, has numerous branches that supply the viscera in the body. When sensory fibers are present in a cranial nerve, the cell bodies of these neurons are located in groups, called **ganglia,** outside the brain. Motor neuron cell bodies are typically located in the gray matter of the brain.

The cranial nerves are designated both by name and by Roman numerals, according to the order in which they appear on the inferior surface of the brain. Most of the nerves have both sensory and motor components. Three of the nerves (I, II, VIII) are associated with the special senses of smell, vision, hearing, and equilibrium and have only sensory fibers. Five other nerves (III, IV, VI, XI, XII) are primarily motor in function but do have some sensory fibers for proprioception. The remaining four nerves (V, VII, IX, X) consist of significant amounts of both sensory and motor fibers. Table 9-8 itemizes the cranial nerves.

Spinal Nerves

Thirty-one pairs of spinal nerves emerge laterally from the spinal cord. Each pair of nerves corresponds to a segment of the cord, and the nerves are named accordingly. This means there are **8 cervical nerves** (C1 to C8), **12 thoracic nerves** (T1 to T12), **5 lumbar nerves** (L1 to L5), **5 sacral nerves** (S1 to S5), and **1 coccygeal nerve** (Co).

Each spinal nerve is connected to the spinal cord by a **dorsal root** and a **ventral root** (see Figure 9-14). The dorsal

root can be recognized by an enlargement, the **dorsal root ganglion.** The dorsal root has only sensory fibers, and the ventral root has only motor fibers. The cell bodies of the sensory neurons are in the dorsal root ganglion, but the motor neuron cell bodies are in the gray matter. The two roots join to form the spinal nerve just before the nerve leaves the vertebral column. Because all spinal nerves have both sensory and motor components, they are all mixed nerves.

Immediately after they leave the vertebral column, the spinal nerves divide into several branches that provide the nerve supply to the muscles and the skin of the body wall. In the thoracic region, the main portions of the nerves go directly to the thoracic wall, where they are called **intercostal nerves.** In other regions, the main portions of the nerves form complex networks called **plexuses** (see Figure 9-13). In the plexus, the fibers are sorted and recombined so that the fibers associated with a particular body part are together even though they may originate from different regions of the cord (Table 9-9).

Autonomic Nervous System
General Features

The **autonomic nervous system** (ANS) is a visceral efferent system, which means it sends motor impulses to the visceral organs. It functions automatically and continuously, without conscious effort, to innervate smooth muscle, cardiac muscle, and glands. It is concerned with heart rate, breathing rate, blood pressure, body temperature, and other

Table 9-8 Summary of Cranial Nerves			
Number	Name	Type	Function
I	Olfactory	Sensory	Sense of smell
II	Optic	Sensory	Vision
III	Oculomotor	Primarily motor	Movement of eyes and eyelids
IV	Trochlear	Primarily motor	Movement of eyes
V	Trigeminal	Mixed	
	Ophthalmic branch		**Sensory fibers** from cornea, skin of nose, forehead, and scalp
	Maxillary branch		**Sensory fibers** from cheek, nose, upper lip, and teeth
	Mandibular branch		**Sensory fibers** from skin over mandible, lower lip, and teeth **Motor fibers** to muscles of mastication
VI	Abducens	Primarily motor	Eye movement
VII	Facial	Mixed	**Sensory fibers** from taste receptors on anterior two thirds of tongue **Motor fibers** to muscles of facial expression, lacrimal glands, and salivary glands
VIII	Vestibulocochlear	Sensory	Hearing and equilibrium
IX	Glossopharyngeal	Mixed	**Sensory fibers** from taste receptors on posterior one third of tongue **Motor fibers** to muscles used in swallowing and to salivary glands
X	Vagus	Mixed	**Sensory fibers** from pharynx, larynx, esophagus, and visceral organs **Somatic motor fibers** to muscles of pharynx and larynx **Autonomic motor fibers** to heart, smooth muscles, and glands to alter gastric motility, heart rate, respiration, and blood pressure
XI	Accessory	Primarily motor	Contraction of trapezius and sternocleidomastoid muscles
XII	Hypoglossal	Primarily motor	Contraction of muscles of tongue

From Applegate E: *The anatomy and physiology learning system,* ed 3, St. Louis, 2006, Saunders.

Table 9-9 Spinal Nerve Plexuses

Plexus	Location	Spinal Nerves Involved	Region Supplied	Major Nerves Leaving Plexus
Cervical	Deep in neck, under sternocleidomastoid muscle	C1 C4	Skin and muscles of neck and shoulder; diaphragm	Phrenic
Brachial	Deep to clavicle, between neck and axilla	C5-C8, T1	Skin and muscles of upper extremity	Musculocutaneous Ulnar Median Radial Axillary
Lumbosacral	Lumbar region of back	T12, L1-L5, S1-S4	Skin and muscles of lower abdominal wall, lower extremity, buttocks, external genitalia	Obturator Femoral Sciatic Pudendal

From Applegate E: *The anatomy and physiology learning system,* ed 3, St. Louis, 2006, Saunders.

Figure 9-17. Preganglionic and postganglionic fibers in the autonomic nervous system. (From Applegate E: *The anatomy and physiology learning system,* ed 3, St. Louis, 2006, Saunders.)

visceral activities that work together to maintain homeostasis.

In the somatic motor pathways, typically there is one neuron that extends from the brain or spinal cord to the effector that is innervated. Autonomic pathways have two neurons between the CNS and the visceral effector (Figure 9-17). The first neuron's cell body is in the brain or spinal cord. Its axon, the **preganglionic fiber,** leaves the CNS and synapses with a second neuron in an **autonomic ganglion.** The cell body of the second neuron is located in the autonomic ganglion. The axon of the second neuron, the **postganglionic fiber,** leaves the ganglion and goes to the effector organ.

The ANS has two parts: the **sympathetic division** and the **parasympathetic division** (Table 9-10). Many visceral organs are supplied with fibers from both divisions **(dual innervation).** In this case, one stimulates and the other inhibits. This antagonistic functional relationship serves as a balance to help maintain homeostasis.

Sympathetic Division

The sympathetic division, illustrated in Figure 9-18, is concerned primarily with preparing the body for stressful or emergency situations. Sometimes called the *fight-or-flight system,* it is an energy-expending system. It stimulates the responses that are necessary to meet the emergency and inhibits the visceral activities that can be delayed momentarily. For example, during an emergency, the sympathetic system increases breathing rate, heart rate, and blood flow to skeletal muscles. At the same time, it decreases activity in the digestive tract because that is not necessary to meet the emergency.

The sympathetic preganglionic fibers arise from the thoracic and lumbar regions of the spinal cord; thus the sympathetic division is sometimes called the **thoracolumbar** (thoar-ah-koh-LUM-bar) **division.** These fibers almost immediately terminate in one of the **paravertebral** (pair-ah-ver-TEE-brull) **ganglia.** A chain of these ganglia, the sympathetic chain, extends longitudinally along each side of the vertebral column. Some fibers synapse in **collateral ganglia** outside the sympathetic chain but still close to the vertebral column. Thus in the sympathetic division, the preganglionic fiber is short, but the postganglionic fiber that makes contact with the effector organ is long.

A sympathetic preganglionic fiber typically synapses with many postganglionic fibers in the ganglion. The

Table 9-10 Comparison of Sympathetic and Parasympathetic Actions on Selected Visceral Effectors

Visceral Effectors	Sympathetic Action	Parasympathetic Action
Pupil of eye	Dilates	Constricts
Lens of eye	Lens flattens for distance vision	Lens bulges for near vision
Sweat glands	Stimulates	No innervation
Arrector pili muscles of hair	Stimulates contraction; goose bumps	No innervation
Heart	Increases heart rate	Decreases heart rate
Bronchi	Dilates	Constricts
Digestive glands	Decreases secretion of digestive enzymes	Increases secretion of digestive enzymes
Digestive tract	Decreases peristalsis	Increases peristalsis
Digestive tract sphincters	Stimulates—closes sphincters	Inhibits—opens sphincters
Blood vessels to digestive organs	Constricts	No innervation
Blood vessels to skeletal muscles	Dilates	No innervation
Blood vessels to skin	Constricts	No innervation
Adrenal medulla	Stimulates secretion of epinephrine	No innervation
Liver	Increases release of glucose	No innervation
Urinary bladder	Relaxes bladder and closes sphincter	Contracts bladder and opens sphincter

From Applegate E: *The anatomy and physiology learning system,* ed 3, St. Louis, 2006, Saunders.

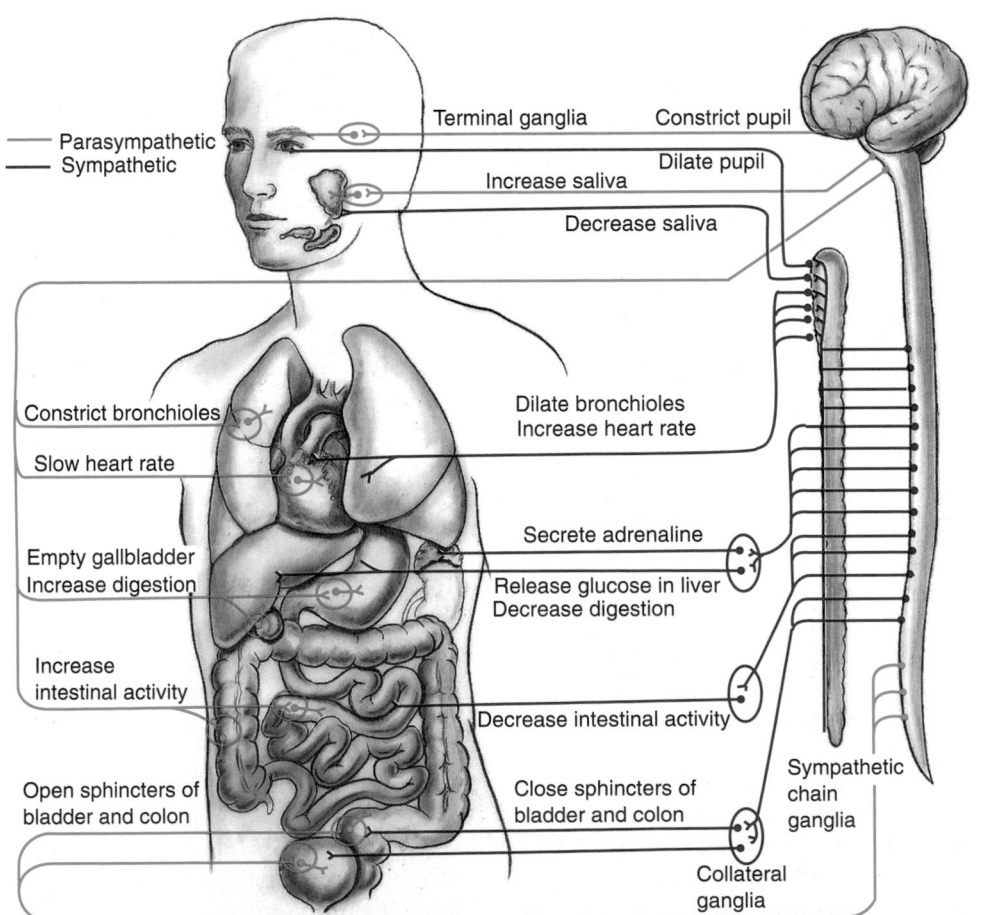

Figure 9-18. Structure and function of autonomic nervous system. (From Applegate E: *The anatomy and physiology learning system,* ed 3, St. Louis, 2006, Saunders.)

postganglionic fibers then go to numerous organs to give a widespread, diffuse effect. At the synapses in the ganglia, the preganglionic fibers release the neurotransmitter **acetylcholine.** For this reason they are called **cholinergic** (koh-lih-NER-jik) **fibers.** Most of the postganglionic fibers release **norepinephrine** (noradrenaline) and are called **adrenergic** (add-rih-NER-jik) **fibers.** Because norepinephrine is inactivated rather slowly, these fibers provide a long-lasting effect. Table 9-11 summarizes the features of the sympathetic nervous system.

Parasympathetic Division

The parasympathetic division is most active under ordinary, relaxed conditions (see Figure 9-18). It also brings the body's systems back to a normal state after an emergency by slowing the heart rate and breathing rate, decreasing blood pressure, decreasing blood flow to skeletal muscles, and increasing digestive tract activity. Sometimes called the *rest-and-repose system,* it is an energy-conserving system.

The parasympathetic preganglionic fibers arise from the brain stem and sacral region of the spinal cord; thus it is

Table 9-11 Some Comparisons between the Sympathetic and Parasympathetic Divisions of the Autonomic Nervous System

Feature	Sympathetic Division	Parasympathetic Division
General effect	Fight or flight; stress and emergency	Rest and repose; normal activity
Extent of effect	Widespread	Localized
Duration of effect	Long lasting	Short duration
Energy	Expends energy	Conserves energy
Origin of outflow	Thoracolumbar	Craniosacral
Ganglia	Paravertebral and collateral	Terminal
Preganglionic fibers	Short	Long
Postganglionic fibers	Long	Short
Neurotransmitters	Preganglionic fibers are cholinergic; most postganglionic fibers are adrenergic	Fibers are all cholinergic
Divergence	Great divergence; a preganglionic fiber synapses with several postganglionic fibers	Little divergence; a preganglionic fiber synapses with few postganglionic fibers

From Applegate E: *The anatomy and physiology learning system,* ed 3, St. Louis, 2006, Saunders.

Highlight on Aging and the Nervous System

Aging of the nervous system is of major importance because changes in this system affect organs in other systems and can cause disturbances of many bodily functions. For example, changes in nerves decrease stimulation of skeletal muscle, which contributes to muscle atrophy with age. Because of its widespread consequences, aging of the nervous system is one of the most distressing aspects of growing old.

Like other cells, nerve cells are lost as a person ages, even in the absence of disease processes. Because neurons are amitotic, those that are lost are not replaced. Loss of neurons is largely responsible for the decrease in brain mass that occurs with aging. Fortunately, the brain has a large reserve supply of neurons, many more than are necessary to carry out its functions, so the decrease in neuron number alone is not devastating. The loss of neurons is not constant in all areas of the brain. For example, about 25% of the specialized cells in the cerebellum, which are responsible for coordinated movements, are lost during aging. This may affect balance and cause difficulty in coordinating fine movements. In other areas of the brain, the number of neurons remains essentially constant throughout life.

It is generally accepted that there is a decline in intelligence with aging, and this is thought to be associated with the loss of neurons. However, it is important to remember that there are wide variations in individuals regarding changes in intellect with age. Because a person is old does not mean that person is "dumb." Many elderly people retain a keen intellect until death. Along with the decline in intelligence, there is a general decline in memory. Again, this varies from person to person. In general, short-term memory seems to be affected more than long-term memory. Intellect and memory appear to be retained better in people who remain mentally and physically active.

Another change observed in older people is a decrease in the rate of impulse conduction along an axon and across a synapse. A reduction in the amount of myelin around the axon probably accounts for the diminished conduction rate along the axon. Decreases in the quantity of neurotransmitter and in the number of receptor sites cause slower conduction across the synapses. These factors contribute to the slower reflexes and the longer time required to process information that are observed in many elderly people. ■

sometimes called the **craniosacral** (kray-nee-oh-SAY-kral) **division.** The ganglia, called **terminal ganglia,** are located near or within the visceral organs. This makes the preganglionic fiber long and the postganglionic fiber short. Typically, a parasympathetic preganglionic fiber synapses with only a few postganglionic fibers, so the effect is localized. Both the preganglionic and the postganglionic fibers are **cholinergic,** which means they secrete acetylcholine at the synapses. Because acetylcholine is readily inactivated, the parasympathetic effect is short term. Table 9-11 summarizes the features of the parasympathetic nervous system and compares them with the features of the sympathetic nervous system.

⟲ TERMINOLOGY REVIEW

Action potential A nerve impulse; a rapid change in membrane potential that involves depolarization and repolarization.

Brain stem The portion of the brain, between the diencephalon and spinal cord, that contains the midbrain, pons, and medulla oblongata.

Cerebellum Second largest part of the human brain, located posterior to the pons and medulla oblongata, and involved in the coordination of muscular movements.

Cerebrum The largest and uppermost part of the human brain; concerned with consciousness, learning, memory, sensations, and voluntary movements.

Diencephalon Part of the brain between the cerebral hemispheres and the midbrain; includes the thalamus, hypothalamus, and epithalamus.

Myelin White, fatty substance that surrounds many nerve fibers.

Neurilemma The layer of Schwann cells that surrounds a nerve fiber in the peripheral nervous system and, in some cases, produces myelin; also called *Schwann's sheath.*

Saltatory conduction Process in which a nerve impulse travels along a myelinated nerve fiber by jumping from one node of Ranvier to the next.

Synapse The region of communication between two neurons.

Threshold stimulus Minimum level of stimulation that is required to start a nerve impulse or muscle contraction; also called *liminal stimulus.*

⬙ ON THE WEB

For Information on the Nervous System:

Inner Body: www.innerbody.com/html/body.html

University of Washington: Nervous System: faculty.washington.edu/chudler/ehc.html

Martindale's: The Virtual Medical Center Brain and Neuro Center: www.martindalecenter.com/MedicalBrain.html

Neuroanatomy and Neuropathology: www.neuropat.dote.hu

Spinal Cord Injury Tracts: www.rexdonald.com/facts.htm

Interactive Brain Atlases: www9.biostr.washington.edu/da.html

The Washington School of Medicine, Neuroscience Tutorial: http://thalamus.wustl.edu/course

---

⚕ PREPARE FOR CERTIFICATION   Visit the Evolve site at http://evolve.elsevier.com/Bonewit/today/ to actively Prepare for your Certification.

---

 *Check out the **Companion CD** bound with the book to access additional interactive activities.*

10

The Senses

LEARNING OBJECTIVES

1. Explain the difference between general senses and special senses, and state examples of each.
2. List and describe the five groups of sense receptors.
3. Identify the sense receptors for touch, pressure, proprioception, temperature, and pain.
4. List and identify the location of the four different taste sensations.
5. Locate the sense receptors for smell, and trace the impulse pathway to the cerebral cortex.
6. Describe the structure of the eye, and explain the function of each structure.
7. Explain how light focuses on the retina.
8. Explain the function of the following photoreceptor cells in the retina: rods and cones.
9. Explain how nerve impulses for sight are initiated in response to light.
10. Describe the structure of the ear, and explain the function of each structure.
11. Explain how nerve impulses for hearing are initiated in response to sound waves.
12. Explain the difference between static equilibrium and dynamic equilibrium.
13. Explain how impulses for static equilibrium and dynamic equilibrium are initiated.

CHAPTER OUTLINE

Introduction to the Senses
Receptors and Sensations
General Senses
  Touch and Pressure
  Proprioception
  Temperature
  Pain
Gustatory Sense
Olfactory Sense
Visual Sense
  Protective Features and Accessory Structures of the Eye

Structure of the Eyeball
Pathway of Light and Refraction
Photoreceptors
Visual Pathway
Auditory Sense
  Structure of the Ear
  Physiology of Hearing
Sense of Equilibrium
  Static Equilibrium
  Dynamic Equilibrium

CAAHEP COMPETENCIES

Content Competencies
Anatomy and Physiology
• Anatomy and physiology of all body systems

• Common pathology/diseases
• Diagnostic/treatment modalities

ABHES COMPETENCIES

Content Competencies
Anatomy and Physiology
• Anatomy and physiology

• Study of diseases and etiology
• All body systems
• Diagnostic/treatment modalities

KEY TERMS

accommodation (ah-kahm-oh-DAY-shun)
chemoreceptor (kee-moh-ree-SEP-tor)
mechanoreceptor (mek-ah-noh-ree-SEP-tor)
nociceptor (noh-see-SEP-tor)

photoreceptor (foh-toh-ree-SEP-tor)
proprioception (proh-pree-oh-SEP-shun)
sensory adaptation (SEN-soh-ree add-dap-TAY-shun)
thermoreceptor (ther-moh-ree-SEP-tor)

Introduction to the Senses

Sense perception depends on sensory receptors that respond to various stimuli. When a stimulus triggers an impulse in a receptor, the action potentials travel to the cerebral cortex, where they are processed and interpreted. Only after this occurs is a particular sensation perceived. Some senses, such as pain, touch, pressure, and proprioception, are widely distributed in the body. These are called **general senses.** Other senses, such as taste, smell, hearing, and sight, are called **special senses** because their receptors are localized in a particular area.

RECEPTORS AND SENSATIONS

Although there are many different kinds of sense receptors, they can be grouped into five types. The basis for these receptor types is the kind of stimulus to which they are sensitive or have a low threshold. The five types of receptors are chemoreceptors, mechanoreceptors, nociceptors, thermoreceptors, and photoreceptors (Table 10-1).

Perceived sensation occurs only after impulses are interpreted by the brain. Steps involved in sensory perception include the following:

1. There must be a **stimulus.**
2. A **receptor** must detect the stimulus and create an action potential.
3. The action potential (impulse) must be **conducted** to the central nervous system (CNS).
4. Within the CNS, the impulse must be **translated** into information.
5. Information must be **interpreted** in the CNS into an awareness or perception of the stimulus.

The impulses from all the receptors are alike. The difference in perception is where they are interpreted in the brain. For example, all impulses going to one particular region are interpreted as sound, whereas those going to another region are interpreted as taste. As the brain interprets a sensation, it projects that sense back to its original source so that the "feeling" seems to come from the receptors that are stimulated. This projection allows us to locate the source of the stimulus.

Some sense receptors, when they are continually stimulated, undergo **sensory adaptation.** They have a decreased sensitivity to a continued stimulus and trigger impulses only if the strength of the stimulus is increased.

GENERAL SENSES

General senses, or **somatic senses,** are those that are found throughout the body. They are associated with the visceral organs, as well as the skin, muscles, and joints, and include the following:

- Touch
- Pressure
- Proprioception
- Temperature
- Pain

Touch and Pressure

As a group, the receptors for touch and pressure are **mechanoreceptors** that are sensitive to forces that deform or displace tissues. They are widely distributed in the skin. Three of the mechanoreceptors involved in touch and pressure are free nerve endings, Meissner's corpuscles, and pacinian corpuscles (Figure 10-1).

Free nerve endings are the dendritic ends of sensory neurons that are interspersed between the cells in epithelial tissue. They do not have a connective tissue covering. They are important in sensing objects, such as clothing, that are in continuous contact with the skin. **Meissner's corpuscles** (MYZE-ners KOAR-pus-als) consist of the ends of sensory nerve fibers surrounded by connective tissue and are specific in localizing tactile sensations. They are located in the dermal papillae, just beneath the epidermis, where they are important in sensing light-discriminative touch stimuli. **Pacinian corpuscles** (pah-SIN-ee-an KOAR-pus-als) are called *lamellated corpuscles* because several layers of connective tissue surround the nerve endings. These are common in deeper dermis and subcutaneous tissues, tendons, and ligaments. They are stimulated by heavy pressure.

Proprioception

Proprioception (proh-pree-oh-SEP-shun) is the sense of position or orientation. It allows us to sense the location and rate of movement of one body part relative to another. **Golgi tendon organs,** found at the junction of a tendon with a muscle, and **muscle spindles,** located in skeletal muscles, are important mechanoreceptors for proprioception. They are illustrated in Figure 10-1.

Temperature

Thermoreceptors are located immediately under the skin and are widely distributed throughout the body. They are

Table 10-1 Types of Sense Receptors

Receptor	Stimulus	Example
Chemoreceptors	Changes in chemical concentration of substances	Taste and smell
Mechanoreceptors	Changes in pressure or movement in fluids	Proprioceptors in joints, receptors for hearing and equilibrium
Nociceptors	Tissue damage	Pain receptors
Thermoreceptors	Changes in temperature	Heat and cold
Photoreceptors	Light energy	Vision

From Applegate E: *The anatomy and physiology learning system,* ed 3, St. Louis, 2006, Saunders.

Highlight on the Senses

ODORS: Nearly everyone is familiar with sensory adaptation in the sense of smell. A particular odor becomes unnoticed after a short time, even though the odor molecules are still present in the air, because the system quickly adapts to the continued stimulation. Odors have the quality of being interpreted as pleasant or unpleasant. Because of this, the sense of smell is as important as taste in the selection of food. For example, a person who has became sick after eating a certain type of food is often nauseated by the smell of that same food at a later occasion.

COLD ADAPTATION: When a person first enters a cool swimming pool on a hot day, there is an abrupt change in temperature; therefore, the cold receptors are strongly stimulated and there is a feeling of discomfort. After a brief time, the receptors adapt, the stimulation fades, and the cool water feels comfortable.

HEADACHE: If there are no pain receptors in the nervous tissue of the brain, what are headaches? Headaches are a type of referred pain, pain that is referred to the surface of the head from deeper structures. The pain stimuli may originate in the meninges or blood vessels within the cranium. Other pain stimuli may originate outside the cranium from muscular spasms, the nasal sinuses, or the eyes.

BITTER TASTE: The taste receptors with the highest degree of sensitivity are those that are stimulated by bitter substances, and a highly intense bitter taste usually causes a person to reject that substance. This is probably an important protective mechanism because many of the deadly toxins found in poisonous plants have an intensely bitter taste.

BLINKING: The eye blinks 6 to 30 times a minute. Blinking stimulates the lacrimal glands to secrete a sterile fluid, or "tears," and helps move the fluid across the eyes.

CORNEAL TRANSPLANT: The cornea was one of the first organs transplanted. Surgical removal of deteriorating corneas and replacement with donor corneas is a common medical procedure for several reasons. The cornea is readily accessible and relatively easy to remove. The tissue is avascular, so there is no bleeding problem or difficulty in establishing circulatory pathways. Corneas are less active than other tissues immunologically and are less likely to be rejected. Long-term success after corneal implant surgery is excellent.

PUPIL SIZE: In addition to regulating the amount of light that enters the eye, pupillary reflexes may also reflect interest or emotional state. For example, frequently the pupils dilate during problem solving or when the subject is appealing. If the subject is boring or repulsive, the pupils constrict.

DETACHED RETINA: Sometimes the sensory portion of the retina breaks away from the pigmented layer, resulting in a **detached retina.** This may be due to trauma, such as a blow to the head, or to certain eye disorders. If allowed to progress, the result is distorted vision and, eventually, blindness. In many cases, the retina can be reattached by laser surgery.

COLOR BLINDNESS: Color blindness occurs because there is an absence or deficiency of one or more of the visual pigments in the cones, and the person cannot distinguish certain colors. In the most common form, red-green color blindness, the cones lack the red pigment and the person is unable to distinguish red from green. Most color blindness is inherited and occurs more frequently in males.

RUPTURED EARDRUM: The eardrum is sometimes ruptured, or perforated, by shock waves from an explosion, scuba diving, trauma, or acute middle ear infections. A perforated eardrum is characterized first by acute pain, then by noise in the affected ear, and then by hearing impairment.

MOTION SICKNESS: Motion sickness is nausea and vomiting resulting from repetitive and excessive stimulation of the equilibrium receptors. Some people are more susceptible than others. ■

most numerous on the lips and are least numerous on some of the broad surfaces of the trunk. Thermoreceptors include at least two types of free nerve endings that are sensitive to temperature changes. In general, there are up to 10 times more **cold receptors** in a given area than **heat receptors.** Extremes in temperature stimulate pain receptors. Below 10°C, pain receptors produce a freezing sensation. As the temperature increases above 10°C, pain impulses cease but **cold receptors** begin to be stimulated. At temperatures about 25°C, **heat receptors** begin to be stimulated and cold receptors fade out. Finally, as temperatures approach 45°C, heat receptors fade out and pain receptors are stimulated to produce a burning sensation. A person determines gradations in temperatures by the degree of stimulation of each

Figure 10-1. General sense receptors. (From Applegate E: *The anatomy and physiology learning system,* ed 3, St. Louis, 2006, Saunders.)

Meissner's corpuscle

Free nerve ending

Golgi tendon organ

Pacinian corpuscle

Muscle spindle

type of receptor. Extreme cold and extreme heat feel almost the same—both are painful—because the pain receptors are being stimulated. Thermoreceptors are strongly stimulated by abrupt changes in temperature and then fade after a few seconds or minutes. In other words, thermoreceptors show rapid **sensory adaptation.**

Pain

The sense of pain is initiated by **nociceptors** (noh-see-SEP-tors), which are free nerve endings that are stimulated by tissue damage. They are widely distributed throughout the skin and in the tissues of the internal organs. The nervous tissue of the brain has no pain receptors; however, other tissues in the head, including the meninges and blood vessels, have an abundant supply. Pain receptors have a protective function because pain is usually perceived as unpleasant and is a signal to locate and remove the source of the tissue damage. Nociceptors usually do not adapt and may continue to send signals after the stimulus is removed.

GUSTATORY SENSE

The **gustatory sense,** or **taste,** is one of the special senses. As previously explained, the senses of taste, smell, hearing, and sight are called *special senses* because their receptors are localized in a particular area.

The organs of taste, the **taste buds,** are localized in the mouth region, primarily on the surface of the tongue, where they lie along the walls of projections called **papillae** (Figure 10-2). The receptors belong to the **chemoreceptor** (kee-moh-ree-SEP-tor) category because they are sensitive to chemicals in the food we eat. In order for these chemicals to be detected by a chemoreceptor, they must be dissolved in water.

Within the taste bud, specialized epithelial cells called **taste cells** or **gustatory cells** are interspersed with supporting cells and nerve fibers (see Figure 10-2). The entire taste

bud opens to the surface through a **taste pore.** Tiny **taste hairs** (microvilli) project from the taste cells through the taste pore, and it is these hairs on the taste cells that function as the receptors.

Although all the taste receptors appear to be alike, there are at least four different types, each one sensitive to a particular kind of stimulus. Consequently, there are four different taste sensations:
* Salty   * Sour
* Sweet   * Bitter

Instead of being evenly distributed over the surface of the tongue, each one of the four tastes is concentrated in a specific region, as illustrated in Figure 10-3.

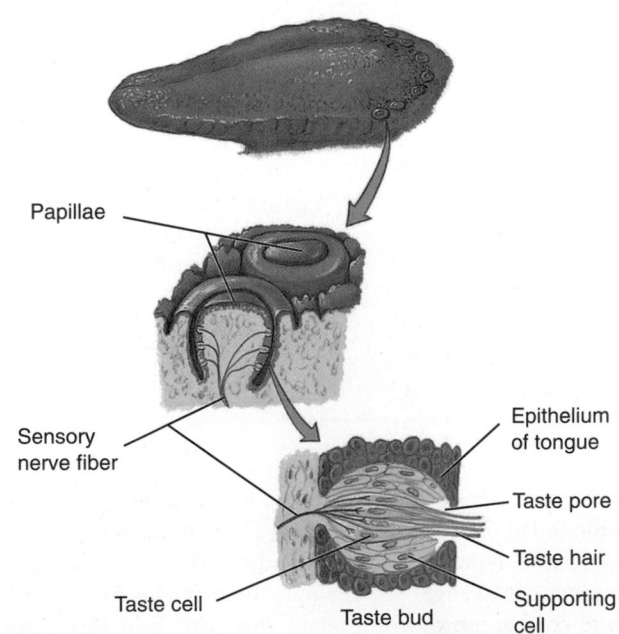

Papillae

Sensory nerve fiber

Taste cell

Epithelium of tongue

Taste pore

Taste hair

Taste bud

Supporting cell

Figure 10-2. Taste buds. (From Applegate E: *The anatomy and physiology learning system,* ed 3, St. Louis, 2006, Saunders.)

When the microvilli, or taste hairs, are stimulated, an impulse is triggered on a nearby nerve fiber. Impulses from the anterior two thirds of the tongue travel along the **facial nerve,** and those from the posterior one third travel along the **glossopharyngeal** (glos-so-fah-RIN-jee-al) **nerve** to the medulla oblongata (see Chapter 9, Table 9-8). From the medulla oblongata they travel to the thalamus, then to the sensory cortex on the parietal lobe, near the lateral sulcus.

OLFACTORY SENSE

The receptors for **olfaction** (sense of smell) are bipolar neurons surrounded by supporting columnar epithelial cells in the **olfactory epithelium** of the nasal cavity (Figure 10-4). The **olfactory neurons** are concentrated in the superior region of the cavity. These neurons have long cilia that extend to the surface and project into the nasal cavity. The cilia are believed to be the sensitive receptors of the neuron.

Like those for taste, the olfactory receptors are **chemoreceptors.** They are stimulated by chemicals dissolved in liquids. In this case, airborne molecules responsible for odors dissolve in the fluid on the surface of the olfactory epithelium and then bind to the receptors and trigger impulses.

Axons from the olfactory neurons pass through foramina in the cribriform plate of the ethmoid bone and enter the **olfactory bulb.** Here they synapse with association neurons that conduct the impulses through the **olfactory tract** to the brain. The olfactory tracts terminate in the **olfactory cortex** in the temporal lobe.

The senses of taste and smell are closely related and complement each other. They often have a combined effect when they are interpreted in the cerebral cortex. This implies that part of what we "taste" is really smell. Also, part of what we "smell" is taste because some airborne molecules move from the nose down to the mouth and stimulate taste buds.

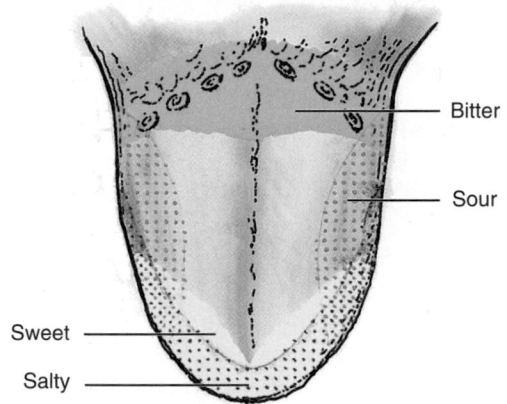

Figure 10-3. Regions of the tongue sensitive to various tastes. (From Applegate E: *The anatomy and physiology learning system,* ed 3, St. Louis, 2006, Saunders.)

Bitter

Sour

Sweet

Salty

VISUAL SENSE

Most of us consider vision to be one of the most important senses we have. The eyes, which contain the photoreceptors, are the organs of vision. They are protected by a bony socket and are assisted in their function of vision by accessory structures that protect and move them.

Protective Features and Accessory Structures of the Eye

Only a small portion of the eye is visible from the exterior. Most of it is surrounded by a protective bony **orbit,** or

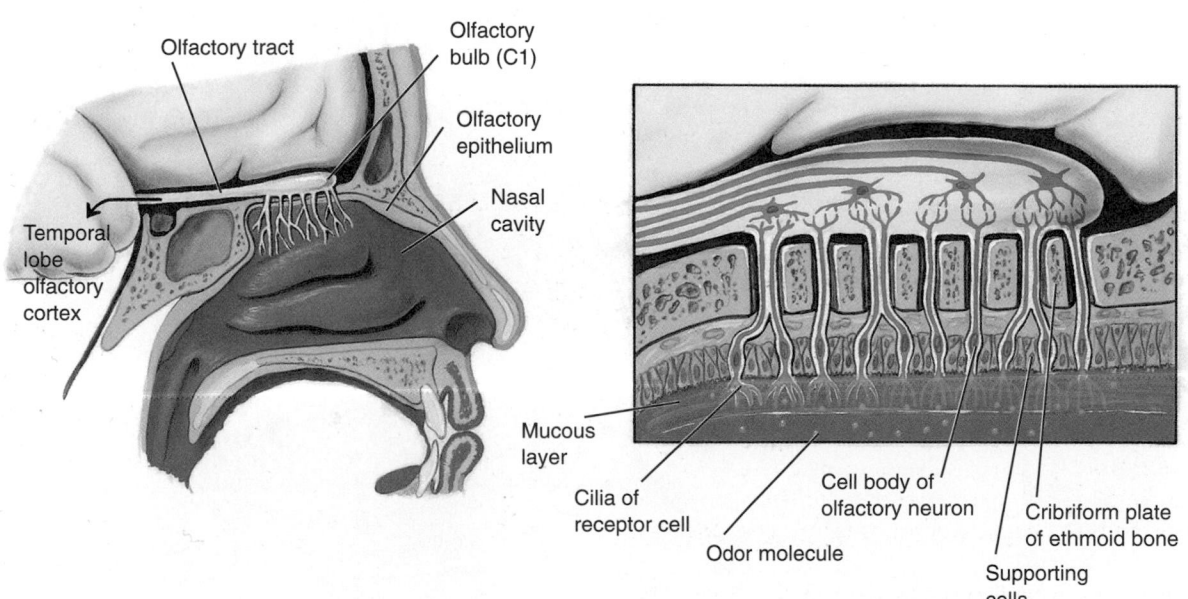

Olfactory tract

Olfactory bulb (C1)

Olfactory epithelium

Nasal cavity

Temporal lobe olfactory cortex

Mucous layer

Cilia of receptor cell

Odor molecule

Cell body of olfactory neuron

Cribriform plate of ethmoid bone

Supporting cells

Figure 10-4. Structure of the olfactory receptors. (From Applegate E: *The anatomy and physiology learning system,* ed 3, St. Louis, 2006, Saunders.)

socket, formed by portions of seven cranial bones: frontal, lacrimal, ethmoid, maxilla, zygomatic, sphenoid, and palatine. It also contains fat, various connective tissues, blood vessels, and nerves.

Eyebrows help to keep perspiration, which can be an irritant, out of the eyes. **Eyelids** function to open and close the eye and to keep foreign objects from entering the eye. The eyelids are composed of skin, connective tissue, muscle, and **conjunctiva** (kon-junk-TYE-vah). The muscles associated with the eyelids are the **orbicularis oculi,** which is a sphincter that closes the eye, and the **levator palpebrae superioris,** which elevates the eyelid to open the eye. The conjunctiva, a thin mucous membrane, lines the eyelid and then folds back to cover the anterior portion of the eyeball, except for the central portion, which is the cornea. Mucus from the conjunctiva helps keep the eye from drying out. **Eyelashes** line the margin of the eyelid and help trap foreign particles. **Sebaceous glands** associated with the eyelashes secrete an oily fluid that helps lubricate the region. Inflammation of the sebaceous glands is called a **stye.**

The **lacrimal** (LACK-rih-mal) **apparatus,** shown in Figure 10-5, consists of the lacrimal gland and various ducts. The **lacrimal gland** is located in the superior and lateral region of the orbit. Tears produced by the lacrimal gland flow through **lacrimal ducts** and across the surface of the eye to the medial side, where they drain into two small **lacrimal canals** (canaliculi). From the lacrimal canals, the tears flow into the **lacrimal sac,** and then into the **nasolacrimal duct,** which opens into the nasal cavity. Tears moisten, lubricate, and cleanse the anterior surface of the eye. They also contain an enzyme (lysozyme) that helps destroy bacteria and prevent infections.

Structure of the Eyeball

The eyeball, or **bulbus oculi** (BUL-bus AHK-yoo-lye), is somewhat spherical, is 2 to 3 cm in diameter, and has an anterior bulge. It is surrounded by orbital fat within the orbital cavity. Figure 10-6 illustrates the structure of the bulbus oculi.

The wall of the eyeball is made up of three concentric coats or tunics. The outermost layer is the **fibrous tunic.** It consists of the white, opaque **sclera** (SKLEE-rah) and the transparent **cornea.** The sclera, the white part of the eye, covers the posterior five sixths of the eyeball, and the muscles that move the eye are attached to it. The transparent cornea, which covers the anterior one sixth of the eyeball, is the "window" of the eye. It helps focus light rays entering the eye.

The middle layer of the eyeball is the **vascular tunic.** It consists of the **choroid** (KOAR-oyd), **ciliary body,** and **iris.** The **choroid** is a highly vascular, brown pigmented layer located between the sclera and the retina in the posterior portion of the eye. It is the largest part of the middle tunic and lines most of the sclera, although it is only loosely con-

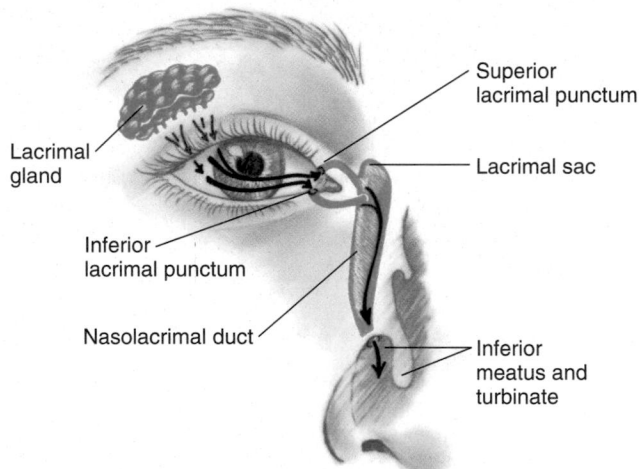

Figure 10-5. Lacrimal apparatus of the eye. (From Jarvis C: *Physical examination and health assessment,* ed 4, St. Louis, 2004, Saunders.)

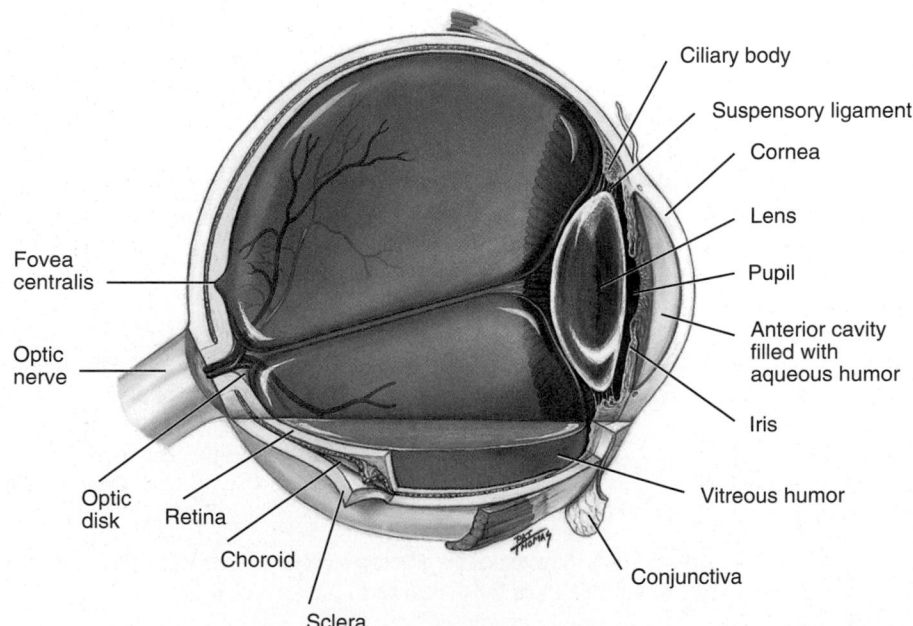

Figure 10-6. Anatomy of the eye. (From Applegate E: *The anatomy and physiology learning system,* ed 3, St. Louis, 2006, Saunders.)

nected to the fibrous coat and can be stripped away easily. The choroid is, however, firmly attached to the retina. The brown pigment in the choroid absorbs excess light rays that might interfere with vision. The blood vessels nourish the interior of the eye. Anteriorly, the choroid is continuous with the **ciliary body.** Numerous finger-like **ciliary processes** within the ciliary body secrete aqueous humor, a fluid in the anterior portion of the eye. The ciliary body also contains the **ciliary muscle. Suspensory ligaments** connect the ciliary body to the transparent, biconvex **lens** of the eye. When the ciliary muscle contracts, the suspensory ligaments relax and the lens bulges to allow focusing for close vision. The **iris** is the conspicuous, colored portion of the eye. It is a doughnut-shaped diaphragm with a central aperture, called the **pupil.** The iris contains two groups of smooth muscles, a radial group and a circular group. When the radial muscles contract, the pupil dilates; when the circular group contracts, the pupil gets smaller. These muscles of the iris continually contract and relax to change the size of the pupil, which regulates the amount of light entering the eye.

The innermost coat of the eyeball is the **nervous tunic,** or **retina** (RET-ih-nah), which is found only in the posterior portion of the eye. It ends at the posterior margin of the ciliary body. The retina contains several layers. The outer layer is deeply pigmented and firmly attached to the choroid. The layer next to the pigmented layer contains the **rods and cones,** which are the receptor (photoreceptor) cells. Other layers consist of bipolar neurons and ganglion cells. The axons of the ganglion cells converge to form the **optic nerve,** which penetrates the tunics at the **optic disk** and passes through the apex of the orbital cavity to reach the brain. Because there are no photoreceptor cells in the optic disk, it is commonly referred to as the "blind spot" of the eye. Just lateral to the optic disk, near the center of the retina, there is a yellow spot called the **macula lutea** (MACK-yoo-lah LOO-tee-ah). The region of the retina that produces the sharpest image is a depression, the **fovea centralis** (FOE-vee-ah sen-TRAL-is), in the center of the macula lutea.

The lens, suspensory ligaments, and ciliary body form a partition that divides the interior of the eyeball into two cavities. The space anterior to the lens, between the cornea and the lens, is the anterior cavity and is filled with **aqueous humor** secreted by the ciliary body. Aqueous humor helps maintain the shape of the anterior part of the eye and nourishes the structures in that region. It is largely responsible for the internal pressure of the eye. The aqueous humor circulates through the anterior cavity and then is reabsorbed into blood vessels at the junction of the sclera and cornea. The posterior cavity, between the lens and the retina, is filled with a colorless, transparent, gel-like **vitreous humor.** The vitreous humor presses the retina firmly against the wall of the eye, supports the internal parts of the eye, and helps maintain its shape.

Pathway of Light and Refraction

Vision depends on light rays. When a person sees an object, light rays from the object enter the eye. Light rays have two important properties—they travel in a straight line and

can be bent. When light rays travel from one substance to another that has a different optical density, the rays bend. The bending of light rays is called **refraction.** When light rays hit a concave surface, they scatter or diverge. When the rays meet a convex surface, they get closer together or converge. The eyes have four refractive surfaces and media. In a normal eye, the cornea, aqueous humor, lens, and vitreous humor bend the light rays so that they focus on the retina. The image that forms on the retina is upside down and backward (Figure 10-7), but somehow the brain turns it around and interprets the image in the correct position.

When an object is at least 20 feet away, the normal relaxed eye is able to focus the image on the retina. When the object is closer than 20 feet, the eye must make adjustments to focus the image. These adjustments are called **accommodation.** The primary action in accommodation, illustrated in Figure 10-8, is changing the shape of the lens. For distance vision, the ciliary muscle is relaxed, the suspensory ligaments are taut, and the lens is flat. When the eyes accommodate for close vision, the ciliary muscle contracts, the suspensory ligaments become loose or relaxed, and the lens bulges or becomes more convex. The closer the object, the more the light rays have to bend to focus and the greater the curvature of the lens.

Photoreceptors

The retina, illustrated in Figure 10-9, contains two kinds of **photoreceptor** cells: rods and cones. These cells are next

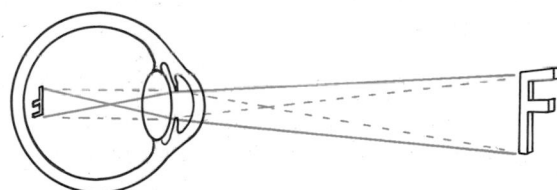

Figure 10-7. Formation of images on the retina. The image on the retina is upside down and backward. (From Applegate E: *The anatomy and physiology learning system,* ed 3, St. Louis, 2006, Saunders.)

Figure 10-8. Accommodation. For distance vision, the ciliary muscles relax, the suspensory ligaments are taut, and the lens is flat. For close vision, the ciliary muscles contract, the suspensory ligaments relax, and the lens becomes more convex. (From Applegate E: *The anatomy and physiology learning system,* ed 3, St. Louis, 2006, Saunders.)

Table 10-2 Comparison of Rods and Cones

Feature	Rods	Cones
Shape	Long, slender projections	Short, thick projections
Location	None in fovea centralis; increase in density away from fovea centralis	Concentrated in fovea centralis; decrease in density away from fovea centralis
Quantity	More numerous than cones	Less numerous than rods
Convergence	High degree of convergence	Less convergence
Pigments	Single pigment, rhodopsin	Three pigments, one each for red, green, blue
Functions	Black and white vision; dim light; night vision; lacks detail	Color vision; bright light; precise vision with fine detail

From Applegate E: *The anatomy and physiology learning system,* ed 3, St. Louis, 2006, Saunders.

Figure 10-9. Structure of the retina showing the rods and cones. (From Applegate E: *The anatomy and physiology learning system,* ed 3, St. Louis, 2006, Saunders.)

to the outermost retina layer of pigmented epithelium. **Rods,** thin cells with slender, rodlike projections, are sensitive to dim light. Even though rods are much more numerous than cones, they are absent in the fovea centralis and their number increases proportionately to the distance away from the fovea centralis. Many rods synapse with a single sensory fiber (convergence); thus vision with rods lacks fine detail. **Cones,** the receptors for color vision and visual acuity, are located primarily in the fovea centralis. They are thicker cells with short, blunt projections. Cones exhibit less convergence than rods, so in addition to color, cones provide sharp images and fine detail. Table 10-2 compares the rods and cones.

Rods contain a substance, **rhodopsin** (roe-DOP-sin) (visual purple), that is very light sensitive. When even small amounts of light focus on the rods, rhodopsin breaks down into its component parts—opsin (a protein) and a derivative of vitamin A, retinal (retinene). This reaction triggers a nerve impulse. Rhodopsin is resynthesized from opsin and retinal to prepare the rods for receiving subsequent stimuli. The more rhodopsin there is in the rods, the greater the sensitivity to light. In bright light, nearly all the rhodopsin in the rods is decomposed. After entering a dimly lit area,

it takes some time for the eyes to adapt to the dim light. During this period, rhodopsin is regenerated in the rods so that they become more sensitive.

Cones function in a manner that is similar to rods. Light-sensitive pigments break down into component parts, and the reaction triggers nerve impulses. Three different types of cones exist, each with a different visual pigment. All the pigments contain retinal, but the protein portion is different. One type responds best to green light, another responds best to blue light, and a third type responds best to red light. The perceived color of an object depends on the quantity and combination of cones that are stimulated. If all the pigments are stimulated, the person senses white. If none are stimulated, the person senses black.

Visual Pathway

Visual impulses generated in the rods and cones of the retina leave the eyes in the axons that form the **optic nerves.** Just anterior to the pituitary gland, these nerves form an X-shaped structure, the **optic chiasma** (OP-tik kye-AZ-mah). Within the optic chiasma, the axons from the medial portion of each retina cross over to enter the **optic tract** on the opposite side (Figure 10-10). The right optic tract contains the fibers from the lateral portion of the right eye and the medial portion of the left eye. The left optic tract contains the fibers from the lateral portion of the left eye and the medial portion of the right eye. The optic tracts lead to the **thalamus.** Just before they reach the thalamus, a few fibers leave the tracts and enter the nuclei that function in visual reflexes (superior colliculi). Most of the fibers enter the thalamus, where they synapse with neurons that carry the impulses in the **optic radiations** to the visual cortex of the occipital lobes. Because some of the fibers cross over to the other side in the optic chiasma, each occipital lobe receives an image of the entire object from each eye but from slightly different perspectives. This enables vision in three dimensions.

AUDITORY SENSE

The **ear** is the organ of hearing (auditory or acoustic organ). It is also the organ for the sense of equilibrium, which is covered later in this chapter. The receptors for hearing,

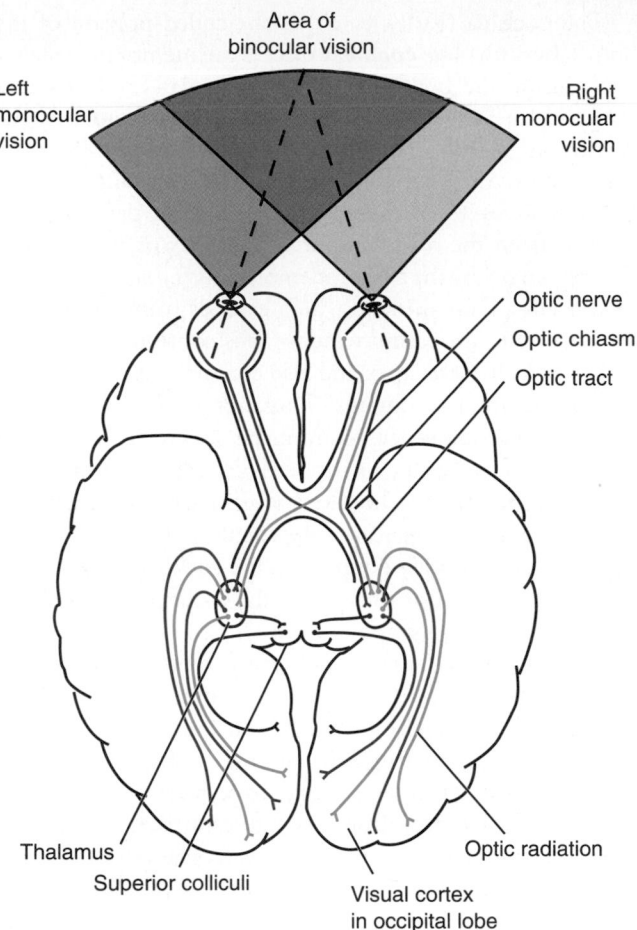

Figure 10-10. Visual pathway. (From Applegate E: *The anatomy and physiology learning system,* ed 3, St. Louis, 2006, Saunders.)

located within the ear, are **mechanoreceptors** (mek-ah-noh-ree-SEP-tors). Physical forces, in the form of sound vibrations, are responsible for initiating impulses that are interpreted as sound.

Structure of the Ear

The "ears" on the sides of the head are only a portion of the actual organ of hearing. A large part of the organ, actually the most important part, lies hidden from view in the temporal bone. Anatomically, the organ of hearing is divided into the external ear, middle ear, and inner ear. The anatomy of the ear is illustrated in Figure 10-11.

External Ear

The **external ear** consists of an auricle, or pinna, and the external auditory canal. The **auricle,** or pinna, is the fleshy part of the external ear that is visible on the side of the head and surrounds the opening into the external auditory meatus. The auricle collects sound waves and directs them toward the auditory canal.

The **external auditory canal** is an S-shaped tube, about 2.5 cm long, that extends from the auricle to the **tympanic membrane.** The skin that lines the external auditory canal has numerous hairs and **ceruminous glands,** which secrete a waxy substance called **cerumen.** The hairs and cerumen help prevent foreign objects from reaching the eardrum. The external ear ends at the tympanic membrane.

Middle Ear

The **middle ear** is an air-filled cavity, called the **tympanic cavity,** in the temporal bone. It begins at the tympanic

Figure 10-11. Anatomy of the ear. (From Jarvis C: *Physical examination and health assessment,* ed 5, St. Louis, 2008, Saunders.)

membrane, contains the auditory ossicles, and has an opening into the eustachian tube. The **oval window** and the **round window** in the medial wall of the middle ear connect the middle ear with the inner ear. The oval window is closed by the stapes, one of the bones in the middle ear. The round window is closed by a membrane.

The **tympanic membrane,** or eardrum, is a thin membrane that separates the external ear from the middle ear. Sound waves cause the tympanic membrane to vibrate.

An **auditory tube** (eustachian tube) connects each middle ear with the throat. Its purpose is to equalize the pressure between the outside air and the middle ear cavity, a condition necessary for normal hearing. Throat infections may spread to the middle ear through the auditory tube.

The **auditory ossicles** are three tiny bones: the **malleus** (hammer), **incus** (anvil), and **stapes** (stirrup). These bones are linked together by tiny ligaments and form a bridge across the space of the tympanic cavity. The malleus is attached to the tympanic membrane, and the stapes is attached to the oval window between the middle ear and the inner ear. The incus is between the malleus and stapes. When the tympanic membrane vibrates, the ossicles transmit the vibrations across the cavity to the oval window, which transfers the motion to the fluids in the inner ear. This fluid motion excites the receptors for hearing.

Inner Ear

The **inner ear** consists of a bony labyrinth and a membranous labyrinth (Figure 10-12). The **bony** (osseous) **labyrinth** is a series of interconnecting chambers in the temporal bone. The **membranous labyrinth,** located inside the bony labyrinth, is a system of membranous tubes that are similar to the bony labyrinth in shape but smaller. A clear fluid called **endolymph** fills the membranous labyrinth. The space between the bony and the membranous labyrinths contains a fluid called **perilymph.** The inner ear is divided into the vestibule, semicircular canals, and cochlea. The vestibule and semicircular canals function in the sense of equilibrium. The cochlea functions in the sense of hearing.

The **cochlea** (KOK-lee-ah) is the coiled portion of the bony labyrinth. The **cochlear duct** is the membranous labyrinth inside the bony labyrinth. Figure 10-13 shows that the inside of the cochlea is divided into three regions by the **vestibular membrane** and the **basilar membrane.** The region above the vestibular membrane is the **scala vestibuli** (SKAY-lah ves-TIB-yoo-lee), which contains perilymph. It extends from the oval window to the apex of the cochlea. The region below the basilar membrane is the **scala tympani** (SKAY-lah TIM-pah-nee), which extends from the apex of the cochlea to the round window. It is continuous with the scala vestibuli at the apex and also contains perilymph. The basilar membrane contains thousands of stiff fibers that gradually increase in length from the base to the apex. The arrangement is similar to the reeds in a harmonica or the bars on a marimba. The fibers vibrate when activated by sound. The middle region of the cochlea, between the scala vestibuli and the scala tympani, is the cochlear duct, which ends as a closed sac at the apex of the cochlea. The cochlear duct contains endolymph.

The **organ of Corti** (KOAR-tee), which contains the receptors for sound, is located on the upper surface of the basilar membrane, within the cochlear duct (Figure 10-14). It consists of **supporting cells** and **hair cells.** The hair cells are specialized sensory cells that have hairlike projections (microvilli) extending from their free surface. The tips of the projections contact a gelatinous **tectorial** (tek-TOE-ree-al) **membrane** that extends over them. Hair cells have no axons, but they are surrounded by sensory nerve fibers that form the **cochlear branch** of the **vestibulocochlear nerve** (cranial nerve VIII).

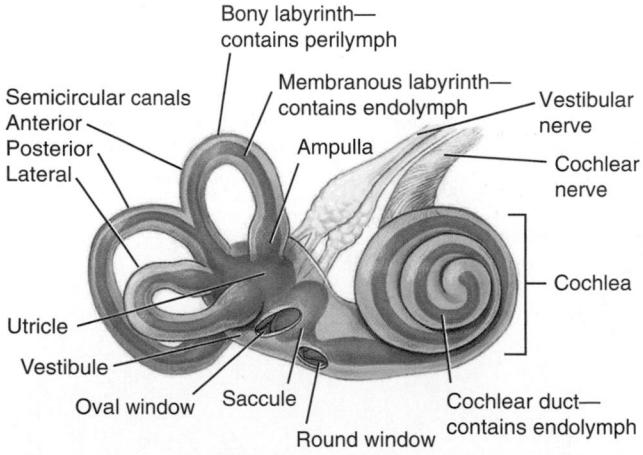

Bony labyrinth—
contains perilymph

Semicircular canals
Anterior
Posterior
Lateral

Membranous labyrinth—
contains endolymph

Ampulla

Vestibular
nerve

Cochlear
nerve

Cochlea

Utricle

Vestibule

Oval window
Saccule
Round window
Cochlear duct—
contains endolymph

Figure 10-12. Labyrinths of the inner ear. (From Applegate E: *The anatomy and physiology learning system,* ed 3, St. Louis, 2006, Saunders.)

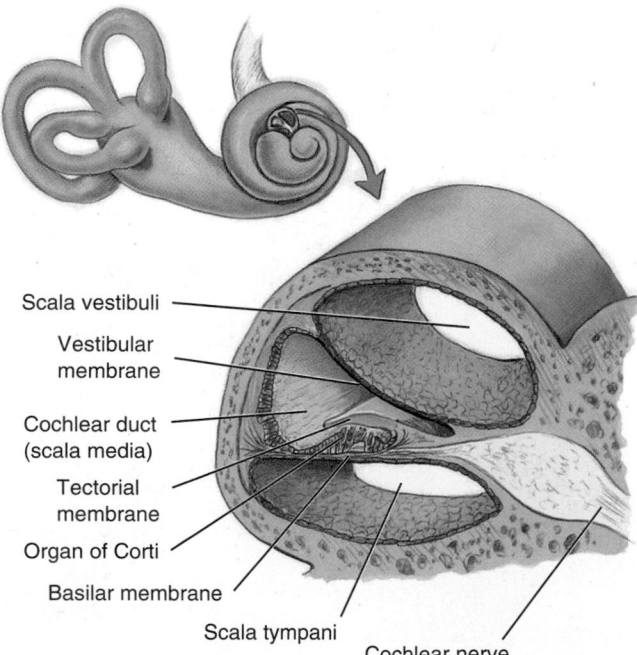

Scala vestibuli

Vestibular
membrane

Cochlear duct
(scala media)

Tectorial
membrane

Organ of Corti

Basilar membrane

Scala tympani

Cochlear nerve

Figure 10-13. Section through the cochlea. (From Applegate E: *The anatomy and physiology learning system,* ed 3, St. Louis, 2006, Saunders.)

Physiology of Hearing

Sound travels through the atmosphere in waves of alternating compressions and decompressions of molecules. Low-pitched tones create low-frequency sound waves; high-pitched tones create high-frequency sound waves. An individual with normal hearing should be able to hear the frequencies of normal speech, which range from 300 to 4000 vibrations per second. Hearing is most acute with frequencies between 2000 and 3000 vibrations per second.

Initiation of Impulses

The process of hearing begins when sound waves enter the external auditory canal. As the waves travel through the external ear, they hit the tympanic membrane and cause it to vibrate. Because the malleus is attached to the membrane, the vibrations are transferred from the tympanic membrane to the malleus, then to the incus, and then to the stapes,

which creates vibrations in the membrane of the oval window. Movement of the oval window passes the vibrations to the perilymph in the inner ear.

Figure 10-15 illustrates an uncoiled cochlea to show the relationships of its components. The vibrations in the perilymph, caused by movement of the oval window, travel through the scala vestibuli, around the apex, and through the scala tympani to the round window. Thus, every time the stapes pushes the oval window inward toward the inner ear, movement in the perilymph pushes the round window outward toward the middle ear to relieve the pressure in the fluid. As vibrations travel through the perilymph, they create corresponding oscillations in the vestibular membrane, which causes movement of the endolymph within the scala media (cochlear duct), and finally the vibrations are transferred to the basilar membrane.

When the basilar membrane moves up and down, the organ of Corti moves with it and the hairs on the hair cells rub against the tectorial membrane. As the hairs contact the membrane, they bend, and this mechanical deformation initiates the nerve impulses that result in hearing. The list below summarizes the sequence of events in the initiation of auditory impulses.

1. The tympanic membrane vibrates in response to sound waves.
2. The malleus, incus, and stapes transfer vibrations to the oval window membrane.
3. Movement of the oval window membrane starts oscillations in the perilymph in the cochlea.
4. Oscillations in the perilymph cause vibrations in the vestibular and basilar membranes.
5. When the basilar membrane moves, the hairs on the hair cells in the organ of Corti rub against the tectorial membrane and bend.
6. Bending of the hairs on the hair cells stimulates the formation of impulses.

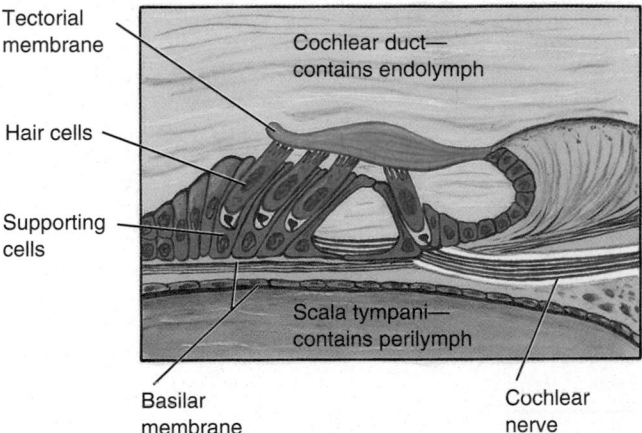

Tectorial membrane
Hair cells
Supporting cells
Cochlear duct—contains endolymph
Scala tympani—contains perilymph
Basilar membrane
Cochlear nerve

Figure 10-14. Organ of Corti. (From Applegate E: *The anatomy and physiology learning system,* ed 3, St. Louis, 2006, Saunders.)

Tympanic membrane
Malleus
Incus
Stapes
Oval window
Scala vestibuli—contains perilymph
Tectorial membrane
Vestibular membrane
Cochlear duct—contains endolymph
Pinna
Apex
Low frequency
High frequency
Round window
Organ of Corti
Basilar membrane
Scala tympani

Figure 10-15. Uncoiled cochlea showing the pathway of pressure waves. (From Applegate E: *The anatomy and physiology learning system,* ed 3, St. Louis, 2006, Saunders.)

7. Impulses are transmitted to the auditory cortex of the temporal lobe on the cochlear branch of cranial nerve VIII, the vestibulocochlear nerve.

Pitch and Loudness

Hair cells along the length of the organ of Corti have varying sensitivities to different frequencies. Also, different regions of the basilar membrane vibrate in response to different frequencies. The portion of the membrane near the base of the cochlea vibrates in response to high frequencies. Near the apex of the cochlea, the basilar membrane responds to low frequencies. Pitch is detected by the portion of the basilar membrane that vibrates in response to the sound and sensitivity of the hair cells.

Loudness is determined by the intensity of the sound waves. The basilar membrane vibrates more (i.e., has a greater magnitude of oscillation) in response to loud sounds. This means that more hair cells are stimulated and more impulses travel to the auditory cortex.

Auditory Pathway

Auditory impulses leave the cochlea on the **cochlear nerve,** a branch of cranial nerve VIII, the **vestibulocochlear nerve.** The fibers synapse in the **medulla,** where some cross over to the opposite side, and then continue to the inferior colliculi of the **midbrain** for auditory reflexes. Next, the impulses are transmitted to the **thalamus,** where they synapse with neurons that transmit the impulses to the auditory cortex of the **temporal lobe.**

SENSE OF EQUILIBRIUM

The sense of equilibrium is a combination of two different senses: the sense of **static equilibrium** and the sense of **dynamic equilibrium.** Static equilibrium is involved in evaluating the position of the head relative to gravity. It occurs when the head is motionless or moving in a straight line. Dynamic equilibrium occurs when the head is moving in a rotational or angular direction.

Static Equilibrium

The organs of static equilibrium are located in the **vestibule** portion of the bony labyrinth of the inner ear. The membranous labyrinth inside the vestibule is divided into two saclike structures, the **utricle** (YOO-trih-kull) and the **saccule** (SACK-yool) (see Figure 10-12). Each of these contains a small structure called a **macula** (MACK-yoo-lah), which is the organ of static equilibrium. The macula consists of sensory hair cells, similar to those in the organ of Corti, and supporting cells (Figure 10-16). The projections, or hairs, of the hair cells are embedded in a gelatinous mass that covers the macula. Grains of calcium carbonate, called **otoliths** (OH-toe-liths), are embedded on the surface of the gelatinous mass.

When the head is in an upright position, the hairs are straight. When the head tilts or bends forward, the otoliths and the gelatinous mass move in response to gravity. As the gelatinous mass moves, it bends some of the hairs on the

Figure 10-16. Structure of the macula. (From Applegate E: *The anatomy and physiology learning system,* ed 3, St. Louis, 2006, Saunders.)

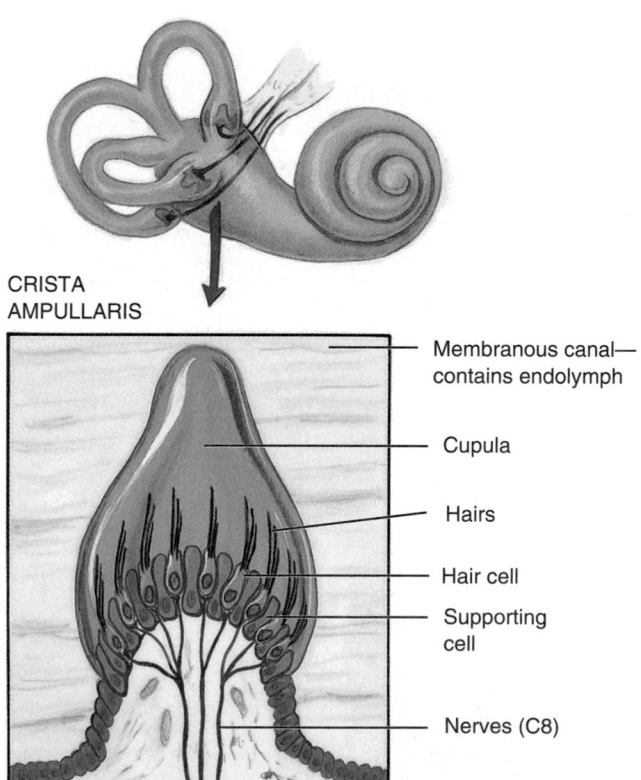

Figure 10-17. Structure of the crista ampullaris. (From Applegate E: *The anatomy and physiology learning system,* ed 3, St. Louis, 2006, Saunders.)

receptor cells. This action initiates an impulse that travels to the CNS by way of the vestibular branch of the vestibulocochlear nerve. The CNS interprets the information and sends motor impulses out to appropriate muscles to maintain balance.

Highlight on Aging and the Senses

As the body ages, a general decline in all of the special senses occurs. The most significant changes in the eye occur in the lens. It tends to become thicker and less elastic, which makes it less able to change shape to accommodate for near vision. This condition, called **presbyopia** or farsightedness of aging, probably is the most common age-related dysfunction of the eye. The lens also tends to become cloudy or opaque, forming cataracts. About 90% of people older than age 70 have some degree of cataract formation; however, it is not always significant enough to affect vision. The cornea tends to become more translucent and less spherical, which contributes to an increase in astigmatism in older people. Older people require more light to see well because atrophy of the muscles in the iris reduces the ability of the pupil to dilate and decreases the amount of light that reaches the retina. The chemical processes that rebuild the visual pigment, rhodopsin, are slower in older people, so dark adaptation takes longer and is not as complete as in young people.

Most age-related changes in the external ear and middle ear have little effect on hearing. A buildup of cerumen, or earwax, in the external ear may contribute to hearing loss in the low-frequency range. The joints between the auditory ossicles in the middle ear may become less movable, which interferes with the transmission of sound waves to the inner ear, but generally it is not clinically significant. Most of the gradual loss of hearing that usually begins by the age of 40 is due to degeneration of the receptor cells in the spiral organ of Corti in the inner ear. Another factor is the decrease in the number of nerve fibers in the vestibulocochlear nerve. The reduction in fibers in the cochlear branch contributes to hearing loss. A decrease in vestibular fibers affects balance and equilibrium.

Taste and smell, both chemical senses, show a decline with age; however, the mechanism is unclear. Diminished perception may be due to degeneration of the receptor cells, to changes in the way the impulses are processed in the brain, or to other factors. It is likely that decreases in sensory perception are due to a combination of several factors. ■

Highlight on Conditions Affecting the Senses

Astigmatism (ah-STIG-mah-tizm) Defective curvature of the cornea or lens of the eye resulting in a distorted image on the retina

Blepharitis (bleff-ahr-EYE-tis) Inflammation of the edges of the eyelid

Glaucoma (glaw-KOH-mah) Disease of the eye characterized by increased intraocular pressure from an accumulation of aqueous humor caused by either increased production or decreased drainage; the increased pressure causes pathologic changes in the optic disk and typical defects in the field of vision; if untreated, glaucoma leads to blindness

Macular degeneration (MACK-yoo-lahr dee-jen-er-A-shun) A gradually progressive condition that results in the loss of central vision because of the breakdown of cells in the macula lutea; frequently affects older people

Meniere's disease (men-ih-ARZ dih-ZEEZ) A chronic disease of the inner ear characterized by recurring attacks of dizziness, tinnitus, and fluctuating hearing loss; attacks vary in duration and frequency

Nyctalopia (nick-tah-LOH-pee-ah) A condition in which the individual has difficulty seeing at night; night blindness

Otosclerosis (oh-toe-sklee-ROH-sis) Progressive formation of bony tissue around the oval window, immobilizing the stapes; results in conduction deafness

Presbycusis (prez-bih-KUS-is) Impairment of hearing resulting from aging

Presbyopia (prez-bih-OH-pee-ah) Impairment of vision caused by aging

Sensorineural deafness (sen-soh-ree NEW-rahl DEFF-nis) Hearing loss as a result of damage along any part of the auditory pathway from the receptor cells in the cochlea to the auditory cortex of the cerebrum; noise-related damage to the receptor cells in the cochlear is this type of deafness

Tinnitus (tin-EYE-tus) A ringing or buzzing sound in the ears

Tympanitis (tim-pan-EYE-tis) Inflammation of the tympanic membrane

Vertigo (VER-tih-goh) A feeling of dizziness, loss of balance, and lightheadedness caused by a disturbance of the semicircular canals, utricle, saccule, or vestibular nerve ■

Dynamic Equilibrium

The sense organs for dynamic equilibrium, the equilibrium of rotational or angular movements, are located in the membranous labyrinth of the **semicircular canals.** Three semicircular canals, positioned at right angles to each other, exist in three different planes (see Figure 10-12). Each membranous canal is surrounded by perilymph and contains endolymph. At the base of each canal, near where it attaches to the utricle, there is a swelling called the **ampulla.** The sensory organs of the semicircular canals are located within the ampullae. Each of these organs, called a **crista ampullaris** (KRIS-tah amp-yoo-LAIR-is), contains sensory hair cells and supporting cells (Figure 10-17). The crista ampullaris is covered by a dome-shaped gelatinous mass called the **cupula** (KEW-pew-lah). The hairs of the hair cells are embedded in the cupula.

When the head turns rapidly, the semicircular canals move with the head but the endolymph tends to remain stationary. The fluid pushes against the cupula, and it tilts to one side. As the cupula tilts, it bends some of the hairs on the hair cells, which triggers a sensory impulse. Because the three canals are in different planes, their cristae are stimulated differently by the same motion. This creates a mosaic of impulses that are transmitted to the CNS on the **vestibular branch** of the **vestibulocochlear nerve.** The CNS interprets the information and initiates appropriate responses to maintain balance. The cerebellum is particularly important in mediating the sense of balance and equilibrium.

TERMINOLOGY REVIEW

Accommodation Mechanism that allows the eye to focus at various distances, primarily achieved by changing the curvature of the lens.

Chemoreceptor A sensory receptor that detects the presence of chemicals; responsible for taste, smell, and monitoring the concentration of certain chemicals in body fluids.

Mechanoreceptor A sensory receptor that responds to a bending or deformation of the cell; examples include receptors for touch, pressure, hearing, and equilibrium.

Nociceptor A sensory receptor that responds to tissue damage; pain receptor.

Photoreceptor A sensory receptor that detects light; located in the retina of the eye.

Proprioception The sense of body position and movements.

Sensory adaptation Phenomenon in which some receptors respond when a stimulus is first applied but decrease their response if the stimulus is maintained; receptor sensitivity decreases with prolonged stimulation.

Thermoreceptor A sensory receptor that detects changes in temperature.

ON THE WEB

For Information on the Senses:

The Joy of Visual Perception: A Web Book: www.yorku.ca/eye

National Eye Institute: www.nei.nih.gov

Ear Nose & Throat: www.entusa.com

The Inner Ear: oto.wustl.edu/cochlea

Vestibular Disorders Association: www.vestibular.org

National Institute on Deafness: www.nidcd.nih.gov

PREPARE FOR CERTIFICATION
Visit the Evolve site at http://evolve.elsevier.com/Bonewit/today/ to actively Prepare for your Certification.

---

 *Check out the **Companion CD** bound with the book to access additional interactive activities.*

11

Endocrine System

CAAHEP COMPETENCIES

Content Competencies
Anatomy and Physiology
• Anatomy and physiology of all body systems

• Common pathology/diseases
• Diagnostic/treatment modalities

ABHES COMPETENCIES

Content Competencies
Anatomy and Physiology
• Anatomy and physiology

• Study of diseases and etiology
• All body systems
• Diagnostic/treatment modalities

KEY TERMS

adenohypophysis (add-eh-noe-hye-PAH-fih-sis)
endocrine gland (EN-doh-krin GLAND)
exocrine gland (EKS-oh-krin GLAND)

hormone (HOAR-mohn)
neurohypophysis (noo-roh-hye-PAH-fih-sis)
target tissue (TAR-get TISH-yoo)

Introduction to the Endocrine System

The organs that make up the endocrine system are the endocrine glands that secrete hormones into the blood. Unlike the organs in other systems, endocrine glands are scattered throughout the body. In addition, they are small and unimpressive; however, as you study this chapter, you will discover that they are extremely important. The study of endocrine glands and hormones is called *endocrinology.*

COMPARISON OF THE ENDOCRINE AND NERVOUS SYSTEMS

The endocrine system, along with the nervous system, functions in the regulation of body activities. The nervous system acts through electrical impulses and neurotransmitters to cause muscle contraction and glandular secretion. The effect is of short duration, measured in seconds, and localized. The endocrine system acts through chemical messengers called *hormones* that influence growth, development, and metabolic activities. The action of the endocrine system is measured in minutes, hours, or weeks and is more generalized than the action of the nervous system.

COMPARISON OF EXOCRINE AND ENDOCRINE GLANDS

The two major categories of glands in the body are **exocrine** and **endocrine.** Exocrine glands have ducts that carry their secretory product to a surface. These have a variety of functions and include the sweat, sebaceous, and mammary glands and the glands that secrete digestive enzymes. The endocrine glands do not have ducts to carry their product to a surface. They are called *ductless glands.* The word "endocrine" is derived from the Greek terms *endo,* meaning "within," and *krine,* meaning "to separate or secrete." The secretory products of endocrine glands are called **hormones** and are secreted directly into the blood and then carried throughout the body where they influence only those cells that have receptor sites for that hormone. Other cells are not affected. Endocrine glands have an extensive network of blood vessels, and organs with the richest blood supply include some of the endocrine glands, such as the thyroid and adrenal glands.

CHARACTERISTICS OF HORMONES

Each hormone produced in the body is unique. Each one is different in its chemical composition, structure, and action. In spite of the differences, there are similarities in these molecules.

Chemical Nature of Hormones

Chemically, hormones may be classified as either **proteins** or **steroids.** All of the hormones in the human body, except the sex hormones and those from the adrenal cortex, are proteins or protein derivatives. This means that their fundamental building blocks are **amino acids.** Protein hormones are difficult to administer orally because they are quickly inactivated by the acid and pepsin in the stomach. These hormones must be administered by injection. Sex hormones and those from the adrenal cortex are steroids, which are lipid derivatives. These lipid-soluble hormones may be taken orally.

Mechanism of Hormone Action

Hormones are potent substances, which means that small amounts of a hormone may have profound effects on metabolic processes. Hormones are carried by the blood throughout the entire body, yet they affect only certain cells. The specific cells that respond to a given hormone have **receptor sites** for that hormone. This is sort of a lock and key mechanism. If the key fits the lock, then the door will open. If a hormone fits the receptor site, then there will be an effect (Figure 11-1). If a hormone and a receptor site do not match, then there is no reaction. All the cells that have receptor sites for a given hormone make up the **target tissue** for that hormone. In some cases, the target tissue is localized in a single gland or organ. In other cases, the target tissue is diffuse and scattered throughout the body so that many areas are affected. Hormones bring about their characteristic effects on target cells by modifying cellular activity.

ENDOCRINE GLANDS AND THEIR HORMONES

The endocrine system is made up of the endocrine glands that secrete hormones. Figure 11-2 illustrates that the eight major endocrine glands are scattered throughout the body; however, they are still considered to be one system because they have similar functions, similar mechanisms of influence, and many important interrelationships.

Some glands also have nonendocrine regions that have functions other than hormone secretion. The pancreas is one of these glands. It has a major exocrine portion that secretes digestive enzymes and an endocrine portion that secretes hormones. The ovaries and testes secrete hormones and also produce the ova and sperm. Some organs, such as the stomach, intestines, and heart, produce hormones, but their primary function is not hormone secretion. These organs are discussed in more detail in the chapters dealing with their predominant function. Table 11-1 summarizes the major endocrine glands and their hormones.

Pituitary Gland

The **pituitary gland** or **hypophysis** is a small gland about 1 cm in diameter, or about the size of a pea. The gland is connected to the hypothalamus of the brain by a slender stalk called the *infundibulum.* The gland has two distinct regions. The anterior portion is called the **adenohypophysis** (add-eh-noe-hye-PAH-fih-sis). The posterior region is called the **neurohypophysis** (noo-roh-hye-PAH-fih-sis).

A cell producing protein hormones

Blood vessels

Protein hormone

A cell producing steroid hormones

Steroid hormone

Target cells

Receptor site

Receptor site

Second messenger

Unmatched hormone and receptor site
No effect

Effect

Effect

Figure 11-1. Hormone-receptor action. (From Applegate E: *The anatomy and physiology learning system,* ed 3, St. Louis, 2006, Saunders.)

Highlight on the Endocrine System

INSULIN: Insulin is a small protein molecule. It cannot be taken by mouth because it is rapidly inactivated by digestive enzymes.

GROWTH HORMONE: Excessive secretion of a hormone is called **hypersecretion.** A deficiency of a hormone is called **hyposecretion.** Usually hyposecretion of growth hormone in the adult poses no problems. However, in rare instances, the deficiency may be so drastic that body tissues atrophy and premature aging appears.

ANTIDIURETIC HORMONE (ADH): Ingestion of alcoholic beverages inhibits ADH secretion and results in increased urine output. Certain drugs, called *diuretics,* counteract the effects of ADH and result in fluid loss. These drugs are sometimes prescribed for patients with high blood pressure or those with edema caused by congestive heart failure because the drugs have the effect of removing fluid from the body.

OXYTOCIN: Oxytocin, or similar synthetic drugs, may be used to hasten the delivery of the placenta, control bleeding after delivery, or stimulate milk ejection.

THYROID FUNCTION: When thyroxine and triiodothyronine, with their incorporated iodine, are released into the blood, more than 99% combines with plasma proteins. This iodine is called **protein-bound iodine** (PBI). The amount of PBI can be measured by a laboratory procedure and is widely used as a test of thyroid function.

CORTISONE: Persons with inflamed joints often receive injections of a pharmaceutic glucocorticoid, cortisone, to relieve the pain and inflammation. Over-the-counter creams and ointments containing hydrocortisone are available to relieve the itching and inflammation of rashes.

GONADOCORTICOIDS: Tumors that result in hypersecretion of gonadocorticoids may have dramatic effects in prepubertal boys and girls. There is a rapid onset of puberty and sex drive in males. Females develop the masculine distribution of body hair, including a beard, and the clitoris enlarges to become more like a penis.

HYPOGLYCEMIA: Hyperinsulinism is usually caused by an overdose of insulin. The result is **hypoglycemia,** or low blood sugar level. The low blood sugar stimulates the secretion of glucagon, epinephrine, and growth hormone, which causes anxiety, nervousness, tremors, and a feeling of weakness. Insufficient glucose levels in the brain lead to disorientation, convulsions, and unconsciousness. Death can occur quickly unless the blood glucose level is raised. The early symptoms can be treated easily by eating sugar.

MELATONIN: Melatonin production appears to be related to the amount of light that enters through the eye. People who work at night and sleep during the day have a reversed cycle of melatonin production. The high melatonin levels occur during the day while they are asleep and the low levels are at night when they are working and light is entering the eye. ■

Table 11-1 Principal Endocrine Glands and Their Hormones

Gland	Hormone	Target Tissue	Principal Actions
Anterior lobe of pituitary	Growth hormone (GH)	Most tissues in body	Stimulates growth by promoting protein synthesis
	Thyroid-stimulating hormone (TSH)	Thyroid gland	Increases secretion of thyroid hormone; increases size of thyroid gland
	Adrenocorticotropic hormone (ACTH)	Adrenal cortex	Increases secretion of adrenocortical hormones, especially glucocorticoids, such as cortisol
	Follicle-stimulating hormone (FSH)	Ovarian follicles in females; seminiferous tubules of testis in males	Follicle maturation and estrogen secretion in females; spermatogenesis in males
	Luteinizing hormone (LH); also called *interstitial cell-stimulating hormone* (ICSH) in males	Ovary in females, testis in males	Ovulation; progesterone production in females; testosterone production in males
	Prolactin	Mammary gland	Stimulates milk production
Posterior lobe of pituitary	Antidiuretic hormone (ADH)	Kidney	Increases water reabsorption (decreases water lost in urine)
	Oxytocin	Uterus; mammary gland	Increases uterine contractions; stimulates ejection of milk from mammary gland
Thyroid gland	Thyroxine and triiodothyronine	Most body cells	Increases metabolic rate; essential for normal growth and development
	Calcitonin	Primarily bone	Decreases blood calcium by inhibiting bone breakdown and release of calcium; antagonistic to parathyroid hormone
Parathyroid gland	Parathyroid hormone (PTH) or parathormone	Bone, kidney, digestive tract	Increases blood calcium by stimulating bone breakdown and release of calcium; increases calcium absorption in digestive tract; decreases calcium lost in urine
Adrenal cortex	Mineralocorticoids (aldosterone)	Kidney	Increases sodium reabsorption and potassium excretion in kidney tubules; secondarily increases water retention
	Glucocorticoids (cortisol)	Most body tissues	Increases blood glucose levels; inhibits inflammation and immune response
	Androgens and estrogens	Most body tissues	Secreted in small amounts so that effect is generally masked by hormones from ovaries and testes
Adrenal medulla	Epinephrine, norepinephrine	Heart, blood vessels, liver, adipose	Helps cope with stress; increases heart rate and blood pressure; increases blood flow to skeletal muscle; increases blood glucose level
Pancreas (islets of Langerhans)	Glucagon	Liver	Increases breakdown of glycogen to increase blood glucose levels
	Insulin	General, but especially liver, skeletal muscle, adipose	Decreases blood glucose levels by facilitating uptake and use of glucose by cells; stimulates glucose storage as glycogen and production of adipose
Testes	Testosterone	Most body cells	Maturation and maintenance of male reproductive organs and secondary sex characteristics
Ovaries	Estrogens	Most body cells	Maturation and maintenance of female reproductive organs and secondary sex characteristics; menstrual cycle
	Progesterone	Uterus and breast	Prepares uterus for pregnancy; stimulates development of mammary gland; menstrual cycle
Pineal gland	Melatonin	Hypothalamus	Inhibits gonadotropin-releasing hormone, which consequently inhibits reproductive functions; regulates daily rhythms, such as sleep and wakefulness

From Applegate E: *The anatomy and physiology learning system,* ed 3, St. Louis, 2006, Saunders.

Highlight on Conditions Affecting the Endocrine System

Acromegaly (ack-roh-MEG-ah-lee) Enlargement of the extremities caused by excessive growth hormone in the adult

Adenoma (add-eh-NOH-mah) A tumor of a gland

Cretinism (KREE-tin-izm) Dwarfism caused by a deficiency of thyroid hormone in childhood and usually accompanied by mental retardation

Cushing's syndrome (KOOSH-ingz SIN-drohm) A group of symptoms caused by prolonged exposure to high levels of cortisol; characterized by excessive deposition of fat in the subscapular area and in the face (moon face), high blood pressure, generalized weakness, and loss of muscle mass because of excessive protein catabolism; may be caused by overproduction of cortisol or by taking glucocorticoid hormone medications to treat inflammatory diseases, such as asthma and rheumatoid arthritis

Diabetes insipidus (di-ah-BEE-teez in-SIP-ih-dus) A metabolic disorder caused by a deficient quantity of antidiuretic hormone, resulting in a large quantity of dilute urine (polyuria) and great thirst (polydipsia)

Diabetes mellitus (di-ah-BEE-teez mell-EYE-tus) Disorder caused by a deficiency of insulin from the beta cells of the pancreatic islets; characterized by a disturbance in the metabolism of blood glucose and manifested by polyuria, polyphagia, and polydipsia

Myxedema (miks-eh-DEE-mah) A condition of swelling attributable to an accumulation of mucus in the skin; results from deficiency of thyroid hormone in the adult

Progeria (pro-JEER-ih-ah) A condition of premature old age occurring in childhood, which may be due to hormone dysfunction ■

Hormones of the Anterior Lobe (Adenohypophysis)
Growth Hormone

Growth hormone (GH) is a protein that stimulates the growth of bones, muscles, and other organs by promoting protein synthesis (Figure 11-3). This hormone drastically affects the appearance of an individual because it influences height. If there is too little of the hormone in a child, that person may become a pituitary dwarf of normal proportions but small stature. An excess of the hormone in a child results in exaggerated bone growth, and the individual becomes

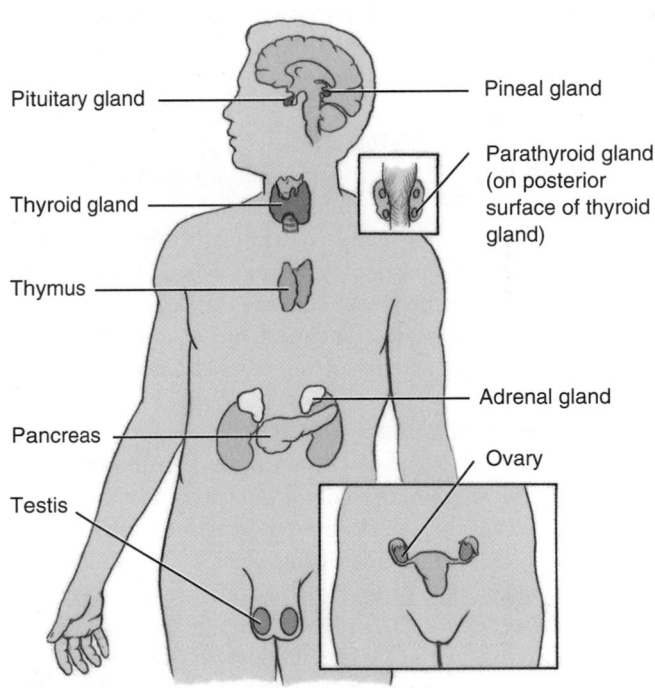

Figure 11-2. Major endocrine glands. (From Applegate E: *The anatomy and physiology learning system,* ed 3, St. Louis, 2006, Saunders.)

Figure 11-3. Effects of hormones from the pituitary gland. *ACTH,* Adrenocorticotropic hormone; *ADH,* antidiuretic hormone; *FSH,* follicle-stimulating hormone; *GH,* growth hormone; *LH,* luteinizing hormone; *OXT,* oxytocin; *PRL,* prolactin; *TSH,* thyroid-stimulating hormone. (From Applegate E: *The anatomy and physiology learning system,* ed 3, St. Louis, 2006, Saunders.)

exceptionally tall or a giant. After ossification is complete and an increase in bone length is no longer possible, excess GH causes an enlargement in the diameter of the bones. The result is a condition called *acromegaly* (ack-roh-MEG-ah-lee), in which the bones of the hands and face become abnormally large.

Thyroid-Stimulating Hormone

Thyroid-stimulating hormone (TSH), or thyrotropin (thye-roh-TROH-pin), causes the glandular cells of the thyroid to secrete thyroid hormone (see Figure 11-3). When there is a hypersecretion of TSH, the thyroid gland enlarges and secretes too much thyroid hormone. Hyposecretion of TSH results in atrophy of the thyroid gland and too little hormone.

Adrenocorticotropic Hormone

Adrenocorticotropic (ah-dree-noh-kor-tih-koh-TROH-pik) hormone (ACTH) reacts with receptor sites in the cortex of the adrenal gland to stimulate the secretion of cortical hormones, particularly cortisol (see Figure 11-3). ACTH also affects the melanocytes in the skin and increases pigmentation. Hypersecretion and hyposecretion of ACTH are reflected in the activity of the adrenal cortex.

Gonadotropic Hormones

Gonadotropic (go-nad-oh-TROH-pik) hormones react with receptor sites in the gonads—ovaries and testes—to regulate the development, growth, and function of these organs. Follicle-stimulating hormone (FSH) stimulates the development of eggs or ova in the ovaries and of sperm in the testes (see Figure 11-3). In addition, it stimulates estrogen production in the female. Luteinizing hormone (LH) causes ovulation and the production and secretion of the female sex hormones—progesterone and estrogen. In the male, LH is sometimes called *interstitial cell-stimulating hormone* (ICSH) because it stimulates the interstitial cells of the testes to produce and secrete the male sex hormone testosterone (see Figure 11-3). Without the gonadotropins FSH and LH, the ovaries and testes decrease in size, ova and sperm are not produced, and sex hormones are not secreted.

Prolactin

Prolactin (PRL) or lactogenic hormone promotes the development of glandular tissue in the female breast during pregnancy and stimulates milk production after the birth of the infant (see Figure 11-3). This hormone does not cause the milk to be ejected from the breast. A hormone from the posterior pituitary and other neural influences are responsible for the ejection of the milk.

Hormones of the Posterior Lobe (Neurohypophysis)
Antidiuretic Hormone

Antidiuretic (ant-eye-dye-yoo-RET-ik) hormone (ADH) promotes the reabsorption of water by the kidney tubules, with the result that less water is lost as urine (see Figure 11-3). This mechanism conserves water for the body. Insufficient amounts of ADH cause excessive water loss in the urine. Large amounts of a dilute urine are produced. This condition is called *diabetes insipidus*. ADH, especially in large amounts, also causes blood vessels to constrict, which increases blood pressure. For this reason, ADH is sometimes called *vasopressin*.

Oxytocin

Oxytocin (ahk-see-TOH-sin) causes contraction of the smooth muscle in the wall of the uterus. It also stimulates the ejection of milk from the lactating breast (see Figure 11-3). A commercial preparation of this hormone, called *Pitocin*, is sometimes used to induce labor.

Thyroid Gland

The thyroid (THYE-royd) gland is a vascular organ that is located in the neck (see Figure 11-2). It consists of two lobes, one on each side of the trachea, just below the larynx or voice box. The two lobes are connected by a narrow band of tissue called the *isthmus.*

Thyroxine and Triiodothyronine

About 95% of the active thyroid hormone is thyroxine, and most of the remaining 5% is triiodothyronine. Both of these require iodine for their synthesis. The iodine is actively transported into the thyroid gland, where its concentration may become as much as 25 times that of the blood, and then it is incorporated into the hormone molecules.

If there is an iodine deficiency, the thyroid cannot make sufficient hormone. This stimulates the thyroid gland to increase in size in a vain attempt to produce more hormone. However, it cannot produce more hormone because it does not have the necessary raw materials, namely, iodine. This type of thyroid enlargement is called *simple goiter* or *iodine deficiency goiter.*

The thyroid hormones containing thyroxine and triiodothyronine help to regulate the metabolism of carbohydrates, proteins, and lipids in the body. They do not have a single target organ; instead, they affect most of the cells in the body. Thyroid hormones increase the rate at which cells release energy from carbohydrates, enhance protein synthesis, are necessary for normal growth and development, and stimulate the nervous system.

In the infant, a deficiency or lack of thyroid hormone, hypothyroidism, results in a condition called *cretinism* (KREE-tin-izm). A cretin is a mentally retarded dwarf with abnormal skeletal features. If the condition is detected early enough, hormone therapy may stimulate growth, prevent the abnormal skeletal features, and increase the metabolic rate. However, therapy must be started within 2 months or less after birth to prevent severe mental retardation. Hypothyroidism in the adult results in a condition called *myxedema* (miks-eh-DEE-mah), which is characterized by lethargy, weight gain, loss of hair, decreased body temperature, low metabolic rate, and slow heart rate. Hormone therapy, in appropriate doses, usually alleviates these symptoms.

Hyperthyroidism results from an enlarged thyroid gland that produces too much hormone. This condition is characterized by a high metabolic rate, hyperactivity, insomnia, nervousness, irritability, and chronic fatigue. An individual with hyperthyroidism often has protruding eyes or exophthalmos (eks-off-THAL-mus) because there is swelling in the tissues behind the eyes. Removal, or destruction by radioactive iodine, of a portion of the thyroid may effectively reduce the symptoms of hyperthyroidism.

Calcitonin

Calcitonin is secreted by the thyroid gland. This hormone opposes the action of the parathyroid glands by reducing the calcium level in the blood. If blood calcium levels become too high, calcitonin is secreted until calcium ion levels decrease to normal. Calcitonin reduces blood calcium levels by reducing the rate at which calcium is released from bone, increasing the rate of calcium excretion by the kidneys, and reducing calcium absorption in the intestines. A deficiency of calcitonin does not seem to increase blood calcium levels.

Parathyroid Glands

Four small masses of epithelial tissue are embedded in the connective tissue capsule on the posterior surface of the thyroid glands. These are the parathyroid glands, and they secrete **parathyroid hormone** (PTH, or parathormone). PTH is the most important regulator of blood calcium levels. The hormone is secreted in response to low blood calcium levels, and its effect is to increase those levels. It does this by increasing osteoclast activity in bones so that calcium is released from the bones into the blood; by increasing calcium reabsorption from the kidney tubules into the blood, which decreases the amount lost in the urine; and by increasing the absorption of dietary calcium in the intestines. Vitamin D is also necessary for dietary calcium to be absorbed in the intestines. PTH is antagonistic to calcitonin from the thyroid gland, meaning it has the opposite effect (Figure 11-4).

Hypoparathyroidism, or insufficient secretion of PTH, leads to increased nerve excitability. The low blood calcium levels trigger spontaneous and continuous nerve impulses, which then stimulate muscle contraction. Tumors of the parathyroid gland may cause excessive secretion of PTH or hyperparathyroidism. This leads to an increased osteoclast activity that removes calcium from the bones and increases the level in the blood. The excess calcium in the blood may precipitate in abnormal locations or cause kidney stones.

Adrenal (Suprarenal) Glands

The adrenal, or suprarenal (soo-prah-REE-null), glands are paired with one gland located near the upper portion of each kidney. The glands are embedded in the fat that surrounds the kidneys. Each gland is divided into an outer region—the adrenal cortex—and an inner region—the adrenal medulla (Figure 11-5).

Hormones of the Adrenal Cortex

The adrenal cortex consists of three different regions, with each region producing a different group or type of hormones. Chemically, all the cortical hormones are steroids.

Mineralocorticoids (min-er-al-oh-KOR-tih-koyds) are secreted by the outermost region of the adrenal cortex. As a group, these hormones help regulate blood volume and the concentration of mineral electrolytes in the blood. The principal mineralocorticoid is **aldosterone** (al-DAHS-

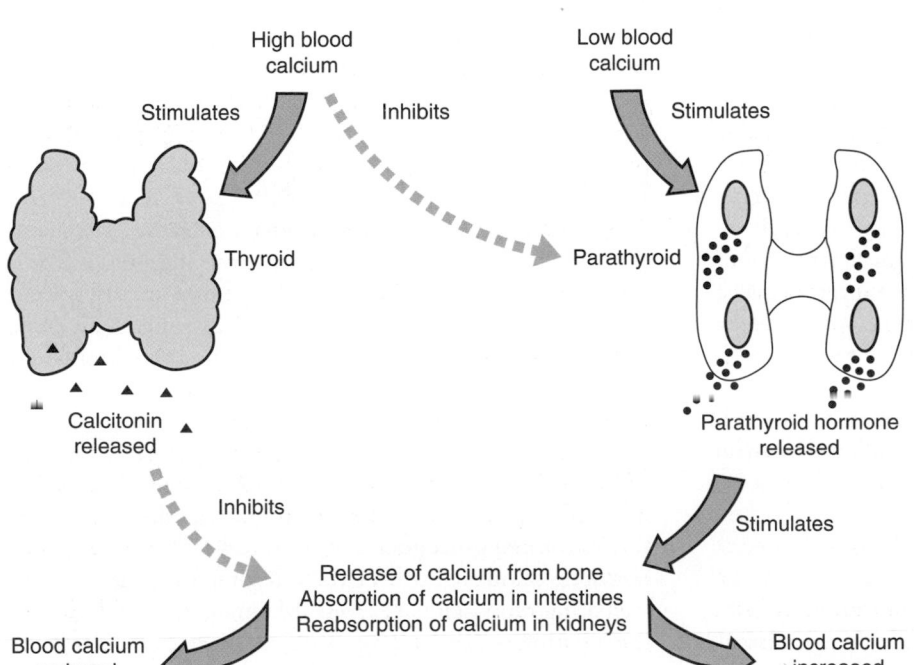

Figure 11-4. Effects of calcitonin and parathyroid hormone on blood calcium levels. (From Applegate E: *The anatomy and physiology learning system,* ed 3, St Louis, 2006, Saunders.)

Figure 11-5. Adrenal gland. (From Applegate E: *The anatomy and physiology learning system,* ed 3, St. Louis, 2006, Saunders.)

ter-ohn). Although aldosterone primarily affects the kidneys, it also acts on the intestines, salivary glands, and sweat glands. In general, its effect is to conserve sodium ions and water in the body and to eliminate potassium ions. Sodium and potassium levels are important in maintaining blood pressure, nerve impulse conduction, and muscle contraction. When the kidney tubules reabsorb sodium ions and excrete potassium in response to aldosterone, they also conserve water and reduce urine output, which increases blood volume. Aldosterone is secreted in direct response to sodium and potassium ions. The rate of aldosterone secretion increases when there is an increase in blood potassium level or a decrease in blood sodium level.

Glucocorticoids (gloo-koh-KOR-tih-koyds) are secreted by the middle region of the adrenal cortex. As a group, these hormones help regulate nutrient levels in the blood. The principal glucocorticoid is **cortisol,** also called *hydrocortisone.* The overall effect of the glucocorticoids is to increase blood glucose levels. Cortisol does this by increasing the cellular metabolism of proteins and fats as energy sources, thus conserving glucose. It also stimulates the liver cells to produce glucose from amino acids and fats. These actions help to maintain appropriate blood glucose levels between meals. In times of prolonged stress, cortisol is secreted in greater than normal amounts to help increase glucose levels to provide energy to respond to the stress. Cortisol also helps to counteract the inflammatory response. For this reason, it is used clinically to reduce the inflammation in certain allergic reactions, bursitis and arthritis, infections, and some types of cancer.

Gonadocorticoids (go-nad-oh-KOR-tih-koyds), or sex hormones, are the third group of steroids secreted by the adrenal cortex. These are secreted by the innermost region. Male hormones, **androgens,** and female hormones, **estrogens,** are secreted in minimal amounts in both sexes by the adrenal cortex, but their effect is usually masked by the hormones from the testes and ovaries. In females, the masculinization effect of androgen secretion may become evident after menopause, when estrogen levels from the ovaries decrease.

Hyposecretion of hormones from the adrenal cortex leads to a condition known as *Addison's disease.* The lack of mineralocorticoids causes low blood sodium levels, high blood potassium levels, and dehydration, while the lack of glucocorticoids causes low blood glucose levels. In addition, there is increased pigmentation in the skin. If untreated, hyposecretion of the adrenal cortex leads to death in a few days.

Hypersecretion of hormones from the adrenal cortex causes Cushing's syndrome. This is characterized by elevated blood glucose levels, retention of sodium ions and water with subsequent puffiness or edema, loss of potassium ions, and, in females, masculinization. These effects are directly related to the actions of the three groups of hormones secreted by the cortex.

Hormones of the Adrenal Medulla

The adrenal medulla secretes two hormones: **epinephrine** (adrenaline) and **norepinephrine** (noradrenaline). About 80% of the medullary secretion is epinephrine. These two hormones are secreted in response to stimulation by sympathetic nerves, particularly during stressful situations (Figure 11-6). Epinephrine, a cardiac stimulator, and norepinephrine, a vasoconstrictor, together cause increases in heart rate, the force of cardiac muscle contraction, and blood pressure. They divert blood supply to the skeletal muscles and decrease the activity of the digestive tract, dilate the bronchioles and increase the breathing rate, and increase the rate of metabolism to provide energy. They prepare the body for strenuous activity and are sometimes called the *fight-or-flight hormones.* Their effect on the body is similar to the sympathetic nervous system, but the effect lasts up to 10 times longer because the hormones are removed from the tissues slowly. The effects of epinephrine are summarized in Figure 11-6.

Pancreas—Islets of Langerhans

The pancreas is a long, soft organ that lies transversely along the posterior abdominal wall, posterior to the stomach, and extends from the region of the duodenum to the spleen. This gland has an exocrine portion that secretes digestive enzymes that are carried through a duct to the duodenum and an endocrine portion that secretes hormones into the blood. The endocrine portion consists of more than 1 million small groups of cells, called *pancreatic islets* or *islets of Langerhans,* that are interspersed throughout the exocrine tissue. The pancreatic islets contain alpha cells that secrete the hormone **glucagon** and beta cells that secrete the hormone **insulin.** Both of these hormones have a role in regulating blood glucose levels. Maintaining blood glucose levels within a normal range is important because this is the primary source of energy for the nervous system. If blood

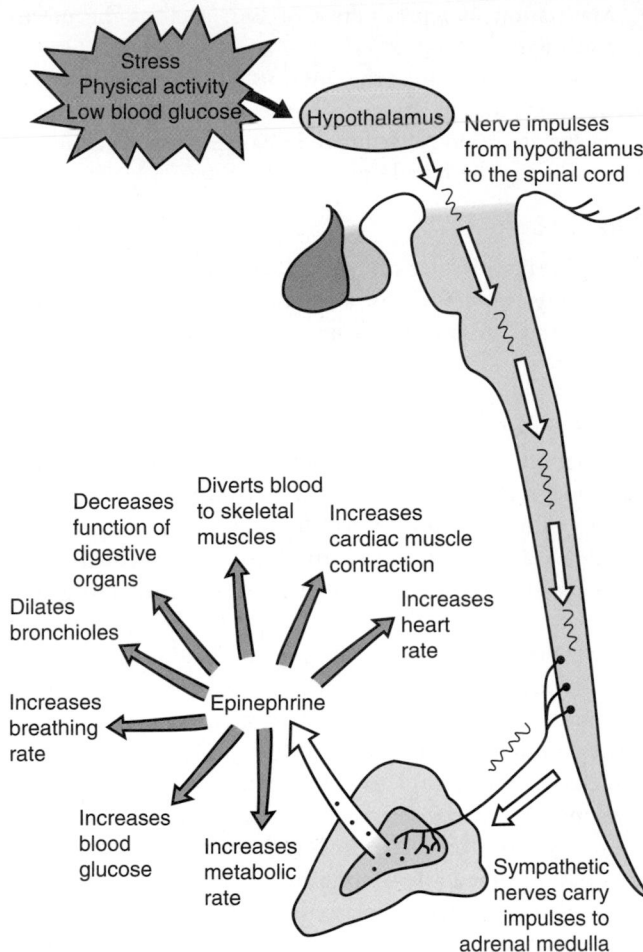

Figure 11-6. Epinephrine—its effects and control of its secretion. (From Applegate E: *The anatomy and physiology learning system,* ed 3, St. Louis, 2006, Saunders.)

glucose levels fall too low, the nervous system does not function properly. If blood glucose levels become too high, the kidneys produce large quantities of urine and dehydration may result.

Glucagon

Alpha cells in the pancreatic islets secrete the hormone glucagon in response to a low concentration of glucose in the blood. Glucagon's principal action is to raise blood glucose levels. It does this by mobilizing glucose and fatty acids from their storage forms. It also stimulates the liver to break down glycogen into glucose and to manufacture glucose from noncarbohydrate sources, such as proteins and fats. These mechanisms prevent hypoglycemia from occurring between meals or when glucose is being used rapidly.

Insulin

Beta cells in the pancreatic islets secrete the hormone insulin in response to a high concentration of glucose in the blood. The action of insulin is opposite of or antagonistic to glucagon. It promotes cellular uptake and use of glucose for energy. It stimulates the liver and muscle to

Highlight on Sir Frederick Banting

Frederick Banting was born in 1891 on a farm near Alliston, Ontario, Canada. While studying at the University of Toronto in 1915, Banting tried to enlist in the Canadian army but was ordered to return to school and complete his medical education. The following year he entered the medical corps as a certified doctor, and in 1919 he was awarded the Military Cross for heroism under fire. At the end of the war, he completed a surgical residency at the Toronto Children's Hospital and then moved to London, Ontario, where he established a medical practice. To supplement his income, he also took a position as a part-time pharmacology lecturer at Western Ontario Medical School.

Trying to stay one step ahead of his students, Banting diligently studied the subject of diabetes for an upcoming lecture. He learned that diabetes was caused by the lack of a protein hormone secreted by the islets of Langerhans in the pancreas. Without this hormone, a person would waste away to a certain death. Autopsies of diabetic patients showed the insular spots on the pancreas were noticeably shriveled. His studies inspired him to propose a research project to his superior, Professor J.J.R. Macleod, who accepted his proposal and assigned Charles Best, a medical graduate with chemistry expertise, to work with Banting.

In their research, the primary problem was how to extract the hormone, which they named *insulin,* from the pancreas without it being destroyed by the proteolytic enzymes of the pancreas. During the summer of 1921, they made their first pancreatic extract with antidiabetic properties from the resected organs of slaughtered cattle. The extract proved to be successful in treating diabetic dogs. Their work then shifted to the problems of purifying the insulin and producing it in useful quantities.

Although insulin is not a cure, its discovery has saved millions of lives worldwide.

In 1922 Banting and Macleod were jointly awarded the Nobel Prize for medicine, and they both shared the prize with their assistants. In 1934 Banting was made a Knight Commander of the Order of the British Empire.

At the outbreak of World War II, Banting again enlisted for military service. He chaired a committee to coordinate medical research and also helped organize the blood supply for transfusions in military hospitals. In 1941, while flying to England to assist the Royal Air Force, he was killed in a plane crash. ∎

remove glucose from the blood and store it as glycogen. When the liver has stored all the glycogen possible, glucose is converted to fat or adipose. Insulin inhibits the manufacture of glucose from noncarbohydrate sources. As a result of these actions, insulin decreases the blood glucose concentration. Hypoactivity of insulin may be caused by insufficient insulin secretion, insufficient receptor sites on target cell membranes, or defective receptor sites that do not recognize insulin. These dysfunctions lead to diabetes mellitus, which is characterized by abnormally high blood glucose levels.

Gonads (Testes and Ovaries)

The gonads, the primary reproductive organs, are the testes in the male and ovaries in the female. These organs are responsible for producing the sperm and ova, but they also secrete hormones and are considered to be endocrine glands. A brief description of their endocrine functions is given here. Reproductive functions and a more thorough discussion of the hormones appear in Chapter 16.

Testes

Male sex hormones, as a group, are called **androgens** (AN-droh-jenz). The principal androgen is **testosterone** (tess-TAHS-ter-ohn), which is secreted by the testes. A small amount is also produced by the adrenal cortex. Production of testosterone begins during fetal development, continues for a short time after birth, nearly ceases during childhood, and then resumes at puberty. This steroid hormone is responsible for the following:

- Growth and development of the male reproductive structures
- Increased skeletal and muscular growth
- Enlargement of the larynx accompanied by voice changes
- Growth and distribution of body hair
- Increased male sexual drive

Ovaries

Two groups of female sex hormones are produced in the ovaries: the **estrogens** (ESS-troh-jenz) and **progesterone** (proh-JESS-ter-ohn). These steroid hormones contribute to the development and function of the female reproductive organs and sex characteristics. At the onset of puberty, estrogens promote the following:

- Development of the breasts
- Distribution of fat evidenced in the hips, legs, and breasts
- Maturation of reproductive organs, such as the uterus and vagina

Progesterone causes the uterine lining to thicken in preparation for pregnancy. Together, progesterone and estrogens are responsible for the changes that occur in the uterus during the female menstrual cycle.

Pineal Gland

The **pineal** (PIE-nee-al) gland, also called *pineal body* or **epiphysis cerebri,** is a small cone-shaped structure that extends posteriorly from the third ventricle of the brain.

The pineal gland consists of portions of neurons, neuroglial cells, and specialized secretory cells called **pinealocytes** (PIE-nee-al-oh-cytes). The pinealocytes synthesize the hormone **melatonin** (mell-ah-TOH-nihn) and secrete it directly into the cerebrospinal fluid, which takes it into the blood. Melatonin secretion is rhythmic in nature, with high levels secreted at night and low levels secreted during the day.

The function of the pineal gland and melatonin in humans has been the subject of controversy and speculation for centuries. Even the ancient Greeks wrote about it. Evidence accumulated during the 1980s indicates that melatonin has a regulatory role in sexual and reproductive development. Melatonin acts on the hypothalamus to inhibit gonadotropin-releasing hormone (GnRH), which then inhibits gonad development.

Another function of melatonin involves the organization and regulation of circadian rhythms, or daily changes in physiologic processes that follow a regular pattern. An example of this is the sleepiness/wakefulness cycle. Increased plasma melatonin levels, which occur at night, are associated with sleepiness. The hormone also seems to play a role in hunger/satiety cycles, mood changes, and jet lag. The high nighttime level of melatonin seems to be a mechanism to daily "reset" the biologic clock.

TERMINOLOGY REVIEW

Adenohypophysis Anterior portion of the pituitary gland.
Endocrine gland Gland that secretes its product directly into the blood; opposite of exocrine gland.
Exocrine gland Gland that secretes its product to a surface or cavity through ducts; opposite of endocrine gland.
Hormone A substance secreted by an endocrine gland.
Neurohypophysis Posterior portion of the pituitary gland.
Target tissue A tissue (cells) that responds to a particular hormone because it has receptor sites for that hormone.

ON THE WEB

For Information on the Endocrine System:

Inner Body: www.innerbody.com

Endocrine Diseases: www.mic.ki.se/diseases/C19.html

Endocrine Web: www.endocrineweb.com

Endocrine System: www.emc.maricopa.edu/faculty/farabee/BIOBK/BiobookENDOCR.html

 PREPARE FOR CERTIFICATION Visit the Evolve site at http://evolve.elsevier.com/Bonewit/today/ to actively Prepare for your Certification.

 Check out the Companion CD bound with the book to access additional interactive activities.

12

Circulatory System

CAAHEP COMPETENCIES

Content Competencies
Anatomy and Physiology
- Anatomy and physiology of all body systems

- Common pathology/diseases
- Diagnostic/treatment modalities

ABHES COMPETENCIES

Content Competencies
Anatomy and Physiology
- Anatomy and physiology

- Study of diseases and etiology
- All body systems
- Diagnostic/treatment modalities

atrioventricular valve (ay-tree-oh-ven-TRIK-yoo-lar VALVE)
cardiac cycle (KAR-dee-ak SYE-kul)
coagulation (koh-ag-yoo-LAY-shun)
conduction myofibers (kon-DUCK-shun my-o-FYE-bers)
diapedesis (dye-ah-peh-DEE-sis)
diastole (dye-AS-toh-lee)
erythrocyte (ee-RITH-roh-syte)
erythropoiesis (ee-rith-roh-POY-eh-sis)

erythropoietin (ee-rith-roh-POY-eh-tin)
hemocytoblast (hee-moh-SYTE-oh-blast)
hematopoiesis (hee-ma-to-poy-EE-sis)
leukocyte (LOO-koh-syte)
semilunar valve (seh-mee-LOO-nar VALVE)
systole (SIS-toh-lee)
thrombocyte (THROM-boh-syte)

Introduction to the Circulatory System

The circulatory system is made up of the heart, blood, and blood vessels. A central pump, the heart, provides the force to move the blood through a system of blood vessels that extend throughout the body. Blood is the primary transport medium that is responsible for meeting the demands of the cells. This chapter focuses on the three components making up the circulatory system: heart, blood, and blood vessels.

HEART

The heart is a muscular pump that provides the force necessary to circulate the blood to all the tissues in the body. Its function is vital because, to survive, the tissues need a continuous supply of oxygen and nutrients, and metabolic waste products must be removed from them. Deprived of these necessities, cells soon undergo irreversible changes that lead to death. Although blood is the transport medium, the heart is the organ that keeps the blood moving through the vessels. The normal adult heart pumps about 5 L of blood every minute throughout life. If it loses its pumping effectiveness for even a few minutes, the individual's life is jeopardized.

Overview of the Heart

Form, Size, and Location of the Heart

Knowledge of the heart's position in the thoracic cavity is important in hearing heart sounds, conducting electrocardiograms (ECGs), and performing cardiopulmonary resuscitation (CPR). The heart, illustrated in Figure 12-1, is located in the thoracic cavity between the two lungs. It is posterior to the sternum and anterior to the vertebral column, and it rests on the diaphragm. About two thirds of the heart mass is to the left of the body's midline and one third is to the right. The **apex,** or pointed end of the heart, extends downward to the level of the fifth intercostal space. The opposite end, the **base,** is larger and less pointed than the apex and has several large vessels attached to it. Its most superior portion is at the level of the second rib. The size of the heart varies with the size of the individual.

On average, it is about 9 cm wide and 12 cm long, which is about the size of a closed fist.

Coverings of the Heart

The heart is enclosed by a loose-fitting, double-layered sac called the **pericardium** (pair-ih-KAR-dee-um), or pericardial sac. The outer layer of the pericardium consists of tough, white fibrous connective tissue and is called the **fibrous pericardium.** The fibrous pericardium is lined with a serous membrane called the **parietal pericardium.** Where the pericardium is attached to the vessels at the base of the heart, the parietal pericardium reflects onto the surface of the heart to form the **visceral pericardium,** or **epicardium.** The small space between the parietal and visceral layers of the pericardium is the **pericardial cavity.** It contains a thin layer of serous fluid that reduces friction between the membranes as they rub against each other during heart contractions.

Structure of the Heart

Layers of the Heart Wall

The heart wall is formed by three layers of tissue: an outer epicardium, a middle myocardium, and an inner endocardium. The **epicardium** (eh-pih-KAR-dee-um) (which is the same as the visceral pericardium) consists of a serous membrane. The epicardium is a thin protective layer that is firmly anchored to the underlying muscle. Blood vessels that nourish the heart wall are located in the epicardium.

The thick middle layer is the **myocardium** (my-oh-KAR-dee-um). It forms the bulk of the heart wall and is composed of cardiac muscle tissue. Refer to Chapter 5 for a review of the different types of muscle tissue. Contractions of the myocardium provide the force that ejects blood from the heart and moves it through the vessels.

The smooth inner lining of the heart wall is the **endocardium** (en-doh-KAR-dee-um). Its smooth surface permits blood to move easily through the heart. The endocardium also forms the valves of the heart and is continuous with the lining of the blood vessels. Figure 12-2 illustrates the layers of the heart wall.

Chambers of the Heart

The internal cavity of the heart is divided into four chambers (Figure 12-3):

Highlight on Conditions and Procedures Affecting the Circulatory System

Conditions

Anemia (ah-NEE-mee-ah) Deficiency in red blood cells (RBCs) or hemoglobin; most common form is iron deficiency anemia caused by a lack of iron to make hemoglobin; other types are aplastic anemia, hemolytic anemia, pernicious anemia, sickle cell anemia, and thalassemia

Angina pectoris (an-JYE-nah PECK-tohr-is) Acute chest pain caused by decreased blood supply to the heart muscle

Arteriosclerosis (ahr-tee-rih-oh-skleh-ROH-sis) A condition of hardening of an artery; an artery becomes less elastic and does not expand under pressure

Atherosclerosis (ath-er-oh-skleh-ROH-sis) A form of arteriosclerosis characterized by the buildup of fatty plaques in the wall of the vessel

Cardiac arrest (KAR-dee-ack ah-REST) Cessation of an effective heartbeat; heart may be completely stopped or quivering ineffectively in fibrillation

Cardiomegaly (kar-dee-oh-MEG-ah-lee) Enlargement of the heart

Cardiomyopathy (kar-dee-oh-my-AHP-ah-thee) Any primary disease of the heart muscle

Congestive heart failure (kahn-JES-tiv HART FAIL-yer) Condition in which the heart's pumping ability is impaired and results in fluid accumulation in vessels and tissue spaces; various stages of difficult breathing occur as fluid accumulates in pulmonary vessels and lung tissue

Ecchymosis (eck-ih-MOH-sis) A blue or purplish patch in the skin caused by intradermal hemorrhage; larger than a petechia; a bruise; plural, ecchymoses

Embolus (EMM-boh-lus) A moving clot or other plug; an object, often a blood clot, that moves in the blood until it obstructs a small vessel and blocks circulation

Fibrillation (fib-rih-LAY-shun) Rapid, random, ineffectual, and irregular contractions of the heart at 350 or more beats per minute

Heart block (HART BLOCK) Impairment of conduction of impulses from the sinoatrial node to heart muscle

Hemophilia (hee-moh-FILL-ih-ah) Excessive bleeding caused by a congenital lack of one or more of the factors necessary for blood clotting; treatment of hemophilia is directed at replacing the missing clotting factors to control and prevent bleeding

Hemorrhoids (HEM-oh-royds) Varicose veins in the anal canal resulting from a persistent increase in venous pressure

Mitral valve prolapse (MY-tral valve PRO-laps) Improper closure of the mitral valve when the heart is pumping blood; also called *floppy valve syndrome*

Myocardial infarction (mye-oh-KAR-dee-ahl in-FARK-shun) Destruction of a region of heart muscle as a result of oxygen deprivation because of a blockage in blood vessels to that area; sometimes called a *heart attack* or *MI*

Petechia (pee-TEE-kee-ah) A pinpoint, purplish red spot in the skin caused by intradermal hemorrhage; plural, petechiae

Phlebitis (fleh-BYE-tis) Inflammation of veins, which may be caused by pooling and stagnation of blood; often leads to the formation of blood clots within the vessel

Polycythemia (pahl-ee-sye-THEE-mee-ah) Any type of increase in the number of RBCs

Purpura (PER-pyoo-rah) A group of disorders characterized by multiple pinpoint hemorrhages and accumulation of blood under the skin

Thrombus (THRAHM-bus) A blood clot

Valvular heart disease (VAL-vyoo-lar HART dih-ZEEZ) Any disorder of the heart valves including insufficiency, stenosis, and prolapse

Varicose veins (VAIR-ih-kohs VANES) Abnormally swollen, distended, and knotted veins, usually in the subcutaneous tissues of the leg

Vasculitis (vas-kew-LYE-tis) Inflammation of a vessel; also called *angiitis*

Procedures

Angioplasty (AN-jih-oh-plas-tee) Surgical repair of a blood vessel or vessels

Arterectomy (ahr-teh-RECK-toh-mee) Surgical removal of an artery

Artificial pacemaker (ahr-tih-FISH-al PAYSE-may-ker) An electronic device that stimulates the initiation of an impulse within the heart

Atherectomy (ath-er-ECK-toh-mee) Surgical removal of plaque from the interior lining of an artery

Cardiac catheterization (KAR-dee-ack kath-eh-ter-ih-ZAY-shun) The process of inserting a thin, flexible tube, called a *catheter,* into a vein or artery and guiding it into the heart for the purpose of detecting pressures and patterns of blood flow

Coronary artery bypass grafting (CABG) A surgical procedure in which a blood vessel from another part of the body is used to bypass the blocked region of a coronary artery

Defibrillation (dee-fib-rih-LAY-shun) A procedure in which an electric shock is applied to the heart with a defibrillator to stop an abnormal heart rhythm

Echocardiography (eck-oh-kar-dee-AHG-rah-fee) A noninvasive clinical procedure using pulses of high-frequency sound waves (ultrasound) that are transmitted into the chest, and echoes returning from the valves, chambers, and surfaces of the heart are plotted and recorded; provides information about valvular or structural defects and coronary artery disease

Plasmapheresis (plaz-mah-feh-REE-sis) The removal of plasma from withdrawn blood with the retransfusion of the formed elements into the donor ■

Highlight on the Circulatory System

PERICARDITIS: Pericarditis is an inflammation of the pericardium. This may interfere with production of the serous fluid that lubricates the surfaces of the parietal and visceral layers. Painful adhesions may form and interfere with contraction of the heart.

DAMAGED HEART VALVES: Sometimes disease processes damage the heart valves so that they are unable to function properly. Incompetent valves permit a "backflow" of blood and the heart has to pump the same blood over and over to get it into the vessels. In valvular stenosis, the valves are stiff and have narrow openings. The heart has to work harder to pump blood out through the small opening. Defective heart valves may result in abnormal heart sounds. For example, if the atrioventricular valves are faulty, a hissing sound may be heard between the first and second heart sounds.

ANGINA PECTORIS: Angina pectoris is chest pain that results when the heart muscle's demand for oxygen exceeds the oxygen supply. Nitroglycerin is sometimes used in the treatment of angina pectoris because it dilates blood vessels, so the patient is less likely to develop a myocardial oxygen deficit.

CORONARY ARTERY BLOCKAGE: If a branch of a coronary artery becomes blocked, blood supply to that region of the heart is cut off and the muscle cells in that area die because of lack of oxygen. This is a **myocardial infarction (MI),** also called a *coronary* or a *heart attack.* The extent of the damage and chances of recovery depend on the location of the blockage and the length of time that elapses before medical intervention occurs.

HEART ENZYMES: When heart muscle is damaged, the dying cells release enzymes into the bloodstream. These enzymes can be measured and are useful in confirming an MI. The enzymes assayed are creatine kinase (CK) and lactate dehydrogenase (LDH).

Variations in normal contraction patterns are called *dysrhythmias* (arrhythmias). One type of dysrhythmia occurs when a conduction myofiber or heart muscle cell independently depolarizes to threshold and triggers a **premature heart contraction.** The cell responsible for the premature contraction is called an **ectopic focus.** Sometimes ectopic foci form feedback loops within the conduction system, causing myocardial contractions to occur at a rapid rate. If not treated properly, this often leads to ventricular tachycardia, fibrillation, and death.

RED BONE MARROW: By the age of 25 years, a person's red bone marrow for **hematopoiesis** is limited to the flat bones of the skull, the iliac crests, ribs, sternum, vertebrae, and the proximal ends of the humerus and femur.

SMOKING: About 20% of a cigarette smoker's hemoglobin is nonfunctional for transporting oxygen because it is bound to carbon monoxide from the cigarette smoke.

RETICULOCYTES: The reticulocyte count in circulating blood gives information about the rate of hematopoiesis. Normally 0.5% to 1.5% of the red blood cells (RBCs) in normal blood are reticulocytes. A number below 0.5% indicates a slowdown in production. Values above 1.5% indicate a greater than normal rate of RBC formation.

VITAMIN K: The K in vitamin K is for *koagulation,* the German word for clotting. In other words, vitamin K is the "koagulation" vitamin. Although this vitamin is necessary in the diet, it is also produced by bacteria in the large intestine and absorbed into the blood.

BLOOD DOPING: Blood doping is a practice reportedly used by some athletes to improve their endurance for aerobic activities such as running, swimming, and cycling. A few weeks before a competition, blood is drawn from the athlete and the RBCs are separated and frozen. Normal hematopoiesis replaces the lost RBCs and brings the blood cell count back to normal. Then, just before the competition, the frozen RBCs are thawed and injected into the athlete. This creates an artificial polycythemia. The idea is that the additional RBCs are able to deliver more oxygen to the muscles and improve aerobic endurance. Whether this occurs is questionable, and the practice is not without danger. All blood transfusions carry some risk. Furthermore, the additional cells increase the viscosity of the blood and put a strain on the heart.

ANEURYSM: An aneurysm is a bulge, or bubble, that develops at a weakened region in the wall of an artery. This is especially dangerous if it is in the aorta or arteries of the brain. If diagnosed soon enough, the aneurysm sometimes may be removed and the vessel surgically repaired. Because the wall is weakened, an aneurysm is subject to rupture. Little can be done when this happens because the massive bleeding usually leads to death before medical care can be obtained.

BLOOD VESSELS: It is estimated that if all the capillaries in the body were placed end to end, they would encircle the earth at the equator two and one-half times! The difference in blood pressure between arteries and veins is obvious when the vessels are cut. Blood flows smoothly and freely from a vein, but it spurts forcefully from an artery.

VARICOSE VEINS: Varicose veins are veins that are twisted and dilated with accumulated blood. These frequently occur in the legs. Conditions that hinder venous return, such as pregnancy, obesity, and standing for long periods of time, allow blood to accumulate in the veins of the extremities. This stretches the veins, so the valve flaps no longer overlap and they permit the backflow of blood. Superficial veins are more susceptible because they receive less support from surrounding tissue.

SUNBATHING: When you are in the sun for an extended period, the cutaneous blood vessels dilate to bring more blood to the skin's surface, which helps keep the body cool. This action decreases the amount of blood in other parts of the body and may diminish the blood supply to the brain. If you are sunbathing and stand up abruptly, you may feel dizzy. This is because the blood momentarily remains in the dilated cutaneous vessels instead of returning to the heart. This causes a decrease in blood pressure. The dizziness is a signal that the brain is not receiving enough oxygen.

RISING RAPIDLY AND DIZZINESS: Sometimes there is a feeling of dizziness when rising rapidly from lying down to a standing position. This is because the body has not had time to respond

Highlight on the Circulatory System—cont'd

to the decrease in blood pressure caused by the downward pull of gravity on the blood. The dizziness is a signal that the brain is not receiving enough blood.

HOLE IN THE HEART: When the foramen ovale between the two atria fails to close after birth, the result is an interatrial septal defect. Because pressure in the right atrium is lower than in the left, blood flows from the left atrium back into the right atrium without going through the systemic circulation. This defect overloads the pulmonary circulation and puts a strain on the heart as it attempts to pump enough blood to maintain adequate supplies to the body tissues. ∎

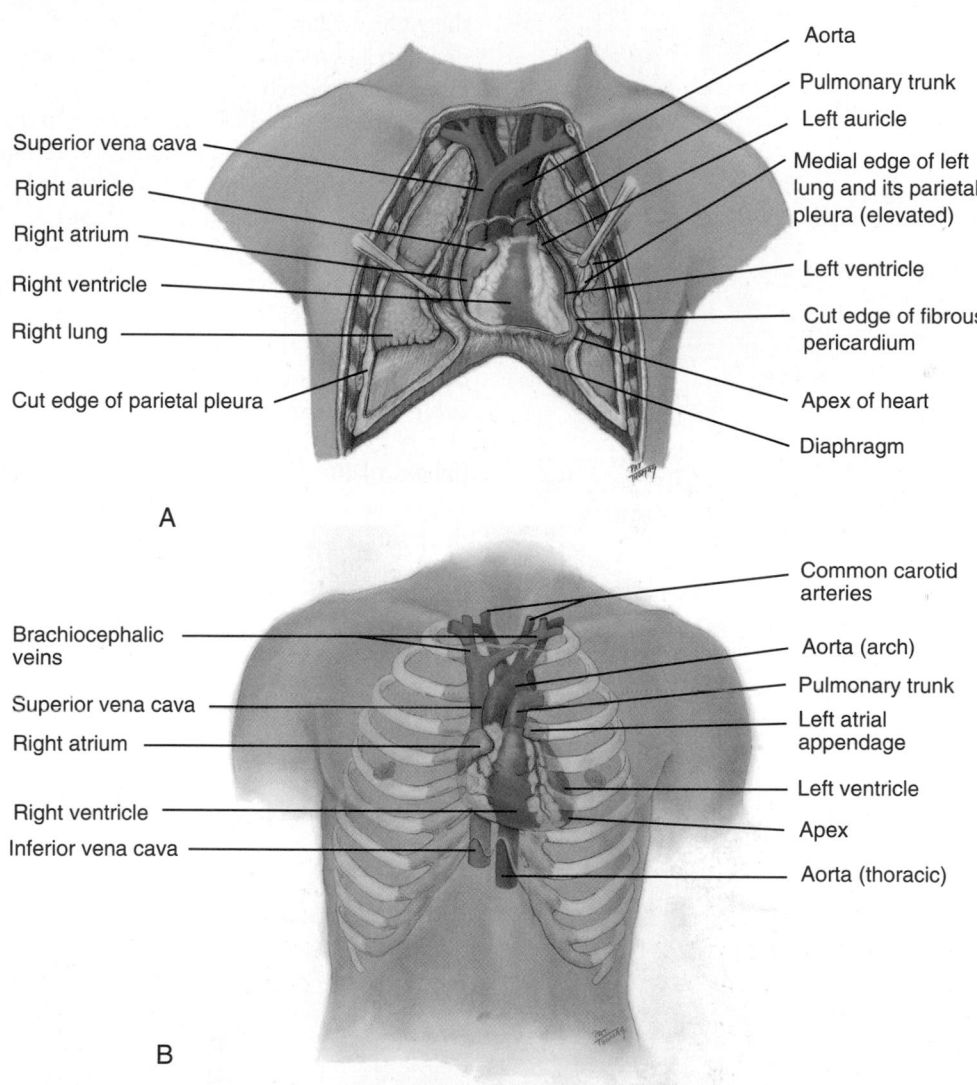

Figure 12-1. **A,** Frontal view of the mediastinum, showing the position of the heart **(B).** (From Jarvis C: *Physical examination and health assessment,* ed 4, Philadelphia, 2004, Saunders.)

- Right atrium
- Right ventricle
- Left atrium
- Left ventricle

The two atria are thin-walled chambers that receive blood from the veins. The two ventricles are thick-walled chambers that forcefully pump blood out of the heart. Differences in thickness of the heart chamber walls are due to variations in the amount of myocardium present, which reflects the amount of force each chamber is required to generate.

The **right atrium** (AY-tree-um) receives deoxygenated blood from the superior vena cava and the inferior vena cava. The superior vena cava returns blood to the heart from the head, neck, and upper extremities. The inferior vena cava returns blood to the heart from the thorax, abdomen,

Endocardium

Myocardium

Visceral pericardium (epicardium)

Parietal pericardium

Fibrous pericardium

Coronary vessels

Pericardial cavity

Figure 12-2. Layers of the heart wall. (From Applegate E: *The anatomy and physiology learning system,* ed 3, St. Louis, 2006, Saunders.)

pelvis, and lower extremities. The **left atrium** receives oxygenated blood from the lungs through four pulmonary veins, two on the right and two on the left. Because the atria are "receiving" chambers rather than "pumping" chambers, their myocardium is relatively thin. The right and left atria are separated by a partition called the **interatrial septum.** A thin region, the **fossa ovalis,** is found in the interatrial septum. This represents an opening, the foramen ovale, that is present between the atria in the fetal heart.

The **right ventricle** (VEN-trih-kull) receives blood from the right atrium and pumps it out to the lungs, where it picks up a new supply of oxygen. The **left ventricle** receives blood from the left atrium and pumps it out to the tissues of the whole body. The ventricles are "pumping" chambers, and this is reflected by a thick myocardium. Because the left ventricle pumps blood to the whole body and the right ventricle only sends blood to the lungs, the left ventricle has to generate a lot more pumping force than the right ventricle. This is reflected in the fact that the left ventricular wall has a thicker myocardium than the right. Both ventricles hold about the same volume of blood. The thick, muscular partition between the right and left ventricles is the **interventricular septum.**

Valves of the Heart

Pumps need a set of valves to keep the fluid flowing in one direction, and the heart is no exception. The heart has two types of valves that keep the blood flowing in the correct direction. The valves between the atria and ventricles are called **atrioventricular (AV)** (ay-tree-oh-ven-TRIK-yoo-

Superior vena cava

Pulmonary arteries

Pulmonic valve

Pulmonary veins

Right atrium

Tricuspid (AV) valve

Right ventricle

Inferior vena cava

Trabeculae carneae

Aorta (thoracic)

Aorta (arch)

Pulmonary trunk

Pulmonary artery

Cut edge of pericardium

Pulmonary veins

Left atrium

Aortic valve

Mitral (AV) valve

Chordae tendineae

Papillary muscle

Left ventricle

Interventricular septum

Figure 12-3. Internal view of the heart showing the chambers. *AV,* Atrioventricular. (From Jarvis C: *Physical examination and health assessment,* ed 4, Philadelphia, 2004, Saunders.)

lar) **valves.** The valves at the base of the large vessels leaving the ventricles are called **semilunar (SL)** (seh-mee-LOO-nar) **valves** (see Figure 12-3).

Atrioventricular Valves

The AV valves permit the flow of blood from the atria into the corresponding ventricle. They also prevent the backflow of blood from the ventricles into the atria. Each valve consists of a fibrous connective tissue ring and double folds of endocardium that form the **cusps** of the valve (Figure 12-4). The valve cusps are attached to the papillary muscles in the ventricles by connective tissue strings called **chordae tendineae** (KOR-dee ten-DIN-ee) (see Figure 12-3). As blood returns to the atria, it pushes the valve cusps open and the blood flows into the ventricles. When the ventricles contract, the force of the blood against the cusps causes them to close and prevents the backward flow of blood into the atria. With myocardial contraction, the papillary muscles exert tension on the chordae tendineae attached to the cusps and prevent the valve from opening back into the atria.

The AV valve between the right atrium and right ventricle has three cusps and is called the **tricuspid valve.** The valve between the left atrium and left ventricle has only two cusps and is called the **bicuspid,** or **mitral, valve** (see Figures 12-3 and 12-4).

Semilunar Valves

The **SL valves** are located at the bases of the large vessels that carry blood from the ventricles (see Figure 12-3). Each valve consists of three cuplike cusps. Contraction of the ventricles increases the pressure of the blood so that it pushes the valves open and the blood leaves the heart. As the ventricles relax and pressure decreases, the blood starts to flow back down the large vessels toward the ventricles.

When the blood flows toward the ventricles, it enters the "cups" of the valve cusps. This closes the opening of the valves and prevents the flow of blood back into the ventricles (see Figure 12-4).

The valve at the exit of the right ventricle is in the base of the pulmonary trunk and is called the **pulmonary SL valve.** The valve at the exit of the left ventricle is in the base of the ascending aorta. It is called the **aortic SL valve** (see Figures 12-3 and 12-4).

Pathway of Blood through the Heart

Although it is convenient to describe the flow of blood through the right side of the heart and then through the left side, it is important to realize that both atria contract at the same time and that both ventricles contract at the same time. The heart functions as two pumps, one on the right and one on the left, that work simultaneously. The "right pump" pumps the blood to the lungs (**pulmonary circulation**) at the same time that the "left pump" pumps blood to the rest of the body (**systemic circulation**). The sequence in which the chambers contract is described in more detail with the cardiac cycle.

The arrows in Figure 12-5 depict the direction that blood flows through the heart. Venous blood from the sys-

Ventricles relaxed— blood flows from atria, opens atrioventricular valves

Tricuspid valve

Bicuspid valve

Ventricles contract— blood leaves ventricles, opens semilunar valves

Opening for coronary artery

Aortic semilunar valve

Pulmonary semilunar valve

Figure 12-4. Valves of the heart as viewed from above. (From Applegate E: *The anatomy and physiology learning system,* ed 3, St. Louis, 2006, Saunders.)

Red = oxygenated blood

Blue = deoxygenated blood

1 = capillary beds of lungs where gas exchange occurs

2 = capillary beds of body tissues where gas exchange occurs

Figure 12-5. Pathway of the blood through the heart. (From Applegate E: *The anatomy and physiology learning system,* ed 3, St. Louis, 2006, Saunders.)

temic circulation is relatively low in oxygen and high in carbon dioxide content. This blood enters the **right atrium** through the superior vena cava and inferior vena cava. It then flows through the **tricuspid valve** into the **right ventricle.** From the right ventricle, it passes through the **pulmonary SL valve** into the **pulmonary trunk** and then into the **pulmonary arteries.** The **pulmonary arteries** carry the blood to the **lungs.** In the lungs, the blood releases carbon dioxide and picks up a new supply of oxygen. **Pulmonary veins** then carry the blood to the **left atrium.** From the left atrium, the blood flows through the **bicuspid valve** into the **left ventricle.** The **blood** then flows through the **aortic SL valve** into the **ascending aorta.** Oxygen-rich blood flowing into the aorta is distributed to all parts of the body through the systemic circulation.

Blood Supply to the Myocardium

The myocardium of the heart wall is working muscle that needs a continuous supply of oxygen and nutrients to function with efficiency. Unlike skeletal muscle, cardiac muscle cannot build up an oxygen debt to be repaid at a later time. It needs a continuous oxygen supply or it dies. For this reason, cardiac muscle has an extensive network of blood vessels to bring oxygen to the contracting cells and to remove waste products.

Two main coronary arteries branch from the ascending aorta just distal to the aortic SL valve. They are the **right and left coronary arteries** (Figure 12-6). The right and left coronary arteries have numerous branches. Blood flow through the coronary arteries is greatest when the myocardium is relaxed. When the ventricles contract, they compress the arteries, which reduces the flow.

Physiology of the Heart

The work of the heart is to pump blood to the lungs through the pulmonary circulation and to the rest of the body through the systemic circulation. This is accomplished by contraction and relaxation of the cardiac muscle in the myocardium.

Conduction System

An effective cycle for productive pumping of blood requires that the heart be synchronized accurately. Both atria need to contract simultaneously, followed by contraction of both ventricles. Contraction of the chambers is coordinated by specialized cardiac muscle cells that make up the **conduction system** of the heart.

Components of the Conduction System

Sinoatrial Node

The conduction system includes several components (Figure 12-7). The first part of the conduction system is the **sinoatrial (SA) node** (sye-noh-AY-tree-al node), which is located in the right atrium, near the entrance of the superior vena cava. Without any neural stimulation, the SA node rhythmically initiates impulses 70 to 80 times per minute. Because it establishes the basic rhythm of the heartbeat, it is called the **pacemaker** of the heart. The impulses from the SA node rapidly travel throughout the atrial myocardium and cause the two atria to contract simultaneously. At the same time, the impulses reach the second part of the conduction system.

Atrioventricular Node

The **AV node,** the second part of the conduction system, is located in the floor of the right atrium, near the interatrial

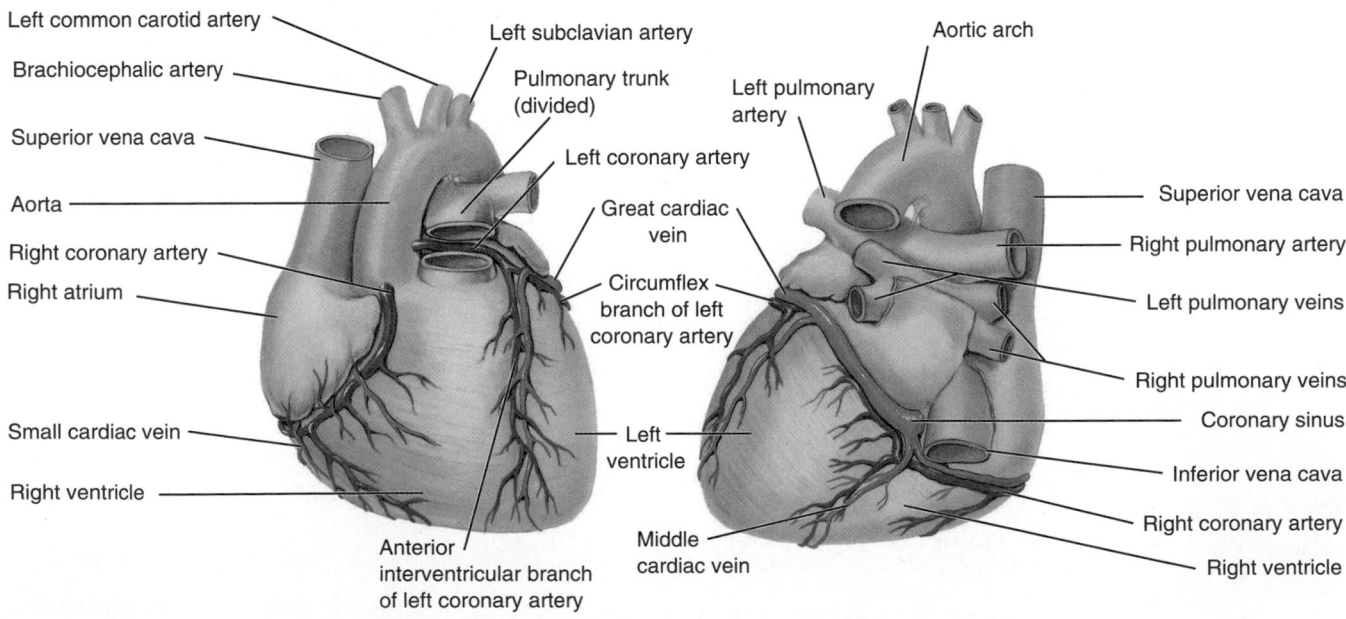

Left common carotid artery
Brachiocephalic artery
Superior vena cava
Aorta
Right coronary artery
Right atrium
Small cardiac vein
Right ventricle
Anterior interventricular branch of left coronary artery

Left subclavian artery
Pulmonary trunk (divided)
Left coronary artery
Great cardiac vein
Circumflex branch of left coronary artery
Left ventricle
Middle cardiac vein

Aortic arch
Left pulmonary artery
Superior vena cava
Right pulmonary artery
Left pulmonary veins
Right pulmonary veins
Coronary sinus
Inferior vena cava
Right coronary artery
Right ventricle

ANTERIOR

POSTERIOR

Figure 12-6. Blood supply to the myocardium. (From Applegate E: *The anatomy and physiology learning system,* ed 3, St. Louis, 2006, Saunders.)

septum. The cells in the AV node conduct impulses more slowly than do other parts of the conduction system, so there is a brief time delay as the impulses travel through the node. This allows time for the atria to finish their contraction phase before the ventricles begin contracting.

Atrioventricular Bundle, Bundle Branches, and Conduction Myofibers

From the AV node, the impulses rapidly travel through the **AV bundle** (bundle of His) to the **right** and **left bundle branches.** The bundle branches extend along the right and left sides of the interventricular septum to the apex. These branch profusely to form **conduction myofibers** (Purkinje fibers) that transmit the impulses to the myocardium. The AV bundle, bundle branches, and conduction myofibers rapidly transmit impulses throughout all the ventricular myocardium so that both ventricles contract at the same time. As the ventricles contract, blood is forced out through

Figure 12-7. Conduction system. (From Applegate E: *The anatomy and physiology learning system,* ed 3, St. Louis, 2006, Saunders.)

the SL valves into the pulmonary trunk and the ascending aorta. After the ventricles complete their contraction phase, they relax and the SA node initiates another impulse to start another cardiac cycle.

Cardiac Cycle

The **cardiac cycle** refers to the alternating contraction and relaxation of the heart chambers during one heartbeat (Figure 12-8). The two atria contract at the same time; then they relax while the two ventricles simultaneously contract. The contraction phase of the chambers is called **systole** (SIS-toh-lee); the relaxation phase is called **diastole** (dye-AS-toh-lee). When the terms *systole* and *diastole* are used alone, they refer to action of the ventricles.

With a heart rate of 75 beats per minute, one cardiac cycle lasts 0.8 second. The cycle begins with **atrial systole,** when both atria contract (see Figure 12-8). During this time, the AV valves are open, the ventricles are in diastole, and blood is forced into the ventricles. Atrial systole lasts for 0.1 second; then the atria relax (**atrial diastole**) for the remainder of the cycle, 0.7 second.

When the atria finish their contraction phase, the ventricles begin contracting. **Ventricular systole** lasts for 0.3 second. Pressure in the ventricles increases as they contract. This closes the AV valves and opens the SL valves, and blood is forced into the pulmonary trunk and ascending aorta that carry blood away from the heart. During this time, the atria are in diastole and are filling with blood returned through the venae cavae. After ventricular systole, when the ventricles relax, the SL valves close, the AV valves open, and blood flows from the atria into the ventricles. All chambers are in simultaneous diastole for 0.4 second, and about 70% of ventricular filling occurs during this period.

Atria contract   Ventricles contract   All chambers relaxed

Figure 12-8. Cardiac cycle. (From Applegate E: *The anatomy and physiology learning system,* ed 3, St. Louis, 2006, Saunders.)

The remaining blood enters the ventricles during atrial systole.

Heart Sounds

The sounds associated with the heartbeat are due to the closure of the valves of the heart. A **stethoscope** is used to listen to these sounds, usually described as lubb-dupp. The **first heart sound,** the lubb, is caused by closure of the AV valves. The **second heart sound,** the dupp, is caused by closure of the SL valves. It has a higher pitch than the first heart sound. There is a pause between the dupp of the first beat and the lubb of the second beat when the entire heart is resting. Therefore the sequence is lubb-dupp, pause, lubb-dupp, pause, lubb-dupp, pause, and so on. Abnormal heart sounds, called **murmurs,** are caused by faulty valves.

BLOOD

The body consists of active cells that need a continuous supply of nutrients and oxygen. Metabolic waste products need to be removed from the cells to maintain a stable cellular environment. Blood is the primary transport medium that is responsible for meeting these cellular demands. A central pump, the heart, provides the force to move the blood through a system of vessels that extend throughout the body. This unit focuses on the blood and how it supports cellular activities.

Functions and Characteristics of Blood

Blood is one of the connective tissues. As a connective tissue, it consists of cells and cell fragments **(formed elements)** suspended in an intercellular matrix **(plasma).** Blood is the only liquid tissue in the body. The total blood volume in an average adult is 4 to 5 L in the female and 5 to 6 L in the male. It accounts for approximately 8% of the total body weight. Blood is slightly heavier and four to five times more viscous than water. It is slightly alkaline with a normal pH range between 7.35 and 7.45.

The activities of the blood may be categorized as **transportation, regulation,** and **protection.** These functional categories overlap and interact as the blood carries out its role in providing suitable conditions for cellular functions. The following activities of blood are transport functions:

- It carries oxygen and nutrients to the cells.
- It transports carbon dioxide and nitrogenous wastes from the tissues to the lungs and kidneys, where these wastes can be removed from the body.
- It carries hormones from the endocrine glands to the target tissues.

The following activities of blood are in the regulation category:

- It helps regulate body temperature by removing heat from active areas, such as skeletal muscles, and transporting it to other regions or to the skin, where it can be dissipated.
- It plays a significant role in fluid and electrolyte balance because the salts and plasma proteins contribute to the osmotic pressure.
- It functions in pH regulation through the action of buffers in the blood.

Functions of the blood that are in the protection category include the following:

- Its clotting mechanisms prevent fluid loss through hemorrhage when blood vessels are damaged.
- Certain cells in the blood, the phagocytic white blood cells, help to protect the body against microorganisms that cause disease by engulfing and destroying the agent.

Highlight on Anatomy and Physiology Pioneers: Karl Landsteiner

Karl Landsteiner was born in Vienna in 1868 and received his medical degree from the University of Vienna in 1891. During his medical training, he became interested in biochemical research. Following his graduation, he spent the next 5 years working at prestigious laboratories in Zurich, Wurzburg, and Munich to obtain additional knowledge in biochemistry. He returned to Vienna in 1896 to continue his studies at the Hygiene Institute, and 2 years later he accepted a position at the Vienna Pathological Institute.

As Landsteiner continued his studies, he became intrigued with the mechanisms of immunity and the nature of antibodies. While in medical school, he observed the frustrations of many surgeons when their patients died from the blood loss that accompanied their surgery. In America and Russia, some surgeons had experimented with blood transfusions with limited success. Many patients died suddenly when blood was transfused into their veins, as though it were poison, but others had no adverse reactions.

Intrigued by this mystery, Landsteiner started experimenting with blood serum from various animals, mixing the blood of one animal with the serum of another. He observed that some combinations of blood and serum turned into a pool of yellow liquid streaked with clumps of blood. As he expanded his research to human blood, he observed that certain combinations were incompatible and that this led to the life-threatening transfusion episodes. In 1901 he showed that there were at least three major types of human blood and that these types were based on the antigens attached to the plasma membrane of the red blood cells. He labeled the types as A, B, and O. The following year he found a fourth type that possessed both antigens A and B, and he called this type AB.

In 1922 Landsteiner accepted a position at the Rockefeller Institute in New York, moved to the United States, and later became an American citizen. While at the Rockefeller Institute, he discovered the additional blood groups M and N and, continuing his research, he identified the Rh factor in 1940. For his discovery of human blood groups, he was awarded the Nobel Prize in physiology or medicine in 1930. ■

- Antibodies in the plasma help protect against disease by their reactions with offending agents.

Composition of Blood

When a sample of blood is spun in a centrifuge, the cells and cell fragments are separated from the liquid part of the blood (Figure 12-9). Because the **formed elements** are heavier than the liquid, they are packed in the bottom of the tube by the centrifugal force. The straw-colored liquid on the top is the **plasma.** Figure 12-9 illustrates that the plasma accounts for about 55% of the blood volume and red blood cells make up the remaining 45% of the volume. The white blood cells and platelets form a thin white layer, called the "buffy coat," between the plasma and red blood cells.

Plasma

Plasma, the liquid portion of the blood, is about 90% water. The remaining portion consists of more than 100 different organic and inorganic solutes dissolved in the water. Table 12-1 summarizes some of the major solutes in plasma. Because plasma is a transport medium, its solutes are continuously changing as substances are added or removed by the cells. With a healthy diet, the plasma is normally in a state of dynamic balance that is maintained by various homeostatic mechanisms.

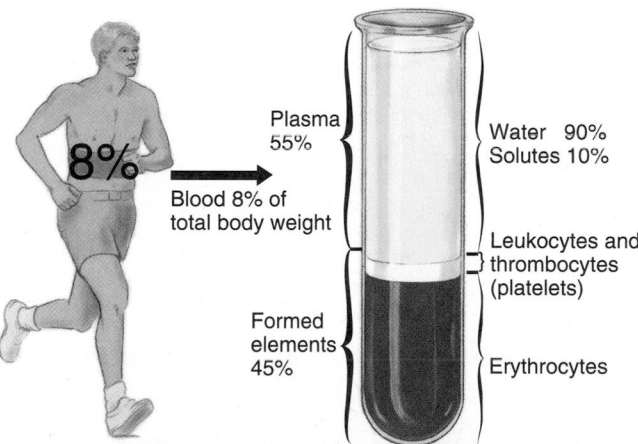

Figure 12-9. Composition of the blood. (From Applegate E: *The anatomy and physiology learning system,* ed 3, St. Louis, 2006, Saunders.)

Table 12-1 Major Solutes in Plasma

Plasma Proteins	Nitrogenous Molecules	Other
Albumins—60%	Amino acids	Nutrients
Globulins—36%	Urea	Hormones
Fibrinogen—4%	Uric acids	Oxygen
		Carbon dioxide
		Electrolytes

From Applegate E: *The anatomy and physiology learning system,* ed 3, St. Louis, 2006, Saunders.

Plasma Proteins

Plasma proteins are the most abundant of the solutes in the plasma. These proteins normally remain in the blood and interstitial fluid and are not used for energy. The three major classes of plasma proteins are as follows:
- Albumins
- Globulins
- Fibrinogen

Many of the plasma proteins are synthesized in the liver, and each one has a different function.

Albumins (al-BYOO-mins) account for about 60% of the plasma proteins. Albumin molecules are produced in the liver and are the smallest of the plasma protein molecules. Because they are so abundant, they contribute to the osmotic pressure of the blood and play an important role in maintaining fluid balance between the blood and interstitial fluid. If the osmotic pressure of the blood decreases, fluid moves from the blood into the interstitial spaces, which results in edema. This also decreases blood volume and, in severe cases, may reduce blood pressure. When blood osmotic pressure increases, fluid moves from the interstitial spaces into the blood and increases blood volume. This increases blood pressure and decreases the amount of water available to the cells.

Globulins (GLOB-yoo-lins) account for about 36% of the plasma proteins. Three types of globulins exist:
- Alpha
- Beta
- Gamma

Alpha and beta globulins are produced in the liver and function in transporting lipids and fat-soluble vitamins in the blood. Gamma globulins are the antibodies that function in immunity. These are produced in lymphoid tissue.

The remaining 4% of the plasma proteins is **fibrinogen** (fye-BRIN-oh-jen), which is the largest of the plasma protein molecules. It is produced in the liver and functions in blood clotting. During the clotting process, a series of reactions converts the soluble fibrinogen into insoluble fibrin, which forms the foundation of a blood clot. When blood clots in a test tube, the liquid that remains is called **serum.** It is similar to plasma but has no fibrinogen because the fibrinogen is converted to fibrin.

Nonprotein Molecules That Contain Nitrogen

Along with the proteins, some other plasma solutes contain nitrogen. These include amino acids, urea, and uric acid. The amino acids are the products of protein digestion. They are absorbed into the blood and are transported to the cells that need them. Urea and uric acid are waste products of protein and nucleic acid catabolism. These molecules are transported to the kidneys for excretion.

Nutrients and Gases

The simple nutrients that are the end products of digestion are transported in the blood so that they form a fraction of the plasma solutes. These nutrients include the amino acids from protein digestion, glucose and other simple sugars from carbohydrate digestion, and fatty acids from lipid digestion.

Oxygen and carbon dioxide are the main respiratory gases that are found as solutes in the plasma. About 3% of the oxygen and 7% to 10% of the carbon dioxide are transported as dissolved gases. Nitrogen is another gas that dissolves in the plasma, but it has little, if any, function in the human body.

Electrolytes

Most of the electrolytes that are solutes in the plasma are inorganic ions, and they contribute to the osmotic pressure of the plasma. In addition, some are important in maintaining membrane potentials and others are significant in regulating the pH of body fluids. Common electrolytes found in the plasma include sodium (Na^+), potassium (K^+), calcium (Ca^{++}), chloride (Cl^-), bicarbonate (HCO_3^-), and phosphate (PO_4^{-3}).

Formed Elements

The formed elements are cells and cell fragments suspended in the plasma. The three classes of formed elements are the **erythrocytes** (ee-RITH-roh-sytes), or red blood cells; the **leukocytes** (LOO-koh-sytes), or white blood cells; and the **thrombocytes** (THROM-boh-sytes), or platelets.

The production of these formed elements, or blood cells, is called **hematopoiesis** (hemopoiesis). Before birth, hematopoiesis (hee-ma-to-poy-EE-sis) occurs primarily in the liver and spleen. After birth, most production is limited to the red bone marrow in specific regions of the body, but some white blood cells are produced in lymphoid tissue. All types of formed elements develop from a single cell type, as illustrated in Figure 12-10. The precursor cell, or stem cell, is called a **hemocytoblast** (hee-moh-SYTE-oh-blast). Seven different cell lines develop from the hemocytoblast.

Erythrocytes
Characteristics and Functions

Erythrocytes (ee-RITH-roh-sytes), or red blood cells (RBCs), are the most numerous of the formed elements. The normal RBC range for an adult female is 4 to 5.5 million RBCs/cubic millimeter (mm^3) of blood. The normal RBC range for an adult male is 4.5 to 6.2 million RBCs/mm^3 of blood.

Figure 12-10. Development of the formed elements. (From Applegate E: *The anatomy and physiology learning system,* ed 3, St. Louis, 2006, Saunders.)

Erythrocytes are tiny **biconcave discs** about 7.5 micrometers (μm) in diameter. They are thin in the middle and thicker around the periphery. The shape of the RBC provides a combination of flexibility for moving through tiny capillaries along with a maximum surface area for the diffusion of gases. Mature RBCs are **anucleate,** meaning they do not have a nucleus. During development the nucleus is lost from the cell, presumably to give the cell more room for hemoglobin. Because the mature cells are anucleate, they cannot undergo mitosis, which means that replacement cells have to develop from the stem cells. Erythrocytes normally move from the bone marrow into the blood while they are still immature, but after they lose the nucleus. These immature erythrocytes that are circulating in the blood are called **reticulocytes.**

The primary function of erythrocytes is to transport oxygen and, to a lesser extent, carbon dioxide. This function is directly related to the **hemoglobin** (hee-moh-GLOH-bin) within the RBC. About one third of each erythrocyte consists of hemoglobin. This molecule has two parts: **heme** and **globin.** The heme portion is formed from a pigment that contains iron. The globin portion is a protein. In the lungs, the heme portion combines with oxygen to form **oxyhemoglobin** (ok-see-hee-moh-GLOH-bin), which is bright red. About 97% of the oxygen used by tissue cells is transported as oxyhemoglobin. In the tissues, the oxygen is released to diffuse into the tissue cells. This produces a type of hemoglobin called **deoxyhemoglobin** (dee-ok-see-hee-moh-GLOH-bin), which is a darker red in color.

Production of Erythrocytes

Erythrocyte production is regulated by a negative feedback mechanism that uses the hormone **erythropoietin** (ee-rith-roh-POY-ee-tin) to stimulate erythrocyte production (Figure 12-11). The liver produces erythropoietin in an inactive form and secretes it into the blood. The kidneys produce a **renal erythropoietic factor** (REF), which activates the erythropoietin. When blood oxygen concentration is low, the kidneys release REF into the blood, which activates the erythropoietin, which then stimulates the red bone marrow to produce RBCs. The additional RBCs combine with oxygen to increase the blood oxygen concentration. As blood oxygen concentration increases, levels of REF and active erythropoietin decrease and RBC production decreases.

Iron, vitamin B_{12}, and folic acid are essential to normal RBC production. The iron is necessary for the synthesis of normal hemoglobin. Iron deficiency anemia results when there is a lack of iron in the diet. This results in a reduced amount of hemoglobin, which decreases the blood's oxygen-carrying capacity. All cells in the body require vitamins B_{12} and folic acid for normal formation. This is especially significant in erythrocytes because of the large numbers produced every day. Certain cells in the stomach produce **intrinsic factor,** a factor necessary for the absorption of vitamin B_{12} in the intestines. Without intrinsic factor, vitamin B_{12} (even though present in the diet) cannot be absorbed. This results in a condition known as **pernicious anemia.**

Destruction of Erythrocytes

Normal erythrocytes live for approximately 120 days. During this time they travel thousands of miles as they circulate throughout the body. Normally the erythrocytes have a flexible cell membrane that allows them to bend and squeeze through the capillaries. As they age, however, their membrane loses its elasticity and becomes fragile. When they are defective or worn out, macrophages, which are phagocytic cells in the spleen and liver, remove them from circulation, and they are replaced by an equal number of new cells. Under typical conditions, more than 2 million erythrocytes are destroyed and replaced every second.

When RBCs are destroyed, the hemoglobin is separated into its heme and globin components (Figure 12-12). The protein portion of the hemoglobin in the erythrocyte is broken down into its constituent amino acids, which are

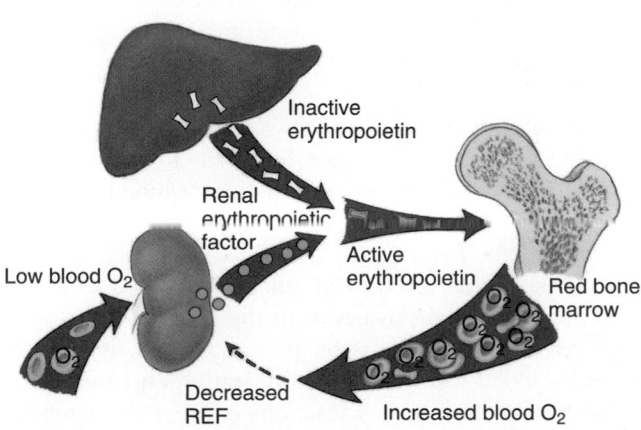

Figure 12-11. Regulation of erythrocyte production. *REF,* Renal erythropoietic factor. (From Applegate E: *The anatomy and physiology learning system,* ed 3, St. Louis, 2006, Saunders.)

Figure 12-12. Life cycle of red blood cells *(RBCs)* and breakdown of hemoglobin. (From Applegate E: *The anatomy and physiology learning system,* ed 3, St. Louis, 2006, Saunders.)

added to the supply of amino acids that are available in the body. The heme portion of the molecule is broken down into an iron compound and bilirubin, a yellow bile pigment. The liver then recycles the iron and sends it to the bone marrow for new hemoglobin. Bilirubin becomes part of the bile, which is secreted by the liver, and is carried in the bile duct to the small intestine.

Leukocytes

Characteristics and Functions

Leukocytes, or white blood cells (WBCs), are generally larger than erythrocytes, but they are fewer in number. A normal WBC count ranges between 4500 and 11,000/mm^3. All leukocytes are derived from hemocytoblast stem cells (see Figure 12-10), but they do not lose their nuclei or accumulate hemoglobin during development. The lack of hemoglobin makes them appear whitish.

Even though they are considered to be blood cells, leukocytes do most of their work in the tissues. They use the blood as a transport medium. Some are phagocytic, others produce antibodies, some secrete histamine and heparin, and others neutralize histamine. Leukocytes are able to move through the capillary walls into the tissue spaces, a process called **diapedesis** (dye-ah-peh-DEE-sis). In the tissue spaces, they provide a defense against organisms that cause disease.

Types of Leukocytes

Blood contains two main groups of leukocytes. The cells that develop granules in the cytoplasm are called **granular leukocytes (granulocytes)** and those that do not have granules are called **nongranular leukocytes (agranulocytes). Neutrophils, eosinophils,** and **basophils** are granular leukocytes. **Monocytes** and **lymphocytes** are nongranular leukocytes. Because WBCs are clear and colorless, they must be stained first with an appropriate dye (usually Wright's stain) before they can be identified under the microscope. The nucleus, cytoplasm, and any granules in the cytoplasm take on the characteristic color of their cell type, which aids in proper identification. The five types of WBCs are described here, along with their reactions to Wright's stain.

Neutrophils   (NOO-troh-fills) are the most common type of leukocyte. Neutrophils make up 50% to 70% of the total number of WBCs. They are characterized by a purple, multilobed nucleus (usually three to five lobes) and many fine granules in the cytoplasm that stain a violet-pink. Immature forms of neutrophils, known as *bands,* can be identified by their curved, nonsegmented nuclei. Normally, 0% to 5% of the neutrophils present are in the immature band form. Neutrophils are the first leukocytes to respond to tissue damage, where they engulf bacteria by phagocytosis. The number of neutrophils and bands increases during acute infections.

Eosinophils   Eosinophils (ee-oh-SIN-oh-fills) make up 1% to 4% of the WBCs. They are characterized by a segmented nucleus, generally of no more than two lobes. Large granules found in the cytoplasm stain a bright reddish orange. Eosinophils neutralize histamine, and their number increases during allergic reactions. They also destroy parasitic worms.

Basophils   Basophils (BAY-soh-fills) are the least numerous of the leukocytes. The normal range for basophils is 0% to 1% of the WBCs. A basophil is about the same size as an eosinophil. Basophils have an **S**-shaped nucleus. The cytoplasm has large, coarse granules that stain a dark bluish-black and almost completely obscure the details of the nucleus. In the tissues, basophils secrete histamine and heparin. Histamine dilates blood vessels to increase blood flow to damaged tissues. It also dilates blood vessels in allergic reactions. Heparin is an anticoagulant that inhibits blood clot formation.

Lymphocytes   Lymphocytes (LIM-foh-sytes) account for 20% to 35% of the WBCs in the blood. Lymphocytes have a large round or slightly indented nucleus that stains a deep purplish blue. A small rim of sky-blue cytoplasm around the nucleus contains few or no granules. Lymphocytes are involved with the immune system and the production of antibodies. An increase in lymphocytes generally occurs with certain viral diseases, including infectious mononucleosis, mumps, chicken-pox, rubella, and viral hepatitis.

Monocytes   Monocytes (MON-oh-sytes) are the largest of the WBCs and make up 3% to 8% of the leukocytes in the blood. Monocytes have a **U**-shaped or kidney-shaped nucleus surrounded by abundant cytoplasm that stains grayish blue. When monocytes leave the blood and enter the tissues, they are called *macrophages* (MACK-roh-fahj-es). In damaged tissues, the macrophages engulf bacteria and cellular debris to finish the cleanup process started by the neutrophils.

Thrombocytes

Thrombocytes, or **platelets,** are not complete cells but small fragments of large cells called **megakaryocytes.** Megakaryocytes (meg-ah-KAIR-ee-oh-sytes) develop from hemocytoblasts in the red bone marrow. Platelets are one third to one half the size of an erythrocyte, and an average platelet count ranges from 150,000 to 500,000 platelets/mm^3 of blood.

Thrombocytes become sticky and clump together to form platelet plugs that close breaks and tears in blood vessels. They also initiate the formation of blood clots.

Hemostasis

Blood vessels that are torn or cut permit blood to escape into the surrounding tissues or to the outside of the body. This has damaging effects on the tissues and, in cases of excessive blood loss, may result in death. Whenever blood vessels are injured, several reactions occur that attempt to minimize blood loss and tissue damage. The stoppage of bleeding is called **hemostasis** (hee-moh-STAY-sis). It includes three separate but interrelated processes:

- Vascular constriction
- Platelet plug formation
- Coagulation

Vascular Constriction

The first response to blood vessel injury is contraction of the smooth muscle in the vessel walls. This creates a **vascular constriction** that restricts the flow of blood through the opening in the vessel. The initial constriction lasts for only a few minutes but allows enough time for the other aspects of hemostasis to begin. As platelets accumulate at the site of the injury, they secrete **serotonin,** a chemical that stimulates smooth muscle contraction and prolongs the vascular constriction.

Platelet Plug Formation

Normally platelets do not stick to each other or to the lining of blood vessel walls. When the lining of the blood vessel breaks, the underlying connective tissue is exposed. The connective tissue attracts platelets and they accumulate in the damaged region, where they adhere to the connective tissue and to each other. This creates a mass of platelets, a **platelet plug,** that obstructs the tear in the vessel. Normal daily activities create numerous tears in minute blood vessels, and these are closed by platelet plugs so that there is no blood loss or damage to surrounding tissues.

Coagulation

The third and most effective mechanism in hemostasis is the formation of a blood clot, or **coagulation** (koh-ag-yoo-LAY-shun). The blood contains factors, called **procoagulants,** that promote clotting. It also contains **anticoagulants** that inhibit clotting. Normally the anticoagulants predominate and override the procoagulants so that the blood remains fluid and does not clot. When vessels are damaged, the procoagulants increase their activity, which results in the formation of a clot.

The formation of a blood clot involves a complex series of chemical reactions and includes numerous clotting factors that are present in the plasma. Even though it is a complex process, it can be summarized in three main steps, as illustrated in Figure 12-13.

1. Platelets and damaged tissues release chemicals that initiate a series of reactions that result in the formation of **prothrombin activator.**
2. In the presence of calcium ions and prothrombin activator, **prothrombin** (pro-THROM-bin) in the plasma is converted from an inactive form to active **thrombin.**
3. Thrombin, in the presence of calcium ions, acts as an enzyme to convert inactive and soluble **fibrinogen** (fye-BRIN-oh-jen) into active and insoluble **fibrin.** The fibrin threads form a mesh that adheres to the damaged tissue and traps blood cells and platelets to form the clot.

Platelets and all the necessary clotting factors must be available for successful clot formation. The liver produces

Figure 12-13. Hemostasis. (From Applegate E: *The anatomy and physiology learning system,* ed 3, St. Louis, 2006, Saunders.)

most of the clotting factors, and many of them require vitamin K for their synthesis. Numerous reactions in the clotting process also require calcium ions. A low platelet count (thrombocytopenia), deficiency of vitamin K or calcium, and liver dysfunction can impair the clotting process.

After a clot has formed, the fibrin strands contract. This process, called **clot retraction,** causes the clot to condense or shrink. Clot retraction pulls the edges of the damaged tissue closer together, reduces the flow of blood to the area, reduces the probability of infection, and enhances healing. Fibroblasts migrate into the clot and form fibrous connective tissue that repairs the damaged area. As healing occurs, the clot is dissolved by a process called **fibrinolysis** (fye-brin-AHL-ih-sis).

Blood Types

ABO Blood Groups

The ABO blood groups are based on the presence or absence of certain antigens on the surface of the RBC membrane. These antigens, A and B, are inherited; consequently, blood types are also inherited. Type A blood has type A antigen; type B blood has type B antigen; type AB blood has both type A and type B antigens; and type O blood has neither type A nor type B antigens (Table 12-2). Certain blood antibodies develop in the plasma shortly after birth. Specifically, a person with type A blood develops B antibodies; a person with type B blood develops A antibodies; a person with both type AB blood develops neither A or B antibodies; and a person with type O blood develops both A and B antibodies (see Table 12-2).

Rh Blood Groups

Even after the ABO blood groups were well established and accurate blood typing procedures were developed, there were still unexplained cases of transfusion reactions. This led to more research, which led to the discovery of the *Rh factor*, so named because it was first studied in the rhesus monkey.

People are Rh positive (Rh+) if they have Rh antigens on the surface of their RBCs. About 85% of people are Rh+. The other 15% do not have the Rh antigens and are Rh negative (Rh−). The presence or absence of Rh antigens is an inherited trait. Normally, neither Rh+ nor Rh− individuals have Rh antibodies. If an Rh− person is exposed to Rh+ blood, either through a blood transfusion or by transfer of blood between a mother and fetus, the Rh− individual develops Rh antibodies. If that individual is exposed to Rh+ blood a second time, a transfusion reaction results. When transfusions are given, it is necessary to match both the Rh type and the ABO type.

BLOOD VESSELS

Blood vessels are the channels through which blood is distributed to body tissues. The vessels make up two closed systems of tubes that begin and end at the heart (Figure 12-14). One system, the **pulmonary vessels,** transports blood from the right ventricle to the lungs and back to the left atrium. The other system, the **systemic vessels,** carries blood from the left ventricle to the tissues in all parts of the body and then returns the blood to the right atrium. Based on their structure and function, blood vessels are classified as either arteries, capillaries, or veins.

Classification and Structure of Blood Vessels
Arteries

Arteries carry blood away from the heart. Pulmonary arteries transport blood that has a low oxygen content from the right ventricle to the lungs. Systemic arteries transport oxygenated blood from the left ventricle to the body tissues. Blood is pumped from the ventricles into large elastic arteries that branch repeatedly into smaller and smaller arteries

---

Highlight on Aging and the Circulatory System

Numerous "age-related" changes occur in the heart. How many of these are due to an actual aging process and how many are due to other factors are questions worth considering. Is it possible to lessen the effects of aging by adjusting lifestyle? Cardiac changes that were once thought to be the result of aging are now believed to be the consequence of a sedentary lifestyle that many consider their "reward" after retirement. Other cardiac changes are due to a lifetime of habits that, while seemingly enjoyable at the time, take their toll later in life. It is difficult to isolate the aging process of the heart because it is so closely related to diet, exercise, and disease processes, but even when these factors are excluded, a clinical pattern of cardiac aging emerges.

In the absence of cardiovascular disease, the heart, particularly the left ventricle, tends to become slightly smaller in elderly people. This is partially due to a decrease in the number and size of cardiac muscle cells and partially due to the reduced demands placed on it by decreasing physical activity. However, because of cardiovascular disease, the heart is often enlarged.

A general thickening of the endocardium and valves of the heart occurs as part of the aging process. The valves tend to become more rigid and incompetent. Thus heart murmurs are detected more frequently in the elderly. Structural changes also occur throughout the conduction system as conducting myofibers are replaced with fibrous tissue. Usually this does not alter the resting pulse rate, but there is a greater than normal increase in heart rate in response to activity. Dysrhythmias are also more frequent.

Numerous disease processes that occur more frequently in the aging individual have an effect on the heart. Most notable of these is arteriosclerosis, or hardening of the arteries. This puts additional stress on the heart and aggravates the normal age-related changes. Although some degree of arteriosclerosis is probably inevitable in the aging process, a significant amount of vascular disease can be prevented by a proper diet, regular walking or other aerobic exercise, and the elimination of cigarette smoking. In other words, lifestyle probably has more effect on the cardiovascular system than aging. ∎

Table 12-2 Antigens and Antibodies in ABO Blood Types		
Blood Type	Antigens on Red Blood Cell	Antibodies in Plasma
A	A	Anti-B
B	B	Anti-A
AB	Both A and B	Neither anti-A nor anti-B
O	Neither A nor B	Both anti-A and anti-B

Modified from Applegate E: *The anatomy and physiology learning system*, ed 3, St. Louis, 2006, Saunders.

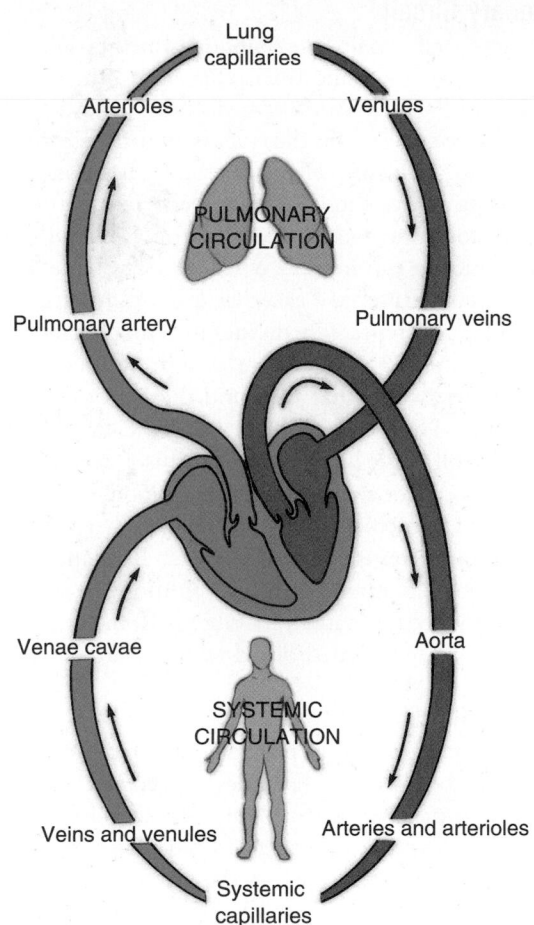

Figure 12-14. Scheme of circulation. (From Applegate E: *The anatomy and physiology learning system,* ed 3, St. Louis, 2006, Saunders.)

Figure 12-15. Structure of blood vessels. (From Applegate E: *The anatomy and physiology learning system,* ed 3, St. Louis, 2006, Saunders.)

until the branching results in microscopic arteries called **arterioles** (ar-TEER-ee-ohlz). The arterioles play a key role in regulating blood flow into the tissue capillaries. About 10% of the total blood volume is in the systemic arterial system at any given time.

The wall of an artery consists of three layers (Figure 12-15). The innermost layer is the **tunica intima** (also called **tunica interna**). The middle layer is the **tunica media,** which consists of smooth muscle and is usually the thickest layer. It not only provides support for the vessel but also changes vessel diameter to regulate blood flow and blood pressure. The outermost layer is the **tunica externa** or **tunica adventitia.**

Capillaries

Capillaries are the smallest and most numerous of the blood vessels. They form the connection between the vessels that carry blood away from the heart (arteries) and the vessels that return blood to the heart (veins). They are the continuation of the smallest arterioles. Arterioles are the smallest vessels with three distinguishable layers in their wall. When the arterioles branch into capillaries, the middle

and outer layers of the wall disappear so that the capillary wall is only a thin endothelium. This thin wall permits the exchange of materials between the blood in the capillary and the adjacent tissue cells. This exchange is the primary function of capillaries.

The diameter of a capillary is so small that erythrocytes must pass through them in single file. This slows the blood flow to allow ample time for the transport of substances across the capillary endothelium.

Veins

Veins carry blood toward the heart. After blood passes through the capillaries, it enters the smallest veins, called

venules. From the venules, it flows into progressively larger and larger veins until it reaches the heart. In the pulmonary circuit, the pulmonary veins transport blood from the lungs to the left atrium of the heart. This blood has a high oxygen content because it has just been oxygenated in the lungs. Systemic veins transport blood from the body tissues to the right atrium of the heart. This blood has a reduced oxygen content because the oxygen has been used for metabolic activities in the tissue cells.

The walls of veins have the same three layers as the arteries (see Figure 12-15). Although all the layers are present, there is less smooth muscle and connective tissue. This makes the walls of veins thinner than those of arteries, which is related to the fact that blood in the veins has less pressure than blood in the arteries. Because the walls of the veins are thinner and less rigid than arteries, veins can hold more blood. Almost 70% of the total blood volume is in the veins at any given time. Medium and large veins have **venous valves,** similar to the SL valves associated with the heart, that help keep the blood flowing toward the heart. Venous valves are especially important in the arms and legs, where they prevent the backflow of blood in response to the pull of gravity.

Circulatory Pathways

The blood vessels of the body are functionally divided into two distinct circuits:
- Pulmonary circuit
- Systemic circuit

The pump for the pulmonary circuit, which circulates blood through the lungs, is the right ventricle. The left ventricle is the pump for the systemic circuit, which provides the blood supply for the tissue cells of the body.

Pulmonary Circuit

The pulmonary circuit takes blood from the right side of the heart to the lungs and then returns it to the left side of the heart (Figure 12-16). Oxygen-poor blood, which has increased levels of carbon dioxide, is returned to the **right atrium** from the tissue cells of the body. It passes through the **tricuspid valve** into the **right ventricle.** During ventricular systole, the blood is ejected through the **pulmonary SL valve** into the **pulmonary trunk,** which divides into the right and left **pulmonary arteries.** Each pulmonary artery enters a lung and repeatedly divides into smaller and smaller vessels until they become capillaries. The **capillaries of the lungs** form networks that surround the air sacs, or alveoli, of the lungs. Here CO_2 diffuses from the capillary blood into the alveoli of the lungs, and O_2 diffuses from the alveoli into the blood. The newly oxygenated blood enters pulmonary venules, which form progressively larger veins, until two **pulmonary veins** emerge from each lung and carry the blood to the **left atrium.** In the pulmonary circuit, the arteries carry deoxygenated blood away from the heart and the veins carry oxygenated blood to the heart.

Systemic Circuit

The systemic circulation provides the functional blood supply to all body tissues. It carries oxygen and nutrients to the cells and picks up carbon dioxide and waste products. Systemic circulation carries oxygenated blood from the left ventricle, through the arteries, to the capillaries in the tissues of the body. The major systemic arteries are illustrated in Figure 12-17. From the tissue capillaries, the deoxygenated blood returns through a system of veins to the right atrium of the heart. The major systemic veins are illustrated in Figure 12-18.

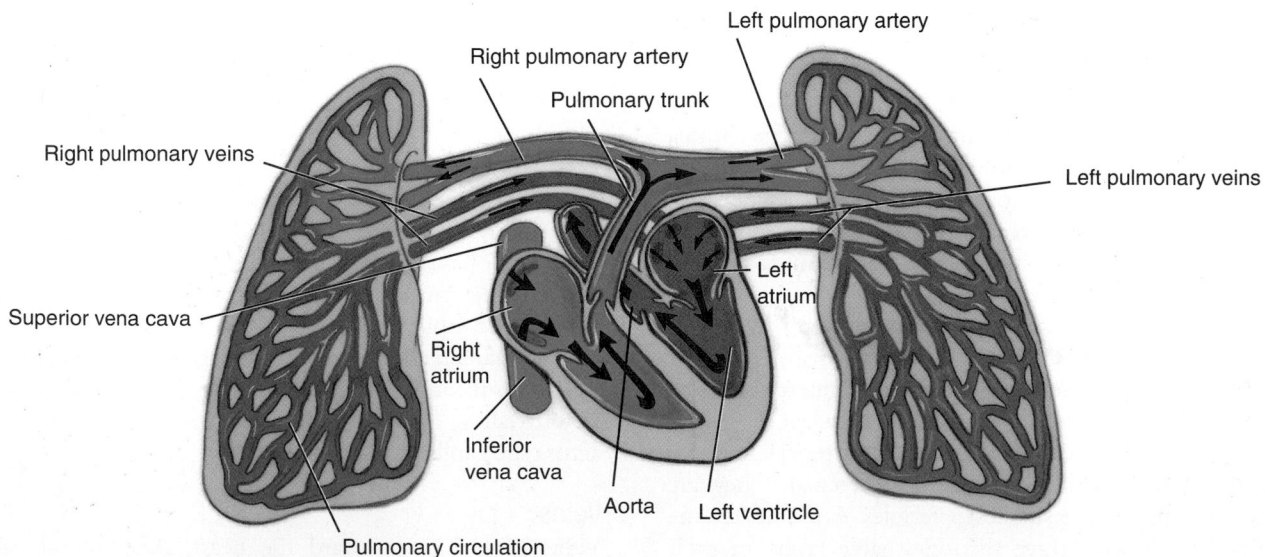

Figure 12-16. Pulmonary circulation. (From Applegate E: *The anatomy and physiology learning system,* ed 3, St. Louis, 2006, Saunders.)

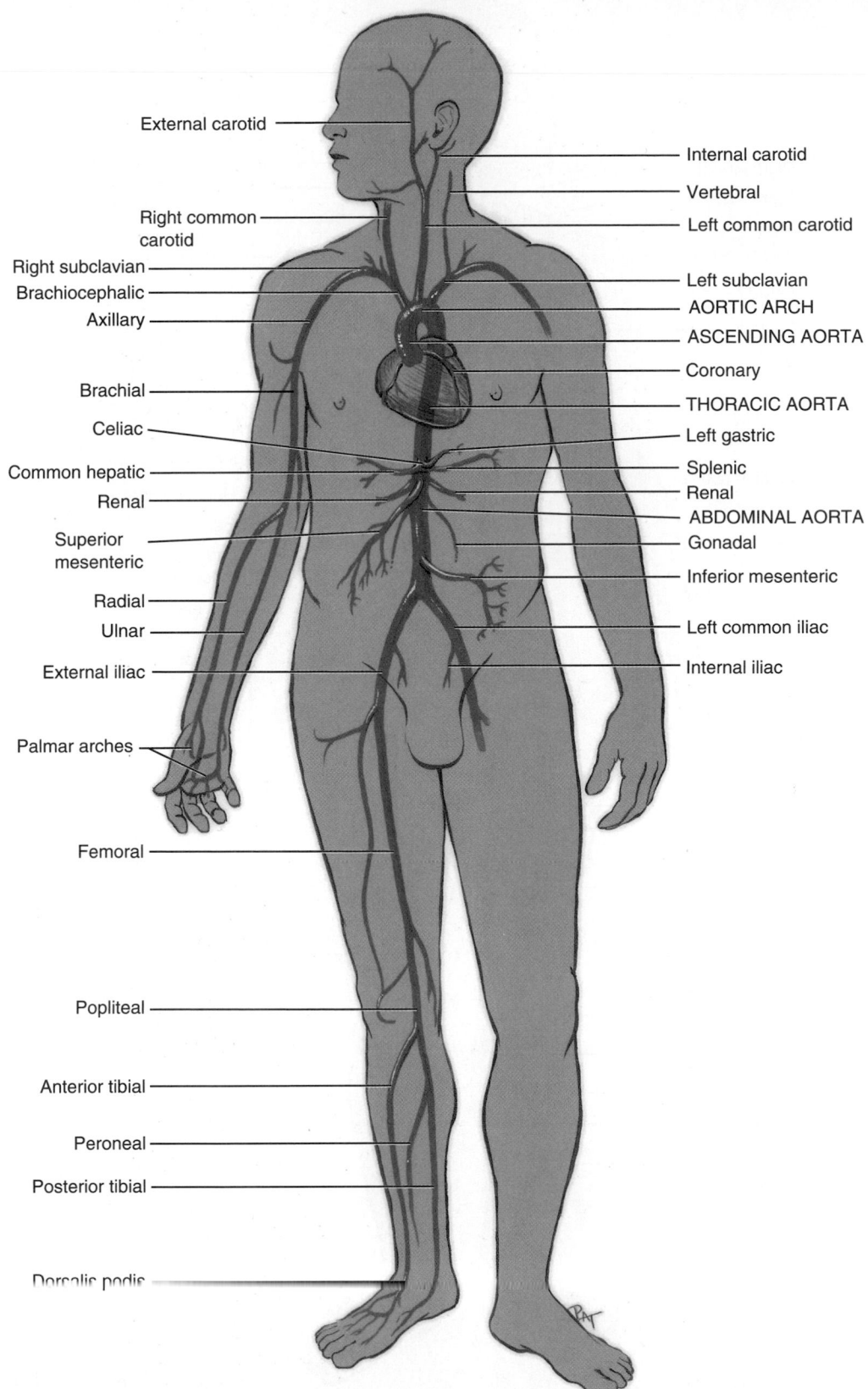

External carotid

Internal carotid

Vertebral

Right common carotid

Left common carotid

Right subclavian

Left subclavian

Brachiocephalic

AORTIC ARCH

Axillary

ASCENDING AORTA

Coronary

Brachial

THORACIC AORTA

Celiac

Left gastric

Common hepatic

Splenic

Renal

Renal

ABDOMINAL AORTA

Superior mesenteric

Gonadal

Inferior mesenteric

Radial

Ulnar

Left common iliac

External iliac

Internal iliac

Palmar arches

Femoral

Popliteal

Anterior tibial

Peroneal

Posterior tibial

Dorsalis pedis

Figure 12-17. Major systemic arteries. (From Applegate E: *The anatomy and physiology learning system,* ed 3, St. Louis, 2006, Saunders.)

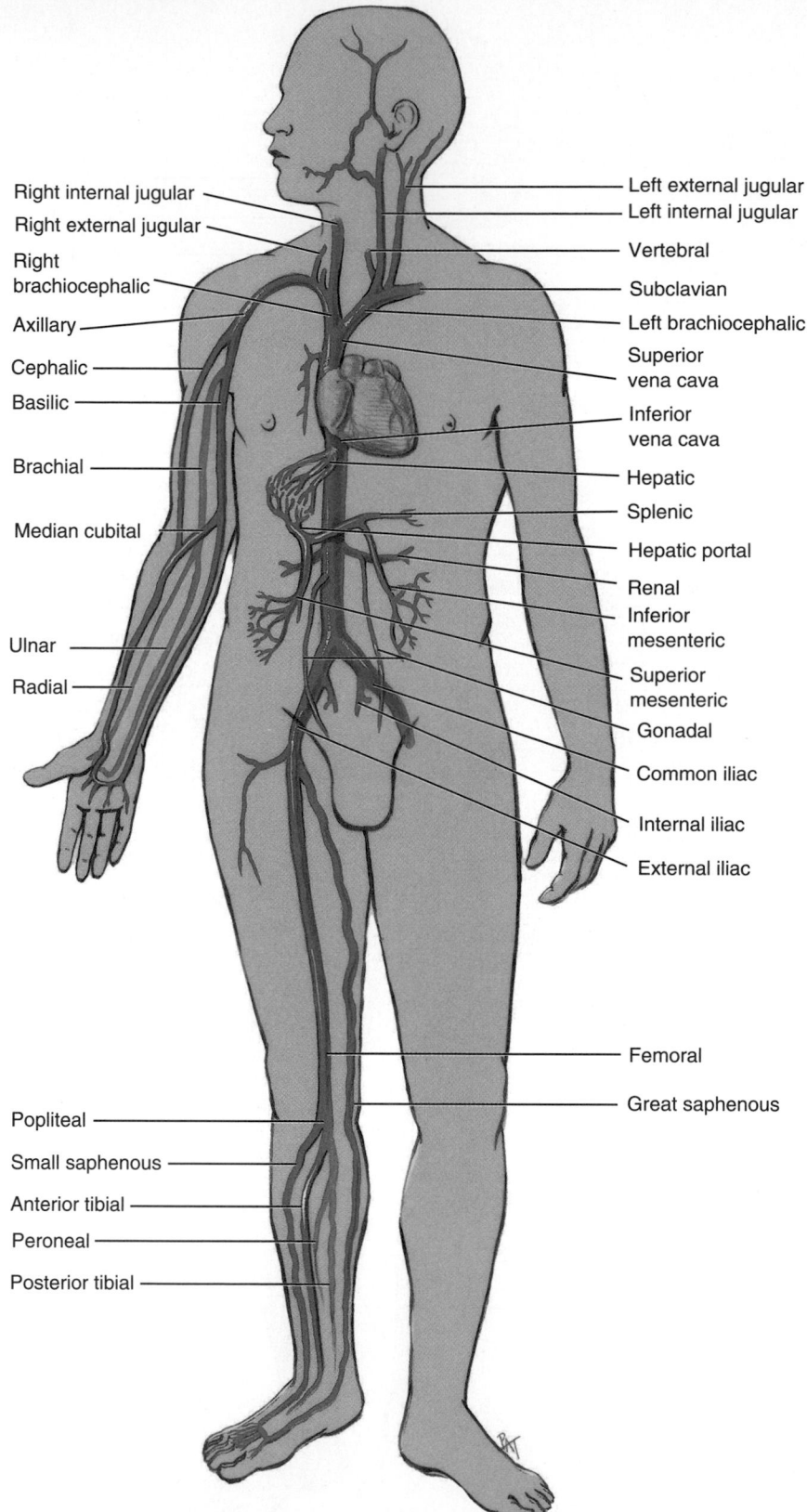

Right internal jugular
Right external jugular
Right brachiocephalic
Axillary
Cephalic
Basilic
Brachial
Median cubital
Ulnar
Radial

Left external jugular
Left internal jugular
Vertebral
Subclavian
Left brachiocephalic
Superior vena cava
Inferior vena cava
Hepatic
Splenic
Hepatic portal
Renal
Inferior mesenteric
Superior mesenteric
Gonadal
Common iliac
Internal iliac
External iliac

Femoral
Great saphenous

Popliteal
Small saphenous
Anterior tibial
Peroneal
Posterior tibial

Figure 12-18. Major systemic veins. (From Applegate E: *The anatomy and physiology learning system,* ed 3, St. Louis, 2006, Saunders.)

TERMINOLOGY REVIEW

Atrioventricular valve Valve between an atrium and a ventricle in the heart.

Cardiac cycle A complete heartbeat consisting of contraction and relaxation of both atria and both ventricles.

Coagulation The process of blood clotting.

Conduction myofibers Cardiac muscle cells specialized for conducting action potentials to the myocardium; part of the conduction system of the heart; also called *Purkinje fibers.*

Diapedesis The process by which white blood cells squeeze between the cells in a vessel wall to enter the tissue spaces outside the blood vessel.

Diastole Relaxation phase of the cardiac cycle; opposite of systole.

Erythrocyte Red blood cell.

Erythropoiesis The process of red blood cell formation.

Erythropoietin A hormone released by the kidneys that stimulates red blood cell production.

Hemocytoblast A stem cell in the bone marrow from which the blood cells arise.

Hematopoiesis Blood cell production, which occurs in the red bone marrow; also called *hemopoiesis.*

Leukocyte White blood cell.

Semilunar valve Valve between a ventricle of the heart and the vessel that carries blood away from the ventricle; also pertains to the valves in veins.

Systole Contraction phase of the cardiac cycle; opposite of diastole.

Thrombocyte One of the formed elements of the blood; functions in blood clotting; also called *platelet.*

ON THE WEB

For Information on the Circulatory System:

The Internet Pathology Laboratory for Medical Education—Hematopathology: library.med.utah.edu/WebPath/ORGAN.html *(Click on "Hematopathology")*

Inner Body: www.innerbody.com/html/body.html

Heart Point: www.heartpoint.com

The Franklin Institute—The Human Heart: www.fi.edu/learn/heart

Cardio Guide: www.mymedline.com/cardio

Human Blood: anthro.palomar.edu/blood

America's Blood Centers: www.americasblood.org

The Franklin Institute—Blood: www.fi.edu/learn/heart/blood/blood.html

 PREPARE FOR CERTIFICATION Visit the Evolve site at http://evolve.elsevier.com/Bonewit/today/ to actively Prepare for your Certification.

 *Check out the **Companion CD** bound with the book to access additional interactive activities.*

13

Respiratory System

LEARNING OBJECTIVES

1. List and describe the structures of the upper respiratory tract.
2. List and describe the structures of the lower respiratory tract.
3. Explain what occurs during inhalation and exhalation.
4. Explain the difference between external respiration and internal respiration.
5. Explain how respiration is regulated by the brain.
6. Identify factors that influence breathing.

CHAPTER OUTLINE

Introduction to the Respiratory System
Functions and Overview of Respiration
Ventilation
   Conducting Passages
   Mechanics of Ventilation
Respiration
   External Respiration

   Internal Respiration
Regulation of Respiration
   Respiratory Center
   Factors That Influence Breathing
   Nonrespiratory Air Movements

CAAHEP COMPETENCIES

Content Competencies
Anatomy and Physiology
- Anatomy and physiology of all body systems

- Common pathology/diseases
- Diagnostic/treatment modalities

ABHES COMPETENCIES

Content Competencies
Anatomy and Physiology
- Anatomy and physiology

- Study of diseases and etiology
- All body systems
- Diagnostic/treatment modalities

KEY TERMS

alveoli (al-VEE-oh-ly)
bronchial tree (BRONG-kee-al TREE)
external respiration (eks-TER-nal res-per-RAY-shun)
internal respiration (in-TER-nal res-per-RAY-shun)

respiratory membrane (RES-per-ah-tor-ee MEM-brayn)
surfactant (sir-FAK-tant)
ventilation (ven-tih-LAY-shun)

Introduction to the Respiratory System

When the respiratory system is mentioned, people generally think of breathing, but this is only one of the activities of the respiratory system. The body cells need a continuous supply of oxygen for the metabolic processes that are necessary to maintain life. The respiratory system works with the circulatory system to provide this oxygen and to remove the waste products of metabolism. The respiratory system also helps to regulate the pH of the blood.

FUNCTIONS AND OVERVIEW OF RESPIRATION

Respiration is the sequence of events that results in the exchange of oxygen and carbon dioxide between the atmosphere and the body cells. Every 3 to 5 seconds nerve impulses stimulate the breathing process, or **ventilation,** which moves air through a series of passages into and out of the lungs. After this, there is an exchange of gases between the lungs and the blood. This is called **external respiration.** The blood **transports** the gases to and from the tissue cells. The exchange of gases between the blood and tissue cells is known as **internal respiration.**

VENTILATION

Ventilation, or breathing, is the movement of air through the conducting passages between the atmosphere and the lungs.

Conducting Passages

The conducting passages are divided into the upper respiratory tract and the lower respiratory tract (Figure 13-1). The **upper respiratory tract** includes the nose, pharynx, and larynx. The **lower respiratory tract** consists of the trachea, bronchial tree, and lungs. These passageways open to the outside and are lined with mucous membrane. In some regions, the membrane has hairs that help filter the air. Other regions may have cilia to propel mucus.

Nose and Nasal Cavities

The framework of the **nose** consists of bone and cartilage. Two small nasal bones and extensions of the maxillae form the bridge of the nose, which is the bony portion. The remainder of the framework is cartilage. This is the flexible portion. Connective tissue and skin cover the framework.

The interior chamber of the nose is the **nasal cavity** (Figure 13-2). It is divided into two parts by the **nasal septum.** Air enters the nasal cavity from the outside through two openings—the **nostrils,** or **external nares** (NAY-reez). The openings from the nasal cavity into the pharynx are the **internal nares.** The **palate** forms the floor of the nasal cavity and separates the nasal cavity from the oral cavity. The anterior portion of the palate is called the **hard palate** because it is supported by bone. The posterior portion has

Highlight on the Respiratory System

RHINITIS: Rhinitis is an inflammation of the nasal mucosa accompanied by excessive mucus production. It can be caused by cold viruses, certain bacteria, and allergens.

PHARYNGITIS AND LARYNGITIS: Inflammation of the pharynx, or a sore throat, is **pharyngitis.** Inflammation of the vocal cords is called **laryngitis.** The inflammation may be caused by overuse of the voice, infection with bacteria or viruses, or inhalation of irritating particles. Laryngitis results in hoarseness or an inability to speak above a whisper.

TRACHEOTOMY: A **tracheotomy** is the creation of an opening into the trachea through the neck and insertion of a tube to facilitate passage of air or removal of secretions.

RESPIRATORY OBSTRUCTION: Foreign objects that become lodged in the larynx or trachea are usually expelled by coughing. If a person cannot speak or make a sound because of the obstruction, it means that the airway is completely blocked. This is a life-threatening situation. The Heimlich maneuver is a procedure in which the air in the person's own lungs is used to forcefully expel the object.

BRONCHOSCOPY: Bronchoscopy is a procedure in which a fiberoptic bundle is inserted into the trachea and directed along the conducting passageways to the smaller bronchi. This allows direct visualization of the inside of the bronchi and collection of specimens for cytologic and bacterial studies.

ASTHMA: Several different forms of asthma exist, all of which have sensitive conducting passages. In many cases the agent that triggers the attack is an allergen in the air. The most obvious and dangerous symptom involves the constriction of the smooth muscle around the bronchial tree. The airways become narrow and breathing is difficult. Treatment includes the use of bronchodilators to dilate the respiratory passages to permit airflow.

PLEURISY: Pleuritis, or pleurisy, is an inflammation of the pleura and is often painful because the sensory nerves in the parietal pleura are irritated. As the condition progresses, the permeability of the membrane changes, which results in an accumulation of fluid in the pleural cavity, making breathing difficult.

PNEUMOTHORAX: The accumulation of air in the pleural cavity is called *pneumothorax.* This condition can occur in pulmonary disease, such as emphysema, carcinoma, tuberculosis, or lung abscesses, when rupture of a lesion allows air to escape from the alveoli into the pleural cavity. It also may follow trauma in which the chest wall is perforated and atmospheric air enters the cavity.

SURFACTANT: Surfactant is not produced until the late stages of fetal life. Newborns who are born prematurely may not have enough surfactant, and the forces of surface tension collapse the alveoli. The newborn must reinflate the alveoli with each breath, which requires tremendous energy. The lack of surfactant accounts for many of the signs and symptoms of infant respiratory distress syndrome (IRDS). The condition is treated by using positive-pressure respirators that maintain pressure within the alveoli to keep them inflated. ∎

Highlight on Conditions Affecting the Respiratory System

Atelectasis (at-eh-LECK-tah-sis) Collapse of the alveoli; the lung is airless

Bronchogenic carcinoma (brong-koh-JEN-ik kar-sin-OH-mah) Cancerous tumors arising from a bronchus; lung cancer; smoking is the primary etiologic agent; spreads readily to the liver, brain, and bones

Chronic obstructive pulmonary disease (COPD) (KRAHN-ik ob-STRUCK-tiv PULL-mon-air-ee dih-ZEEZ) A chronic condition of obstructed airflow through the bronchial tubes and lungs, usually accompanied by dyspnea; includes emphysema and chronic bronchitis

Coryza (koh-RYE-zah) The common cold, characterized by sneezing, nasal discharge, coughing, and malaise; caused by a rhinovirus

Croup (KROOP) Acute respiratory syndrome in infants and children, characterized by obstruction of the larynx, barking cough, and strained, high-pitched, noisy breathing

Hemoptysis (hee-MAHP-tih-sis) Spitting of blood as a result of bleeding from any part of the respiratory tract

Pertussis (per-TUSS-is) Whooping cough; a highly contagious bacterial infection of the pharynx, larynx, and trachea; characterized by explosive coughing spasms ending in a "whooping" sound

Pneumoconiosis (new-moh-koh-nee-OH-sis) General term for lung pathology that occurs after long-term inhalation of pollutants, characterized by chronic inflammation, infection, and bronchitis

Pneumothorax (new-moh-THOH-raks) Accumulation of air or gas in the pleural space, resulting in collapse of the lung on the affected side

Pulmonary edema (PULL-mon-air-ee eh-DEE-mah) Swelling and fluid in the air sacs and bronchioles; often caused by inability of the heart to pump blood; the blood then backs up in the pulmonary blood vessels and fluid seeps into the alveoli and bronchioles

Smoker's respiratory syndrome (SMOH-kers reh-SPY-rah-tor-ee SIN-drohm) A group of respiratory symptoms seen in smokers; includes coughing, wheezing, vocal hoarseness, pharyngitis, dyspnea, and susceptibility to respiratory infections ∎

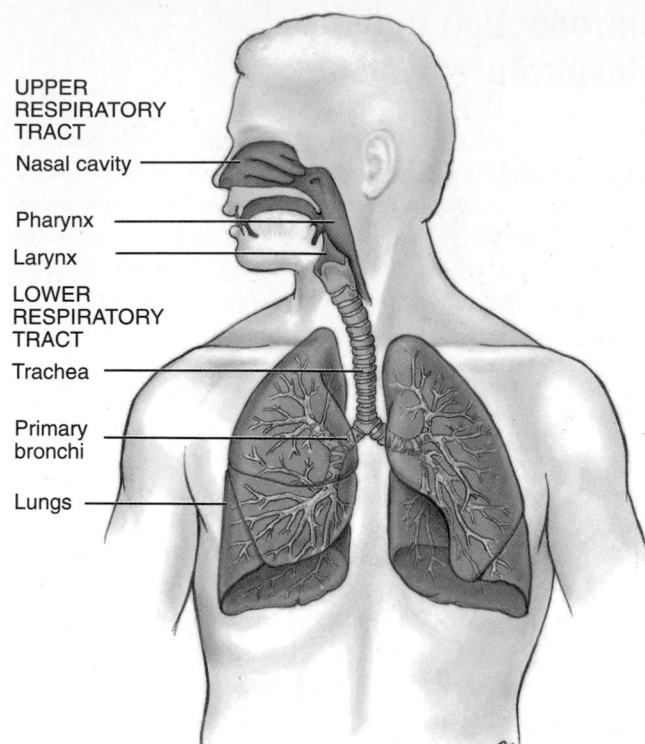

Figure 13-1. Conducting passages of the respiratory system. (From Applegate E: *The anatomy and physiology learning system,* ed 3, St. Louis, 2006, Saunders.)

Paranasal sinuses are air-filled cavities in the frontal, maxillae, ethmoid, and sphenoid bones. These sinuses surround the nasal cavity and open into it. They function to reduce the weight of the skull, produce mucus, and influence voice quality by acting as resonating chambers. The sinuses are lined with mucous membrane that produces mucus, which drains into the nasal cavity. During infections and allergies, the membranes in the passages that drain the sinuses become inflamed and swollen. The swelling may block the passages and cause the mucus to accumulate in the sinuses. As the mucus accumulates, pressure within the sinuses increases, resulting in a sinus headache.

As air passes through the nasal cavity, it is filtered, warmed, and moistened. The mucous membrane that lines most of the nasal cavity is **ciliated pseudostratified columnar epithelium.** Goblet cells in the mucous membrane produce mucus. The **mucus** traps microorganisms, dust, and other foreign particles. The **cilia** attached to the epithelium propel the mucus with the trapped particles toward the pharynx, where it is swallowed. Acid in the gastric juice destroys most of the microorganisms that are swallowed. An extensive capillary network under the mucous membrane warms and moistens the air before it reaches the rest of the respiratory tract.

Pharynx

The **pharynx** (FAIR-inks), commonly called the *throat,* is a passageway about 13 cm long. It serves both the respira-

no bony support, so it is called the **soft palate.** The soft palate terminates in a projection called the **uvula** (YOO-vyoo-lah), which helps direct food into the oropharynx.

Nasal conchae (KONG-kee) are bony ridges that project into the nasal cavity (see Figure 13-2). The three nasal conchae function by increasing the surface area of the nasal cavity to warm and moisten the air. They also help direct air flow through the nasal cavity. Dust and other particles in the air tend to become trapped in the mucous membrane around the nasal conchae.

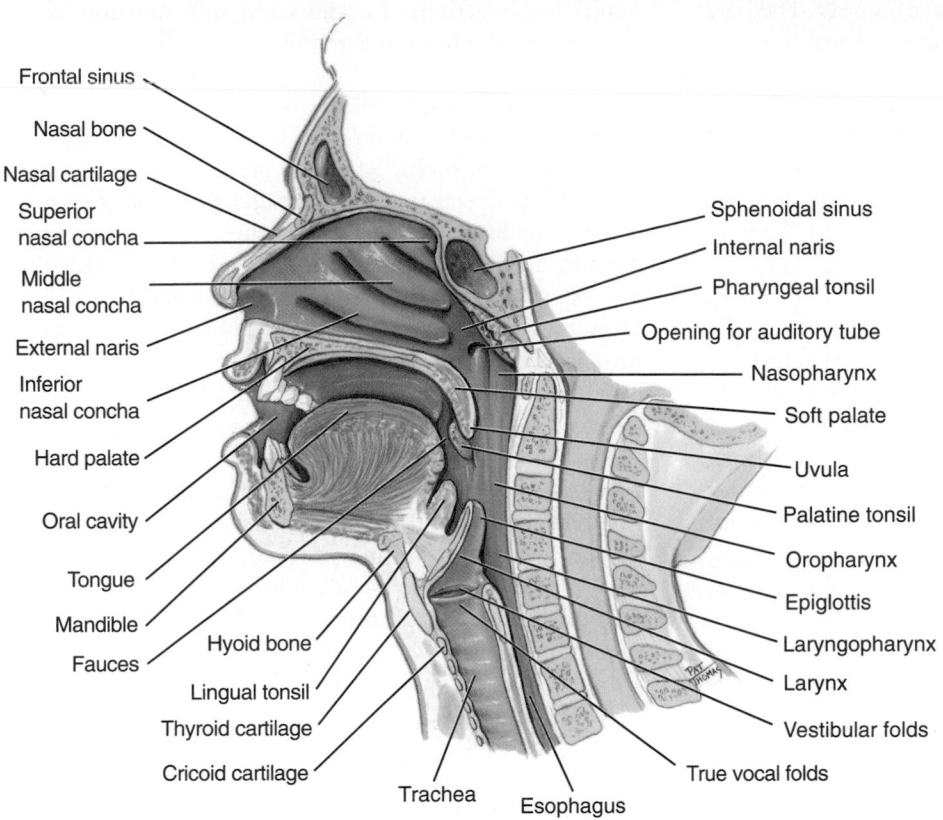

Frontal sinus
Nasal bone
Nasal cartilage
Superior nasal concha
Middle nasal concha
External naris
Inferior nasal concha
Hard palate
Oral cavity
Tongue
Mandible
Fauces
Hyoid bone
Lingual tonsil
Thyroid cartilage
Cricoid cartilage
Trachea
Esophagus

Sphenoidal sinus
Internal naris
Pharyngeal tonsil
Opening for auditory tube
Nasopharynx
Soft palate
Uvula
Palatine tonsil
Oropharynx
Epiglottis
Laryngopharynx
Larynx
Vestibular folds
True vocal folds

Figure 13-2. Features of the upper respiratory tract. (From Applegate E: *The anatomy and physiology learning system,* ed 3, St. Louis, 2006, Saunders.)

tory and digestive systems by receiving air from the nasal cavity and air, food, and water from the oral cavity. Inferiorly, it opens into the larynx and esophagus. The pharynx is divided into three regions according to location: nasopharynx, oropharynx, and laryngopharynx (see Figure 13-2).

The **nasopharynx** (nay-zoh-FAIR-inks) is the portion of the pharynx that is posterior to the nasal cavity and extends to the uvula. Air enters this region from the nasal cavity through the internal nares. The mucous membrane in the nasopharynx is similar to the lining of the nasal cavity. The **auditory** (eustachian) **tubes** from the two middle ear cavities open into the nasopharynx. The auditory tubes help to equalize the air pressure on both sides of the tympanic membrane. Collections of lymphoid tissue, called **pharyngeal tonsils** (or **adenoids**), are located in the posterior wall of the nasopharynx.

The **oropharynx** (ohr-oh-FAIR-inks) is the portion of the pharynx that is posterior to the oral cavity. It receives air, food, and water from the oral cavity. During swallowing, the soft palate and uvula move upward to prevent the material from going into the nasopharynx. The opening between the oral cavity and oropharynx is called the **fauces** (FAW-seez). The fauces is bordered by masses of lymphoid tissue called **tonsils.** The **palatine tonsils** are in the lateral walls of the oropharynx, adjacent to the fauces. The **lingual tonsils** are located on the surface of the posterior portion of the tongue, also in the region of the fauces. The tonsils

in the pharynx function in immune responses and help prevent infections.

The most inferior portion of the pharynx is the **laryngopharynx** (lah-ring-goh-FAIR-inks) (see Figure 13-2). Both the oropharynx and laryngopharynx are lined with a mucous membrane of stratified squamous epithelium.

Larynx

The **larynx** (LAIR-inks), commonly called the *voice box,* is the passageway for air between the pharynx and the trachea. It is about 5 cm long and formed by nine pieces of cartilage that are connected to each other by muscles and ligaments.

The three largest cartilaginous portions of the larynx are the thyroid cartilage, cricoid cartilage, and epiglottis (see Figure 13-2). The **thyroid cartilage** forms a projection in the neck called the *Adam's apple.* The projection is more pronounced in males than in females. The **cricoid** (KRY-koyd) **cartilage** forms the base of the larynx and is attached to the trachea. The **epiglottis** (eh-pih-GLOT-is) is a long, leaf-shaped structure. During swallowing, the epiglottis covers the opening into the larynx to prevent food and water from entering the trachea.

The larynx houses two pairs of ligaments. The upper pair are the **vestibular folds,** or **false vocal cords.** They work with the epiglottis to prevent particles from entering the lower respiratory tract. The lower pair are the **true vocal cords,** which function in sound production. Muscles control the length and tension of the true vocal cords. They are relaxed during normal breathing. When the vocal cords are under tension, exhaled air moving by them causes them to vibrate and produce sound. The length of the vocal cords determines the pitch of the sound, and the force of the moving air regulates the loudness. The opening between the true vocal cords is the **glottis,** which leads to the trachea.

Trachea

The **trachea** is commonly called the *windpipe.* The trachea consists of a tube that extends from the larynx and into the mediastinum, where it divides into the right and left bronchi (Figure 13-3). It is about 12 to 15 cm long. The walls of the trachea are supported by 15 to 20 C-shaped pieces of hyaline cartilage that hold the trachea open despite the pressure changes that occur during breathing. The posterior open part of the C-shaped cartilage is closed by smooth muscle and connective tissue and is next to the esophagus. During swallowing, the esophagus bulges into the soft part of the trachea.

The mucous membrane that lines the trachea is ciliated epithelium similar to that in the nasal cavity and nasopharynx. Goblet cells located in the mucous membrane produce mucus that traps airborne particles and microorganisms. The cilia propel the mucus upward, where it is either swallowed or expelled. Continued irritation from cigarette smoke and other air pollutants damages the cilia, and the mucus with the trapped particles is not removed. Microorganisms thrive in the accumulated mucus, which results in respiratory infections. Irritation and inflammation of the mucous membrane stimulate the cough reflex.

Bronchi and Bronchial Tree

In the mediastinum, the trachea divides into the **right** and **left primary bronchi.** After the bronchi enter the lungs, they branch several times into smaller and smaller passages to form the **bronchial tree** (see Figure 13-3). The primary bronchi divide to form **secondary (lobar) bronchi;** then the secondary bronchi branch into **tertiary (segmental) bronchi.** The branching continues, finally giving rise to the **bronchioles.** The terminal bronchioles branch into smaller respiratory bronchioles, which lead into microscopic **alveolar ducts.** Alveolar ducts terminate in clusters of tiny air sacs called **alveoli.**

The alveolar ducts and alveoli consist primarily of **simple squamous epithelium,** which permits rapid diffusion of oxygen and carbon dioxide. Exchange of gases between the air in the lungs and the blood in the capillaries occurs across the walls of the alveolar ducts and alveoli.

Lungs

The two **lungs** occupy most of the space in the thoracic cavity (Figure 13-4). The lungs are soft and spongy because they are mostly air spaces surrounded by the alveolar cells and elastic connective tissue. They are separated from each other by the mediastinum, which contains the heart. Each lung is roughly cone shaped, rests on the diaphragm, and extends upward just above the midpoint of the clavicle.

Figure 13-3. Features of the lower respiratory tract. (From Applegate E: *The anatomy and physiology learning system,* ed 3, St. Louis, 2006, Saunders.)

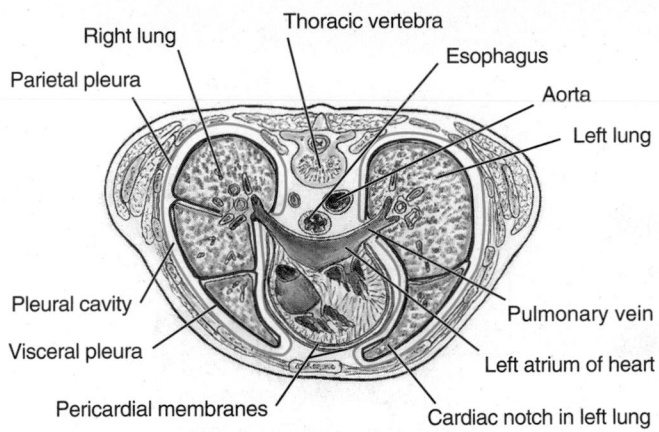

Figure 13-4. Features of the lungs and pleura. (From Applegate E: *The anatomy and physiology learning system,* ed 3, St. Louis, 2006, Saunders.)

The **right lung** is shorter, is broader, and has a greater volume than the left lung. It is divided into three lobes (superior, middle, and inferior) by two fissures. The **left lung** is longer and narrower than the right lung. It has an indentation, called the **cardiac notch,** on its medial surface for the apex of the heart. The left lung is divided into two lobes by a single fissure.

Each lung is enclosed by a double-layered **serous membrane** called the **pleura** (see Figure 13-4). The **visceral pleura** is firmly attached to the surface of the lung. The visceral pleura is continuous with the **parietal pleura** that lines the wall of the thorax. The small space between the visceral and parietal pleurae is the **pleural cavity.** It contains a thin film of serous fluid that is produced by the pleura. The fluid acts as a lubricant to reduce friction as the two layers slide against each other.

Mechanics of Ventilation

Pulmonary ventilation is commonly referred to as *breathing.* It is the process of air flowing into the lungs during inhalation and out of the lungs during exhalation. Air flows because of pressure differences between the atmosphere and the gases inside the lungs. Under normal conditions, the average adult takes 12 to 20 breaths per minute. A breath is one complete respiratory cycle that consists of one inhalation and one exhalation. The amount of air that is exchanged during one cycle varies with age, sex, size, and physical condition.

Inhalation

Inhalation (or inspiration) is the process of taking air into the lungs. It is the active phase of ventilation because it is the result of muscle contraction. In normal, quiet breathing, the primary muscle involved in inhalation is the diaphragm. The **diaphragm** is a dome-shaped muscle that separates the thoracic cavity from the abdominal cavity. When the diaphragm contracts, it drops, or becomes flatter. This increases the size (volume) of the thoracic cavity. When the thoracic volume increases, the pressure within the lungs decreases

below atmospheric pressure. This causes air to flows from the region of higher atmospheric pressure outside the body into the region of lower pressure within the lungs. Air continues to flow into the lungs until the pressure equals atmospheric pressure.

Exhalation

Exhalation (or **expiration**) is the process of letting air out of the lungs during the breathing cycle. When the diaphragm relaxes, the volume of the thoracic cavity decreases to its normal resting size. This decrease in lung volume causes an increase in the pressure of the lungs. Air now flows from the region of higher pressure within the lungs to the region of lower atmospheric pressure outside the body until the two pressures are equal.

As air leaves the lungs during exhalation, the alveoli become smaller. The interior surfaces of the alveoli are coated with a thin layer of fluid. The fluid molecules are attracted to each other, which tends to cause the surfaces to adhere to each other. This makes it harder to inflate the lungs during inhalation and creates a tendency for the lungs to collapse. Normally this is prevented by a substance called **surfactant** (sir-FAK-tant). Surfactant is a substance that is produced by certain cells within the lung tissue that reduces the attraction between the fluid molecules. Without surfactant, the alveoli collapse and become nonfunctional.

RESPIRATION

External Respiration

External respiration is the exchange of oxygen and carbon dioxide between the lungs and the blood in the surrounding capillaries. Oxygen diffuses from the alveoli of the lungs into the blood, and carbon dioxide diffuses from the blood into the air in the alveoli. The surfaces in the lungs where diffusion occurs constitute the **respiratory membrane.**

The respiratory membrane consists of the layers that the gases must travel through to get into or out of the alveoli (Figure 13-5). These layers are as follows:
- Thin layer of fluid that lines the alveolus
- Simple squamous epithelium in the alveolar wall
- Basement membrane of the epithelium
- Small interstitial space
- Basement membrane of capillary epithelium
- Simple squamous epithelium (endothelium) of the capillary wall

The rate of gaseous exchange across the respiratory membrane depends on the surface area of the membrane, thickness of the membrane, solubility of the gas, and difference in pressure of the gas on the two sides of the membrane. Most of the approximately 70 square meters of surface area included in the respiratory membrane comes from the more than 300 million alveoli present in healthy adult lungs.

Internal Respiration

Internal respiration is the exchange of gases between the tissue cells and the blood in the tissue capillaries. After the

Figure 13-5. Components of the respiratory membrane. (From Applegate E: *The anatomy and physiology learning system,* ed 3, St. Louis, 2006, Saunders.)

blood picks up oxygen in the lungs, the blood returns to the left side of the heart, which pumps it to the tissue capillaries. The oxygen is given off to the cells and the carbon dioxide is picked up by the blood to be transported as a waste product to the lungs.

REGULATION OF RESPIRATION

The normal breathing rate in adults averages between 12 and 20 breaths per minute. The rate is higher, up to 40 breaths per minute, in children. The basic rate is established by the respiratory center in the brain stem, but environmental conditions and emotions influence variations in the rate.

Respiratory Center

Groups of neurons in the **pons** and **medulla oblongata** (regions of the brain stem) make up the **respiratory center.** This center controls the rate and depth of breathing and contains both inhalation and exhalation areas. The inhalation area sends impulses along the **phrenic nerve** to the diaphragm. This causes the diaphragm to contract and inhalation results. The inhalation neurons fatigue quickly and quit sending impulses to the diaphragm. When the impulses cease, the muscles of the diaphragm relax and exhalation occurs. If the respiratory center in the brain stem is damaged, the impulses cease and breathing stops.

Factors That Influence Breathing

Even though the respiratory center establishes the basic rhythm of breathing, it is influenced by the following factors that cause variations in the rate and depth of breathing.

Chemoreceptors

Chemoreceptors in the medulla are sensitive to changes in carbon dioxide concentrations in the blood and cerebrospinal fluid. They are not sensitive to changes in oxygen levels. If carbon dioxide concentrations increase, the receptors stimulate the respiratory center to increase the rate and depth of breathing. This decreases the concentrations back to normal levels. In contrast, low carbon dioxide levels decrease the rate and depth of breathing. Breathing may even stop for brief periods of time until concentrations increase to normal levels.

Stimulus from Higher Brain Centers

Impulses from higher brain centers may override the respiratory center temporarily. These impulses may be either voluntary or involuntary; however, the voluntary controls are limited. For example, if you try to voluntarily hold your breath, you can do so for only a limited time. When carbon dioxide levels reach a certain critical point, the impulses from the higher brain centers are ignored and the respiratory center resumes regular breathing.

Involuntary impulses from higher brain centers may stimulate rapid breathing in response to emotions, such as anxiety or excitement. Chronic pain also may result in involuntary stimulation from the higher brain centers. In contrast, sudden pain or sudden cold may cause a gasp or a momentary cessation of breathing.

Temperature

An increase in body temperature caused by a fever or strenuous physical exercise increases the breathing rate. The increased body temperature is associated with increased

Highlight on Aging and the Respiratory System

Various harmful substances, including cigarette smoke, air pollution, and pathogens, continually bombard the respiratory system and take their toll. There is no way to avoid all of these irritants except to stop breathing! Some irritants, like cigarette smoke, can be decreased, but others are inescapable.

Because of the continual contact between the respiratory system and the environment, it is difficult to distinguish between the changes in the tissues of the breathing apparatus, including the lungs, that are due to aging and those that are the result of disease or other factors outside the body. Modifications in the lining of the respiratory tract probably are caused by environmental, rather than solely aging, factors. Long-term exposure to irritants results in deterioration of the cilia, which hinders their cleansing action and movement of mucus. As a consequence, the occurrence of emphysema and chronic bronchitis increases with age. Diminishing effectiveness of the immune system makes the elderly more susceptible to pneumonia and other microbial diseases. However, excluding external influences, there are changes that take place as a result of "normal" aging.

One of the most common signs of respiratory aging, in general, is when a person is unable to maintain the same level of physical activity that was experienced in younger years. This is a gradual decline and may not be noticeable until phrases like, "I used to be able to . . ." become part of the conversation. The cardiovascular and muscular systems have an effect on endurance, and the skeletal system has an effect on thoracic volume, but the major change is a decreased ability of the respiratory system to acquire and deliver oxygen to the blood.

The impairment in oxygen delivery is the result of structural changes that take place in the respiratory tissues. One type of change is a loss of elasticity in the tissues of the respiratory system. The cartilage in the walls of the trachea and bronchi undergoes a progressive calcification. Smooth muscle fibers in the bronchioles are replaced by fibrous tissue, so they are less able to stretch and contract. Modifications in lung tissue cause the alveoli to lose some of their elastic recoil. The cumulative effect of these changes is a gradual decrease in respiratory volume and capacity and an increase in the volume of residual air in the lungs. Another change is deterioration of the walls between adjacent alveoli. This increases the size of each individual alveolus but reduces the total surface area of the respiratory membrane for diffusion of gases. A lower percentage of the oxygen in alveolar air is able to diffuse into the lung capillaries. These changes result in a decreased ability to acquire and deliver oxygen to the blood, which reduces the capacity for physical activity. ■

Table 13-1 Nonrespiratory Air Movements	
Movement	**Description**
Sneezing	Spasmodic contraction of exhalation muscles that forces air through nose and mouth
Coughing	Long inhalation followed by closure of glottis; then a strong exhalation forces glottis open and sends a blast of air through upper respiratory tract
Sighing	Long inhalation followed by a shorter but forceful exhalation
Hiccupping	Spasmodic contraction of diaphragm followed by sudden closure of glottis to produce a sharp sound
Crying	An inhalation followed by many short exhalations; glottis remains open and vocal cords vibrate; usually accompanied by tears and characteristic facial expressions
Laughing	Same basic movements as crying but facial expressions differ; may be indistinguishable from crying
Yawning	A deep inhalation through a widely opened mouth

From Applegate E: *The anatomy and physiology learning system,* ed 3, St. Louis, 2006, Saunders.

metabolism, which uses more oxygen and generates more carbon dioxide. When body temperature decreases, metabolic rate diminishes and breathing rate also decreases.

Nonrespiratory Air Movements

In addition to normal air movements that occur during breathing and result in pulmonary ventilation, there are a number of modifications called **nonrespiratory air movements.** Some of these are reflexes that clear air passages, others are voluntary, and some express emotions. These nonrespiratory air movements are outlined in Table 13-1.

TERMINOLOGY REVIEW

Alveoli Microscopic dilations of terminal bronchioles in the lungs, where diffusion of gases occurs; air sacs in the lungs.

Bronchial tree The bronchi and all their branches that function as passageways between the trachea and the alveoli.

External respiration Exchange of gases between the lungs and the blood.

Internal respiration Exchange of gases between the blood and tissue cells.

Respiratory membrane Any surface in the lungs where diffusion occurs; consists of the layers that the gases must pass through to get into or out of the alveoli.

Surfactant A substance, produced by certain cells in lung tissue, that reduces surface tension between fluid molecules that line the respiratory membrane and helps keep the alveolus from collapsing.

Ventilation Movement of air into and out of the lungs; breathing.

ON THE WEB

For Information on the Respiratory System:

The Internet Pathology Laboratory for Medical Education—Gastrointestinal Pathology: library.med.utah. edu/WebPath/ORGAN.html *(Click on "Pulmonary Pathology")*

Chronic Obstructive Pulmonary Diseases: www.priory. com/cmol/copd.htm

 PREPARE FOR CERTIFICATION   Visit the Evolve site at http://evolve.elsevier.com/Bonewit/today/ to actively Prepare for your Certification.

 Check out the **Companion CD** *bound with the book to access additional interactive activities.*

14

Digestive System

LEARNING OBJECTIVES

1. Identify the components of the digestive tract and the accessory organs.
2. List six functions of the digestive system.
3. Describe the general histology of the four layers in the digestive tract wall.
4. Describe the features and function of the oral cavity, teeth, pharynx, and esophagus.
5. List and describe the location of the three salivary glands.
6. Explain the function of saliva.
7. Describe the structure and features of the stomach and its role in digestion.
8. Describe the structure and features of the small intestine and its role in digestion and absorption.
9. Describe the structure, features, and function of the large intestine.
10. Describe the structure and function of the liver, gallbladder, and pancreas.
11. Explain how substances are absorbed into the body through the small intestine.

CHAPTER OUTLINE

Introduction to the Digestive System
Functions of the Digestive System
General Structure of the Digestive Tract
Components of the Digestive Tract
  Mouth
  Pharynx
  Esophagus
  Stomach
  Small Intestine
  Large Intestine

Accessory Organs of Digestion
  Liver
  Gallbladder
  Pancreas
Chemical Digestion
  Carbohydrate Digestion
  Protein Digestion
  Lipid Digestion
Absorption

CAAHEP COMPETENCIES

Content Competencies
Anatomy and Physiology
• Anatomy and physiology of all body systems

• Common pathology/diseases
• Diagnostic/treatment modalities

ABHES COMPETENCIES

Content Competencies
Anatomy and Physiology
• Anatomy and physiology

• Study of diseases and etiology
• All body systems
• Diagnostic/treatment modalities

KEY TERMS

absorption (ab-SOARP-shun)
chyme (KYME)
mesentery (MEZ-en-tair-ee)

peristalsis (pair-ih-STALL-sis)
plicae circulares (PLY-kee sir-kyoo-LAIR-eez)
rugae (ROO-jee)

Introduction to the Digestive System

The digestive system includes the **digestive tract** and its **accessory organs.** The function of the digestive system is to process food into molecules that can be absorbed and used by the cells of the body (Figure 14-1). Food is broken down, bit by bit, until the molecules are small enough to be absorbed and the waste products are eliminated. The digestive tract (also called the **alimentary canal** or **gastrointestinal [GI] tract**) consists of a long, continuous tube that extends from the mouth to the anus. It includes the mouth, pharynx, esophagus, stomach, small intestine, and large intestine. The tongue and teeth are accessory structures located in the mouth. The salivary glands, liver, gallbladder, and pancreas are not part of the digestive tract but are major accessory organs that have a role in digestion. These secrete fluids into the digestive tract.

FUNCTIONS OF THE DIGESTIVE SYSTEM

Food undergoes three types of processes in the body:
- Digestion
- Absorption
- Metabolism

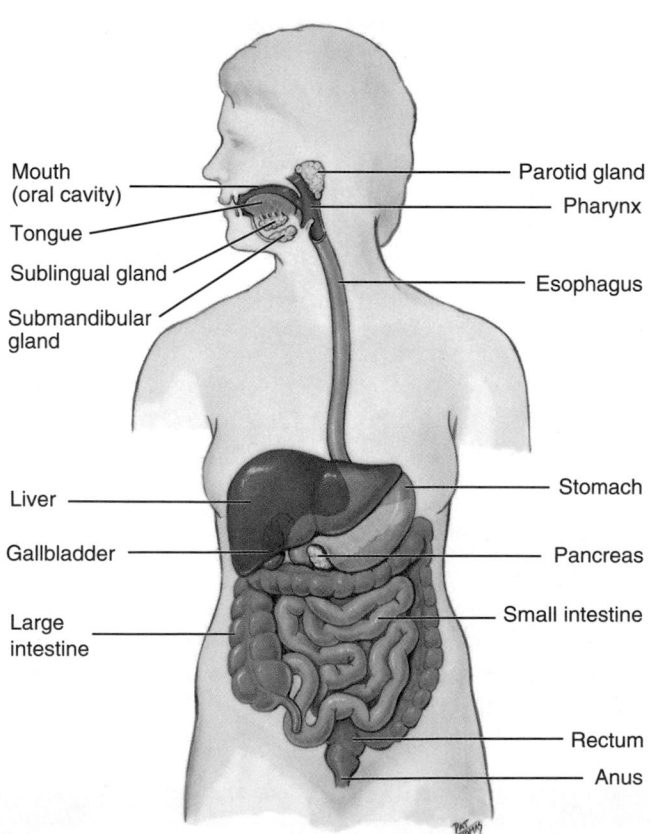

Mouth (oral cavity)
Tongue
Sublingual gland
Submandibular gland
Parotid gland
Pharynx
Esophagus
Liver
Gallbladder
Large intestine
Stomach
Pancreas
Small intestine
Rectum
Anus

Figure 14-1. Organs of the digestive system. (From Applegate E: *The anatomy and physiology learning system,* ed 3, St. Louis, 2006, Saunders.)

Digestion and absorption occur in the digestive tract. After the nutrients are absorbed, they are available to all cells in the body and are used by the cells in metabolism.

The digestive system prepares nutrients for use by the body's cells through the following six activities:
- **Ingestion**—The first activity of the digestive system is to take in food. This process is called *ingestion.* Ingestion has to take place before anything else can happen.
- **Mechanical digestion**—The large pieces of food that are ingested have to be broken into smaller particles that can be acted on by various enzymes. This is called *mechanical digestion.* Mechanical digestion begins in the mouth with chewing, or **mastication** (mas-tih-KAY-shun), and continues with churning and mixing actions in the stomach.
- **Chemical digestion**—The complex molecules of carbohydrates, proteins, and fats are transformed by chemical digestion into smaller molecules that can be absorbed and used by the cells. Chemical digestion uses water to break down the complex molecules. This process is known as **hydrolysis. Digestive enzymes** speed up the hydrolysis process, which is otherwise slow.
- **Movements**—After ingestion and mastication, the food particles move from the mouth into the pharynx, and then into the esophagus. This movement is called **deglutition** (dee-gloo-TISH-un), or swallowing. **Mixing movements** occur in the stomach as a result of smooth muscle contraction. These repetitive contractions mix the food particles with enzymes and other fluids. The movements that propel the food particles through the digestive tract are called **peristalsis.** These are rhythmic waves of contractions that move the food particles through the various regions in which mechanical and chemical digestion takes place.
- **Absorption**—The simple molecules that are produced from chemical digestion pass through the lining of the small intestine into the blood. This process is called *absorption.*
- **Elimination**—The food molecules that cannot be digested need to be eliminated from the body. The removal of indigestible wastes through the anus, in the form of feces, is **defecation** (def-eh-KAY-shun).

GENERAL STRUCTURE OF THE DIGESTIVE TRACT

The **digestive tract** is a long, continuous tube that is about 9 m (30 ft) in length. It opens to the outside at both ends, through the mouth at one end and through the anus at the other. Although there are variations in each region, the basic structure of the wall is the same throughout the entire length of the tube.

The wall of the digestive tract has four layers or **tunics** (Figure 14-2):
- Mucosa
- Submucosa
- Muscular layer (muscularis)
- Serous layer or serosa

Highlight on the Digestive System

COLD SORES: Cold sores, or fever blisters, are small fluid-filled blisters that itch and are painful, usually appearing around the lips and in the mouth. They are caused by recurring infections with the herpes simplex virus. After the initial infection, the virus remains dormant in a cutaneous nerve until it is activated by stress, fever, or ultraviolet radiation.

CLEFT PALATE: Cleft palate is a condition in which the bones in the hard palate do not fuse completely during prenatal development. This leaves an opening between the nasal and oral cavities. An infant with this problem has difficulty creating enough suction for proper feeding. Cleft palate can usually be corrected surgically.

TONGUE TIED: A person with a short frenulum linguae is "tongue tied." The movement of the tongue is abnormally limited, which causes difficulties in speech. Surgically cutting the frenulum corrects this problem.

WISDOM TEETH: The third molars are the last teeth to erupt. These are sometimes called "wisdom teeth" because they usually erupt between the ages of 17 and 25 years, when one is supposed to be wise. These teeth may remain embedded in the jawbone. If this happens, they are said to be impacted. In some cases, wisdom teeth are absent altogether.

GINGIVITIS: Gingivitis is an inflammation of the gingiva, or gum. The gums become sore and red and may bleed. This condition is reversible if it is not neglected and if corrective action is taken. Periodontal disease results when gingivitis is neglected and bacteria invade the bone around the tooth. This is a major cause of tooth loss in adults.

CAVITIES: Caries, or dental cavities, are caused by the demineralization of the teeth resulting from the action of bacteria that live in the mouth. The bacteria metabolize sugars in the mouth, producing acids that dissolve the calcium salts of the tooth. If the bacteria reach the pulp cavity, it is necessary to perform a root canal procedure. In this procedure, the pulp cavity with its nerve is destroyed, and the cavity is completely filled with a solid filling material.

MUMPS: Mumps is a viral infection of the parotid glands. The infection causes inflammation in the gland, which makes opening the mouth and chewing difficult. If the disease occurs in postadolescent males, the infection may spread to the testes, which, in severe cases, may result in sterility.

BAD BREATH: Halitosis, commonly called "bad breath," results from an overabundance of bacteria in the mouth. In some cases it may be due to poor oral hygiene. In others, it may be caused by a disease process that reduces the secretion of saliva for cleansing the mouth and moving food particles to the pharynx for swallowing. As a result, some food particles remain in the mouth and decompose, which provides a growth medium for the bacteria.

HIATAL HERNIA: A hiatal hernia occurs when a portion of the stomach protrudes into the thoracic cavity through a weakened area of the diaphragm. Frequently it develops when a small region of the fundus balloons backward through the esophageal hiatus. Symptoms of this condition include pain in the upper abdomen and "heartburn" caused by the reflux of stomach acid into the esophagus, especially when the person is lying down.

VOMITING: Vomiting is the forceful ejection of the stomach contents through the mouth. It can be initiated by extreme stretching of the stomach or by the presence of irritants such as bacterial toxins, alcohol, spicy foods, and certain drugs. The vomiting action is a coordinated reflex controlled by the vomiting center of the medulla oblongata.

LACTOSE INTOLERANCE: Lactose intolerance is caused by a deficiency of the intestinal enzyme lactase, which acts on lactose, a sugar found in milk. When people with lactose intolerance drink milk, this sugar is not digested properly. Bacterial action on the undigested sugar causes gas and a bloated feeling. The undigested lactose also prevents absorption of water from the small intestine, which leads to diarrhea. The solution to this problem is to avoid milk and milk products.

APPENDICITIS: Appendicitis is an inflammation that sometimes occurs when infectious material becomes trapped inside the appendix. If the inflamed appendix ruptures and releases the infectious contents into the abdominal cavity, the peritoneum may become involved, resulting in a potentially life-threatening inflammation of the peritoneum, called *peritonitis*. Treatment for appendicitis is usually the surgical removal of the appendix.

CIRRHOSIS: Cirrhosis is a chronic liver disease that may develop as a result of chronic alcoholism or severe hepatitis. The hepatic cells of the liver are destroyed and replaced with fibrous connective tissue such that the liver no longer functions properly. One consequence of cirrhosis is the buildup of bilirubin in the blood because it is not properly incorporated into the bile and excreted. The word *cirrhosis* means "orange-colored condition," which refers to the discoloration of the liver in this disease.

GALLSTONES: Gallstones are formed in the gallbladder when cholesterol precipitates from the bile and hardens into stones because there is a lack of bile salts. Problems develop when the stones leave the gallbladder and lodge in the bile duct. This obstructs the flow of bile into the small intestine and interferes with fat absorption. Surgery may be required to remove the gallstones. ■

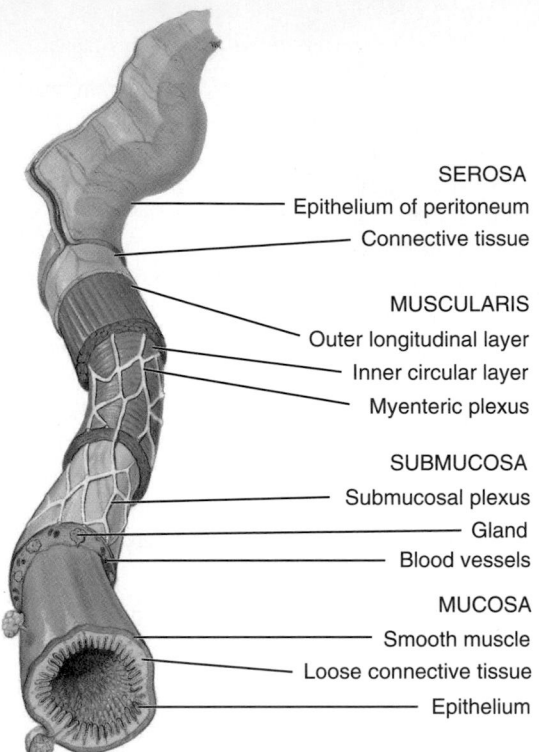

SEROSA
Epithelium of peritoneum
Connective tissue

MUSCULARIS
Outer longitudinal layer
Inner circular layer
Myenteric plexus

SUBMUCOSA
Submucosal plexus
Gland
Blood vessels

MUCOSA
Smooth muscle
Loose connective tissue
Epithelium

Figure 14-2. Basic histology of the digestive tract. (From Applegate E: *The anatomy and physiology learning system,* ed 3, St. Louis, 2006, Saunders.)

Lips
Gingiva (gums)
Hard palate
Soft palate
Uvula
Palatine tonsil
Papillae of tongue
Fauces
Tongue

Figure 14-3. Features of the oral cavity. (From Applegate E: *The anatomy and physiology learning system,* ed 3, St. Louis, 2006, Saunders.)

Mucosa The mucosa, or mucous membrane layer, is the innermost tunic of the wall. It lines the lumen of the digestive tract. The mucosa consists of epithelium, an underlying loose connective tissue layer, and a thin layer of smooth muscle. In certain regions, the mucosa develops folds that increase the surface area. Certain cells in the mucosa secrete mucus, digestive enzymes, and hormones. Ducts from other glands pass through the mucosa to the lumen of the digestive tract. In the mouth and anus, where thickness for protection against abrasion is necessary, the epithelium is stratified squamous. The stomach and intestines have a thin, simple columnar epithelial layer to enhance secretion and absorption.

Submucosa The submucosa is a thick layer of loose connective tissue that surrounds the mucosa. This layer also contains blood and lymphatic vessels, nerves, and some glands. Abundant blood vessels supply necessary nourishment to the surrounding tissues. Blood and lymph carry away absorbed nutrients that are the end products of digestion. The nerves in the submucosa form a network called the *submucosal plexus* that provides autonomic nerve impulses to the muscle layers of the digestive tract.

Muscle layer The muscular layer (labeled *muscularis* in Figure 14-2) consists of two layers of smooth muscle. The inner circular layer has fibers arranged in a circular manner around the circumference of the tube. When these muscles contract, the diameter of the tube is decreased. In the outer longitudinal layer the fibers run

lengthwise along the long axis of the tube. When these fibers contract, their length decreases and the tube shortens. A network of autonomic nerve fibers, called the *myenteric* (mye-en-TAIR-ik) *plexus,* exists between the circular and longitudinal muscle layers. The myenteric plexus, along with the submucosal plexus, is important for controlling the movements and secretions of the digestive tract. In general, parasympathetic impulses stimulate movement and secretion in the gastrointestinal tract and sympathetic impulses inhibit these activities.

Serosa or Adventitia The fourth and outermost layer in the wall of the digestive tract is called the *adventitia* if it is above the diaphragm and the *serosa* if it is below the diaphragm. The adventitia is composed of connective tissue. The serosa, which is below the diaphragm, has a layer of epithelium covering the connective tissue. It is actually the visceral peritoneum and secretes serous fluid for lubrication. The serous fluid allows the abdominal organs to move smoothly against each other without friction.

COMPONENTS OF THE DIGESTIVE TRACT
Mouth

The mouth, or **oral cavity,** is the first part of the digestive tract. It is adapted to perform the following: receive food by ingestion, break it into small particles by mastication, and mix it with saliva. The lips, cheeks, and palate form the boundaries of the mouth. The oral cavity contains the teeth and tongue and receives the secretions from the salivary glands (Figure 14-3).

Lips and Cheeks

The lips and cheeks help hold food in the mouth and keep it in place for chewing. They are also used in the formation of words for speech.

The lips are folds of skeletal muscle covered with a thin transparent epithelium. Their reddish color is due to the many blood vessels underlying the epithelium. The lips contain numerous sensory receptors that are useful for judging the temperature and texture of foods.

The cheeks form the lateral boundaries of the oral cavity. The main component of the cheeks is the **buccinator muscle** and other muscles of facial expression. On the outside, the muscles are covered by skin and subcutaneous tissue. Inside the oral cavity, the muscles are lined with a moist mucous membrane of stratified squamous epithelium. The multiple layers of epithelium provide protection against abrasion from food particles.

Palate

The **palate** is the roof of the oral cavity. It separates the oral cavity from the nasal cavity. The anterior portion, the **hard palate,** is supported by bone. The posterior portion, the **soft palate,** is skeletal muscle and connective tissue. The soft palate ends in a projection called the **uvula.** During swallowing, the soft palate and uvula move upward to direct food away from the nasal cavity and into the oropharynx.

Tongue

The largest and most movable organ in the oral cavity is the **tongue.** Most of the tongue consists of skeletal muscle. The major attachment for the tongue is the posterior region, or **root,** which is anchored to the hyoid bone. The anterior portion is relatively free but is connected to the floor of the mouth, in the midline, by a membranous fold of tissue called the **frenulum linguae.** The dorsal surface of the tongue is covered by tiny projections called **papillae.** The papillae provide friction for manipulating food in the mouth, and they also contain the taste buds (see Chapter 10). The **lingual tonsils** are embedded in the posterior surface of the tongue. The lingual tonsils provide defense against bacteria that enter the mouth.

The muscles in the tongue allow the tongue to perform the following: manipulate the food in the mouth for mastication, move the food around to mix it with saliva, shape it into a ball-like mass called a *bolus,* and direct it toward the pharynx for swallowing. It is a major sensory organ for taste and is one of the major organs used in speech.

Teeth

Two different sets of teeth develop in the mouth. The first set begins to appear at approximately 6 months of age and continues to develop until about 2½ years of age. This set is known as the **primary** or **deciduous teeth.** The primary teeth contain 10 teeth in each jaw for a total of 20 teeth. Figure 14-4A illustrates the types of primary teeth. Starting at 6 years of age, the primary teeth begin to fall out and are replaced by the **secondary** or **permanent teeth.** This set contains 16 teeth in each jaw for a total of 32 teeth. These teeth are illustrated in Figure 14-4B.

Different teeth are shaped to handle food in different ways. The **incisors** are chisel shaped and have sharp edges for biting food. **Cuspids (canines)** are cone shaped and have points for grasping and tearing food. **Bicuspids (premolars)** and **molars** have flat surfaces with rounded projections for crushing and grinding. Note the location of each type of tooth in Figure 14-4. Table 14-1 summarizes the number and types of teeth in the primary and secondary sets. They are listed in the sequence in which they erupt. There is considerable variation in the ages at which teeth erupt and when the deciduous teeth are shed. The times listed represent an average range and there may be exceptions.

Although the different types of teeth have different shapes, each tooth has three parts:
- A crown
- A neck
- A root

The **crown** is the visible portion of the tooth, covered by **enamel.** The **root** is the portion that is embedded in the sockets (alveolar processes) of the mandible and maxilla.

Second molar

First molar

Canine

Lateral incisor

Central incisor

Third molar (wisdom tooth)

Second molar

First molar

Second premolar (bicuspid)

First premolar (bicuspid)

Canine

Lateral incisor

Central incisor

A   B

Figure 14-4. Deciduous **(A)** and permanent **(B)** teeth. (From Applegate E: *The anatomy and physiology learning system,* ed 3, St. Louis, 2006, Saunders.)

Table 14-1 Ages at Which Teeth Erupt and Are Shed		
Tooth Type	Age at Eruption	Age at Shedding
Deciduous Teeth		
Central incisors	6-8 mo	5-7 yr
Lateral incisors	8-10 mo	6-8 yr
First molars	12-16 mo	9-11 yr
Canines	16-20 mo	8-11 yr
Second molars	20-30 mo	9-11 yr
Permanent Teeth		
First molars	6-7 yr	
Central incisors	6-8 yr	
Lateral incisors	7-9 yr	
Canines	9-10 yr	
First premolars	9-11 yr	
Second premolars	10-12 yr	
Second molars	11-13 yr	
Third molars	15-25 yr	

From Applegate E: *The anatomy and physiology learning system,* ed 3, St. Louis, 2006, Saunders.

Figure 14-5. Longitudinal section of a tooth. (From Applegate E: *The anatomy and physiology learning system,* ed 3, St. Louis, 2006, Saunders.)

The **neck** is a small region in which the crown and root meet and is adjacent to the **gingiva,** or **gum.**

The central core of a tooth is the **pulp cavity.** It contains the **pulp,** which consists of connective tissue, blood vessels, and nerves. In the root, the pulp cavity is called the **root canal.** Nerves and blood vessels enter the root through an **apical foramen.** The pulp cavity is surrounded by **dentin,** which forms the bulk of the tooth. Dentin is a living cellular substance similar to bone. In the root, the dentin is surrounded by a thin layer of calcified connective tissue called **cementum,** which attaches the root to the **periodontal ligaments.** The ligaments have fibers that firmly anchor the root in the alveolar process. **Enamel** surrounds the dentin in the crown of the tooth. Enamel is the hardest substance in the body. Figure 14-5 shows a longitudinal section of a tooth and illustrates the major features.

Salivary Glands

Three pairs of **salivary glands** secrete saliva into the oral cavity. The saliva is mixed with food during mastication (Figure 14-6). The **parotid glands** are the largest of the salivary glands. One gland is located on each side of the head just in front of the ear. **Submandibular glands** are located on the floor of the mouth. Small **sublingual glands** are also located in the floor of the mouth, anterior to the submandibular glands, and under the tongue.

Saliva contains water, mucus, and the enzyme **amylase.** Functions of saliva include the following:
- It has a cleansing action on the teeth.
- It moistens and lubricates food during mastication and swallowing.
- It dissolves certain molecules so that foods can be tasted.
- It begins the chemical digestion of starches.

Pharynx

The **pharynx** is a passageway that connects the nasal and oral cavities to the larynx and esophagus (see Figure 13-2). It serves both the respiratory and digestive systems as a channel for air and food. The upper region is the **nasopharynx** and is posterior to the nasal cavity. It contains the **pharyngeal tonsils,** also known as the **adenoids.** The nasopharynx functions as a passageway for air but has no function in the digestive system. The middle region posterior to the oral cavity is the **oropharynx.** This is the region food enters when it is swallowed. The opening from the oral cavity into the oropharynx is called the **fauces.** Masses of lymphoid tissue, the **palatine tonsils,** are near the fauces. The lower region of the pharynx is the **laryngopharynx.** The laryngopharynx opens into both the esophagus and the larynx.

Food is forced into the pharynx by the tongue. When food reaches the opening (fauces), sensory receptors around the fauces respond and initiate an involuntary swallowing reflex. This reflex action has several parts. The uvula is elevated to prevent food from entering the nasopharynx. The epiglottis drops downward to prevent food from entering the larynx and to direct the food into the esophagus. Peristaltic movements propel the food from the pharynx into the esophagus.

Esophagus

The **esophagus** is a collapsible muscular tube, about 25 cm long, that serves as a passageway for food between the pharynx and stomach. It lies behind the trachea and in front of the vertebral column. It passes through an opening in

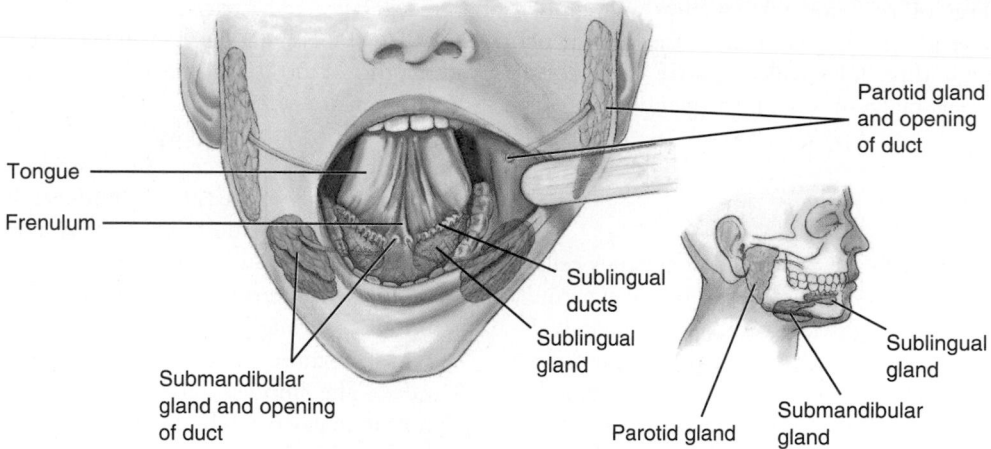

Figure 14-6. Salivary glands. (From Jarvis C: *Physical examination and health assessment,* ed 4, Philadelphia, 2004, Saunders.)

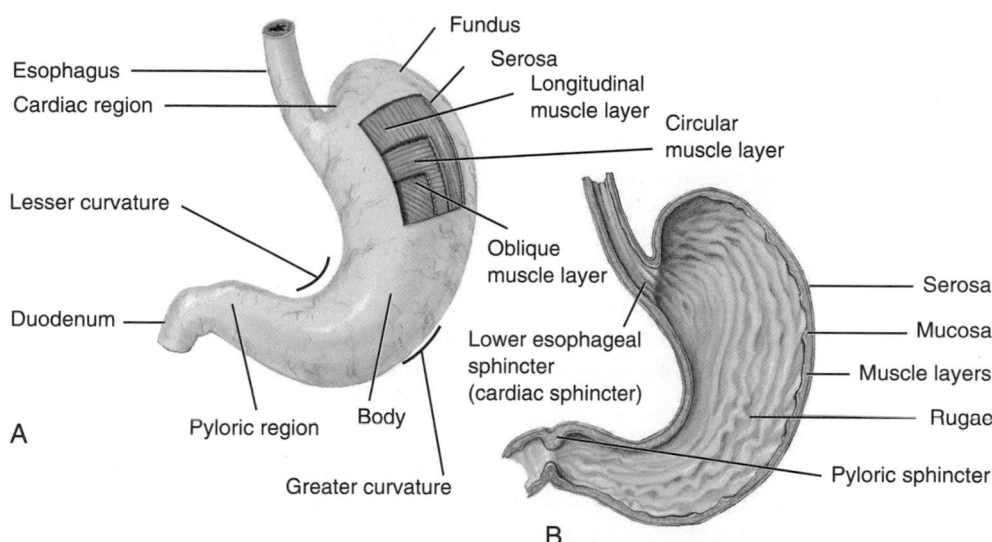

Figure 14-7. Features of the stomach. **A,** External view. **B,** Internal view. (From Applegate E: *The anatomy and physiology learning system,* ed 3, St. Louis, 2006, Saunders.)

the diaphragm and then empties into the stomach. The mucosa has glands that secrete mucus to keep the lining of the esophagus moist and well lubricated. This functions to ease the passage of food through the esophagus. The lower **esophageal sphincter** (sometimes called the **cardiac sphincter**) controls the movement of food between the esophagus and the stomach.

Stomach

The **stomach** receives food from the esophagus and is located in the upper left quadrant of the abdomen. Its capacity varies, but in the adult it averages about 1.5 L, although in some individuals it may hold up to 4 L.

Structure

The stomach is divided into the cardiac, fundic, body, and pyloric regions (Figure 14-7). The **cardiac region** is

a small region around the opening from the esophagus. The **fundus** is the most superior region. It balloons above the cardiac region to form a temporary storage area. The **body** is the main portion of the stomach. The body of the stomach curves to the right, creating two curvatures. The **lesser curvature** is concave and the **greater curvature** is convex. As the body approaches the exit from the stomach, it narrows into the **pyloric region.** A circular band of smooth muscle forms the **pyloric sphincter,** which acts as a valve between the stomach and small intestine.

The muscular layer in the wall of the stomach provides mixing movements to mix the food with enzymes and other fluids. When the stomach is empty, the mucosa and submucosa exhibit longitudinal folds, called **rugae** (ROO-jee). These folds allow the stomach to expand, and as it fills the rugae become less apparent.

Gastric Secretions

The mucosal lining of the stomach contains numerous **gastric glands.** The gastric glands open to the surface of the mucosa through tiny holes called **gastric pits.** Four different types of cells make up the gastric glands:

- Mucous cells
- Parietal cells
- Chief cells
- Endocrine cells

Exocrine gastric glands are composed of mucous cells, parietal cells, and chief cells. The secretions of the exocrine gastric glands make up the **gastric juice.** Approximately 2 to 3 L of gastric juice are produced every day. The products of the endocrine cells are secreted directly into the bloodstream and are not a part of the gastric juice.

Mucous cells produce two types of **mucus** in the stomach. One type is thick and alkaline and forms a protective coating for the stomach lining. The other type is thin and watery. It mixes with the food and creates a fluid medium for chemical reactions. **Parietal cells** secrete **hydrochloric acid** and **intrinsic factor.** The hydrochloric acid kills bacteria and provides an acidic environment for the action of enzymes in the stomach. Intrinsic factor aids in the absorption of vitamin B_{12}. **Chief cells** secrete **pepsinogen.** Pepsinogen is an inactive form of the enzyme pepsin. Hydrochloric acid converts the inactive pepsinogen into the active enzyme pepsin, which begins the chemical digestion of proteins.

The **endocrine cells** secrete the hormone **gastrin,** which functions in the regulation of gastric activity. Table 14-2 summarizes the various cells and secretions of the gastric glands.

The churning action of the muscles in the stomach wall breaks the food particles of the bolus that was swallowed into smaller sizes and mixes them with the gastric juice. This produces a semifluid mixture called **chyme** (KYME), which leaves the stomach through the pyloric sphincter and enters the small intestine.

Table 14-2 Secretions of Gastric Glands		
Cell Type	**Secretion**	**Function**
Mucous cells	Mucus (thick, alkaline)	Protects stomach lining
	Mucus (thin, watery)	Medium for chemical reactions
Parietal cells	Hydrochloric acid	Kills bacteria; activates pepsinogen
	Intrinsic factor	Absorption of vitamin B_{12}
Chief cells	Pepsinogen (active form is pepsin)	Begins digestion of proteins into polypeptides
Endocrine cells	Gastrin (a hormone)	Stimulates gastric gland secretion

From Applegate E: *The anatomy and physiology learning system,* ed 3, St. Louis, 2006, Saunders.

Regulation of Gastric Secretions

The regulation of gastric secretions is accomplished through neural and hormonal mechanisms. Gastric juice is produced all the time, but the amount varies based on certain factors. Regulation of gastric secretions may be divided into cephalic, gastric, and intestinal phases (Figure 14-8).

Cephalic phase The cephalic phase begins when an individual thinks pleasant thoughts about food or sees, smells, or tastes food. This phase anticipates food and prepares the stomach to receive it. The sensory input stimulates centers in the medulla oblongata, which sends impulses through the vagus nerve to the stomach. These impulses cause an increase in the secretion of gastric juice. The impulses also increase the secretion of the hormone gastrin, which enters the blood and circulates back to the stomach to increase the activity of the gastric glands.

Gastric phase The gastric phase accounts for more than two thirds of the gastric juice secretion. The gastric phase begins when food reaches the stomach. The presence of food in the stomach and the distention of the stomach wall stimulate reflexes that result in gastrin secretion. Gastrin, in turn, stimulates the secretion of gastric juice, which contains hydrochloric acid and pepsinogen. The hydrochloric acid acidifies the stomach contents and activates the pepsinogen into pepsin, which breaks down proteins. Stomach distention also sends signals to the brain, which responds by transmitting impulses back to the gastric glands through the vagus nerve.

Intestinal phase The passage of chyme through the pyloric sphincter into the first part (duodenum) of the small intestine triggers the intestinal phase of regulation. Distention and the presence of acid chyme in the duodenum stimulate the secretion of intestinal hormones, which in turn inhibit gastric secretions. These factors also initiate responses in the medulla oblongata that inhibit gastric secretions. These inhibitory responses help prevent excess acid chyme from entering the small intestine. When the chyme is neutralized and moves away from the duodenum, the inhibitory responses stop and gastric secretion is again stimulated. The intestinal phase regulates the entry of chyme into the small intestine.

Stomach Emptying

Peristalsis in the stomach pushes chyme toward the pyloric region. As the chyme accumulates, the pyloric sphincter relaxes and a small amount of chyme is pumped into the small intestine. The rate at which the stomach empties depends on the nature of the contents and the receptivity of the small intestine. The stomach is usually empty within 4 hours after a meal. Liquids tend to pass through the stomach quickly. Solids stay in the stomach until they are well mixed with gastric juice. Carbohydrates move through rather quickly, proteins take a little longer, and fatty foods may stay in the stomach as long as 4 to 6 hours.

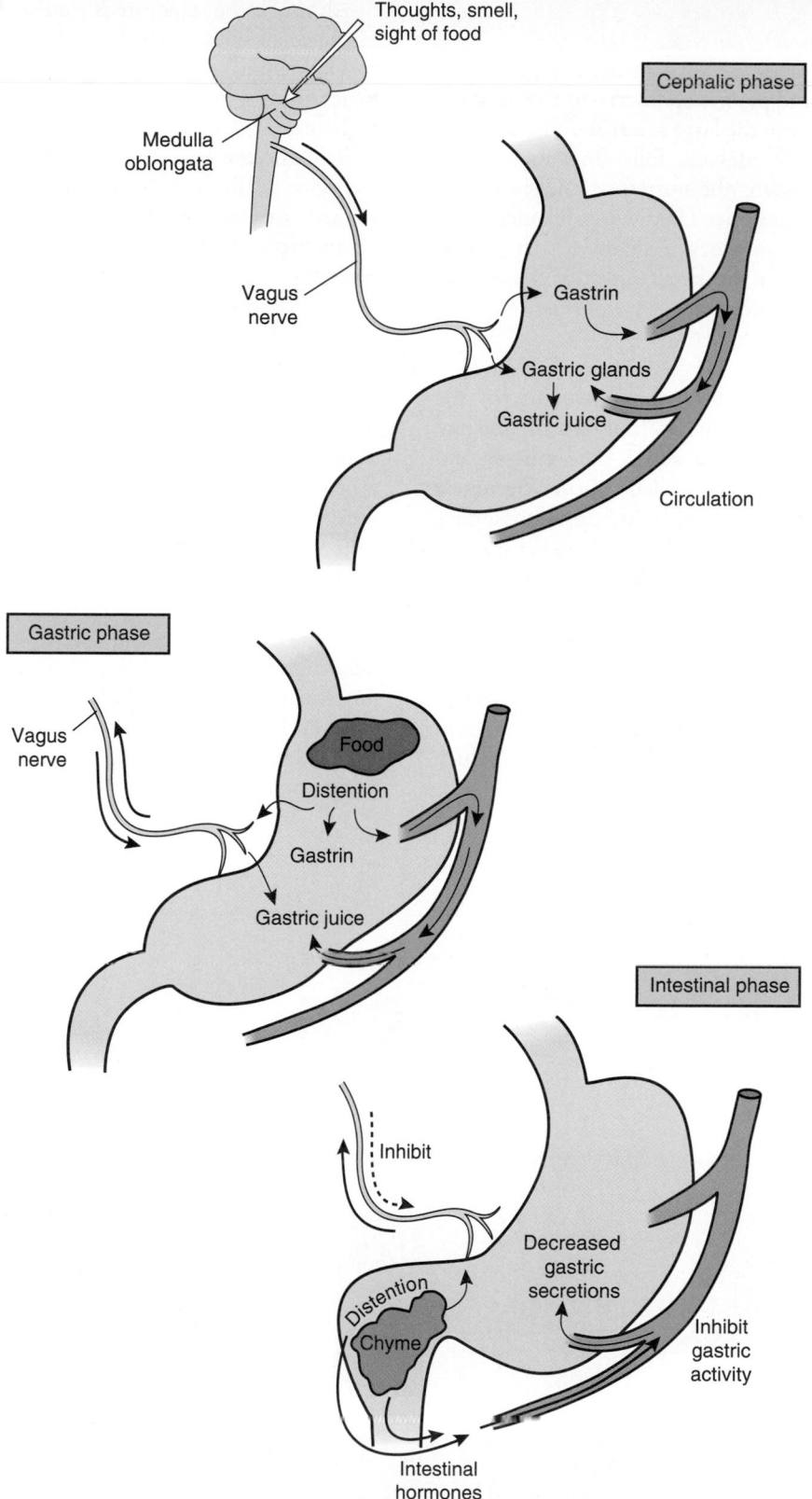

Figure 14-8. Regulation of gastric secretions. (From Applegate E: *The anatomy and physiology learning system,* ed 3, St. Louis, 2006, Saunders.)

Small Intestine

The small intestine is about 2.5 cm in diameter and 6 m long. It extends from the pyloric sphincter to the ileocecal valve, where it empties into the large intestine. The function of the small intestine includes the following: finishes the process of digestion, absorbs the nutrients, and passes the residue on to the large intestine. The liver, gallbladder, and pancreas are accessory organs of the digestive system that are closely associated with the small intestine. These are described later in this chapter.

Structure

The small intestine follows the general structure of the digestive tract in that the wall has four layers: mucosa, submucosa, smooth muscle, and serosa. The mucosa and submucosa have circular folds, called **plicae circulares** (PLY-kee sir-kyoo-LAIR-eez), which increase the surface area for absorption (Figure 14-9). Finger-like extensions of the mucosa, called **villi,** project from the circular folds, and this further increases the surface area. Each villus surrounds a blood capillary network and a lymph capillary, or **lacteal.** These function in the absorption of nutrients. **Intestinal glands** extend downward between adjacent villi. The surface epithelium on the villi has tiny hairlike cytoplasmic extensions, called **microvilli,** that form a **brush border,** which again increases surface area.

Although the structure is similar throughout, the length of the small intestine is divided into three regions:

- Duodenum
- Jejunum
- Ileum

The **duodenum** is the first part and is about 25 cm long. It begins at the pyloric sphincter and continues in a C-shaped curve to the jejunum. The duodenum receives the chyme from the stomach and secretions from the liver and pancreas.

The second portion of the small intestine is the **jejunum,** which is about 2.5 m long. This is continuous with the third portion, the **ileum,** which is about 3.5 m long. No distinct separation exists between the jejunum and ileum. They are similar in structure and are suspended from the abdominal wall by a fold of peritoneum, called **mesentery.** There is a gradual decrease in the number and length of the villi and an increase in the number of goblet cells in the mucosa from the beginning of the jejunum to the terminal portion of the ileum.

Secretions of the Small Intestine

Intestinal glands secrete large amounts of watery fluid that is neutral or slightly alkaline in pH. It keeps the chyme in a liquid form and provides both an appropriate environment for the many chemical reactions of digestion and a

Figure 14-9. Wall of the small intestine. (From Applegate E: *The anatomy and physiology learning system,* ed 3, St. Louis, 2006, Saunders.)

fluid medium for the absorption of nutrients. The fluid is readily reabsorbed by the capillaries in the microvilli.

Mucus is secreted by the wall of the small intestine. The alkaline mucus protects the intestinal wall from the acid chyme and digestive enzymes.

Digestive enzymes are located in the microvilli of the mucosal epithelial cells. These enzymes include the following: **peptidase,** which acts on segments of proteins called *peptides;* **maltase, sucrase,** and **lactase,** which act on disaccharides (double sugars); and an **intestinal lipase,** which acts on neutral fats. **Enterokinase** (en-ter-oh-KYE-nayz), although not actually a digestive enzyme, is produced by the mucosal epithelial cells. This enzyme activates a protein-splitting enzyme from the pancreas.

In addition to mucus and digestive enzymes, intestinal cells secrete at least two hormones—secretin and cholecystokinin. **Secretin** (see-KREE-tin) stimulates the pancreas to secrete a fluid that has a high bicarbonate ion concentration. This fluid helps to neutralize chyme so that the intestinal enzymes can function. **Cholecystokinin** (koh-lee-sis-toh-KYE-nin) stimulates the release of bile from the gallbladder and the secretion of digestive enzymes from the pancreas. It also inhibits gastric motility and secretions.

The most important factor for regulating secretions in the small intestine is the presence of chyme. This is largely a local reflex action in response to chemical and mechanical irritation from the chyme and in response to distention of the intestinal wall. This is a direct reflex action; thus the greater the amount of chyme, the greater the secretion.

Large Intestine

The **large intestine** is larger in diameter than the small intestine but is only about 1.5 m long (Figure 14-10). It begins at the **ileocecal** (ill-ee-oh-SEE-kul) **junction,** where the ileum enters the large intestine, and ends at the anus. The ileocecal junction has a circular band of smooth muscle fibers—the **ileocecal sphincter**—and a valve—the **ileocecal valve.**

Characteristics

The wall of the large intestine has the same types of tissue that are found in other parts of the digestive tract, but there are some distinguishing characteristics. The mucosa has large numbers of goblet cells but does not have any villi. The longitudinal muscle layer, although present, is incomplete. The longitudinal muscle is limited to three distinct bands, called **teniae coli** (TEE-nee-aye KOH-lye), that run the entire length of the colon. Contraction of the teniae coli exerts pressure on the wall and creates a series of pouches, called **haustra** (HAWS-trah), along the colon. **Epiploic** (ep-ih-PLOH-ik) **appendages,** pieces of fat-filled connective tissue, are attached to the outer surface of the colon.

Regions of the Large Intestine

The large intestine consists of the cecum, colon, rectum, and anal canal (see Figure 14-10).

Cecum   The cecum is the proximal portion of the large intestine. It is a blind pouch that extends from the ileocecal junction. The vermiform appendix is attached to the cecum. In humans, the appendix has no function in digestion but does contain some lymphatic tissue.

Colon   The colon is the longest portion of the large intestine and is divided into ascending, transverse, descending, and sigmoid portions. The ascending colon begins at the ileocecal junction and travels upward on the right side, until it reaches the liver. Here it turns to the left, becomes the transverse colon, and continues across the abdomen toward the spleen on the left side. Here the colon turns sharply downward and travels along the posterior abdominal wall as the descending colon. The descending colon makes an S-shaped curve, called the *sigmoid colon,* and then becomes the rectum. The curve between the ascending and transverse portions is the hepatic flexure. The curve between the transverse and descending portions is the splenic flexure.

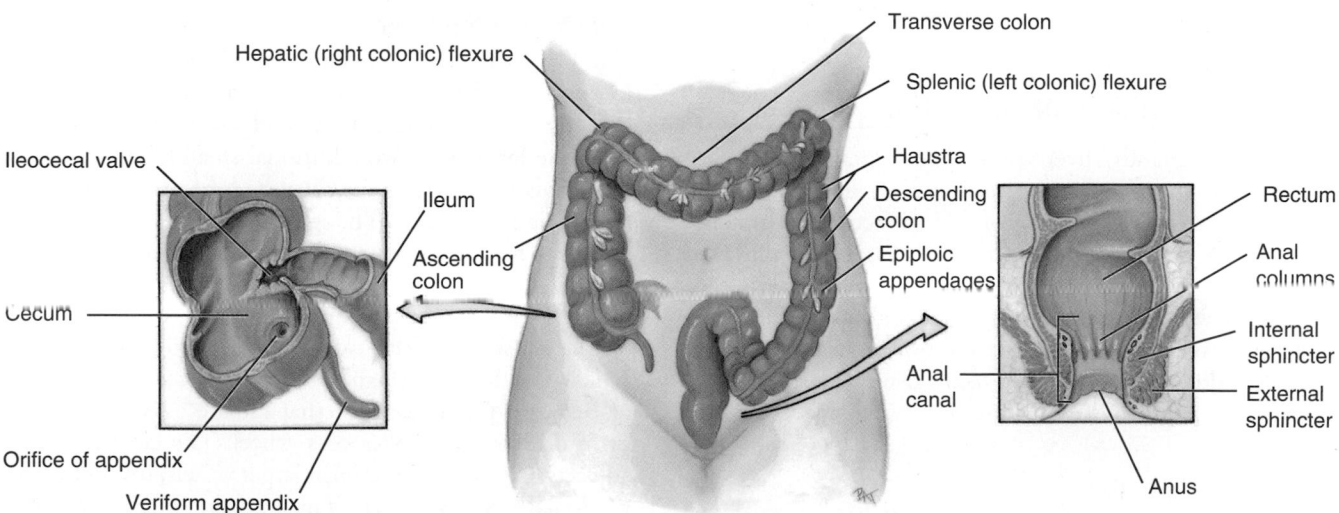

Figure 14-10. Features of the large intestine. (From Applegate E: *The anatomy and physiology learning system,* ed 3, St. Louis, 2006, Saunders.)

Rectum The rectum continues from the sigmoid colon to the anal canal and has a thick muscular layer.

Anal canal The last 2 to 3 cm of the digestive tract comprise the anal canal, which opens to the outside at the anus. The mucosa of the rectum is folded to form longitudinal anal columns. The smooth muscle layer is thick and forms the internal anal sphincter at the superior end of the anal canal. This sphincter is under involuntary control. At the inferior end of the anal canal is the external anal sphincter. This sphincter is composed of skeletal muscle and is under voluntary control.

Functions of the Large Intestine

The large intestine produces no digestive enzymes. Chemical digestion is completed in the small intestine before the chyme reaches the large intestine. There are no villi for the absorption of nutrients. This process is also accomplished in the small intestine. The primary functions of the large intestine are the absorption of fluid and electrolytes and the elimination of waste products.

The chyme that enters the large intestine contains materials that were not digested or absorbed in the small intestine—water, electrolytes, and bacteria. Some of the water and electrolytes are absorbed in the cecum and ascending colon. Although the quantity is relatively small, this absorptive function of the large intestine is important in maintaining fluid balance in the body. The residue that remains from the chyme becomes the feces.

The large intestine has the same types of mixing and peristaltic movements as occur in other parts of the digestive tract, but they are more sluggish and occur less frequently. They are more likely to occur after a meal as a result of reflexes initiated in the small intestine. As the rectum fills with feces, the defecation reflex is triggered and the waste products are eliminated.

The only secretory product in the large intestine is mucus from the numerous goblet cells. The mucus protects the intestinal wall against abrasion and irritation from the chyme. It also helps hold the particles of fecal matter together.

ACCESSORY ORGANS OF DIGESTION

The salivary glands, liver, gallbladder, and pancreas are not part of the digestive tract, but they have a role in digestive activities and are considered accessory organs. Because the salivary glands are so closely associated with the mouth and their primary function is performed in the mouth, they are considered part of the oral cavity. The liver and pancreas have functions in addition to digestion, and the gallbladder is closely related to the liver; thus these three organs are described as separate accessory organs in this section.

Liver

The liver is a large, reddish-brown organ. It is the largest gland in the body and is located in the right hypochondriac

---

Highlight on Conditions Affecting the Digestive System

Anorexia (ann-oh-REK-see-ah) Lack or loss of appetite for food

Aphagia (ah-FAY-jee-ah) Inability to swallow

Ascites (ah-SYE-teez) An accumulation of serous fluid in the peritoneal cavity

Borborygmus (bor-boh-RIG-mus) Rumbling noise caused by propulsion of gas through the intestines

Bulimia (boo-LIM-ee-ah) An emotional disorder characterized by binge eating and often terminating in self-induced vomiting

Cholecystitis (kohl-ee-sis-TYE-tis) Inflammation of the gallbladder; sometimes caused by obstruction of the cystic duct with gallstones

Cholelithiasis (kohl-ee-lith-EYE-ah-sis) Formation of gallstones

Cirrhosis (sih-ROH-sis) A chronic liver disease marked by degeneration of liver cells with eventual resistance to blood flow through the organ

Diarrhea (dye-ah-REE-ah) Frequent passage of unformed watery feces

Diverticula (dye-ver-TICK-yoo-lah) Pouchlike herniations through the muscular wall of a tubular organ, such as the colon

Dysphagia (dis-FAY-jee-ah) Difficulty in swallowing because of inflammation, paralysis, or obstruction

Emesis (EM-eh-sis) Vomiting

Hematemesis (hee-mat-EM-eh-sis) Blood in the vomit

Pyrosis (pye-ROH-sis) Regurgitation of stomach acid into the esophagus; heartburn

Volvulus (VAHL-vyoo-lus) A twisting of the bowel on itself that causes an obstruction ■

---

and epigastric regions of the abdomen, just beneath the diaphragm.

Structure of the Liver

The liver is divided into two major lobes and two minor lobes. The **falciform** (FALL-sih-form) **ligament** attaches the liver to the abdominal wall and separates the **right lobe** from the **left lobe.** Two additional small lobes are evident on the visceral surface: the **caudate lobe** and the **quadrate lobe** (Figure 14-11). The **porta** is also on the visceral surface. The porta is where the **hepatic artery** and **hepatic portal vein** enter the liver and where the **hepatic ducts** exit.

The substance of the liver is divided into functional units called **liver lobules** (Figure 14-12). A liver lobule consists of **hepatocytes** (liver cells) that radiate outward from the **central vein** like spokes of a wheel. The central veins of adjacent lobules unite to form larger vessels, until they form the **hepatic veins,** which drain into the inferior vena cava. Tiny channels, called **bile canaliculi,** are interwoven with the liver cells and carry the bile that is produced by the

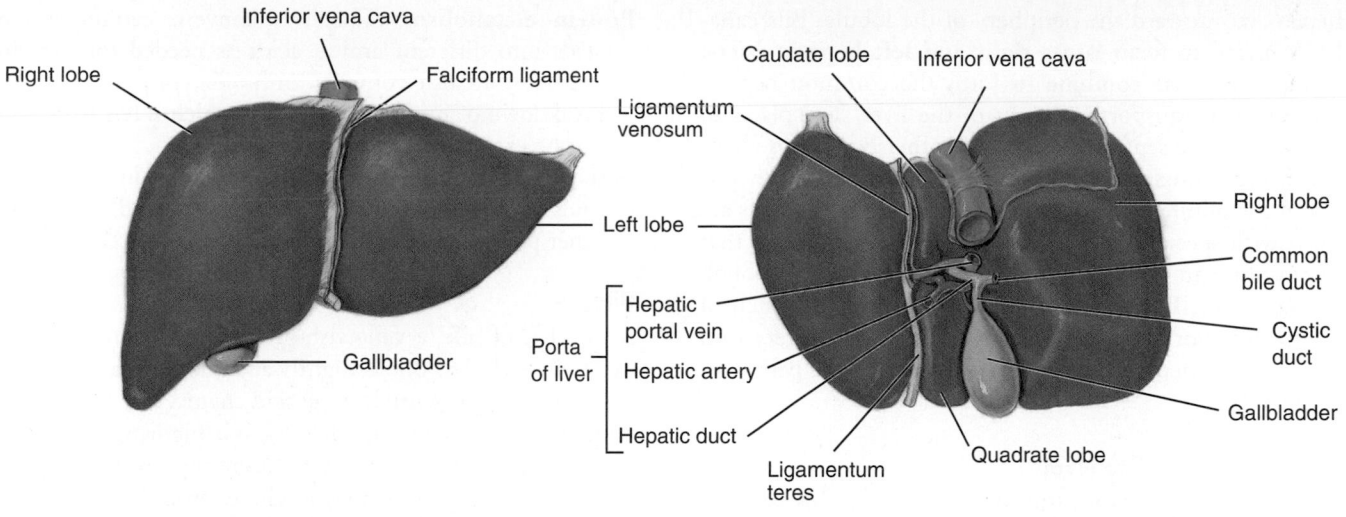

Figure 14-11. Features of the liver. (From Applegate E: *The anatomy and physiology learning system,* ed 3, St. Louis, 2006, Saunders.)

Figure 14-12. Liver lobules. (From Applegate E: *The anatomy and physiology learning system,* ed 3, St. Louis, 2006, Saunders.)

hepatocytes toward the periphery of the lobule. Bile canaliculi merge to form larger **right and left hepatic ducts.** These two ducts combine to form the common hepatic duct, which transports bile out of the liver. The plates of hepatocytes are separated from each other by venous channels, called **sinusoids,** which carry blood from the periphery of the lobule toward the central vein. The sinusoids are lined with special phagocytic cells, called *Kupffer cells,* that remove foreign particles from the blood as it flows through the sinusoids. **Portal triads,** which consist of a branch of the hepatic portal vein, a branch of the hepatic artery, and a branch of a hepatic duct, are located around the periphery of the lobule.

Blood Supply to the Liver

The liver receives blood from two sources. Freshly oxygenated blood is brought to the liver by the **common hepatic artery.** Blood that is rich in nutrients from the digestive tract is carried to the liver by the **hepatic portal vein.** Venous blood from the hepatic portal vein and arterial blood from the hepatic arteries mix together as the blood flows through the sinusoids toward the **central vein.** The central veins of the liver lobules merge to form larger **hepatic veins** that drain into the inferior vena cava.

Functions of the Liver

The liver has a wide variety of functions, many of which are vital to life. Hepatocytes (liver cells) perform most of the functions attributed to the liver, but the phagocytic Kupffer cells that line the sinusoids are responsible for cleansing the blood. Liver functions include the following:

Secretion   The liver produces and secretes bile.

Synthesis of bile salts   Bile salts are produced in the liver and facilitate fat digestion and the absorption of fats and fat-soluble vitamins.

Synthesis of plasma proteins   The liver synthesizes albumin, fibrinogen, globulins, and clotting factors.

Storage   The liver stores glucose in the form of glycogen and also stores iron and vitamins A, B_{12}, D, E, and K.

Detoxification   The liver alters the chemical composition of toxic compounds to make them less harmful. It also changes the configuration of certain drugs, such as penicillin, and excretes them in the bile to remove them from the body.

Excretion   Hormones, drugs, cholesterol, and bile pigments from the breakdown of hemoglobin are excreted in the bile.

Carbohydrate metabolism   The liver has a major role in maintaining blood glucose levels. It removes excess glucose from the blood and converts it to glycogen for storage; it breaks down glycogen into glucose when more is necessary; and it converts noncarbohydrate molecules into glucose.

Lipid metabolism   The liver functions in the breakdown of fatty acids, in the synthesis of cholesterol and phospholipids, and in the conversion of excess carbohydrates and proteins into fats.

Protein metabolism   The liver converts certain amino acids into different amino acids as needed for protein synthesis. It also converts ammonia, produced in the breakdown of proteins, into urea, which is less toxic and can be excreted in the bile.

Filtering   The phagocytic Kupffer cells that line the sinusoids remove bacteria, damaged red blood cells, and other particles from the blood.

Bile

About 1 L of bile, a yellowish-green fluid, is produced by liver cells each day. Bile is slightly alkaline, with a pH of 7.6 to 8.6, so it helps neutralize the acid chyme. The main components of bile are water, bile salts, bile pigments, and cholesterol. The bile salts are useful secretory products of the liver, but the bile pigments and cholesterol are waste products excreted in the bile and eliminated from the body.

Bile salts function in the digestion of fats. Bile salts act as **emulsifying agents** that break large fat globules into tiny fat droplets. This increases the surface area of the fat and allows for more efficient enzyme action in fat digestion. Bile salts also facilitate the absorption of fat-soluble vitamins and the end products of fat digestion.

Bile pigments are produced in the breakdown of hemoglobin from damaged red blood cells. The hemoglobin is broken down into heme, which contains iron, and globin, a protein. The liver recycles the iron from the heme and the globin. The remainder of the heme portion is converted into bile pigments, which are normally excreted in the bile. Bile pigments are responsible for the color of the urine and feces. The principal bile pigment is **bilirubin** (bill-ih-ROO-bin).

Cholesterol is a product of lipid metabolism. Bile salts act on cholesterol to make it soluble; then it is excreted in the bile.

Gallbladder

The **gallbladder** is a pear-shaped sac that is attached to the liver by the **cystic duct** (see Figure 14-11). The cystic duct joins the **hepatic duct** from the liver to form the **common bile duct.** The common bile duct empties into the duodenum. When the gallbladder contracts, bile is ejected from the gallbladder into the cystic duct.

The principal functions of the gallbladder are to store and concentrate bile. Bile is continuously produced by the liver and then travels through the hepatic duct and common bile duct to the duodenum. There is a sphincter (sphincter of Oddi) where the common bile duct enters the duodenum. If the small intestine is empty, the sphincter is closed and the bile backs up through the cystic duct into the gallbladder for concentration and storage until it is needed. When chyme with fatty contents enters the duodenum, the hormone **cholecystokinin** (koh-lee-sis-toh-KYE-nin) stimulates the gallbladder to contract and the sphincter to open. This permits bile to flow from the gallbladder, through the cystic duct and common bile duct, and then into the duodenum.

Pancreas

The **pancreas** is an elongated and flattened organ that is located along the posterior abdominal wall (Figure 14-13). One end of the pancreas, the **head,** is on the right side within the curve of the duodenum; the other end, the **tail,** is on the left side next to the spleen.

The pancreas has both endocrine and exocrine functions. The endocrine portion consists of the scattered **islets of Langerhans,** which secrete the hormones insulin and glucagon into the blood. These hormones and their functions are discussed in Chapter 11. The exocrine portion is the major part of the gland. It consists of **pancreatic acinar** (AS-ih-nar) **cells** that secrete digestive enzymes into tiny ducts interwoven between the cells. These tiny ducts merge to form the main **pancreatic duct,** which extends the full length of the pancreas and empties into the duodenum. The pancreatic duct usually joins the common bile duct to form a single point of entry into the duodenum. Both ducts are controlled by the hepatopancreatic sphincter (sphincter of Oddi).

Pancreatic juice has a high concentration of bicarbonate ions and contains digestive enzymes that act on carbohydrates, proteins, and lipids. **Pancreatic amylase** acts on starch and other complex carbohydrates to break them into simpler sugars called *disaccharides.* Protein-splitting enzymes from the pancreas include trypsin. **Trypsin** breaks the proteins into shorter chains of amino acids, called *peptides.* Like other enzymes that act on proteins, trypsin is secreted in an inactive form, **trypsinogen.** Trypsinogen is activated by enterokinase when it reaches the duodenum. The pancreas also secretes peptidase enzymes that break peptides into amino acids. **Pancreatic lipase** breaks fats into fatty acids and monoglycerides.

Pancreatic secretion of digestive juice is regulated by the nervous system and by hormones. When parasympathetic impulses from the nervous system stimulate secretion of gastric juice, some impulses go to the pancreas and stimulate the secretion of pancreatic juice. When acid chyme enters the duodenum, the intestinal mucosa produces the hormone **secretin,** which travels in the blood to the pancreas. Secretin stimulates the pancreas to produce a fluid that has a high concentration of bicarbonate ions to neutralize the acids in the duodenum. Proteins and fats in the chyme stimulate the intestinal mucosa to secrete the hormone **cholecystokinin,** which also travels in the blood to the pancreas. This hormone stimulates the pancreas to produce a pancreatic juice that is rich in digestive enzymes. These digestive enzymes travel through the pancreatic duct to the duodenum, where they perform their actions.

CHEMICAL DIGESTION

Chemical digestion breaks down large complex molecules into smaller molecules that can be absorbed by the cells of the intestinal mucosa. The reactions in chemical digestion are **hydrolysis** reactions, which use water to split molecules. These reactions proceed at a slow rate. The purpose of the various digestive enzymes is to speed up the hydrolysis reactions of chemical digestion. The enzymes do not alter the reactions; they just make them occur more rapidly. Table

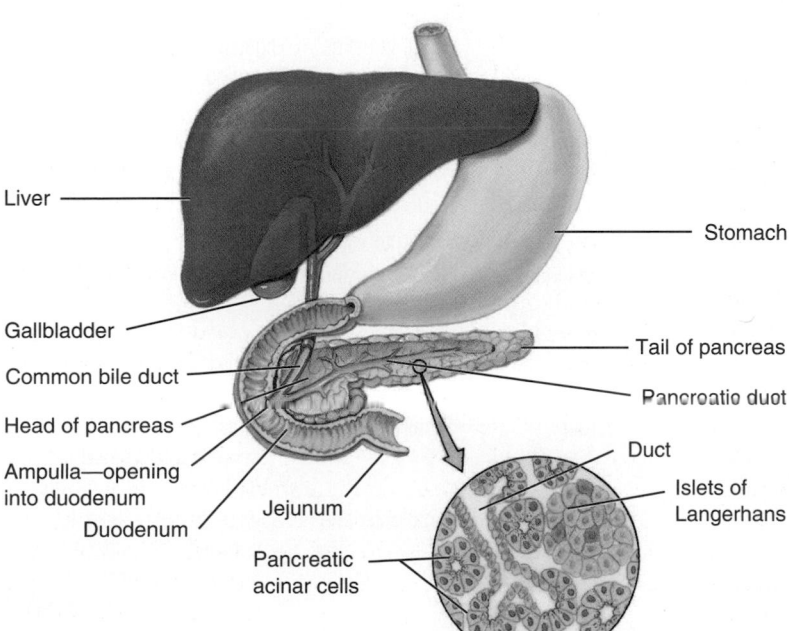

Liver
Gallbladder
Common bile duct
Head of pancreas
Ampulla—opening into duodenum
Duodenum
Jejunum
Pancreatic acinar cells
Stomach
Tail of pancreas
Pancreatic duct
Duct
Islets of Langerhans

Figure 14-13. Location and features of the pancreas. (From Applegate E: *The anatomy and physiology learning system,* ed 3, St. Louis, 2006, Saunders.)

Highlight on Anatomy and Physiology Pioneers: William Beaumont

William Beaumont was born in Lebanon, Connecticut, in 1785. His father was a farmer who had fought in the American Revolutionary War. At the age of 22, Beaumont moved to Champlain, New York, to become the town's schoolmaster and secretary for the local debating society.

A few years later, Beaumont decided to pursue a medical career. At that time in the United States, there were few medical schools and it was common practice for a potential doctor to be trained by studying textbooks and serving an apprenticeship under an established physician. Beaumont followed this path and was approved to practice surgery by the Third Medical Society of Vermont in 1812. In September of that year, he enlisted as a surgeon's mate in the U.S. Army and served during the War of 1812, often working for as long as 2 days straight, treating the wounded, amputating arms and legs, and boring holes in fractured skulls to relieve pressure on the brain.

After the war's end, Beaumont established a private medical practice in Plattsburgh, New York. Then in 1819 he closed his practice and reentered the army, this time as a post surgeon at Fort Mackinac, which was located on a small island in Lake Michigan near the Canadian border. While serving at Fort Mackinac, he treated a French-Canadian voyageur named Alexis St. Martin, who had been shot by a musket at close range. His wound was large and affected part of a lung, two ribs, and the stomach. Beaumont diligently treated the severe wounds but could not get the hole in the stomach to completely close. It had to be repeatedly bandaged to prevent food and drink from coming out. Because Alexis could no longer work as a voyageur, Beaumont hired him as the family's live-in handyman.

Beaumont then began to carefully study digestion. He tied small pieces of food with silk string and dangled them through the hole into Alexis's stomach, removing the items at 1-hour intervals to observe the process of digestion. These experiments showed that gastric juice had solvent properties and that exercise helped the production and release of gastric juice. Before Beaumont's experiments, there was a great deal of argument in the medical community as to the nature of gastric juice and the control of its secretion. He showed that it was not produced continuously, but in response to the presence or anticipation of food in the stomach. He also confirmed that the acid made by the stomach was hydrochloric acid, and additional experiments showed the inflammatory results of alcohol abuse. Despite having a hole in his stomach and being subjected to these experiments, Alexis St. Martin lived for 58 years after being wounded.

In 1833 Beaumont returned to Plattsburgh, New York, and published his observations in a book, *Experiments and Observations of the Gastric Juice and the Physiology of Digestion.* Beaumont stated, "Facts are more persuasive than arguments." It was widely recognized that he had made considerable advances in the understanding of digestion. His book was translated into many languages and was the basis for the descriptions of digestive physiology found in most medical textbooks. ∎

14-3 reviews the hormones and digestive enzymes that have been discussed in previous sections of this chapter.

Carbohydrate Digestion

Starches and other complex carbohydrates are first broken down into disaccharides, or double sugars, by the action of salivary amylase and pancreatic amylase. The disaccharides **sucrose, maltose,** and **lactose** are the result of this stage of digestion. Sucrase, maltase, and lactase—enzymes from the small intestine—act on the disaccharides to convert them to monosaccharides, or simple sugars, that can be absorbed. The digestion of maltose yields two molecules of glucose; sucrose produces one molecule of glucose and one of fructose; lactose yields 1 molecule each of glucose and galactose. The end products of complete carbohydrate digestion are the monosaccharides **glucose, fructose,** and **galactose.**

Table 14-3 Enzymes and Hormones of the Digestive System		
Secretion	**Source**	**Action**
Enzymes		
Amylase	Salivary glands	Digestion of complex carbohydrates into disaccharides
	Pancreas	
Pepsin	Stomach	Digestion of proteins into polypeptides
Sucrase	Small intestine	Digestion of disaccharides into glucose, fructose, and galactose
Maltase		
Lactase		
Peptidase	Small intestine	Digestion of peptides into amino acids
	Pancreas	
Lipase	Small intestine	Digestion of fats into monoglycerides and fatty acids
	Pancreas	
Enterokinase	Small intestine	Activates trypsinogen
Hormones		
Gastrin	Stomach	Stimulates activity of gastric glands
Secretin	Small intestine	Stimulates pancreas to secrete bicarbonate ions to neutralize acid chyme
Cholecystokinin	Small intestine	Stimulates gallbladder to contract and release bile; stimulates pancreas to secrete digestive enzymes

From Applegate E: *The anatomy and physiology learning system,* ed 3, St. Louis, 2006, Saunders.

Protein Digestion

The first digestive enzyme to act on proteins is pepsin in the stomach. Pepsin is secreted by the gastric glands in an inactive form, pepsinogen, which is activated by hydrochloric acid. When chyme reaches the duodenum, trypsin from the pancreas acts on the proteins. Trypsin is secreted in the inactive form, trypsinogen, which is activated by enterokinase in the small intestine. Pepsin and trypsin break down proteins into shorter chains of amino acids called **peptides.** Peptidase enzymes from the small intestine and pancreas break the peptide bonds to produce **amino acids.** The amino acids are the absorbable end products of protein digestion.

Lipid Digestion

The small intestine is the only place in which lipid (fat) digestion occurs because the necessary enzymes are produced by the pancreas and enter the small intestine through the pancreatic duct. Triglycerides are the most abundant dietary fats. Fat molecules tend to attract each other to form large globules, which reduces the surface area for enzyme action. After the fats enter the duodenum, they are **emulsified** by bile. Emulsification does not break any chemical bonds, but it reduces the attraction between molecules so that they disperse. Pancreatic lipases act on the surfaces of the emulsified fat droplets. Lipase action breaks two fatty acid chains from the triglyceride molecules, yielding **monoglycerides** and **free fatty acids.**

ABSORPTION

Approximately 10 L of food, beverage, and secretions enter the digestive tract every day. Usually less than 1 L enters the large intestine. The other 9 L or more are absorbed in the small intestine. Absorption takes place along the entire length of the small intestine, but most of it occurs in the jejunum. By the time the chyme reaches the distal part of the ileum and large intestine, all that remains is some water, indigestible materials, and bacteria.

⟳ TERMINOLOGY REVIEW

Absorption The passage of digestive end products from the gastrointestinal tract into the blood or lymph.

Chyme The semifluid mixture of food and gastric juice that leaves the stomach through the pyloric sphincter.

Mesentery Extensions of peritoneum that are associated with the intestine.

Peristalsis Rhythmic contractions of the intestine that move food along the digestive tract.

Plicae circulares Circular folds in the mucosa and submucosa of the small intestine.

Rugae Longitudinal folds in the mucosa of the stomach.

⌇ ON THE WEB

For Information on the Digestive System:

The Internet Pathology Laboratory for Medical Education—Gastrointestinal Pathology: library.med.utah.edu/WebPath/ORGAN.html *(Click on "Gastrointestinal Pathology")*

The Internet Pathology Laboratory for Medical Education—Hepatic Pathology: library.med.utah.edu/WebPath/ORGAN.html *(Click on "Hepatic Pathology")*

Inner Body: www.innerbody.com/html/body.html

Atlas of Gastrointestinal Endoscopy: www.endoatlas.com

The Helicobacter Foundation: www.helico.com

National Institute of Health Digestive Diseases: digestive.niddk.nih.gov

Pathophysiology of the Digestive System: arbl.cvmbs.colostate.edu/hbooks/pathphys/digestion/

National Institute of Health—Office of Dietary Supplements: dietary-supplements.info.nih.gov

American Dietetic Association: www.eatright.org

 PREPARE FOR CERTIFICATION   Visit the Evolve site at http://evolve.elsevier.com/Bonewit/today/ to actively Prepare for your Certification.

 *Check out the **Companion CD** bound with the book to access additional interactive activities.*

15

Urinary System

LEARNING OBJECTIVES

1. State six functions of the urinary system.
2. Describe the location and structural features of the kidneys.
3. Draw and label the parts of a nephron.
4. State the two parts of the juxtaglomerular apparatus.
5. Describe the location, structure, and function of the ureter, urinary bladder, and urethra.
6. List and describe the three steps in urine formation.
7. Identify the hormones that affect kidney function, and explain how they affect kidney function.
8. Explain the function of renin.

CHAPTER OUTLINE

Introduction to the Urinary System
Components of the Urinary System
  Kidneys
  Ureters
  Urinary Bladder
  Urethra

Urine Formation
  Glomerular Filtration
  Tubular Reabsorption
  Tubular Secretion
  Regulation of Urine Concentration and Volume
  Micturition

CAAHEP COMPETENCIES

Content Competencies
Anatomy and Physiology
- Anatomy and physiology of all body systems

- Common pathology/diseases
- Diagnostic/treatment modalities

ABHES COMPETENCIES

Content Competencies
Anatomy and Physiology
- Anatomy and physiology

- Study of diseases and etiology
- All body systems
- Diagnostic/treatment modalities

KEY TERMS

glomerular capsule (gloh-MER-yoo-lar KAP-sool)
juxtaglomerular apparatus (juks-tah-gloh-MER-yoo-lar
  ap-pah-RAT-us)

nephron (NEFF-rahn)
renal tubule (REE-nal TOOB-yool)

Introduction to the Urinary System

The overall function of the **urinary system** is to maintain the volume and composition of body fluids within normal limits. The urinary system accomplishes this by ridding the body of waste products that accumulate as a result of cellular metabolism. Because of this, the urinary system is sometimes referred to as the *excretory system*. Although the urinary system has a major role in excretion, other organs contribute to the excretory function. Some waste products, such as carbon dioxide and water, are excreted by the lungs through the respiratory system. The skin is another excretory organ that rids the body of wastes through the sweat glands. The liver and intestines excrete bile pigments that result from the destruction of hemoglobin. The major task of excretion, however, still belongs to the urinary system. If the urinary system fails, the other organs cannot take over and compensate adequately. In addition to ridding the body of waste products, the urinary system maintains an appropriate fluid volume. It does this by regulating the amount of water that is excreted in the urine. Other functions of the urinary system include regulating the concentrations of various electrolytes in the body fluids and maintaining normal pH of the blood.

In addition to maintaining fluid balance in the body, the urinary system controls red blood cell production by secreting the hormone **erythropoietin** (ee-rith-roh-poy-EE-tin). The urinary system also plays a role in maintaining normal blood pressure by secreting the enzyme **renin.**

COMPONENTS OF THE URINARY SYSTEM

The **urinary system** consists of the kidneys, ureters, urinary bladder, and urethra. The kidneys produce the urine and account for the other functions (described earlier) performed by the urinary system. The ureters transport the urine away from the kidneys to the urinary bladder. The urinary bladder stores the urine until it is excreted from the body. The urethra is a tubular structure that carries the urine from the urinary bladder to the outside of the body. The components of the urinary system are illustrated in Figure 15-1.

Kidneys

The **kidneys** are the primary organs of the urinary system. They are the organs that filter the blood, remove the wastes, and excrete the wastes in the urine. They are the organs that perform the functions of the urinary system. The other components of the urinary system are accessory structures to help eliminate the urine from the body.

Location

The kidneys are located between the twelfth thoracic and third lumbar vertebrae, one on each side of the vertebral column. The right kidney is usually slightly lower than the left because the liver displaces it downward. The kidneys

Highlight on the Urinary System

HANGOVER: Alcohol inhibits the secretion of antidiuretic hormone, so when people drink alcohol, they experience diuresis, or excessive urination. Experts believe that the dehydration caused by diuresis contributes to "hangover" symptoms.

KIDNEY STONES: Kidney stones develop when uric acid or calcium salts precipitate instead of remaining dissolved in the urine. The stones usually form in the renal pelvis, but they may also develop in the urinary bladder. If small enough, they may pass naturally with urine flow but usually cause a lot of discomfort. If kidney stones cause a serious obstruction, they may need to be surgically removed. A newer method of treatment called *lithotripsy* uses high-frequency sound waves to break the stone into small pieces so that it may pass naturally. The formation of stones in the urine is called **urolithiasis.**

NEPHRONS: The number of nephrons does not increase after birth. Growth of the kidney is due to enlargement of the individual nephrons. When nephrons are damaged they are not replaced.

NEPHROPTOSIS: Nephroptosis, commonly referred to as a *floating kidney,* occurs when the kidney is no longer held in place by the renal fascia and it drops out of its normal position. This may make the kidney more vulnerable to injury if it is no longer protected by the ribs. Another danger is that the ureter may become twisted and block the flow of urine. Nephroptosis occurs more frequently in horseback riders, truck drivers, and people who ride motorcycles.

POLYCYSTIC KIDNEY DISEASE: This inherited condition affects the tubular portion of the nephrons. Swelling or cysts develop along the tubules, and as the cysts enlarge they displace and damage functional kidney tissue. This eventually leads to a total loss of kidney function. When this occurs in both kidneys, a transplant is necessary.

UREMIA: When the kidneys do not function properly and fail to remove the waste products from the blood, uremia may result. Uremia is a condition in which there is a toxic level of urea in the blood.

URINARY INCONTINENCE: Urinary incontinence is the inability to control urination and to retain urine in the bladder. Temporary incontinence may result when the muscles around the bladder and urethra become weakened and lose muscle tone. This is sometimes caused by stretching of the muscles during childbirth. Because these muscles help restrict the outlet of the bladder, their weakness contributes to a leakage of urine. A cough or sneeze may increase pressure within the bladder sufficiently to force urine to escape. Permanent incontinence is usually caused by damage to the central nervous system or by extensive damage to the bladder or urethra.

URINARY TRACT INFECTION (UTI): UTIs occur more frequently in women than in men because of differences in the urethra. In females the urethral opening is in close proximity to the anal opening, which gives intestinal bacteria easier access to the urethra. The female urethra is short, which allows any infection to spread to the urinary bladder. An infection of the urethra is called *urethritis,* and one of the urinary bladders is called *cystitis.* ■

Highlight on Anatomy and Physiology Pioneers: Joseph Murray

Joseph Murray was born in Milford, Massachusetts, in 1919, the son of a district court judge and a school teacher. Both of his parents stressed the value of education, and at an early age Murray decided he wanted to be a surgeon. He attended Harvard Medical School and received his degree in 1943. Following his graduation, he joined the military and was stationed at Valley Forge General Hospital in Pennsylvania.

Many of the military patients at Valley Forge Hospital were suffering from severe burns, and sometimes the injuries were so extensive that donor sites from their own bodies were not available for skin grafts. To save lives, the necessary skin was taken from other people and used as a temporary surface cover. These foreign grafts were eventually rejected, some more slowly than others. A surgeon colleague, Colonel Brown, postulated that the closer the genetic relationship between the skin donor and the recipient, the slower the rejection. Colonel Brown told Murray about identical twins that he had cross–skin-grafted as an experiment in 1937. The grafts had permanently survived in both twins.

After the war, Murray joined a team of doctors studying kidney failure at Brigham and Women's Hospital in Boston. Much of their research centered on the possibility of transplanting a kidney from one person to another. Previous research had shown that blood vessels and organs could be transplanted within an individual without harm, but not between individuals because of the strong biologic force that caused foreign tissue to be rejected. Murray was not discouraged by this because he believed that the immunologic barrier was not present in identical twins. He experimented with dogs to develop the necessary surgical techniques for kidney transplantation and showed that a kidney transplanted from one dog to another could be induced to function.

In December 1954 Murray had an opportunity to try his techniques on human identical twins. One twin had diseased kidneys and would soon die without a new functional kidney. His twin brother had two healthy kidneys. To make sure the twins were identical, Murray performed numerous blood tests and even had the Boston police department document their fingerprint patterns. This first human kidney transplant was successful, and the twin brothers lived productive lives for several years following the transplant.

Murray then began research on drugs that would temporarily suppress the body's immune system so that transplanted organs would have a chance to survive. During the 1960s there were many breakthroughs that contributed to successful transplants. No longer did the donor and recipient have to be identical twins.

In 1990 Murray was awarded the Nobel Prize in physiology or medicine for his accomplishments. Today about 20,000 kidney transplants are performed each year, and more than 100,000 patients are presently leading better lives because of Murray's pioneering efforts. ■

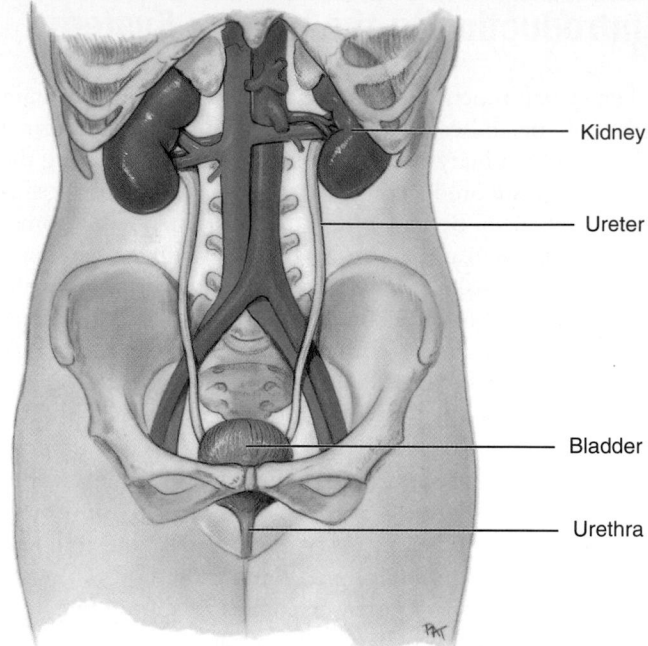

Figure 15-1. Components of the urinary system. (From Applegate E: *The anatomy and physiology learning system,* ed 3, St. Louis, 2006, Saunders.)

are partially protected by the lower ribs and lie in shallow depressions against the posterior abdominal wall. Each kidney is held in place by connective tissue, called **renal fascia.**

A thick layer of adipose tissue surrounds each kidney. This is called *perirenal fat* and it helps to protect the kidney. A tough, fibrous connective tissue encases each kidney and is called the *renal capsule.* The renal capsule provides support for the soft tissue that is inside.

Macroscopic Structure

In the adult, each kidney is approximately 3 cm thick, 6 cm wide, and 12 cm long. The kidney is bean shaped with an indentation, called the **hilum.** The hilum leads to a large cavity within the kidney called the **renal sinus.** The **ureter** and **renal vein** leave the kidney at the hilum, and the **renal artery** enters the kidney at the hilum.

The macroscopic internal structure of the kidney is illustrated in Figure 15-2. The outer, reddish region is the **renal cortex.** The renal cortex surrounds a darker reddish brown region called the **renal medulla.** The renal medulla consists of a series of **renal pyramids.** The renal pyramids appear striated because they contain straight tubular structures and blood vessels. The wide bases of the pyramids are adjacent to the cortex. The pointed ends of the pyramids, called **renal papillae,** are directed toward the center of the kidney. Portions of the renal cortex extend into the spaces between adjacent pyramids to form **renal columns.** The cortex and medulla make up the functional tissue of the kidney.

The central region of the kidney contains the **renal pelvis,** which is continuous with the ureter. The renal pelvis is a large cavity that collects the urine as it is produced. The periphery of the renal pelvis is interrupted by cuplike projections called **calyces.** A **minor calyx** surrounds the renal papillae of each pyramid and collects urine from that pyramid. Several minor calyces converge to form a **major calyx.** From the major calyces the urine flows into the renal pelvis and from there into the ureter.

Nephrons

Each kidney contains more than 1 million functional units, called **nephrons,** located in the cortex and medulla. A nephron consists of the following two parts (Figure 15-3):

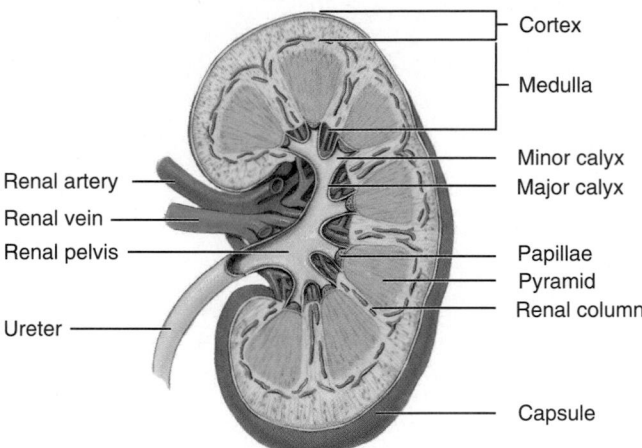

Figure 15-2. Coronal (frontal) section through the kidney. (From Applegate E: *The anatomy and physiology learning system,* ed 3, St. Louis, 2006, Saunders.)

- Renal corpuscle
- Renal tubule

The **renal corpuscle** consists of a cluster of capillaries, called the **glomerulus** (gloh-MER-yoo-lus). The glomerulus is surrounded by a double-layered epithelial cup, called the **glomerular capsule (Bowman's capsule).** Blood enters the glomerulus through an **afferent arteriole** and is filtered in the glomerulus. The blood then leaves the glomerulus through an **efferent arteriole** (Figure 15-4). As the blood is filtered, the filtrate enters the glomerular capsule, which is continuous with the renal tubule. Renal corpuscles are located in the cortex of the kidney and give it a granular appearance.

The **renal tubule,** which carries fluid away from the glomerular capsule, consists of three regions:

1. Proximal convoluted tubule
2. Nephron loop (Henle's loop)
3. Distal convoluted tubule

The first portion of the tubule is highly coiled and is known as the **proximal convoluted tubule.** Next the tubule straightens and dips into the medulla, makes a U-turn, and ascends back toward the cortex. This forms the **nephron loop** (Henle's loop). The portion of the loop that descends from the proximal convoluted tubule into the medulla is the **descending limb,** and the part that ascends back toward the cortex is the **ascending limb.** The final region of the tubule, which is also coiled and found in the cortex, is known as the **distal convoluted tubule** (see Figure 15-4).

Collecting Ducts

Urine passes from the nephrons into **collecting ducts.** The distal convoluted tubules from several nephrons join with

Figure 15-3. Nephron illustrating the regions in the cortex and the regions in the medulla. (From Applegate E: *The anatomy and physiology learning system,* ed 3, St. Louis, 2006, Saunders.)

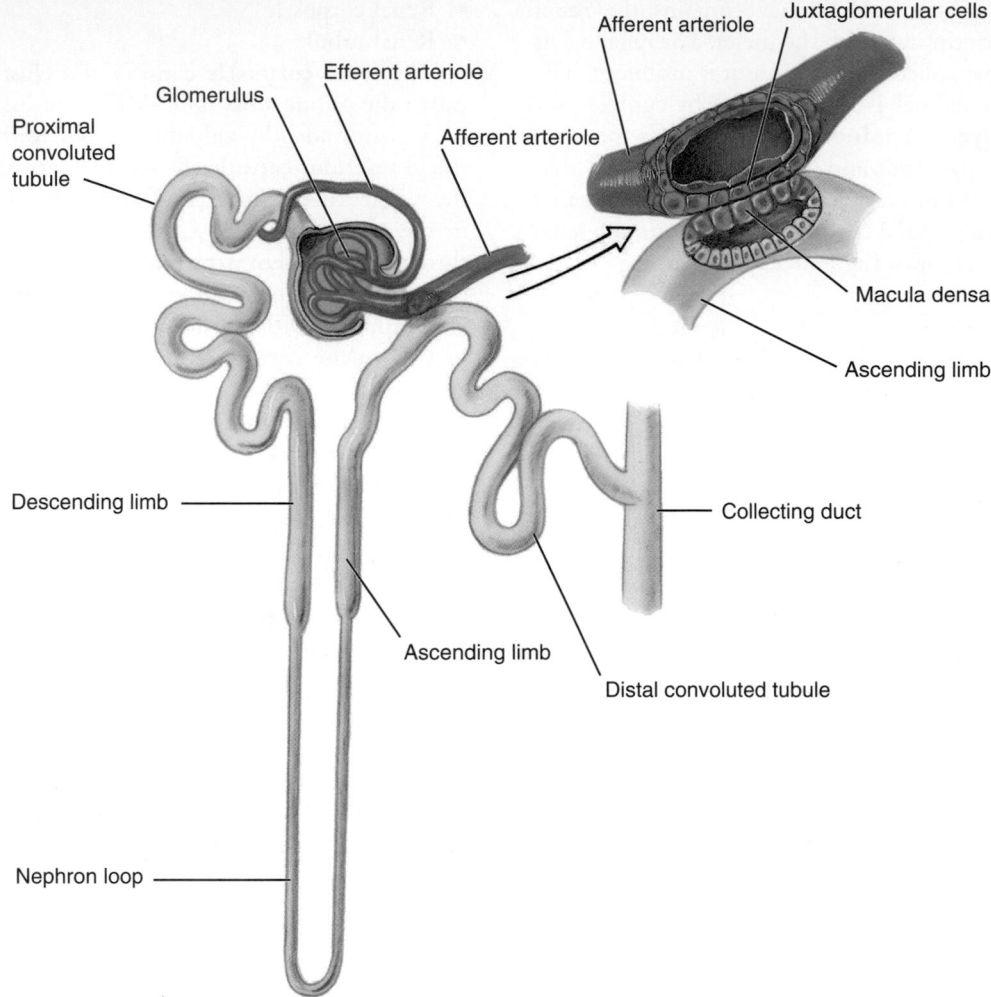

Figure 15-4. Juxtaglomerular apparatus and its relationship to the nephron. (From Applegate E: *The anatomy and physiology learning system,* ed 3, St. Louis, 2006, Saunders.)

each collecting duct. The collecting ducts extend from the base of the pyramids to the renal papillae. These straight tubules, with the nephron loops and blood vessels, give the medulla its striated appearance. Fluid flows from the collecting ducts into the minor calyces that surround the renal papillae.

Juxtaglomerular Apparatus

The ascending limb of the nephron loop, in the region where it continues into the distal convoluted tubule, comes into contact with the glomerular afferent arteriole of the same nephron (Figure 15-4). In the region of contact, the cells of the ascending limb are modified to form the **macula densa,** and those in the afferent arteriole are modified to form the **juxtaglomerular** (juks-tah-gloh-MER-you-lar) **cells.** The macula densa monitors sodium chloride concentration in the urine and also influences the juxtaglomerular cells. In the afferent arteriole, the juxtaglomerular cells produce the enzyme **renin,** which has a role in the regulation of blood pressure. Together, the macula densa and

juxtaglomerular cells make up the **juxtaglomerular apparatus.**

Blood Flow through the Kidney

Blood flows through the kidneys at an approximate rate of 1200 ml per minute. This is about one fourth of the total cardiac output. Blood is brought to the kidneys by the renal arteries, which are branches from the abdominal aorta.

Ureters

Each **ureter** is a small tube, about 25 cm long, that carries urine from the renal pelvis to the urinary bladder. It descends from the renal pelvis and enters the urinary bladder on the posterior inferior surface.

The wall of the ureter consists of three layers (Figure 15-5). The outer layer is a supporting layer of fibrous connective tissue known as the **fibrous coat.** The middle layer is known as the **muscular coat.** It consists of smooth muscle. The main function of this layer is peristalsis to propel the urine through the ureter. The inner layer is the

Figure 15-5. Ureter, urinary bladder, and urethra. **A,** Urinary tract. **B,** Cross section through the ureter. **C,** Cross section of the bladder wall. **D,** Regions of the male urethra. (From Applegate E: *The anatomy and physiology learning system,* ed 3, St. Louis, 2006, Saunders.)

mucosa. This layer secretes mucus, which coats and protects the surface of the cells.

Urinary Bladder

The **urinary bladder** is located in the pelvic cavity and is a temporary storage reservoir for urine (see Figure 15-5). The size and shape of the urinary bladder vary with the amount of urine it contains and with the pressure from surrounding organs.

The inner lining of the urinary bladder consists of a **mucous membrane.** When the bladder is empty, the mucosa has numerous folds called **rugae.** The rugae allow the bladder to expand as it fills. The second layer in the wall of the bladder is the **submucosa.** It is composed of connective tissue with elastic fibers. The next layer is the **muscularis,** which is composed of smooth muscle. The smooth muscle fibers are interwoven in all directions, and collectively these are called the **detrusor** (dee-TROO-sor) **muscle.** Contraction of this muscle expels urine from the bladder.

A triangular area, called the **trigone,** is formed by three openings in the floor of the urinary bladder. Two of the openings are from the ureters and form the base of the trigone. Small flaps of mucosa cover these openings and act as valves that allow urine to enter the bladder but prevent it from backing up from the bladder into the ureters. The third opening, at the apex of the trigone, is the opening into

the urethra. A band of the detrusor muscle encircles this opening to form the **internal urethral sphincter.**

Urethra

The final passageway for the flow of urine is the **urethra.** The urethra consists of a thin-walled tube that conveys urine from the floor of the urinary bladder to outside of the body (see Figure 15-5). The opening to the outside is known as the **external urethral orifice.**

The beginning of the urethra, where it leaves the urinary bladder, is surrounded by the **internal urethral sphincter.** This sphincter is smooth (involuntary) muscle. Another sphincter, the **external urethral sphincter,** is skeletal (voluntary) muscle and encircles the urethra where it passes through the pelvic floor. These two sphincters control the flow of urine through the urethra.

In females the urethra is short, only 3 to 4 cm (about 1.5 inches) long. The external urethral orifice opens to the outside just anterior to the opening for the vagina.

In males the urethra is much longer, about 20 cm (7 to 8 inches) in length, and transports both urine and semen. The first part of the male urethra passes through the prostate gland and is called the **prostatic urethra.** The second part is a short region that penetrates the pelvic floor and enters the penis. This short region is known as the **membranous urethra.** The third part of the male urethra is the longest region and is called the **spongy urethra.** This portion of the urethra extends the entire length of the penis, and the external urethral orifice opens to the outside at the tip of the penis.

URINE FORMATION

The work of the kidneys, performed by the nephrons, is to maintain the volume and composition of body fluids, regulate the pH of the blood, and remove waste products from the blood. The result of this work is the formation of urine. As urine is excreted to the outside of the body, it carries with it the wastes, excess water, and excess electrolytes. At the same time, the kidneys conserve other electrolytes to maintain the appropriate balance. The formation of urine involves three basic steps:

• Glomerular filtration
• Tubular reabsorption
• Tubular secretion

Glomerular Filtration

The first step in the formation of urine is **glomerular filtration.** During this process, blood plasma moves across the **filtration membrane** in the renal corpuscle and enters the glomerular capsule. The filtration membrane consists of the capillary endothelium of the glomerulus and the endothelium of the capsule. The force that moves the fluid across the membrane is **filtration pressure,** and the fluid that enters the capsule is the **filtrate.**

Blood flows through the kidneys at an average rate of 1200 ml per minute. As the blood passes through the glomeruli, about 19% of the plasma enters the glomerular capsule as filtrate. This is equivalent to forming filtrate at a rate of 125 ml per minute, or 180 L per day. This is the total value for all the nephrons in both kidneys. The filtration membrane acts as a barrier that prevents blood cells and protein molecules from entering the capsule; therefore they are absent from the filtrate.

Tubular Reabsorption

If the volume and composition of the filtrate in the glomerular capsule are compared with the volume and composition of urine, it is obvious that changes occur after filtration. First of all, about 180 L (45 gallons) of filtrate are formed in a 24-hour period. This volume is reduced to 1 to 2 L of urine. Glucose is present in the filtrate but normally absent in the urine. Urea and uric acid are present in higher concentrations in the urine than in the filtrate.

Tubular reabsorption is the first process that changes the volume and composition of the filtrate. Tubular reabsorption is the movement of substances from the filtrate in the kidney tubules into the blood. Only about 1% of the filtrate remains in the tubules and becomes urine. In general, water and other substances that are useful to the body are reabsorbed. Wastes remain in the filtrate and are excreted in the urine.

About 65% of the reabsorption takes place in the proximal convoluted tubule, 15% in the nephron loop (loop of Henle), and 19% in the distal convoluted tubule and collecting duct. This leaves about 1% of the filtrate to be excreted as urine. Figure 15-6 illustrates tubular reabsorption and the specific substances that are reabsorbed into the blood from each part of the tubule of the nephron.

Tubular Secretion

The final process in the formation of urine is the transport of molecules and ions into the filtrate. This is called **tubular secretion.** Most of these substances are waste products of cellular metabolism that become toxic if allowed to accumulate in the body. Tubular secretion is the method by which some drugs, such as penicillin, are removed from the body. The tubular secretion of hydrogen ions plays an important role in regulating the pH of the blood. Other molecules and ions that may enter the filtrate by tubular secretion include potassium ions, creatinine, and histamine.

The final product, urine, produced by the nephrons consists of the substances that are filtered, minus the substances that are reabsorbed in the tubules, plus the substances that are added by tubular secretion.

Regulation of Urine Concentration and Volume

The concentration and volume of urine depend on conditions in the internal environment of the body. Cells in the hypothalamus are sensitive to changes in the composition of the blood and initiate appropriate responses that affect the kidneys. If the concentration of solutes in the blood increases above normal, the kidneys excrete a small volume of concentrated urine. This conserves water in the body and gets rid of solutes to restore the blood to normal. If the blood solute concentration decreases below normal, the kidneys conserve solutes and get rid of water by producing large quantities of dilute urine. Urine production plays an important role in maintaining homeostasis of blood concentration and volume. By regulating blood volume, the kidneys also play a role in regulating blood pressure because volume is directly related to pressure.

Three hormones—**aldosterone, antidiuretic hormone, and atrial natriuretic hormone**—influence urine concentration and volume. Aldosterone, secreted by cells of the adrenal cortex, acts on the kidney tubules to increase the reabsorption of sodium. When sodium is reabsorbed, water follows by osmosis. This reduces urine output.

Antidiuretic hormone (ADH) is produced by cells in the hypothalamus and is released from the posterior lobe of the pituitary gland. ADH makes the distal convoluted tubule and collecting duct more permeable to water. When ADH is present, more water is reabsorbed, which reduces the volume of urine and makes it more concentrated. Water is conserved in the body. In the absence of ADH, the tubules are less permeable to water and there is less reabsorption. This results in large quantities of dilute urine, and water is lost from the body.

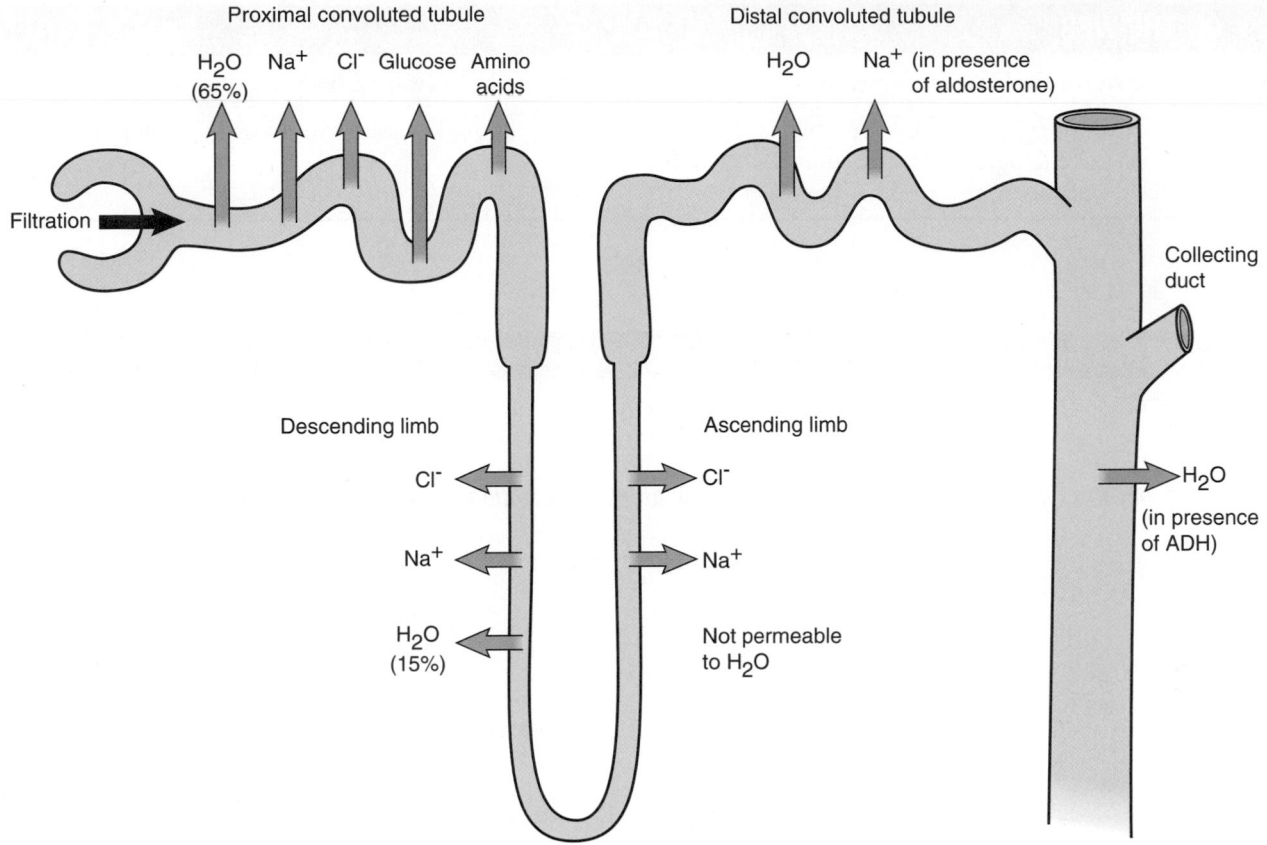

Figure 15-6. Tubular reabsorption. *ADH,* Antidiuretic hormone. (From Applegate E: *The anatomy and physiology learning system,* ed 3, St. Louis, 2006, Saunders.)

Special cells in the heart produce a hormone called *atrial natriuretic hormone,* or *atriopeptin,* which is secreted when the atrial cells are stretched. This hormone promotes the excretion of sodium and water by acting directly on the kidney tubules and by inhibiting the secretion of ADH, renin, and aldosterone. The result of atrial natriuretic hormone is a decrease in both blood volume and blood pressure.

Renin is an enzyme that is produced by the juxtaglomerular cells in the kidney in response to low blood pressure or decreased blood sodium concentration. Renin promotes the production of **angiotensin II** in the blood. Angiotensin II is a powerful vasoconstrictor, which increases the blood pressure. Angiotensin II also stimulates the adrenal gland to secrete aldosterone, which acts on the kidney tubules to conserve sodium and water. This increases blood volume and, consequently, increases blood pressure.

Micturition

Micturition (mik-too-RISH-un), commonly called *urination* or *voiding,* is the act of expelling urine from the bladder. The bladder can hold up to a liter of urine, but normally when it contains 200 to 400 ml, stretch receptors in the bladder wall trigger impulses that initiate the **micturition reflex.** This is an automatic and involuntary response that is coordinated in the spinal cord. Impulses are transmitted along parasympathetic nerves to the detrusor muscle. Even though the micturition reflex is involuntary, it can be inhibited or stimulated by higher brain centers.

⟲ TERMINOLOGY REVIEW

Glomerular capsule Double-layered epithelial cup that surrounds the glomerulus in a nephron; also called *Bowman's capsule.*

Juxtaglomerular apparatus Complex of modified cells in the afferent arteriole and the ascending limb/distal tubule in the kidney; helps regulate blood pressure by secreting renin; consists of the macula densa and juxtaglomerular cells.

Nephron Functional unit of the kidney consisting of a renal corpuscle and a renal tubule.

Renal tubule Tubular portion of the nephron that carries the filtrate away from the glomerular capsule; site where tubular reabsorption and secretion occur.

ON THE WEB

For Information on the Urinary System:

The Internet Pathology Laboratory for Medical Education—Renal Pathology: library.med.utah.edu/Web Path/ORGAN.html *(Click on "Renal Pathology")*

Inner Body: www.innerbody.com/html/body.html

Urinary Incontinence: www.seekwellness.com/incontinence

PREPARE FOR CERTIFICATION

Visit the Evolve site at http://evolve.elsevier.com/Bonewit/today/ to actively Prepare for your Certification.

*Check out the **Companion CD** bound with the book to access additional interactive activities.*

16

Reproductive System

LEARNING OBJECTIVES

Male Reproductive System
1. Distinguish between primary and secondary reproductive organs.
2. Describe the location and structure of each component of the male reproductive system.
3. Explain the process by which spermatids become mature sperm.
4. Trace the pathway of sperm from the testes to the outside of the body.
5. Outline the physiologic events in the male sexual response.
6. Describe the roles of gonadotropin-releasing hormone (GnRH), follicle-stimulating hormone (FSH), luteinizing hormone (LH), and testosterone in male reproductive functions.

Female Reproductive System
1. Identify each component of the female reproductive system, including the mammary glands.
2. Describe oogenesis.
3. Describe the development of ovarian follicles.
4. Outline the physiologic events in the female sexual response.
5. Describe the roles of GnRH, FSH, LH, estrogen, and progesterone in female reproductive functions.
6. Describe what happens in each phase of the ovarian and uterine cycles, when each phase occurs, and how the cycles interact.

CHAPTER OUTLINE

Introduction to the Reproductive System
Male Reproductive System
  Testes
  Duct System
  Accessory Glands
  Penis
  Male Sexual Response
  Hormonal Control

Female Reproductive System
  Ovaries
  Genital Tract
  External Genitalia
  Female Sexual Response
  Hormonal Control
  Mammary Glands

CAAHEP COMPETENCIES

Content Competencies
Anatomy and Physiology
• Anatomy and physiology of all body systems

• Common pathology/diseases
• Diagnostic/treatment modalities

ABHES COMPETENCIES

Content Competencies
Anatomy and Physiology
• Anatomy and physiology

• Study of diseases and etiology
• All body systems
• Diagnostic/treatment modalities

gametes (GAM-eets)
gonads (GO-nads)
oogenesis (oh-oh-JEN-eh-sis)
ovarian cycle (oh-VAIR-ee-an SYE-kul)

ovarian follicle (oh-VAIR-ee-an FAHL-ih-kul)
spermatogenesis (spur-mat-oh-JEN-eh-sis)
spermiogenesis (spur-mee-oh-JEN-eh-sis)
uterine cycle (YOO-ter-in SYE-kul)

Introduction to the Reproductive System

The major function of the reproductive system is to produce offspring. The reproductive system is responsible for the following four functions:

- To produce egg and sperm cells
- To transport and sustain these cells
- To nurture the developing offspring
- To produce hormones

These functions are divided between the **primary reproductive organs** and the **secondary** (or **accessory**) **reproductive organs.** The primary reproductive organs are called **gonads.** They include the ovaries and testes. These gonads are responsible for producing the egg and sperm cells known as **gametes.** The gonads are also responsible for producing hormones. These hormones function in the maturation of the reproductive system and the development of sexual characteristics. The hormones also play important roles in regulating the normal physiology of the reproductive system. All other organs, ducts, and glands in the reproductive system are considered secondary, or accessory, reproductive organs. These structures transport and sustain the gametes and nurture the developing offspring.

MALE REPRODUCTIVE SYSTEM

The male reproductive system produces, sustains, and transports sperm; introduces the sperm into the female vagina; and produces hormones. Figure 16-1 illustrates the organs of the male reproductive system.

Testes

The **testes** (or **testicles**) are the male gonads. The testes begin their development high in the abdominal cavity, near the kidneys. During the last 2 months before birth, or shortly after birth, the testes descend into the **scrotum.** The scrotum is a pouch that extends below the abdomen and behind the penis. The location of the testes outside the abdominal cavity may seem to make them vulnerable to injury. However, this location provides a temperature about 3°C below normal body temperature. This lower temperature is necessary for the production of viable sperm. The scrotum consists of skin and subcutaneous tissue. A vertical septum, or partition, of subcutaneous tissue in the center of the scrotum divides it into two parts, each containing one testis. Smooth muscle fibers, called the **dartos muscle,** are located in the subcutaneous tissue. The dartos muscle contracts to give the scrotum its wrinkled appearance. When this muscle is relaxed, the scrotum is smooth. Another muscle known as the **cremaster muscle** is located in the spermatic cord. The cremaster controls the position of the scrotum and testes. When it is cold or a man is sexually aroused, this muscle contracts to pull the testes closer to the body for warmth.

Structure

Each testis is an oval structure about 5 cm long and 3 cm in diameter (Figure 16-2). A tough, white fibrous connective tissue capsule, known as the **tunica albuginea** (TOO-nik-ah al-byoo-JIN-ee-ah), surrounds each testis. The tunica albuginea extends inward to form **septa** that partition the testis into **lobules.** Each testis contains about 250 lobules. Each lobule contains one to four highly coiled **seminiferous** (seh-mye-NIFF-er-us) **tubules** that converge to form a single **straight tubule.** The straight tubule leads into the **rete testis** (REE-tee TEST-is), which is a tubular network on one side of the testis. Short efferent ducts exit the testes. **Interstitial cells** (cells of Leydig) are located between the seminiferous tubules within a lobule. Interstitial cells produce male sex hormones.

Spermatogenesis

Sperm are produced within the seminiferous tubules. The process of sperm formation is known as **spermatogenesis** (spur-mat-oh-JEN-eh-sis). The seminiferous tubules are packed with cells in various stages of spermatogenesis (Figure 16-3). Interspersed with these cells are large cells that extend from the periphery of the tubule to the lumen. These large cells are the **supporting cells** (Sertoli cells), which support and nourish the other cells.

Early in embryonic development, **primordial germ cells** enter the testes and differentiate into **spermatogonia** (spur-mat-oh-GOH-nee-ah). Spermatogonia are immature cells that remain dormant until puberty. Spermatogonia are located around the periphery of the seminiferous tubules. They are diploid cells, meaning that they contain 46 chromosomes (23 pairs). At puberty, hormones stimulate these cells to begin dividing by mitosis. Some of the daughter cells produced by mitosis remain at the periphery as spermatogonia. Others are pushed toward the lumen and undergo some changes to become **primary spermatocytes.**

Highlight on the Reproductive System

INGUINAL HERNIA: The inguinal canal is a weak area in the abdominal wall that may rip open, resulting in an inguinal hernia. A portion of the intestine may pass through the opening into the scrotum. This is painful and potentially dangerous if the blood supply to the intestine is constricted. This condition is more common in men than in women. Inguinal hernias are frequently repaired by surgery.

UNDESCENDED TESTICLES: The condition in which the testes do not descend into the scrotum is called **cryptorchidism.** *Crypt* means "hidden" and *orchid* refers to the testis, so the term means "hidden testis." Cryptorchidism results in sterility if it is not corrected before puberty because the cooler temperature of the scrotum is necessary for sperm production.

VASECTOMY: A vasectomy is a surgical procedure, usually accomplished through a tiny incision in the scrotum, that severs the vas deferens. A bilateral vasectomy results in sterility because it interrupts the pathway of the sperm to the outside of the body.

ENLARGED PROSTATE GLAND: Benign prostatic hyperplasia is a common condition in older men. In this condition, the prostate enlarges and compresses the urethra, making urination difficult. This situation results in urine retention in the bladder, which makes the individual more susceptible to urinary tract infections.

PROSTATE CANCER: Cancer of the prostate is a common cancer in men. It usually starts in one of the secretory glands, and as it continues, it produces a lump on the surface of the prostate. In many cases by the time the lump can be palpated through the wall of the rectum, the cancer has metastasized to other areas of the body. It is hoped that using blood screening techniques (e.g., prostate-specific antigen [PSA]) in addition to rectal palpation will result in earlier detection of the tumor so that treatment can begin before metastasis occurs.

CIRCUMCISION: Circumcision is the surgical removal of the prepuce of the penis. Sometimes this is done to correct **phimosis,** a condition in which the prepuce is too tight and obstructs urine flow. In certain cultures, circumcision is performed as a religious rite or an ethnic custom. For others, it is a matter of family preference. The medical benefits of circumcision are a subject of debate in the medical community. Some believe it is practical for hygienic reasons. Evidence indicates that circumcision may reduce the risk of penile cancer.

IMPOTENCE: Impotence is the inability to achieve an erection. Psychological stresses are often blamed for impotence, but other causes can lead to the difficulty. Impotence may result from an abnormality of the erectile tissue or failure of the parasympathetic reflexes that produce an erection. Drugs and alcohol may cause temporary impotence because they can interfere with the nerve and blood vessel actions that are necessary for an erection.

OVARIAN CANCER: Carcinomas of the ovary account for more deaths than those of cervical and uterine cancers together. Because there are no screening tests and few symptoms in the early stages, ovarian carcinomas are usually in an advanced stage when they are discovered. Surgery, radiation therapy, and chemotherapy are used as therapeutic measures.

TUBAL LIGATION: Tubal ligation is a surgical procedure in which the uterine tubes are burned or severed and tied off. This is a permanent method of birth control because sperm are unable to reach the egg for fertilization. The technique involves making a small incision in the abdomen and inserting a small tube through which the ligation instruments can be introduced.

ECTOPIC PREGNANCY: An ectopic pregnancy occurs when a fertilized egg implants in some site other than the uterus. Ectopic pregnancies may occur in the uterine tubes. Because the tubes are not equipped to sustain and nourish the developing embryo, miscarriages often occur. The uterine tubes are unable to expand like the uterus and may rupture with subsequent hemorrhage. Surgery may be indicated to remove the implant and to preserve the uterine tube before rupture occurs.

MITTELSCHMERZ: Mittelschmerz is a distress that some women experience during ovulation. Typical symptoms include one sided lower abdominal pain, which may switch sides from one month to another, at or around the time of ovulation. The pain is usually described as sharp or cramping and lasts from 24 to 48 hours. There is no known prevention, and treatment consists of analgesics.

FIBROCYSTIC DISEASE: Fibrocystic disease is a common benign condition of the breast. Small sacs of tissue and fluid develop in the breast tissue, and the patient notices lumps in the breast often associated with premenstrual tenderness. Mammography and surgical biopsy may be indicated to differentiate between fibrocystic disease and carcinoma of the breast. ■

Because they are produced by mitosis, primary spermatocytes are diploid and have 46 chromosomes.

Each primary spermatocyte goes through the first meiotic division (meiosis I) to produce two **secondary spermatocytes.** Each secondary spermatocyte contains 23 chromosomes (haploid). Just before this division, the genetic material is replicated so that each chromosome consists of two strands, called **chromatids,** that are joined by a centromere. During meiosis I, one chromosome (consisting of two chromatids) goes to each secondary spermatocyte. In the second meiotic division (meiosis II), each secondary spermatocyte divides to produce two **spermatids.** There is no replication of genetic material in this division, but the centromere divides so that a single-stranded chromatid goes to each cell.

As a result of the two meiotic divisions, each primary spermatocyte produces four spermatids (Figure 16-4). During spermatogenesis there are two cellular divisions but

Figure 16-1. Structures in the male reproductive system. (From Applegate E: *The anatomy and physiology learning system,* ed 3, St. Louis, 2006, Saunders.)

Bladder
Pubic symphysis
Ductus deferens
Prostate
Spongy urethra
Penis

Ureter
Seminal vesicle
Rectum
Prostatic urethra
Ejaculatory duct
Membranous urethra
Bulbourethral gland
Epididymis
Testis
Scrotum

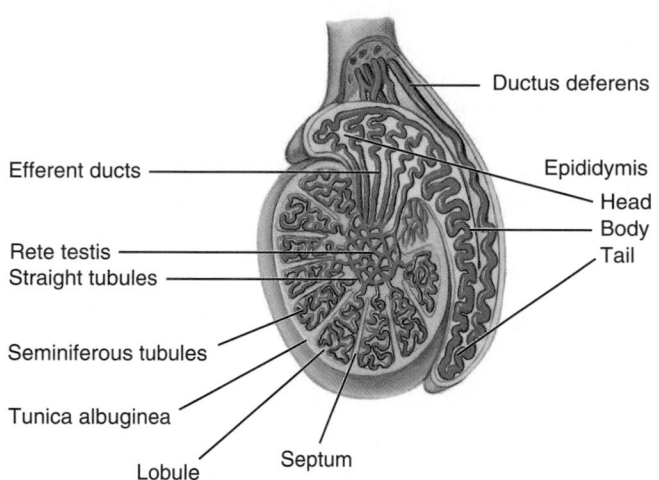

Ductus deferens
Efferent ducts
Epididymis
Head
Body
Tail
Rete testis
Straight tubules
Seminiferous tubules
Tunica albuginea
Septum
Lobule

Figure 16-2. Sagittal section of a testis. (From Applegate E: *The anatomy and physiology learning system,* ed 3, St. Louis, 2006, Saunders.)

only one replication of DNA, so each spermatid has 23 chromosomes (haploid), one from each pair in the original primary spermatocyte. Each successive stage in spermatogenesis is pushed toward the center of the tubule. This results in the more immature cells at the periphery and the more differentiated cells are nearer the center (see Figure 16-3).

Spermatogenesis (and oogenesis in the female) differs from mitosis (review Chapter 5) because the resulting cells have only half the number of chromosomes as the original cell. When the sperm cell nucleus unites with an egg cell nucleus, the full number of chromosomes is restored. If sperm and egg cells were produced by mitosis, then each successive generation would have twice the number of chromosomes as the preceding one.

The final step in the development of sperm is called **spermiogenesis** (spur-mee-oh-JEN-eh-sis). In this process,

the spermatids formed from spermatogenesis become mature spermatozoa, or sperm. The mature sperm cell has a **head, midpiece,** and **tail** (see Figure 16-3). The head contains the 23 chromosomes surrounded by a nuclear membrane. The tip of the head is covered by an **acrosome** (AK-roh-sohm). The acrosome contains enzymes that help the sperm penetrate the female gamete. The midpiece contains mitochondria that provide adenosine triphosphate (ATP). The tail, also called the *locomotor region,* is a typical flagellum for locomotion. The sperm are released into the lumen of the seminiferous tubule, where they leave the testes and enter the epididymis. In the epididymis the sperm undergo final maturation and become capable of fertilizing a female gamete.

Sperm production begins at puberty and continues throughout the life of a male. The entire process, beginning with a primary spermatocyte, takes about 74 days. After ejaculation, the sperm can live for about 48 hours in the female reproductive tract.

Duct System

Sperm cells pass through a series of ducts to reach the outside of the body. After they leave the testes, the sperm pass through the epididymis, ductus deferens, ejaculatory duct, and urethra.

Epididymis

Sperm leave the testes through a series of efferent ducts that enter the **epididymis** (ep-ih-DID-ih-mis) (see Figure 16-2). The epididymis is a long tube that is tightly coiled to form a comma-shaped organ. When the sperm leave the testes, they are immature and incapable of fertilizing ova. They complete their maturation process and become fertile as they move through the epididymis. Mature sperm are stored in the lower portion of the epididymis.

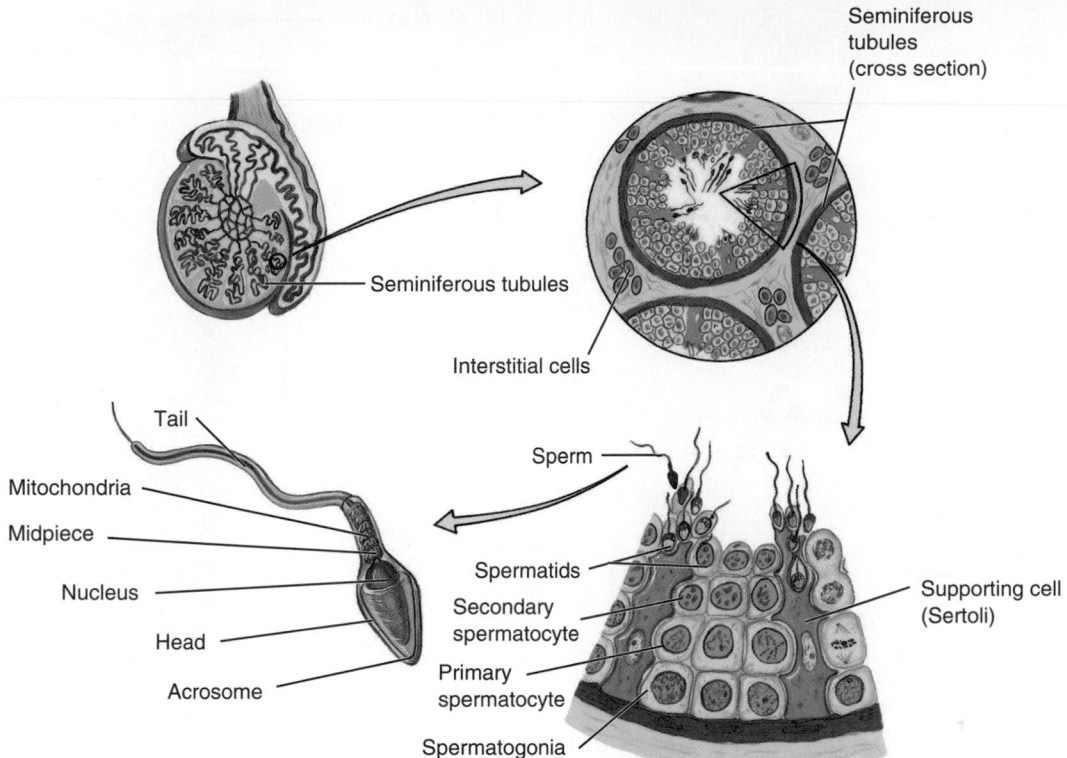

Figure 16-3. Cross section of a seminiferous tubule showing the different cell types. (From Applegate E: *The anatomy and physiology learning system,* ed 3, St. Louis, 2006, Saunders.)

Ductus Deferens

The **ductus deferens** (also called **vas deferens**) is a tube that is continuous with the epididymis (see Figure 16-2). The ductus deferens enters the abdominopelvic cavity and passes along the lateral pelvic wall. It crosses over the ureter and posterior portion of the urinary bladder and then descends along the posterior wall of the bladder toward the prostate gland (see Figure 16-1). Sperm are stored in the ductus deferens, near the epididymis, and peristaltic movements propel the sperm through the tube.

The proximal portion of the ductus deferens is a component of the **spermatic cord,** which contains vascular and neural structures that supply the testes. The spermatic cord contains the ductus deferens, testicular artery and veins, lymph vessels, testicular nerve, cremaster muscle (which elevates the testes for warmth and at times of sexual stimulation), and a connective tissue covering.

Ejaculatory Duct

Each ductus deferens joins the duct from the adjacent seminal vesicle to form a short **ejaculatory** (ee-JAK-yoo-lah-to-ree) **duct** (see Figure 16-1). Each ejaculatory duct passes through the prostate gland and empties into the urethra.

Urethra

The **urethra** (yoo-REE-thrah) extends from the urinary bladder to the external urethral orifice at the tip of the penis.

It is a passageway for sperm and fluids from the reproductive system and for urine from the urinary system. While reproductive fluids are passing through the urethra, sphincters contract tightly to keep urine from entering the urethra.

The male urethra is divided into three regions (see Figure 16-1). The **prostatic urethra** is the portion that passes through the prostate gland. It receives the ejaculatory duct and numerous ducts from the prostate gland. The next portion, the **membranous urethra,** is a short region that passes through the pelvic floor. The longest portion is the **penile urethra** (also called *spongy urethra*), which extends the length of the penis and opens to the outside at the external urethral orifice. The ducts from the bulbourethral glands open into the penile urethra.

Accessory Glands

The accessory glands of the male reproductive system include the seminal vesicles, prostate gland, and bulbourethral glands. These glands secrete fluids that enter the urethra.

Seminal Vesicles

The paired **seminal vesicles** are saclike glands (see Figure 16-1). Each gland has a short duct that joins with the ductus deferens to form an ejaculatory duct. The ejaculatory ducts empty into the urethra. The seminal vesicles secrete a fluid that is viscous and contains fructose. The fructose provides an energy source for the spermatozoa.

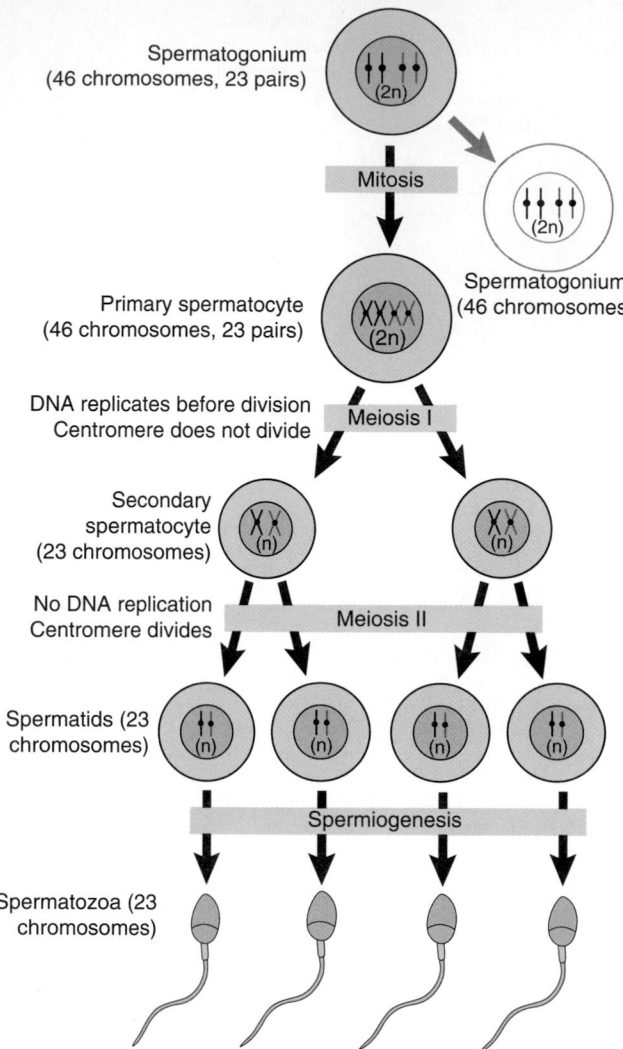

Figure 16-4. Spermatogenesis. (From Applegate E: *The anatomy and physiology learning system,* ed 3, St. Louis, 2006, Saunders.)

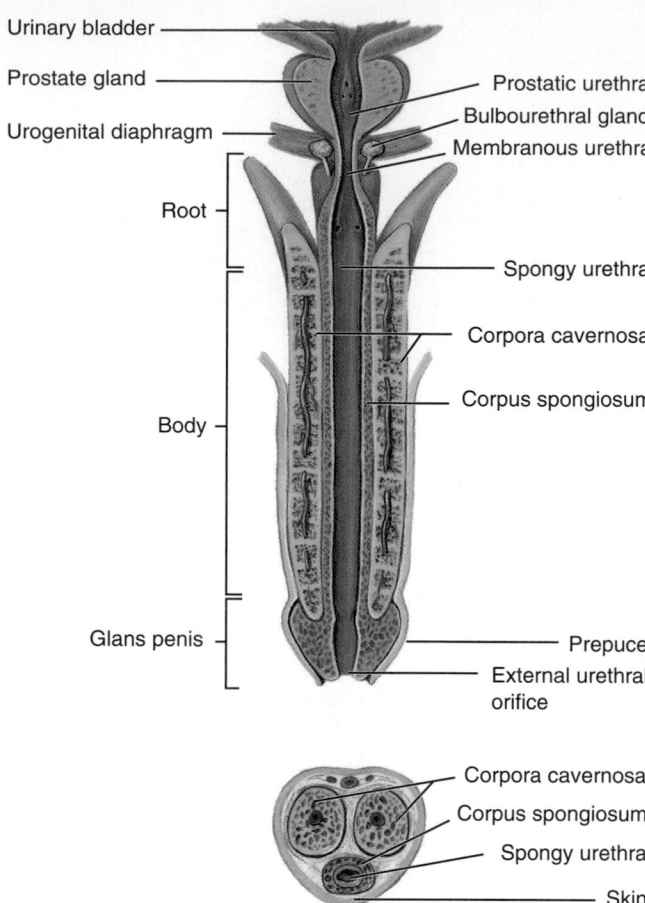

Figure 16-5. Structure of the penis. (From Applegate E: *The anatomy and physiology learning system,* ed 3, St. Louis, 2006, Saunders.)

Prostate

The **prostate gland** is a firm, dense structure that is located just behind the urinary bladder (see Figure 16-1). It is about the size of a walnut and encircles the urethra as it leaves the urinary bladder. Numerous short ducts from the prostate gland empty into the prostatic urethra. The secretions of the prostate are thin, milky colored, and alkaline. They function to enhance the motility of the sperm.

Bulbourethral Glands

The paired **bulbourethral (Cowper's) glands** (see Figure 16-1) are small, about the size of a pea, and are located near the base of the penis. A short duct from each gland enters the penile urethra. In response to sexual stimulation, the bulbourethral glands secrete an alkaline, mucus-like fluid. This fluid performs the following functions: neutralizes the acidity of the urine residue in the urethra, helps to neutralize the acidity of the vagina, and provides some lubrication for the tip of the penis during intercourse.

Seminal Fluid

Seminal fluid (or **semen**) consists of a slightly alkaline (pH 7.5) mixture of sperm cells and secretions from the accessory glands. Secretions from the seminal vesicles make up about 60% of the **semen.** Most of the remaining semen consists of secretions from the prostate gland. Spermatozoa and secretions from the bulbourethral glands contribute only a small volume to the semen.

The volume of semen in a single ejaculation varies from 1.5 to 6 ml. There are usually between 50 and 150 million sperm per milliliter of semen. Sperm counts below 10 to 20 million per milliliter usually cause fertility problems. Although only one spermatozoon actually penetrates and fertilizes an ovum, it takes several million spermatozoa in an ejaculation to ensure that fertilization will take place.

Penis

The **penis** is the male copulatory organ located in front of the scrotum. The penis functions in transferring sperm to the vagina. The penis consists of three columns of erectile tissue that are wrapped in connective tissue and covered with skin (Figure 16-5). There are two dorsal columns known as the **corpora cavernosa** (KOR-por-ah kav-er-NOH-sah). A single, midline ventral column surrounds the urethra and is called the **corpus spongiosum** (KOR-pus spun-jee-OH-sum).

The penis has a root, body, and glans penis. The **root** of the penis attaches it to the pubic arch. The **body** (or **shaft**) of the penis is the visible, pendant portion. The corpus spongiosum expands at the end of the penis to form the **glans penis.** The urethra opens through the external urethral orifice at the tip of the glans penis. A loose fold of skin, called the **prepuce** (PREE-pyoos), or **foreskin,** covers the glans penis.

Male Sexual Response

In the absence of sexual arousal, the erectile tissue of the penis contains only a small volume of blood, causing the penis to be flaccid. During sexual excitement, arterioles that supply blood to the erectile tissue dilate. As a result, the spaces in the erectile tissue become engorged with blood, causing the penis to enlarge and become rigid. This is called **erection** and is necessary to allow the penis to enter the female vagina. The erection reflex may be initiated by stimuli such as anticipation, memory, and visual sensations. It may also be the result of stimulation of touch receptors on the glans penis and skin of the genital area. Emotions and thoughts can inhibit erection.

Continued sexual stimulation causes the reflexes that promote an erection to become more and more intense until a level is reached that prompts a surge of impulses to the genital organs. These impulses stimulate rhythmic contractions of the epididymides, vasa deferentia, and ejaculatory ducts. The impulses also cause contractions of the accessory glands. This results in **emission,** which is the forceful discharge of semen into the urethra. **Ejaculation** immediately follows emission and is the forceful expulsion of semen from the urethra to the exterior. Concurrently with emission and ejaculation, the sphincters of the urinary bladder constrict to prevent semen from entering the bladder and to inhibit the flow of urine from the bladder.

The rhythmic muscle contractions of ejaculation are accompanied by feelings of intense pleasure, increased heart rate, elevated blood pressure, and increased respiration. Together, these physiologic activities are referred to as **climax,** or **orgasm.** This is quickly followed by relaxation, and blood leaves the penis so that it becomes flaccid. After orgasm, there is a latent period, lasting from several minutes to several hours, during which another erection is impossible.

Hormonal Control

The hypothalamus, anterior pituitary, and testes have significant roles in the hormonal control of male reproductive functions. Puberty in males usually begins between the ages of 10 and 12 and continues until ages 16 to 18. During this period the male reproductive organs become sexually mature. The sequence of events that triggers the onset of puberty is unknown. It begins when certain unknown stimuli cause the hypothalamus to start secreting **gonadotropin-releasing hormone** (GnRH), which enters the blood and goes to the anterior pituitary gland.

In response to GnRH, the anterior pituitary secretes luteinizing hormone and follicle-stimulating hormone. **Luteinizing hormone** (LH) promotes the growth of the interstitial cells (cells of Leydig) in the testes and stimulates the cells to secrete **testosterone. Follicle-stimulating hormone** (FSH) binds with receptor sites on the sustentacular cells (Sertoli cells) in the seminiferous tubules. This action makes the spermatogenic cells respond to stimulation by testosterone. Testosterone and FSH act together to stimulate spermatogenesis in the seminiferous tubules. Figure 16-6 summarizes the hormonal control of testicular functions.

Male sex hormones are collectively called **androgens.** The most abundant androgen is testosterone. Before birth, testosterone from the adrenal cortex stimulates the development of the male reproductive organs. Between birth and puberty, testosterone levels are low. Then at puberty, under the influence of LH, the interstitial cells begin secreting high levels of testosterone. The adrenal cortex continues to secrete small amounts of androgens. The increase in testosterone levels at puberty promotes the maturation of the male reproductive organs, stimulates spermatogenesis, and

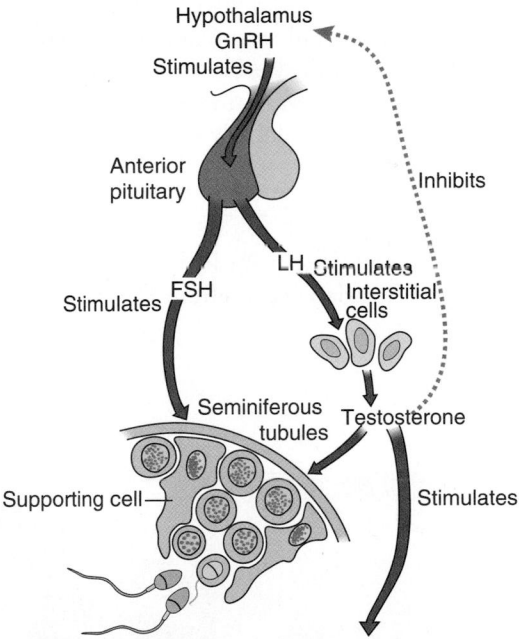

Figure 16-6. Hormonal regulation of testicular function. *FSH,* Follicle-stimulating hormone; *GnRH,* gonadotropin-releasing hormone; *LH,* luteinizing hormone. (From Applegate E: *The anatomy and physiology learning system,* ed 3, St. Louis, 2006, Saunders.)

promotes the development of the male secondary sex characteristics.

After puberty, testosterone production is controlled by a negative feedback mechanism that involves the hypothalamus (see Figure 16-6). High blood testosterone levels inhibit GnRH. This removes the stimulus for LH, which reduces the testosterone level back to normal. Testosterone production continues from puberty throughout the rest of a man's life, although there is some decline in quantity in old age.

FEMALE REPRODUCTIVE SYSTEM

The organs of the female reproductive system perform the following functions: produce and sustain the female sex cells (egg cells, or ova), transport these cells to a site where they may be fertilized by sperm, provide a favorable environment for the developing offspring, move the offspring to the outside at the end of the development period, and produce the female sex hormones. The female reproductive system includes the ovaries, uterine tubes, uterus, vagina, accessory glands, and external genital organs (Figure 16-7).

Ovaries

The primary reproductive organs in the female are the paired **ovaries.** Each ovary is a solid, ovoid structure about the size and shape of an almond (approximately 3.5 cm in length, 2 cm wide, and 1 cm thick). The ovaries are located in shallow depressions, called **ovarian fossae,** one on each side of the uterus. They are held loosely in place by peritoneal ligaments.

Structure

The ovaries are covered on the outside by a layer of epithelium called **germinal (ovarian) epithelium** (Figure 16-8).

Underneath this layer there is a dense connective tissue capsule known as the **tunica albuginea.** The substance of the ovaries is indistinctly divided into an outer **cortex** and an inner **medulla.** The cortex appears more dense and granular because of the presence of numerous **ovarian follicles** in various stages of development. Each of the follicles contains a female germ cell known as an **oocyte.** The medulla consists of loose connective tissue with abundant blood vessels, lymphatic vessels, and nerve fibers.

Oogenesis

Female sex cells (or gametes) develop in the ovaries by a form of meiosis called **oogenesis** (oh-oh-JEN-eh-sis). The sequence of events in oogenesis is similar to the sequence in spermatogenesis, but the timing and final result are different (Figure 16-9). Early in fetal development, primitive germ cells in the ovaries differentiate into **oogonia** (oh-oh-GO-nee-ah). The oogonia divide rapidly to form thousands of cells that have a full complement of 46 chromosomes (23 pairs). Oogonia then enter a growth phase, enlarge, and become **primary oocytes.** The primary oocytes (with 46 chromosomes) replicate their DNA and begin the first meiotic division. This process stops in prophase and the cells remain in this suspended state until puberty. Many of the primary oocytes degenerate before birth. Even with this decline, the two ovaries together contain approximately 700,000 oocytes at birth. This is the lifetime supply, and no more will develop. This is quite different than the male in whom spermatogonia and primary spermatocytes continue to be produced throughout the reproductive lifetime. By puberty the number of primary oocytes has further declined to about 400,000.

Beginning at puberty, several primary oocytes start to grow again each month. One of the primary oocytes seems

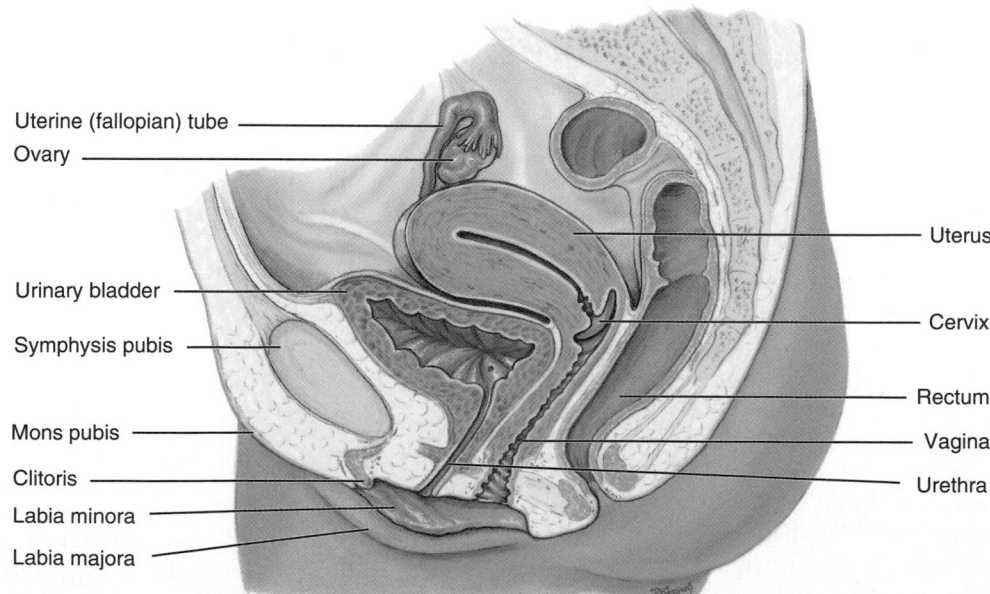

Figure 16-7. Organs of the female reproductive system. (From Applegate E: *The anatomy and physiology learning system,* ed 3, St. Louis, 2006, Saunders.)

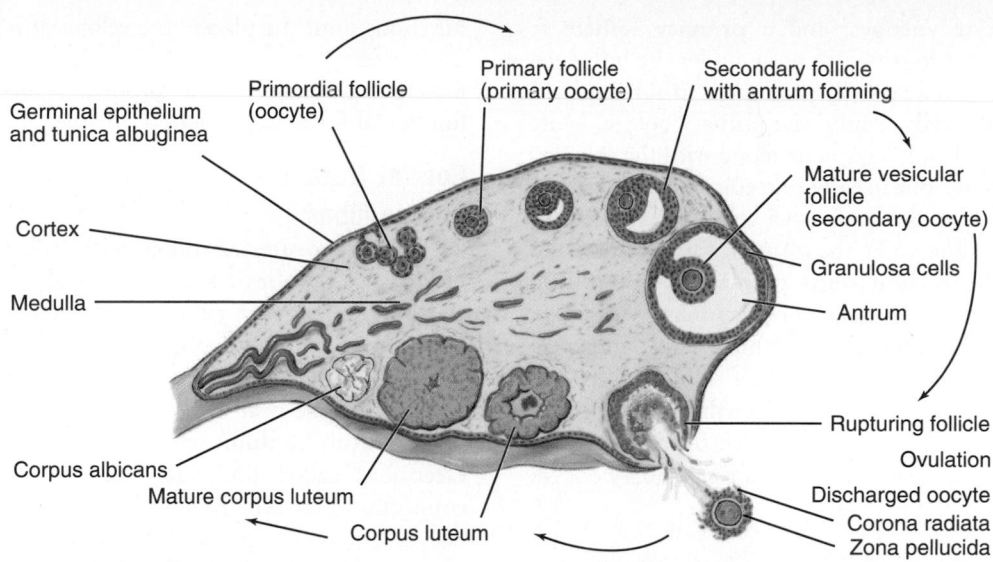

Figure 16-8. Structure of an ovary illustrating the stages in follicle development and corpus luteum formation. (From Applegate E: *The anatomy and physiology learning system,* ed 3, St. Louis, 2006, Saunders.)

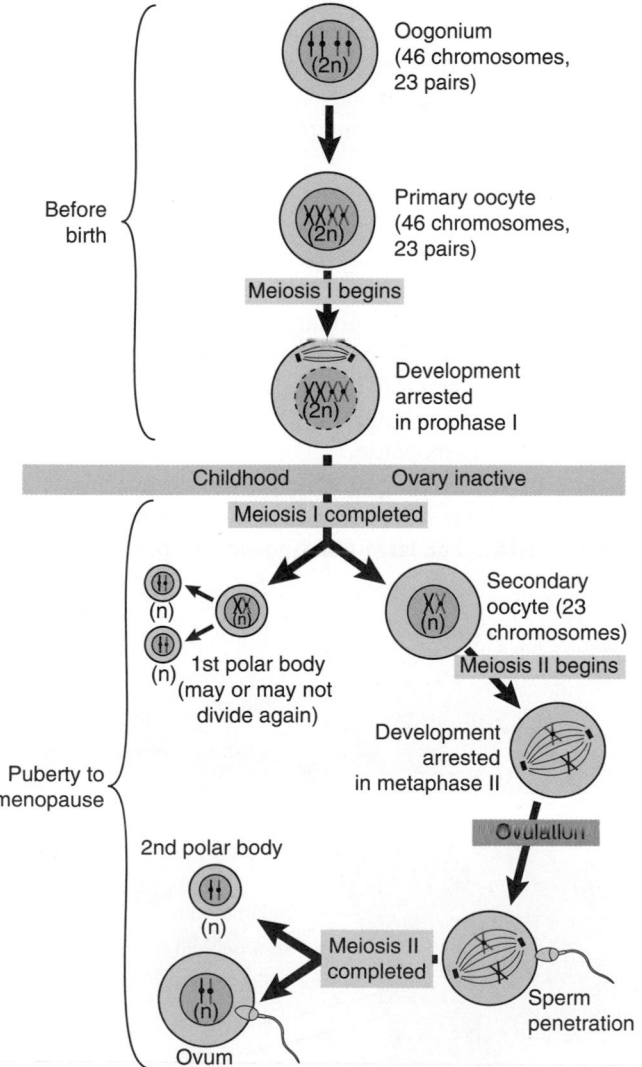

Figure 16-9. Oogenesis. (From Applegate E: *The anatomy and physiology learning system,* ed 3, St. Louis, 2006, Saunders.)

to outgrow the others, and it resumes meiosis I. The other cells degenerate. The large cell undergoes an unequal division so that nearly all the cytoplasm, organelles, and half the chromosomes go to one cell, which becomes a **secondary oocyte.** The remaining half of the chromosomes go to a smaller cell called the **first polar body.** The secondary oocyte begins the second meiotic division, but the process stops in metaphase. At this point, ovulation occurs. If fertilization occurs, meiosis II continues. Again this is an unequal division with all of the cytoplasm going to the ovum, which has 23 single-stranded chromosomes. The smaller cell from this division is a **second polar body.** The first polar body also usually divides in meiosis II to produce two even smaller polar bodies. If fertilization does not occur, the second meiotic division is never completed and the secondary oocyte degenerates. Here again there are obvious differences between the male and female. In spermatogenesis, four functional spermatozoa develop from each primary spermatocyte. In oogenesis, only one functional fertilizable cell develops from a primary oocyte. The other three cells are polar bodies and they degenerate.

Ovarian Follicle Development

An ovarian follicle consists of a developing oocyte surrounded by one or more layers of cells called **follicular cells.** At the same time the oocyte is progressing through meiosis, corresponding changes are taking place in the follicular cells (see Figure 16-8). **Primordial follicles,** which consist of a primary oocyte surrounded by a single layer of flattened cells, develop in the fetus and are the stage that is present in the ovaries at birth and throughout childhood.

Beginning at puberty FSH stimulates changes in the primordial follicles. The follicular cells become cuboidal, the primary oocyte enlarges, and a **primary follicle** is created. The follicles continue to grow under the influence of FSH, and the follicular cells proliferate to form several layers of **granulosa cells** around the primary oocyte. Most of these primary follicles degenerate along with the primary oocytes within them, but usually one continues to develop each month. The granulosa cells start secreting estrogen. In addition, a cavity, known as the *antrum,* forms within the follicle. When the antrum starts to develop, the follicle becomes a **secondary follicle.** The granulosa cells also secrete a substance that forms a clear membrane, known as the **zona pellucida** (ZOH-nah peh-LOO-sih-dah), around the oocyte. After about 10 days of growth the follicle is a mature vesicular (graafian) follicle, which forms a "blister" on the surface of the ovary. It contains a secondary oocyte ready for ovulation.

Ovulation

Ovulation occurs when the mature follicle at the surface of the ovary ruptures and releases the secondary oocyte into the peritoneal cavity. The ovulated secondary oocyte is ready for fertilization. It is still surrounded by the zona pellucida and a few layers of cells called the **corona radiata** (koh-ROH-nah ray-dee-AH-tah). If it is not fertilized, the secondary oocyte degenerates in a couple of days. If a spermatozoon passes through the corona radiata and zona pellucida and enters the cytoplasm of the secondary oocyte, the second meiotic division resumes to form a polar body and a mature ovum.

After ovulation, the portion of the follicle that remains in the ovary enlarges and is transformed into a **corpus luteum** (see Figure 16-8). The corpus luteum is a glandular structure that secretes progesterone and some estrogens. Its fate depends on whether fertilization occurs. If fertilization does not take place, the corpus luteum remains functional for about 10 days and then begins to degenerate into a **corpus albicans.** This structure is primarily scar tissue, and its hormone output ceases. If fertilization occurs, the corpus luteum persists. The corpus luteum continues its hormone functions until the placenta develops sufficiently to secrete the necessary hormones. Again, the corpus luteum ultimately degenerates into a corpus albicans; it just remains functional for a longer period of time.

Genital Tract

Uterine Tubes

There are two **uterine tubes** (also called **fallopian** [fah-LOH-pee-an] **tubes**). Each tube is about 4 cm long and about 1 cm in diameter and extends laterally from the upper portion of the uterus to the region of the ovary on that side (Figure 16-10). One tube is associated with each ovary. The end of the tube near the ovary expands to form a funnel-shaped **infundibulum,** which is surrounded by finger-like extensions called **fimbriae.** Because there is no direct connection between the infundibulum and the ovary, the oocyte enters the peritoneal cavity before it enters the uterine tube. At the time of ovulation, the fimbriae increase their activity and create currents in the peritoneal fluid that help propel the oocyte into the uterine tube. Once inside the uterine tube, the oocyte is moved along by the rhythmic beating of cilia on the epithelial lining and by the peristaltic action of the smooth muscle in the wall of the tube. The journey through the uterine tube takes about 7 days. Because the oocyte is fertile for only 24 to 48 hours, fertilization usually occurs in the uterine tube.

Uterus

The **uterus** is a muscular organ that receives the fertilized oocyte and provides an appropriate environment for the developing offspring. It is located in the pelvic cavity, between the rectum and urinary bladder (see Figure 16-7). Before the first pregnancy, the uterus is about the size and shape of a pear, with the narrow portion directed inferiorly. After childbirth, the uterus is usually larger, and then regresses after menopause.

The upper, bulging surface of the uterus, above the entrance of the uterine tubes, is known as the **fundus** (see Figure 16-10). The large main portion of the uterus is the

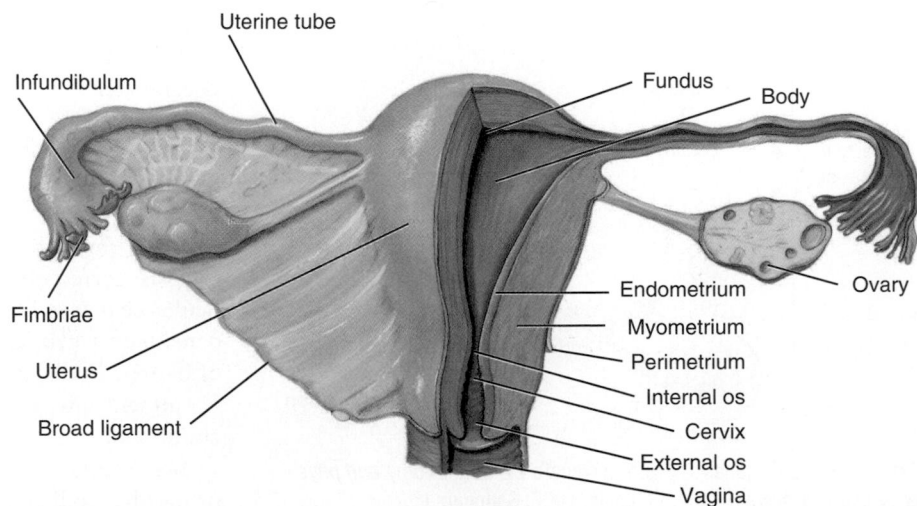

Figure 16-10. Uterus and uterine tubes. (From Applegate E: *The anatomy and physiology learning system,* ed 3, St. Louis, 2006, Saunders.)

body. The narrow region of the uterus that is directed into the vagina is the **cervix.** The opening between the body and cervix is known as the **internal os,** and the opening from the cervix into the vagina is the **external os.** Several ligaments hold the uterus in place. The largest of these is the **broad ligament,** which drapes over the uterus like a sheet and extends laterally to the lateral pelvic wall. The broad ligament also encloses the uterine tubes.

The wall of the uterus consists of perimetrium, myometrium, and endometrium. The outer serous layer is known as the **perimetrium.** The thick middle layer is known as the **myometrium.** The myometrium consists of smooth muscle and makes up the bulk of the uterine wall. The inner layer is called the **endometrium.** It is a mucous membrane that is subdivided into two regions. The **stratum functionale** of the endometrium is the portion that is sloughed off during menstruation. The deeper, thinner **stratum basale** is more constant and provides the materials to rebuild the stratum functionale after menstruation.

Vagina

The **vagina** is a fibromuscular tube, about 10 cm long, that extends from the cervix of the uterus to the outside. It is located between the rectum and urinary bladder. The vagina provides a passageway for menstrual flow to reach the outside, receives the penis and semen during sexual intercourse (coitus), and serves as the birth canal during the birth of a baby. The smooth muscle and mucosal lining of the vaginal wall are capable of stretching to accommodate the erect penis and to permit passage of a baby. The opening of the vagina to the outside is known as the **vaginal orifice.** The vaginal orifice may be incompletely covered by a thin fold of mucous membrane called the **hymen.**

External Genitalia

The external genitalia are accessory structures of the female reproductive system that are outside the vagina. They are also referred to as the **vulva.** The external genitalia include the labia majora, mons pubis, labia minora, clitoris, and glands within the vestibule (Figure 16-11).

The **labia majora** are two large fat-filled folds of skin that enclose the other external genitalia. Anteriorly the labia majora merge to form the **mons pubis.** The mons pubis is a rounded elevation of fat that overlies the pubic symphysis.

After puberty the mons pubis and labia majora are covered with coarse pubic hair. The **labia minora** are two smaller folds of skin medial to the labia majora.

The area between the two labia minora is called the **vestibule.** At the anterior end of the vestibule (where the two labia minora meet), there is a small mass of erectile tissue called the **clitoris** (KLY-toh-ris). The clitoris becomes erect in response to sexual stimulation. The labia minora merge and form a hood over the clitoris known as the **prepuce.** Posterior to the clitoris, the urethra and vagina open into the vestibule. **Paraurethral glands** open into the vestibule on each side of the urethral orifice. These glands secrete mucus. The **greater vestibular glands** (Bartholin's glands) open into the vestibule next to the vaginal orifice. These glands produce a mucus-like secretion for lubrication during sexual intercourse.

Female Sexual Response

The female sexual response is similar to that of the male and consists of erection and orgasm. The body's responses to sexual stimuli produce increased blood flow to the erectile tissue in the clitoris, the vaginal mucosa, breasts, and nipples. The clitoris and nipples become rigid and erect. The breasts and vaginal mucosa enlarge. Glands in the cervix and the vestibular glands secrete fluids that lubricate the vaginal mucosa and aid the entry of the penis.

With continued stimulation, the female response culminates in orgasm. This is accompanied by rhythmic contractions of the uterus and muscles of the pelvic floor. This helps the movement of sperm through the uterus toward the uterine tubes. The rhythmic muscle contractions are accompanied by feelings of intense pleasure, increased heart rate, elevated blood pressure, and increased respiration rate. This is followed by a general relaxation and feeling of warmth throughout the body.

Hormonal Control

As in the male, the hypothalamus, anterior pituitary, and gonads secrete hormones that have significant roles in the control of reproductive functions (Figure 16-12). The hypothalamus secretes GnRH, the anterior pituitary secretes FSH and LH, and the ovaries secrete the sex hormones **estrogen** and **progesterone.** Unlike the male, the secretion of these hormones follows monthly cyclic patterns that

Clitoris

Labium minorus

Labium majorus

Anus

Mons pubis

Prepuce

Urethral orifice

Openings for paraurethral glands

Vagina

Opening for greater vestibular gland

Vestibule

Figure 16-11. Female external genitalia. (From Applegate E: *The anatomy and physiology learning system,* ed 3, St. Louis, 2006, Saunders.)

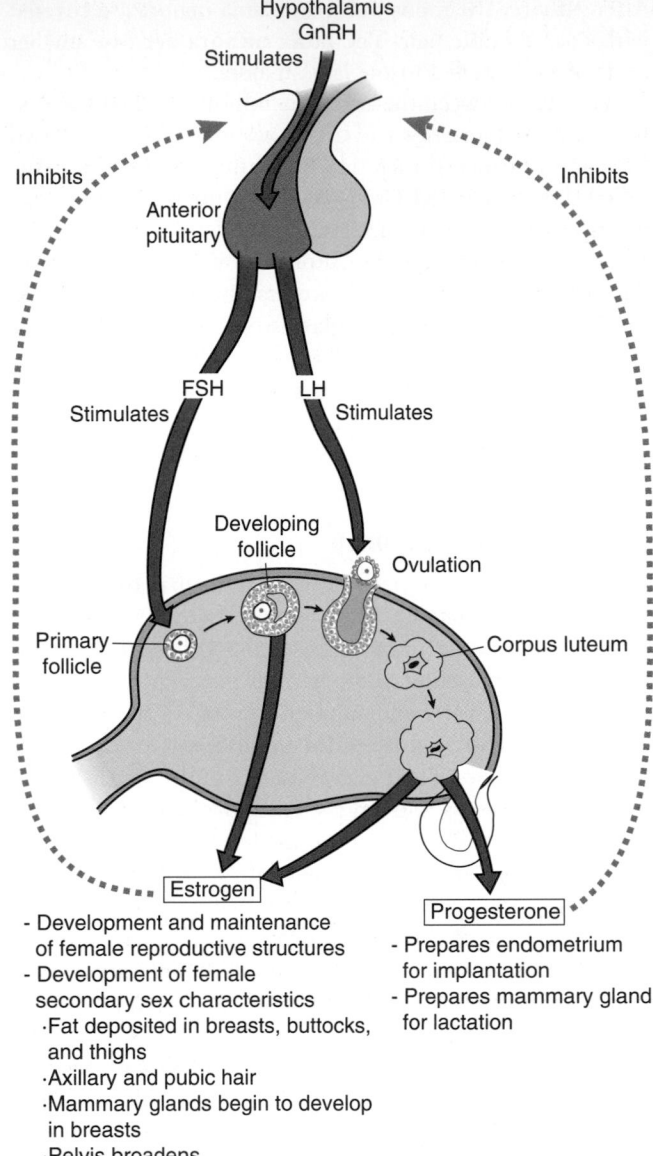

Figure 16-12. Hormonal regulation of ovarian functions. *FSH,* Follicle-stimulating hormone; *GnRH,* gonadotropin-releasing hormone; *LH,* luteinizing hormone. (From Applegate E: *The anatomy and physiology learning system,* ed 3, St. Louis, 2006, Saunders.)

Figure 16-13. Correlation of events in the ovarian and uterine cycles. *FSH,* Follicle-stimulating hormone; *LH,* luteinizing hormone. (From Applegate E: *The anatomy and physiology learning system,* ed 3, St. Louis, 2006, Saunders.)

affect the ovaries and uterus. These cycles, referred to as the **ovarian cycle** and the **menstrual** (uterine) **cycle,** begin at puberty and continue for about 40 years.

At puberty certain stimuli cause the hypothalamus to start secreting GnRH. This hormone enters the blood and goes to the anterior pituitary gland, where it stimulates the secretion of FSH and LH. These hormones, in turn, affect the ovaries and uterus, and the monthly cycles begin. In females, the beginning of puberty is marked by the first period of menstrual bleeding, called **menarche** (meh-NAHR-kee). After this the cycles continue, more or less regularly, until the late 40s or early 50s. At this time, the cycles become increasingly irregular until they finally stop. **Menopause** is the cessation of the reproductive cycles.

Ovarian Cycle

The ovarian cycle includes the changes that occur within the ovaries as the follicles develop (follicular phase), ovulation occurs (ovulatory phase), and the corpus luteum develops (luteal phase) (Figure 16-13).

Follicular phase   The follicular phase of the cycle begins when GnRH from the hypothalamus stimulates increased secretion of FSH from the anterior pituitary. FSH stimulates growth of the ovarian follicles. As the follicles enlarge, estrogen secretion increases. Low levels of estrogen exert a negative feedback effect on the hypothalamus and anterior pituitary but also increase the effect of FSH on the follicle. The follicle continues to grow and mature until the middle of the cycle.

Ovulatory phase The ovulatory phase is the result of high levels of estrogen from the mature follicles. Low levels of estrogen have a negative feedback effect on the pituitary, but high levels have a positive feedback effect. This results in a surge of LH and a smaller increase in FSH. The surge of LH stimulates resumption of meiosis in the oocyte and causes the rupture of the follicle, and estrogen levels decline.

Luteal phase The luteal phase occurs when the surge of LH stimulates the development of the corpus luteum from the ruptured follicle. LH also stimulates the corpus luteum to secrete progesterone and some estrogen. These have a negative feedback effect on the hypothalamus and anterior pituitary so that FSH and LH levels decline. As the LH level declines, corpus luteum activity declines and the inhibitory effect is removed. The cycle starts over.

Uterine (Menstrual) Cycle

The uterine (menstrual) cycle reflects changes in the endometrium of the uterus. These changes occur to the thick outer layer of the endometrium, known as the *stratum functionale*. Changes in estrogen and progesterone levels are responsible for the changes in the uterus. The **uterine cycle** is divided into the menstrual phase, proliferative phase, and secretory phase (see Figure 16-13).

Menstrual phase The menstrual phase begins on the first day of the cycle and continues for 3 to 5 days. The thick stratum functionale detaches from the uterine wall and passes through the vagina as the menstrual flow. During this time, follicles are growing in the ovary.

Proliferative phase The proliferative phase begins with the end of the menstrual phase and lasts for about 8 days. The growing follicles in the ovary secrete increasing levels of estrogen. The estrogen stimulates repair of the endometrium in the uterus. The endometrium thickens, glands develop, and blood vessels grow in the new tissue. Ovulation occurs at the end of this uterine phase.

Secretory phase During the secretory phase, progesterone is being secreted by the corpus luteum. The progesterone stimulates continued growth and thickening of the endometrium. Arteries and glands grow and enlarge. The glands secrete glycogen, which will nourish a developing embryo if fertilization occurs. If fertilization does not occur, the corpus luteum in the ovary begins to degenerate. This leads to menstruation, and the cycle starts over again.

Menopause

Menopause is the cessation of the female reproductive cycles. Even though menopause is marked by the lack of menstrual cycles, the first changes occur in the ovary. By the age of 45 or 50, ovarian follicles cease responding to FSH and LH from the pituitary gland. As a result, the follicle cells do not produce estrogen and there is no ovulation, no corpus luteum, and no progesterone. Without estrogen and progesterone, the cyclic changes in the uterus stop and menstruation ceases. This is the visible evidence of menopause. As estrogen and progesterone levels decline, FSH and LH increase because of the lack of ovarian hormone feedback. These high levels of pituitary hormones with the low levels of ovarian hormones are believed to be responsible for a variety of symptoms associated with the onset of menopause. Some women experience hot flashes, sweating, depression, headaches, irritability, and insomnia. However, many women experience few, if any, of these symptoms.

Mammary Glands

The mammary glands are the organs of milk production. Mammary glands are located in the breast overlying the pectoralis major muscles. They are present in both sexes but usually functional only in the female.

Each breast has a raised **nipple,** which is surrounded by a circular pigmented area called the **areola** (ah-REE-oh-lah). The nipples are sensitive to touch, and they contain smooth muscle that contracts and causes them to become erect in response to stimulation.

The adult female breast contains 15 to 20 lobes of glandular tissue that radiate around the nipple (Figure 16-14). The **lobes** are separated by connective tissue and adipose. The connective tissue helps support the breast. Some bands of connective tissue, called **suspensory** (Cooper's) **ligaments,** extend through the breast from the skin to the underlying muscles. The amount and distribution of the adipose determines the size and shape of the breast. Each lobe consists of **lobules** that contain the glandular units. A **lactiferous** (lak-TIFF-er-us) **duct** collects the milk from the lobules within each lobe and carries it to the nipple. Just before the nipple, the lactiferous duct enlarges to form a **lactiferous sinus (ampulla),** which serves as a reservoir for milk. After the sinus, the duct again narrows and each duct opens independently on the surface of the nipple.

Mammary gland function is regulated by hormones. At puberty, increasing levels of estrogen stimulate the development of glandular tissue in the female breast. Estrogen also causes the breasts to increase in size through the accumulation of adipose tissue. Progesterone stimulates the development of the duct system. During pregnancy these hormones further enhance development of the mammary glands. Prolactin from the anterior pituitary stimulates the production of milk within the glandular tissue, and oxytocin causes the ejection of milk from the glands.

Lactiferous duct

Lactiferous sinus

Lobule

Lobe

2nd rib

Pectoralis major muscle

Adipose tissue

Cooper's ligaments

Figure 16-14. Breast and mammary glands. (From Jarvis C: *Physical examination and health assessment,* ed 4, St. Louis, 2004, Saunders.)

Highlight on Aging and the Reproductive System

Men normally do not experience a sudden decline in reproductive function comparable to menopause in women. Instead, they experience a gradual and subtle decline over many years. After age 50, men have some testicular atrophy, partially caused by a decrease in the size of the seminiferous tubules and partially a result of a reduction in the number of interstitial cells. These changes are accompanied by a decline in sperm and testosterone production. Both the seminal vesicles and the prostate show a decrease in secretory activity, which results in a reduction in the volume of semen. The portion of the prostate gland that surrounds the urethra often enlarges and may constrict the urethra, making urination difficult. The penis may undergo some atrophy and become smaller with age. The blood vessels and erectile tissue in the penis become less elastic, which hinders the ability to attain an erection. Although there is a general decline in the aging male reproductive system, many men are capable of achieving erection and ejaculation into old age.

After menopause, there is a gradual decline in the female reproductive system. Most of the changes are believed to be due to the reduction in estrogen. The ovaries undergo progressive atrophy. The uterus becomes smaller, and fibrous connective tissue replaces much of the myometrium. The vagina becomes narrower and shorter, and its walls become thin and less elastic.

Glands that lubricate the vagina reduce their secretory activity, and the vagina becomes dry. The vaginal secretions that remain are less acidic, which makes older women more susceptible to vaginal infections. The external genitalia and mammary glands undergo atrophic changes. The lack of estrogen also affects nonreproductive organs. This is particularly true in the case of bone metabolism, which is indicated by the increased prevalence of osteoporosis in postmenopausal women. There is also increased cardiovascular disease.

Estrogen replacement therapy is prescribed for many women to combat osteoporosis and other symptoms of menopause. However, there is controversy about the risks involved with this treatment, particularly the risks of uterine and breast cancer. Consideration should be given to the risks and benefits before beginning estrogen replacement therapy. Current practice often prescribes progesterone in conjunction with estrogen, which seems to reduce some of the risks.

There is a growing awareness that elderly people have sexual needs and enjoy sexual relations. Although age-related physical and hormonal changes that take place in the reproductive system may alter these needs and sexual functioning, studies demonstrate that sexuality remains important to many older people. ■

TERMINOLOGY REVIEW

Gametes Sex cells: sperm and ova.

Gonads Primary reproductive organs; organs that produce the gametes: testes in the male and ovaries in the female.

Oogenesis Process of meiosis in the female in which one ovum and three polar bodies are produced from one primary oocyte.

Ovarian cycle Monthly cycle of events that occur in the ovary from puberty to menopause; occurs concurrently with the uterine cycle.

Ovarian follicle An oocyte surrounded by one or more layers of cells within the ovaries.

Spermatogenesis Process of meiosis in the male in which four spermatids are produced from one primary spermatocyte.

Spermiogenesis Morphologic changes that transform a spermatid into a mature sperm.

Uterine cycle Monthly cycle of events that occur in the uterus from puberty to menopause; also called the *menstrual cycle;* occurs concurrently with the ovarian cycle.

ON THE WEB

For Information on the Reproductive System:

The Internet Pathology Laboratory for Medical Education—Female Reproductive Pathology: library.med.utah.edu/WebPath/ORGAN.html *(Click on "Female Genital Tract Pathology")*

Inner Body: www.innerbody.com/html/body.html

The Internet Pathology Laboratory for Medical Education—Male Reproductive Pathology: library.med.utah.edu/WebPath/ORGAN.html *(Click on "Male Reproductive Pathology")*

Department of Health and Human Services, The Office of Women's Health: www.4women.gov/COE

Gene School: library.thinkquest.org/28599/index.htm

The Visible Embryo: visembryo.com

PREPARE FOR CERTIFICATION   Visit the Evolve site at http://evolve.elsevier.com/Bonewit/today/ to actively Prepare for your Certification.

CD   *Check out the **Companion CD** bound with the book to access additional interactive activities.*

17

Medical Asepsis and the OSHA Standard

LEARNING OBJECTIVES	PROCEDURES
Microorganisms and Medical Asepsis	
1. Define a microorganism, and give examples of types of microorganisms.	Handwashing
2. Explain the difference between a nonpathogen and a pathogen.	
3. Define medical asepsis.	
4. List the six basic requirements for growth and multiplication of microorganisms.	
5. Outline the infection process and cycle, including the following:	
Give examples of the means of entry of microorganisms into the body.	
Give examples of the means of transmission of microorganisms from one person to another.	
Give examples of the means of exit of microorganisms from the body.	
List and explain the protective mechanisms the body uses to prevent the entrance of microorganisms.	
6. Explain the difference between resident flora and transient flora.	
7. State when each of the following is performed: handwashing, antiseptic handwashing, and alcohol-based hand rub.	Applying an alcohol-based hand rub
8. Identify medical aseptic practices that should be followed in the medical office.	
9. Explain how proper handwashing helps prevent the transmission of microorganisms.	
10. List examples of when to wear clean disposable gloves.	Application and removal of clean disposable gloves
OSHA Bloodborne Pathogens Standard	
1. Explain the purpose of OSHA.	Adhere to the OSHA Bloodborne Pathogens Standard.
2. Describe the purpose of the Needlestick Safety and Prevention Act.	
3. List and describe the elements that must be included in the OSHA exposure control plan.	
4. Explain the purpose of the following OSHA requirements: labeling requirements and sharps injury log.	
5. Define and give examples of each of the following: engineering controls, work practice controls, personal protective equipment, and housekeeping procedures.	
6. Identify the guidelines for use of personal protective equipment.	
Regulated Medical Waste	
1. List examples of medical waste and how to discard each type of waste.	Prepare regulated waste for pickup by an infectious waste service.
2. Explain how to handle and dispose of regulated medical waste.	

Bloodborne Diseases
1. Explain how hepatitis B and C are transmitted in the health care setting.
2. Describe postexposure prophylaxis for hepatitis B.
3. Explain what occurs when HIV gains entrance into the body.

CHAPTER OUTLINE

Introduction to Medical Asepsis and the OSHA Standard

Microorganisms and Medical Asepsis
Growth Requirements for Microorganisms
Infection Process Cycle
Protective Mechanisms of the Body
Medical Asepsis in the Medical Office

OSHA Bloodborne Pathogens Standard
Purpose of the Standard
Needlestick Safety and Prevention Act
OSHA Terminology

Components of the OSHA Standard
Control Measures
Regulated Medical Waste
Handling Regulated Medical Waste
Disposal of Regulated Medical Waste
Bloodborne Diseases
Hepatitis B
Hepatitis C
Acquired Immune Deficiency Syndrome

CAAHEP COMPETENCIES

Clinical Competencies
Fundamental Procedures
- Perform handwashing.
- Dispose of biohazardous materials.
- Practice Standard Precautions.

General Competencies
Legal Concepts
- Identify and respond to issues of confidentiality.
- Perform within legal and ethical boundaries.
- Demonstrate knowledge of federal and state health care legislation and regulations.

Patient Instruction
- Identify community resources.

ABHES COMPETENCIES

Clinical Duties
- Apply principles of aseptic techniques and infection control.
- Dispose of biohazardous materials.
- Practice standard precautions.

Legal Concepts
- Monitor legislation related to current healthcare issues and practices.

Instruction
- Teach patients methods of health promotion and disease prevention.

KEY TERMS

aerobe (AIR-obe)
anaerobe (AN-er-obe)
antiseptic
asepsis (ay-SEP-sis)
cilia (SIL-ee-ya)
contaminated (kon-TAM-in-ated)
decontamination (DEE-kon-tam-in-AY-shun)
hand hygiene
infection
medical asepsis
microorganism (MYE-kroe-OR-gan-iz-um)
nonintact (NON-in-takt) skin
nonpathogen (non-PATH-oh-jen)

opportunistic (OP-pore-tune-IS-tik) infection
optimum (OP-tuh-mum) growth temperature
parenteral (pare-EN-ter-al)
pathogen (PATH-oh-jen)
perinatal (pare-ee-NAY-tul)
pH (PEE-AYCH)
postexposure prophylaxis (proe-fil-ACKS-is) (PEP)
regulated medical waste (RMW)
reservoir (REZ-er-vwar) host
resident flora (FLOE-ruh)
susceptible (sus-SEP-tih-bul)
transient (TRAN-zee-ent) flora

Introduction to Medical Asepsis and the OSHA Standard

Medical **asepsis** and **infection** control are crucial in preventing the spread of disease. The medical assistant should always practice good medical aseptic techniques to provide a safe and healthy environment in the medical office. The Occupational Safety and Health Administration (OSHA) Bloodborne Pathogens Standard is important for infection control. This standard is required by the federal government to reduce the exposure of health care employees to infectious diseases. This chapter presents a thorough discussion of medical asepsis, infection control, and the OSHA Bloodborne Pathogens Standard.

MICROORGANISMS AND MEDICAL ASEPSIS

Microorganisms are tiny living plants or animals that cannot be seen with the naked eye, but instead must be viewed with the aid of a microscope. Common types of microorganisms include bacteria, viruses, protozoa, fungi, and animal parasites. Most microorganisms are harmless and do not cause disease. They are termed **nonpathogens.** Other microorganisms, known as **pathogens,** are harmful to the body and can cause disease.

In the medical office, practices must be employed to reduce the number and hinder the transmission of pathogenic microorganisms. These practices are known as *medical asepsis.* **Medical asepsis** means that an object or area is clean and free from infection. Nonpathogens would still be present on a clean or medically aseptic substance or surface, but all the pathogens would have been eliminated.

Growth Requirements for Microorganisms

For microorganisms to survive, certain growth requirements must be present in the environment, as follows:

1. **Proper nutrition.** Microorganisms that use inorganic or nonliving substances as a source of food are known as *autotrophs.* Microorganisms that use organic or living substances for food are known as *heterotrophs.*
2. **Oxygen.** Most microorganisms need oxygen to grow and multiply and are termed **aerobes.** Other microorganisms, known as **anaerobes,** grow best in the absence of oxygen.
3. **Temperature.** Each microorganism has a temperature at which it grows best, known as the **optimum growth temperature.** Most microorganisms grow best at 98.6°F (37°C), the human body temperature.
4. **Darkness.** Microorganisms grow best in darkness.
5. **Moisture.** Microorganisms need moisture for cell metabolism and to carry away wastes.
6. **pH.** Most microorganisms prefer a neutral pH. If the environment of the microorganisms becomes too acidic or too basic, they die.

If growth requirements are taken away from the environment of microorganisms, they are unable to survive. Eliminating these conditions is one way to reduce the growth and transmission of pathogens in the medical office.

Infection Process Cycle

For a pathogen to survive and produce disease, a continuous cycle must be followed; this is known as the *infection process cycle* (Figure 17-1). If the cycle is broken at any point, the pathogen dies. The medical assistant has a responsibility to help break this cycle in the medical office by practicing good techniques of medical asepsis. These techniques are discussed in the next section.

Protective Mechanisms of the Body

The body has protective mechanisms to help prevent the entrance of pathogens, and these help break the infection process cycle. Protective mechanisms of the body are as follows:

1. The skin is the body's most important defense mechanism; it serves as a protective barrier against the entrance of microorganisms.
2. The mucous membranes of the body, which line the nose and throat and respiratory, gastrointestinal, and genital tracts, help protect the body from invasion by microorganisms.
3. Mucus and cilia in the nose and respiratory tract fight off pathogens. Mucus traps the smaller microorganisms that enter the body, and the hairlike **cilia** constantly beat toward the outside to remove them from the body.
4. Coughing and sneezing help force pathogens from the body.
5. Tears and sweat are secretions that aid in the removal of pathogens from the body.
6. Urine and vaginal secretions are acidic. Pathogens cannot grow in an acidic environment.
7. The stomach secretes hydrochloric acid, which helps in the process of digestion. This acidic environment discourages the growth of pathogens that enter the stomach.

Medical Asepsis in the Medical Office

Hand Hygiene

Hand hygiene refers to the process of cleansing or sanitizing the hands. Hand hygiene is considered the most important medical aseptic practice in the medical office for preventing the spread of infection. Specific techniques for sanitizing the hands in the medical office include the following:

- Handwashing with a detergent soap and water
- Handwashing with an antimicrobial soap and water
- Applying an alcohol-based hand rub

The Centers for Disease Control and Prevention (CDC) issued new recommendations for hand hygiene in health care settings. The purpose of these guidelines is to promote improved hand hygiene practices and to reduce transmission of pathogenic microorganisms to patients and employees in health care settings. The CDC guidelines for hand

1. **RESERVOIR HOST** is one that becomes infected by the pathogen and also serves as a source of transfer of the pathogen. The host provides nourishment for a microorganism to grow and multiply. Examples include people and animals.

5. **SUSCEPTIBLE HOST** is one that is capable of being infected by the pathogen. The resistance or ability to fight off disease of the host is low. Factors that contribute to low resistance and increased susceptibility include poor health, poor hygiene, poor nutrition, and stress.

2. **MEANS OF EXIT** from the reservoir host include the mouth, nose, throat, ears, eyes, intestinal tract, urinary tract, reproductive tract, and open wounds.

4. **MEANS OF ENTRY** into the host include the mouth, nose, throat, ears, eyes, intestinal tract, reproductive tract, open wounds and breaks in the skin, and mucous membranes.

3. **MEANS OF TRANSMISSION** from one person to another include direct contact with an infected person or discharge. Indirect transfer includes water vapor from the lungs, as when a person coughs or sneezes; contaminated hands and equipment; contaminated food and water; and insects that carry pathogens.

Figure 17-1. The infection process cycle. (From Bonewit-West K: *Clinical procedures for medical assistants,* ed 7, St. Louis, 2008, Saunders.)

hygiene as they apply to the medical office are outlined in Box 17-1. They are also discussed further in this section.

Resident and Transient Flora

Microorganisms on the hands are classified into the following categories: resident flora and transient flora. **Resident flora** (also known as *normal flora*) normally reside and grow in the epidermis and deeper layers of the skin known as the *dermis*. Resident flora are generally harmless and nonpathogenic. Because resident flora are attached to the deeper skin layers, they are difficult to remove from the skin.

Transient flora live and grow on the superficial skin layers, or epidermis. They are picked up on the hands in the course of daily activities. In the medical office, this may include contact with an infected patient, contaminated equipment, or contaminated surfaces. Transient flora are often pathogenic, but because they are attached loosely to the skin, they can be removed easily with proper handwashing or by applying an alcohol-based hand rub.

Handwashing

Handwashing refers to washing the hands with a detergent soap and water. Detergent soap (commonly known as *plain*

Putting It All into Practice

My name is Jennifer Hawk, and I work for a large group of physicians in a multispecialty clinic. I work in both the front and back areas of the office. I really enjoy experiencing all of these areas of the office, and I definitely never get bored.

The most interesting experience I have had as a practicing medical assistant is seeing the impact that I make on patients' lives. They rely on you and look to you first for help in their health care situation. You are most often the first person they come into contact with in the office, and they look to you for understanding and empathy. Especially patients who come to your office on a regular basis see you as a kind of family member. They appreciate a familiar face and smile. Most often, you are the individual giving the patient instructions concerning testing they will be having done or medication they will be taking. Patients truly do count on your knowledge and assistance throughout their course of care. I was genuinely surprised at what an impact I could have on others. ■

Prepare for Success

BOX 17-1 CDC Guidelines for Hand Hygiene in Health Care Settings

Wash Hands with a Detergent Soap or an Antimicrobial Soap

- When the hands are visibly soiled with dirt or body fluids (e.g., blood, feces, urine, respiratory secretions)
- Before eating
- After using the restroom

Apply an Alcohol-Based Hand Rub (or Wash Hands)

- Before and after patient contact
- Before applying and after removing gloves
- After contact with body fluids or excretions, mucous membranes, nonintact skin, and wound dressings as long as the hands are not visibly soiled
- When moving from a contaminated body site to a clean body site during patient care
- After contact with inanimate objects (e.g., medical equipment) when providing health care to a patient

General Recommendations

- Keep natural nail tips less than ¼-inch long. Avoid wearing artificial nails.
- Do not add soap to a partially empty liquid soap dispenser. The practice of "topping off" dispensers can lead to bacterial contamination of the soap. The correct procedure is either to dispose of an empty dispenser or rinse an empty dispenser thoroughly and then refill it.
- Disposable paper towels are recommended for drying the hands after handwashing. Multiple-use cloth towels are not recommended.
- Use hand lotions or creams to minimize the occurrence of dermatitis associated with frequent handwashing.
- Change gloves during patient care if moving from a contaminated body site to a clean body site.
- Remove gloves after caring for a patient. Do not wear the same pair of gloves for the care of more than one patient.

From Bonewit-West K: *Clinical procedures for medical assistants*, ed 7, St. Louis, 2008, Saunders.

Figure 17-2. **A,** Antimicrobial soap. **B,** Alcohol-based hand rubs. (From Bonewit-West K: *Clinical procedures for medical assistants*, ed 7, St. Louis, 2008, Saunders.)

This is because repeated handwashing tends to dry out the hands, leading to irritation, chapping, and dermatitis.

Antiseptic Handwashing

Washing the hands with an antimicrobial soap is termed *antiseptic handwashing*. Antimicrobial soaps contain an **antiseptic,** which is an agent that functions to kill or inhibit the growth of microorganisms (Figure 17-2A). Antiseptic handwashing sanitizes the hands through the mechanical scrubbing action and through the action of the antiseptic. Proper handwashing with an antimicrobial soap removes all soil and transient flora from the hands. Most antimicrobial soaps also deposit an antibacterial film on the skin that discourages bacterial growth. Antiseptic handwashing should be performed by the medical assistant before assisting with a minor office surgery. Examples of antiseptics contained in antimicrobial soaps include triclosan, chlorhexidine, hexachlorophene, iodine, and chloroxylenol.

Alcohol-Based Hand Rubs

The CDC guidelines recommend the use of an alcohol-based hand rub for sanitizing the hands when they are not visibly soiled (see Box 17-1). Alcohol-based hand rubs consist of 60% to 90% alcohol (ethanol or isopropanol) and come in the form of gels, lotions, and foams (Figure 17-2B). Studies have shown that hand rubs are more effective than traditional soap-and-water handwashing in removing transient flora and reducing bacterial counts on the hands. The advantages that alcohol-based hand rubs offer over traditional handwashing are as follows:

- Alcohol-based hand rubs are usually more accessible than sinks.
- They do not require rinsing; water or hand drying with a towel is not necessary.
- Less time is required to perform hand hygiene. It takes 20 to 30 seconds to sanitize the hands with an alcohol-based hand rub compared with 1 to 2 minutes to perform proper handwashing.

soap) contains agents that help break down and emulsify dirt and oil present on the skin. Soap is used to sanitize the hands through the physical removal of dirt and transient flora. It is important to use adequate friction during handwashing to ensure the removal of all transient flora. Procedure 17-1 outlines the handwashing procedure.

The CDC hand hygiene guidelines recommend that handwashing be performed when the hands are visibly soiled with dirt or body fluids, before eating, and after using the restroom (see Box 17-1). If the hands are not visibly soiled, the CDC recommends that an alcohol-based hand rub be used to sanitize the hands rather than handwashing.

- Most alcohol-based hand rubs contain emollients, which help prevent the skin of the hands from overdrying. As the alcohol dries, protective fats and oils remain on the hands.

Alcohol-based hand rubs have disadvantages. They are more expensive than plain soap. They also cause a brief stinging sensation if they are applied to broken skin such as a cut or abrasion on the hand. Procedure 17-2 describes the proper steps for performing an alcohol-based hand rub.

Infection Control

In addition to hand hygiene, other good aseptic practices in the medical office include the following:

1. Follow the OSHA Bloodborne Pathogens Standard (presented in this chapter).
2. Keep the medical office free from dirt and dust, which can collect and carry microorganisms.
3. Ensure that the reception area and examining rooms are well ventilated. Stuffy rooms encourage microorganisms to settle on objects.
4. Keep the reception area and examining rooms bright and airy. Light discourages the growth of microorganisms.
5. Eliminate insects by the use of insecticides or window screens. Insects are a means of transmission of microorganisms.
6. Carefully dispose of wastes, such as urine, feces, and respiratory secretions; all wastes should be handled as though they contain pathogens.
7. Do not let soiled items touch clothing.
8. Avoid coughs and sneezes of patients. The water vapor expelled from the lungs with coughing and sneezing may contain pathogens.
9. Use discretion in the amount of jewelry worn; wear minimal jewelry or no jewelry at all. Microorganisms can become lodged in the grooves and crevices of jewelry and serve as a means of transmission of pathogens.
10. Teach patients aseptic practices to control the spread of infection at home.

Gloves

The CDC recommends that clean disposable gloves be worn when the medical assistant is likely to come in contact with any body substance, such as blood, urine, feces, mucous membranes, and nonintact skin. Clean disposable gloves should be worn when administering an injection, performing a venipuncture, or performing a urinalysis.

Gloves reduce hand contamination by 70% to 80%, reduce cross-contamination between patients, and protect patients and health care workers from infection. It is important for the medical assistant to change gloves before and after contact with each patient. Sterile gloves are used to perform sterile procedures, such as a dressing change or to assist the physician during minor office surgery, which is described in more detail in Chapter 25. Procedure 17-3 presents the proper method for applying and removing clean disposable gloves.

Text continued on p. 277

PROCEDURE **17-1** Handwashing

Outcome Perform handwashing.

Equipment/Supplies

- Liquid or bar soap
- Paper towels
- Waste container

---

1. **Procedural Step.** Remove your watch or push it up on the forearm so that the wrist is clear. Avoid wearing rings. If you wear rings, remove all except a plain wedding band and put them in a safe place.
   Principle. Microorganisms can lodge in the crevices and grooves of rings.
2. **Procedural Step.** Stand at the sink, making sure clothing does not touch the sink.
   Principle. The sink is considered contaminated, and if the uniform touches the sink, it may pick up microorganisms and transfer them.
3. **Procedural Step.** Turn on the faucets using a paper towel.
   Principle. The faucets are considered contaminated because they harbor microorganisms.

Turn on the faucets using a paper towel. (From Bonewit-West K: *Clinical procedures for medical assistants,* ed 7, St. Louis, 2008, Saunders.)

Continued

PROCEDURE **17-1** Handwashing—cont'd

4. **Procedural Step.** Adjust the water temperature. The water should be warm to make the best suds.
   Principle. Water that is too hot or too cold tends to dry the skin, causing chapping and cracking and making it easy for pathogens to enter the body or be transferred to patients.

5. **Procedural Step.** Discard the paper towel in the waste container.
   Principle. The paper towel is considered contaminated after touching the faucets.

6. **Procedural Step.** Wet the hands and forearms thoroughly with water. The hands should be held lower than the elbows at all times. Do not touch the inside of the sink because it is also contaminated.
   Principle. When you hold the hands lower than the elbows, bacteria and debris are carried away from the arms and body and into the sink.

7. **Procedural Step.** Apply soap to the hands. If you use liquid soap, apply 1 teaspoon of soap (approximately the size of a nickel). If you use bar soap, it must be retained in the hands during sudsing up. Rinse the bar soap before returning it to the soap dish. The soap dish should have drainage holes so that the soap can dry out—moisture encourages the growth of microorganisms.
   Principle. Microorganisms and debris accumulate on the soap during the handwashing procedure. Rinsing the soap helps carry these away.

8. **Procedural Step.** Wash the palms and backs of the hands with 10 circular motions. Use friction along with the circular motions to wash the palm and back of each hand.
   Principle. Friction helps dislodge and remove microorganisms from the hands.

Wash the back of the hands. (From Bonewit-West K: *Clinical procedures for medical assistants,* ed 7, St. Louis, 2008, Saunders.)

9. **Procedural Step.** Wash the fingers with 10 circular motions. Interlace the fingers and thumbs, and use friction and circular motions while rubbing the fingers back and forth.

Apply soap to the hands. (From Bonewit-West K: *Clinical procedures for medical assistants,* ed 7, St. Louis, 2008, Saunders.)

Interlace the fingers and use friction. (From Bonewit-West K: *Clinical procedures for medical assistants,* ed 7, St. Louis, 2008, Saunders.)

Principle. This kind of movement helps remove microorganisms and debris that have accumulated between the fingers.

10. Procedural Step. Rinse well, making sure to hold the hands lower than the elbows.

Principle. Running water helps rinse away dirt and microorganisms.

Rinse well, holding the hands lower than the elbows. (From Bonewit-West K: *Clinical procedures for medical assistants,* ed 7, St. Louis, 2008, Saunders.)

11. Procedural Step. Wash the wrists and forearms, using friction along with circular motions. (*Note:* The hands are washed first because they are the most contaminated; microorganisms and dirt are washed away and not spread to the wrists and forearms.)

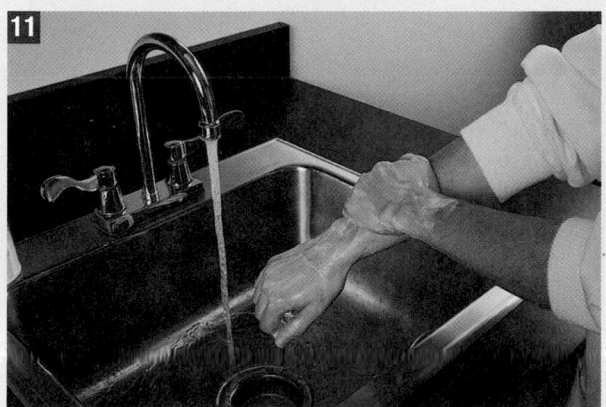

Wash wrists and forearms using friction. (From Bonewit-West K: *Clinical procedures for medical assistants,* ed 7, St. Louis, 2008, Saunders.)

12. Procedural Step. Clean the fingernails with a manicure stick. The fingernails should be cleaned at least once daily, preferably during initial handwashing (i.e., handwashing performed just after arriving at the medical office to begin your day).

Principle. Dirt and microorganisms collect underneath the fingernails.

13. Procedural Step. Rinse the arms and hands.

Principle. The running water rinses away the dirt and microorganisms.

14. Procedural Step. Repeat the handwashing procedure. For initial handwashing or when the hands come into contact with blood or other potentially infectious materials, the handwashing procedure should be repeated. This is to ensure removal of all pathogens.

15. Procedural Step. Dry the hands gently and thoroughly, and discard the paper towel.

Principle. Drying the hands gently prevents them from becoming chapped. Microorganisms can lodge in the crevices of chapped hands. Ensure the hands are dried completely because wet skin also may cause chapping.

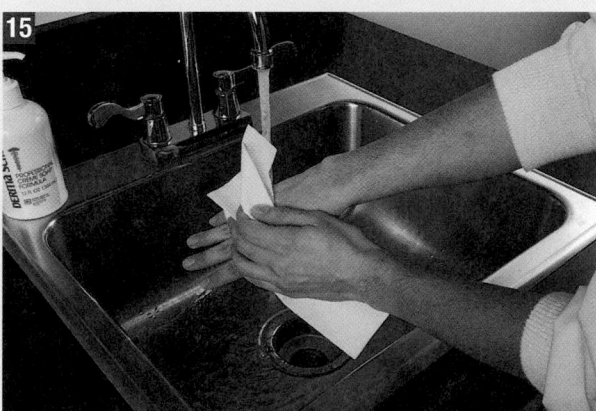

Dry the hands gently and thoroughly. (From Bonewit-West K: *Clinical procedures for medical assistants,* ed 7, St. Louis, 2008, Saunders.)

16. Procedural Step. Turn off the water, using a paper towel, and discard the paper towel in a waste container.

Principle. The faucet is considered contaminated, whereas the hands are medically aseptic or clean.

17. Procedural Step. Do not touch the sink with the bare hands.

Principle. The hands are now medically aseptic, and the sink is considered contaminated.

PROCEDURE 17-1

PROCEDURE **17-2**   Applying an Alcohol-Based Hand Rub

Outcome Apply an alcohol-based hand rub.

Equipment/Supplies

• Alcohol-based hand rub

1. **Procedural Step.** Inspect the hands to ensure they are not visibly soiled. Hands that are visibly soiled must be washed with soap and water.
   Principle. Alcohol-based hand rubs are not intended for the removal of visible soil.
2. **Procedural Step.** Remove your watch or push it up on the forearm. Avoid wearing rings. If you wear rings, remove all except a plain wedding band and put them in a safe place.
   Principle. Microorganisms can lodge in the crevices and grooves of rings.
3. **Procedural Step.** Apply the alcohol-based hand rub to the palm of one hand as follows:
   Gel or Lotion. Apply approximately 1 ml of the gel or lotion, which is an amount approximately equal to the size of a dime.
   Foam. Apply 3 g of foam, which is an amount approximately equal to the size of a walnut.
   Principle. Using more than the recommended amount results in a prolonged (and unnecessary) period of time for your hands to dry.
4. **Procedural Step.** Thoroughly spread the hand rub over all surfaces of both hands (and fingers) up to ½ inch above the wrist. Spread the hand rub around and under your fingernails.
   Principle. Failure to cover all surfaces can leave areas of the hands contaminated. Microorganisms tend to collect around and underneath the fingernails.

Apply lotion equal to the size of a dime. (From Bonewit-West K: *Clinical procedures for medical assistants,* ed 7, St. Louis, 2008, Saunders.)

Apply foam equal to the size of a walnut. (From Bonewit-West K: *Clinical procedures for medical assistants,* ed 7, St. Louis, 2008, Saunders.)

5. Procedural Step. Rub the hands together until they are dry, which usually takes 10 to 30 seconds. Allow your hands to dry completely before touching anything. The hands are now medically aseptic.

Note: After cleaning your hands 5 to 10 times with a hand rub, a buildup of emollients may occur on your hands. The emollients can be easily removed by washing your hands with soap and water.

Principle. If you have applied a sufficient amount of hand rub, it should take at least 10 to 30 seconds for your hands to feel dry. Your hands will still feel a little wet at first. Let them dry completely before touching anything.

Rub the hands together until they are dry. (From Bonewit-West K: *Clinical procedures for medical assistants,* ed 7, St. Louis, 2008, Saunders.)

see DVD

PROCEDURE **17-3**   Application and Removal of Clean Disposable Gloves

Outcome Apply and remove clean disposable gloves.

Equipment/Supplies

- Clean disposable gloves

Applying Clean Disposable Gloves

No special technique is required when clean disposable gloves are applied. This is because the hands are clean and the gloves are clean; the medical assistant can touch any part of the gloves during application without contaminating them.

1. Procedural Step. Remove all rings, and sanitize your hands. Handwashing should be performed if the hands are visibly soiled. If this is not the case, use an alcohol-based hand rub to sanitize the hands. Ensure your hands are completely dry.

Principle. Rings may cause the gloves to tear. The warm, moist environment inside gloves provides ideal growing conditions for the multiplication of transient microorganisms present on the hands. Sanitizing the hands removes these microorganisms and prevents the transmission of pathogens. Moisture encourages the growth of microorganisms.

2. Procedural Step. Choose the appropriate size of gloves; they should not be too small or too large. The gloves should fit snugly but not be too tight. Apply the gloves, and adjust them so that they fit comfortably.

Principle. If your gloves are too small, they may rip as you are applying them or become uncomfortable to wear. If they are too large, you may find it difficult to perform your tasks.

Apply the gloves. (From Bonewit-West K: *Clinical procedures for medical assistants,* ed 7, St. Louis, 2008, Saunders.)

3. Procedural Step. Inspect the gloves for tears. If a tear is present, a new pair of gloves must be applied.

Removing Clean Disposable Gloves

Gloves must be removed in a manner that protects the medical assistant from contaminating his or her clean hands with pathogens that may be present on the outside of the gloves. This is accomplished by not allowing the bare hands to come in contact with the outside of the gloves.

Continued

PROCEDURE **17-3** Application and Removal of Clean Disposable Gloves—cont'd

1. Procedural Step. Grasp the outside of the left glove 1 to 2 inches from the top with your gloved right hand. (*Note:* It does not matter which glove is removed first. You may start with the right glove if you prefer.)

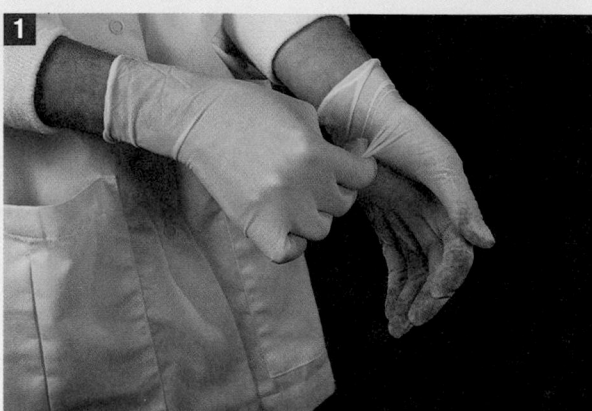

Grasp the glove 1 to 2 inches from the top of the glove. (From Bonewit-West K: *Clinical procedures for medical assistants,* ed 7, St. Louis, 2008, Saunders.)

2. Procedural Step. Slowly pull the left glove off the hand. It will turn inside out as it is removed from your hand.

3. Procedural Step. Pull the left glove free, and scrunch it into a ball with your gloved right hand.

Scrunch the glove into a ball. (From Bonewit-West K: *Clinical procedures for medical assistants,* ed 7, St. Louis, 2008, Saunders.)

4. Procedural Step. Place the index and middle finges of the left hand on the inside of the right glove. Do not allow your clean hand to touch the outside of the glove.

5. Procedural Step. Pull the glove off the right hand. It will turn inside out as it is removed from your hand, enclosing the balled-up left glove. Discard both gloves in an appropriate container. If your gloves are visibly contaminated with blood or other potentially infectious materials, discard them in a biohazard waste con-

tainer. Otherwise, they can be discarded in a regular waste container.

Place the index and middle fingers inside the glove. (From Bonewit-West K: *Clinical procedures for medical assistants,* ed 7, St. Louis, 2008, Saunders.)

Discard both gloves in an appropriate container. (From Bonewit-West K: *Clinical procedures for medical assistants,* ed 7, St. Louis, 2008, Saunders.)

6. Procedural Step. Sanitize your hands to remove any microorganisms that may have come in contact with your hands.

OSHA BLOODBORNE PATHOGENS STANDARD

Purpose of the Standard

The federal government established OSHA to assist employers in providing a safe and healthy working environment for their employees. To provide a safe working environment for health care workers, OSHA developed a comprehensive set of regulations known as the *OSHA Occupational Exposure to Bloodborne Pathogens Standard.*

These regulations went into effect in 1992 and are designed to reduce the risk to employees of exposure to infectious diseases.

The OSHA Bloodborne Pathogens Standard must be followed by any employee with occupational exposure to pathogens, regardless of the place of employment. In addition to medical assistants, employees with occupational exposure include physicians, nurses, dentists, dental hygienists, medical laboratory personnel, and emergency medical technicians. Employees who may have less obvious occupational exposure are correctional and law enforcement officers, firefighters, hospital laundry workers, morticians, and custodians.

Failure by employers to comply with the OSHA standard could result in a citation carrying a maximum penalty of $7000 for each violation and a maximum penalty of $70,000 for repeat violations.

Needlestick Safety and Prevention Act

Since the adoption of the OSHA Bloodborne Pathogens Standard, needlestick injuries among health care workers have continued to be a problem because of their high frequency of occurrence and the severity of the health effects associated with exposure to bloodborne pathogens. To address this problem, Congress passed the Needlestick Safety and Prevention Act (NSPA). The NSPA directed OSHA to revise the Bloodborne Pathogens Standard to incorporate stronger measures to reduce needlesticks and other sharps injuries among health care workers. In response to this mandate, the primary measure instituted by OSHA was to establish detailed requirements that employers identify and make use of safer medical devices. This revised

OSHA Bloodborne Pathogens Standard went into effect in 2001 and is described in detail in this chapter.

OSHA Terminology

The following definitions help clarify terms relating to the OSHA Bloodborne Pathogens Standard.

Occupational exposure Occupational exposure is reasonably anticipated skin, eye, mucous membrane, or parenteral contact with blood or other potentially infectious materials that may result from the performance of an employee's duties.

Parenteral *Parenteral* refers to the piercing of the skin barrier or mucous membranes, such as through needlesticks, human bites, cuts, and abrasions.

Blood *Blood* means human blood, human blood components, and products made from blood. Blood components include plasma, serum, platelets, and serosanguineous fluid (e.g., exudates from wounds). An example of a blood product is a medication derived from blood, such as immune globulins.

Bloodborne pathogens Bloodborne pathogens are pathogenic microorganisms in human blood that can cause disease in humans. Bloodborne pathogens include, but are not limited to, hepatitis B virus (HBV), hepatitis C virus (HCV), and human immunodeficiency virus (HIV).

Other potentially infectious materials Other potentially infectious materials (OPIM) include the following:
- Semen and vaginal secretions
- Cerebrospinal, synovial, pleural, pericardial, peritoneal, and amniotic fluids
- Any body fluid that is visibly contaminated with blood
- Any body fluid that has not been identified
- Saliva in dental procedures
- Any unfixed human tissue
- Any tissue culture, cells, or fluid known to be HIV infected

Contaminated *Contaminated* is defined as the presence or reasonably anticipated presence of blood or OPIM on an item or surface.

Decontamination Decontamination is the use of physical or chemical means to remove, inactivate, or destroy pathogens on a surface or item to the point that they are no longer capable of transmitting infectious particles, and the surface or item is rendered safe for handling, use, or disposal.

Nonintact skin Nonintact skin is skin that has a break in the surface. It includes, but is not limited to, skin with dermatitis, abrasions, cuts, burns, hangnails, chapping, and acne.

Exposure incident *Exposure incident* is defined as a specific eye, nose, mouth, other mucous membrane, nonintact skin, or parenteral contact with blood or OPIM that results from an employee's duties.

What Would You Do? What Would You *Not* Do?

Case Study 1

Petra Meyer has come in for her annual gynecologic examination. She notices that alcohol-based hand rubs are being used in the medical office. She says that she has seen them in the grocery store and wants to know if they are as good as regular soap and water for washing hands. Petra wants to know how much to use and how long to rinse the hands after applying them. Petra says she likes to garden and wants to know if hand rubs are effective in removing ground-in soil from the hands. Petra also is curious to know why they are now being used so much in health care settings. ■

Components of the OSHA Standard

The OSHA Bloodborne Pathogens Standard is presented on the following pages as it pertains to the medical office and includes the following categories:

- Exposure control plan
- Safer medical devices
- Labeling requirements
- Communication of hazards to employees
- Record-keeping

Exposure Control Plan

The OSHA standard requires that the medical office develop an exposure control plan (ECP) (Figure 17-3). The ECP is a written document stipulating the protective measures that must be followed in that medical office to eliminate or minimize employee exposure to bloodborne pathogens and OPIM. The ECP must be made available for review by all medical office staff. The ECP must include the following elements:

1. **An exposure determination.** The purpose of this section of the ECP is to identify employees who must receive training, protective equipment, hepatitis vaccination, and other protections required by the Bloodborne Pathogens Standard. The exposure determination must include (1) a list of all job classifications in which *all* employees are likely to have occupational exposure, such as physicians, medical assistants, and laboratory technicians, and (2) a list of job classifications in which only *some* employees have occupational exposure, such as custodians. For the second classification of jobs, the determination must include a list of tasks in which occupational exposure may occur, such as emptying the trash.

2. **The method of compliance.** The method of compliance section of the ECP must document the specific health and safety control measures that are taken in the medical office to eliminate or minimize the risk of occupational exposure. These measures are extremely important in reducing the risk of the medical assistant to infectious diseases and are discussed in more detail later in this section (see Control Measures).

3. **Postexposure evaluation and follow-up procedures.** The postexposure evaluation and follow-up must specify the procedures to follow in the event of an exposure incident in the medical office, including the method of documenting and investigating an exposure incident and the postexposure evaluation, medical treatment, and follow-up that would be made available to the employee. (Refer to the *OSHA Postexposure Evaluation and Follow-Up Procedures* box.)

OSHA requires employers to review and update their ECP at least annually to ensure that the plan remains current with the latest information on eliminating or reducing exposure to bloodborne pathogens. The ECP also must be updated whenever necessary to reflect new or modified tasks and procedures that affect occupational exposure.

Labeling Requirements

The OSHA Bloodborne Pathogens Standard requires that containers and appliances containing biohazardous materials be labeled with a *biohazard warning label*. The biohazard warning label must be fluorescent orange or orange-red and contain the biohazard symbol and the word "BIOHAZARD" in a contrasting color (Figure 17-4A).

A warning label must be attached to the following: (1) containers of regulated waste; (2) refrigerators and freezers used to store blood and OPIM; and (3) containers and bags used to store, transport, or ship blood or OPIM (Figure 17-4B). Red bags or red containers may be substituted for biohazard warning labels. The labeling requirement is designed to alert employees to possible exposure, particularly in situations where the nature of the material or contents is not readily identifiable as blood or OPIM.

Communicating Hazards to Employees

According to the OSHA standard, employers must ensure that all medical office employees with risk of occupational exposure participate in a training program. The program must present the ECP for the medical office, focusing on the measures that employees are to take for their safety. Training must be provided at the time an employee is initially assigned to tasks in which occupational exposure may occur and at least annually thereafter.

The employer must maintain records of the training sessions, which must include presentation dates, content of

Figure 17-3. Example of an exposure control plan. (From Bonewit-West K: *Clinical procedures for medical assistants,* ed 7, St. Louis, 2008, Saunders.)

OSHA Postexposure Evaluation and Follow-Up Procedures

An exposure incident is a specific eye, nose, mouth, other mucous membrane, nonintact skin, or parenteral contact with blood or other potentially infectious materials (OPIM) that results from an employee's duties. In the event of an exposure incident to bloodborne pathogens or OPIM, OSHA requires the following steps to be performed:

1. Perform initial first aid measures immediately (e.g., wash a needlestick injury thoroughly with soap and water).
2. Document the route of exposure and the conditions and circumstances of the exposure incident. This includes such information as the engineering controls, work practice controls, and personal protective equipment being used at the time of the incident.
3. Identify and document the source individual (unless the employer can establish that identification is not feasible or is prohibited by state or local law). A source individual is any person, living or dead, whose blood or OPIM may be a source of occupational exposure to the health care worker.
4. Obtain consent to test the source individual's blood. Test it as soon as possible to determine HBV, HCV, and HIV infectivity. The following guidelines apply to this requirement:
   - If consent is not obtained, the employer must document that legally required consent cannot be obtained.
   - If the source individual's consent is not required by law, the source individual's blood (if available) must be tested and the results documented.
   - If the source individual is already known to be infected with HBV, HCV, or HIV, testing does not need to be repeated.
5. Provide the exposed employee with the source individual's test results. Inform the employee of applicable laws and regulations concerning disclosure of the identity and infectious status of the source individual.
6. Obtain consent to test the employee's blood. Collect and test the blood of the employee as soon as possible for HBV, HCV, and HIV serologic status. If the employee does not give consent for HIV serologic testing, the baseline blood sample must be preserved for at least 90 days. If the employee elects to have the baseline sample tested during the 90-day waiting period, such testing must be done as soon as feasible.
7. When medically indicated, provide the employee with appropriate postexposure prophylaxis as recommended by the U.S. Public Health Service.

the sessions, names and qualifications of the trainers, and names and job titles of employees who attended. These records must be maintained for 3 years from the date of the training session.

Record-Keeping

The OSHA Bloodborne Pathogens Standard requires that the following records be maintained:

Figure 17-4. A, Biohazard warning label. **B,** Biohazard bag used to hold and transport blood or other potentially infectious materials. (From Bonewit-West K: *Clinical procedures for medical assistants,* ed 7, St. Louis, 2008, Saunders.)

1. **OSHA medical record.** The OSHA standard requires that the employer maintain an accurate OSHA record of every medical office employee at risk for occupational exposure. These records must be kept confidential except for review by OSHA officials and as required by law. The record must include the following: employee's name; Social Security number; hepatitis B vaccination status, including dates of vaccination; results of any postexposure examinations, medical testing, and follow-up procedures; and a written evaluation of any exposure incident along with a copy of the exposure incident report. The employer is required to maintain records for the duration of employment plus 30 years.

2. **Sharps injury log.** Employers with more than 10 employees at risk for occupational exposure are required to maintain a log of injuries from contaminated sharps. The log must be maintained in a way that protects the confidentiality of injured employees (e.g., removal of personal identification). The purpose of the log is to help employers and employees keep track of all needlestick injuries. This tracking helps identify problem areas that need attention and ineffective devices that need to be replaced. The sharps injury log must contain the following information:

- Type and brand of device involved in the injury
- Location of the incident (i.e., work area)
- Explanation of how the incident occurred

Control Measures

Specific health and safety control measures are required by OSHA to eliminate or minimize the risk of occupational exposure in the medical office. These measures are divided into six categories: engineering controls, work practice controls, personal protective equipment, housekeeping, hepatitis B vaccination, and universal precautions.

Engineering Controls

The medical office must use engineering controls to eliminate or minimize the risk of occupational exposure. *Engineering controls* include all control measures that isolate or remove health hazards from the workplace. Engineering controls must be examined and maintained or replaced as required to ensure their effectiveness. Examples of engineering controls include the following:

- Readily accessible handwashing facilities
- Safer medical devices

- Biohazard sharps containers and biohazard bags
- Autoclaves

Safer Medical Devices

Safer medical devices are one example of an engineering control. A *safer medical device* is a device that, based on reasonable judgment, would make an exposure incident involving a contaminated sharp less likely. *Reasonable judgment* refers to the judgment of the health care worker who would be using the device.

Safer medical devices include sharps with engineered sharps injury protection and needleless systems. A *sharp with engineered sharps injury protection* (SESIP) is a non-needle sharp or a needle device with a built-in safety feature used for procedures that involve the risk of a sharps injury. Examples of SESIPs include safety engineered syringes and phlebotomy devices (Figure 17-5).

A *needleless system* is a device that does not use a needle for (1) the administration of medication or other fluids, (2) the collection or withdrawal of body fluids after initial access to a vein or artery is established, or (3) any other procedure involving the potential for occupational exposure to bloodborne pathogens as a result of percutaneous injuries from contaminated sharps. An example of a needleless system is a jet injection syringe, which uses compressed air to administer an injection rather than a needle.

Employers are required to evaluate and implement commercially available safer medical devices and other engineering controls that eliminate occupational exposure to the lowest extent feasible. Input from employees involved in direct patient care must be taken into consideration in making this determination. This helps to ensure that the individuals who are using the devices have the opportunity for input. As part of the annual review of the exposure

Figure 17-5. A, Safety engineered syringe. **B,** Safety engineered phlebotomy device. (From Bonewit-West K: *Clinical procedures for medical assistants,* ed 7, St. Louis, 2008, Saunders.)

control plan, the following information must be documented: (1) safer medical devices that reflect changes in technology are being evaluated and implemented in the workplace, and (2) input was obtained from employees in selecting safer medical devices.

Work Practice Controls

Work practice controls reduce the likelihood of exposure by altering the manner in which the technique is performed. It is important that the medical assistant consistently adhere to these safety rules, which include the following:

1. Perform all procedures involving blood or OPIM in a manner that minimizes splashing, spraying, spattering, and generation of droplets of these substances.
2. Observe warning labels on biohazard containers and appliances. Bags or containers that bear a biohazard warning label or are color-coded red indicate that they hold blood or OPIM. Refrigerators, freezers, and other appliances that contain hazardous materials also must bear a biohazard warning label.
3. Bandage cuts and other lesions on the hands before gloving.
4. Sanitize the hands after removing gloves, regardless of whether or not the gloves are visibly contaminated.
5. If your hands or other skin surfaces come in contact with blood or OPIM, thoroughly wash the area as soon as possible with soap and water.
6. If your mucous membranes (e.g., eyes, mouth, nose) come in contact with blood or OPIM, flush them with water as soon as possible.
7. Do not break or shear contaminated needles.
8. Do not remove, recap, or bend a contaminated needle except in unusual circumstances when no other alternative is possible or when it is required by a specific medical procedure. Such actions must be performed by a method other than the traditional two-handed procedure. Needle removal can be accomplished with a one-handed technique using a sharps container with a well-designed unwinder. Recapping must be performed through the use of a one-handed technique; using a two-handed technique is strictly prohibited. The one-handed recapping technique involves holding the syringe in the dominant hand and picking up the needle with the cap using a scooping motion. The cap is secured onto the needle by pushing it against a hard surface. (*Note:* Sterile needles may be recapped, such as after the withdrawal of medication from a vial or ampule.)
9. Immediately after use, place contaminated sharps in a puncture-resistant, leakproof container that is appropriately labeled or color-coded. *Contaminated sharps* are contaminated objects that can penetrate the skin, including (but not limited to) needles, lancets, scalpels, broken glass, and capillary tubes.
10. Do not eat, drink, smoke, apply cosmetics or lip balm, or handle contact lenses in areas where you may be exposed to blood or OPIM.
11. Do not store food or drink in refrigerators, freezers, or cabinets or on shelves or countertops where blood or OPIM are present.
12. Place blood specimens or OPIM in containers that prevent leakage during collection, handling, processing, storage, transport, or shipping. Ensure the containers are closed before being stored, transported, or shipped and are labeled or color-coded for easy identification.
13. Before any equipment that might be contaminated is serviced or shipped for repair or cleaning, such as a centrifuge, it must be inspected for blood or OPIM. If such material is present, the equipment must be decontaminated. If it cannot be decontaminated, it must be appropriately labeled to indicate clearly the contamination site, to enable those coming into contact with the equipment to take appropriate precautions.
14. If you are exposed to blood or OPIM, perform first aid measures immediately (e.g., wash a needlestick injury thoroughly with soap and water). After taking these measures, report the incident to your physician-employer as soon as possible so that postexposure procedures can be instituted. (See the box titled *OSHA Postexposure Evaluation and Follow-Up Procedures*.) The most obvious exposure incident is a needlestick, but any eye, mouth, or other mucous membrane, nonintact skin, or parenteral contact with blood or OPIM constitutes an exposure incident and should be reported.

Personal Protective Equipment

The OSHA standard specifies that personal protective equipment must be used in the medical office whenever occupational exposure remains after instituting engineering and work practice controls. *Personal protective equipment* is clothing or equipment that protects an individual from contact with blood or OPIM; examples include gloves, chin-length face shields, masks, protective eyewear, laboratory coats, and gowns. The type of protective equipment appropriate for a given task depends on the degree of exposure that is anticipated, as outlined here:

1. Wear gloves when it is reasonably anticipated that your hands will have contact with blood and OPIM, mucous membranes, or nonintact skin; when performing vascular access procedures; and when handling or touching contaminated surfaces or items. Gloves cannot prevent a needlestick or other sharps injury, but they can prevent a pathogen from entering the body through a break in the skin, such as a cut, abrasion, burn, or rash.

Figure 17-6. Jennifer wears a combination mask and eye-protection device and a laboratory coat to protect against splashes, spray, spatter, and droplets of blood. (From Bonewit-West K: *Clinical procedures for medical assistants,* ed 7, St. Louis, 2008, Saunders.)

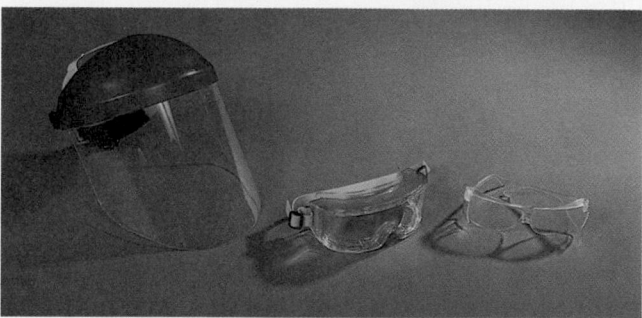

Figure 17-7. Examples of eye-protection devices. *Left,* Face shield; *center,* goggles; *right,* glasses with solid side shields. (From Bonewit-West K: *Clinical procedures for medical assistants,* ed 7, St. Louis, 2008, Saunders.)

2. Wear chin-length face shields or masks in combination with eye-protection devices whenever splashes, spray, spatter, or droplets of blood or OPIM may be generated, posing a hazard through contact with the eyes, nose, or mouth (e.g., removing a stopper from a tube of blood, transferring serum from whole blood) (Figure 17-6).

3. Wear appropriate protective clothing, such as gowns, aprons, and laboratory coats, when gross contamination can reasonably be anticipated during performance of a task or procedure (e.g., laboratory testing procedure). The type of protective clothing depends on the task and degree of exposure anticipated.

Personal Protective Equipment Guidelines

Certain guidelines must be followed when using protective equipment:

1. Protective equipment must not allow blood or OPIM to pass through or reach the skin, underlying garments (e.g., scrubs, street clothes, undergarments), eyes, mouth, or other mucous membranes under normal conditions of use and for the duration of time the protective equipment is used.

2. The employer must provide appropriate personal protective equipment at no cost to you. The employer is responsible for ensuring the equipment is available in appropriate sizes, is readily accessible, and is used correctly. In addition, the employer must ensure that the equipment is cleaned, laundered, repaired, replaced, or disposed of as needed to ensure its effectiveness.

3. Alternatives must be provided for employees who are allergic to the gloves normally provided. Examples of alternatives include hypoallergenic gloves and powderless gloves.

4. If gloves become contaminated, torn, or punctured, replace them as soon as practical.

What Would You Do? What Would You *Not* Do?

Case Study 2

Tracy Smith is pregnant and is at the medical office to have her blood drawn for a prenatal profile. Tracy says she does not understand why gloves have to be worn when her blood is drawn. She says that it makes her feel like a leper, and she is absolutely sure that she does not have any diseases. Tracy says she has been reading information about the hepatitis B vaccine because she knows her baby will be given this vaccine soon after birth. She wants to know why it is recommended that an infant be immunized for hepatitis B. Tracy says that infants are not at risk for contracting hepatitis B because the way it is transmitted is mostly through sexual contact and illegal drug use. ■

5. All eye-protection devices must have solid side shields; chin-length face shields, goggles, and glasses with solid side shields are acceptable (Figure 17-7); standard prescription eyeglasses are unacceptable as eye protection.

6. If a garment is penetrated by blood or OPIM, it must be removed as soon as possible and placed in an appropriately designated container for washing.

7. All personal protective equipment must be removed before leaving the medical office.

8. When protective equipment is removed, it must be placed in an appropriately designated area or container for storage, washing, decontamination, or disposal.

9. Utility gloves may be decontaminated and reused unless they are cracked, peeling, torn, or punctured or no longer provide barrier protection.

10. If you believe using protective equipment would prevent proper delivery of health care or would pose an increased hazard to your safety or that of a coworker, in extenuating circumstances you may temporarily and briefly decline its use. After such an incident, the circumstances must be investigated to determine whether the situation could be prevented in the future.

Housekeeping

The OSHA standard requires that specific housekeeping procedures be followed to ensure that the work site is maintained in a clean and sanitary condition. The medical office must develop and implement a written schedule for cleaning and decontaminating each area where exposure occurs. The cleaning and decontamination method must be specified for each task and should be based on the type of surface to be cleaned, the type of soil present, and the tasks or procedures being performed in that area. Housekeeping procedures include the following:

1. Clean and decontaminate equipment and work surfaces after completing procedures that involve blood or OPIM. Cleaning is accomplished using a detergent soap, and decontamination is performed using an appropriate disinfectant (Figure 17-8).
2. Clean and decontaminate all equipment and work surfaces as soon as possible after exposure to blood or OPIM. For the decontamination of blood spills, OSHA recommends the use of a 10% solution of sodium hypochlorite (household bleach) in water (1 part bleach to 10 parts water).
3. Inspect and decontaminate all reusable receptacles, such as bins, pails, and cans, on a regular basis. If contamination is visible, the item must be cleaned and decontaminated as soon as possible.
4. Do not pick up broken, contaminated glassware with the hands, even if gloves are worn. Use mechanical means, such as a brush and dustpan, tongs, and forceps (Figure 17-9).
5. Protective coverings, such as plastic wrap and aluminum foil, may be used to cover work surfaces or equipment, but they must be removed or replaced if contamination occurs.
6. Handle contaminated laundry as little as possible and with appropriate personal protective equipment. Place all contaminated laundry in leakproof bags that are properly labeled or color-coded. Contaminated laundry must not be sorted or rinsed at the medical office.
7. If the outside of a biohazard container becomes contaminated, it must be placed in a second suitable container.
8. Biohazard sharps containers (Figure 17-10) must be closable, puncture resistant, and leakproof. They must bear a biohazard warning label and be color-coded red to ensure identification of the contents as hazardous. To ensure effectiveness, the following guidelines must be observed:
   - Locate the sharps container as close as possible to the area of use to avoid the hazard of transporting a contaminated needle through the workplace.

Figure 17-9. Use mechanical means to pick up broken contaminated glass. (From Bonewit-West K: *Clinical procedures for medical assistants,* ed 7, St. Louis, 2008, Saunders.)

Figure 17-8. Clean and decontaminate work surfaces with an appropriate disinfectant after completing procedures involving blood and other potentially infectious materials. (From Bonewit-West K: *Clinical procedures for medical assistants,* ed 7, St. Louis, 2008, Saunders.)

Figure 17-10. Biohazard sharps containers. (From Bonewit-West K: *Clinical procedures for medical assistants,* ed 7, St. Louis, 2008, Saunders.)

- Maintain sharps containers in an upright position to keep liquid and sharps inside.
- Do not reach into the sharps container with your hand.
- Replace sharps containers on a regular basis, and do not allow them to overfill. (Experts recommend that sharps containers be replaced when they are three-quarters full.)

Hepatitis B Vaccination

The OSHA standard requires physicians to offer the hepatitis B vaccination series free of charge to all medical office personnel who have occupational exposure. The vaccination must be offered within 10 working days of initial assignment to a position with occupational exposure, unless the following factors exist: (1) The individual has previously received the hepatitis B vaccination series, (2) antibody testing has revealed that the individual is immune to hepatitis B, or (3) the vaccine is contraindicated for medical reasons.

Medical office personnel who decline vaccination must sign a hepatitis B waiver form documenting refusal. This form must be filed in the employee's OSHA record (Figure 17-11). Employees who decline vaccination may request the vaccination later, which the employer must then provide according to the aforementioned criteria.

Universal Precautions

Before the release of the OSHA standard, the CDC issued recommendations for health care workers known as the *Universal Precautions.* According to the concept of Universal Precautions, all human blood and certain human body fluids are treated as though known to be infectious for HIV, HBV, HCV, and other bloodborne pathogens. The OSHA standard states that the Universal Precautions must be observed; these precautions form the heart of the OSHA standard itself.

REGULATED MEDICAL WASTE

Medical waste is generated in the medical office through the diagnosis, treatment, and immunization of patients. Some of this waste poses a threat to health and safety and is known as **regulated medical waste (RMW).** The OSHA Bloodborne Pathogens Standard defines RMW as follows:
- Any liquid or semiliquid blood or OPIM
- Items contaminated with blood or OPIM that would release these substances in a liquid or semiliquid state if compressed
- Items that are caked with dried blood or OPIM and are capable of releasing these materials during handling
- Contaminated sharps
- Pathologic and microbiologic wastes that contain blood or OPIM

RMW must be discarded properly so as not to become a source of transfer of disease. According to the OSHA definition, a dressing saturated with blood is considered RMW and must be discarded in a biohazard bag. A bandage with a spot of blood on it is not considered RMW and can be discarded in a regular waste container. Box 17-2 gives the guidelines for discarding medical waste in the medical office.

Highlight on OSHA Bloodborne Pathogens Standard

General Information

The exposure control plan (ECP) must be made available to OSHA on request.

OSHA inspectors are responsible for determining whether the medical office meets the Bloodborne Pathogens Standard. This is accomplished through a careful review of the ECP, interviews with the medical office employer and employees, and observation of work activities.

Feces, nasal secretions, saliva, sputum, sweat, tears, urine, and vomitus are not considered by OSHA to be potentially infectious material unless they contain blood.

Control Measures

Employees must be trained in the proper use of the following: engineering controls (including safer medical devices), work practice controls, and personal protective equipment.

General work clothes, such as scrubs, uniforms, pants, shirts, and blouses, are not intended to function as protection against a hazard and are not considered personal protective equipment.

Employees are not permitted to launder contaminated clothing at home; it is the employer's responsibility to have contaminated clothing laundered.

If an employee is allergic to the standard latex gloves, the employer must provide a suitable alternative, such as hypoallergenic gloves.

Needlestick Injuries

The CDC estimates that every year 600,000 to 800,000 health care workers in the United States experience needlestick and other sharps injuries, and 1000 of these individuals contract serious infections as a result of these injuries. The CDC estimates that 62% to 88% of sharps injuries can be prevented by the use of safer medical devices.

A wide variety of commercially available safer medical devices have been developed to reduce the risk of needlestick and other sharps injuries.

Safer medical devices that eliminate exposure to the lowest extent feasible must be evaluated and implemented in the health care setting. The lack of injuries on the sharps injury log does *not* exempt the employer from this provision. ∎

HEPATITIS B VACCINE REFUSAL

I understand that due to my occupational exposure to blood or other potentially infectious materials, I may be at risk of acquiring hepatitis B virus (HBV) infection. I have been given the opportunity to be vaccinated with hepatitis B vaccine at no charge to myself. However, I decline hepatitis B vaccination at this time. I understand that by declining this vaccine I continue to be at risk of acquiring hepatitis B, a serious disease. If in the future I continue to have occupational exposure to blood or to other potentially infectious materials and I want to be vaccinated with hepatitis B vaccine, I can receive the vaccination series at no charge to me.

_____

Employee Name (printed)

_____   _____

Employee Signature   Date

_____   _____

Witness Signature   Date

Figure 17-11. Hepatitis B vaccine waiver form. This form must be signed by an employee with occupational exposure who declines hepatitis B vaccination. (From Bonewit-West K: *Clinical procedures for medical assistants,* ed 7, St. Louis, 2008, Saunders.)

BOX 17-2 Guidelines for Discarding Medical Waste in the Medical Office

Regular Waste Container

The following items that have been used for health care are not considered regulated medical waste (RMW) and can be discarded in a covered waste container lined with a regular trash bag.

- Disposable drapes
- Disposable patient gowns
- Examining table paper
- Disposable clean or sterile gloves
- Gauze tinged with blood or other body fluids
- Disposable probe covers for thermometers
- Tongue depressors
- Tissues with respiratory secretions
- Disposable ear speculums
- Empty urine containers
- Urine testing strips
- Disposable diapers
- Feminine hygiene products

Biohazard Sharps Container

The following items are sharps. They are considered RMW and must be discarded in a biohazard sharps container.

- Hypodermic syringes and needles
- Venipuncture needles
- Lancets
- Razor blades
- Scalpel blades
- Suture needles
- Blood tubes
- Capillary pipets

- Microscope slides and coverslips
- Broken glassware

Biohazard Bag Waste Container

The following items are considered RMW. They are not sharps and can be discarded in a covered waste container lined with a biohazard bag.

- Any item saturated or dripping with blood or other potentially infectious materials (OPIM) (e.g., dressings, gauze, cotton balls, paper towels, and tissues that are saturated or dripping with blood)
- Any item caked with dried blood or OPIM, such as dressings and sutures
- Disposable clean or sterile gloves contaminated with blood or OPIM
- Disposable vaginal speculums and collection devices (swabs, spatulas, brushes)
- Tissue or fluid removed during minor office surgery
- Microbiologic waste, such as specimen cultures and collection devices
- Discarded live and attenuated vaccines

Sanitary Sewer

Disposal of small quantities of blood and other body fluids to the sanitary sewer is considered a safe method of disposing of these waste materials. The following fluids can be carefully poured down a utility sink, drain, or toilet. (*Note:* State regulations may dictate the maximum volume allowable for discharge of blood or body fluids into the sanitary sewer.)

- Blood
- Body excretions such as urine
- Body secretions such as sputum

From Bonewit-West K: *Clinical procedures for medical assistants,* ed 7, St. Louis, 2008, Saunders.

Handling Regulated Medical Waste

RMW must be handled carefully to prevent an exposure incident. The OSHA Bloodborne Pathogens Standard outlines specific actions to take when handling RMW, as follows:

1. Separate regulated waste from the general refuse at its point of origin. Disposable items containing RMW should be placed directly into biohazard containers and not mixed with the regular trash.
2. Ensure that biohazard containers are closable, leakproof, and suitably constructed to contain the contents during handling, storage, and transport. These containers include biohazard bags and sharps containers.
3. To prevent spillage or protrusion of the contents, close the lid of a sharps container before removing it from an examining room. Never open, empty, or clean a contaminated sharps container. If there is a chance of leakage from the sharps container, the medical assistant should place it in a second container that is closable, leakproof, and appropriately labeled or color-coded.
4. Securely close biohazard bags before removing them from an examining room. To provide additional protection, some medical offices double-bag by placing the primary bag inside a second biohazard bag.
5. Transport full biohazard containers to a secured area away from the general public, using personal protective equipment (e.g., gloves).

Disposal of Regulated Medical Waste

Each state is responsible for developing policies for disposal of RMW. To avoid noncompliance, it is important for the medical assistant to know and understand the specific regulated waste policies and guidelines set forth in his or her state.

Most medical offices use a commercial medical waste service to dispose of RMW. The service is responsible for picking up and transporting the medical waste to a treatment facility for incineration to destroy pathogens and render it harmless. The waste can then be safely disposed of in a sanitary landfill. Regulated waste treatment facilities must be licensed and hold permits issued by the Environmental Protection Agency (EPA), allowing them to dispose of RMW.

A series of steps must be followed for preparing and storing RMW for pickup by the service. Although these steps may vary slightly from state to state, general measures required by most states include the following:

1. Place biohazard bags and sharps containers into a receptacle provided by the medical waste service. The receptacle is usually a cardboard box (Figure 17-12). The box should be securely sealed with packing tape, and a biohazard warning label must appear on two opposite sides of the box.
2. Store the biohazard boxes in a locked room inside the facility or in a locked collection container outside for pickup by the medical waste service. This step is aimed

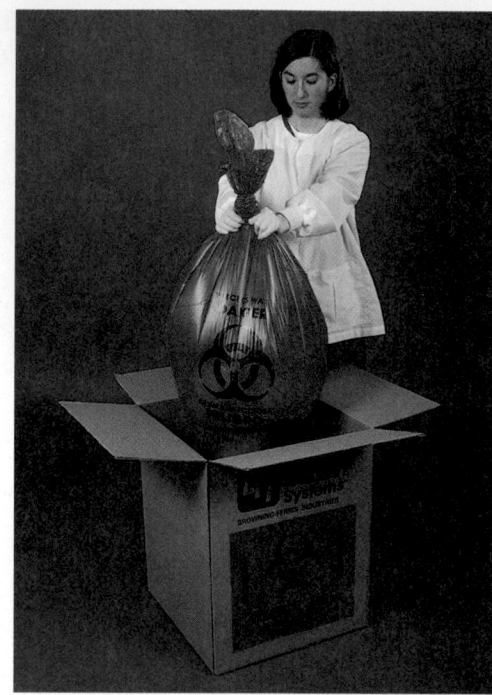

Figure 17-12. Jennifer places a biohazard bag inside a cardboard box in preparation for pickup by the medical waste service. (From Bonewit-West K: *Clinical procedures for medical assistants,* ed 7, St. Louis, 2008, Saunders.)

What Would You Do? What Would You *Not* Do?

Case Study 3

Giles Lee is 45 years old and is at the medical office. Twenty-five years ago, he was in a serious car accident and had to have a blood transfusion. He says that he donated blood for the first time 2 months ago. Last week he received a letter saying that his blood tested positive for hepatitis C and that he should see his physician. Giles says that he must have gotten hepatitis C from the blood transfusion he received when he was 20. He does not understand how that could have happened because the blood supply is tested for these types of diseases. Giles wants to know why he has not had any symptoms. He also wants to know if he can give hepatitis C to his wife and teenage children. ∎

at preventing unauthorized access to items such as needles and syringes. The regulated waste storage area should be labeled with one of the following:
- "Authorized Personnel Only" sign
- International biohazard symbol
3. Many states require that a tracking record be completed when the waste is picked up by the medical waste service. The form includes such information as the type and quantity of waste (weighed in pounds) and where it is being sent. The form must be signed by a representative of the medical waste service and the medical office. After the waste has been destroyed at the regulated waste treatment facility, a record documenting its disposal is mailed to the medical office.

BLOODBORNE DISEASES

The biggest threats to health care workers from occupational exposure are HBV, HCV, and HIV. Hepatitis is much easier to transmit than is HIV. After a needlestick exposure to blood infected with HBV, health care workers who are not immune to hepatitis B have a 6% to 30% chance of developing the disease. The risk of infection after a needlestick exposure to blood infected with HCV is approximately 2%. After a needlestick exposure to HIV-infected blood, a health care worker has a 0.3% chance of developing AIDS; he or she has a 0.09% chance of developing AIDS after a mucous membrane exposure.

Hepatitis B

Hepatitis B is an infection of the liver caused by HBV. The most common means of transmitting hepatitis B in the health care setting are blood and blood components, such as serum and plasma.

Health care workers are most likely to contract hepatitis B through needlesticks and cuts with contaminated sharps. The virus is also spread in the health care setting, but less effectively, through blood splashes to the eyes, mouth, and nonintact skin and through body fluids such as semen and vaginal secretions.

The number of health care workers who contract hepatitis in the workplace has declined dramatically since the development of the OHSA standard and the hepatitis B vaccine. Statistics show that in 1983, there were more than 10,000 health care workers who contracted hepatitis B in the workplace, but by 2001, that number had decreased to fewer than 400 health care workers. Preventive treatment is available for individuals exposed to hepatitis B who have not been vaccinated.

Postexposure Prophylaxis

Postexposure prophylaxis (PEP) refers to treatment administered to an individual after exposure to an infectious disease to prevent the disease. The PEP for unvaccinated individuals exposed to hepatitis B involves the administration of a passive and an active immunizing agent. It is important to administer both of these agents as soon as possible after an exposure incident—preferably within 24 hours, but no later than 7 days.

The passive immunizing agent provides temporary immunity to hepatitis B, giving the active agent a chance to take effect. The passive agent is hepatitis B immune globulin (HBIG), which contains antibodies that provide immunity to hepatitis B for 1 to 3 months.

The *active immunizing agent* in the hepatitis B vaccine (Figure 17-13) is produced from genetically altered yeast cells; brand names are Recombivax HB and Engerix-B. The hepatitis B vaccine is administered intramuscularly in a series of three doses. The second dose is given 1 month after the first dose, and the third dose is administered 6 months after the first dose (i.e., 0, 1 month, and 6 months). Mild side effects, such as soreness at the injection site, may

Highlight on Hepatitis B Vaccine

The hepatitis B vaccine became available in 1982 and is 95% effective in providing immunity.

The hepatitis B vaccine is well tolerated by most patients. The most common side effect is soreness at the injection site, including induration, erythema, and swelling. Occasionally, a low-grade fever, headache, and dizziness occur.

Current data show that the vaccine-induced antibodies may decline over time, but the immune system memory that programs the body to produce these antibodies remains intact indefinitely. Because of this, an individual with declining antibodies is still protected against hepatitis B. At present, the CDC does not recommend a booster dose once an individual has received the initial (three-dose) vaccine series.

The hepatitis B vaccine is recommended for all infants, children, and adolescents who are 18 years old or younger. It also is recommended for adults older than 18 years who are at increased risk for developing hepatitis B. This population includes employees with occupational exposure (e.g., health care workers), hemodialysis patients, hemophiliacs, individuals with multiple sex partners, homosexually active men, injection drug users, and household and sexual contacts of individuals with chronic hepatitis B.

The number of individuals contracting hepatitis B has decreased sharply since the development of the hepatitis B vaccine. As more people become immune to hepatitis B through the immunization of infants, the goal of eliminating hepatitis B in the United States may be realized. ∎

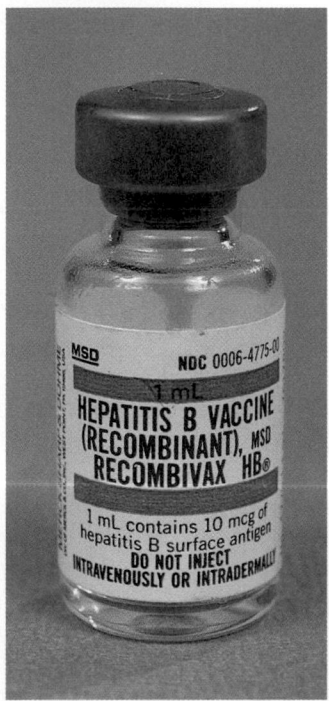

Figure 17-13. Hepatitis B vaccine. (From Bonewit-West K: *Clinical procedures for medical assistants*, ed 7, St. Louis, 2008, Saunders.)

occur, but serious reactions to the vaccine are extremely rare.

As previously discussed, the OSHA standard recommends that all health care workers receive the hepatitis B vaccine (an active immunizing agent) as a preventive measure against hepatitis B. After an exposure incident, a medical assistant who has previously been vaccinated probably would not require further treatment, unless laboratory tests reveal that his or her antibody level is low. In this case, a booster dose of the vaccine is recommended.

Hepatitis C

Hepatitis C is an infection of the liver caused by HCV. Currently, no vaccine is available for the prevention of hepatitis C. In the medical office, the most likely means of contracting hepatitis C is through needlesticks and other sharps injuries. The chance of contracting hepatitis C in the health care setting is much lower than that of contracting hepatitis B.

Most individuals with acute hepatitis C have no symptoms; if symptoms do occur, they are mild and flulike.

Highlight on Viral Hepatitis

In the United States, there are an estimated 150,000 new cases of hepatitis each year. Approximately 42% of these infections are caused by hepatitis B, 40% are caused by hepatitis A, and 18% are caused by hepatitis C.

Symptoms common to all types of hepatitis include fatigue, nausea, loss of appetite, abdominal pain, and jaundice.

Hepatitis A, B, and C are designated as nationally notifiable diseases by the CDC. When the physician diagnoses a case of hepatitis A, B, or C, a reportable disease form must be completed and filed with the local public health department.

In recent years, antiviral drugs have been developed to treat the chronic forms of hepatitis B and C; however, not all infected individuals are candidates for treatment. These drugs, which must be taken for a prolonged time, are effective in removing the virus from approximately 40% of chronically infected patients.

Hepatitis B

The most common means of transmission of hepatitis B is through sexual contact with an infected individual and by sharing needles for injection drug use with an infected individual. Hepatitis B is not spread by sneezing, coughing, hugging, kissing, casual contact, breastfeeding, food, water, or sharing eating utensils or drinking glasses.

The highest rate of new hepatitis B infections occur in 20- to 49-year-olds. The greatest decline has occurred among children and adolescents as a result of routine hepatitis B immunization.

It is estimated that more than 1.25 million people in the United States are infected with chronic hepatitis B; this means that these individuals are carriers of hepatitis B and capable of transmitting the disease to others. Many of these individuals do not know that they are carriers.

Every year, approximately 5000 Americans die as a result of the long-term consequences of chronic hepatitis B, such as cirrhosis and liver cancer.

Whether or not an HBV-infected individual goes on to develop chronic hepatitis B depends primarily on age. After being infected with acute viral hepatitis B, chronic infection develops in 90% of infants infected by their mothers at birth, 30% of children infected between ages 1 and 5 years, and 6% of individuals infected after age 5 years.

Hepatitis B can survive outside the body in a dried state for at least 1 week and still be capable of causing infection. Examples of surfaces that could harbor dried blood or body fluids infected with HBV include contaminated worktables, equipment, and instruments.

Hepatitis C

Chronic hepatitis C is the most common chronic viral infection in the United States. Approximately 3 million Americans have been diagnosed with chronic hepatitis C, and each year it causes an estimated 10,000 to 12,000 deaths resulting from cirrhosis and liver cancer.

The most common means of transmission of hepatitis C is by sharing needles for injection drug use with an infected individual. Hepatitis C is not spread by casual contact, such as sneezing, coughing, hugging, sharing food or water, or sharing eating utensils or drinking glasses. It is rarely transmitted through sexual contact.

Individuals infected with hepatitis C should not share personal items that may have blood on them with other members of the household (e.g., toothbrushes, nail-grooming equipment, razors).

Chronic hepatitis C is known as "an epidemic that occurred in the past." Numerous individuals became infected with hepatitis C more than 25 years ago and are now being diagnosed with it. This is because the symptoms of chronic hepatitis C often do not appear until 10 to 30 years after infection, and many times the first symptoms come only with advanced liver disease. Chronic hepatitis C surpasses alcoholism as the leading cause of liver cirrhosis and liver transplantation in the United States.

By 2015, the CDC predicts that there will be a fourfold increase in the number of individuals diagnosed with chronic hepatitis C and a threefold increase in the annual death toll by 2010.

Before 1992, a blood test to determine the presence of hepatitis C did not exist. Because of this, a significant number of people contracted hepatitis C from HCV-infected blood transfusions. The CDC has begun a campaign to encourage people who received blood transfusions before July 1992 to ask their physicians if they should be tested for hepatitis C.

Postexposure prophylaxis with immune globulin is not effective in preventing hepatitis C, and no vaccine exists yet to prevent hepatitis C. Vaccines are difficult to develop for hepatitis C because the virus mutates so frequently. The only way to control the disease is by preventing exposure to the hepatitis C virus. ■

Approximately 55% to 85% of individuals with acute hepatitis C develop chronic hepatitis C. After 10 to 30 years, about 20% of these individuals develop serious liver disease, including cirrhosis of the liver and cancer of the liver. Ultimately, 1% to 5% of individuals with chronic hepatitis C die from liver failure (see the box titled *Highlight on Viral Hepatitis*). Antiviral drugs have also been developed to treat chronic hepatitis C and are effective in 40% of cases.

Acquired Immune Deficiency Syndrome

Acquired immune deficiency syndrome (AIDS) is a chronic disorder of the immune system that eventually destroys the body's ability to fight off infection. AIDS is caused by a retrovirus known as *human immunodeficiency virus* (HIV), which is most frequently transmitted through sexual contact and sharing drug needles. The following description helps to clarify the difference between these two terms. The virus and the infection itself are known as *HIV*, whereas the term *AIDS* is used to refer to the last stage of HIV infection. Simply put, the terms *HIV infection* and *AIDS* refer to different stages of the same disease.

When HIV gains entrance into the body, it begins to attack and destroy certain white blood cells known as *CD4⁺ T cells,* which are involved in protecting the body against viral, fungal, and protozoal infections. As more and more CD4⁺ T cells are destroyed, the immune system is gradually weakened. After a period of time, which may last 10 years or more, the body's immune system becomes so ravaged by the attack that it succumbs to the diseases associated with AIDS.

AIDS is characterized by the presence of severe and life-threatening opportunistic infections and unusual cancers (known as *AIDS-defining conditions*) that rarely affect individuals with healthy immune systems. An **opportunistic infection** is an infection that results from a defective immune system that cannot defend itself from pathogens normally found in the environment. Opportunistic infections are extremely difficult to treat because the infection tends to recur quickly after a course of therapy is completed.

Memories *from* Externship

Jennifer Hawk: As a student, I was extremely nervous to go out on externship. I was so scared to think that I was actually going to be in a medical office setting and would have to put everything I had learned into practice. Would I remember everything? Would I do something wrong and hurt the patient? It was such an overwhelming feeling! But to my relief, I had a very good experience. The office staff was so friendly and helpful to me, and I surprised myself at how easily everything I had learned stayed with me. It was so exciting to see that I was actually functioning as a team member in the health care field. I could not have had better training. ∎

Prepare for Success

Highlight on AIDS

Prevalence

AIDS was first reported in the United States in 1981, but most likely it existed here and in other parts of the world for many years before that. Since 1981, more than 950,000 cases of AIDS have been reported in the United States, and every year 40,000 people in the United States are infected with HIV. Since 1981, there have been an estimated 530,000 deaths in the United States from AIDS.

The epidemic is growing most rapidly among women 25 to 44 years old and minority populations. There also has been an increase in the number of AIDS cases among individuals who are age 50 and older. This increase may be due to the fact that members of this age group do not think of themselves as at risk for contracting AIDS and may not practice safe sex.

Transmission

HIV can be transmitted through sexual contact and sharing drug needles. Scientific evidence shows that HIV is not spread through casual, everyday contact. There is no evidence that HIV is spread by sharing facilities or equipment, such as telephones, computers, food utensils, bedding, doorknobs, and bathrooms. Because HIV is not passed through the air, it is not spread through coughing and sneezing. HIV is also not spread through tears, sweat, shaking hands, hugging, or by donating blood.

Most individuals infected with HIV show no symptoms and may not develop full-blown AIDS for 10 years or more. After infection with HIV, the individual is infected for life.

Women can transmit HIV to their fetuses during pregnancy or birth. Approximately one quarter to one third of pregnant women infected with HIV who are not being treated with antiretroviral drugs pass the infection to their infants. HIV also can be spread to infants through the breast milk of mothers infected with the virus. The CDC recommends that all pregnant women be offered voluntary HIV testing as a routine part of prenatal care.

Worldwide, more than 700,000 infants are infected with HIV each year. If antiretroviral drugs are taken during pregnancy and the infant is delivered by cesarean section, the chance of transmitting HIV to the infant is reduced significantly. In developing countries, such as sub-Saharan Africa, women seldom know their HIV status, and treatment is often unavailable.

Continued

Highlight on AIDS—cont'd

Diagnostic Tests

The enzyme immune assay (EIA) test and the enzyme-linked immunosorbent assay (ELISA) test are used as screening tests for the presence of HIV. Because of the possibility of a false-positive result, a second screening test is always performed if a blood specimen tests positive. If the second test also is positive, a more specific test, such as the Western blot test, is performed to confirm the test results. An individual who tests positive for HIV is seropositive.

A negative HIV test is not conclusive for the absence of HIV infection. If an individual has recently been infected with HIV, the antibodies may not have had time to develop. It generally takes 3 to 6 months for the antibodies to appear in the blood.

CDC Definition of AIDS

As scientists have learned more about the disease, the CDC's definition of AIDS has changed several times since the beginning of the AIDS epidemic. The current AIDS definition includes the presence of one or both of the following conditions:

1. HIV positive and a CD4+ T cell count below 200 cells/μL (normal CD4+ T cell count for a healthy individual ranges from 500 to 1500 cells/μL)
2. Presence of one or more AIDS-defining conditions (opportunistic infections and unusual cancers)

Treatment

There is no cure for AIDS; there is no vaccine to prevent it. Powerful antiviral drugs have been developed that slow the reproduction of the virus and reduce the viral load in the body. In many patients, these drugs have dramatically delayed HIV from progressing to full-blown AIDS. These drugs can have serious side effects, and they do not prevent the spread of the disease to someone else. Numerous drugs also are available to treat the opportunistic infections and cancers that occur with AIDS. ■

PATIENT TEACHING   Acquired Immune Deficiency Syndrome

Teach patients the ways in which AIDS is transmitted

- Having unprotected sex (vaginal, anal, or oral) with someone who is infected with HIV. The virus is most commonly found in semen, blood, and vaginal secretions.
- Sharing needles for injection drug use with someone who is infected with HIV. This occurs as follows: If an HIV-infected individual uses a needle to pierce his or her skin, there will be a tiny amount of blood left on the needle. If another person uses the same needle, the person will be injecting the HIV-infected blood into his or her body.
- Transmitting in utero. A pregnant woman with HIV can pass it on to her fetus. Infants born with HIV usually develop AIDS by 2 years of age.
- Receiving a blood transfusion or blood products (before 1985) from someone infected with HIV. (In 1985, blood banks began screening blood for AIDS, so this is largely a problem of blood received before then.)
- There is a greater risk of contracting AIDS if you already have another sexually transmitted disease, such as chlamydia, gonorrhea, syphilis, herpes, or bacterial vaginosis.

Teach patients how to prevent AIDS

- Know your sexual partner(s) and their sexual history and drug use.
- Use a latex condom during sexual intercourse to minimize the risk of infection. HIV cannot pass through the latex if the condom does not break and is used properly. If a lubricant is used with the condom, it should be water based, such as K-Y jelly, because an oil-based lubricant such as petroleum jelly could break down the latex.
- Avoid sexual practices that involve the exchange of body fluids, such as semen or vaginal secretions.
- If you think that you could have HIV, never let your blood, semen, or vaginal fluid enter another person's body.
- Do not share needles for injectable drug use.

Teach patients to recognize the symptoms of AIDS

- Unexplained fatigue
- Weight loss of 10 to 15 lb in less than 2 months, but without dieting
- Unexplained fever, chills, and sweating at night for more than 2 weeks
- Unexplained swollen glands for more than 1 month
- Unexplained diarrhea or bloody stools for more than 2 weeks
- Unexplained persistent dry cough, shortness of breath, or difficulty in breathing
- White patches on the tongue or mouth that cannot be scraped off

Explain to patients that these symptoms also could be signs of other diseases. If they have any of these symptoms, however, they should consider having an HIV test. The earlier the infection is detected, the earlier treatment can begin that may delay the onset of other symptoms. ■

Table 17-1 Forms of Viral Hepatitis

	Hepatitis A (HAV)	Hepatitis B (HBV)	Hepatitis C (HCV)	Hepatitis D (HDV)	Hepatitis E (HEV)
Incubation period	2-6 wk	6 wk to 6 mo	2 wk to 6 mo	2 wk to 5 mo	3-6 wk
Means of transmission	Caused by a virus found in the feces of HAV-infected individuals. Transmitted almost exclusively by the fecal-oral route through practices of poor hygiene; also transmitted by the consumption of food and water contaminated with human feces	Caused by a virus found in the blood and certain body fluids of HBV-infected individuals. Transmitted by exposure to contaminated semen and vaginal secretions by personal contact, especially sexual contact; parenteral exposure to contaminated blood and blood components, such as through injecting drugs using contaminated needles and accidental needlestick injuries by health care workers; **perinatally** from an infected mother to her infant during birth	Caused by a virus found in the blood of HCV-infected individuals. Parenteral exposure to contaminated blood or blood components, primarily from injecting drugs using contaminated needles. It is possible to transmit HCV during intercourse, but it is uncommon	Same as hepatitis B	Fecal-oral route through practices of poor hygiene; consumption of food and water contaminated with feces
Characteristics	Usually occurs in children and young adults, especially in environments of poor sanitation and overcrowding; often a mild disease with symptoms similar to the flu and lasting 1-2 wk; there is a vaccine available to prevent hepatitis A	Symptoms usually last 1-4 wk, but it may be 6 mo before the individual fully recovers; there is a vaccine available to prevent hepatitis B	At risk are individuals who received a blood transfusion before 1992; currently a vaccine does not exist for hepatitis C	Affects only those already infected with hepatitis B; a person who has received the hepatitis B vaccine also is protected from hepatitis D	Rare in the United States; generally seen in developing countries; usually occurs in epidemics rather than sporadic cases
Symptoms	Symptoms include fever, malaise, fatigue, anorexia, nausea, vomiting, and abdominal discomfort, followed in some people by dark urine, clay-colored stools, and mild jaundice	Symptoms include fatigue, headache, loss of appetite, nausea, vomiting, malaise, and muscle and joint pain, followed in some people by dark urine, clay-colored stools, abdominal pain, and jaundice	Symptoms are similar to those of hepatitis B	Occurs as a coinfection or superinfection with hepatitis B and intensifies the symptoms of hepatitis B	Symptoms are similar to those of hepatitis B

Continued

Table 17-1 Forms of Viral Hepatitis—cont'd

	Hepatitis A (HAV)	Hepatitis B (HBV)	Hepatitis C (HCV)	Hepatitis D (HDV)	Hepatitis E (HEV)
Prognosis	Most people recover fully within 6-10 wk and become immune to the virus; rarely fatal; chronic hepatitis does not develop; carrier states do not develop	Most people recover fully and become immune to this disease; some people (10%) go on to develop chronic hepatitis and may develop cirrhosis and liver cancer; these people also are carriers of hepatitis B. Eventually 25% of people with chronic hepatitis B die from liver failure	Approximately 55-85% of people infected with hepatitis C are unable to clear the virus from their body and develop chronic hepatitis, which may lead to liver damage, such as cirrhosis and liver cancer. These people are also carriers of hepatitis C. Eventually 1% to 5% of people with chronic hepatitis C die from liver failure	Frequently leads to chronic hepatitis; high fatality rate (30% of chronic hepatitis patients)	Does not progress to chronic hepatitis; hepatitis E is particularly dangerous if contracted by pregnant women (10-20% fatality rate in these individuals)

From Bonewit-West K: *Clinical procedures for medical assistants,* ed 7, St. Louis, 2008, Saunders.

MEDICAL PRACTICE *and the* LAW

Three behaviors are crucial in protecting yourself from a lawsuit:
1. Establish a rapport. If patients believe that you truly care about them and have their best interests at heart, they rarely sue, even if you make a mistake.
2. Follow all procedures according to your procedures manual. If you do everything right, and the patient has an adverse outcome, you will not likely be found liable.
3. Document everything you do objectively. Lawsuits often come to court years after the incident, and nobody's memory is as good as written documentation. Document only facts, not your opinion. Document the patient's reaction to treatments.

Ethics and Law

Ethics is the highest standard of behavior and is loosely based on the Golden Rule. No law can force you to behave ethically, but most major professions have a written code of ethics, including the American Association of Medical Assistants (AAMA). Ethics uses words such as *should* and *may.* If you are angry with someone, ethically, you should not yell at him or her. This is not against the law, but it is unethical.

Law is the lowest standard of behavior and is enforced by federal, state, and local law enforcement personnel. Laws use words such as *must* and *shall.* If you are angry with someone, legally, you must not hit him or her. This behavior is illegal, and you could be charged with assault and battery.

Regarding medical asepsis and infection control, you have a duty and a responsibility to protect yourself, your coworkers, and, most important, your patients. Follow specific guidelines established by OSHA and the CDC to prevent the transmission of pathogens. ▪

What Would You Do? What Would You *Not* Do? RESPONSES

Case Study 1
Page 277

What Did Jennifer Do?
❏ Told Petra that the hand sanitizers (alcohol-based hand rubs) are as good, if not better, than soap and water for removing germs from the hands.
❏ Explained to Petra that an amount of gel equal to the size of a dime should be rubbed on her hands until the gel dries. Told Petra that she did not need to rinse her hands afterward.
❏ Stressed to Petra that hand sanitizers are not designed to remove soil from the hands and that she should wash her hands with soap and water when they are visibly soiled.
❏ Explained that the Centers for Disease Control and Prevention now recommends that hand sanitizers be used in health care settings to help prevent the spread of disease.

What Did Jennifer Not *Do?*
❏ Did not tell Petra that she should switch from soap and water to hand sanitizers.

What Would You Do/What Would You *Not* Do? Review Jennifer's response and place a checkmark next to the information you included in your response. List additional information you included in your response.

_____

_____

_____

_____

What Would You Do? What Would You *Not* Do?   RESPONSES—cont'd

Case Study 2
Page 282

What Did Jennifer Do?

❑ Explained to Tracy that a federal agency known as the *Occupational Safety and Health Administration* (OSHA) requires gloves be worn when drawing a patient's blood in the office. Told her that the office could be fined if they were not worn.

❑ Told Tracy that having her infant immunized for hepatitis B is an investment in her child's future. Explained that her child could come into contact with the virus anytime in his or her life. Stressed that if a young child becomes infected with hepatitis B, the child has a higher risk of developing chronic hepatitis, which can cause serious liver problems later in life.

❑ Gave Tracy a brochure on hepatitis B to take home.

What Did Jennifer Not Do?

❑ Did not discourage Tracy from having her baby immunized for hepatitis B.

What Would You Do/What Would You *Not* Do? Review Jennifer's response and place a checkmark next to the information you included in your response. List additional information you included in your response.

_____

_____

_____

_____

Case Study 3
Page 286

What Did Jennifer Do?

❑ Explained to Giles that the blood supply was not tested for hepatitis C until 1992 because a test to detect the presence of hepatitis C was not developed until then.

❑ Told Giles that it is possible for someone to have hepatitis C and not exhibit any symptoms.

❑ Told Giles that he should ask the physician his question about giving hepatitis C to others.

What Did Jennifer Not Do?

❑ Did not automatically assume that Giles had hepatitis C because he had not yet been seen by the physician. It would be up to the physician to make a diagnosis of hepatitis C.

❑ Did not tell Giles about the serious complications of hepatitis C. If Giles is diagnosed with hepatitis C, it would be the physician's responsibility to relay this information.

What Would You Do/What Would You *Not* Do? Review Jennifer's response and place a checkmark next to the information you included in your response. List additional information you included in your response.

_____

_____

_____

_____

TERMINOLOGY REVIEW

Aerobe A microorganism that needs oxygen to live and grow.

Anaerobe A microorganism that grows best in the absence of oxygen.

Antiseptic An agent that inhibits the growth of or kills microorganisms.

Asepsis Free from infection or pathogens; the actions practiced to make and maintain an area or object free from infection or pathogens.

Cilia Slender, hairlike projections that constantly beat toward the outside to remove microorganisms from the body.

Contaminate To soil or to make impure. An aseptic object is contaminated when it touches something that is not clean.

Decontamination The use of physical or chemical means to remove, inactivate, or destroy pathogens on a surface or item to the point where they are no longer capable of transmitting infectious particles; the surface or item is rendered safe for handling, use, or disposal.

Hand hygiene The process of cleansing or sanitizing the hands.

Infection The condition in which the body, or part of it, is invaded by a pathogen.

Medical asepsis Practices that are employed to reduce the number and hinder the transmission of pathogens.

Microorganism A microscopic plant or animal.

Nonintact skin Skin that has a break in the surface. It includes, but is not limited to, abrasions, cuts, hangnails, paper cuts, and burns.

Nonpathogen A microorganism that does not normally produce disease.

Opportunistic infection An infection that results from a defective immune system that cannot defend the body from pathogens normally found in the environment.

Optimum growth temperature The temperature at which an organism grows best.

Parenteral Taken into the body through the piercing of the skin barrier or mucous membranes, such as through needlesticks, human bites, cuts, and abrasions.

Pathogen A disease-producing microorganism.

Perinatal Relating to the period shortly before and after birth.

pH The degree to which a solution is acidic or basic.

Continued

TERMINOLOGY REVIEW—cont'd

Postexposure prophylaxis (PEP) Treatment administered to an individual after exposure to an infectious disease to prevent the disease.

Regulated medical waste (RMW) Medical waste that poses a threat to health and safety.

Reservoir host The organism that becomes infected by a pathogen and serves as a source of transfer of the pathogen to others.

Resident flora Harmless, nonpathogenic microorganisms that normally reside on the skin and usually do not cause disease. Also known as *normal flora*.

Susceptible Easily affected; lacking resistance.

Transient flora Microorganisms that reside on the superficial skin layers and are picked up in the course of daily activities. They are often pathogenic but can be removed easily from the skin by sanitizing the hands.

ON THE WEB

For Information on Federal Regulations and Recommendations for Infection Control:

Occupational Safety and Health Administration (OSHA): www.osha.gov

Centers for Disease Control and Prevention (CDC): www.cdc.gov

National Institute for Occupational Safety and Health (NIOSH): www.cdc.gov/niosh

CDC Recommendations for Hand Hygiene in the Healthcare Setting: www.cdc.gov/handhygiene

Food and Drug Administration (FDA): www.fda.gov

Environmental Protection Agency: www.epa.gov

Association for the Advancement of Medical Instrumentation (AAMI): www.aami.org

Division of Healthcare Quality Promotion (DHQP): www.cdc.gov/ncidod/dhqp

Epidemiology Program Office: www.cdc.gov/epo

Morbidity and Mortality Weekly Report: www.cdc.gov/mmwr

For Information on Hepatitis:

CDC National Center for Infectious Diseases: www.cdc.gov/hepatitis

Hepatitis Foundation International: www.hepfi.org

Hepatitis B Foundation: www.hepb.org

National Institute of Allergy and Infectious Diseases: www.niaid.nih.gov

HealthTalk: www.healthtalk.com

For Information on AIDS:

CDC National Center for HIV, STD, and TB Prevention: www.cdc.gov/ncidod/diseases

AIDS Education Global Information System: www.aegis.com

AIDS Research Information Center: www.critpath.org/aric

AIDS Information: www.aidsinfo.nih.gov

The Body—AIDS and HIV Information Resource: www.thebody.com

About AIDS: aids.about.com

HIV Positive.Com: www.hivpositive.com

HIV Insite: www.hivinsite.ucsf.edu

Mayo Clinic: www.mayoclinic.com

 PREPARE FOR CERTIFICATION Visit the Evolve site at http://evolve.elsevier.com/Bonewit/today/ to actively Prepare for your Certification.

 Check out the **Companion CD** *bound with the book to access additional interactive activities.*

18

Sterilization and Disinfection

Hazard Communication Standard

1. Explain the purpose of the Hazard Communication Standard.
2. List and describe the information that must be included on the label of a hazardous chemical.
3. List and describe the information that must be included in a material safety data sheet (MSDS).

Read and interpret an MSDS.

Sanitization

1. State the purpose of sanitization.
2. State the advantages of using an ultrasonic cleaner to clean instruments.
3. List and describe the guidelines that should be followed when sanitizing instruments.

Sanitize instruments.

Disinfection

1. State the use of the three levels of disinfection: high, intermediate, and low.
2. Explain the differences among the following: critical item, semicritical item, and noncritical item.
3. List and describe the primary use of disinfectants in the medical office.

Sterilization

1. Explain how the autoclave functions to sterilize articles.
2. List the components of a sterilization monitoring program.
3. List and describe types of sterilization indicators.
4. Identify the advantages and disadvantages of the following types of wraps: sterilization paper, sterilization pouches, and muslin.
5. List the guidelines that should be followed when the autoclave is loaded.
6. Identify the sterilization times for each of the following categories: unwrapped articles, wrapped articles, liquids, and large wrapped packs.
7. Describe the method for storing wrapped articles.
8. Describe the daily, weekly, and monthly maintenance of the autoclave.

Wrap articles to be autoclaved.
Sterilize articles in the autoclave.
Maintain the autoclave.

Other Sterilization Methods

1. State the primary use of the following types of sterilization methods: dry heat, ethylene oxide gas, chemicals, and radiation.

CAAHEP COMPETENCIES

Clinical Competencies
Fundamental Procedures
- Wrap items for autoclaving.
- Perform sterilization techniques.

ABHES COMPETENCIES

Clinical Duties
- Wrap items for autoclaving.
- Perform sterilization techniques.

KEY TERMS

antiseptic (an-tih-SEP-tik)
autoclave (AU-toe-klave)
contaminate (kon-TAM-in-ate)
critical item
decontamination (DEE-kon-tam-in-AY-shun)
detergent
disinfectant (dis-in-FEK-tant)
hazardous chemical
incubate (IN-kyoo-bate)

load
material safety data sheet (MSDS)
noncritical item
sanitization (san-ih-tih-ZAY-shun)
semicritical item
spore
sterilization (stare-ill-ih-ZAY-shun)
thermolabile (ther-moe-LAH-bul)

Introduction to Sterilization and Disinfection

The air and all objects around us contain microorganisms. The medical assistant is responsible for helping to reduce and eliminate microorganisms to prevent the spread of disease. This can be accomplished by practicing good techniques of medical and surgical asepsis (see Chapters 17 and 25).

Physical and chemical agents are used to destroy microorganisms in the medical office. The agent selected depends on the intended use of the article. Articles that penetrate sterile tissue or the vascular system, such as surgical instruments, must be sterilized. Articles that come in contact with

the skin, such as stethoscopes, blood pressure cuffs, and percussion hammers, should be disinfected.

Sanitization, disinfection, and sterilization involve hazardous chemicals. It is essential for the medical assistant to know the precautions that are required when working with hazardous chemicals.

DEFINITION OF TERMS

Terms that aid in understanding this chapter are listed and defined here.

Sanitization Sanitization is a process that removes organic material and reduces the number of microorganisms to a safe level as determined by public health requirements. Sanitization removes all organic material, such as blood, body fluids, and tissue, from an article. For articles that are used in examinations, treatments, and office surgery to be properly sterilized or disinfected, they must first be sanitized.

Decontamination *Decontamination* refers to the use of physical or chemical means to remove or destroy pathogens on an item so that it is no longer capable of transmitting disease; this makes the item safe to handle.

Detergent A detergent is an agent that cleanses by emulsifying dirt and oil.

Disinfectant A disinfectant is an agent used to destroy pathogenic microorganisms; however, it does not kill the resistant bacterial spores. Disinfectants are generally applied to inanimate objects.

Spore A spore is a hard, thick-walled capsule that some bacteria form by losing moisture and condensing their contents to contain only the essential parts of the protoplasm of the cell. Spores represent a resting and protective stage of the bacterial cell and are more resistant to drying, sunlight, heat, and disinfectants than is the vegetative form of the bacterium. Favorable conditions cause the spore to germinate into a vegetative bacterium again, capable of reproducing. Two examples of species of bacteria that form spores are *Clostridium botulinum,* which causes botulism, and *Clostridium tetani,* which causes tetanus.

Sterilization Sterilization is the process of destroying all forms of microbial life, including bacterial spores. An object that is *sterile* is free of all living microorganisms and spores. There can be no relative degrees of sterility— an object is either sterile or not sterile. The device most commonly used to sterilize articles in the medical office is the autoclave.

HAZARD COMMUNICATION STANDARD

The Hazard Communication Standard (HCS) is a requirement of the Occupational Safety and Health Administration (OSHA). The purpose of the HCS is to ensure that employees are informed of the hazards associated with chemicals in their workplaces. Chemicals can be in the form of a liquid, solid, or gas. A **hazardous chemical** is any chemical that presents a threat to the health and safety of an individual coming into contact with it. Hazardous chemicals are those that are corrosive, toxic, irritating, carcinogenic, flammable, or reactive.

The HCS is based on the concept that employees have a right to know about the hazardous chemicals in their workplace and the precautions to take to protect themselves when working with hazardous chemicals. In the medical office, sanitization, disinfection, and sterilization procedures involve the use of hazardous chemicals; the medical assistant must have a thorough knowledge of the HCS.

The HCS consists of the following components:

- Development of a hazard communication program
- Inventory of hazardous chemicals
- Labeling requirements
- Material safety data sheet requirements
- Employee information and training

Hazard Communication Program

As part of the HCS, employers are required to develop a hazard communication program. The hazard communication program consists of a written plan that describes what the facility is doing to meet the requirements of the HCS. The information in the plan must be made available and communicated to all employees who work with hazardous chemicals.

Inventory of Hazardous Chemicals

The employer must develop and maintain a list of hazardous chemicals that are used and stored in the workplace. The list must include the name of the chemical, the name of the manufacturer, the hazardous ingredients, and the health and safety ratings of the chemical. The list must be updated as new chemicals are introduced into the workplace. In the medical office, hazardous chemicals often include the following:

- Products used for sanitization, disinfection, and sterilization (e.g., chemical disinfectants, autoclave cleaner)
- Chemicals used for laboratory testing (e.g., laboratory testing reagents, developing solutions, controls)
- Pharmaceutical products such as local anesthetics (e.g., lidocaine [Xylocaine])
- Front office products (e.g., toner for copying machine and laser printer)
- Cleaning products (e.g., drain cleaner)

Labeling of Hazardous Chemicals

The HCS requires that each container of a hazardous chemical be labeled by the manufacturer with a warning to alert the user that the chemical is dangerous (Figure 18-1). The label must include the possible hazards of the chemical and the steps that can be taken to protect against those risks. The hazard warnings can use words, pictures, or symbols to provide the user with an understanding of the physical and health hazards of the chemical. If a label falls off a product or is damaged or obscured, a replacement label must be applied. If a chemical is transferred to a new container, a label with all the required information must be attached to the new container.

Container Label Requirements

The HCS requires that manufacturers label the containers of hazardous chemicals they produce with specific information. This information allows the user of the chemical to tell at a glance the hazards of using the chemical and the basic steps to take to protect oneself. The information required by the HCS includes the following:

1. **Name of the chemical.** The name of the chemical must be clearly indicated on the label.
2. **Manufacturer information.** The name, address, and emergency phone number of the company that manufactures the chemical must be stated on the label.

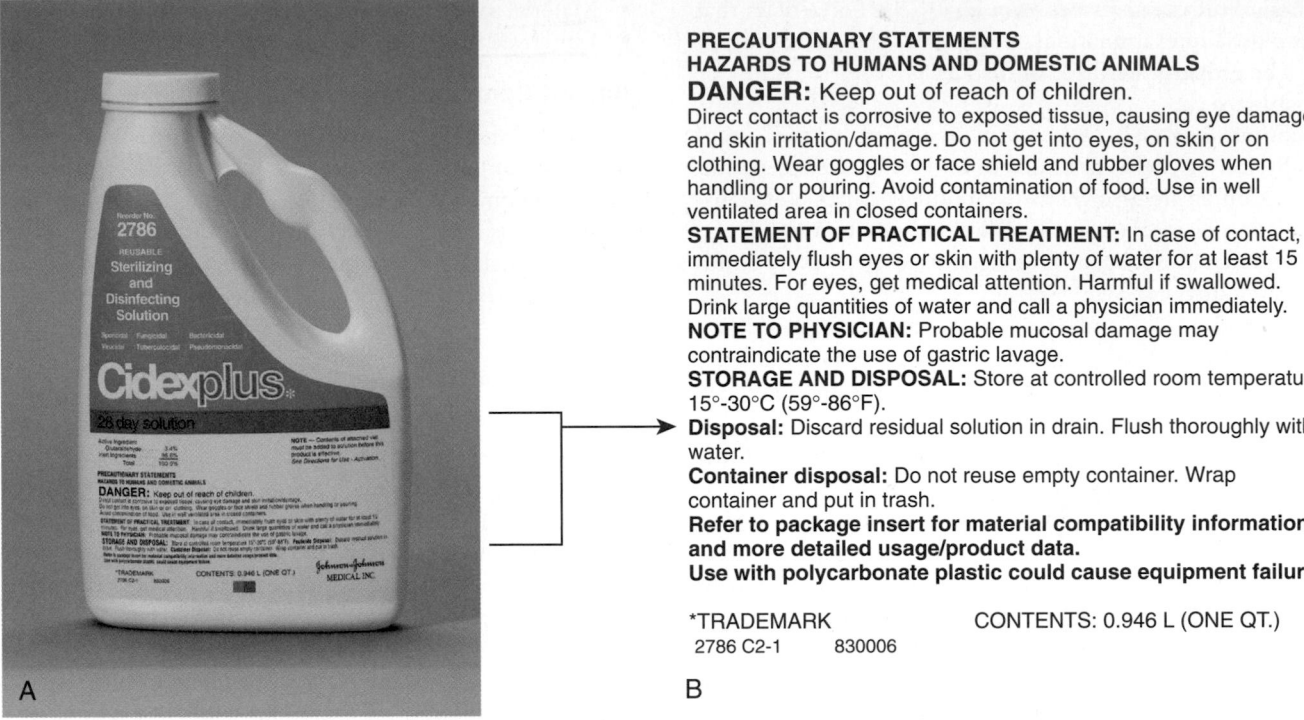

PRECAUTIONARY STATEMENTS
HAZARDS TO HUMANS AND DOMESTIC ANIMALS
DANGER: Keep out of reach of children.
Direct contact is corrosive to exposed tissue, causing eye damage and skin irritation/damage. Do not get into eyes, on skin or on clothing. Wear goggles or face shield and rubber gloves when handling or pouring. Avoid contamination of food. Use in well ventilated area in closed containers.
STATEMENT OF PRACTICAL TREATMENT: In case of contact, immediately flush eyes or skin with plenty of water for at least 15 minutes. For eyes, get medical attention. Harmful if swallowed. Drink large quantities of water and call a physician immediately.
NOTE TO PHYSICIAN: Probable mucosal damage may contraindicate the use of gastric lavage.
STORAGE AND DISPOSAL: Store at controlled room temperature 15°-30°C (59°-86°F).
Disposal: Discard residual solution in drain. Flush thoroughly with water.
Container disposal: Do not reuse empty container. Wrap container and put in trash.
Refer to package insert for material compatibility information and more detailed usage/product data.
Use with polycarbonate plastic could cause equipment failure.

*TRADEMARK   CONTENTS: 0.946 L (ONE QT.)
2786 C2-1   830006

A   B

Figure 18-1. A, Hazardous chemical container label. **B,** The label must indicate the possible hazards of the chemical. (From Bonewit-West K: *Clinical procedures for medical assistants,* ed 7, St. Louis, 2008, Saunders.)

3. **Physical hazards of the chemical.** Physical hazards that must be stated include the potential of the chemical to catch fire, explode, or react with other chemicals or materials.
4. **Health hazards of the chemical.** Health hazards include the potential of the chemical to cause irritation to tissue, cancer, a sensitivity reaction, or a toxic or corrosive reaction.
5. **Safety precautions.** The protective clothing, equipment, and procedures that are recommended when working with the chemical must be stated on the label. Examples include gloves, protective eyewear, and working with the chemical in a well-ventilated area.
6. **Storing, handling, and disposal of the chemical.** Information on how the chemical should be stored, handled, and disposed of must be stated on the label.

Material Safety Data Sheets

A **material safety data sheet (MSDS)** provides more detailed information than the container label regarding the chemical, its hazards, and measures to take to prevent injury and illness when handling the chemical (Figure 18-2). The HCS requires that a current MSDS be kept on file for each hazardous chemical used or stored in the workplace. MSDS must be readily accessible to employees and provided to them on request. Importantly, the medical assistant should review the MSDS before working with a hazardous chemical.

Companies that manufacture and distribute hazardous chemicals must provide an MSDS with every product. A hazardous chemical should never be used unless an MSDS

What Would You Do? What Would You *Not* Do?

Case Study 1
Elba Cordera has brought her daughter Maria in for a well-baby visit. Maria is 9 months old and is just starting to crawl. Mrs. Cordera is taking precautions to baby-proof her house to protect Maria from accidents. Mrs. Cordera wants to know how to tell whether a cleaning product is poisonous. She also wants to know what she should do if Maria gets into a cleaning product and spills it on herself or swallows it. ■

is available. In the event of an accidental exposure, information on the MSDS must be readily available as a reference for emergency treatment. If an MSDS is missing, the supplier or the manufacturer of that chemical should be contacted for a replacement.

An MSDS does not have to be kept on file for a hazardous chemical that is used in the workplace in the same way that a household consumer would use it. For example, correction fluids, such as Wite-Out and Liquid Paper, contain a hazardous chemical. If the medical assistant uses it in the same way, however, that a household consumer would use it (i.e., to correct errors on a document), an MSDS does not need to be kept on file. If household bleach (sodium hypochlorite) is used to decontaminate blood spills in the medical office, an MSDS would need to be kept on file because the bleach is not being used in the same way that a household consumer would use it.

MATERIAL SAFETY DATA SHEET (MSDS)		
Date of Issue: 4/28/04		**Date of Revision: 8/8/09**

SECTION 1   IDENTIFICATION

GENERIC NAME: Glutaraldehyde	**INFORMATION TELEPHONE NUMBER: 1 (800) 733-8690**
BRAND NAME: Aldecide	**EMERGENCY TELEPHONE NUMBER:**
MANUFACTURER'S NAME: Brennan Corporation	**1 (800) 331-0766**
MFG. ADDRESS: P.O. Box 93	
CITY: Camden STATE: NJ ZIP: 08106	

SECTION 2   COMPOSITION OF INGREDIENTS

CAS NUMBER	CHEMICAL NAME OF INGREDIENTS	PERCENT	PEL	TLV
111-30-8	Glutaraldehyde	2.5	0.2 ppm	0.2 ppm
7732-18-5	Water	97.4	None	None
7632-00-0	Sodium Nitrite	<1	None	None

SECTION 3   PHYSICAL AND CHEMICAL PROPERTIES

BOILING POINT: 212° F	**SPECIFIC GRAVITY (H$_2$O = 1): 1.004**
VAPOR PRESSURE (mm Hg): 0.20 at 20° C	**VAPOR DENSITY (AIR = 1): 1.1**
ODOR: Sharp odor	**pH: 7.5-8.5**
SOLUBILITY IN WATER: Complete (100%)	**MELTING POINT: n/a**
APPEARANCE: Bluish-green liquid	**FREEZING POINT: 32° F**
EVAPORATION RATE: 0.98 (Water = 1)	**ODOR THRESHOLD: 0.04 ppm**

SECTION 4   FIRE AND EXPLOSION HAZARD DATA

FLASH POINT: Not flammable (aqueous solution)	**NFPA Rating:**
FLAMMABILITY LIMITS: LEL: n/a	**Health: 2**
EXTINGUISHING MEDIA: n/a (aqueous solution)	**Flammability: 0**
SPECIAL FIRE FIGHTING PROCEDURES: n/a	**Reactivity: 0**
UNUSUAL FIRE/EXPL HAZARDS: None	

SECTION 5   REACTIVITY DATA

STABILITY: Stable under recommended storage conditions.
CONDITIONS TO AVOID: Avoid direct sunlight and temperatures above 104° F (40° C).
INCOMPATIBILITY (MATERIAL TO AVOID): Strong acids and alkalines will neutralize active ingredient.
HAZARDOUS DECOMPOSITION BYPRODUCTS: None
HAZARDOUS POLYMERIZATION: Will not occur

Figure 18-2. Material safety data sheet. (From Bonewit-West K: *Clinical procedures for medical assistants,* ed 7, St. Louis, 2008, Saunders.)

Continued

Material Safety Data Sheet Requirements

The HCS requires that manufacturers of hazardous chemicals include the following information on MSDS (see Figure 18-2):

1. **Identification.** This section provides information used to identify the chemical and must include the chemical's generic name and its brand name; the name, address, and emergency phone number of the manufacturer; and the date the MSDS was prepared.

2. **Composition of ingredients.** This section provides a list of the ingredients in the hazardous chemical and exposure limits of each chemical.

3. **Physical and chemical properties.** Physical and chemical properties of the chemical must be listed in this section, such as appearance, odor, boiling point, and freezing point.

4. **Fire and explosion data.** Some hazardous chemicals may cause a fire or explosion if used improperly. This

MATERIAL SAFETY DATA SHEET

SECTION 6   HEALTH HAZARD DATA

ROUTE OF ENTRY: SKIN: yes   **EYES: yes**   **INHALATION: yes**   **INGESTION: yes**

SIGNS AND SYMPTOMS OF OVEREXPOSURE:

SKIN: Moderate irritation. May aggravate existing dermatitis.

EYES: Serious eye irritant. May cause irreversible damage which could permanently impair vision.

INHALATION: Vapors may be severely irritating and cause stinging sensations in the eyes, nose, throat, and lungs. May aggravate pre-existing asthma.

INGESTION: May cause irritation or chemical burns of the mouth, throat, esophagus, and stomach. May cause vomiting, diarrhea, epigastric distress, headache, dizziness, faintness, mental confusion, and general systemic illness.

CARCINOGENICITY DATA: **NTP: No**   **AIRC: No**   **OSHA: No**

SECTION 7   EMERGENCY FIRST AID PROCEDURES

SKIN: Wash skin with soap and water for 15 minutes. If skin redness or irritation persists, seek medical attention. Remove contaminated clothing and wash before reuse.

EYES: Immediately flush with water for 15 minutes. Seek medical attention.

INHALATION: Remove to fresh air. If irritation persists, seek medical attention.

INGESTION: Do not induce vomiting. Seek medical attention immediately. Call a physician or Poison Control Center.

SECTION 8   PRECAUTIONS FOR SAFE HANDLING AND USE

SPILL PROCEDURES: Ventilate area, wear protective gloves and eye gear. Wipe with sponge, mop, or towel. Flush with large quantities of water. Collect liquid and discard it.

WASTE DISPOSAL METHOD: Container must be triple rinsed and disposed of in accordance with federal, state, and/or local regulations. Used solution should be flushed thoroughly with water into sewage disposal system in accordance with federal, state, and/or local regulations.

PRECAUTIONS IN HANDLING AND STORAGE: Store in a cool, dry place (59-86° F) away from direct sunlight or sources of intense heat. Keep container tightly closed when not in use.

SECTION 9   CONTROL MEASURES

VENTILATION: Ensure adequate ventilation to maintain recommended exposed limit.

RESPIRATORY PROTECTION: None normally required for routine use.

SKIN PROTECTION: Wear chemical resistant protective gloves. Butyl rubber, nitrile rubber, polyethylene, or double-gloved latex.

EYE PROTECTION: Safety goggles or safety glasses

WORK/HYGIENE PRACTICES: Prompt rinsing of hands after contact. Handle in accordance with good personal hygiene and safety practices. These practices include avoiding unnecessary exposure.

Figure 18-2, cont'd.

section indicates under what circumstances this may occur and what to do if it does occur, including recommended extinguishing agents.

5. **Reactivity data.** Some chemicals react when combined with other chemicals or materials. The reactivity data list the substances and conditions that the chemical should be kept away from to prevent a dangerous reaction. This information helps in determining where and how to store the chemical.

6. **Health hazard data.** This section is one of the most important areas for health care workers and includes the following information:

- Route of entry, which indicates how the chemical can enter the body, including skin contact, eye contact, inhalation, and ingestion
- Signs and symptoms of overexposure (e.g., burning eyes, nausea, dizziness, difficulty in breathing)
- Medical conditions that are aggravated by exposure to the chemical (e.g., asthma, dermatitis)
- Acute and chronic health hazards that could result from overexposure (e.g., skin irritation, eye damage, lung damage)

This section also indicates whether the hazardous chemical has been identified as a potential carcinogen by the National Toxicology Program (NTP), the International Agency for Research on Cancer (IARC), and OSHA.

7. **Emergency first-aid procedures.** This section identifies the first-aid measures to take if exposed to the chemical (e.g., in case of eye contact, immediately flush eyes with water for 15 minutes).

8. **Precautions for safe handling and use.** This section tells what to do for a spill or leak, the method of disposal of the chemical, and how to handle and store the chemical.

9. **Control measures.** This section lists engineering controls, work practice controls, and personal protective equipment that should be used to protect oneself from the hazardous chemical. Examples of these measures include using chemical-resistant gloves and eye protection and working in a well-ventilated area.

Employee Information and Training

The HCS requires that employees be provided with information and training regarding hazardous chemicals in the workplace. The training session must be offered at the time of an employee's initial assignment to a work area where hazardous chemicals are present and whenever a new chemical hazard is introduced into the work area. The training program must be an ongoing activity, and each training session must be documented. The HCS requires that the following information be relayed to employees who work with hazardous chemicals:

1. The requirements making up the HCS
2. Physical and health hazards associated with exposure to chemicals in the workplace
3. Measures the employees can take to protect themselves from injury or illness from hazardous chemicals
4. Emergency procedures to carry out in the event of exposure to a hazardous chemical or a chemical spill
5. The meaning of the information on container labels and how to use that information
6. The meaning of the information on MSDS and how to use that information
7. The location of the following: hazard communication program plan, list of hazardous chemicals in the workplace, and MSDS for each chemical in the workplace

SANITIZATION

Sanitization involves a series of steps designed to remove organic material from an article and to reduce the number of microorganisms on the article to a safe level (Procedure 18-1). Organic material on an article may result in incomplete sterilization or disinfection. This is because the organic material acts as a physical barrier preventing the physical or chemical agent from reaching the surface of the article to kill microorganisms.

Sanitizing Instruments

The most frequent items sanitized in the medical office are medical and surgical instruments. This section focuses on

Putting It All into Practice

My name is Kara VanDyke, and I work for two physicians in a family practice medical office. As a medical assistant, one of the situations you deal with on an almost daily basis is drug representatives who come to the office to promote their products. Their job is anything but easy. The waiting and the frequent rejections would make most people think twice before applying for the job.

One winter day, I am sure I made one drug representative really think twice about his career choice. As the representative stopped at our office, he, being a polite young man, let a patient enter the building first with wet, snow-covered feet. Trying to make a good impression with a new suit and dress shoes, he soon found himself doing a "Spanish fandango" while trying to maintain his balance and eventually crashed to the floor.

I thought I would help by mopping up the snow-tracked floor. What I did not know was the mop had wax on it. Needless to say, when he returned with the requested drug samples, we were not able to keep him from falling a second time! ∎

Prepare for Success

the theory and procedure for sanitizing instruments. The general steps in the sanitization procedure of instruments are as follows:

1. *Rinse* the instruments to prevent organic material from drying on the instruments.
2. *Decontaminate* the instruments with a chemical disinfectant to remove pathogenic microorganisms, making the instrument safe to handle.
3. *Clean* the instruments to remove all organic matter.
4. *Thoroughly rinse* the instruments to remove all detergent residue.
5. *Dry* the instruments to prevent stains on the instruments.
6. *Check the instruments* for defects and working condition.
7. *Lubricate* hinged instruments to make the instruments function well and last longer.

Cleaning Instruments

Two methods can be used to perform the cleaning step (step 3 in the preceding list) of the sanitization procedure: the manual method and the ultrasound method.

Manual Method

The manual method is used most often in the medical office. It involves the manual cleaning of instruments using a cleaning solution and a brush. Manual cleaning is recommended for delicate instruments because vibrations that occur with the ultrasound method may damage these instruments.

Figure 18-3. Ultrasonic cleaner. (From Bonewit-West K: *Clinical procedures for medical assistants,* ed 7, St. Louis, 2008, Saunders.)

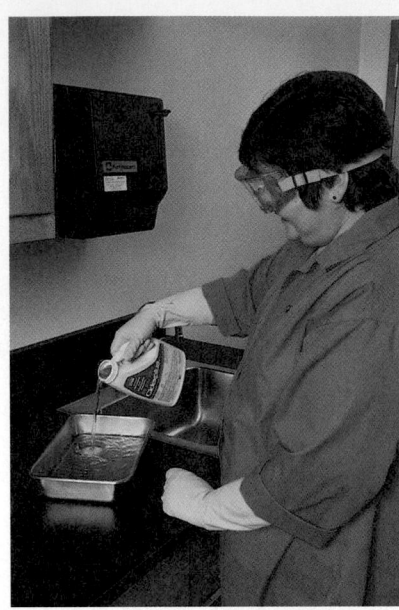

Figure 18-4. Kara wears utility gloves and safety goggles to protect herself from the irritating effects of glutaraldehyde. (From Bonewit-West K: *Clinical procedures for medical assistants,* ed 7, St. Louis, 2008, Saunders.)

Ultrasound Method

The ultrasound method uses a machine known as an *ultrasonic cleaner* (Figure 18-3). The ultrasound method offers a safety advantage in that instruments do not have to be handled during the cleaning process. This decreases the incidence of an accidental puncture or cut from a sharp instrument. An ultrasonic cleaner works by converting sound waves into mechanical energy, which creates small bubbles all over the instruments. When the bubbles burst, vibrations occur that loosen and remove debris from the instruments. Ultrasonic cleaners are especially good at removing debris from hard-to-reach areas, such as box locks of hemostats and screw locks of scissors.

Before the instruments are placed in the ultrasonic cleaner, they should be separated according to the type of metal (e.g., stainless steel, aluminum, brass). Instruments made of dissimilar metals should not be cleaned together in the ultrasonic cleaner. When different metals are in close contact, the ions from one metal can flow to another. This may result in a permanent blue-black stain on an instrument, which can be removed only by having the instrument refinished.

Guidelines for Sanitizing Instruments

The following guidelines should be followed when sanitizing surgical instruments:

1. **Wear gloves during the sanitization process.** Following the OSHA Bloodborne Pathogens Standard, the medical assistant should wear disposable gloves during the entire sanitization procedure. This protects the medical assistant from bloodborne pathogens and other potentially infectious materials. The medical assistant should be especially careful when working with hazardous chemicals and when handling sharp instruments. Heavy-duty utility gloves should be worn over the disposable gloves to provide protection from the irritating effects of chemical agents and accidental punctures or cuts from sharp instruments.

2. **Handle instruments carefully.** Instruments are expensive and delicate, yet durable. They can last for many years if handled and maintained properly. Dropping an instrument on the floor or throwing an instrument into a basin may damage it. Instruments should never be piled in a heap because they become entangled and may be damaged when separated. Keep sharp instruments separate from other instruments to prevent damaging or dulling the cutting edge. Also, keep delicate instruments separate to protect them from damage.

3. **Follow instructions on labels of chemical agents.** Before using a chemical agent, such as a chemical disinfectant, an instrument cleaner, or an autoclave cleaner, review the product's MSDS and carefully read the label on the container. Check the label to determine the use, mixing, and storage of the chemical agent. Read and observe precautions listed on the label regarding personal safety, such as the use of gloves and eye protection (Figure 18-4). Also, check the expiration date on the label of the chemical agent. Chemicals tend to lose their potency over time and should not be used past the expiration date.

4. **Use a proper cleaning agent.** A low-sudsing detergent with a neutral pH should be used to clean the instruments. Commercially available instrument cleaners meet these criteria (Figure 18-5). These cleaners usually come in a concentrated liquid or powder form and must be diluted with water before use. Never substitute any other type of detergent, such as dishwasher detergent or laundry detergent; these detergents may not be low-sudsing or have the proper pH for sanitizing instruments. If a detergent with an alkaline pH is used and not completely rinsed off, it could leave a residue on the instrument. This could result in an orange-brown stain on the instru-

Figure 18-5. Commercially available surgical instrument cleaners. *Left,* Instrument cleaner; *center,* stain remover; *right,* spray lubricant. (From Bonewit-West K: *Clinical procedures for medical assistants,* ed 7, St. Louis, 2008, Saunders.)

ment that resembles rust. Using an acid detergent also can cause staining and permanent corrosion.

5. **Use proper cleaning devices.** Proper cleaning devices should be used for the manual cleaning of surgical instruments. A stiff nylon brush should be used to clean the surface of the instrument. A stainless-steel wire brush can be used to clean grooves, crevices, or serrations. A stain on an instrument often can be removed using a commercial instrument stain remover (see Figure 18-5). Never use steel wool or other abrasives to remove stains because damage could occur to the instrument.

6. **Carefully inspect each instrument for defects and proper working condition.** After cleaning, rinsing, and drying the instrument, it is important to check it for defects and proper working condition as follows:
   - The blades of an instrument should be straight and not bent.
   - The tips of an instrument should approximate tightly and evenly when the instrument is closed.
   - An instrument with a box lock (e.g., hemostatic forceps, needle holders) should move freely but must not be too loose. The pin that holds the box lock together should be flush against the instrument.
   - An instrument with a spring handle (e.g., thumb and tissue forceps) should have sufficient tension to grasp objects tightly.
   - The cutting edge of a sharp instrument should be smooth and devoid of nicks.
   - Scissors should cut cleanly and smoothly. To test for this, the medical assistant should cut into a thin piece of gauze. The scissors are in proper working condition if they cut all the way to the end of the blade without catching on the gauze.

7. **Lubricate hinged instruments.** Lubricate box locks, screw locks, scissor blades, and any other moving part of each instrument. The lubricant makes the instrument function better and last longer. Use a lubricant that can be penetrated by steam, such as a commercial spray lubricant or a lubricant bath (see Figure 18-5). Lubricate after performing the final rinse (and drying of the instrument); otherwise the lubricant would be rinsed off the instrument. Never use industrial oils or silicon sprays. These substances are not steam penetrable and can build up on the instrument, affecting its working condition.

PROCEDURE 18-1

PROCEDURE 18-1   Sanitization of Instruments

Outcome Sanitize instruments.

Equipment/Supplies

- Sink
- Disposable gloves
- Heavy-duty utility gloves
- Contaminated instruments
- Environmental Protection Agency (EPA)-approved chemical disinfectant and MSDS
- Disinfectant container
- Cleaning solution and MSDS
- Basin
- Stiff nylon brush
- Stainless-steel wire brush
- Paper towels
- Cloth towel
- Instrument lubricant

1. **Procedural Step.** Review the MSDS for the hazardous chemicals you will be using in the sanitization process.
   Principle. The MSDS provides information regarding the chemical, its hazards, and measures to take to

prevent injury and illness when handling the disinfectant.

2. **Procedural Step.** Apply disposable gloves. Transport the contaminated instruments to the cleaning area as soon as possible after use. The instruments should be

Continued

PROCEDURE 18-1 Sanitization of Instruments—cont'd

carried in a covered basin from the examining room to the cleaning area.

Principle. Disposable gloves act as a barrier to protect the medical assistant from infectious materials. Transporting contaminated instruments in a covered basin promotes infection control.

3. **Procedural Step.** Apply heavy-duty utility gloves over the disposable gloves.

   Principle. Utility gloves help protect the hands from the irritating effects of chemical solutions.

4. **Procedural Step.** Separate sharp instruments and delicate instruments from other instruments.

   Principle. Separating sharp instruments from others prevents damage to or dulling of the cutting edge of these instruments. Delicate instruments should be separated to protect them from damage.

5. **Procedural Step.** Immediately rinse the instruments thoroughly under warm, not hot, running water (≈110°F [44°C]) to remove organic material, such as blood, body fluids, tissue, and other debris.

   Principle. Rinsing the instruments as soon as possible prevents organic material from drying on the instruments, making it difficult to remove later. Hot water may cause coagulation of organic material, making it more difficult to remove.

Rinse instruments under warm water to remove organic matter. (From Bonewit-West K: *Clinical procedures for medical assistants,* ed 7, St. Louis, 2008, Saunders.)

6. **Procedural Step.** Decontaminate the instruments by disinfecting them in an EPA-approved chemical disinfectant as follows:

   a. Select the proper chemical disinfectant; check the expiration date on the container label.

   b. Observe all personal safety precautions listed on the label of the disinfectant (e.g., wearing safety goggles).

   c. Follow the manufacturer's directions on the label for proper mixing and use of the disinfectant.

   d. Label the plastic or stainless steel disinfecting container with the name of the disinfectant and the date when the disinfectant is no longer effective and must be discarded (reuse life).

   e. Pour the disinfectant into the labeled container and immerse the articles into the disinfectant. Ensure the articles are completely submerged in the disinfectant.

   f. Cover the container that holds the chemical disinfectant.

   g. Disinfect the articles for 10 minutes.

   Principle. Decontaminating the instruments removes pathogenic microorganisms from them, making them safe to handle. A disinfectant past its expiration date loses its potency and should not be used. An EPA-approved disinfectant has been determined by the EPA to be effective when used as directed, without causing an unreasonable risk to the public or the environment. The container must be kept covered to prevent the escape of toxic fumes and to prevent evaporation of the disinfectant, which could change its potency.

7. **Procedural Step.** Clean the instruments. The instruments can be cleaned using the manual method or the ultrasound method as follows:

Manual Method for Cleaning Instruments

   a. Obtain the instrument cleaning solution; check its expiration date.

   b. Observe all personal safety precautions listed on the label of the cleaning agent.

   c. Follow the directions on the manufacturer's label for proper mixing and use of the cleaning agent. The detergent may need to be diluted with water.

   d. Remove the articles from the chemical disinfectant and place them in the basin containing the cleaning solution.

   e. Use a stiff nylon brush to clean the surface of each instrument. Scrub all parts of the instrument thoroughly. Brush delicate instruments carefully to prevent damaging them.

   f. Use a stainless-steel wire brush to clean grooves, crevices, or serrations where contaminants such as blood and tissue may collect.

   g. If there is a stain on the instrument, attempt to remove it using a damp cloth or sponge to which a commercial stain remover has been applied.

h. Scrub each instrument until it is visibly clean and free from organic material and stains.

Clean the surface of the instrument with a stiff nylon brush. (From Bonewit-West K: *Clinical procedures for medical assistants,* ed 7, St. Louis, 2008, Saunders.)

Clean grooves, crevices, or serrations with a wire brush. (From Bonewit-West K: *Clinical procedures for medical assistants,* ed 7, St. Louis, 2008, Saunders.)

Principle. A cleaning agent past its expiration date loses its potency and should not be used. Taking appropriate precautions with cleaning agents prevents harm to the medical assistant from hazardous chemicals. All organic material must be removed from the instruments to ensure complete sterilization in the autoclave.

Ultrasound Method for Cleaning Instruments

a. Using a cleaning agent recommended by the manufacturer, prepare the cleaning solution in the ultrasonic cleaner. Observe all personal safety precautions listed on the label.

b. Remove the articles from the chemical disinfectant, and separate instruments made of dissimilar metals, such as stainless steel, aluminum, and bronze.

c. Place the instruments in the ultrasonic cleaner with hinged instruments in an open position.

d. Ensure that sharp instruments do not touch other instruments.

e. Ensure that all instruments are fully submerged in the cleaning solution.

f. Place the lid on the ultrasonic cleaner.

Completely submerge instruments in the cleaning solution. (From Bonewit-West K: *Clinical procedures for medical assistants,* ed 7, St. Louis, 2008, Saunders.)

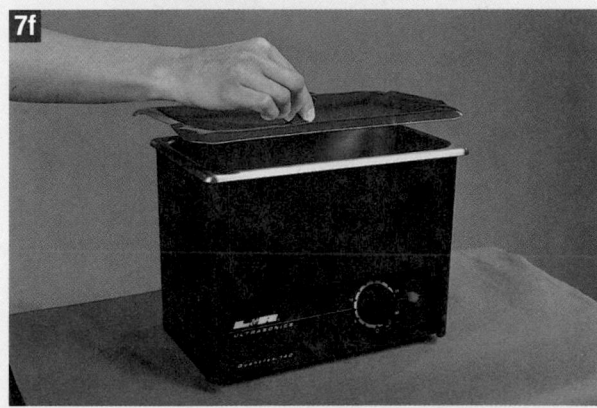

Place the lid on the ultrasonic cleaner. (From Bonewit-West K: *Clinical procedures for medical assistants,* ed 7, St. Louis, 2008, Saunders.)

g. Turn on the ultrasonic cleaner, and clean the instruments for the length of time recommended by the manufacturer.

h. After completion of the cleaning cycle, remove the instruments from the machine.

Principle. Taking appropriate precautions with chemical agents prevents harm to the medical assistant from hazardous chemicals. Mixing dissimilar

Continued

PROCEDURE 18-1

PROCEDURE **18-1** Sanitization of Instruments—cont'd

metals together could result in permanent stains on the instruments. Instruments must be completely submerged with hinged instruments in an open position so that the solution can reach all parts of the instrument.

8. Procedural Step. Rinse each instrument thoroughly with warm, not hot, water (110°F [44°C]) for at least 20 to 30 seconds to remove all traces of the detergent. Open and close hinged instruments while rinsing to ensure the solution is completely rinsed out of every part of the instrument.

Principle. Detergent residue left on the instrument could cause stains, which could build up and interfere with the proper functioning of the instrument. Using warm water helps to remove the cleaning solution and facilitates the drying process.

Dry the instrument with a paper towel. (From Bonewit-West K: *Clinical procedures for medical assistants,* ed 7, St. Louis, 2008, Saunders.)

10. Procedural Step. Check each instrument for defects and proper working condition. Scissors should cut all the way to the end of a thin piece of gauze without catching. If defects are noted, or if the instrument is not working properly, it must be discarded or sent to the manufacturer for repair.

Principle. Instruments that have defects or are not in proper working condition are unsafe to use on a patient during a medical or surgical procedure.

Rinse thoroughly with warm water. (From Bonewit-West K: *Clinical procedures for medical assistants,* ed 7, St. Louis, 2008, Saunders.)

9. Procedural Step. Dry each instrument with a paper towel, and place the instrument on a cloth towel for additional air drying.

Principle. If the instrument is not completely dry, stains may occur on the instrument.

Check the instrument for defects and proper working order. (From Bonewit-West K: *Clinical procedures for medical assistants,* ed 7, St. Louis, 2008, Saunders.)

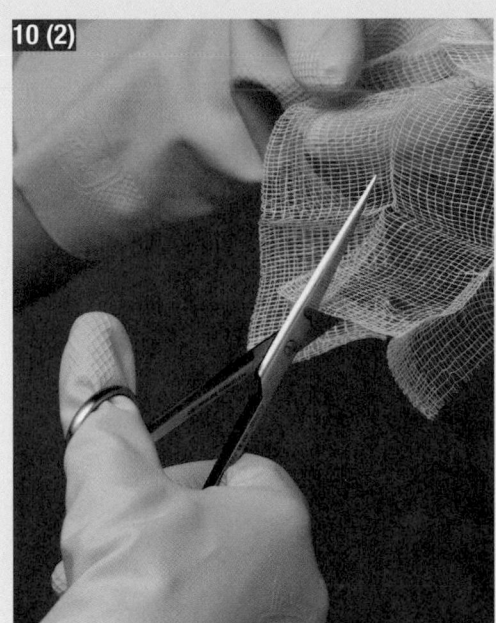

Scissors should cut through gauze without catching. (From Bonewit-West K: *Clinical procedures for medical assistants,* ed 7, St. Louis, 2008, Saunders.)

11. **Procedural Step.** Lubricate hinged instruments using a steam-penetrable lubricant as follows:
  a. Apply the lubricant to a hinged instrument in its open position.
  b. Open and close the instrument after applying the lubricant so that it reaches all parts of the hinged area.
  c. Place the instrument back on the towel, and allow it to drain. Rinsing or wiping are unnecessary.
  Principle. Lubricating an instrument makes it function better and last longer.

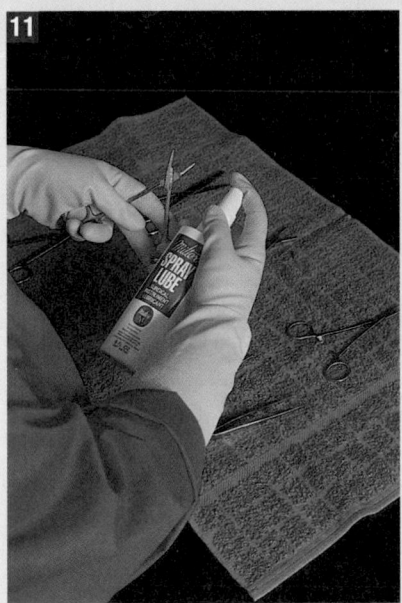

Lubricate hinged instruments. (From Bonewit-West K: *Clinical procedures for medical assistants,* ed 7, St. Louis, 2008, Saunders.)

12. **Procedural Step.** Dispose of the cleaning solution according to the manufacturer's instructions. Remove both sets of gloves, and sanitize your hands.
13. **Procedural Step.** Wrap the instruments and sterilize them in the autoclave according to the medical office policy.

PROCEDURE 18-1

DISINFECTION

Disinfection is the process of destroying pathogenic microorganisms, but it does not kill bacterial spores. Disinfection is accomplished in the medical office through the use of liquid chemical agents that are applied to inanimate objects. Chemical disinfection has been discussed with respect to its role in the sanitization process to decontaminate surgical instruments and make them safe to handle. This section discusses the use of chemical disinfection to disinfect semicritical and noncritical items so that they can be used for patient care. Table 18-1 lists disinfectants most frequently used in the medical office, along with common names and uses for each.

Levels of Disinfection

Disinfection can be classified according to three levels of disinfection based on killing action.

High-Level Disinfection

High-level disinfection is a process that destroys all microorganisms with the exception of bacterial spores. High-level disinfection is used to disinfect semicritical items. A **semicritical item** is an item that comes in contact with nonintact skin or intact mucous membranes, such as a flexible fiberoptic sigmoidoscope. A frequently used high-level disinfectant is 2% glutaraldehyde (e.g., Cidex, MetriCide). A newer high-level disinfectant that is growing in popularity is Cidex OPA (ortho-phthalaldehyde). Cidex OPA does not contain glutaraldehyde, which means it is less toxic and safer to handle.

Intermediate-Level Disinfection

Intermediate-level disinfection is a process that inactivates tubercle bacilli (the causative agent of tuberculosis), all veg-

Table 18-1 Disinfectants Used in the Medical Office

Disinfectant	Common Names	Use in the Medical Office
Glutaraldehyde	Cidex MetriCide ProCide Omnicide Wavicide	Disinfection of flexible fiberoptic sigmoidoscopes
Alcohol	Isopropyl alcohol	Disinfection of stethoscopes, blood pressure cuffs, tuning forks, and percussion hammers; isopropyl alcohol wipes are used to disinfect rubber stoppers of multiple-dose medication vials
Chlorine and chlorine compounds	Sodium hypochlorite (household bleach)	Recommended by OSHA for decontamination of blood spills
Phenolics	Carbolic acid Hydroxybenzene Phenic acid Phenyl hydroxide Phenylic acid	Disinfection of walls, furniture, floors, and laboratory work surfaces
Quaternary ammonium compounds	Benzalkonium chloride	Disinfection of walls, furniture, floors, and laboratory work surfaces

From Bonewit-West K: *Clinical procedures for medical assistants,* ed 7, St. Louis, 2008, Saunders.

What Would You Do? What Would You *Not* Do?

Case Study 2

Alecia Scout brings in her 2-year-old son, Benjamin, for a preschool physical examination. Benjamin is unhappy and crying loudly. Mrs. Scout says that Benjamin is upset because she would not let him play with the toys in the waiting room. She is afraid that he will catch a disease from a sick child who has played with the toys. Mrs. Scout is visibly annoyed and says that medical offices should not keep toys in the waiting room because they might spread disease and cause problems for parents who do not want their children to play with the toys. ■

Memories *from* Externship

Kara VanDyke: During my externship experience, I was placed in a pediatrician's office. I wanted to go to a pediatric site because I love being around children. One day I was in the examining room with my patient, a 4-year-old boy who was there with his mother. It was standard procedure at this office to take every patient's temperature. I started getting out our electronic thermometer to take his temperature when I noticed he looked a little frightened. He was looking at the thermometer funny, and he said, "Can you do it in my ear?" I said I was sorry but we didn't have that kind of thermometer. I told him I could do it under his arm or under his tongue. His mom looked at him, and he said, "But I want it in my ear." He finally agreed to let me do it under his arm. When I was finished taking his temperature, he smiled and said, "You're the nicest doctor!" ■

Prepare for Success

---

etative bacteria, most viruses, and most fungi, but it does not kill bacterial spores. Intermediate-level disinfection is used to disinfect noncritical items. **Noncritical items** are items that come in contact with intact skin but not mucous membranes, including stethoscopes, blood pressure cuffs, tuning forks, percussion hammers, and crutches. A common intermediate-level disinfectant is isopropyl alcohol, which is frequently used in the form of alcohol wipes.

Low-Level Disinfection

Low-level disinfection is a process that kills most bacteria, some viruses, and some fungi, but it cannot be relied on to kill resistant microorganisms, such as tubercle bacilli, and it cannot kill bacterial spores. Low-level disinfectants typically are used to disinfect surfaces such as examining tables, laboratory countertops, and walls. Low-level disinfectants used in the medical office include sodium hypochlorite (household bleach) and phenolics.

STERILIZATION

Sterilization is the process of destroying all forms of microbial life, including bacterial spores. An item that is sterile is free of all living microorganisms and spores. Sterilization must be used to process all critical items. A **critical item** is an item that comes in contact with sterile tissue or the vascular system.

As previously described, a semicritical item (one that comes in contact with nonintact skin or with intact mucous membranes) can be chemically disinfected using a high-level disinfectant. Most offices prefer instead to sterilize semicritical items in the autoclave (e.g., vaginal specula, nasal specula). The autoclave provides a convenient, efficient, safe, and inexpensive method for destroying microorganisms. Chemical disinfectants are not only more expensive to use, but also are more hazardous and create problems regarding their proper disposal. The exception is any semicritical item that is heat sensitive. Flexible fiberoptic sigmoidoscopes would be damaged by the heat of an autoclave and must be chemically disinfected.

Sterilization Methods

Sterilization involves the use of physical or chemical methods. Each method of sterilization has advantages and disadvantages. The method used to achieve sterility depends primarily on the nature of the item to be sterilized. The most common physical and chemical sterilization methods include the following:

Physical Methods	Chemical Methods
Steam under pressure (autoclave)	Ethylene oxide gas
Hot air (dry heat oven)	Cold sterilization (chemical agents)
Radiation	

The most common method for sterilizing articles in the medical office is steam under pressure using an autoclave. The autoclave is discussed in detail in this chapter; the other methods of sterilization are briefly described.

Autoclave

The autoclave is dependable, efficient, and economical and can be used to sterilize items that are not harmed by moisture or high temperature. Refer to the box titled *Items Sterilized in the Autoclave* for a list of heat-resistant items that can be sterilized in the autoclave.

An **autoclave** consists of an outer jacket surrounding an inner sterilizing chamber. Under pressure, distilled water is converted to steam, which fills the inner sterilizing chamber. The pressure plays no direct part in killing microorganisms; rather, it functions to attain a higher temperature than could be reached by the steam from boiling water (212°F [100°C]). The cooler, drier air already in the chamber is forced out through the air exhaust valve.

It is important that all the air in the chamber be replaced by steam. When air is present, the temperature in the autoclave is reduced and a temperature that is adequate for sterilization is not reached. When all the air has been removed, the air exhaust valve seals off the inner chamber and the temperature in the autoclave begins to increase.

Items Sterilized in the Autoclave

Surgical instruments	Brushes
Medical instruments	Dressings
Minor office surgery trays	Glassware
Liquids	Reusable syringes

During the sterilization process, the steam penetrates materials in the sterilizing chamber. The materials are cooler, so the steam condenses into moisture on them, giving up its heat. This heat serves to kill all microorganisms and their spores.

The autoclave is usually operated at approximately 15 lb of pressure per square inch (psi) at a temperature of 250°F (121°C). Vegetative forms of most microorganisms are killed in a few minutes at temperatures ranging from 130°F to 150°F (54°C to 65°C), but certain bacterial spores can withstand a temperature of 240°F (115°C) for more than 3 hours. No organism, however, can survive direct exposure to saturated steam at 250°F (121°C) for 15 minutes or longer.

The sterilization process using the autoclave is discussed in this section (with the exception of sanitization, which was already presented). The sterilization process consists of the following components:
- Monitoring program
- Sanitizing articles
- Wrapping articles
- Operating the autoclave (autoclave cycle)
- Handling and storing packs
- Maintaining the autoclave

Monitoring Program

To ensure that instruments and supplies are sterile when used, the Centers for Disease Control and Prevention (CDC) recommends that the medical office establish and maintain a monitoring program of the sterilization process. The monitoring program should consist of the following:
1. Written policies and procedures for each step of the sterilization process
2. Sterilization indicators to ensure that minimum sterilizing conditions have been achieved
3. Records for each cycle maintained in an autoclave log (Figure 18-6)

The information that should be recorded for each autoclave cycle includes the following:
- Date and time of the cycle
- Description of the **load**
- Exposure time
- Exposure temperature
- Results of the sterilization indicator
- Initials of the operator

Some autoclaves have recorders that automatically print out a portion of this information at the end of the cycle (Figure 18-7).

Sterilization Indicators

Materials that are being sterilized must be exposed to steam at a sufficient temperature and for a proper length of time. Sterilization indicators are available to determine the effectiveness of the procedure and to check against improper wrapping of articles, improper loading of the autoclave, and faulty operation of the autoclave.

An article is not considered sterile unless the steam has penetrated to its center; most sterilization indicators are

AUTOCLAVE LOG

Date/Time	Description of the Load	Cycle Time (min)	Temperature (°F)	Indicator* (+/−)	Initials	Comments
7/25/10 4:00 PM	Surgical instruments	20	250	−	KV	
7/26/10 3:00 PM	MOS tray setups	30	250	−	KV	

*Indicator Interpretation:
Positive (+): Spores not killed, indicating sterilization conditions have not been met.
Negative (−): Spores killed, indicating sterilization conditions have been met.

MAINTENANCE: (Indicate date, vendor name, service, etc.)

Figure 18-6. Example of an autoclave log. (From Bonewit-West K: *Clinical procedures for medical assistants,* ed 7, St. Louis, 2008, Saunders.)

placed in the center of the article. The medical assistant should carefully read the instructions that come with the sterilization indicators. The most reliable indicators check for the attainment of the proper temperature and indicate the duration of the temperature.

If an indicator does not change properly, a problem may be present in the sterilization technique or in the working condition of the autoclave. The manufacturer's guidelines for proper sterilization techniques should be reviewed, and the articles should be resterilized following these guidelines. If the indicator still does not change properly, the autoclave is in need of repair and should not be used until it has been serviced.

Sterilization indicators should be stored in a cool, dry area. Excessive heat or moisture can damage the indicator. The most common sterilization indicators are chemical indicators and biologic indicators, which are described next.

What Would You Do? What Would You *Not* Do?

Case Study 3

Cassie Augusta is in the examining room and is being prepared for the removal of a sebaceous cyst. Cassie is concerned about the instruments that the physician will be using to perform the procedure. She wants to know if they are "safe." Cassie says that her friend Mackenzie got a tattoo several years ago and developed hepatitis 3 weeks later. Mackenzie thinks she got hepatitis from the instruments that were used for her tattoo procedure. Cassie wants to know if it is possible for an instrument to give someone hepatitis. She says she heard that hepatitis can cause liver cancer and wants to know if this is true. Cassie also wants to know if there is a vaccine to prevent hepatitis. ■

```
READY

BEGIN

SET TEMP:      270 F      Temperature
SET TIME:      015    ←—  Time
RUN #          011    ←—  Cycle number

DATE   7/25/10

HEAT UP
DEG      PSI      MIN
066      00.0     000
066      00.0     002
074      00.0     004
164      00.0     006     Heat-up
219      04.1     008     phase
234      09.4     010
261      22.6     012

STERILIZE
DEG      PSI      MIN
272      30.2     000
272      30.7     001
273      31.3     002
274      31.0     003
273      30.7     004
273      30.4     005
273      30.1     006
272      30.0     007     Sterilization
272      30.1     008     phase
272      30.4     009
272      30.4     010
272      30.7     011
273      31.0     012
273      30.8     013
274      31.0     014
273      30.7     015

VENT
COMPLETE
```

Figure 18-7. Example of a printout of an autoclave cycle. (From Bonewit-West K: *Clinical procedures for medical assistants,* ed 7, St. Louis, 2008, Saunders.)

Figure 18-8. Autoclave tape. *Top,* Autoclave tape as it appears before the sterilization process. *Bottom,* Diagonal lines appear on the tape during autoclaving and indicate that the wrapped article has been autoclaved. (From Bonewit-West K: *Clinical procedures for medical assistants,* ed 7, St. Louis, 2008, Saunders.)

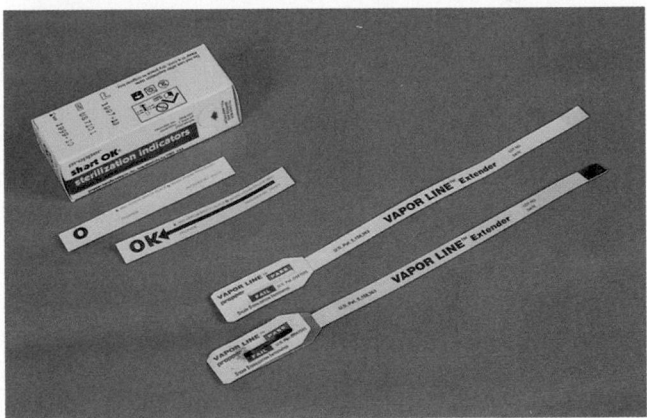

Figure 18-9. Sterilization strips. Sterilization strips contain a thermolabile dye and change color when exposed to steam under pressure for a certain length of time. (From Bonewit-West K: *Clinical procedures for medical assistants,* ed 7, St. Louis, 2008, Saunders.)

Chemical Indicators

Chemical indicators are impregnated with a **thermolabile** dye that changes color when exposed to the sterilization process. If the chemical reaction of the indicator does not show the expected results, the item may not be sterile and must be resterilized. Chemical indicators include autoclave tape and sterilization strips.

Autoclave Tape. Autoclave tape contains a chemical that changes color if it has been exposed to steam. The tape is available in a variety of colors, can be written on, and is useful for closing and identifying the wrapped article (Figure 18-8). Autoclave tape has some limitations as an indicator. Because it is placed on the outside of the pack, it cannot ensure that steam has penetrated to the center of the pack. It also does not ensure that the item has been sterilized; it merely indicates that an article has been in the autoclave and that a high temperature has been attained.

Sterilization Strips. Sterilization strips are commercially prepared paper or plastic strips that contain a thermolabile dye and that change color when exposed to steam under pressure for a certain length of time (Figure 18-9). Most sterilization strips are designed to change color after being exposed to a temperature of 250°F (121°C) for 15 minutes. The indicator strip should be placed in the center of the wrapped pack, with the end containing the dye placed in an area of the pack considered to be the hardest for steam to penetrate.

Biologic Indicators

Biologic indicators are the best means available for determining the effectiveness of the sterilization procedure. The CDC recommends that medical office personnel use a biologic indicator to monitor all autoclaves at least once a week.

A biologic indicator is a preparation of living bacterial spores. Biologic indicators are commercially available in the form of dry spore strips in small glassine envelopes. Biologic monitoring of an autoclave requires the use of a preparation of spores of *Bacillus stearothermophilus,* which is a microorganism with spores particularly resistant to moist heat.

Each biologic testing unit includes two spore tests that are sterilized and one spore control that is not sterilized (Figure 18-10). The biologic indicator is placed in the center of two wrapped articles. The articles are placed in areas of the autoclave that are the least accessible to steam penetration, such as on the bottom tray of the autoclave, near the front of the autoclave, and in the back of the autoclave.

After the indicators have been exposed to sterilization conditions, they must be processed before the results can be obtained. The two methods for processing results are the in-house method and the mail-in method.

In-House Method. The in-house method involves processing and interpreting the results at the medical office. After sterilization, the processed spores are **incubated** for 24 to 48 hours. If sterilization conditions have been met, the color or condition of the processed spores is different from those of the control and the spore test is interpreted as negative. If sterilization conditions have not been met, the processed spores and the unprocessed control display the same color or condition and the spore test is interpreted as positive.

Mail-in Method. With this method, the processed bacterial spores and the (unprocessed) control are mailed to a processing laboratory. The test is performed by the laboratory, and the results are returned to the medical office.

If spores are not killed in routine spore tests, the autoclave should be checked immediately for proper use and function and the spore test should be repeated. If the spore test remains positive, the autoclave should not be used until it is serviced.

Wrapping Articles

Articles to be sterilized in the autoclave first must be thoroughly sanitized (see Procedure 18-1). Next, the articles are prepared for autoclaving by wrapping them. The purpose of wrapping articles is to protect them from recontamination during handling and storage. Articles that are wrapped and handled correctly remain sterile after autoclaving until the package seal is broken.

The wrapping material should be made of a substance that is not affected by the sterilization process and should allow steam to penetrate while preventing contaminants, such as dust, insects, and microorganisms, from entering during handling and storage. It should not tear or puncture easily and should allow the sterilized package to be opened without contamination of the contents. A wrapper should not be used if it is torn or has a hole. Examples of wrapping material used for autoclaving are sterilization paper, sterilization pouches, and muslin.

Sterilization Paper

Sterilization paper is a disposable and inexpensive wrapping material. It consists of square sheets of paper of different sizes (Figure 18-11). The most common sizes (in inches) are 12 × 12, 15 × 15, 18 × 18, 24 × 24, 30 × 30, and 36 × 36. Articles must be wrapped in such a way that they do not become contaminated when the pack is opened. The proper method for wrapping instruments using sterilization paper is outlined in Procedure 18-2. This method of wrapping can be used for all types of instruments and supplies.

The disadvantage of sterilization paper is that it is difficult to spread open for removal of the contents. It has a "memory" and tends to flip back easily, so it may not open flat to provide a sterile field. (*Memory* is the ability of a material to retain a specific shape or configuration.) Because sterilization paper is opaque, it is impossible to view the contents of a pack before opening it.

Figure 18-10. Biologic indicator. A biologic indicator includes two spore tests that are sterilized *(top right)* and one spore control that is not sterilized *(bottom right).* (From Bonewit-West K: *Clinical procedures for medical assistants,* ed 7, St. Louis, 2008, Saunders.)

Figure 18-11. Sterilization paper wraps. Sterilization paper consists of square sheets of paper that are available in different sizes. (From Bonewit-West K: *Clinical procedures for medical assistants,* ed 7, St. Louis, 2008, Saunders.)

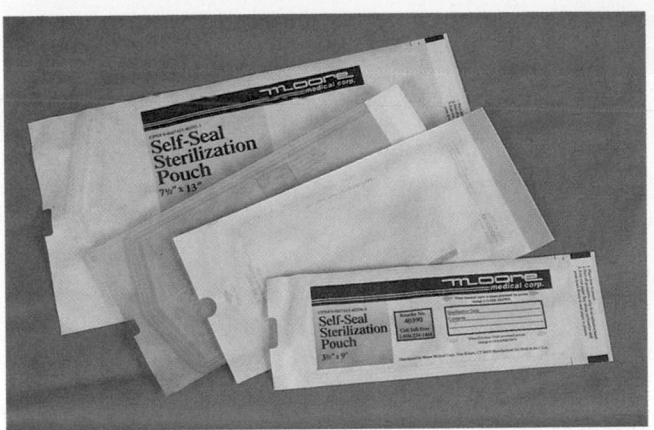

Figure 18-12. Sterilization pouches. Sterilization pouches consist of a combination of paper and plastic and are available in different sizes. (From Bonewit-West K: *Clinical procedures for medical assistants,* ed 7, St. Louis, 2008, Saunders.)

Sterilization Pouches

Sterilization pouches typically consist of a combination of paper and plastic; paper comprises one side of the pouch, and a plastic film comprises the other side (Figure 18-12). Sterilization pouches are available in different sizes; the most common sizes (in inches) are 3 × 9, 5 × 10, and 7 × 12.

Most pouches have a peel-apart seal on one end that is used later to open the pouch for removal of the sterile item. The other end of the pouch is open and is used to insert the item into the pouch. When the article has been inserted, this end is sealed with heat or adhesive tape. The proper method for wrapping an instrument using a pouch is outlined in Procedure 18-3.

Sterilization pouches provide good visibility of the contents on the plastic side. Most manufacturers include a sterilization indicator on the outside of the pouch. After removing a pouch from the autoclave, the medical assistant should check the indicator for proper color change. If the indicator does not change to the appropriate color (specified by the manufacturer), the contents of the pouch must be resterilized.

Muslin

Muslin is a reusable woven fabric and is available in different sizes. Muslin is flexible and easy to handle and is considered the most economical sterilization wrap because it can be reused. Because of its durability, muslin is frequently used to wrap large packs, such as tray setups for minor office surgery. Muslin is "memory free," so it lies flat when opened. A pack wrapped in muslin may be opened on a table so that the wrapper becomes a sterile field. The procedure for wrapping an article with muslin is the same as that for sterilization paper (see Procedure 18-2).

 PROCEDURE 18-2   Wrapping Instruments Using Paper or Muslin

Outcome Wrap an instrument for autoclaving.

Equipment/Supplies

- Sanitized instrument
- Appropriate-sized wrapping material (sterilization paper or muslin)
- Sterilization indicator strip
- Autoclave tape
- Permanent marker

1. **Procedural Step.** Sanitize your hands.
2. **Procedural Step.** Assemble the equipment. Select the appropriate-sized wrapping material for the instrument being wrapped. Check the expiration date on the sterilization indicator box. If the sterilization strips are outdated, do not use them.
   Principle. Instruments are wrapped so that they are protected from recontamination after they have been sterilized. Outdated strip indicators may not provide accurate test results.
3. **Procedural Step.** Place the wrapping material on a clean, flat surface. Turn the wrap in a diagonal position to your body so that it resembles a diamond shape.

Turn the wrap in a diagonal position. (From Bonewit-West K: *Clinical procedures for medical assistants,* ed 7, St. Louis, 2008, Saunders.)

Continued

4. Procedural Step. Place the instrument in the center of the wrapping material with the longest part of the instrument pointing toward the two side corners. If the instrument has a movable joint, place it on the wrap in a slightly open position. If necessary, a gauze square can be used to hold the instrument in an open position.

Principle. Instruments with movable joints must be in an open position to allow steam to reach all parts of the instrument. If the instrument is in a closed position, heat exposure could cause the instrument to crack at its weakest part, such as the lock area.

5. Procedural Step. Place a sterilization indicator in the center of the pack next to the instrument.

Principle. Sterilization indicators assess the effectiveness of the sterilization process.

Place a sterilization indicator in the center of the pack next to the instrument. (From Bonewit-West K: *Clinical procedures for medical assistants,* ed 7, St. Louis, 2008, Saunders.)

6. Procedural Step. Fold the wrapping material up from the bottom, and double-back a small corner, creating a flap. This flap will later be used to open the sterile pack without contaminating the instrument.

Fold the wrapping material up from the bottom, and double-back a small corner. (From Bonewit-West K: *Clinical procedures for medical assistants,* ed 7, St. Louis, 2008, Saunders.)

7. Procedural Step. Fold over one edge of the wrapping material, and double-back the corner.

8. Procedural Step. Fold over the other edge of the wrapping material, and double-back the corner.

Fold over the other edge of the wrapping material, and double-back the corner. (From Bonewit-West K: *Clinical procedures for medical assistants,* ed 7, St. Louis, 2008, Saunders.)

9. Procedural Step. Fold the pack up from the bottom, pull the top flap down, and secure it with autoclave tape. Ensure that the pack is firm enough for handling but loose enough to permit proper circulation of steam.

Principle. Instruments must be wrapped properly to permit full penetration of steam and to prevent contaminating them when the wrap is opened. Using autoclave tape indicates that the pack has been through the autoclave cycle and prevents mix-ups with packs that have not been processed.

Fold the pack up from the bottom. (From Bonewit-West K: *Clinical procedures for medical assistants,* ed 7, St. Louis, 2008, Saunders.)

10. Procedural Step. Label the pack according to its contents. Mark the pack with the date of sterilization and your initials.

Principle. Dating the pack ensures that the most recently sterilized packs are stored in back of previously sterilized packs.

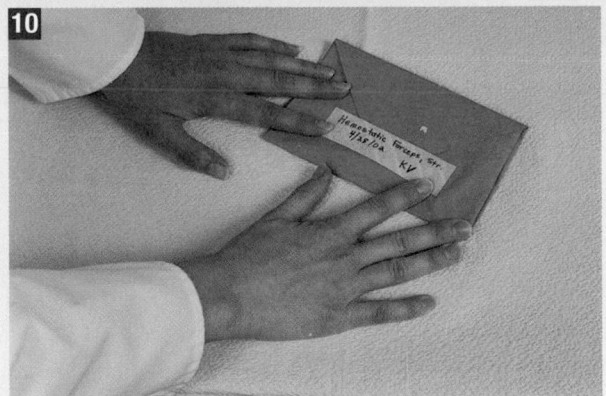

Label and date the pack. Include your initials. (From Bonewit-West K: *Clinical procedures for medical assistants,* ed 7, St. Louis, 2008, Saunders.)

PROCEDURE 18-3 Wrapping Instruments Using a Pouch

Outcome Wrap an instrument for autoclaving.

Equipment/Supplies

- Sanitized instrument
- Appropriate-sized sterilization pouch
- Permanent marker

1. Procedural Step. Sanitize your hands.

2. Procedural Step. Assemble the equipment. Select the appropriate-sized sterilization pouch for the instrument being wrapped. For hinged instruments, use a bag wide enough so that the instrument can be placed in a slightly open position inside the bag.

Principle. Instruments are wrapped so that they are protected from recontamination after they have been sterilized.

3. Procedural Step. Place the sterilization pouch on a clean, flat surface.

4. Procedural Step. Label the pack according to its contents. Mark the pack with the date of sterilization and your initials.

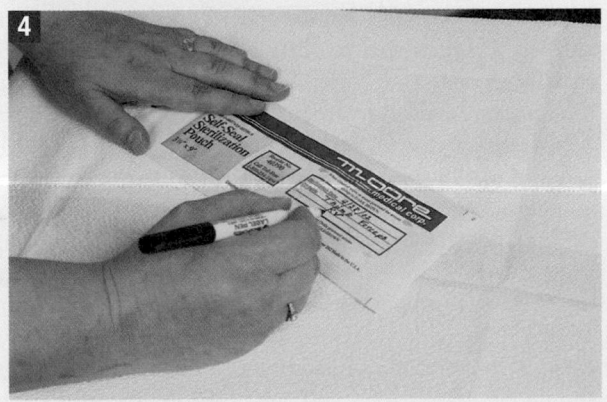

Label and date the pack. Include your initials. (From Bonewit-West K: *Clinical procedures for medical assistants,* ed 7, St. Louis, 2008, Saunders.)

Principle. Dating the pack ensures that the most recently sterilized packs are stored in back of previously sterilized packs.

5. Procedural Step. Insert the instrument to be sterilized into the unsealed, open end of the pouch. If the instrument has a movable joint, place it in the pouch in a slightly open position. If necessary, a gauze square can be used to hold the instrument in an open position.

Insert the instrument into the pouch. (From Bonewit-West K: *Clinical procedures for medical assistants,* ed 7, St. Louis, 2008, Saunders.)

6. Procedural Step. Seal the open end of the pouch as follows:

Adhesive Closure. Peel off the paper strip located above the perforation to expose the adhesive. Fold along the

Continued

PROCEDURE 18-3

PROCEDURE 18-3   Wrapping Instruments Using a Pouch—cont'd

6a

Peel off the paper strip. (From Bonewit-West K: *Clinical procedures for medical assistants,* ed 7, St. Louis, 2008, Saunders.)

6b

Press firmly to seal the pack. (From Bonewit-West K: *Clinical procedures for medical assistants,* ed 7, St. Louis, 2008, Saunders.)

perforation and press firmly to seal the paper to the plastic. Ensure that the seal is secure by running fingers back and forth on both sides of the pouch over the entire sealing area.

Heat Closure. Seal the pouch using a heat-sealing device.

7. Procedural Step. Sterilize the pack in the autoclave.

Operating the Autoclave

The autoclave must be operated according to the manufacturer's instructions. The medical assistant should read the operating manual carefully before running the autoclave for the first time. Thereafter, the manual should be kept in an accessible location so that it is available if needed as a reference. Procedure 18-4 outlines a general procedure for sterilizing articles in the autoclave.

The steps involved in achieving sterilization using an autoclave are known as the *autoclave cycle.* Accomplishment of each step varies based on whether the autoclave is operated manually or automatically. Figure 18-13 illustrates the autoclave cycle for manual and automatic autoclave operation.

Guidelines for Autoclave Operation

Location of the Autoclave

The autoclave must be placed on a level surface to ensure that the chamber fills correctly. The front of the autoclave should be near the front of the support surface so that water can be easily drained from the drain tube into a container when the autoclave is being flushed.

Filling the Water Reservoir

Distilled water is used to fill the water reservoir of the autoclave. Normal tap water contains minerals, such as chlorine, which have corrosive effects on the stainless-steel chamber of the autoclave. In addition, using tap water may cause a mineral buildup that can block the air exhaust valve. This causes air pockets, which prevent the temperature from increasing in the autoclave. The water reservoir is filled to the proper level as indicated in the operating manual. An

autoclave malfunction may occur if the reservoir is overfilled or if there is not enough water in the reservoir.

Loading the Autoclave

For an item to attain sterility, steam must penetrate every fiber and reach every surface of the item at a required temperature and for a specified time. To accomplish this, all packs must be positioned in the chamber to allow free circulation and penetration of steam. The following guidelines should be followed when loading the autoclave:

1. Small packs are best because steam penetrates them more easily; it takes longer for steam to reach the center of a large pack to ensure sterilization. A pack should be no larger than 12 × 12 × 20 inches.

2. To allow for proper steam penetration, the packs should be packed as loosely as possible inside the autoclave, with approximately 1 to 3 inches between small packs and 2 to 4 inches between large packs. Packs should not be allowed to touch surrounding walls, and at least 1 inch should separate the autoclave trays. Placing the articles too close together retards the flow of steam (Figure 18-14).

3. Jars and glassware should be placed on their sides in the autoclave with their lids removed. If they are placed upright, air may be trapped in them and they would not be sterilized. Trapped air must flow out and be replaced by steam during the sterilization process (Figure 18-15).

4. Packs that contain layers of fabric, such as dressings, should be placed in a vertical position. Because steam flows from top to bottom, this method allows the steam to penetrate the layers of fabric.

AUTOMATIC OPERATION		MANUAL OPERATION
	The autoclave is turned on	
Set the sterilization program Press start button		
Chamber automatically fills with water	The chamber is filled with water	Fill manually using control
The automatic timer begins a timing countdown	Temperature reaches desired temperature and pressure (usually 250° F, 15 lb pressure)	Set timer using control
	Packs are subjected to steam at a specified temperature and duration of time	
Autoclave automatically vents	Steam is vented from the chamber	Manually vent steam using control
Door automatically opens slightly, and audible beep sounds when completed	The load is dried	Crack the door Set timer for appropriate drying time

Figure 18-13. The autoclave cycle for manual and automatic operation. (From Bonewit-West K: *Clinical procedures for medical assistants,* ed 7, St. Louis, 2008, Saunders.)

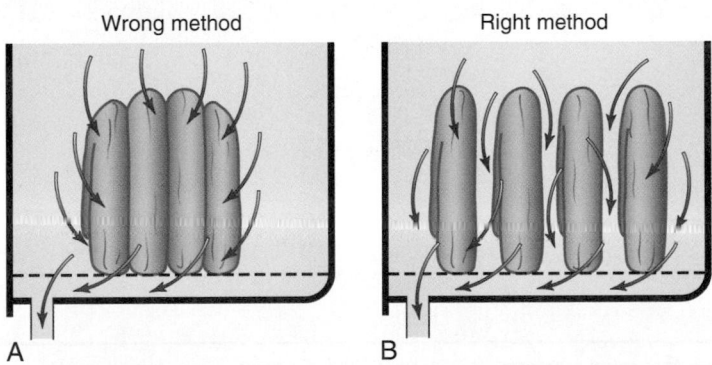

Wrong method   Right method

A   B

Figure 18-14. Arrangement of packs in the autoclave. **A,** Improper arrangement of packs in the autoclave. This arrangement prevents adequate penetration of steam, resulting in failure to sterilize the portions in the center of the mass. **B,** Proper arrangement of packs in the autoclave. The packs are separated from each other, and steam can now permeate each pack quickly and in the much shorter period of exposure needed. (Courtesy/modified from AMSCO/American Sterilizer Company, Erie, Pa.)

5. Sterilization pouches should be positioned on their sides to maximize steam circulation and to facilitate the drying process. Pouches can also be placed on the autoclave tray with the paper side up and the plastic side down.

Timing the Load

The autoclave is operated at approximately 15 psi with a temperature of 250°F (121°C). The length of time required for sterilization varies according to the item that is being sterilized (Table 18-2). Steam can easily reach the surfaces of hard, nonporous items such as unwrapped instruments (e.g., vaginal specula) to kill microorganisms; these items require approximately 15 minutes of sterilization time. A large minor office surgery pack requires a longer sterilization time, about 30 minutes, because more time is needed for steam to penetrate to the center of the pack. Rubber goods may be damaged, however, by exposure to excessive heat. To prevent this, the medical assistant should sterilize rubber items for only the prescribed amount of time.

The sterilizing time should not begin until the desired temperature in the autoclave has been reached. Timing the load is accomplished automatically or manually. Autoclaves with automatic operation begin timing the load automatically when the desired temperature has been reached. With the manual method of operation, the medical assistant must set the timer by hand using a timing control on the front of the autoclave. The medical assistant should not set the timer until the temperature gauge reaches the desired temperature. The articles in the load are not considered sterile unless they have been subjected to steam for the proper length of time at the proper temperature.

Drying the Load

The sterilized articles are moist and must be allowed to dry before they are removed from the autoclave. Microorganisms can move quickly through the moisture on a wet wrap and onto the sterile article inside, resulting in contamination.

When the load has been subjected to steam for the proper length of time and temperature, the chamber must be vented of steam. Venting the chamber permits the pressure in the autoclave to decrease to zero and the chamber to cool, making it safe for the door to be opened. Most autoclaves are designed to vent automatically, which eliminates having to vent them manually.

The door of the autoclave should be opened approximately ½ inch but no more than 1 inch. Opening the door more than 1 inch causes cold air from the outside to rush into the autoclave, resulting in condensation of water on the packs. Cracking the door allows the moisture on the articles to change from a liquid to a vapor and to escape through the crack. The residual heat in the inner chamber also helps to dry the articles. The load should be allowed to dry for 15 to 60 minutes, depending on the type of autoclave and the load. Loads that contain large packs require

Figure 18-15. Jars and glassware should be placed on their sides in the autoclave with their lids removed. (Courtesy AMSCO/American Sterilizer Company, Erie, Pa.)

Table 18-2 Minimum Sterilizing Times		
Items (Manual Operation)*	Program (Automatic Operation)†	Time (min at 250°F [121°C])
Unwrapped nonsurgical instruments	Unwrapped	15
Open glass or metal canisters		
Nonsurgical rubber tubing		
Wrapped instruments	Wrapped	20
Fabric or muslin		
Wrapped trays of loose instruments		
Rubber tubing		
Minor office surgery tray setup (wrapped)	Packs	30
Liquids or gels	Liquids	30

From Bonewit-West K: *Clinical procedures for medical assistants,* ed 7, St. Louis, 2008, Saunders.

*Manual operation: The sterilizing time is selected based on the items being sterilized, as indicated in this column. The sterilizing time is set using the manual timing control when the autoclave has reached a temperature of 250°F (121°C).

†Automatic operation: The sterilization program selected from this column is based on the item being autoclaved. The program is selected by pressing the appropriate program button on the front of the autoclave (i.e., unwrapped, wrapped, packs, liquids). The autoclave automatically begins the proper timing countdown when it reaches 250°F (121°C).

a longer drying time than loads with smaller packs. The medical assistant should follow the manufacturer's recommendations for proper drying times of various loads.

Handling and Storing Packs

Sterilized wrapped articles should be handled carefully and as little as possible. If a wrapped article is crushed, compressed, or dropped, the sterility of the contents cannot be assumed, and the pack must be resterilized. This is known as *event-related sterility*, meaning that a sterile pack is considered sterile indefinitely, unless an event occurs that interferes with the sterility of the article.

Sterilized packs should be stored in clean, dry areas that are free from dust, insects, and other sources of contamination. Wrapped articles should be stored with the most recently sterilized articles placed in the back. The medical assistant should thoroughly check each sterilized pack at least twice: before storing it and before using it. If the pack is torn or opened, or if it is wet, it is no longer sterile and must be rewrapped and resterilized.

Maintaining the Autoclave

For the autoclave to work efficiently, it must be maintained properly. The operating manual that accompanies the autoclave provides specific information for the care and maintenance of that type of autoclave.

Safety precautions should be followed when performing maintenance procedures. Before proceeding with preventive maintenance, the autoclave must be cool, the pressure gauge at zero, and the power cord disconnected from the wall socket. Autoclave maintenance is performed on a daily, weekly, and monthly basis as follows:

Daily Maintenance

1. Wipe the outside of the autoclave with a damp cloth and a mild detergent.
2. Wipe the interior of the autoclave and the trays with a damp cloth.
3. Clean the rubber gasket on the door of the autoclave with a damp cloth.
4. Inspect the rubber door gasket for damage that could prevent a good seal.

Weekly Maintenance

1. Wash the inside of the chamber and the trays with a commercial autoclave cleaner according to the manufacturer's instructions, observing all personal safety precautions. This usually involves the following steps: The water reservoir must be drained first. A soft cloth or a soft brush should be used to clean the chamber. Do not use steel wool or a steel brush or other abrasive agents because they can damage the chamber. When the chamber is clean, it should be rinsed thoroughly with distilled water. The chamber must be dried thoroughly and the door left open overnight.
2. Wash the metal shelves with an autoclave cleaner, and rinse them thoroughly with distilled water.

Monthly Maintenance

1. Flush the system to remove any buildup of residue, which could cause corrosion of the chamber lines. Carefully follow the manufacturer's directions in the instruction manual to perform this procedure.
2. Check the air trap jet to ensure it is functioning properly. The air trap jet prevents air pockets from occurring in the chamber, to ensure adequate sterilization.
3. Check the safety valve to ensure it is functioning properly. The safety valve releases pressure in the chamber if it gets too high.

Other Sterilization Methods

In addition to the autoclave, other methods can be used to sterilize articles. These methods are not generally used in the medical office and are discussed only briefly in this chapter.

Dry Heat Oven

Dry heat ovens are used to sterilize articles that cannot be penetrated by steam or may be damaged by it. Dry heat is less corrosive than moist heat for instruments with sharp edges; it does not dull their sharp edges. Oil, petroleum jelly, and powder cannot be penetrated by steam and must be sterilized in a dry heat oven. Moist heat sterilization tends to erode the ground-glass surfaces of reusable syringes, whereas dry heat does not.

Dry heat ovens operate similar to an ordinary cooking oven. A longer exposure period is necessary with dry heat because microorganisms and spores are more resistant to dry heat than to moist heat and because dry heat penetrates more slowly and unevenly than moist heat. The most commonly used temperature for dry heat sterilization is 320°F (160°C) for 1 to 2 hours, depending on the article being sterilized. The recommended wrapping material for dry heat sterilization is aluminum foil because it is a good conductor of heat, and it protects against recontamination during handling and storage. Dry heat sterilization indicators are available to determine the effectiveness of the sterilization process.

Ethylene Oxide Gas Sterilization

Ethylene oxide is a colorless gas that is toxic and flammable. It is used to sterilize heat-sensitive items that cannot be sterilized in an autoclave. After items are sterilized with this gas, they must be aerated to remove the toxic residue of the ethylene oxide.

Ethylene oxide sterilization is a more complex and expensive process than steam sterilization. It is frequently used in the medical manufacturing industry for producing prepackaged, presterilized disposable items, such as syringes, sutures, catheters, and surgical packs.

Cold Sterilization

Cold sterilization involves the use of a chemical agent for an extended length of time. Only chemicals that are designated *sterilants* by the EPA can be used for sterilizing articles. If a chemical agent holds this status, the word *sterilant* is printed on the front of the container.

The item to be sterilized must be completely submerged in the chemical for a long time (6 to 24 hours depending on the manufacturer's instructions). Prolonged immersion of instruments can damage them. In addition, each time an instrument is added to the instrument container, the clock must be restarted for the entire amount of time. For these reasons, and because this method involves the use of a haz-

ardous chemical, cold sterilization should be used only when an autoclave, gas, or a dry heat oven are not indicated or are unavailable.

Radiation

Radiation uses high-energy ionizing radiation to sterilize articles. Medical manufacturers use radiation to sterilize prepackaged surgical equipment and instruments that cannot be sterilized by heat or chemicals.

PROCEDURE 18-4   Sterilizing Articles in the Autoclave

Outcome Sterilize a load of contaminated articles in the autoclave.

Equipment/Supplies

- Autoclave and instruction manual
- Distilled water

- Wrapped articles
- Heat-resistant gloves

1. **Procedural Step.** Assemble the equipment.
2. **Procedural Step.** Check the level of water in the autoclave and add distilled water, if needed.
   Principle. Water contained in the water reservoir of the autoclave is converted to steam during the sterilization process. Distilled water is used to prevent corrosion of the stainless-steel chamber of the autoclave.

If needed, add distilled water to the autoclave. (From Bonewit-West K: *Clinical procedures for medical assistants,* ed 7, St. Louis, 2008, Saunders.)

3. **Procedural Step.** Properly load the autoclave following these guidelines:
   a. Do not overload the chamber. Small packs should be placed 1 to 3 inches apart, and large packs should be placed 2 to 4 inches apart. The packs should not touch the chamber walls.
   b. Ensure that at least 1 inch separates the autoclave trays.
   c. Place jars and glassware on their sides.
   d. Place dressings in a vertical position.
   e. When sterilizing dressings and hard goods together, place dressings on the top shelf and hard goods on the lower shelf.

Properly load the autoclave. (From Bonewit-West K: *Clinical procedures for medical assistants,* ed 7, St. Louis, 2008, Saunders.)

   f. When using sterilization pouches, set the pouches on their sides to maximize steam circulation and to facilitate drying.
   Principle. The autoclave must be loaded properly to ensure adequate steam penetration of all articles.
4. **Procedural Step.** Operate the autoclave according to the procedure described in the instruction manual. A general procedure for the manual and the automatic methods of operation follows.

Manually Operated Autoclave

   a. Determine the sterilizing time for the type of articles being autoclaved (see Table 18-2).
   b. Turn on the autoclave.
   c. Fill the chamber with water using the appropriate control.
   d. Securely close and latch the door of the autoclave.
   e. Set the timing control when the temperature gauge reaches the desired temperature (usually 250°F

[121°C]). At the end of the steam exposure time, an indicator light usually comes on or a beeper sounds.

Set the timing control. (From Bonewit-West K: *Clinical procedures for medical assistants,* ed 7, St. Louis, 2008, Saunders.)

f. If the autoclave does not vent automatically, use the appropriate control to release steam from the chamber.

g. Dry the load by cracking open the door approximately ½ inch but no more than 1 inch. Set the drying time using the timing control. The drying time varies between 15 and 60 minutes, depending on the autoclave and the type of load.

Principle. To ensure sterilization, the load should not be timed until the proper temperature has been reached. The sterility of wrapped packs cannot be ensured unless the wrapped articles are allowed to dry fully. Microorganisms can move through the moisture on a wet wrap and **contaminate** the sterile article inside.

Crack the door to dry the load. (From Bonewit-West K: *Clinical procedures for medical assistants,* ed 7, St. Louis, 2008, Saunders.)

Automatically Operated Autoclave

a. Securely close and latch the door of the autoclave.

b. Turn on the autoclave.

c. Determine the sterilization program according to what is being autoclaved (see Table 18-2). Press the appropriate program button on the front of the

autoclave to select the program. Press the start button.

d. Indicators on the front of the autoclave tell you what is happening (automatically) in the autoclave:

Automatic autoclave buttons and indicators. (From Bonewit-West K: *Clinical procedures for medical assistants,* ed 7, St. Louis, 2008, Saunders.)

Filling Indicator. Lights up when the chamber is filling with water

Sterilizing Indicator. Lights up during the heat-up and sterilization phases of the cycle

Temperature Display. Digital display of the temperature in the autoclave

Time Display. Digital countdown of the time remaining in the sterilization program

Drying Indicator. Lights up during the drying phase of the cycle

Complete or Ready Indicator. Illuminates when the autoclave has completed the cycle and sterilized articles can be removed from the autoclave

5. Procedural Step. Turn off the autoclave. Wearing heat-resistant gloves, remove the load. Do not touch the inner chamber of the autoclave with your bare hands.

Remove the load with heat-resistant gloves. (From Bonewit-West K: *Clinical procedures for medical assistants,* ed 7, St. Louis, 2008, Saunders.)

Continued

PROCEDURE **18-4** Sterilizing Articles in the Autoclave—cont'd

PROCEDURE 18-4

Principle. Heat-resistant gloves protect the medical assistant's hands when the warm packs from the chamber of the autoclave are being removed. The inner chamber of the autoclave is hot and could burn bare skin.

6. **Procedural Step.** Inspect the packs as you take them out of the autoclave. If the packs show any damage, such as holes or tears, the articles should be rewrapped and resterilized.

7. **Procedural Step.** Check the sterilization indicators located on the outside of the pack to ensure the proper response has occurred.

Principle. Autoclave tape only indicates that the article has been through the autoclave cycle; it does not ensure that sterilization has taken place. Sterilization is determined when the pack is opened for use and the sterilization strip indicator in the center of the pack is checked for its proper response.

Check the sterilization indicator on the outside of the pack. (From Bonewit-West K: *Clinical procedures for medical assistants,* ed 7, St. Louis, 2008, Saunders.)

8. **Procedural Step.** Record monitoring information in the autoclave log. Include the date and time of the cycle, a description of the load, the exposure time, and the temperature. If a biologic indicator has been included in the load, process it according to the medical office policy and record results on the autoclave log.

9. **Procedural Step.** Store the packs in a clean, dustproof area with the most recently sterilized packs placed behind previously sterilized packs.

10. **Procedural Step.** Maintain appropriate daily care of the autoclave, following the manufacturer's recommendations. The daily care of the autoclave includes the following:
    a. Wipe the outside of the autoclave with a damp cloth and a mild detergent.
    b. Wipe the interior of the autoclave and the trays with a damp cloth.
    c. Clean the rubber gasket located on the door of the autoclave with a damp cloth.
    d. Inspect the rubber door gasket for damage that could prevent a good seal.

    Principle. For the autoclave to work efficiently, it must be properly maintained.

Clean the rubber gasket with a damp cloth. (From Bonewit-West K: *Clinical procedures for medical assistants,* ed 7, St. Louis, 2008, Saunders.)

MEDICAL PRACTICE *and the* **LAW**

If not performed properly, sterilization and disinfection can adversely affect patients, which can make the medical assistant and other office personnel liable for resultant injuries. Meticulous care must be taken to ensure that all procedures are performed correctly and completely.

Sterilization and disinfection procedures include the use of hazardous chemicals. These chemicals must be stored, used, and disposed of in specific ways mandated by law. The autoclave can be a dangerous machine if it is not used correctly, and it could harm others with hot steam. If you use the autoclave without proper instruction, you could be liable for injuries or accidents resulting from misuse.

Whenever you are dealing with contaminated articles, you have a duty to protect yourself, other employees, patients, and other articles from cross-contamination. ■

What Would You Do? What Would You *Not* Do? RESPONSES

Case Study 1
Page 298

What Did Kara Do?

❑ Complimented Mrs. Cordera for her concern and efforts to baby-proof her home.

❑ Gave Mrs. Cordera a patient information brochure on baby-proofing the home.

❑ Told Mrs. Cordera that she should assume that all cleaning products are poisonous. Got out a disinfectant container and showed Mrs. Cordera the information on the label that tells what to do in case of an accidental poisoning.

❑ Gave the National Poison Control hotline number (1-800-222-1222) to Mrs. Cordera and told her that was the fastest way to obtain information on what to do in case of an accidental poisoning. Told her to keep this number by her phone.

What Did Kara Not *Do?*

❑ Did not take Mrs. Cordera's question lightly.

What Would You Do/What Would You *Not* Do? Review Kara's response and place a checkmark next to the information you included in your response. List additional information you included in your response.

_____

_____

_____

_____

Case Study 2
Page 308

What Did Kara Do?

❑ Explained to Mrs. Scout that toys are in the waiting room for children to play with to make their visit more comfortable and less stressful.

❑ Reassured Mrs. Scout that the medical office personnel do everything they can to prevent the spread of germs in the office and that the toys are sanitized every day.

❑ Relayed to Mrs. Scout that only toys that can be sanitized are kept in the medical office.

❑ Told Mrs. Scout that her concern would be brought up at the weekly office meeting.

What Did Kara Not *Do?*

❑ Did not get defensive because Mrs. Scout was just being concerned about her child's health.

What Would You Do/What Would You *Not* Do? Review Kara's response and place a checkmark next to the information you included in your response. List additional information you included in your response.

_____

_____

_____

_____

Case Study 3
Page 310

What Did Kara Do?

❑ Told Cassie through verbal and nonverbal behavior that her concern was valid.

❑ Told Cassie that hepatitis can be transmitted through dirty instruments.

❑ Reassured Cassie that all instruments are sterilized in the autoclave, which has special indicators to ensure all germs have been killed.

❑ Gave Cassie a patient information brochure on hepatitis. Told her that individuals with chronic hepatitis can develop liver cancer and that the best way to avoid hepatitis is through measures and behaviors recommended for prevention.

❑ Told Cassie that a vaccine is available to prevent hepatitis B, but not hepatitis C.

What Did Kara Not *Do?*

❑ Did not dismiss her concern about dirty instruments as unimportant.

❑ Did not overly alarm her about the consequences of chronic hepatitis.

What Would You Do/What Would You *Not* Do? Review Kara's response and place a checkmark next to the information you included in your response. List additional information you included in your response.

_____

_____

_____

TERMINOLOGY REVIEW

Antiseptic A substance that kills disease-producing microorganisms but not their spores. An antiseptic is usually applied to living tissue.

Autoclave An apparatus for the sterilization of materials, using steam under pressure.

Contaminate To soil, stain, or pollute; to make impure.

Critical item An item that comes in contact with sterile tissue or the vascular system.

Decontamination The use of physical or chemical means to remove or destroy pathogens on an item so that it is no longer capable of transmitting disease; this makes the item safe to handle.

Detergent An agent that cleanses by emulsifying dirt and oil.

Disinfectant An agent used to destroy pathogenic microorganisms but not their spores. Disinfectants are usually applied to inanimate objects.

Hazardous chemical Any chemical that presents a threat to the health and safety of an individual coming into contact with it.

Incubate To provide proper conditions for growth and development.

Load The articles that are being sterilized.

Material safety data sheet (MSDS) A sheet that provides information regarding a chemical, its hazards, and measures to take to prevent injury and illness when handling the chemical.

Noncritical item An item that comes into contact with intact skin, but not mucous membranes.

Sanitization A process to remove organic matter from an article and to reduce the number of microorganisms to a safe level as determined by public health requirements.

Semicritical item An item that comes into contact with nonintact skin or intact mucous membranes.

Spore A hard, thick-walled capsule formed by some bacteria that contains only the essential parts of the protoplasm of the bacterial cell.

Sterilization The process of destroying all forms of microbial life, including bacterial spores.

Thermolabile Easily affected or changed by heat.

ON THE WEB

For Information on Infection Control in the Health Care Setting:

Centers for Disease Control and Prevention: www.cdc.gov

Environmental Protection Agency: www.epa.gov

National Institute of Environmental Health Sciences: www.niehs.nih.gov

National Institute for Occupational Safety and Health: www.cdc.gov/niosh

Infection Control Today: www.infectioncontroltoday.com

Association for Professionals in Infection Control and Epidemiology: www.apic.com

To Locate a Material Data Safety Sheet:

MSDS Search: www.msdssearch.com

HazCom: www.hazard.com/msds

 PREPARE FOR CERTIFICATION Visit the Evolve site at http://evolve.elsevier.com/Bonewit/today/ to actively Prepare for your Certification.

 Check out the **Companion CD** *bound with the book to access additional interactive activities.*

19

Vital Signs

LEARNING OBJECTIVES	PROCEDURES

Temperature

1. Define a vital sign.
2. Explain the reason for taking vital signs.
3. Explain how body temperature is maintained.
4. List examples of how heat is produced in the body.
5. List examples of how heat is lost from the body.
6. State the normal body temperature range and the average body temperature.
7. List and explain factors that can cause variation in the body temperature.
8. List and describe the three stages of a fever.
9. List the sites for taking body temperature, and explain why these sites are used.
10. List and describe the guidelines for using a tympanic membrane thermometer.

Measure oral body temperature.
Measure axillary body temperature.
Measure rectal body temperature.
Measure aural body temperature.
Measure temporal artery body temperature.

Pulse

1. Explain the mechanism of pulse.
2. List and explain the factors that affect the pulse rate.
3. Identify a specific use of each of the eight pulse sites.
4. State the normal range of pulse rate for each age group.
5. Explain the difference between pulse rhythm and pulse volume.

Measure radial pulse.
Measure apical pulse.

Respiration

1. Explain the purpose of respiration.
2. State what occurs during inhalation and exhalation.
3. State the normal respiratory rate for each age group.
4. List and explain the factors that affect the respiratory rate.
5. Explain the difference between the rhythm and depth of respiration.
6. Describe the character of the following abnormal breath sounds: crackles, rhonchi, wheezes, and pleural friction rub.

Measure respiration.

Pulse Oximetry

1. Explain the purpose of pulse oximetry.
2. State the normal oxygen saturation level of a healthy individual.
3. List and describe the function of the controls, indicators, and displays on a pulse oximeter.
4. Describe the difference between a reusable and a disposable oximeter probe.
5. List and describe factors that may interfere with an accurate pulse oximetry reading.

Perform pulse oximetry.

Blood Pressure

1. Define blood pressure.
2. State the normal range of blood pressure for an adult.
3. List and describe factors that affect the blood pressure.
4. Identify the different parts of a stethoscope and a sphygmomanometer.
5. Identify the Korotkoff sounds.
6. Explain how to prevent errors in blood pressure measurement.

Measure blood pressure.
Determine systolic pressure by palpation.

CAAHEP COMPETENCIES

Clinical Competencies
Patient Care
- Obtain vital signs.
- Prepare and maintain examination and treatment areas.

General Competencies
Professional Communications
- Recognize and respond to verbal communications.
- Recognize and respond to nonverbal communications.

Patient Instruction
- Provide instruction for health maintenance and disease prevention.

Operational Functions
- Perform routine maintenance of administrative and clinical equipment.

ABHES COMPETENCIES

Communication
- Recognize and respond to verbal and nonverbal communication.
- Principles of verbal and nonverbal communication.

Clinical Duties
- Take vital signs.

Office Management
- Operate and maintain facilities and perform routine maintenance of administrative and clinical equipment safely.

Instruction
- Teach patients methods of health promotion and disease prevention.

KEY TERMS

adventitious (ad-ven-TISH-us) sounds
afebrile (uh-FEB-ril)
alveolus (al-VEE-uh-lus)
antecubital (AN-tih-CYOO-bi-tul) space
antipyretic (AN-tih-pye-REH-tik)
aorta (ay-OR-tuh)
apnea (AP-nee-uh)
axilla (aks-ILL-uh)
bounding pulse
bradycardia (BRAY-dee-CAR-dee-uh)
bradypnea (BRAY-dip-NEE-uh)
Celsius (SELL-see-us) scale
conduction (kon-DUK-shun)
convection (kon-VEK-shun)
crisis
cyanosis (sye-an-OH-sus)
diastole (dye-AS-toe-lee)
diastolic (DYE-uh-STOL-ik) pressure
dyspnea (DISP-nee-uh)
dysrhythmia (dis-RITH-mee-uh)
eupnea (YOOP-nee-uh)
exhalation (EKS-hal-AY-shun)
Fahrenheit (FAIR-en-hite) scale

febrile (FEH-bril)
fever
frenulum linguae (FREN-yoo-lum LIN-gway)
hyperpnea (HYE-perp-NEE-uh)
hyperpyrexia (HYE-per-pye-REK-see-uh)
hypertension (HYE-per-TEN-shun)
hyperventilation (HYE-per-ven-til-AY-shun)
hypopnea (hye-POP-nee-uh)
hypotension (HYE-poe-TEN-shun)
hypothermia (HYE-poe-THER-mee-uh)
hypoxemia (hye-pok-SEE-mee-uh)
hypoxia (hye-POKS-ee-uh)
inhalation (IN-hal-AY-shun)
intercostal (IN-ter-KOS-tul)
Korotkoff (kuh-ROT-kof) sounds
malaise (mal-AYZE)
manometer (man-OM-uh-ter)
meniscus (men-IS-kus)
orthopnea (orth-OP-nee-uh)
pulse oximeter
pulse oximetry
pulse pressure
pulse rhythm

pulse volume
radiation (RAY-dee-AY-shun)
SaO₂
sphygmomanometer (SFIG-moe-man-OM-uh-ter)
SpO₂
stethoscope (STETH-uh-skope)

systole (SIS-toe-lee)
systolic (sis-TOL-ik) pressure
tachycardia (TAK-ih-KAR-dee-uh)
tachypnea (TAK-ip-NEE-uh)
thready pulse

Introduction to Vital Signs

Vital signs are objective guideposts that provide data to determine a person's state of health. The vital signs include temperature, pulse, respiration (collectively called *TPR*), and blood pressure (BP). Another indicator of a patient's health status is pulse oximetry. Although some physicians order this measurement routinely on all patients as part of the patient workup, most physicians only order this vital sign when the patient complains of respiratory problems (e.g., shortness of breath).

The normal ranges of the vital signs are finely adjusted, and any deviation from normal may indicate disease. During the course of an illness, variations in the vital signs may occur. The medical assistant should be alert to any significant changes and report them to the physician because they indicate a change in the patient's condition. When patients visit the medical office, vital signs are routinely checked to establish each patient's usual state of health and establish baseline measurements against which future measurements can be compared. The medical assistant should have a thorough knowledge of the vital signs and attain proficiency in taking them to ensure accurate findings.

General guidelines that the medical assistant should follow when measuring the vital signs are as follows:

1. Be familiar with the normal ranges for all vital signs. Keep in mind that normal ranges vary based on the different age groups (infant, child, adult, elder).
2. Make sure that all equipment for measuring vital signs is in proper working condition to ensure accurate findings.
3. Eliminate or minimize factors that affect the vital signs, such as exercise, food and beverage consumption, and emotional states.
4. Use an organized approach when measuring the vital signs. If all of the vital signs are ordered, they are usually measured starting with temperature, followed by pulse, respiration, blood pressure, and pulse oximetry.

TEMPERATURE

Regulation of Body Temperature

Body temperature is maintained within a fairly constant range by the hypothalamus, which is located in the brain. The hypothalamus functions as the body's thermostat. It normally allows the body temperature to vary only about 1° to 2° Fahrenheit (F) throughout the day.

Body temperature is maintained through a balance of the heat produced in the body and the heat lost from the body (Figure 19-1). A constant temperature range must be maintained for the body to function properly. When minor changes in the temperature of the body occur, the hypothalamus senses this and makes adjustments as needed to ensure that the body temperature stays within a normal and safe range. If an individual is playing tennis on a hot day, the body's heat-cooling mechanism is activated to remove excess heat from the body through perspiration.

Heat Production

Most of the heat produced in the body is through voluntary and involuntary muscle contractions. Voluntary muscle contractions involve the muscles over which a person has control (e.g., the moving of legs or arms). Involuntary muscle contractions involve the muscles over which a person has no control; examples are physiologic processes such as digestion, the beating of the heart, and shivering.

Body heat is also produced by cell metabolism. Heat is produced when nutrients are broken down in the cells. Fever and strong emotional states also can increase heat production in the body.

Heat Loss

Heat is lost from the body through the urine and feces and in water vapor from the lungs. Perspiration also contributes to heat loss. Perspiration is the excretion of moisture through the pores of the skin. When the moisture evaporates, heat is released and the body is cooled.

Radiation, conduction, and convection all cause loss of heat from the body. **Radiation** is the transfer of heat in the form of waves; body heat is continually radiating into cooler surroundings. **Conduction** is the transfer of heat from one object to another by direct contact; heat can be transferred by conduction from the body to a cooler object it touches. **Convection** is the transfer of heat through air currents; cool air currents can cause the body to lose heat. These processes are illustrated in Figure 19-2.

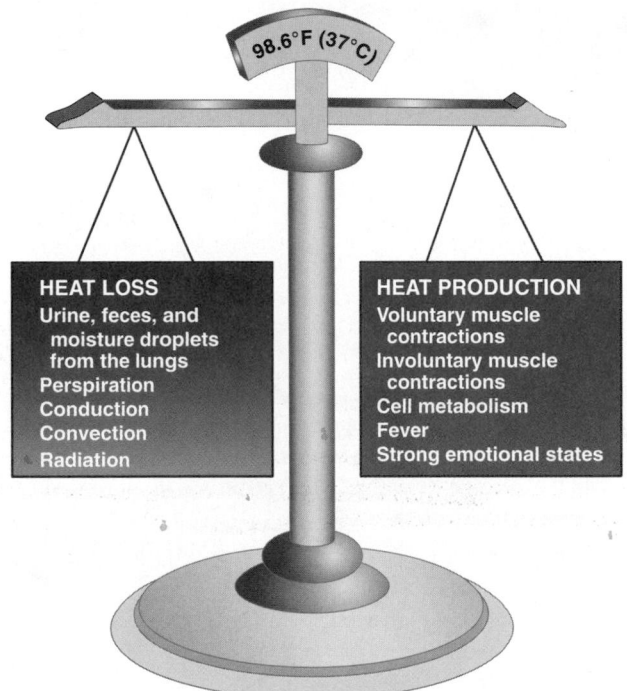

Figure 19-1. Body temperature represents a balance between the heat produced in the body and the heat lost from the body. (From Bonewit-West K: *Clinical procedures for medical assistants,* ed 7, St. Louis, 2008, Saunders.)

Body Temperature Range

The purpose of measuring body temperature is to establish the patient's baseline temperature and to monitor an abnormally high or low body temperature. The normal body temperature range is 97°F to 99°F (36.1°C to 37.2°C), the average temperature being 98.6°F (37°C). Body temperature is usually recorded using the Fahrenheit system of measurement. Table 19-1 lists comparable **Fahrenheit** and **Celsius** temperatures and explains how to convert temperatures from one scale to the other.

Alterations in Body Temperature

A body temperature greater than 100.4°F (38°C) indicates a **fever,** or *pyrexia.* If the body temperature falls between 99°F (37.2°C) and 100.4°F (38°C), it is termed a *low-grade fever.* When an individual has a fever, the heat that the body is producing is greater than the heat the body is losing. A temperature reading greater than 105.8°F (41°C) is known as **hyperpyrexia.** Hyperpyrexia is a serious condition, and a temperature greater than 109.4°F (43°C) is generally fatal.

A body temperature less than 97°F (36.1°C) is classified as subnormal, or **hypothermia.** This means that the heat the body is losing is greater than the heat it is producing. A person usually cannot survive with a temperature less than 93.2°F (34°C). Terms used to describe alterations in body temperature are illustrated in Figure 19-3.

Variations in Body Temperature

During the day-to-day activities of an individual, normal fluctuations occur in the body temperature. The body temperature rarely stays the same throughout the course of a day. The medical assistant should take the following

Figure 19-2. Heat loss from the body. With radiation, the body gives off heat in the form of waves to the cooler outside air. With conduction, the chair becomes warm as heat is transferred from the individual to the chair. With convection, air currents move heat away from the body. (From Bonewit-West K: *Clinical procedures for medical assistants,* ed 7, St. Louis, 2008, Saunders.)

Table 19-1 Equivalent Fahrenheit and Celsius Temperatures

Fahrenheit	Celsius
93.2	34
95	35
96.8	36
97.7	36.5
98.6	37
99.5	37.5
100.4	38
101.3	38.5
102.2	39
104	40
105.8	41
107.6	42
109.4	43
111.2	44

Temperature Conversion

1. Celsius to Fahrenheit: To convert Celsius to Fahrenheit, multiply by 9/5 and add 32:

$$°F = (°C \times 9/5) + 32$$

2. Fahrenheit to Celsius: To convert Fahrenheit to Celsius, subtract 32 and multiply by 5/9:

$$°C \times (°F - 32) \times 5/9$$

From Bonewit-West K: *Clinical procedures for medical assistants*, ed 7, St. Louis, 2008, Saunders.

Figure 19-3. Terms that describe alterations in body temperature (adult oral temperature). (From Bonewit-West K: *Clinical procedures for medical assistants*, ed 7, St. Louis, 2008, Saunders.)

points into consideration when evaluating a patient's temperature.

1. **Age.** Infants and young children normally have a higher body temperature than adults because their thermoregulatory system is not yet fully established. Elderly individuals usually have a lower body temperature owing to factors such as loss of subcutaneous fat, lack of exercise, and loss of thermoregulatory control. Table 19-2 shows the normal ranges of body temperature according to age group.

2. **Diurnal variations.** During sleep, body metabolism slows down, as do muscle contractions. The body's temperature is lowest in the morning before metabolism and muscle contractions begin increasing.

3. **Emotional states.** Strong emotions, such as crying and extreme anger, can increase the body temperature. This is important to consider when working with young children, who frequently cry during examination procedures or when they are ill.

4. **Environment.** Cold weather tends to decrease the body temperature, whereas hot weather increases it.

5. **Exercise.** Vigorous physical exercise causes an increase in voluntary muscle contractions, which elevates the body temperature.

6. **Patient's normal body temperature.** Some patients normally run a low or high temperature. The medical

Table 19-2 Variations in Body Temperature by Age

Age	Site	Average Temperature	
Newborn	Axillary	97-100°F	36.1-37.8°C
1 yr	Oral	99.7°F	37.6°C
5 yr	Oral	98.6°F	37°C
Adult	Oral	98.6°F	37°C
	Rectal	99.6°F	37.5°C
	Axillary	97.6°F	36.4°C
	Aural	98.6°F	37°C
Elderly (older than 70 yr)	Oral	96.8°F	36°C

From Bonewit-West K: *Clinical procedures for medical assistants*, ed 7, St. Louis, 2008, Saunders.

assistant should review the patient's past vital sign recordings.

7. **Pregnancy.** Cell metabolism increases during pregnancy, which elevates body temperature.

Fever

Fever, or pyrexia, denotes that a patient's temperature has increased to greater than 100.4°F (38°C). An individual who has a fever is said to be **febrile;** one who does not have a fever is **afebrile.**

Fever is a common symptom of illness, particularly inflammation and infection. When there is an infection in the body, the invading pathogen functions as a *pyrogen*, which is any substance that produces fever. Pyrogens reset the hypothalamus, causing the body temperature to increase above normal. Fever is not an illness itself, but rather a sign that the body may have an infection. Most fevers are self-limiting; that is, the body temperature returns to normal after the disease process.

Stages of a Fever

A fever can be divided into the following three stages:

1. The *onset* is when the temperature first begins to increase. The increase may be slow or sudden, the patient often experiences coldness and chills, and the pulse and respiratory rate increase.
2. During the *course of a fever*, the temperature rises and falls in one of the following three fever patterns: continuous, intermittent, or remittent. Fever patterns are described and illustrated in Table 19-3. During this stage, the patient has an increased pulse and respiratory rate and feels warm to the touch. The patient also may experience one or more of the following: flushed appearance, increased thirst, loss of appetite, headache, and malaise. **Malaise** refers to a vague sense of body discomfort, weakness, and fatigue.
3. During the *subsiding stage*, the temperature returns to normal. It can return to normal gradually or suddenly (known as a **crisis**). As the body temperature is returning to normal, the patient usually perspires and may become dehydrated.

Assessment of Body Temperature

Assessment Sites

Five sites are available for measuring body temperature: mouth, **axilla**, rectum, ear, and forehead. The locations in

Highlight on Fever

Although most fevers indicate an infection, not all do. Noninfectious causes of fever include heatstroke, drug hypersensitivity, neoplasms, and central nervous system damage.

A fever is usually not harmful if it remains less than 102°F (38.9°C). Research suggests that fever may serve as a defense mechanism to destroy pathogens that are unable to survive above the normal body temperature range.

The level of the fever is not related to the seriousness of the infection. A patient with a temperature of 104°F (40°C) may not be any sicker than a patient with a temperature of 102°F (38.9°C).

In children, fever often is one of the first signs of illness and has a tendency to become highly elevated. In contrast, in elderly patients, fever may be elevated only 1°F to 2°F above normal, even with a severe infection.

During a fever, the body's basal metabolism increases 7% for each degree of temperature elevation. Heart and respiratory rates also increase to meet this metabolic demand.

Chills during a fever result when the hypothalamus has been reset at a higher temperature. In an attempt to reach this temperature, involuntary muscle contractions (chills) occur, which produce heat, causing the temperature of the body to increase. After the higher temperature has been reached, the chills subside and the individual then feels warm.

Increased perspiration during a fever occurs when the hypothalamus has been reset at a lower temperature (e.g., after taking an **antipyretic** or after the cause of the fever has been removed). To cool the body and reach this lower temperature, the body perspires, often profusely; profuse perspiration is known as *diaphoresis*. ■

Table 19-3 Fever Patterns		
Pattern	**Description**	**Illustration**
Continuous fever	Body temperature fluctuates minimally but always remains elevated *Occurs with:* Scarlet fever Pneumococcal pneumonia	98.6°F (37°C)
Intermittent fever	Body temperature alternately rises and falls and at times returns to normal or becomes subnormal *Occurs with:* Bacterial infections Viral infections	98.6°F (37°C)
Remittent fever	Wide range of temperature fluctuations occur, all of which are above normal *Occurs with:* Influenza Pneumonia Endocarditis	98.6°F (37°C)

From Bonewit-West K: *Clinical procedures for medical assistants*, ed 7, St. Louis, 2008, Saunders.

which temperatures are taken should have an abundant blood supply so that the temperature of the entire body is obtained, not the temperature of only a part of the body. In addition, the site must be as closed as possible to prevent air currents from interfering with the temperature reading. The site chosen for measuring a patient's temperature depends on the patient's age, condition, and state of consciousness; the type of thermometer available; and the medical office policy.

Oral Temperature

The oral method is a convenient and one of the most common means for measuring body temperature. When the medical assistant records a temperature, the physician assumes it has been taken through the oral route, unless it is otherwise noted. A rich blood supply is found under the tongue in the area on either side of the **frenulum linguae.** The thermometer should be placed in this area to receive the most accurate reading. The patient must keep the mouth closed during the procedure to provide a closed space for the thermometer.

Axillary Temperature

Axillary temperature is recommended as a site for measuring temperature in toddlers and preschoolers. The axillary

site also should be used for mouth-breathing patients and for patients with oral inflammation or who have had oral surgery.

The temperature obtained through the axillary method measures approximately 1°F lower than the same person's temperature taken through the oral route (see Table 19-2). The medical assistant should make a notation to tell the physician that the temperature was taken through the axillary route.

Rectal Temperature

The rectal temperature provides an extremely accurate measurement of body temperature because few factors can alter the results. The rectum is highly vascular and, of the five sites, provides the most closed cavity. The temperature obtained through the rectal route measures approximately 1°F higher than the same person's temperature taken through the oral route (see Table 19-2). The medical assistant should make a notation on the patient's chart if the temperature has been taken rectally.

The rectal method is generally used for infants and young children, unconscious patients, and mouth-breathing patients and when greater accuracy in body temperature is desired. The rectal site should not be used with newborns because of the danger of rectal trauma.

Aural Temperature

The aural (ear) site is used with the tympanic membrane thermometer. The ear provides a closed cavity that is easily accessible. Tympanic membrane thermometers provide instantaneous results, are easy to use, and are comfortable for the patient. They make it easier to measure the temperature of children younger than 6 years, uncooperative patients, and patients who are unable to have their temperatures taken orally.

Forehead Temperature

The temporal artery is a major artery of the head that runs laterally across the forehead and down the side of the neck. In the area of the forehead, it is located approximately 2 mm below the surface of the skin. Because the temporal artery is located so close to the skin surface and is easily accessible, the forehead provides an ideal site for obtaining a body temperature measurement. In addition, the temporal artery has a constant steady flow of blood, which assists in providing an accurate measurement of the patient's body temperature.

The forehead site can be used to measure body temperature using a temporal artery thermometer in individuals of all ages (newborns, infants, children, adults, elderly). The results compare in accuracy with other methods used to measure body temperature. The temperature obtained through the forehead site is about the same as a rectal temperature measurement. The temporal artery reading measures approximately 1 degree higher than oral body temperature and 2 degrees higher than axillary temperature on the Fahrenheit scale.

Putting It All into Practice

My name is Sergio Martinez, and I am a registered medical assistant. I work in a large clinic that is associated with a medical school. At present, I work in the family medicine department, but I also have worked in dermatology and internal medicine. Family medicine is the area I enjoy most because of the wide variety of tasks that are performed. There is rarely a dull moment.

I focus primarily on clinical medical assisting. Taking vital signs is a big part of my job responsibilities. It is routine at my clinic to take height, weight, temperature, pulse, respiration, and blood pressure on every patient seen at the clinic, no matter what the reason for his or her visit. I assist the physician with various procedures, examinations, and minor office surgery, and I administer injections, run electrocardiograms, and perform various laboratory tests.

Taking vital signs and length and weight on small children can be very challenging at times. Some children start to cry as soon as they are put on the scale. Taking a temperature on an uncooperative toddler can be very difficult. I try to calm the child as much as possible, and for good behavior, I give a lot of praise. Stickers also are a great reward for cooperative behavior. Usually when small children learn that they can trust you, they are not as frightened by the experience. It is rewarding when a child learns not to be afraid of being evaluated for routine vital signs. ■

Prepare for Success

Types of Thermometers

The four types of thermometers available for measuring body temperature are electronic thermometers, tympanic membrane thermometers, temporal artery thermometer, and chemical thermometers. Mercury glass thermometers, previously commonly used in medical offices, are no longer used because they break easily and release mercury. Mercury is a chemical that is dangerous to the human body because it can cause damage to the nervous system. If mercury is released into the environment, it can be harmful to wildlife. Many cities have banned the sale or use of mercury because of its potential hazards.

Electronic Thermometer

An electronic thermometer is frequently used in the medical office to measure body temperature. Electronic thermometers are portable and measure oral, axillary, and rectal temperatures ranging from 84°F to 108°F (28.9°C to 42.2°C).

An electronic thermometer measures body temperature in a brief time; the time varies between 4 and 20 seconds, depending on the brand of thermometer. The temperature results are digitally displayed on an LCD screen. An electronic thermometer consists of interchangeable oral and rectal probes attached to a battery-operated portable unit (Figure 19-4). The probes are color-coded for ease in identifying them. The oral probe is color-coded with blue on its collar and is used to take oral and axillary temperatures; the rectal probe is color-coded with red on its collar and is used to take rectal temperatures only.

A disposable plastic cover is placed over the probe to prevent the transmission of microorganisms among patients. Depending on the method of taking the temperature, the probe is inserted in the mouth, axilla, or rectum and is left in place until an audible tone is emitted from the thermometer. When the tone sounds, the patient's temperature in degrees Fahrenheit is displayed on the screen. The medical assistant ejects the plastic probe cover into a regular waste container.

The casing, probes, and attached cords of the electronic thermometer should be periodically cleaned with a soft cloth slightly dampened with a solution of warm water and a disinfectant cleaner.

Procedures 19-1, 19-2, and 19-3 outline the methods for measuring oral, axillary, and rectal temperature using an electronic thermometer.

Tympanic Membrane Thermometer

The tympanic membrane thermometer is used at the aural site. The tympanic membrane thermometer functions by detecting thermal energy that is naturally radiated from the body. As with the rest of the body, the tympanic membrane gives off heat waves known as *infrared waves*. The tympanic thermometer functions like a camera by taking a "picture" of these infrared waves, which are considered a documented indicator of body temperature (Figure 19-5). The thermometer calculates the body temperature from the energy generated by the waves and converts it to an oral or rectal equivalent.

The tympanic membrane thermometer is battery operated and consists of a small handheld device with a sensor probe (Figure 19-6). To operate the thermometer, the probe

Figure 19-4. Electronic thermometer. (From Bonewit-West K: *Clinical procedures for medical assistants,* ed 7, St. Louis, 2008, Saunders.)

Figure 19-5. The tympanic membrane thermometer functions by detecting thermal energy that is naturally radiated from the tympanic membrane. (From Bonewit-West K: *Clinical procedures for medical assistants,* ed 7, St. Louis, 2008, Saunders.)

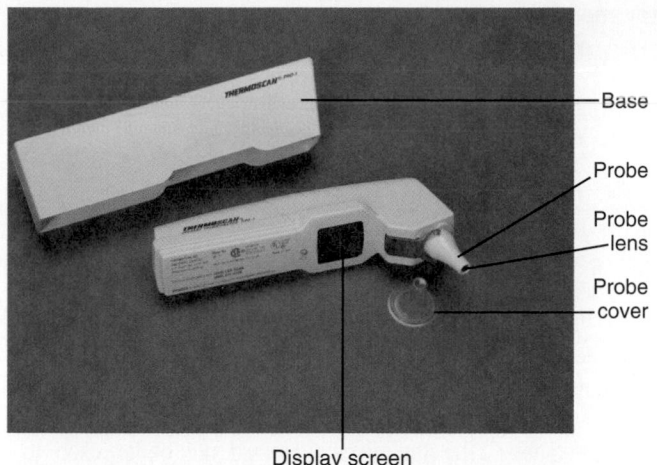

Base

Probe

Probe lens

Probe cover

Display screen

Figure 19-6. Tympanic membrane thermometer. (From Bonewit-West K: *Clinical procedures for medical assistants,* ed 7, St. Louis, 2008, Saunders.)

is covered with a disposable soft plastic cover and placed in the outer third of the external ear canal. An activation button is depressed momentarily, and the results are displayed in 1 to 2 seconds on a digital screen. The probe cover is ejected into a regular waste container. The procedure for taking aural body temperature using a tympanic membrane thermometer is presented in Procedure 19-4.

Temporal Artery Thermometer

Measuring temperature using a temporal artery thermometer is the newest method for assessing body temperature. A temporal artery thermometer is an electronic device consisting of a probe attached to a portable unit (Figure 19-7).

To perform the procedure, a scan button is continually depressed while the probe is gently and slowly moved across the patient's forehead. During this process, the probe sensor scans the forehead for the infrared heat given off by the temporal artery. The probe sensor captures the highest

Guidelines for Using a Tympanic Membrane Thermometer

The following guidelines help ensure accurate aural temperature measurement with a tympanic membrane thermometer.

1. **Determine whether a tympanic thermometer can be used to measure the patient's temperature.** The tympanic thermometer should not be used on a patient with inflammation of the external ear canal (e.g., otitis externa) or when the ear contains a discharge, such as blood or pus. The presence of otitis media and tympanostomy tubes does not significantly affect the temperature reading; a normal amount of cerumen also has no effect. An excessive buildup of cerumen that occludes the ear canal can result in a falsely low temperature reading.

2. **Determine whether external factors are present that may influence the temperature reading.** If any of these factors are present, remove the individual from the situation and wait 20 minutes before taking the temperature. External factors include an individual who has been lying on one ear or the other; who has had the ears covered (e.g., hat, ear muffs); who has been exposed to very hot or very cold temperatures; or who has been recently swimming or bathing.

3. **Select the temperature measurement system desired.** The temperature of a tympanic membrane thermometer can be displayed in degrees Fahrenheit or degrees Celsius. Follow the manufacturer's instructions to change from one measurement to the other.

4. **Place the probe properly in the patient's ear.** The most important factor in obtaining an accurate temperature is the proper placement of the probe in the patient's ear, which is outlined as follows.
   - **Straighten the ear canal.** The ear canal has an S shape that obstructs the view of the tympanic membrane. To obtain an accurate temperature measurement, the ear canal must be straightened before inserting the probe. This allows the probe sensor to obtain a clear picture of the tympanic membrane.
   - **Seal the opening of the ear.** The probe must be inserted tightly enough to seal the opening of the ear without causing patient discomfort. If the probe does not seal the ear canal, cooler external air can cause the thermometer to register a lower temperature.
   - **Correctly position the probe.** Position the tip of the probe toward the opposite temple (approximately midway between the opposite ear and eyebrow). This allows the sensor to obtain the best possible picture of the tympanic membrane. If the tip is positioned incorrectly, it may be aimed at the ear canal, which results in a falsely low reading.

5. **Verify the accuracy of the temperature reading, if needed.** If you need to take the patient's temperature again, you can use the other ear. Slight but insignificant differences occur between the temperature readings in the right ear and the left ear. Before using the same ear, however, you must wait 2 minutes to allow the aural temperature to stabilize.

6. **Check the probe lens before taking the temperature.** The end of the probe is covered with a lens that is transparent to heat waves. To ensure a high level of accuracy, it is extremely important to keep this lens clean and intact. Before taking a temperature, always check to ensure that the lens is shiny and clear. Fingerprints, cerumen, and dust reduce the transparency of the lens, resulting in falsely low temperature readings. If the lens is dirty, it must be cleaned before taking the patient's temperature. If the lens is damaged, the thermometer cannot be used and must be repaired.

Continued

Guidelines for Using a Tympanic Membrane Thermometer—cont'd

7. **Respond appropriately to digital messages.** A message to alert the user is displayed in the digital screen under the following circumstances:
   - An attempt is made to take a temperature without changing the cover after the last temperature.
   - An attempt is made to take a temperature with no probe cover in place.
   - The battery is low.
   - The thermometer is in need of repair.
8. Care for the tympanic thermometer properly.
   - **Probe lens.** Dust and other minute particles of environmental debris can build up on the probe lens during normal use. The lens should be cleaned as part of routine maintenance or when it becomes dirty. To clean the lens, gently wipe its surface with an antiseptic wipe and immediately wipe it dry with a cotton swab. After cleaning, allow at least 5 minutes before taking a temperature.
   - **Thermometer casing.** Clean the casing of the thermometer periodically by wiping it dry with a soft cloth slightly dampened with a solution of warm water and a disinfectant cleaner. Make sure the cloth is damp but not wet to prevent the disinfectant solution from running inside the thermometer, which could damage it.
9. **Store the thermometer properly.** Keep the thermometer away from temperature extremes, which could damage the thermometer. The thermometer should not be exposed to excessive heat (greater than 95°F [35°C]) or excessive cold (less than 60°F [15.6°C]).

Figure 19-7. Temporal artery thermometer. (From Bonewit-West K: *Clinical procedures for medical assistants*, ed 7, St. Louis, 2008, Saunders.)

temperature or *peak temperature* in the area being scanned. The peak temperature represents the temperature given off by the temporal artery or body temperature.

Along with measuring the peak temperature, the probe sensor automatically measures the *ambient temperature*, which is the surrounding air temperature. This is done because there is a small heat loss from the forehead as a result of cooling by ambient temperature. The thermometer's computer determines and automatically corrects for any effect from ambient temperature. An accurate body temperature reading is digitally displayed on the screen on the thermometer. The procedure for measuring temperature using a temporal artery thermometer is presented in Procedure 19-5.

Earlobe Temperature Measurement

Sweating of the forehead can cause an inaccurate temporal artery temperature reading. This is because perspiration causes the skin of the forehead to cool, resulting in a falsely low temperature reading. Sweating of the forehead occurs when a patient's fever breaks. It also occurs when a patient's skin is clammy; in this instance, forehead sweating may be present but not readily visible. To avoid this problem, the temperature of the neck area located just behind the earlobe also must be measured.

The area behind the earlobe is less affected by sweating than the forehead. During sweating, the blood vessels behind the earlobe dilate, resulting in a constant, steady flow of blood, which provides an accurate measurement of body temperature. After scanning the forehead, the medical assistant must place the probe of the thermometer in the soft depression of the neck just below the mastoid process of the ear. If the patient's forehead has cooled from sweating, the earlobe temperature automatically registers as the peak temperature, thereby overriding the forehead temperature.

The area behind the earlobe does not normally provide an accurate body temperature measurement and supersedes the forehead measurement only when the patient is in a diaphoretic state. Additional guidelines for temporal artery temperature measurement are presented in Box 19-1.

Care and Maintenance

The temporal artery thermometer should be stored in a clean, dry area. The thermometer must be protected from extremes in temperature, direct sunlight, and dust. The casing of the thermometer should be cleaned periodically with a soft cloth moistened with a solution of warm water and a disinfectant cleaner; never splash water on or immerse the unit in water because this could damage the internal components of the thermometer.

To obtain an accurate measurement, the probe lens must be clean and shiny. Dust and other minute particles of environmental debris can build up on the probe lens during normal use, preventing the probe sensor from getting an accurate "view" of the heat emitted by the temporal artery

BOX 19-1 Temporal Artery Thermometer Guidelines

1. The operating environmental temperature for a temporal artery thermometer is 60°F to 104°F (15.5°C to 40°C).
2. Do not take temperature over scar tissue, open sores, or abrasions.
3. Ensure that the side of the head to be measured is exposed to the environment. Anything covering the area to be measured (e.g., hair, hat, wig, bandages) traps body heat, resulting in a falsely high reading.

4. A falsely low temporal artery reading can result from the following:
   - A dirty probe lens
   - Sweating of the forehead (in this instance, the earlobe measurement becomes the overriding temperature reading)
   - Scanning the forehead too quickly
   - Not keeping the button depressed while scanning the forehead and area behind the earlobe

From Bonewit-West K: *Clinical procedures for medical assistants,* ed 7, St. Louis, 2008, Saunders.

Figure 19-8. Disposable chemical single-use thermometers. **A,** The thermometer is removed from the wrapper by pulling on the handle. **B,** The thermometer is inserted under the tongue and left in place for 60 seconds. **C,** The thermometer is read by noting the highest reading among the dots that have changed color. (From Bonewit-West K: *Clinical procedures for medical assistants,* ed 7, St. Louis, 2008, Saunders.)

and resulting in a falsely low reading. The lens should be cleaned if it becomes dirty and as part of routine maintenance. The lens is cleaned by gently wiping its surface with an antiseptic wipe and immediately wiping it dry with a cotton-tipped applicator stick.

Chemical Thermometers

Chemical thermometers contain chemicals that are heat sensitive and include disposable chemical single-use thermometers and temperature-sensitive strips. They are used most often by patients at home to measure body temperature. Although chemical thermometers are less accurate than other types of thermometers, they assist in providing a general assessment of body temperature. Because of their chemical makeup, they should be stored in a cool area, preferably colder than 86°F (30°C), and should not be

exposed to direct sunlight because heat may cause the thermometer to register a higher temperature. Each type of chemical thermometer is described here.

Disposable Chemical Single-Use Thermometers

The disposable chemical single-use thermometer has small chemical dots at one end that respond to body heat by changing color (Figure 19-8A and B). Each thermometer comes in its own wrapper. The protective wrapper must be peeled back to expose the handle of the thermometer. The thermometer is removed from the wrapper by pulling on the handle, taking care not to touch the dotted area. The thermometer is inserted under the tongue and left in place for the duration of time recommended by the manufacturer (generally 60 seconds). After removal of the thermometer, the dots are observed for a change in color. The thermometer is read by noting the highest reading among the dots that have changed color (Figure 19-8C). The thermometer is discarded after use.

Temperature-Sensitive Strips

A temperature-sensitive strip consists of a reusable plastic strip that contains heat-sensitive liquid crystals designed to measure body temperature. The plastic strip is pressed onto the forehead and held in place until the colors stop changing, generally 15 seconds. The results are read by observing the color change and noting the corresponding temperature indicated on the strip (Figure 19-9).

Text continued on p. 346

Figure 19-9. Temperature-sensitive strip. The plastic strip is pressed onto the forehead and held in place until the color stops changing (generally 15 seconds). The results are read by observing the color and noting the corresponding temperature indicated on the strip. (From Bonewit-West K: *Clinical procedures for medical assistants,* ed 7, St. Louis, 2008, Saunders.)

What Would You Do? What Would You *Not* Do?

Case Study 1

Marcela Mason comes in with Olivia, her 5-year-old daughter. Olivia has had a fever and sore throat for the past 2 days. Olivia's aural temperature is taken in her left ear, and it measures 103.3°F. Mrs. Mason says that she has an ear thermometer at home, but when she took Olivia's temperature with it, the readings were always below 97°F. She knew that could not be right because Olivia felt so warm. Mrs. Mason would like to be able to use her ear thermometer, but she thinks that it might be broken because of the low readings. Mrs. Mason says that she is thinking of switching back to a mercury glass thermometer, but she has heard that it is not a good idea to use this type of thermometer anymore and wants to know why. ■

PROCEDURE 19-1   Measuring Oral Body Temperature—Electronic Thermometer

Outcome Measure oral body temperature.

Equipment/Supplies

- Electronic thermometer
- Oral probe (blue collar)
- Plastic probe cover
- Waste container

---

1. **Procedural Step.** Sanitize your hands, and assemble the equipment.
2. **Procedural Step.** Remove the thermometer unit from its storage base, and attach the oral (blue collar) probe to it. This is accomplished by inserting the latching plug (at the end of the coiled cord of the oral probe) to the plug receptacle on the thermometer unit until it clicks into place. Insert the probe into the face of the thermometer.
   Principle. The oral probe is color-coded with a blue collar for ease in identifying it.
3. **Procedural Step.** Greet the patient and introduce yourself. Identify the patient and explain the procedure. If the patient has recently ingested hot or cold food or beverages or has been smoking, you must wait 15 to 30 minutes before taking the temperature.

Principle. Ingestion of hot or cold food or beverages and smoking changes the temperature of the mouth, which could result in an inaccurate reading.

4. **Procedural Step.** Grasp the probe by the collar, and remove it from the face of the thermometer. Slide the probe into a disposable plastic probe cover until it locks into place.
   Principle. Removing the probe from the thermometer automatically turns on the thermometer. The probe cover prevents the transfer of microorganisms from one patient to another.
5. **Procedural Step.** Take the patient's temperature by inserting the probe under the patient's tongue in the pocket located on either side of the frenulum linguae. Instruct the patient to keep the mouth closed.

PROCEDURE 19-1

Principle. There is a good blood supply in the tissue under the tongue. The mouth must be kept closed to prevent cooler air from entering and affecting the temperature reading.

Attach the oral probe to the thermometer. (From Bonewit-West K: *Clinical procedures for medical assistants,* ed 7, St. Louis, 2008, Saunders.)

Slide the probe into a probe cover. (From Bonewit-West K: *Clinical procedures for medical assistants,* ed 7, St. Louis, 2008, Saunders.)

Insert the probe under the patient's tongue. (From Bonewit-West K: *Clinical procedures for medical assistants,* ed 7, St. Louis, 2008, Saunders.)

6. Procedural Step. Hold the probe in place until you hear the tone. At that time, the patient's temperature appears as a digital display on the screen. Make a mental note of the temperature reading. (The temperature indicated on this thermometer is 98.2°F [36.8°C]).

The patient's temperature appears as a digital display on the screen. (From Bonewit-West K: *Clinical procedures for medical assistants,* ed 7, St. Louis, 2008, Saunders.)

Continued

PROCEDURE 19-1

PROCEDURE 19-2

PROCEDURE **19-1**   Measuring Oral Body Temperature—Electronic Thermometer—cont'd

7. **Procedural Step.** Remove the probe from the patient's mouth. Discard the probe cover by firmly pressing the ejection button while holding the probe over a regular waste container. Do not allow your fingers to come in contact with the probe cover.

Principle. The probe cover should not be touched so as to prevent the transfer of microorganisms from the patient to the medical assistant. Saliva is not considered regulated medical waste; the probe can be discarded in a regular waste container.

8. Procedural Step. Return the probe to its stored position in the thermometer unit. Return the thermometer unit to its storage base.

Principle. Returning the probe to the unit automatically turns off and resets the thermometer.

9. Procedural Step. Sanitize your hands, and chart the results. Include the date, time, and temperature reading.

Principle. Patient data must be recorded properly to aid the physician in the diagnosis and to provide future reference.

Discard the probe cover by pressing the ejection button. (From Bonewit-West K: *Clinical procedures for medical assistants,* ed 7, St. Louis, 2008, Saunders.)

CHARTING EXAMPLE

Date	
10/15/10	2:15 p.m. T: 98.2° F. ——S. Martinez, RMA

PROCEDURE **19-2**   Measuring Axillary Body Temperature—Electronic Thermometer

Outcome Measure axillary body temperature. *Note:* Many of the principles for taking temperature already have been stated and are not included in this procedure.

Equipment/Supplies

- Electronic thermometer
- Oral probe (blue collar)

- Plastic probe cover
- Waste container

1. Procedural Step. Sanitize your hands, and assemble the equipment.

2. Procedural Step. Remove the thermometer unit from its storage base, and attach the oral (blue collar) probe to it. This is accomplished by inserting the latching plug (on the end of the coiled cord of the oral probe) to the plug receptacle on the thermometer unit until it locks into place. Insert the probe into the face of the thermometer.

3. Procedural Step. Greet the patient and introduce yourself. Identify the patient and explain the procedure.

4. Procedural Step. Remove clothing from the patient's shoulder and arm. Ensure that the axilla is dry. If it is wet, pat it dry with a paper towel or a gauze pad.

Principle. Clothing removal provides optimal exposure of the axilla for proper placement of the thermometer. Rubbing the axilla causes an increase in the temperature in that area owing to friction, resulting in an inaccurate temperature reading.

5. Procedural Step. Grasp the probe by the collar, and remove it from the face of the thermometer. Slide the probe into a disposable probe cover until it locks into place.

6. Procedural Step. Take the patient's temperature by placing the probe in the center of the patient's axilla. Instruct the patient to hold the arm close to the body. Hold the arm in place for small children and other patients who cannot maintain the position themselves.

Principle. Interference from outside air currents is reduced when the arm is held in the proper position.

Place the probe in the center of the patient's axilla. (From Bonewit-West K: *Clinical procedures for medical assistants,* ed 7, St. Louis, 2008, Saunders.)

7. Procedural Step. Hold the probe in place until you hear the tone. At that time, the patient's temperature appears as a digital display on the screen. Make a mental note of the temperature reading.

8. Procedural Step. Remove the probe from the patient's axilla. Discard the probe cover by firmly pressing the ejection button while holding the probe over a regular waste container. Do not allow your fingers to come in contact with the probe cover.

9. Procedural Step. Return the probe to its stored position in the thermometer unit. Return the thermometer unit to its storage base.

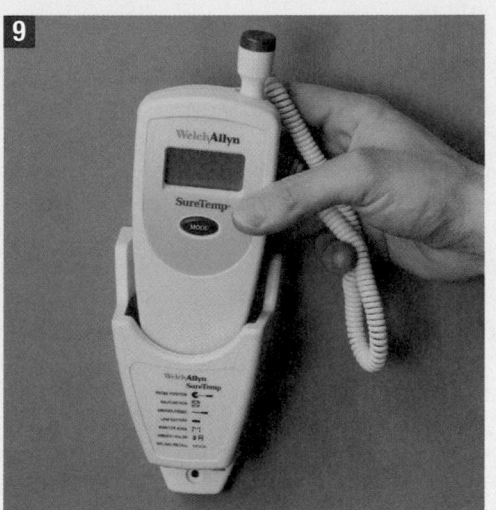

Return the thermometer to its base. (From Bonewit-West K: *Clinical procedures for medical assistants,* ed 7, St. Louis, 2008, Saunders.)

10. Procedural Step. Sanitize your hands, and chart the results. Include the date, time, and axillary temperature reading. The symbol Ⓐ must be charted next to the temperature reading to tell the physician that an axillary reading was taken.

CHARTING EXAMPLE	
Date	
10/15/10	9:30 a.m. T: 97.4° F Ⓐ —S. Martinez, RMA

PROCEDURE 19-3   Measuring Rectal Body Temperature— Electronic Thermometer

Outcome Measure rectal body temperature.

Equipment/Supplies

- Electronic thermometer
- Rectal probe (red collar)
- Plastic probe cover
- Lubricant

- Disposable gloves
- Tissues
- Waste container

1. **Procedural Step.** Sanitize your hands, and assemble the equipment.

2. **Procedural Step.** Remove the thermometer unit from its storage base. Attach the rectal (red collar) probe to it. This is accomplished by inserting the latching plug (on the end of the coiled cord of the rectal probe) to the plug receptacle on the thermometer unit. Insert the probe into the face of the thermometer.
   Principle. The rectal probe is color-coded with a red collar for ease in identifying it.

3. **Procedural Step.** Greet the patient and introduce yourself. Identify the patient and explain the procedure. If a patient is a child or an adult, provide him or her with a patient gown. Instruct the patient to remove enough clothing to provide access to the anal area and to put on the gown with the opening in the back. If the patient is an infant, ask the parent to remove his or her diaper.
   Principle. It is important to explain what you will be doing because body temperature may be higher in a fearful or apprehensive patient. The patient gown provides the patient with modesty and comfort.

4. **Procedural Step.** Apply gloves. Position the patient. ***Adults and children:*** Position the patient in the Sims position, and drape the patient to expose only the anal area. ***Infants:*** Position the infant on his or her abdomen.
   Principle. Gloves protect the medical assistant from microorganisms in the anal area and feces. Correct positioning allows clear viewing of the anal opening and provides for proper insertion of the thermometer. Draping reduces patient embarrassment and provides warmth.

5. **Procedural Step.** Grasp the probe by the collar, and remove it from the face of the thermometer. Slide the probe into a disposable plastic probe cover until it locks into place. Apply a lubricant to the tip of the probe cover up to a level of 1 inch.
   Principle. A lubricated thermometer can be inserted more easily and does not irritate the delicate rectal mucosa.

Apply a lubricant to the tip of the probe cover. (From Bonewit-West K: *Clinical procedures for medical assistants,* ed 7, St. Louis, 2008, Saunders.)

6. **Procedural Step.** Instruct the patient to lie still. Separate the buttocks to expose the anal opening, and gently insert the thermometer probe approximately 1 inch into the rectum of an adult, ⅝ inch in children, and ½ inch in infants. Do not force insertion of the probe. Hold the probe in place until the temperature registers.

Gently insert the probe ½ inch into the rectum. (From Bonewit-West K: *Clinical procedures for medical assistants,* ed 7, St. Louis, 2008, Saunders.)

Principle. The probe must be inserted correctly to prevent injury to the tissue of the anal opening. The probe should be held in place to prevent damage to the rectal mucosa.

7. Procedural Step. Hold the probe in place until you hear the tone. At that time, the patient's temperature appears as a digital display on the screen. Make a mental note of the temperature reading.

8. Procedural Step. Gently remove the probe from the rectum in the same direction as it was inserted. Avoid touching the probe cover. Discard the probe cover by firmly pressing the ejection button while holding the probe over a regular waste container. Return the probe to its stored position in the thermometer unit. Return the thermometer unit to its storage base.

Principle. Fecal material is not considered regulated medical waste; the probe can be discarded in a regular waste container.

9. Procedural Step. Wipe the patient's anal area with tissues to remove excess lubricant. Dispose of the tissues in a regular waste container.

Principle. Wiping the anal area makes the patient more comfortable.

10. Procedural Step. Remove gloves, and sanitize your hands. Chart the results. Include the date, time, and rectal temperature reading. The symbol Ⓡ must be charted next to the temperature reading to tell the physician that a rectal reading was taken.

CHARTING EXAMPLE

Date	
10/15/10	11:15 a.m. T: 99.8° F Ⓡ — S. Martinez, RMA

PROCEDURE 19-4   Measuring Aural Body Temperature—Tympanic Membrane Thermometer

Outcome Measure aural body temperature.

Equipment/Supplies

- Tympanic membrane thermometer
- Probe cover
- Waste container

1. Procedural Step. Sanitize your hands, and assemble the equipment.

Principle. Your hands should be clean and free from contamination.

2. Procedural Step. Greet the patient and introduce yourself. Identify the patient and explain the procedure.

Principle. It is important to explain what you will be doing because body temperature may be higher in a fearful or apprehensive patient.

3. Procedural Step. Remove the thermometer from its storage base. Ensure that the probe lens is clean and intact.

Principle. A dirty or damaged probe lens could result in a falsely low temperature reading.

4. Procedural Step. Place a cover on the probe by pressing the probe tip straight down into the cover box. You will be able to see and feel the cover snap securely into place on the probe. This procedure automatically turns on the thermometer.

Principle. The probe cover protects the lens and provides infection control. The cover must be seated securely on the probe to activate the thermometer.

Place a cover on the probe. (From Bonewit-West K: *Clinical procedures for medical assistants,* ed 7, St. Louis, 2008, Saunders.)

Continued

PROCEDURE 19-4   Measuring Aural Body Temperature—Tympanic Membrane Thermometer—cont'd

5. **Procedural Step.** Pull the probe straight up from the cover box. Look at the digital display to see if the thermometer is ready to use.

When the thermometer is ready, it displays the word "READY." (From Bonewit-West K: *Clinical procedures for medical assistants,* ed 7, St. Louis, 2008, Saunders.)

6. Procedural Step. Hold the thermometer in your dominant hand. If you are right handed, you should take the temperature in the patient's right ear. If you are left handed, take the temperature in the patient's left ear.
Principle. Taking the temperature with the dominant hand assists in the proper placement of the probe in the patient's ear.

7. **Procedural Step.** Straighten the patient's external ear canal with your nondominant hand, as follows:
Adults and Children Older Than 3 Years Old. Gently pull the ear auricle upward and backward.
Children Younger Than 3 Years Old. Gently pull the ear pinna downward and backward.
Principle. Straightening the ear canal allows the probe sensor to obtain a clear picture of the tympanic membrane, resulting in an accurate temperature measurement.

Straighten the canal of adults and children older than 3 years by pulling the ear auricle upward and backward. (From Bonewit-West K: *Clinical procedures for medical assistants,* ed 7, St. Louis, 2008, Saunders.)

Straighten the canal of children younger than 3 years by pulling the ear auricle downward and backward. (From Bonewit-West K: *Clinical procedures for medical assistants,* ed 7, St. Louis, 2008, Saunders.)

8. Procedural Step. Insert the probe into the patient's ear canal tightly enough to seal the opening, but without causing patient discomfort. Point the tip of the probe toward the opposite temple (approximately midway between the opposite ear and eyebrow).
Principle. Sealing the ear canal prevents cooler external air from entering the ear, which could result in a falsely low reading. Correct positioning of the probe optimizes the sensor's view of the tympanic membrane, leading to an accurate temperature reading.

9. Procedural Step. Ask the patient to remain still. Hold the thermometer steady, and depress the activation button. Depending on the brand of the thermometer, perform one of the following:

a. Hold the button down for one full second, and then release it, *or*

b. Hold down the button down until an audible tone is heard.

Principle. The thermometer cannot take a temperature unless the activation button is depressed for 1 full second. When the button is depressed, the infrared sensor in the probe scans the thermal energy radiated by the tympanic membrane.

10. Procedural Step. Remove the thermometer from the ear canal. Turn the digital display of the thermometer toward you, and read the temperature. Make a mental note of the temperature reading. If the temperature seems to be too low, repeat the procedure to ensure that you have used the proper technique. The temperature indicated on this thermometer is 98°F (37.2°C).

Principle. The temperature remains on the display screen until another cover is inserted on the probe. Improper technique can result in a falsely low temperature reading.

Read the temperature on the digital display. (From Bonewit-West K: *Clinical procedures for medical assistants,* ed 7, St. Louis, 2008, Saunders.)

11. Procedural Step. Dispose of the probe cover by ejecting it into a regular waste container.

Dispose of the probe cover. (From Bonewit-West K: *Clinical procedures for medical assistants,* ed 7, St. Louis, 2008, Saunders.)

12. Procedural Step. Replace the thermometer in its storage base.

Principle. The thermometer should be stored in its base to protect the probe lens from damage and dirt.

13. Procedural Step. Sanitize your hands.

14. Procedural Step. Chart the results. Include the date, time, aural temperature reading, and which ear was used to take the temperature (AD: right ear; AS: left ear). Using these abbreviations, the physician knows that the temperature was taken through the aural route.

CHARTING EXAMPLE	
Date	
10/15/10	3:00 p.m. T: 98° F, AD — S. Martinez, RMA

PROCEDURE 19-4

PROCEDURE 19-5   Measuring Temporal Artery Body Temperature

Outcome Measure temporal artery body temperature.

Equipment/Supplies

- Temporal artery thermometer
- Probe cover
- Antiseptic wipe
- Waste container

1. **Procedural Step.** Sanitize your hands, and assemble the equipment.
2. **Procedural Step.** Greet the patient and introduce yourself. Identify the patient and explain the procedure.
3. **Procedural Step.** Examine the probe lens of the temporal artery thermometer to ensure that the lens is clean and intact.
   Principle. A dirty or damaged probe lens could result in a falsely low temperature reading.
4. **Procedural Step.** Place a disposable cover over the probe. If the thermometer does not use disposable covers, clean the probe with an antiseptic wipe and allow it to dry.
   Principle. Applying a probe cover or cleaning the probe with an antiseptic wipe provides infection control.

Place a disposable probe cover on the thermometer. (From Bonewit-West K: *Clinical procedures for medical assistants,* ed 7, St. Louis, 2008, Saunders.)

5. **Procedural Step.** Select an appropriate site; the right or left forehead can be used. The site selected should be fully exposed to the environment.
   Principle. The temporal artery is located in the center of each side of the forehead, approximately 2 mm below the surface of the skin.
6. **Procedural Step.** Prepare the patient by brushing away any hair that is covering the side of the forehead to be scanned and the area behind the earlobe on the same side.
   Principle. Hair covering the area to be measured traps body heat, resulting in a falsely high temperature reading.

7. **Procedural Step.** Hold the thermometer in your dominant hand with your thumb on the scan button.
8. **Procedural Step.** Gently position the probe of the thermometer on the center of the patient's forehead, midway between the eyebrow and the hairline.

Position the probe on the center of the patient's forehead. (From Bonewit-West K: *Clinical procedures for medical assistants,* ed 7, St. Louis, 2008, Saunders.)

9. **Procedural Step.** Depress the scan button, and keep it depressed for the entire measurement.
   Principle: Not keeping the scan button depressed can result in a falsely low temperature reading.
10. **Procedural Step.** Slowly and gently slide the probe straight across the forehead, midway between the eyebrow and the upper hairline. Continue until the hairline is reached. Keep the scan button depressed and the probe flush (flat) against the forehead. During this time, a beeping sound occurs and a red light blinks to indicate a measurement is taking place. Rapid beeping and blinking indicate a rise to a higher temperature. A slow beeping indicates that the thermometer is still scanning but not finding a higher temperature.
    Principle. The thermometer continually scans for the peak temperature as long as the scan button is depressed. The probe must be held flat against the forehead to ensure accurate scanning of the temporal artery.

Slowly slide the probe straight across the patient's forehead. (From Bonewit-West K: *Clinical procedures for medical assistants,* ed 7, St. Louis, 2008, Saunders.)

11. Procedural Step. Keeping the button depressed, lift the probe from the forehead, and gently place the probe behind the earlobe in the soft depression of the neck just below the mastoid process. Hold the probe in place for 1 to 2 seconds.
Principle. Taking the patient's temperature behind the earlobe prevents an error in temperature measurement in the event that the patient is sweating.

Place the probe behind the ear lobe. (From Bonewit-West K: *Clinical procedures for medical assistants,* ed 7, St. Louis, 2008, Saunders.)

12. Procedural Step. Release the scan button on the digital display, and read the temperature. Make a mental note of the temperature reading (The temperature indicated on this thermometer is 99.1°F [37.3°C]). The reading remains on the display for approximately 15 to 30 seconds after the button is released. The thermometer shuts off automatically after 30 seconds. To turn the thermometer off imme-

diately, press and release the scan button quickly. If the patient's temperature needs to be taken again, wait 60 seconds or use the opposite side of the forehead. *Principle.* Taking a measurement cools the skin, and taking another measurement too soon may result in an inaccurate reading.

Read the temperature. (From Bonewit-West K: *Clinical procedures for medical assistants,* ed 7, St. Louis, 2008, Saunders.)

13. Procedural Step. Dispose of the probe cover by pushing it off the probe with your thumb and ejecting it into a regular waste container. Wipe the probe with an antiseptic wipe, and allow it to dry.

Wipe the probe with an antiseptic wipe. (From Bonewit-West K: *Clinical procedures for medical assistants,* ed 7, St. Louis, 2008, Saunders.)

PROCEDURE 19-5

Continued

PROCEDURE 19-5   Measuring Temporal Artery Body Temperature—cont'd

14. Procedural Step. Sanitize your hands, and chart the results. Include the date, time, and temperature reading. The symbol (TA) must be charted next to the temperature reading to tell the physician that a temporal artery reading was taken. Store the thermometer in a clean, dry area.

CHARTING EXAMPLE

Date	
10/15/10	9:15 a.m. T: 99.1° F (TA)— S. Martinez, RMA

Table 19-4 Pulse Rates of Various Age Groups

Age Group	Pulse Range (beats/min)	Average Pulse (beats/min)
Infant (birth to 1 yr)	120-160	140
Toddler (1-3 yr)	90-140	115
Preschool child (3-6 yr)	80-110	95
School-age child (6-12 yr)	75-105	90
Adolescent (12-18 yr)	60-100	80
Adult (after 18th yr)	60-100	80
Adult (after 60th yr)	67-80	74
Well-trained athletes	40-60	50

From Bonewit-West K: *Clinical procedures for medical assistants*, ed 7, St. Louis, 2008, Saunders.

PULSE

Mechanism of the Pulse

When the left ventricle of the heart contracts, blood is forced from the heart into the **aorta,** which is the major trunk of the arterial system of the body. The aorta is already filled with blood and must expand to accept the blood being pushed out of the left ventricle. This creates a pulsating wave that travels from the aorta through the walls of the arterial system. This wave, known as the *pulse,* can be felt as a light tap by an examiner. The pulse rate is measured by counting the number of "taps," or beats per minute. The heart rate can be determined by taking the pulse rate.

Factors Affecting Pulse Rate

Pulse rate can vary depending on many factors. The medical assistant should take each of the following into consideration when measuring pulse:

1. **Age.** The pulse varies inversely with age. As the age increases, the pulse rate gradually decreases. Table 19-4 lists the pulse rates of the various age groups.
2. **Gender.** Women tend to have a slightly faster pulse rate than men.
3. **Physical activity.** Physical activity, such as jogging and swimming, increases the pulse rate temporarily.
4. **Emotional states.** Strong emotional states, such as anxiety, fear, excitement, and anger, temporarily increase the pulse rate.

5. **Metabolism.** Increased body metabolism, such as occurs during pregnancy, increases the pulse rate.
6. **Fever.** Fever increases the pulse rate.
7. **Medications.** Medications may alter the pulse rate. For example, digitalis decreases the pulse rate, and epinephrine increases it.

Pulse Sites

The pulse is felt most strongly when a superficial artery is held against a firm tissue, such as bone. The locations of the sites used for measuring the pulse are shown in Figure 19-10 and are described next.

Radial   The most common site for measuring the pulse is the radial artery, which is located in a groove on the inner aspect of the wrist just below the thumb. The radial pulse is easily accessible and can be measured with no discomfort to the patient. This site is also used by individuals at home monitoring their own heart rates, such as athletes, patients taking heart medication, and individuals starting an exercise program. The procedure for measuring radial pulse is outlined in Procedure 19-6.

Apical   The apical pulse has a stronger beat and is easier to measure than the other pulse sites. If the medical assistant is having difficulty feeling the radial pulse or if the radial pulse is irregular or abnormally slow or rapid, the apical pulse should be taken (Procedure 19-7). This pulse site is often used to measure pulse in infants and in children up to 3 years old because the other sites are difficult to palpate accurately in these age groups. The apical pulse is measured using a stethoscope. The chest piece of the stethoscope is placed lightly over the apex of the heart, which is located in the fifth **intercostal** (between the ribs) space at the junction of the left midclavicular line (Figure 19-11).

Brachial   The brachial pulse is in the **antecubital space,** which is the space located at the front of the elbow. This site is used to take blood pressure, to measure pulse in infants during cardiac arrest, and to assess the status of the circulation to the lower arm.

Ulnar   The ulnar pulse is located on the ulnar (little finger) side of the wrist. It is used to assess the status of circulation to the hand.

Temporal   The temporal pulse is located in front of the ear and just above eye level. This site is used to measure

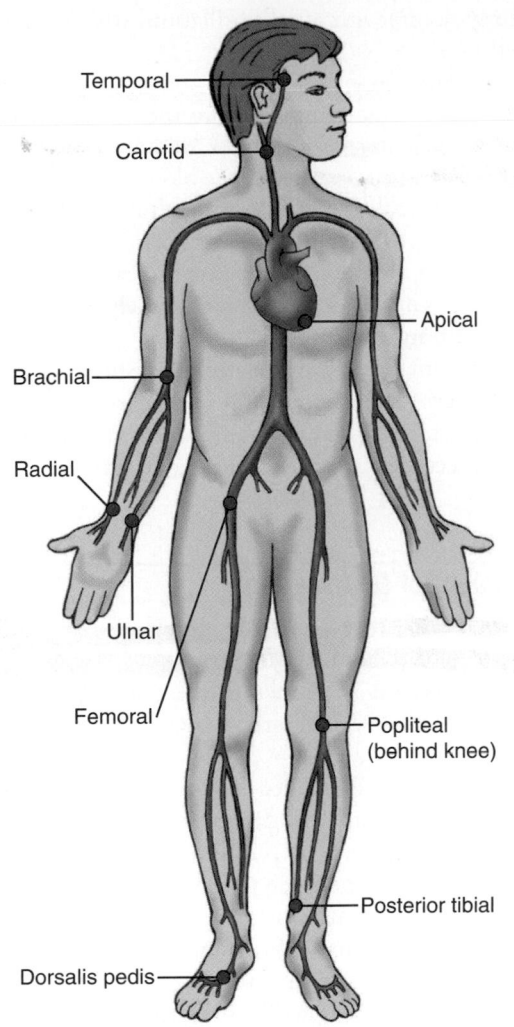

Figure 19-10. Pulse sites. (From Bonewit-West K: *Clinical procedures for medical assistants*, ed 7, St. Louis, 2008, Saunders.)

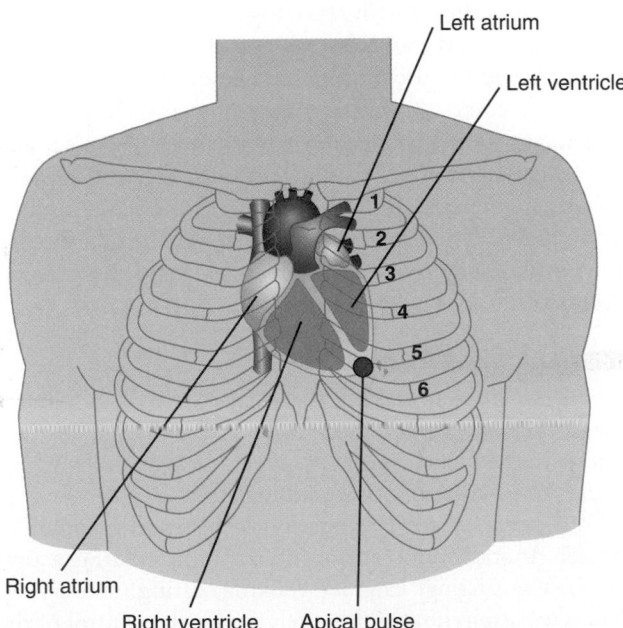

Figure 19-11. The apical pulse is found over the apex of the heart, which is located in the fifth intercostal space at the junction of the left midclavicular line. (From Bonewit-West K: *Clinical procedures for medical assistants*, ed 7, St. Louis, 2008, Saunders.)

pulse when the radial pulse is inaccessible. It is also an easy access site to assess pulse in children.

Carotid The carotid pulse is located on the anterior side of the neck, slightly to one side of the midline, and is the best site to find a pulse quickly. This site is used to measure pulse in children and adults during cardiac arrest. The carotid site also is commonly used by individuals to monitor pulse during exercise.

Femoral The femoral pulse is in the middle of the groin. This site is used to measure pulse in infants and children and in adults during cardiac arrest and to assess the status of the circulation to the lower leg.

Popliteal The popliteal pulse is at the back of the knee and is detected most easily when the knee is slightly flexed. This site is used to measure blood pressure when the brachial pulse is inaccessible and to assess the status of the circulation to the lower leg.

Posterior Tibial The posterior tibial pulse is located on the inner aspect of the ankle just posterior to the ankle bone. This site is used to assess the status of circulation to the foot.

Dorsalis Pedis The dorsalis pedis pulse is located on the upper surface of the foot, between the first and second metatarsal bones. This site is used to assess the status of circulation to the foot.

Assessment of Pulse

The purpose of measuring pulse is to establish the patient's baseline pulse rate and to assess the pulse rate after special procedures, medications, or disease processes that affect heart functioning. Pulse is measured using palpation at all of the pulse sites except the apical site.

Memories *from* Externship

Sergio Martinez: One experience that really stands out in my memory occurred during my externship at a family practice medical office. I needed to take the blood pressure of a small 6-year-old boy. After I put the cuff on his arm, his eyes started filling up with tears. I stopped, removed the cuff, and asked him if something was wrong. He said he was afraid that, when I started squeezing that thing around his arm, his hand would fall off. I sat down next to him, spent some time talking with him, and reassured him that his hand would be perfectly fine and would not fall off. I put the cuff on my arm and pumped it up to show him that he would be safe. He then agreed to let me take his blood pressure. After I took his blood pressure, he wiggled his hand, gave me a big smile, and said that it didn't hurt at all. That situation made me realize that children may have a lot of fears about what might happen to them at the medical office. Since that experience, I always take the time to explain procedures to children before I perform them. ∎

Prepare for Success

A pulse is palpated by applying moderate pressure with the sensitive pads located on the tips of the three middle fingers. The pulse should not be taken with the thumb because the thumb has a pulse of its own. This could result in a measurement of the medical assistant's pulse rather than the patient's pulse. Excessive pressure should not be applied when measuring pulse because it could obliterate, or close off, the pulse. It may not be possible to detect the pulse if too little pressure is applied, however. An accurate assessment of pulse includes a determination of the pulse rate, the pulse rhythm, and the pulse volume.

Pulse Rate

The pulse rate is the number of heart pulsations or heartbeats that occur in 1 minute; therefore, pulse rate is measured in beats per minute. Normal pulse rates vary widely in the various age groups, as shown in Table 19-4. For a healthy adult, the normal resting pulse rate ranges from 60 to 100 beats per minute, with the average falling between 70 and 80 beats per minute.

An abnormally fast heart rate of more than 100 beats per minute is known as **tachycardia.** Tachycardia may indicate disease states, such as hemorrhaging or heart disease. An individual's pulse rate may normally exceed 100 beats per minute, however, during vigorous exercise or during strong emotional states.

Bradycardia is an abnormally slow heart rate, less than 60 beats per minute. A pulse rate less than 60 beats per minute may occur normally during sleep. Trained athletes often have low pulse rates. If a patient exhibits tachycardia or bradycardia during radial pulse measurement, the apical pulse should also be measured.

Pulse Rhythm and Volume

In addition to measuring the pulse rate, the medical assistant should determine the rhythm and volume of the pulse. The **pulse rhythm** denotes the time interval between heartbeats; a normal rhythm has the same time interval between beats. Any irregularity in the heart's rhythm is known as a **dysrhythmia** (also termed *arrhythmia*) and is characterized by unequal or irregular intervals between the heartbeats. If a dysrhythmia is present, the physician may order one or more of the following: an apical-radial pulse, an electrocardiogram, or Holter monitoring.

An *apical-radial pulse* is performed to determine whether a pulse deficit is present. Taking an apical-radial pulse involves measuring the apical pulse at the same time as the radial pulse for a duration of 1 full minute. A *pulse deficit* exists when the radial pulse rate is less than the apical pulse rate. If one medical assistant measures an apical pulse rate of 88 beats per minute, and another medical assistant simultaneously measures a radial pulse rate of 76 beats per minute, this results in a pulse deficit of 12 beats. A pulse deficit means that not all of the heartbeats are reaching the peripheral arteries. A pulse deficit is caused by an inefficient contraction of the heart that is not strong enough to transmit a pulse wave to the peripheral pulse site. A pulse deficit

frequently occurs with atrial fibrillation, which is a type of dysrhythmia.

The **pulse volume** refers to the strength of the heartbeat. The amount of blood pumped into the aorta by each contraction of the left ventricle should remain constant, making the pulse feel strong and full. If the blood volume decreases, the pulse feels weak and may be difficult to detect. This type of pulse is usually accompanied by a fast heart rate and is described as a **thready pulse.** An increase in the blood volume results in a pulse that feels extremely strong and full, known as a **bounding pulse.**

Any abnormalities in the rhythm or volume of the pulse should be recorded accurately in the patient's chart by the medical assistant. A pulse that has a normal rhythm and volume is recorded as being regular and strong.

RESPIRATION
Mechanism of Respiration

The purpose of respiration is to provide for the exchange of oxygen and carbon dioxide between the atmosphere and the blood. Oxygen is taken into the body to be used for vital body processes, and carbon dioxide is given off as a waste product.

Each respiration is divided into two phases: **inhalation** and **exhalation** (Figure 19-12). During inhalation, or inspiration, the diaphragm descends and the lungs expand, causing air containing oxygen to move from the atmosphere into the lungs. Exhalation, or expiration, involves the removal of carbon dioxide from the body. The diaphragm ascends, and the lungs return to their original state so that air containing carbon dioxide is expelled. One complete respiration is composed of one inhalation and one exhalation.

Respiration can be classified as *external* or *internal*. External respiration involves the exchange of oxygen and carbon dioxide between the **alveolus** (thin-walled sacs) of the lungs and the blood (Figure 19-13). The blood, located in small capillaries, comes in contact with the alveoli, picks up oxygen, and carries it to the cells of the body. At this point, the oxygen is given off to the cells and carbon dioxide is picked up by the blood to be transported as a waste product to the lungs. The exchange of oxygen and carbon dioxide between the body cells and the blood is known as *internal respiration.*

Control of Respiration

The medulla oblongata, located in the brain, is the control center for involuntary respiration. A buildup of carbon dioxide in the blood sends a message to the medulla, which triggers respiration to occur automatically.

To a certain extent, respiration is also under voluntary control. An individual can control respiration during activities such as singing, laughing, talking, eating, and crying. Voluntary respiration is ultimately under the control of the medulla oblongata. The breath can be held for only a certain length of time, after which carbon dioxide begins to build

PATIENT TEACHING Aerobic Exercise

Answer questions patients have about aerobic exercise.

What is aerobic exercise?

Aerobic exercise increases, sustains, and decreases your pulse over time. Aerobic exercise is accomplished through a steady, nonstop activity, such as walking, jogging, cycling, or swimming. Each workout should include a warm-up and cool-down period of at least 5 minutes each. This is to prevent muscle or joint injuries.

What are the benefits of an aerobic exercise program?

The benefits of an aerobic exercise program include strengthening of the heart, a slower resting pulse rate, reduction of stress, increased energy, lowering of body fat, a decrease of "bad" (low-density lipoprotein) cholesterol, and an increase of "good" (high-density lipoprotein) cholesterol. The key to a safe and effective aerobic exercise program is the target heart rate (THR).

What is target heart rate?

Your THR is a safe and effective exercise pulse range that indicates you are exercising at the right level for your age and for what you are trying to accomplish with exercise. Exercising at a level below your THR does little to promote fitness; exercising at a level above your THR may not be safe.

How do I determine my target heart rate?

The following formula is used to determine your THR:

1. Subtract your age from 220 to determine your maximum heart rate (MHR), which is the fastest your heart can beat safely for your age. The MHR of a 40-year-old person is calculated as follows:

$$220 - 40 \text{ years old} = 180 \text{ (MHR)}$$

2. Determine the lower end of your THR range by multiplying your MHR by 0.6. For our example:

$$180 \times 0.60 = 108 \text{ (low end of THR)}$$

3. Determine the upper end of your THR range by multiplying your MHR by 0.8. For our example:

$$180 \times 0.80 = 144 \text{ (upper end of THR)}$$

Always exercise within your THR range. The 40-year-old person in our example should exercise with a THR between 108 and 144.

How often should aerobic exercise be performed?

A report from the American Cancer Society recommends that adults spend at least 30 minutes or more, at least 5 days a week, in moderately intense exercise to obtain the maximum benefits for heart health. Researchers say that this exercise recommendation is based on studies of the amount of energy burned by people who maintain a healthy weight. They stress that there are many ways to accomplish this goal, such as through playing with your children, doing housework, gardening, mowing the grass, walking the dog, bicycling, golfing, swimming, and other day-to-day activities. The American Cancer Society further recommends that children and adolescents engage in at least 60 minutes per day of moderate to vigorous physical activity at least 5 days a week. ■

What Would You Do? What Would You *Not* Do?

Case Study 2

Alex Jacoby is 18 years old and a senior in high school. He comes to the office complaining of severe pain in his left shoulder. Alex is an outstanding competitive swimmer and is currently ranked first in the state in the 100-yard butterfly. Alex has a big meet coming up and must do well because he has a chance of getting an athletic scholarship to the University of Florida. He says he thinks he can take 2 seconds off his best time at this meet and he does not want anything to interfere with that. Alex wants the physician to do whatever he can to make his shoulder better and thinks that a steroid injection and OxyContin might be the answer. His vital signs are as follows: temperature 98.5°F, pulse 48 beats/min, respirations 12 breaths/min, and blood pressure 108/68 mm Hg. Alex asks why his pulse is so slow and wants to know if there is any medication he can take to make it faster. ■

up in the body, resulting in a stimulus to the medulla that causes respiration to occur involuntarily. Small children may voluntarily hold their breath during a temper tantrum. A parent who does not understand the principles of respiration may be concerned that the child would cease breathing. The medical assistant should be able to explain that involuntary respiration would eventually occur and the child would resume breathing.

Assessment of Respiration

Because an individual can control his or her respiration, the medical assistant should measure respirations without the patient's knowledge. Patients may change their respiratory rate unintentionally if they are aware that they are being measured. An ideal time to measure respiration is after the pulse is taken. Procedure 19-6 outlines the procedures for taking pulse and respiration in one continuous procedure.

Respiratory Rate

The respiratory rate of a normal healthy adult ranges from 12 to 20 respirations per minute. With most adults, there is a ratio of one respiration for every four pulse beats. If the

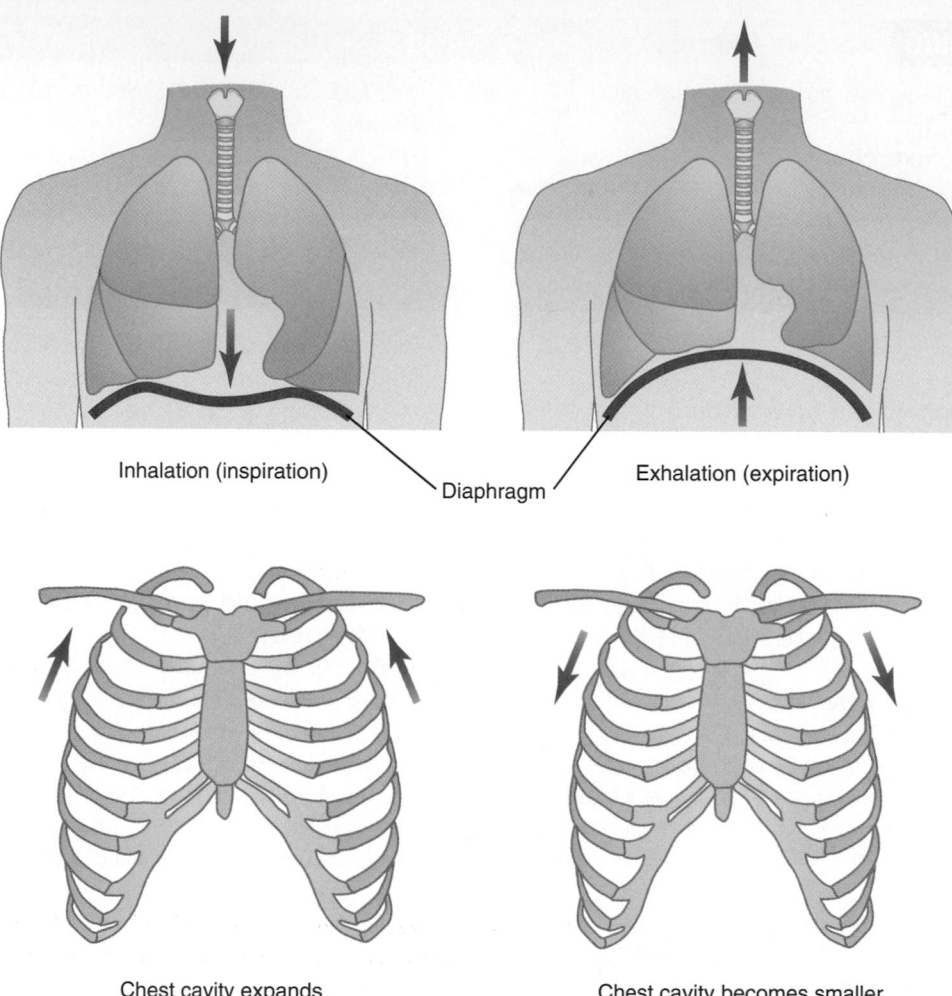

Inhalation (inspiration)   Exhalation (expiration)

Diaphragm

Chest cavity expands   Chest cavity becomes smaller

Figure 19-12. Inhalation and exhalation. (From Bonewit-West K: *Clinical procedures for medical assistants,* ed 7, St. Louis, 2008, Saunders.)

respiratory rate is 18, the pulse rate would be approximately 72 beats per minute. An abnormal increase in the respiratory rate of more than 20 respirations per minute is referred to as **tachypnea.** An abnormal decrease in the respiratory rate of less than 12 respirations per minute is known as **bradypnea.** When measuring the respiratory rate, the medical assistant should take into consideration the following factors:

1. **Age.** As age increases, the respiratory rate decreases. The respiratory rate of a child would be expected to be faster than that of an adult. Table 19-5 provides a chart of the respiratory rates for the various age groups.
2. **Physical activity.** Physical activity increases the respiratory rate temporarily.
3. **Emotional states.** Strong emotional states temporarily increase the respiratory rate.
4. **Fever.** A patient with a fever has an increased respiratory rate. One way that heat is lost from the body is through the lungs; a fever causes an increased respiratory rate as the body tries to rid itself of the excess heat.

Table 19-5 Respiratory Rates of Various Age Groups

Age Group	Average Respiratory Range (breaths/min)	Respiratory Average (breaths/min)
Infant (birth to 1 yr)	30-40	35
Toddler (1-3 yr)	23-35	30
Preschool child (3-6 yr)	20-30	25
School-age child (6-12 yr)	18-26	22
Adolescent (12-18 yr)	12-20	16
Adult (after 18th yr)	12-20	16

From Bonewit-West K: *Clinical procedures for medical assistants,* ed 7, St. Louis, 2008, Saunders.

5. **Medications.** Certain medications increase the respiratory rate, and others decrease it. If the medical assistant is unsure of what effect a particular drug may have on the respiratory rate, he or she should consult a drug reference, such as the *Physician's Desk Reference* (PDR).

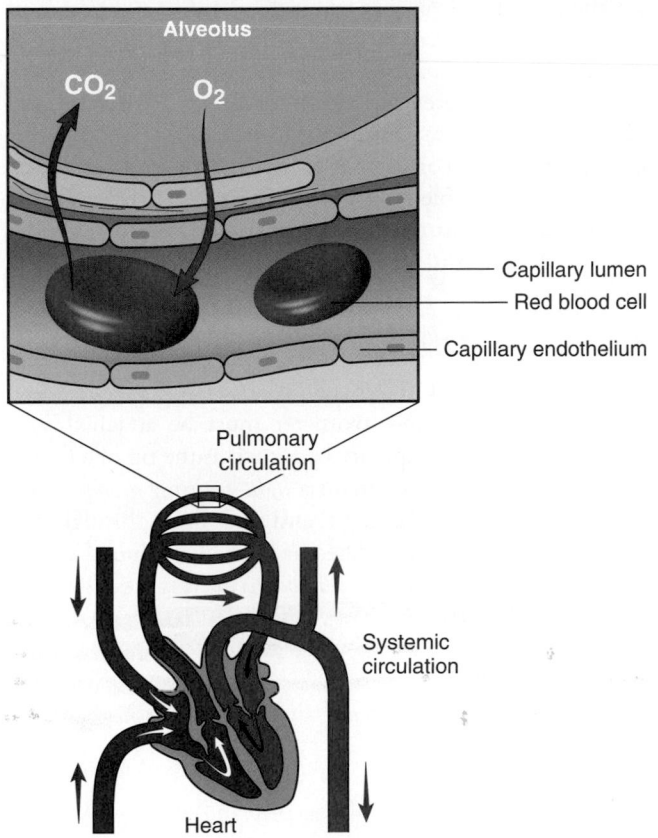

External Respiration

Alveolus

CO_2 O_2

Capillary lumen
Red blood cell
Capillary endothelium

Pulmonary
circulation

Systemic
circulation

Heart

Figure 19-13. Exchange of oxygen and carbon dioxide between the alveoli of the lungs and the blood. (From Bonewit-West K: *Clinical procedures for medical assistants,* ed 7, St. Louis, 2008, Saunders.)

Rhythm and Depth of Respiration

The *rhythm* and *depth* should be noted when measuring respiration. Normally the rhythm should be even and regular, and the pauses between inhalation and exhalation should be equal. The depth of respiration indicates the amount of air that is inhaled or exhaled during the process of breathing. Respiratory depth is generally described as normal, deep, or shallow and is determined by observing the amount of movement of the chest. For normal respirations, the depth of each respiration in a resting state is approximately the same. Deep respirations are those in which a large volume of air is inhaled and exhaled, whereas shallow respirations involve the exchange of a small volume of air. Normal respiration is referred to as **eupnea.** The rate is approximately 12 to 20 respirations per minute, the rhythm is even and regular, and the depth is normal.

Hyperpnea is an abnormal increase in the rate and depth of the respirations. A patient with hyperpnea exhibits a deep, rapid, and labored respiration. Hyperpnea occurs normally with exercise and abnormally with pain and fever. It also can occur with any condition in which the supply of oxygen is inadequate, such as heart disease and lung disease.

Hyperventilation is an abnormally fast and deep type of breathing that is usually associated with acute anxiety conditions, such as panic attacks. An individual who is hyperventilating is "overbreathing," which usually causes dizziness and weakness.

Hypopnea is a condition in which a patient's respiration exhibits an abnormal decrease in the rate and depth. The depth is approximately half that of normal respiration. Hypopnea often occurs in individuals with sleep disorders.

PATIENT TEACHING | Chronic Obstructive Pulmonary Disease

Answer questions that patients have about chronic obstructive pulmonary disease (COPD).

What is COPD?
COPD is a chronic airway obstruction that results from emphysema, chronic bronchitis, or asthma, or any combination of these conditions. COPD is a chronic, debilitating, irreversible, and sometimes fatal disease.

How many people have COPD?
COPD affects an estimated 16 million Americans, and its incidence is increasing. It is the fourth leading cause of death in the United States behind heart disease, cancer, and stroke. Although COPD is much more common in men than in women, the greatest increase of death rates is occurring in women.

What causes COPD?
Cigarette smoking for a period of many years is the leading cause of COPD. Other causes include air pollution and occupational exposure to irritating inhalants, such as noxious dusts, fumes, and vapors.

What types of tests might the physician order?
Respiratory tests to diagnose COPD include various types of pulmonary function tests. Examples of pulmonary function tests are spirometry, lung volumes, diffusion capacity, arterial blood gas studies, pulse oximetry, and cardiopulmonary exercise tests.

What treatment might the physician prescribe?
Treatment is focused on improving breathing difficulties and may include bronchodilator drug therapy, breathing exercises, and oxygen therapy.
1. Encourage patients with COPD to comply with therapy prescribed by the physician.
2. Provide the patient with information about smoking, asthma, emphysema, and chronic bronchitis. Educational materials are available from the American Lung Association, American Heart Association, and American Cancer Society. ■

Color of the Patient

The patient's color should be observed while the respiration is being measured. A reduction in the oxygen supply to the tissues (hypoxia) results in a condition known as **cyanosis,** which causes a bluish discoloration of the skin and mucous membranes. Cyanosis is first observed in the nail beds and lips because in these areas the blood vessels lie close to the surface of the skin. Cyanosis typically occurs in patients with advanced emphysema and in patients during cardiac arrest.

Apnea is a temporary absence of respirations. Some individuals experience apnea during sleep; this condition is known as *sleep apnea.* Apnea can be a serious condition if the individual's breathing ceases for more than 4 to 6 minutes because brain damage or death could occur.

Respiratory Abnormalities

A patient who is having difficulty breathing or shortness of breath has a condition known as **dyspnea.** Dyspnea may occur normally during vigorous physical exertion and abnormally in patients with asthma and emphysema. A patient with dyspnea may find it easier to breathe while in a sitting or standing position. This state is called **orthopnea** and occurs with disorders of the heart and lungs, such as asthma, emphysema, pneumonia, and congestive heart failure.

Breath Sounds

Breath sounds are caused by air moving through the respiratory tract. Normal breath sounds are quiet and barely audible. Abnormal breath sounds are referred to as **adventitious sounds** and generally signify the presence of a respiratory disorder. The cause and character of abnormal breath sounds are presented in Table 19-6.

PULSE OXIMETRY

Pulse oximetry is a painless and noninvasive procedure used to measure the oxygen saturation of hemoglobin in arterial blood. Hemoglobin is a complex compound found in red blood cells that functions in transporting oxygen in the body. Pulse oximetry provides the physician with infor-

mation on a patient's cardiorespiratory status—in particular, the amount of oxygen being delivered to the tissues of the body. The procedure for performing pulse oximetry is presented in Procedure 19-8.

A **pulse oximeter** is the device used to measure and display the oxygen saturation of the blood. It is a computerized device that consists of a two-sided, cliplike probe connected by a cable to a monitor (Figure 19-14). A pulse oximeter also measures the patient's pulse rate in beats per minute. A constant-pitched audible beep is emitted with each pulse beat.

Assessment of Oxygen Saturation

Mechanism of Action

The probe of the pulse oximeter must be attached to a peripheral pulsating capillary bed, such as the tip of a finger. One side of the probe contains a *light-emitting diode* (LED) that transmits infrared light and red light through the patient's tissues to a light detector located on the other side of the probe, known as the *photodetector* (Figure 19-15).

Hemoglobin that is bright red in color has a high oxygen content (*oxygen-rich*) and absorbs more of the infrared light emitted by the LED. Hemoglobin that is dark red in color is low in oxygen (*oxygen-poor*) and absorbs more of the red

Figure 19-14. Pulse oximeter. (From Bonewit-West K: *Clinical procedures for medical assistants,* ed 7, St. Louis, 2008, Saunders.)

Table 19-6 Abnormal Breath Sounds		
Type	Cause	Character
Crackles* (rales)	Air moving through airways that contain fluid	Dry or wet intermittent sounds that vary in pitch (this sound can be duplicated by rubbing hair together next to ear)
Rhonchi*	Thick secretions, tumors, or spasms that partially obstruct air flow through large upper airways	Deep, low-pitched, rumbling sound more audible during expiration
Wheezes	Severely narrowed airways caused by partial obstruction in smaller bronchi and bronchioles; common symptom of asthma	Continuous, high-pitched, whistling musical sounds heard during inspiration and expiration
Pleural friction rub*	Inflamed pleura rubbing together	High, grating sound similar to rubbing leather pieces together; heard on inspiration and expiration

From Bonewit-West K: *Clinical procedures for medical assistants,* ed 7, St. Louis, 2008, Saunders.
*Audible only through a stethoscope.

Figure 19-15. The probe of the pulse oximeter is attached to a peripheral capillary bed in the fingertip. The LED transmits light through the capillary bed to a light detector (photodetector) located on the other side of the probe to measure the oxygen saturation of hemoglobin. (From Bonewit-West K: *Clinical procedures for medical assistants,* ed 7, St. Louis, 2008, Saunders.)

light. The oximeter's computer compares and calculates the light transmitted from the oxygen-rich hemoglobin and the oxygen-poor hemoglobin and, from this ratio, is able to determine the oxygen saturation of the patient's hemoglobin. This measurement is converted to a percentage and displayed as a digital readout on the screen of the monitor. Because the pulse oximeter measures the oxygen saturation of peripheral capillaries, the abbreviation **SpO$_2$** *(saturation of peripheral oxygen)* is used to record the reading.

A more complete but invasive measurement of oxygen saturation is arterial blood gas analysis, which requires drawing a blood specimen from an artery. The abbreviation for this type of arterial oxygen saturation measurement is **SaO$_2$** *(saturation of arterial oxygen).*

Interpretation of Results

The pulse oximetry reading represents the percentage of hemoglobin that is saturated (filled) with oxygen. Each molecule of hemoglobin can carry four oxygen molecules. If 100 molecules of hemoglobin were fully saturated with oxygen, they would be carrying 400 molecules of oxygen and the oxygen saturation reading would be 100%. If these same 100 molecules of hemoglobin were carrying only 360 molecules of oxygen, however, the oxygen saturation reading would be 90%. The more hemoglobin that is saturated with oxygen, the higher the oxygen saturation of the blood.

The oxygen saturation level of most healthy individuals is 95% to 99%. Because the air we breathe is only 21% saturated with oxygen, it is unusual for an individual's hemoglobin to be fully or 100% saturated with oxygen. Patients on supplemental oxygen sometimes have a reading of 100%, however.

An oxygen saturation level less than 95% typically results in an inadequate amount of oxygen reaching the tissues of the body, although patients with chronic pulmonary disease are sometimes able to tolerate lower saturation levels. Respiratory failure, resulting in tissue damage, usually occurs when the oxygen saturation decreases to a level between 85% and 90%. Cyanosis typically appears when an individ-

ual's oxygen saturation reaches a level of 75%, and an oxygen saturation less than 70% is life-threatening.

A decrease in the oxygen saturation of the blood (less than 95%) is known as **hypoxemia.** Hypoxemia can lead to a more serious condition known as hypoxia. **Hypoxia** is defined as a reduction in the oxygen supply to the tissues of the body, and if not treated, it can lead to tissue damage and death. The first symptoms of hypoxia include headache, mental confusion, nausea, dizziness, shortness of breath, and tachycardia. The tissues most sensitive to hypoxia are the brain, heart, pulmonary vessels, and liver.

Purpose of Pulse Oximetry

In the medical office, pulse oximetry is often performed on patients complaining of respiratory problems (e.g., dyspnea). A decreased pulse oximetry reading (along with further testing and the patient's clinical signs and symptoms) assists the physician in proper diagnosis and treatment, which may include drug therapy and oxygen therapy.

Conditions that can cause a decreased SpO$_2$ value (hypoxemia) include the following:

- Acute pulmonary disease (e.g., pneumonia)
- Chronic pulmonary disease (e.g., emphysema, asthma, bronchitis)
- Cardiac problems (e.g., congestive heart failure, coronary artery disease)

In addition to assisting the physician in diagnosing a patient's condition, pulse oximetry is used to assess the following:

- Effectiveness of oxygen therapy
- Patient's tolerance to activity
- Effectiveness of treatment (e.g., bronchodilators)
- Patient's tolerance to analgesia and sedation

In the medical office, pulse oximetry is most often used as a "spot-check" measurement—in other words, as a single measurement of oxygen saturation. Occasionally, pulse oximetry may be used for the short-term *continuous monitoring* of a patient in the office for the following: to monitor a patient experiencing an asthmatic attack or to monitor a sedated patient during minor office surgery.

Components of the Pulse Oximeter

Most medical offices use a handheld pulse oximeter (see Figure 19-14), which is portable, lightweight, and battery operated. This is in contrast to a stand-alone oximeter, which is more apt to be used in a hospital setting for the continuous bedside monitoring of a patient's oxygen saturation level. A pulse oximeter not only measures oxygen saturation, but also measures the pulse rate in beats per minute. The two main parts of the pulse oximeter, the monitor and probe, are described in more detail next.

Monitor

The monitor contains controls, indicators, and displays (Figure 19-16). These may vary slightly depending on the brand of oximeter. Those that are found on most handheld pulse oximeters include the following:

Figure 19-16. Pulse oximeter monitor: controls, indicators, and displays. (From Bonewit-West K: *Clinical procedures for medical assistants,* ed 7, St. Louis, 2008, Saunders.)

1. **On/off control.** Turns the oximeter on and off.
2. **SpO₂% display.** A digital display of the patient's oxygen saturation expressed as a percent. This number is updated with each pulse beat.
3. **Pulse rate display.** This display indicates the patient's pulse rate in beats per minute. This number is updated with each pulse beat. Most oximeters emit a constant-pitched audible beep with each pulse beat.
4. **Pulse strength bar graph indicator.** This indicator provides a visual display of the patient's pulse strength at the probe placement site. The pulse strength indicator consists of a segmented display of bars. The pulse strength indicator "sweeps" with each pulse beat, and the stronger the pulse, the more segments that light up on the bar graph.
5. **Pulse search indicator.** This indicator lights when the oximeter is searching for the patient's pulse.
6. **Adjustable volume control.** This control is used to adjust the beep that sounds with each pulse beat. In most oximeters, the settings are high, low, and off.
7. **Low battery indicator.** This indicator is used to warn that the battery is getting low. The indicator lights up and the monitor sounds an alarm when approximately 30 minutes of battery use remain.
8. **Alarm messages.** Alarm messages indicate a problem or condition that may affect the reading. Alarm messages must not be ignored and must be corrected before continuing.

When the pulse oximeter is turned on, it automatically performs a power-on self-test (POST), which takes approximately 3 to 5 seconds. During the POST, the oximeter checks its internal systems to ensure they are functioning properly. If the oximeter detects a problem, an alarm sounds and the monitor displays an error code. If this occurs, the medical assistant should refer to the troubleshooting section of the user's manual for interpretation of the error code and the necessary action that should be taken.

When the POST is completed, the oximeter begins searching for a pulse. During this time, the pulse search indicator lights up. It takes several seconds for the oximeter to locate a pulse and to calculate and display the SpO₂ reading. If the oximeter is unable to detect a pulse, or if the pulse is too weak to provide the necessary data needed to calculate oxygen saturation, the oximeter is unable to make

Figure 19-17. Disposable *(top)* and reusable *(bottom)* probes for the pulse oximeter. (From Bonewit-West K: *Clinical procedures for medical assistants,* ed 7, St. Louis, 2008, Saunders.)

a measurement. In this case, an alarm sounds and the oximeter may automatically shut off. If this occurs, the medical assistant should reposition the probe or move the probe to another finger and perform the procedure again.

Probe

The probe of the pulse oximeter may be reusable or disposable (Figure 19-17). Most offices use reusable clip-on probes. Reusable probes are convenient to use and easy to apply, but they are more susceptible to inaccurate readings owing to patient movement. Reusable probes must be cleaned and disinfected after each use. Disposable probes are expensive to use and are generally employed for the long-term monitoring of a patient's oxygen saturation level in a hospital setting. Disposable probes are made of an adhesive, bandage-like material and are discarded after use.

It is important to handle reusable probes carefully. Hitting a probe against a hard object or dropping it may damage it. It is also important to use the probe designed for the pulse oximeter being used. Mixing probes from different manufacturers can result in an inaccurate reading.

The probe must be attached to the patient at a peripheral site that is highly vascular and where the skin is thin. The most common site to apply a probe is the tip of a finger (Figure 19-18); other acceptable sites include the toe and earlobe. A specially designed probe is available for application to the earlobe; it is smaller than a finger probe and has a curved ear attachment to hold it in place.

A cable connects the probe to the monitor. The probe may be permanently attached to the cable, or it may be a separate device that requires connection to the cable. The pulse oximeter monitor should never be lifted or carried by the cable because this could damage the cable connections

Figure 19-18. Applying a probe at the tip of a finger. (From Bonewit-West K: *Clinical procedures for medical assistants*, ed 7, St. Louis, 2008, Saunders.)

or cause the cable to disconnect from the monitor and possibly drop on the floor or fall on the patient.

Factors Affecting Pulse Oximetry

Although pulse oximetry is an easy procedure to perform, the medical assistant must be aware of certain factors that may interfere with an accurate reading. These factors are listed along with guidelines for correcting or preventing them.

1. **Incorrect positioning of the probe.** As previously discussed, the oximeter probe consists of two parts: an LED and a photodetector. Because light is transmitted from the LED through the tissues to the photodetector, it is important that these two components be aligned directly opposite to each other during the measurement. In most cases, this automatically occurs when the clip-on probe is applied. Proper alignment of the probe may be impossible, however, with patients who have small fingers (e.g., a thin patient or a child) or patients who have large fingers (e.g., an obese patient). To obtain an accurate reading, another site must be used, such as the earlobe. In addition, pediatric probes are available for use with thin patients or children.

2. **Fingernail polish or artificial nails.** A dark, opaque coating on the fingernail may result in a falsely low reading. This is because the coating interferes with proper light transmission through the finger. The darker the coating, the more likely that the SpO_2 reading will be affected. Blue, black, and green nail polishes tend to cause the most problems. If the patient is wearing fingernail polish, it should be removed with acetone or fingernail polish remover. If the patient has artificial fingernails, another site should be used to take the measurement, such as the earlobe or toe. Oil, dirt, and grime on the fingertip can also interfere with proper light transmission. If the patient's fingertip is dirty, cleanse the site

with soap and water and allow it to dry. Areas with bruises, burns, stains, or tattoos should be avoided as a probe placement site. Darkly pigmented skin and jaundice do not usually affect the ability of the oximeter to obtain an accurate reading.

3. **Poor peripheral blood flow.** A pulse oximeter works best when there is a good strong pulse in the finger to which the probe is applied. Poor peripheral blood flow may cause the pulse to be so weak that the oximeter cannot obtain a reading. Conditions resulting in poor blood flow include peripheral vascular disease, vasoconstrictor medications, severe hypotension, and hypothermia. In these situations, the medical assistant should try using the earlobe because it is less affected by decreased blood flow. Sometimes patients with cold fingers (but who are not hypothermic) may have enough constriction of the peripheral capillaries that it interferes with obtaining a reading. To solve this problem, the medical assistant should ask the patient to warm his or her fingers by rubbing the hands together. The probe should never be attached to the finger of an arm to which an automatic blood pressure cuff is applied because blood flow to the finger would be cut off when the cuff inflates, resulting in loss of the pulse signal.

4. **Ambient (surrounding) light.** Ambient light shining directly on the probe, such as bright fluorescent light, direct sunlight, or an overhead examination light, may result in an inaccurate reading. This is because some of the ambient light may be picked up by the probe's photodetector and alter the reading. This problem can be corrected by one of the following: turning off the light, moving the patient's hand away from the light source, or covering the probe with an opaque material such as a washcloth.

5. **Patient movement.** Patient movement is a common cause of an inaccurate reading. Motion affects the ability of the light to travel from the LED to the photodetector and prevents the probe from picking up the pulse signal. To avoid this problem, it is important that the medical assistant instruct the patient to remain still and not move during the procedure. Occasionally, patient movement cannot be eliminated, such as when the patient has tremors of the hands. In these instances, the oxygen saturation level should be measured at a site that is less affected by motion, such as the toe or earlobe.

Pulse Oximeter Care and Maintenance

The pulse oximeter monitor and cable should be cleaned periodically using a damp cloth slightly dampened with a solution of warm water and a disinfectant cleaner. The medical assistant should make sure that the cloth is not too wet to prevent the solution from running into the monitor, which could damage the internal components. The probe should be cleaned periodically with a soft cloth moistened with warm water and a disinfectant cleaner. Cleaning the probe removes dirt and grime that could interfere with proper light transmission, leading to an inaccurate reading. The probe also should be disinfected after each use by wiping it thoroughly with an antiseptic wipe and allowing it to dry. The probe should never be soaked or immersed in a liquid solution because this would damage it. The probe is heat-sensitive and cannot be autoclaved. The pulse oximeter should be stored at room temperature in a dry environment.

Text continued on p. 361

PROCEDURE 19-6   Measuring Pulse and Respiration

Outcome Measure pulse and respiration.

Equipment/Supplies

- Watch with a second hand

---

1. **Procedural Step.** Sanitize your hands. Greet the patient and introduce yourself. Identify the patient and explain the procedure. Observe the patient for any signs that might affect the pulse or respiratory rate.
   Principle. Pulse rate can vary according to the factors listed on p. 387.

2. **Procedural Step.** Have the patient sit down. Position the patient's arm in a comfortable position. The forearm should be slightly flexed to relax the muscles and tendons over the pulse site.
   Principle. Relaxed muscles and tendons over the pulse site make it easier to palpate the pulse.

3. **Procedural Step.** Place your three middle fingertips over the radial pulse site. Never use your thumb to take a pulse. The radial pulse is located in a groove on the inner aspect of the wrist just below the thumb.
   Principle. The thumb has a pulse of its own; using the thumb results in a measurement of the medical assistant's pulse and not the patient's pulse.

4. **Procedural Step.** Apply moderate, gentle pressure directly over the site until you feel the pulse. If you cannot feel the pulse, it may be caused by:
   a. Incorrect location of the radial pulse: Move your fingers to a slightly different location in the groove of the wrist until you feel the pulse.
   b. Applying too much pressure or not enough pressure: Vary the depth of your hold until you can feel the pulse.
   Principle. A normal pulse can be felt with moderate pressure. The pulse cannot be felt if not enough pressure is applied, whereas too much pressure applied to the radial artery closes it off, and no pulse is felt.

5. **Procedural Step.** Count the pulse for 30 seconds and make a mental note of this number. Note the rhythm and volume of the pulse. If abnormalities occur in the rhythm or volume, count the pulse for 1 full minute.
   Principle. A longer time ensures an accurate assessment of abnormalities.

Place the three middle fingers over the radial pulse site. (From Bonewit-West K: *Clinical procedures for medical assistants,* ed 7, St. Louis, 2008, Saunders.)

Count the pulse for 30 seconds. (From Bonewit-West K: *Clinical procedures for medical assistants,* ed 7, St. Louis, 2008, Saunders.)

6. **Procedural Step.** After taking the pulse, continue to hold three fingers on the patient's wrist with the same amount of pressure, and measure the respirations. This helps to ensure that the patient is unaware that respirations are being monitored.

Principle. If the patient is aware that respiration is being measured, the breathing may change.

Count the number of respirations for 30 seconds. (From Bonewit-West K: *Clinical procedures for medical assistants,* ed 7, St. Louis, 2008, Saunders.)

7. Procedural Step. Observe the rise and fall of the patient's chest as the patient inhales and exhales.

Principle. One complete respiration includes one inhalation and one exhalation.

8. Procedural Step. Count the number of respirations for 30 seconds, and make a mental note of this number; note the rhythm and depth of the respirations. Also observe the patient's color. If abnormalities occur in the rhythm or depth, count the respiratory rate for 1 full minute.

9. Procedural Step. Sanitize your hands, and chart the results. If you counted the pulse and respirations for 30 seconds, multiply each of the numbers counted by 2. This will give you the pulse rate and respiratory rate for 1 full minute. Include the date; time; pulse rate, rhythm, and volume; and respiratory rate, rhythm, and depth.

CHARTING EXAMPLE

Date	
10/15/10	2:30 p.m. P: 74. Reg and strong. R: 18. Even and reg. ————— S. Martinez, RMA

PROCEDURE 19-7

PROCEDURE 19-7　Measuring Apical Pulse

Outcome Measure apical pulse.

Equipment/Supplies

- Watch with a second hand
- Stethoscope
- Antiseptic wipe

1. Procedural Step. Sanitize your hands. Greet the patient and introduce yourself. Identify the patient and explain the procedure. Observe the patient for any signs that might increase or decrease the pulse rate.

2. Procedural Step. Assemble the equipment. If the stethoscope's chest piece consists of a diaphragm and a bell, rotate the chest piece to the bell position. Clean the earpieces and chest piece of the stethoscope with an antiseptic wipe.

Principle. The bell position allows better auscultation of heart sounds. Cleaning the earpieces helps prevent the transmission of microorganisms.

3. Procedural Step. Ask the patient to unbutton or remove his or her shirt. Have the patient sit or lie down (supine).

Principle. A sitting or supine position allows access to the apex of the heart.

4. Procedural Step. Warm the chest piece of the stethoscope with your hands. Insert the earpieces of the stethoscope into your ears, with the earpieces directed slightly forward, and place the chest piece over the apex of the patient's heart. The apex of the heart is located in the fifth intercostal space at the junction of the left midclavicular line.

Principle. Warming the chest piece reduces the discomfort of having a cold object placed on the chest. In addition, a cold chest piece could startle the patient, resulting in an increase in the pulse rate. The earpieces should be directed forward to follow the direction of the ear canal, which facilitates hearing.

Continued

Insert the earpieces into your ears with the earpieces directed slightly forward. (From Bonewit-West K: *Clinical procedures for medical assistants,* ed 7, St. Louis, 2008, Saunders.)

Count the number of beats for 30 seconds, and multiply by 2. (From Bonewit-West K: *Clinical procedures for medical assistants,* ed 7, St. Louis, 2008, Saunders.)

5. **Procedural Step.** Listen for the heartbeat, and count the number of beats for 30 seconds (and multiply by 2) if the rhythm and volume are normal or if the apical pulse is being taken on an infant or child. If abnormalities occur in the rhythm or volume, count the pulse for 1 full minute. You will hear a "lubb-dupp" sound through the stethoscope. This sound is the closing of the heart's valves. Each "lubb-dupp" is counted as one beat.

6. **Procedural Step.** Sanitize your hands, and chart the results. Include the date, time, and the apical pulse rate, rhythm, and volume.

7. **Procedural Step.** Clean the earpieces and the chest piece of the stethoscope with an antiseptic wipe.

CHARTING EXAMPLE

Date	
10/15/10	10:15 a.m. AP: 68. Reg and strong.————
	———————— S. Martinez, CMA (AAMA)

PROCEDURE **19-8**   **Performing Pulse Oximetry**

Outcome Perform pulse oximetry.

Equipment/Supplies

- Handheld pulse oximeter
- Reusable finger probe
- Antiseptic wipe

1. **Procedural Step.** Sanitize your hands.
2. **Procedural Step.** Assemble the equipment. Handle the probe carefully, and perform the following:
   a. Carefully inspect the probe to ensure it opens and closes smoothly. Inspect the probe windows (LED and photodetector) to ensure they are clean and free of lint.
   b. Disinfect the probe windows and surrounding platforms with an antiseptic wipe, and allow them to dry.

Disinfect the probe with an antiseptic wipe. (From Bonewit-West K: *Clinical procedures for medical assistants,* ed 7, St. Louis, 2008, Saunders.)

   c. If necessary, connect the probe to the cable.
   d. Connect the cable to the monitor by plugging it into the port on the monitor. Do not lift or carry the monitor by the cable.

Connect the cable to the monitor by plugging it into the port on the monitor. (From Bonewit-West K: *Clinical procedures for medical assistants,* ed 7, St. Louis, 2008, Saunders.)

Principle. Misuse or improper handling of the probe could damage it. Dirt or lint on the probe windows could interfere with proper light transmission, leading to an inaccurate reading. Cross-contamination among patients is prevented by disinfecting the probe. Lifting the monitor by the cable could damage the cable connections.

3. **Procedural Step.** Greet the patient and introduce yourself. Identify the patient and explain the procedure. Explain to the patient that the clip-on probe does not hurt and feels similar to a clothespin attached to the finger. If the patient seems fearful, place the probe on your own finger first to reassure the patient it is not painful.
4. **Procedural Step.** Seat the patient comfortably in a chair with the lower arm firmly supported and the palm facing down.
   Principle. Supporting the lower arm helps prevent patient movement during the procedure.
5. **Procedural Step.** Select an appropriate finger to apply the probe. Use the tip of the patient's index, middle, or ring finger. If the patient's fingers are very small or very large, and the probe cannot seem to be aligned properly, use the earlobe to take the measurement. If the patient exhibits tremors of the hands, use the earlobe to obtain the reading.
   Principle. The probe must be applied to a peripheral site with thin skin that is highly vascular. Very small or very large fingers may not allow for proper positioning of the probe on the finger.
6. **Procedural Step.** Observe the patient's fingernail. If the patient is wearing dark fingernail polish, ask her to remove it with acetone or nail polish remover. If the patient is wearing artificial nails, choose another probe site, such as the toe or earlobe.
   Principle. An opaque coating on the fingernail may interfere with proper light transmission through the finger, leading to an inaccurate reading.
7. **Procedural Step.** Check to ensure the patient's fingertip is clean. If it is dirty, cleanse the site with soap and water and allow it to dry. Ensure that the patient's finger is not cold. If it is cold, ask the patient to rub his or her hands together.
   Principle. Oils, dirt, or grime on the finger can interfere with the proper light transmission through the finger, leading to an inaccurate reading. Sometimes patients with cold fingers may have enough constriction of the capillaries that it interferes with obtaining a reading.
8. **Procedural Step.** Ensure that ambient light does not interfere with the measurement. Position the probe securely on the fingertip as follows:
   a. Ensure that the probe window is fully covered by placing the finger over the LED window with the fleshy tip of the finger covering the window. The tip of the finger should touch the end of the probe stop.

Continued

PROCEDURE 19-8   Performing Pulse Oximetry—cont'd

Position the probe securely on the fingertip. (From Bonewit-West K: *Clinical procedures for medical assistants,* ed 7, St. Louis, 2008, Saunders.)

Allow several seconds for the pulse oximeter to detect the pulse. (From Bonewit-West K: *Clinical procedures for medical assistants,* ed 7, St. Louis, 2008, Saunders.)

  b. Ensure that the LED and the photodetector are aligned opposite to each other.

  c. Allow the cable to lie across the back of the hand and parallel to the arm of the patient.

  Principle. Ambient light can be picked up by the probe and alter the reading. Proper alignment of the LED and photodetector is necessary for an accurate reading.

9. **Procedural Step.** Instruct the patient to remain still and to breathe normally. Turn on the oximeter by pressing the on/off control. Wait while the oximeter goes through its power-on self-test (POST). If the monitor fails the POST, refer to the troubleshooting section of the user manual for interpretation of the error code and necessary action that should be taken.

  Principle. Patient movement may lead to an inaccurate reading. The monitor automatically conducts a POST to ensure it is functioning properly.

10. **Procedural Step.** Allow several seconds for the pulse oximeter to detect the pulse and calculate the oxygen saturation of the blood. Ensure that the pulse strength indicator fluctuates with each pulsation and that the pulse signal is strong. If the oximeter sounds an alarm indicating it was unable to locate a pulse, reposition the probe on the patient's finger or move the probe to another finger and perform the procedure again.

  Principle. The reading takes several seconds to display. The pulse strength indicator provides a quick assessment of pulse quality. If the oximeter is unable to locate a pulse, it will be unable to obtain a reading.

11. **Procedural Step.** Leave the probe in place until the oximeter displays a reading. Read the oxygen saturation value and pulse rate, and make a mental note of these readings. On this pulse oximeter, the oxygen saturation reading is 99% and the pulse rate is 69. If the SpO_2 reading is less than 95%, reposition the probe on the finger and perform the procedure again.

Read the oxygen saturation value and pulse rate. (From Bonewit-West K: *Clinical procedures for medical assistants,* ed 7, St. Louis, 2008, Saunders.)

  Principle. A low SpO_2 reading may be caused by improper positioning of the probe on the finger.

12. **Procedural Step.** Remove the probe from the patient's finger, and turn off the oximeter.

13. **Procedural Step.** Sanitize your hands, and chart the results. Include the date, time, SpO_2 reading, and pulse rate.

14. **Procedural Step.** Disconnect the cable from the monitor. Disinfect the probe with an antiseptic wipe. Properly store the monitor in a clean, dry area.

CHARTING EXAMPLE	
Date	
10/15/10	2:30 p.m. SpO_2: 99%. P: 69. ————
	———————— S. Martinez, RMA

BLOOD PRESSURE

Mechanism of Blood Pressure

Blood pressure (BP) is a measurement of the pressure or force exerted by the blood on the walls of the arteries in which it is contained. Each time the ventricles contract, blood is pushed out of the heart and into the aorta and pulmonary aorta, exerting pressure on the walls of the arteries. This phase in the cardiac cycle is known as **systole,** and it represents the highest point of blood pressure in the body, or the **systolic pressure.** The phase of the cardiac cycle in which the heart relaxes between contractions is referred to as **diastole.** The **diastolic pressure** (recorded during diastole) is lower because the heart is relaxed. Contraction and relaxation of the heart result in two different pressures, systolic and diastolic.

Interpretation of Blood Pressure

Blood pressure measurement is expressed as a fraction. The numerator is the systolic pressure, and the denominator is the diastolic pressure. The standard unit for measuring blood pressure is millimeters of mercury (mm Hg). A blood pressure reading of 110/70 mm Hg means that there was enough force to raise a column of mercury 110 mm during systole and 70 mm during diastole.

Based on guidelines from the National Heart, Lung, and Blood Institute (NHLBI), a blood pressure less than 120/80 mm Hg is classified as normal, whereas a blood pressure reading of 120/80 is classified as *prehypertension.* These guidelines were issued as a result of scientific studies showing that the risk of heart disease begins at a blood pressure reading lower than previously thought. The NHLBI guidelines are outlined in Table 19-7.

Blood pressure should be taken during every office visit to allow the physician to compare the patient's readings over time. This is a good preventive measure in guarding against serious illness. A single blood pressure reading taken on one occasion does not characterize an individual's blood pressure accurately. Several readings, taken on different occasions, provide a good index of an individual's baseline blood pressure.

Blood pressure readings should always be interpreted using a patient's baseline blood pressure. An increase or decrease of 20 to 30 mm Hg in a patient's baseline blood pressure is significant, even if it is still within the normal accepted blood pressure range.

The most common condition that causes an abnormal blood pressure reading is **hypertension.** Hypertension, or high blood pressure, results from excessive pressure on the walls of the arteries. Hypertension is determined by a sustained systolic blood pressure reading of 140 mm Hg or greater or a sustained diastolic reading of 90 mm Hg or greater. See Table 19-7 for the NHLBI classifications for hypertension. **Hypotension,** or low blood pressure, results from reduced pressure on the arterial walls. Hypotension is determined by a blood pressure reading less than 95/60 mm Hg.

Table 19-7 Classification of Blood Pressure for Adults Age 18 and Older

Blood Pressure Classifications	Systolic Blood Pressure (mm Hg)		Diastolic Blood Pressure (mm Hg)
Normal	Less than 120	*and*	Less than 80
Prehypertension*	120-139	*or*	80-89
Hypertension*			
Stage 1	140-159	*or*	90-99
Stage 2	160 or higher	*or*	100 or higher

From National Heart, Lung, and Blood Institute: *The seventh report of the Joint National Committee on Detection, Evaluation, and Treatment of High Blood Pressure, NIH Publication No. 03-5231,* Bethesda, Md, 2003, U.S. Department of Health and Human Services.
*Based on the average of two or more properly measured, seated blood pressure readings taken at each of two or more visits.

Pulse Pressure

The difference between systolic and diastolic pressure is the **pulse pressure.** It is determined by subtracting the smaller number from the larger. If the blood pressure is 110/70 mm Hg, the pulse pressure would be 40 mm Hg. A pulse pressure between 30 and 50 mm Hg is considered to be within normal range.

Factors Affecting Blood Pressure

Blood pressure does not remain at a constant value. Numerous factors may affect it throughout the course of the day. An understanding of these factors helps to ensure an accurate interpretation of blood pressure readings.

1. **Age.** Age is an important consideration when determining whether a patient's blood pressure is normal. As age increases, the blood pressure gradually increases: A 6-year-old child may have a normal reading of 90/60 mm Hg, whereas a young, healthy adult may have a blood pressure reading of 116/76 mm Hg, and it would not be unusual for a 60-year-old man to have a reading of 130/90 mm Hg. As an individual gets older, there is a loss of elasticity in the walls of the blood vessels, causing this increase in pressure to occur. Table 19-8 is a chart of the average optimal blood pressure readings for various age groups.

2. **Gender.** After puberty, women usually have a lower blood pressure than men of the same age. After menopause, women usually have a higher blood pressure than men of the same age.

3. **Diurnal variations.** Fluctuations in an individual's blood pressure are normal during the course of a day. When one awakens, the blood pressure is lower as a result of the decreased metabolism and physical activity during sleep. As metabolism and activity increase during the day, the blood pressure rises.

4. **Emotional states.** Strong emotional states, such as anger, fear, and excitement, increase the blood pressure. If the medical assistant observes such a reaction, an attempt

Table 19-8 Average Optimal Blood Pressure for Age

Age	Blood Pressure (mm Hg)
Newborn (6.6 lb)	40 (mean)
1 mo	85/54
1 yr	95/65
6 yr*	105/65
10-13 yr*	110/65
14-17 yr*	120/75
Adult	Less than 120/80

From National High Blood Pressure Education Program (NHBPEP); National Heart, Lung, and Blood Institute; National Institutes of Health: The seventh report of the Joint National Committees on Detection, Evaluation, and Treatment of High Blood Pressure, *JAMA* 239:2560, 2003.
*In children and adolescents, hypertension is defined as blood pressure that is, on repeated measurement, at the 95th percentile or greater adjusted for age, height, and gender (NHBPEP, 1997).

What Would You Do? What Would You *Not* Do?

Case Study 3

Tyrone Jackson, 45 years old, is at the office to have his blood pressure checked. Three months ago, Tyrone started taking a diuretic and an antihypertensive prescribed by the physician to reduce his blood pressure. The last recording in his chart indicates that Tyrone's blood pressure decreased from 180/112 mm Hg to 126/84 mm Hg; however, his blood pressure at this visit is 158/98 mm Hg. Tyrone says that he has not been very good at taking his medication lately. He says it is really hard to remember to take all those pills every day. He also says that he felt just fine before being put on blood pressure pills, but when he started taking them, he felt awful. He had to urinate more often; when he got up fast, he felt dizzy; and he had some problems with headaches. Tyrone says that he decided to cut back on his pills to see if these problems got better, and sure enough, they went away altogether. Tyrone wants to know if there is anything he can do to lower his blood pressure other than taking pills. ■

should be made to calm the patient before taking blood pressure.

5. **Exercise.** Physical activity temporarily increases the blood pressure. To ensure an accurate reading, a patient who has been involved in physical activity should be given an opportunity to rest for 20 to 30 minutes before blood pressure is measured.

6. **Body position.** The blood pressure of a patient who is in a lying or standing position is usually different from that measured when the patient is sitting. A notation should be made on the patient's chart if the reading was obtained in any position other than sitting, using the following abbreviations: *L* (lying) and *St* (standing).

7. **Medications.** Many medications may increase or decrease the blood pressure. Because of this factor, it is important to record in the patient chart all prescription and over-the-counter medications that the patient is taking.

8. **Other factors.** Other factors that may increase the blood pressure include pain, a recent meal, smoking, and bladder distention.

Assessment of Blood Pressure

The equipment needed to measure blood pressure includes a stethoscope and a sphygmomanometer. The **stethoscope** amplifies sounds produced by the body and allows the medical assistant to hear them.

Stethoscope

The most common type of stethoscope used in the medical office is the acoustic stethoscope. It consists of four parts: earpieces, sidepieces known as *binaurals,* plastic or rubber tubing, and a chest piece (Figure 19-19A).

Stethoscope Chest Piece

Two types of chest pieces exist: a *diaphragm,* which is a large, flat disc, and a bell, which has a bowl-shaped appear-

Figure 19-19. A, Parts of a stethoscope. **B,** Types of chest pieces. (From Bonewit-West K: *Clinical procedures for medical assistants,* ed 7, St. Louis, 2008, Saunders.)

ance (Figure 19-19B). The chest piece of a stethoscope consists of a diaphragm and a bell, or just a diaphragm. If a chest piece consists of a diaphragm and a bell, the medical assistant must ensure the desired piece is rotated into position before use. Failure to do so would not allow the medical assistant to hear sound through the earpieces.

PATIENT TEACHING   Hypertension

Answer questions patients have about hypertension.

What is high blood pressure?

Blood pressure is the force of blood against the walls of the arteries. High blood pressure, also called **hypertension,** means the pressure in the arteries is consistently above normal (140/90 mm Hg), resulting in excessive pressure on the walls of the arteries. Hypertension is the most common life-threatening disease among Americans. An estimated one in four Americans has high blood pressure. The incidence of hypertension in the United States has increased dramatically as a result of an aging population and increased incidence of obesity.

What are the symptoms of high blood pressure?

Approximately one third of people who have high blood pressure are unaware of it because there are few or no symptoms and, as a result, an individual with hypertension may go undiagnosed for many years. If symptoms do occur, they may include one or more of the following: headaches, dizziness, flushed face, fatigue, epistaxis (nosebleed), excessive perspiration, heart palpitations, frequent urination, and leg claudication (cramping in the legs with walking). The only way to know for sure whether you have high blood pressure is to have it checked regularly.

What causes high blood pressure?

In about 90% of cases, the precise cause of high blood pressure is unknown. This type of hypertension is known as *essential or primary hypertension.* Certain factors seem to increase the risk of developing essential hypertension, however, including:

- **Heredity.** A family history of high blood pressure increases an individual's risk of developing high blood pressure.
- **Weight.** Individuals who are overweight or obese are two to six times more likely than the general population to develop high blood pressure.
- **Ethnicity.** Research has shown that more black than white Americans develop high blood pressure.
- **Age.** Blood pressure normally increases as one grows older.
- **Sodium intake.** Sodium, found in salt and processed, canned, and most snack foods, does not cause high blood pressure; however, it can aggravate high blood pressure. Most Americans consume more sodium than they need. The current recommendation is to consume less than 2.4 g (2400 mg) of sodium per day. This is equivalent to 6 g (about 1 teaspoon) of salt.
- **Chronic stress.** Research indicates that people who are under continuous stress tend to develop more heart and circulatory problems than people who are not under stress.

- **Smoking.** Smoking tobacco constricts blood vessels, causing an increase in blood pressure.
- **Alcohol consumption.** Heavy alcohol consumption may increase the blood pressure.

The remaining 10% of individuals with hypertension have *secondary hypertension.* This means that the high blood pressure can be linked to a known cause, which includes chronic kidney disease, adrenal and thyroid disease, narrowing of the aorta, steroid therapy, oral contraceptives, and preeclampsia associated with pregnancy.

What can happen if high blood pressure is not treated?

If high blood pressure is not brought under control, it can cause severe damage to vital organs, such as the heart, brain, kidneys, and eyes. This damage can result in a heart attack or heart failure, stroke, kidney damage, or damaged vision. Early detection and treatment of high blood pressure can prevent these complications. High blood pressure is often discovered during a routine medical examination or (less commonly) when an individual experiences one of the complications of hypertension caused by damage to a vital organ.

Can high blood pressure be cured?

Essential hypertension cannot be cured, but many treatments are used to bring it under control. These include lifestyle modifications, such as weight reduction, a healthy diet rich in fruits and vegetables and low in saturated fat, limitation of salt intake, regular aerobic exercise, cessation of smoking, limitation or elimination of alcohol consumption, and stress management. If lifestyle modifications alone are not enough, medications are available for reducing blood pressure, allowing the patient to lead a normal, healthy, active life.

How long will I undergo treatment?

Treatment for essential hypertension is usually lifelong. Even if you feel fine, you will probably have to continue treatment for the rest of your life to maintain your blood pressure in a healthy range. If you discontinue your diet and lifestyle changes or stop taking your medication, your blood pressure will increase again.

- Encourage patients with hypertension to adhere to the treatment prescribed by the physician. Help patients remember to take their medication by telling them to associate their medication schedule with a daily routine, such as brushing their teeth or having meals.
- Provide the patient with educational materials on high blood pressure available from sources such as the American Heart Association. ■

The diaphragm chest piece is more useful for hearing high-pitched sounds, such as lung and bowel sounds, whereas the bell chest piece is more useful for hearing low-pitched sounds, such as those produced by the heart and vascular system. Before using a stethoscope, the medical assistant should ensure that it is in proper working condition.

Sphygmomanometers

The **sphygmomanometer** is an instrument that measures the pressure of blood within an artery. It consists of a **manometer,** an inner inflatable bladder surrounded by a covering known as the *cuff,* and a pressure bulb with a control valve to inflate and deflate the inner bladder. The

Highlight on Stethoscopes

The stethoscope was first introduced in the 1800s by a French physician named René Laënnec. This early stethoscope consisted of a simple wooden tube with a bell-shaped opening at one end.

The selection of a stethoscope is an individual decision. One hears sounds differently when using different stethoscopes. The primary consideration in choosing a stethoscope should be that it is well made and fits well in your ears. Stethoscopes are available from uniform shops and medical supply companies.

The usual length of tubing on a stethoscope is 12 to 16 inches (30 to 40 cm), but you may prefer the longer 22-inch tubing. An argument against long tubing is that it transmits sound less efficiently. Research has shown, however, that 6 to 8 more inches of tubing does not significantly alter the transmission of most sounds.

The stethoscope should have metal binaurals. The binaurals should allow you to angle the earpieces firmly to follow the direction of your ear canal. Binaurals that are too tight are uncomfortable, and binaurals that are too loose do not allow you to hear as well as you should.

The earpieces should fit comfortably and snugly in the ear canal. If you can understand what someone is saying in the same room, they are too loose, which would interfere with effective auscultation. Some stethoscopes come with removable ear tips in different sizes. This offers the advantage of selecting an ear tip that fits your ear canal. Flexible ear tips of soft rubber are usually more comfortable than nonflexible tips of hard rubber or plastic.

The chest piece should be a key factor in the selection of a stethoscope. A stethoscope with a diaphragm and a bell offers the most versatility for listening to different types of sounds. Many stethoscopes have a rubber or plastic rim around the diaphragm and bell to avoid chilling the patient with a cold chest piece and to decrease air leaks between the chest piece and the patient.

The most common problem with use of stethoscopes is air leaking. Air leaks interfere with effective sound transmission and allow environmental noise to enter the stethoscope. Air leaks may result from a cracked earpiece, a cracked or chipped chest piece, or a break in the tubing.

Stethoscopes must be cared for properly to ensure proper functioning and to prevent the transmission of disease in the medical office. The earpieces should be removed and cleaned regularly with a cotton-tipped applicator moistened with alcohol to remove cerumen. The chest piece should be cleaned with an antiseptic wipe to remove dirt, dust, lint, and oils. The tubing should be cleaned with a paper towel using an antimicrobial soap and water. Alcohol should not be used to clean the tubing because it can dry out the tubing and cause it to crack over time. ∎

Figure 19-20. The parts of an aneroid sphygmomanometer. (From Bonewit-West K: *Clinical procedures for medical assistants,* ed 7, St. Louis, 2008, Saunders.)

Figure 19-21. The scale of the gauge of an aneroid sphygmomanometer. (From Bonewit-West K: *Clinical procedures for medical assistants,* ed 7, St. Louis, 2008, Saunders.)

manometer contains a scale for registering the pressure of the air in the bladder.

The two types of sphygmomanometers are the aneroid and mercury. The *aneroid sphygmomanometer* is lightweight and portable, but the *mercury sphygmomanometer* is more accurate.

Aneroid Sphygmomanometer

The aneroid sphygmomanometer (Figure 19-20) has a manometer gauge with a round scale. The scale is calibrated in millimeters, with a needle that points to the calibrations (Figure 19-21). To ensure an accurate reading, the needle

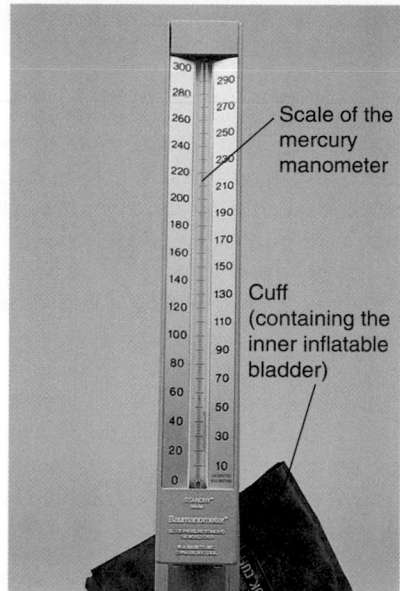

Figure 19-22. The parts of a mercury sphygmomanometer. (From Bonewit-West K: *Clinical procedures for medical assistants,* ed 7, St. Louis, 2008, Saunders.)

Figure 19-23. Blood pressure cuffs: child, adult, and thigh. (From Bonewit-West K: *Clinical procedures for medical assistants,* ed 7, St. Louis, 2008, Saunders.)

Table 19-9 Types of Blood Pressure Cuffs			
Cuff	Bladder Length (cm)	Bladder Width (cm)	Acceptable Circumference (cm)
Child arm	21	8	16-21
Small adult arm	24	10	22-26
Adult arm	30	13	27-34
Large adult arm	38	16	35-44
Adult thigh	42	20	45-52

From Bonewit-West K: *Clinical procedures for medical assistants,* ed 7, St. Louis, 2008, Saunders.

must be positioned initially at zero. The manometer must be placed in the correct position for proper viewing. The medical assistant should be no farther than 3 feet from the scale on the gauge of the manometer, and the manometer should be placed so that it can be viewed directly. At least once a year, an aneroid sphygmomanometer should be recalibrated to ensure its accuracy.

Mercury Sphygmomanometer

The mercury sphygmomanometer (Figure 19-22) has a vertical tube calibrated in millimeters that is filled with mercury. Although more accurate than the aneroid sphygmomanometer, the use of the mercury sphygmomanometer is being discouraged because mercury is a hazardous chemical.

If a mercury manometer is used to measure blood pressure, it must be placed in the correct position for proper viewing. The medical assistant should be no farther than 3 feet from the scale of the manometer. A portable mercury manometer should be placed on a flat surface so that the mercury column is in a vertical position. The wall model mercury manometer is mounted securely against a wall, placing the mercury column in a vertical position.

The following guidelines must be followed when measuring blood pressure with a mercury sphygmomanometer. Before the blood pressure reading is obtained, the mercury must be even with the zero level at the base of the calibrated tube. Pressure created by inflation of the inner bladder causes the mercury to rise in the tube. The top portion of the mercury column, the **meniscus,** curves slightly upward. The blood pressure should be read at the top of the meniscus, with the eye at the same level as the meniscus of the mercury column.

Cuff Sizes

Blood pressure cuffs come in a variety of sizes and are measured in centimeters (cm) (Figure 19-23). The size of a cuff refers to its inner inflatable bladder, rather than its cloth cover. Table 19-9 lists the types of cuffs available and the size of the inner bladder of each cuff.

For accurate blood pressure measurement, the inner bladder of the cuff should encircle at least 80% of the arm circumference and be wide enough to cover two thirds of the distance from the axilla to the antecubital space (Figure 19-24). Child cuffs often must be used for adults with thin arms. The adult cuff is used for the average-sized adult arm, and the thigh cuff is used for taking blood pressure from the thigh or for adults with large arms. If the cuff is too small, the reading may be falsely high, as it would be, for example, when an adult cuff is used on a patient with a large arm. If the cuff is too large, the reading may be falsely low, as it would be when an adult cuff is used with a patient with a thin arm. The cuff should fit snugly and should be applied so that the center of the inflatable bag is directly over the brachial artery to allow for complete compression of the artery. The cuff has an interlocking, self-sticking

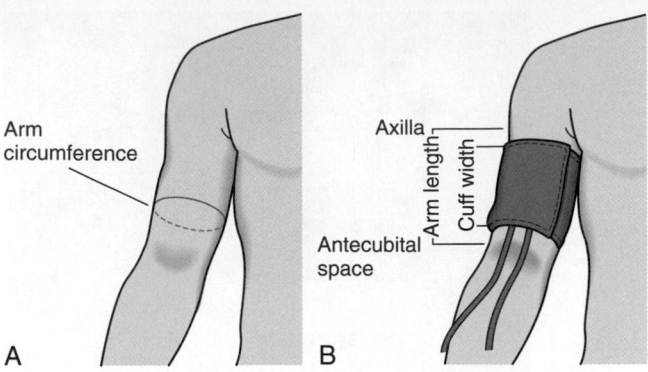

Figure 19-24. Determination of proper cuff size. **A,** The bladder of the cuff should be long enough to encircle 80% of the arm. **B,** The cuff should be wide enough to cover two thirds of the distance from the axilla to the antecubital space. (From Bonewit-West K: *Clinical procedures for medical assistants,* ed 7, St. Louis, 2008, Saunders.)

substance (Velcro) that facilitates closing and fastening the cuff in place temporarily.

Korotkoff Sounds

Korotkoff sounds are used to determine the systolic and diastolic blood pressure readings. When the bladder of the cuff is inflated, the brachial artery is compressed so that no audible sounds are heard through the stethoscope. As the cuff is deflated, at a rate of 2 to 3 mm Hg per second, the sounds become audible until the blood flows freely and they can no longer be heard (Table 19-10). The medical assistant should practice listening to these sounds and be able to identify the various phases.

Procedure 19-9 outlines the procedure for taking blood pressure using an aneroid sphygmomanometer. Procedure 19-10 outlines the procedure for determining systolic pressure by palpation.

Table 19-10 Korotkoff Sounds

Phase	Description	Illustration
	Inflation of cuff compresses and closes off brachial artery so that no blood flows through artery	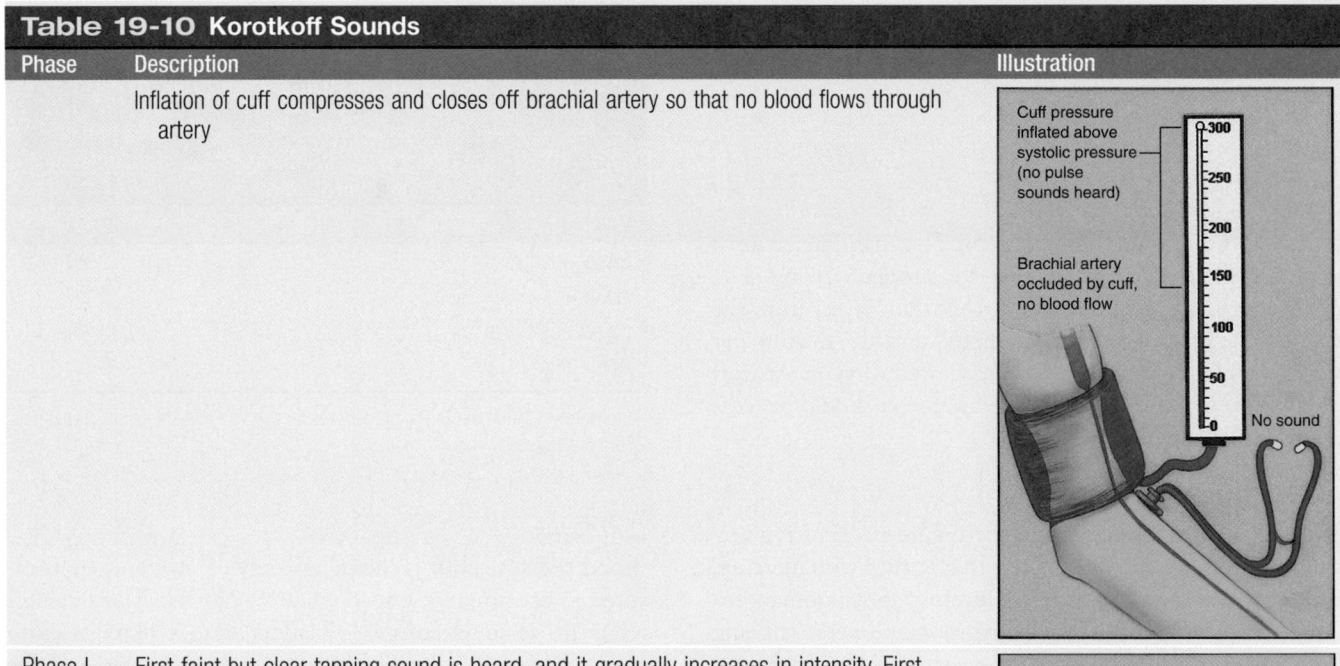
Phase I	First faint but clear tapping sound is heard, and it gradually increases in intensity. First tapping sound is systolic pressure	

Table 19-10 Korotkoff Sounds—cont'd

Phase	Description	Illustration
Phase II	As cuff continues to deflate, sounds have murmuring or swishing quality	
Phase III	With further deflation, sounds become crisper and increase in intensity	
Phase IV	Sounds become muffled and have soft, blowing quality. According to the American Heart Association, onset of muffled sounds is best index of diastolic pressure in children. Pressure in cuff is released at moderate steady rate of 2-3 mm Hg per second	
Phase V	Sounds disappear. This is typically recorded as diastolic pressure for an adult. Some authorities believe that adult diastolic pressure falls midway between phases IV and V; some physicians want the medical assistant to record phases IV and V as the diastolic pressure (e.g., 120/84/80)	

From Bonewit-West K: *Clinical procedures for medical assistants,* ed 7, St. Louis, 2008, Saunders.

Prevention of Errors in Blood Pressure Measurement

The following guidelines should be followed to prevent errors in blood pressure measurement:

1. **Instruct the patient** not to consume caffeine or use tobacco for 30 minutes before blood pressure measurement.

2. **The patient should be seated** in a quiet room for at least 5 minutes before blood pressure is taken. Patient anxiety and apprehension can cause a spasm of the brachial artery, which can increase the blood pressure reading by as much as 30 to 50 mm/Hg. This is known as the "white coat effect," which refers to the white laboratory coat worn by the physician.

3. **Always use the proper cuff size.** If the cuff is too small, it may come loose as the cuff is inflated, or the reading may be falsely high. If the cuff is too large, the reading may be falsely low. The inner inflatable bladder of the cuff should encircle at least 80% of the patient's arm and cover two thirds of the distance from the axilla to the antecubital space.

4. **Never take blood pressure over clothing.** Clothing interferes with the ability to hear the Korotkoff sounds, which could result in an inaccurate blood pressure reading. Roll up the patient's sleeve approximately 5 inches above the elbow. If the sleeve is too tight after being rolled up, remove the arm from the sleeve. A tight sleeve causes partial compression of the brachial artery, resulting in an inaccurate reading.

5. **Position the patient's arm properly.** Position the arm at heart level, and ensure it is well supported with the palm facing upward. If the arm is above heart level, the blood pressure reading may be falsely low. If the arm is not supported or placed below heart level, the blood pressure reading may be falsely high.

6. **Avoid extraneous sounds from the cuff.** Position the cuff approximately 1 to 2 inches above the bend in the elbow. The cuff should be up far enough to prevent the stethoscope from touching it; otherwise, extraneous sounds, which could interfere with an accurate measurement, may be picked up.

7. **Compress the brachial artery completely.** Center the inner bladder of the cuff directly over the artery to be compressed. Most cuffs are labeled with arrows indicating the center of the bladder for the right and left arms. Centering the inner bladder allows for complete compression of the brachial artery.

8. **Apply equal pressure over the brachial artery.** The cuff should be applied so that it fits smoothly and snugly around the patient's arm. This prevents bulging or slipping and permits application of an equal pressure over the brachial artery. A loose-fitting cuff can cause a falsely high reading.

9. **Position the earpieces so that you can hear the sounds clearly.** Place the earpieces of the stethoscope in your ears with the earpieces directed slightly forward. This allows the earpieces to follow the direction of the ear canal, which facilitates hearing.

10. **Avoid extraneous sounds from the tubing.** Make sure the tubing of the stethoscope hangs freely and is not permitted to rub against any object. If the stethoscope tubing rubs against an object, extraneous sounds may be picked up, which could interfere with an accurate measurement.

11. **Position the chest piece properly.** Palpate the brachial pulse to provide good positioning of the chest piece over the brachial artery. Place the chest piece firmly, but gently, over the brachial artery to assist in transmitting clear and audible sounds. Do not allow the chest piece to touch the cuff to prevent extraneous sounds from being picked up, which could interfere with an accurate measurement.

12. **Release the pressure at a moderate steady rate.** Release the pressure in the cuff at a rate of 2 to 3 mm Hg/sec to ensure an accurate blood pressure measurement. Releasing the pressure too slowly is uncomfortable for the patient and could cause a falsely high diastolic reading. Releasing the pressure too quickly could cause a falsely low systolic reading.

Continued

Prevention of Errors in Blood Pressure Measurement—cont'd

13. **Avoid venous congestion.** If you need to take the blood pressure in the same arm again, wait 1 to 2 minutes to allow blood trapped in the veins (venous congestion) to be released. Venous congestion can result in a falsely high systolic reading and a falsely low diastolic reading.

14. **Measure and record the blood pressure in both arms during the initial blood pressure assessment of a new patient.** There may normally be a difference of 5 to 10 mm Hg between the two arms. During return visits, the blood pressure should be measured in the arm with the higher initial reading.

PROCEDURE **19-9**   Measuring Blood Pressure

Outcome Measure blood pressure.

Equipment/Supplies

- Stethoscope
- Sphygmomanometer
- Antiseptic wipe

1. Procedural Step. Sanitize your hands, and assemble the equipment. If the chest piece consists of a diaphragm and a bell, rotate it to the diaphragm position. Clean the earpieces and chest piece of the stethoscope with the antiseptic wipe.

Principle. The chest piece must be rotated to the proper position for sound to be heard through the earpieces.

Rotate the chest piece to the diaphragm position. (From Bonewit-West K: *Clinical procedures for medical assistants,* ed 7, St. Louis, 2008, Saunders.)

2. Procedural Step. Greet the patient and introduce yourself. Identify the patient and explain the procedure. Explain to the patient that measuring blood pressure may normally cause a little numbing and tingling in the arm when the cuff is inflated. While explaining the procedure, observe the patient for signs that might influence the reading, such as anger, fear, pain, and recent physical activity. If it is not possible

to reduce or eliminate these influences, list them in the patient's chart. Determine how high to pump the cuff by checking the patient's chart for previously measured systolic reading, or determine the patient's systolic pressure by palpation (see Procedure 19-10).

3. Procedural Step. Have the patient sit quietly in a comfortable position for at least 5 minutes before measuring his or her blood pressure. Roll up the patient's sleeve approximately 5 inches above the elbow. If the sleeve does not roll up or is too tight after being rolled up, remove the arm from the sleeve. The arm should be positioned at heart level and well supported, with the palm facing up.

Principle. Patient anxiety can cause a significant increase in blood pressure. Clothing interferes with the ability to hear the Korotkoff sounds, which could result in an inaccurate blood pressure reading. A tight sleeve causes partial compression of the brachial artery, resulting in an inaccurate reading. The position of the arm allows easy access to the brachial artery. Placing the arm above heart level may cause the reading to be falsely low. Not supporting the arm or placing it below heart level may cause the reading to be falsely high.

4. Procedural Step. Select the proper cuff size. The inner inflatable bladder of the cuff should be long enough to encircle at least 80% of the patient's arm and wide enough to cover two thirds of the distance from the axilla to the antecubital space.

Principle. The appropriate size cuff must be used to ensure an accurate measurement. If the cuff is too small, it may come loose as the cuff is inflated or the reading may be falsely high. If the cuff is too large, the reading may be falsely low.

The inner bladder should encircle at least 80% of the patient's arm. (From Bonewit-West K: *Clinical procedures for medical assistants,* ed 7, St. Louis, 2008, Saunders.)

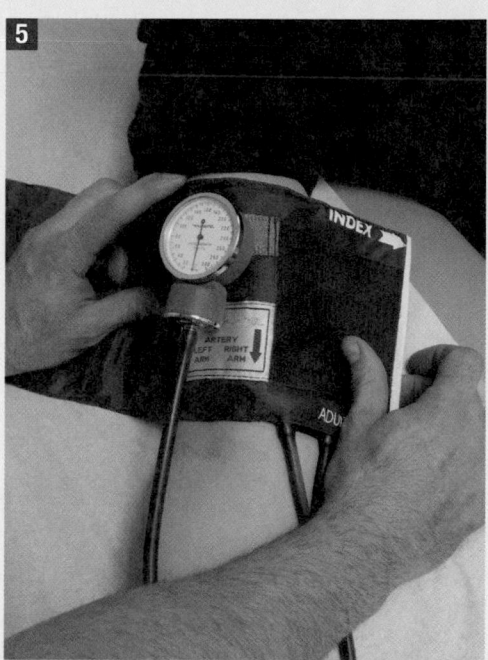

Center the inner bladder over the brachial pulse site. (From Bonewit-West K: *Clinical procedures for medical assistants,* ed 7, St. Louis, 2008, Saunders.)

5. Procedural Step. Locate the brachial pulse with the fingertips. The brachial pulse is located near the center of the antecubital space but slightly to the little finger side of the arm. Center the inner bladder over the brachial pulse site. (*Note:* Place the cuff on the patient's arm so that the lower edge of the cuff is approximately 1 to 2 inches above the bend in the elbow. Most cuffs are labeled with a right and left arrow indicating the center of the bladder. The right arrow should be placed over the brachial pulse site when you are using the right arm, and the left arrow should be placed over the brachial pulse site when you are using the left arm.)
Principle. The cuff should be placed high enough to prevent the stethoscope from touching it; otherwise, extraneous sounds, which could interfere with an accurate measurement, may be picked up. Centering the inner bladder over the pulse site allows complete compression of the brachial artery.

6. Procedural Step. Wrap the cuff smoothly and snugly around the patient's arm, and secure the end of it.
Principle. Applying the cuff properly prevents it from bulging or slipping. This technique permits application of an equal pressure over the brachial artery.

7. Procedural Step. Position the manometer for direct viewing and at a distance of no more than 3 feet.
Principle. The medical assistant may have trouble seeing the scale on the manometer if it is placed more than 3 feet away.

8. Procedural Step. Place the earpieces of the stethoscope in your ears, with the earpieces directed slightly forward. During the blood pressure measurement, the tubing of the stethoscope should hang freely and should not be permitted to rub against any object.
Principle. The earpieces should be directed forward, permitting them to follow the direction of the ear canal, which facilitates hearing. If the stethoscope tubing rubs against an object, extraneous sounds may be picked up, which would interfere with an accurate measurement.

9. Procedural Step. Making sure the arm is well extended, locate the brachial pulse again and place the diaphragm of the stethoscope over the brachial pulse site. The diaphragm should be positioned to make a tight seal against the patient's skin. Enough pressure should be exerted to leave a temporary ring on the patient's skin when the disk is removed. Do not allow the chest piece to touch the cuff.
Principle. A well-extended arm allows easier palpation of the brachial pulse. Locating the brachial pulse again is necessary for proper positioning of the chest piece over the brachial artery. Proper positioning of the diaphragm and good contact of the diaphragm with the skin helps transmit clear and audible Korotkoff sounds through the earpieces of the stethoscope. If the diaphragm touches the cuff, extraneous sounds may be picked up, which would interfere with an accurate measurement.

Continued

PROCEDURE 19-9 Measuring Blood Pressure—cont'd

Locate the brachial pulse again before placing the diaphragm over the site. (From Bonewit-West K: *Clinical procedures for medical assistants,* ed 7, St. Louis, 2008, Saunders.)

diastolic reading. Releasing the pressure too quickly could cause a falsely low systolic reading. The systolic pressure is the point at which the blood first begins to spurt through the artery as the cuff pressure begins to decrease; it represents the pressure that occurs on the walls of the arteries during systole.

Pump air into the cuff as rapidly as possible. (From Bonewit-West K: *Clinical procedures for medical assistants,* ed 7, St. Louis, 2008, Saunders.)

10. Procedural Step. Close the valve on the bulb by turning the thumbscrew clockwise (to the right) with the thumb and forefinger of your dominant hand until it feels tight but can still be loosened with the thumb and forefinger of one hand when you need to deflate the cuff. Pump air into the cuff as rapidly as possible to a level of 20 to 30 mm Hg above the previously measured or palpated systolic pressure.
Principle. Inflation of the cuff compresses and closes off the brachial artery so that no blood flows through the artery. If the patient has had the blood pressure measured previously at the medical office, the recorded systolic pressure can be used to determine how high to inflate the cuff. A preliminary determination of the systolic pressure by palpation allows the medical assistant to estimate how high to inflate the cuff.

11. Procedural Step. Release the pressure at a moderately steady rate of 2 to 3 mm Hg/sec by slowly turning the thumbscrew counterclockwise (to the left) with the thumb and forefinger. This opens the valve and allows the air in the cuff to escape slowly. Listen for the first clear tapping sound (phase I of the Korotkoff sounds). This represents the systolic pressure. Note this point on the scale of the manometer.
Principle. Releasing the pressure too slowly is uncomfortable for the patient and could cause a falsely high

Release the pressure at a moderately steady rate. (From Bonewit-West K: *Clinical procedures for medical assistants,* ed 7, St. Louis, 2008, Saunders.)

12. **Procedural Step.** Continue to deflate the cuff while listening to the Korotkoff sounds. Listen for the onset of the muffled sound that occurs during phase IV. Continue to deflate the cuff, and note the point on the scale at which the sound ceases (phase V). Continue to steadily deflate the cuff for another 10 mm/Hg to ensure there are no more sounds.

    Principle. Phase V marks the diastolic pressure (which represents the pressure that occurs on the walls of the arteries during diastole); the cuff pressure is reduced, and blood is flowing freely through the brachial artery.

13. **Procedural Step.** Quickly and completely deflate the cuff to zero. If you could not obtain an accurate blood pressure reading, wait 1 to 2 minutes before taking another measurement on the same arm. Remove the earpieces of the stethoscope from your ears, and carefully remove the cuff from the patient's arm.

Principle. Venous congestion results when blood pressure is taken, which alters a second reading if it is taken too soon on the same arm.

14. **Procedural Step.** Sanitize your hands, and chart the results. Include the date, time, and blood pressure reading. Blood pressure is recorded using even numbers. Make a notation in the patient's chart if the lying or standing position was used to take blood pressure. Abbreviations that can be used are *L* (lying) and *St* (standing).

15. **Procedural Step.** Clean the earpieces and the chest piece of the stethoscope with an antiseptic wipe, and replace the equipment properly.

CHARTING EXAMPLE

Date	
10/20/10	2:30 p.m. BP: 106/74.—S. Martinez, RMA

PROCEDURE **19-10**   Determining Systolic Pressure by Palpation

Outcome Determine systolic pressure by palpation.

Equipment/Supplies

- Sphygmomanometer

1. **Procedural Step.** Sanitize your hands, and assemble the equipment.
2. **Procedural Step.** Locate the brachial pulse with the fingertips. Place the cuff on the patient's arm so that the inner bladder is centered over the brachial pulse site.
3. **Procedural Step.** Wrap the cuff smoothly and snugly around the patient's arm, and secure the end of it.
4. **Procedural Step.** Position the manometer for direct viewing and at a distance of no more than 3 feet.
5. **Procedural Step.** Locate the radial pulse with your fingertips.
6. **Procedural Step.** Close the valve on the bulb, and pump air into the cuff until the pulsation ceases.
7. **Procedural Step.** Release the valve at a moderate rate of 2 to 3 mm Hg per heartbeat while palpating the artery with your fingertips.
8. **Procedural Step.** Record the point at which the pulsation reappears as the palpated systolic pressure.
9. **Procedural Step.** Deflate the cuff completely, and wait 15 to 30 seconds before checking the blood pressure.

Release the valve while palpating the radial artery. (From Bonewit-West K: *Clinical procedures for medical assistants,* ed 7, St. Louis, 2008, Saunders.)

MEDICAL PRACTICE and the LAW

Measurement of vital signs is standard procedure for almost every patient in the physician's office. Because vital sign measurements are performed so frequently, the medical assistant may tend to minimize their importance. Changes in vital signs may be the first indicator of disease or illness, so meticulous attention must be paid to the performance and documentation of vital signs and to comparing the current measurements with past measurements for each patient.

Most patients want to know their vital signs, especially their blood pressure or temperature if febrile. Although the patient owns the information that you collect, be aware that you may not give this information to family members without the patient's consent. Some offices have a policy that indicates specific information the medical assistant can give the patient; some physicians prefer to disclose this information themselves and discuss it with their patients.

Often the measurement of vital signs is the first contact the patients have with the medical assistant. The most important factor in determining whether a patient will sue is not the skill of the practitioner, but the level of rapport with the patient. In everything you do, convey your caring and concern to every patient. ■

What Would You Do? What Would You *Not* Do? RESPONSES

Case Study 1
Page 336

What Did Sergio Do?
❑ Told Mrs. Mason that sometimes ear thermometers can be a little tricky to use.
❑ Showed Mrs. Mason how to use the ear thermometer and let her practice by taking Olivia's temperature.
❑ Explained how to care for and maintain the ear thermometer to prevent inaccurate readings.
❑ Explained to Mrs. Mason that the use of mercury is being discouraged because it can be toxic to humans and animals.

What Did Sergio Not *Do?*
❑ Did not ask Mrs. Mason if she had read the directions that came with her ear thermometer.
❑ Did not tell Mrs. Mason that she should switch back to the mercury thermometer.
❑ Did not ask Mrs. Mason why she waited so long to bring Olivia to the office.

What Would You Do/What Would You *Not* Do? Review Sergio's response and place a checkmark next to the information you included in your response. List the additional information you included in your response.

_____
_____
_____
_____

Case Study 2
Page 349

What Did Sergio Do?
❑ Recognized and congratulated Alex on his swimming achievements.
❑ Told Alex that it is normal for his pulse to be that slow because of his athletic training and it shows that he is in good shape.

❑ Assured Alex that the physician will do everything he can to help Alex.
❑ Stressed to Alex how important it is to follow the physician's advice so that his shoulder heals as soon as possible.

What Did Sergio Not *Do?*
❑ Did not comment on Alex's request for a steroid injection or OxyContin. Made sure to chart the information so that the physician could handle the situation.
❑ Did not criticize Alex for putting a swim meet before his health.

What Would You Do/What Would You *Not* Do? Review Sergio's response and place a checkmark next to the information you included in your response. List the additional information you included in your response.

_____
_____
_____
_____

Case Study 3
Page 362

What Did Sergio Do?
❑ Empathized with Tyrone about having to take so many pills. Suggested that he get a daily pill container to help him remember.
❑ Stressed to Tyrone the importance of taking his blood pressure medication. Explained to him that high blood pressure is a "silent disease." He may feel fine, but damage to his body organs can still be taking place if he does not take his pills.
❑ Gave Tyrone a brochure about high blood pressure and went over the long-term effects of hypertension and lifestyle changes that could help lower blood pressure.
❑ Encouraged Tyrone to call the office when he experiences side effects from medications because the physician may be able to do something to help.

What Would You Do? What Would You *Not* Do?   RESPONSES—cont'd

What Did Sergio Not *Do?*

❑ Did not tell him it was all right to discontinue his medication.

What Would You Do/What Would You *Not* **Do?** Review Sergio's response and place a checkmark next to the information you included in your response. List the additional information you included in your response.

TERMINOLOGY REVIEW

Adventitious sounds Abnormal breath sounds.

Afebrile Without fever; the body temperature is normal.

Alveolus A thin-walled air sac of the lungs in which the exchange of oxygen and carbon dioxide takes place.

Antecubital space The space located at the front of the elbow.

Antipyretic An agent that reduces fever.

Aorta The major trunk of the arterial system of the body. The aorta arises from the upper surface of the left ventricle.

Apnea The temporary cessation of breathing.

Axilla The armpit.

Bounding pulse A pulse with an increased volume that feels strong and full.

Bradycardia An abnormally slow heart rate (less than 60 beats per minute).

Bradypnea An abnormal decrease in the respiratory rate of less than 10 respirations per minute.

Celsius scale A temperature scale on which the freezing point of water is 0° and the boiling point of water is 100°; also called the *centigrade scale.*

Conduction The transfer of energy, such as heat, from one object to another by direct contact.

Convection The transfer of energy, such as heat, through air currents.

Crisis A sudden falling of an elevated body temperature to normal.

Cyanosis A bluish discoloration of the skin and mucous membranes.

Diastole The phase in the cardiac cycle in which the heart relaxes between contractions.

Diastolic pressure The point of lesser pressure on the arterial wall, which is recorded during diastole.

Dyspnea Shortness of breath or difficulty in breathing.

Dysrhythmia An irregular rhythm; also termed *arrhythmia.*

Eupnea Normal respiration. The rate is 16 to 20 respirations per minute, the rhythm is even and regular, and the depth is normal.

Exhalation The act of breathing out.

Fahrenheit scale A temperature scale on which the freezing point of water is 32° and the boiling point of water is 212°.

Febrile Pertaining to fever.

Fever A body temperature that is above normal; synonym for *pyrexia.*

Frenulum linguae The midline fold that connects the undersurface of the tongue with the floor of the mouth.

Hyperpnea An abnormal increase in the rate and depth of respiration.

Hyperpyrexia An extremely high fever.

Hypertension High blood pressure.

Hyperventilation An abnormally fast and deep type of breathing, usually associated with acute anxiety conditions.

Hypopnea An abnormal decrease in the rate and depth of respiration.

Hypotension Low blood pressure.

Hypothermia A body temperature that is below normal.

Hypoxemia A decrease in the oxygen saturation of the blood. Hypoxemia may lead to hypoxia.

Hypoxia A reduction in the oxygen supply to the tissues of the body.

Inhalation The act of breathing in.

Intercostal Between the ribs.

Korotkoff sounds Sounds heard during the measurement of blood pressure that are used to determine the systolic and diastolic blood pressure readings.

Malaise A vague sense of body discomfort, weakness, and fatigue that often marks the onset of a disease and continues through the course of the illness.

Manometer An instrument for measuring pressure.

Meniscus The curved surface on a column of liquid in a tube.

Orthopnea The condition in which breathing is easier when an individual is in a sitting or standing position.

Continued

TERMINOLOGY REVIEW—cont'd

Pulse oximeter A computerized device consisting of a probe and monitor used to measure the oxygen saturation of arterial blood.

Pulse oximetry The use of a pulse oximeter to measure the oxygen saturation of arterial blood.

Pulse pressure The difference between the systolic and diastolic pressures.

Pulse rhythm The time interval between heartbeats.

Pulse volume The strength of the heartbeat.

Radiation The transfer of energy, such as heat, in the form of waves.

SaO_2 (saturation of arterial oxygen) Abbreviation for the percentage of hemoglobin that is saturated with oxygen in arterial blood.

Sphygmomanometer An instrument for measuring arterial blood pressure.

SpO_2 (saturation of peripheral oxygen) Abbreviation for the percentage of hemoglobin that is saturated with

oxygen in arterial blood as measured by a pulse oximeter.

Stethoscope An instrument for amplifying and hearing sounds produced by the body.

Systole The phase in the cardiac cycle in which the ventricles contract, sending blood out of the heart and into the aorta and pulmonary aorta.

Systolic pressure The point of maximum pressure on the arterial walls, which is recorded during systole.

Tachycardia An abnormally fast heart rate (greater than 100 beats per minute).

Tachypnea An abnormal increase in the respiratory rate of more than 20 respirations per minute.

Thready pulse A pulse with a decreased volume that feels weak and thin.

ON THE WEB

For Information on Hypertension:

American Heart Association: www.americanheart.org

National Heart, Lung, and Blood Institute: www.nhlbi.nih.gov

Cardiology Channel: www.cardiologychannel.com

Hypertension Education Foundation: www.hypertension-foundation.org

American Society of Hypertension: www.ash-us.org

For Information on Lung Disease:

American Lung Association: www.lungusa.org

Pulmonology Channel: www.pulmonologychannel.com

Lung Cancer Online: www.lungcanceronline.org

 PREPARE FOR CERTIFICATION Visit the Evolve site at http://evolve.elsevier.com/Bonewit/today/ to actively Prepare for your Certification.

 *Check out the **Companion CD** bound with the book to access additional interactive activities.*

20

The Physical Examination

CAAHEP COMPETENCIES

Clinical Competencies
Patient Care
- Prepare and maintain examination and treatment areas.
- Prepare patient for and assist with routine and specialty examinations.

General Competencies
Patient Instruction
- Instruct individuals according to their needs.
- Provide instruction for health maintenance and disease prevention.
- Identify community resources.

Operational Functions
- Perform an inventory of supplies and equipment.
- Perform routine maintenance of administrative and clinical equipment.

ABHES COMPETENCIES

Clinical Duties
- Prepare patients for procedures.
- Prepare and maintain examination and treatment area.
- Prepare patient for and assist physician with routine and specialty examinations and treatments and minor office surgeries.

Office Management
- Maintain physical plant.
- Operate and maintain facilities and perform routine maintenance of administrative and clinical equipment safely.
- Inventory equipment and supplies.

Instruction
- Teach patients methods of health promotion and disease prevention.

KEY TERMS

audiometer (aw-dee-OM-eh-ter)
auscultation (os-kul-TAY-shun)
bariatrics (BAR-ee-AT-riks)
clinical diagnosis
diagnosis
differential (diff-er-EN-shul) diagnosis
inspection
mensuration (men-soo-RAY-shun)

ophthalmoscope (off-THAL-meh-skope)
otoscope (AH-toe-skope)
palpation (pal-PAY-shun)
percussion (per-KUSH-un)
percussion hammer
prognosis
speculum (SPEK-yoo-lum)
symptom

Introduction to the Physical Examination

A complete patient examination consists of three parts: *health history, physical examination* of each body system, and *laboratory and diagnostic tests.* The physician uses the results to determine the patient's general state of health, arrive at a diagnosis and prescribe treatment, and observe any change in a patient's illness after treatment has been instituted.

An important and frequent responsibility of the medical assistant is to assist with a physical examination. Because health-promotion and disease-prevention activities have become an important focus of health care, individuals are becoming more aware of the need for a yearly physical examination to detect early signs of illness and prevent serious health problems. Also, a physical examination may be a prerequisite for employment, participation in sports, attendance at summer camp, and admission to school. The physical examination is explained in detail in this chapter. Taking the health history, collecting specimens, and performing laboratory and diagnostic tests are discussed in other chapters.

DEFINITION OF TERMS

The medical assistant should know and understand the following terms relating to the patient examination:

Final diagnosis Often simply called the **diagnosis,** this term refers to the scientific method of determining and identifying a patient's condition through the evaluation of the health history, the physical examination, laboratory tests, and diagnostic procedures. A final diagnosis is crucial because it provides a logical basis for treatment and prognosis.

Clinical diagnosis The clinical diagnosis is an intermediate step in the determination of a final diagnosis. The clinical diagnosis of a patient's condition is obtained

Highlight on Health Screening

The chance of developing certain diseases is greater at different ages. Periodic health screening is recommended for the detection and early treatment of disease.

Test or Procedure	Gender	Recommended Frequency
Beginning at age 20 years		
Blood pressure	M & F	Every year
Cholesterol level	M & F	Every 5 years
Blood glucose level	M & F	Every 3-5 years
Breast self-examination	F	Every month
Beginning at the age specified		
Clinical breast examination (by a physician)	F	Every 3 years beginning at age 29, and every year beginning at age 40
Pap test and pelvic examination	F	Begin within 3 years of the onset of vaginal intercourse or at age 21, whichever comes first, then every 1 to 2 years
Testicular self-examination	M	Every month beginning at age 15
Rectal examination	M & F	Every year beginning at age 40
Fecal occult blood test	M & F	Every year starting at age 50
Sigmoidoscopy	M & F	Every 5 years beginning at age 50
Prostate cancer screening	M	Every year beginning at age 50
Mammography	F	Every year beginning at age 40
Electrocardiogram	M & F	One baseline recording starting at age 40

through the evaluation of the health history and the physical examination without the benefit of laboratory or diagnostic tests. Outside laboratories provide a space to specify the clinical diagnosis on the laboratory request form; this information assists the laboratory in correlating the clinical laboratory data and the physician's needs. When the physician has analyzed the test results, a final diagnosis usually can be established.

Differential diagnosis   Two or more diseases may have similar **symptoms.** The differential diagnosis involves determining which of these diseases is producing the patient's symptoms so that a final diagnosis can be established. For example, streptococcal sore throat and pharyngitis have similar symptoms. A differential diagnosis is made by obtaining a throat specimen and performing a strep test.

Prognosis   The prognosis is the probable course and outcome of a patient's condition and the patient's prospects for recovery.

Risk factor   A risk factor is a physical or behavioral condition that increases the probability that an individual will develop a particular condition; examples are genetic factors, habits, environmental conditions, and physiologic conditions. The presence of a risk factor for a certain disease does not mean that the disease will develop; it means only that a person's chances of developing that disease are greater than those of a person without the risk factor. For example, cigarette smoking is a risk factor for developing lung cancer and heart disease. A person who smokes has a higher risk of developing lung cancer than a person who does not or who has stopped smoking.

Acute illness   An acute illness is characterized by symptoms that have a rapid onset, are usually severe and intense, and subside after a relatively short time. In some cases, the acute episode progresses into a chronic illness. Examples of acute illness include influenza, strep throat, and chickenpox.

Chronic illness   A chronic illness is characterized by symptoms that persist for more than 3 months and show little change over a long time. Examples of chronic illness include diabetes mellitus, hypertension, and emphysema.

Therapeutic procedure   A therapeutic procedure is performed to treat a patient's condition with the goal of eliminating it or promoting as much recovery as possible. Examples of therapeutic procedures include the administration of medication, ear and eye irrigations, and therapeutic ultrasound.

Diagnostic procedure   A diagnostic procedure is a procedure performed to assist in the diagnosis of a patient's condition; examples include electrocardiography, x-ray examination, and sigmoidoscopy.

Laboratory testing   Laboratory testing involves the analysis and study of specimens obtained from patients to assist in diagnosing and treating disease.

PREPARATION OF THE EXAMINING ROOM

Proper preparation of the examining room provides a comfortable and healthy environment for the patient and facilitates the physical examination. The following guidelines should be followed in preparing the examining room:

1. Ensure the examining room is free of clutter and well lit.
2. Check the examining rooms daily to ensure there are ample supplies. Restock supplies that are getting low.
3. Empty waste receptacles frequently.
4. Replace biohazard containers as needed. When removing biohazard containers from the examining room (see Chapter 17), follow the OSHA Bloodborne Pathogens Standard.
5. Make sure the room is well ventilated, and install an air freshener to eliminate odors.
6. Maintain room temperatures that are comfortable not only for a fully clothed individual, but also for an individual who has disrobed.
7. Clean and disinfect examining tables, countertops, and faucets daily.
8. Remove dust and dirt from furniture and towel dispensers.
9. Change the examining table paper after each patient by unrolling a fresh length. Check to ensure there is an ample supply of gowns and drapes ready for use.
10. Ensure that the examining room door is closed during the examination because patient privacy is paramount.
11. Properly clean and prepare equipment, instruments, and supplies that are used for patient examinations so that they are ready for use by the physician. Table 20-1 lists the equipment and supplies, along with their uses, that may be employed during a physical examination.
12. Check equipment and instruments regularly to verify that they are in proper working condition. This protects the patient from harm caused by faulty equipment.
13. Have the equipment and supplies ready for the examination and arranged for easy access by the physician. The equipment and supplies needed for the physical examination vary according to the type of examination and the physician's preference (Figure 20-1).
14. Know how to operate and care for each piece of equipment and each instrument. The manufacturer includes an operating manual, which should be read carefully and thoroughly and kept available for reference.

Table 20-1 Equipment and Supplies for the Physical Examination

Item	Description and Purpose
Patient examination gown	Gown made of disposable paper or cloth that provides patient modesty, comfort, and warmth
Drape	A length of disposable paper or cloth to cover patient or parts of patient to provide comfort and warmth and reduce exposure
Sphygmomanometer	Instrument used to measure blood pressure
Stethoscope	Instrument used to auscultate body sounds, such as blood pressure and lung and bowel sounds
Thermometer	Instrument used to measure body temperature
Upright balance scale	Device used to measure weight and height
Otoscope	Lighted instrument with lens, used to examine external ear canal and tympanic membrane
Tuning fork	Small metal instrument consisting of stem and two prongs, used to test hearing acuity
Ophthalmoscope	Lighted instrument with lens, used for examining interior of eye
Tongue depressor	Flat wooden blade used to depress patient's tongue during examination of mouth and pharynx
Antiseptic wipe	Disposable pad saturated with antiseptic, such as alcohol, that is used to cleanse skin
Tape measure	Flexible device calibrated in inches on one side and centimeters on other side, used to measure patient (e.g., diameter of limb, head circumference)
Percussion hammer	Instrument with rubber head, used for testing neurologic reflexes
Speculum	Instrument for opening body orifice or cavity for viewing (e.g., ear speculum, nasal speculum, vaginal speculum)
Disposable gloves	Gloves, usually latex, that are worn only once to provide protection from bloodborne pathogens and other potentially infectious materials
Lubricant	Agent applied to physician's gloved hand or speculum that reduces friction between parts to make insertion easier
Specimen container	Container in which body specimen is placed for transport to laboratory (after it has been labeled)
Tissues	Used for wiping body secretions
Cotton-tipped applicator	Small piece of cotton wrapped around the end of a slender wooden stick, used for collection of specimen from body
Overhead examination light	Light mounted on flexible movable stand to focus light on area for good visibility
Basin	Container in which used instruments are deposited
Biohazard container	Specially made container used for receiving items that contain infectious waste
Waste receptacle	Container for used disposable articles that do not contain infectious waste

From Bonewit-West K: *Clinical procedures for medical assistants*, ed 7, St. Louis, 2008, Saunders.

Clean gloves   Gauze   Lubricant   Tape measure

Fecal occult blood testing supplies

Specimen collection system

Antiseptic wipe   Percussion hammer   Tongue depressor   Tuning forks   Otoscope   Ophthalmoscope

Figure 20-1. Common instruments and supplies used for the physical examination. (From Bonewit-West K: *Clinical procedures for medical assistants,* ed 7, St. Louis, 2008, Saunders.)

Highlight on Patient Teaching

The purpose of patient teaching is to help the patient develop habits, attitudes, and skills that enable the individual to maintain and improve his or her own health.

Fact: Patients who are active, informed participants in their health care are more apt to follow the physician's instructions than patients who are passive recipients of medical services.

Action: Provide patients with information on health care. Every patient interaction is an opportunity for teaching.

Fact: Adult learners are goal oriented and performance centered. They need and want information that would assist them in managing and improving their health.

Action: Review the information that you provide to patients, and determine whether it is nice to know or necessary to know. Select subject matter that is practical and useful and relates directly to the patient's needs.

Fact: The more information that is presented, the more the patient is likely to forget. Approximately half of information presented to the patient is forgotten in the first 5 minutes after giving it.

Action: When teaching, use the following pointers to help patients learn and retain information:

- Keep it short and be specific.
- Speak in terms the patient can understand.
- Focus on "how," rather than "why."
- Repeat and reinforce important information.
- Give practical examples, and provide ample time for patient practice.

- Ask for feedback from the patient to determine whether he or she understands the information.
- Provide the patient with written information.

Fact: Each individual has a distinct style of learning and learns best when using his or her preferred learning style. The three main learning styles are reading, listening, and doing. People often use more than one style for learning.

Action: Use a variety of teaching strategies to engage the various learning styles of patients. Examples of teaching strategies include explanations, printed handouts, audiovisual aids, demonstrations, and discussions.

Fact: Only two thirds of patients comply with health care instructions prescribed by the physician. Factors that influence compliance include the patient's adaptation to illness, motivation to change, physical capability, and support systems.

Action: The following help increase patient compliance with prescribed treatment:

- Address the patient by his or her name of choice. (Keep in mind that many patients object to being called by their first name by strangers.)
- Encourage the patient to take an active role in personal health care.
- Help the patient set goals and objectives for change.
- Encourage care and support from family members.
- Make the patient aware of outside resources.
- Give positive reinforcement when the patient makes healthful changes. ∎

PREPARATION OF THE PATIENT

The medical assistant is responsible for preparing the patient for the physical examination. After escorting the patient to the examining room, the medical assistant should identify the patient by his or her name and date of birth. This avoids mistaking one patient for another. If the medical assistant performs a procedure on the wrong patient by mistake, he or she could be held liable. The medical assistant then takes vital signs and measures the weight and height of the patient. The results of these procedures are charted in the patient's medical record.

The medical assistant can reduce a patient's apprehension and embarrassment by addressing the patient by his or her name of choice; by adopting a friendly and supportive attitude; and by speaking clearly, distinctly, and slowly. The medical assistant should explain the purpose of the examination and offer to answer any questions. This also facilitates the physical examination of the patient.

The patient should be asked whether he or she needs to empty the bladder before the examination. An empty bladder makes the examination easier and is more comfortable for the patient. If a urine specimen is needed, the patient is requested to void.

Instructions on disrobing for the examination should be specific so that the patient understands what items of clothing to remove and where to place the clothing. The disrobing facility should be comfortable and provide privacy. It is helpful to have a place for the patient to sit to make it easier to remove clothing and shoes. The facility also should be equipped with hooks for hanging clothing. Instructions for putting on the examination gown and for locating the gown opening reduce patient confusion. If the medical assistant senses that the patient will have trouble undressing, assistance should be offered. Elderly and disabled patients sometimes have difficulty removing clothing.

The medical assistant is responsible for making the patient's medical record available for review by the physician. The medical office has a designated location where the record is placed, such as a small shelf mounted on the wall next to the outside of the examining room door or in a chart holder mounted on the outside of the examining room door. The medical assistant should ensure that the medical record is placed so that patient-identifiable information is not visible. This is required by the Health Insurance Portability and Accountability Act (HIPAA) Privacy Rule to protect a patient's health information.

The physical examination is performed with the patient positioned on an examining table, which is specially constructed to facilitate the examination. For safety, it is advisable to help the patient on and off the examining table.

MEASURING WEIGHT AND HEIGHT

The medical assistant routinely measures the weight and height of many types of patients. The process of measuring the patient is **mensuration.** A change in weight may be

---

What Would You Do? What Would You *Not* Do?

Case Study 1

Abbey Auden, 35 years old, is at the medical office. Her husband got a backyard trampoline for their two school-age children, and she decided to try it out. Abbey landed wrong on the trampoline and hurt her back and neck. For the past 5 days she has been having headaches and back pain. Abbey refuses to have her weight taken because she has gained weight over the past several years and does not want to know how much she's gained. She does not understand why weight has to be taken at an office visit in the first place. Abbey says that many times when she should go to the doctor, she does not, just to avoid being weighed. She says she would not even be here now except that her husband insisted that she come. ■

Putting It All into Practice

My name is Hope Fauber, and I am a certified medical assistant. I work in a medical clinic with a family medicine department of 10 physicians and 10 residents and interns. My duties cover a broad spectrum, from pediatrics to geriatrics, and include prenatal care, allergy injections, minor office surgery, electrocardiograms, colposcopies, immunizations, and wound care.

At our clinic, many of the patients are elderly. I occasionally come across geriatric patients who are not very cooperative and are "set in their ways." One 90-year-old woman, in particular, had a reputation in the office of being cantankerous and difficult to work with. One day when the physician ordered laboratory work on her, I prepared to draw blood from her tiny, frail body, praying that everything would go smoothly. As I helped her up after a successful "stick," she, of all people, reached to give me a hug and said to me, "I like you. That didn't even hurt!" She continued to hold my hand and talk to me as I walked her out of the office. This turned out to be the last time I would see her because she moved out of town, but not out of my heart, leaving a lasting impression on my life. ■

Prepare for Success

---

significant in the diagnosis of a patient's condition and in prescribing the course of treatment. Underweight and overweight patients who follow a diet therapy program should be weighed at regular intervals to determine their progress. Prenatal patients are weighed during each prenatal visit to assist in the assessment of fetal development and of the mother's health. Procedure 20-1 describes how to measure height and weight.

An adult's weight is usually measured during each office visit; an adult's height is typically measured only during the first visit or when a complete physical examination of the

Highlight on Cultural Diversity

Culture consists of the values, beliefs, and practices of a particular group of people. Culture is deeply rooted and is passed on from one generation to the next through communication. It includes areas such as religion, dietary practices, family lines of authority, family life patterns, beliefs, and health practices.

As the demographics of the United States continue to change, the medical assistant is faced with the challenge of providing care to an increasing number of cultural groups. It is important for the medical assistant to learn as much as possible about the cultural values of the patients coming to the medical office. This is known as *cultural awareness* and can be accomplished by carefully observing and listening to patients to acquire knowledge of their cultural values.

Cultural sensitivity is the respect and appreciation for cultural diversity, whereas *cultural competence* is understanding and using the cultural background of a patient to assist with the resolution of a problem. Because health practices are part of a patient's culture, changing them may have a negative impact on the patient. Whenever possible, the medical assistant should incorporate factors from a patient's cultural background into his or her health care.

Guidelines for Achieving Cultural Competence

The following guidelines help the medical assistant in developing cultural awareness and sensitivity and in achieving cultural competence:

1. **Respect the patient's values, beliefs, and practices.** Even if you do not agree with them, it is important to respect the patient's right to hold these values and not dismiss them as strange or odd. Cultural values play an important role in a patient's lifestyle. Patients from some cultures believe that losing blood depletes the body's strength and provides a route for the soul to leave the body. If a blood specimen is necessary, these patients may become highly distressed or refuse to have their blood drawn. Members of some cultural groups believe that illness results when the body's natural balance or harmony is disturbed. To restore the balance, alternative forms of medicine, such as herbal remedies and aromatherapy, are used.

2. **Refrain from cultural stereotypes.** Not all people of a cultural group have the same beliefs, practices, and values. Assuming that all members of a cultural group are alike is known as *stereotyping* and should be avoided. Just as one would never assume that all people in the United States like hamburgers and baseball, every individual must be approached according to his or her specific beliefs and practices.

3. **Always address patients by their last names (and Mr., Mrs., Miss or Ms.) unless they give you permission to use other names.** In many cultures, using a first name to address anyone other than family or friends is considered disrespectful. Most older people in the United States dislike being called by their first name and feel it shows a lack of respect.

4. **Speak slowly and clearly.** Communicating with a patient may be difficult if the patient has a limited knowledge of English. With these patients, you should speak slowly and clearly in a normal tone and volume of voice. Speaking loudly does not help the patient understand any better and may be offensive to the patient.

5. **Show respect for cultural lines of authority.** In many cultures, respect is given based on age and gender. In certain cultures, elders are considered the holders of the culture's wisdom and are highly respected. In other cultures, youth is valued over age. In certain cultures, the male dominates, and women have very little status. Because of this, a female patient from this type of culture may not be permitted to give her own health history or answer questions. In addition, a male patient from this culture may not accept instructions from a female medical assistant.

6. **Use appropriate eye contact.** In most cultures, direct eye contact is important and generally shows that the other is attentive and listening. It conveys self-confidence, openness, interest, and honesty, whereas the lack of eye contact may be interpreted as secretiveness, shyness, guilt, or lack of interest. Other cultures consider eye contact impolite or an invasion of privacy; these patients show respect by avoiding direct eye contact.

7. **Be aware of cultural responses to illness.** The conditions under which an individual assumes the role of a (sick) patient and the way he or she performs in that role vary with culture. Individuals of some cultures resist the sick role and blame sickness on external forces as a means of punishment. These individuals may deny their illness and fail to provide much information when the medical assistant takes their symptoms. In other cultures, individuals take an optimistic view of the outcome of health care and, because of this, are more likely to elicit information and follow the physician's instructions.

8. **Learn to appreciate the richness of diversity as an asset, rather than a hindrance, to communication and effective interaction with patients.** ■

patient is requested. Children are weighed and their height (or length) is measured during each office visit to observe their pattern of growth and calculate medication dosage.

The patient's height is used to interpret body weight (see the box *Highlight on Interpreting Body Weight*). The weight and height are compared against a standardized chart that serves as a general guide to determine whether the patient's weight falls within normal limits (Figure 20-2).

Text continued on p. 388

What Would You Do? What Would You *Not* Do?

Case Study 2

Karen Steiner drops her 17-year-old daughter, Mikayla, off at the office for her sports physical examination. Mikayla is captain of the varsity cheerleading squad and getting ready to start her senior year in high school. Mikayla's vital signs are normal, and she measures 5 feet 6 inches tall and weighs 105 lb. With some reluctance, Mikayla admits that she's been having problems with heartburn, and she's pretty sure she knows what's causing it. She says that she has to keep her weight down for cheerleading and after eating dinner with her family, she makes herself vomit to get rid of the food in her stomach. Mikayla is not too concerned about doing this because a lot of the popular girls at school are doing the same thing. She says it's the easy way to stay slim, and she would like to lose another 10 lb before football season starts. Mikayla wants some prescription drug samples to help with the heartburn because the over-the-counter pills that she's been taking are not working anymore. She does not want her parents to know about any of this because she's afraid that they would not understand and might make her drop out of cheerleading. ■

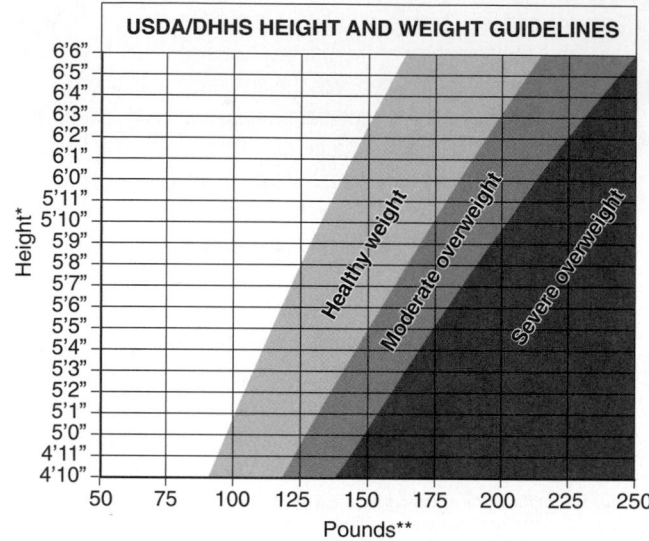

* Without shoes.
**Without clothes. The higher weights apply to people with more muscle and bone, such as many men.

Figure 20-2. U.S. Department of Agriculture/Department of Health and Human Services height and weight guidelines. (From *Report of the Dietary Guidelines Advisory Committee on the dietary guidelines for Americans,* Washington, DC, 1995, U.S. Department of Health and Human Services.)

PATIENT TEACHING   Health Promotion and Disease Prevention

Teach patients the essentials of health promotion and disease prevention. Help patients become aware of the following patterns of behavior that promote and support health:
- Keeping up to date with immunizations
- Eating nutritiously from the food pyramid
- Exercising regularly
- Maintaining normal weight
- Managing stress
- Maintaining high self-esteem
- Avoiding tobacco and drugs
- Using alcohol wisely

- Understanding how the environment affects health and taking appropriate action to improve it
- Knowing the facts about cardiovascular disease, cancer, infections, sexually transmitted diseases, and accidents, and using this knowledge to protect against them
- Understanding the changes that occur through the natural processes of aging
- Developing a sense of responsibility for health by taking an active role in establishing and maintaining a healthy lifestyle ■

Guidelines for Measuring Weight and Height

When using an upright balance scale to measure weight and height, use the following guidelines.

Weight

1. **Locate the scale to provide privacy for the patient.** Place the scale on a hard, level surface in a private location. Many patients are self-conscious about having their weight measured and prefer that it be done in privacy. Do not make weight-sensi-

tive comments during the procedure. This is especially important for patients with weight control problems, such as obesity and eating disorders.

2. **Balance the scale before measuring weight.** If the scale is not balanced, the weight measurement will be inaccurate. The scale is balanced when the upper and lower weights are on zero and the indicator point comes to a rest at the center of the balance area.

Guidelines for Measuring Weight and Height—cont'd

3. **Assist the patient.** Assist the patient on and off the scale platform. The scale platform moves slightly and may cause the patient to become unsteady.

4. **Obtain an accurate weight.** Always ask the patient to remove his or her shoes. Measure weight with the patient in normal clothing. Ask the patient to remove heavy outer clothing, such as a sweater or a jacket.

5. **Interpret the calibration markings accurately.** The lower calibration bar is divided into 50-lb increments (Figure 20-3A). The upper calibration bar is divided into pounds and quarter pounds. The longer calibration lines indicate pound increments, and the shorter calibration lines indicate quarter-pound and half-pound increments (Figure 20-3B).

6. **Determine the patient's weight correctly.** Add the measurement on the lower scale to the measurement on the upper scale. The result should be rounded to the nearest quarter pound. Occasionally, the patient's weight may need to be converted to kilograms, which is the metric unit of measurement for weight. This may be required when determining medication dosage. The following formulas are used to convert weight and height measurements from one system to another.

Weight Conversion

Pounds to Kilograms. Divide the number of pounds by 2.2:

$$136 \text{ lb} \div 2.2 = 61.8 \text{ kg}$$

Kilograms to Pounds. Multiply the number of kilograms by 2.2:

$$75 \text{ kg} \times 2.2 = 165 \text{ lb}$$

Height Conversion

Inches to Centimeters. Multiply the number of inches by 2.5:

$$64 \text{ inches} \times 2.5 = 160 \text{ cm}$$

Centimeters to Inches. Divide the number of centimeters by 2.5:

$$185 \text{ cm} \div 2.5 = 74 \text{ inches (or 6 feet 2 inches)}$$

Height

1. **Provide for the patient's safety.** Follow the proper procedure when measuring the patient's height. An error in technique could result in injury. If a patient is placed on the scale in a forward position, the measuring bar could fall into the patient's face when he or she steps off of the scale, causing a facial injury.

2. **Determine the calibration markings accurately.** Depending on the brand of scale, the calibration markings are divided into inches or feet and inches. (Figure 20-4 is an example of a scale divided into feet and inches.) The calibration rod is also calibrated into centimeters, which is the metric unit of measurement for height. This unit of measurement is not typically used to measure height in the United States.

3. **Read the measurement correctly.** The height measurement is read from the top of the bar down and should be read to the nearest quarter inch. For most patients, you can read the height measurement at the junction of the stationary calibration rod and the movable calibration rod (Figure 20-5A). If the patient's height is less than the top value of the stationary calibration rod, however, you must read the measurement from the bottom of the bar up directly on the stationary rod. For example, on most scales the highest calibration on the stationary rod is 50 inches; patients with a height of 50 inches or less would have their height read directly from the stationary rod (Figure 20-5B).

Figure 20-3. Calibration markings for measuring weight on an upright balance scale. **A,** The upper calibration bar is divided into pounds and quarter pounds. **B,** The longer calibration lines indicate pound increments, and the shorter calibration lines indicate quarter-pound and half-pound increments. (From Bonewit-West K: *Clinical procedures for medical assistants,* ed 7, St. Louis, 2008, Saunders.)

Continued

Guidelines for Measuring Weight and Height—cont'd

4. **Record the height measurement correctly.** Record the height measurement in feet and inches. If the scale is calibrated in inches, convert the reading to feet and inches by dividing the number of inches by 12. A height measurement of 60 inches is recorded as 5 feet (60 inches ÷ 12 = 5). If the patient's height measurement is 64 inches, the results would be recorded as 5 feet, 4 inches.

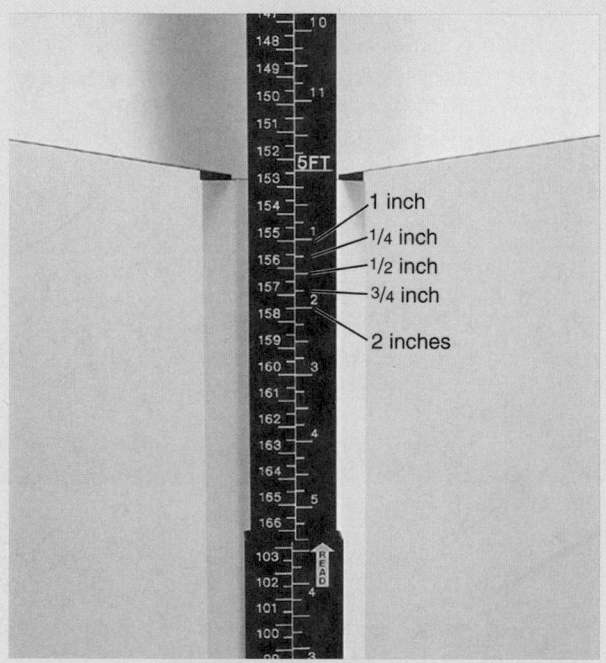

Figure 20-4. Calibration markings for measuring height on an upright balance scale. (From Bonewit-West K: *Clinical procedures for medical assistants,* ed 7, St. Louis, 2008, Saunders.)

Figure 20-5. A, Reading a height measurement at the junction of the stationary calibration rod and the movable calibration rod. The height measurement in this illustration is 6 feet, 1 inch. **B(1),** Reading a height measurement on the stationary calibration rod. *Note:* The measuring bar must first be released and moved down to the stationary bar to measure the patient's height. **B(2),** Reading the height at the junction of the bar and the rod. The height measurement in this illustration is 3 feet, 2 inches. (From Bonewit-West K: *Clinical procedures for medical assistants,* ed 7, St. Louis, 2008, Saunders.)

Highlight on Interpreting Body Weight

The two common methods to interpret body weight are weight in relation to standard tables and calculation of the body mass index (BMI).

Height and Weight Tables

One way to interpret body weight is through the use of standardized height and weight tables. In 1959, the Metropolitan Life Insurance Company (MET) issued a set of tables indicating desirable height and weight ranges for men and women. In 1983, MET issued revised tables for men and women that showed height and weight ranges higher than those in the 1959 table. Many health experts believe that the desirable weight ranges of the revised tables are too high and do not represent healthy body weight.

In 1995, the U.S. Department of Agriculture (USDA) and the Department of Health and Human Services (DHHS) issued a set of weight guidelines (see Figure 20-2) that are lower than those of the MET tables. The USDA/DHHS guidelines do not distinguish between weights of men and women and must be interpreted by each individual as follows. Women usually have smaller bones and less muscle than men, so they should use the lower end of the range. Men and large-boned, muscular women should use the higher end of the weight range to find their healthy body weights.

Body Mass Index

Another method for interpreting body weight is the BMI. The BMI expresses the correlation of an individual's weight to his or her height. Except for trained athletes, the BMI strongly correlates with total body fat content in adults. This provides an indication of the risk of developing chronic health conditions associated with obesity. Many health experts believe that the BMI is a more accurate standard for interpreting body weight than height and weight tables.

Method for Calculating BMI

a. Use the following website to have your BMI calculated automatically: www.cdc.gov/nccdphp/dnpa/bmi
b. Use the following steps to calculate your BMI:
  1. Multiply your weight in pounds (without clothes or shoes) by 703. For an individual who weighs 135 lb:

$$135 \times 703 = 94{,}905$$

  2. Divide this number by your height in inches. If this individual is 66 inches tall:

$$94{,}905 \div 66 = 1438$$

  3. Divide this amount again by your height in inches, and round off to the nearest whole number:

$$1438 \div 66 = 21.79, \text{ or } 22$$

The BMI of this individual is 22.

Interpretation of the BMI

In June 1998, the National Heart, Lung, and Blood Institute (NHLBI), a federal health agency, issued a set of guidelines for the classification of body weight in adults. One of these guidelines relates to the interpretation of the BMI, as is outlined here.

BMI	Interpretation
Below 18.5	Underweight
18.5-24.9	Healthy weight
25-29.9	Overweight
30-39.9	Obesity
40 or more	Morbid obesity

The NHLBI recommends that the BMI be determined in all adults. People of normal weight should have their BMI reassessed every 2 years.

Adult Obesity

The incidence of obesity in the United States has increased markedly, and obesity is now one of the most common problems encountered by primary care physicians. According to a report released by the U.S. Surgeon General's office, more than 61% of Americans are overweight, and 30% of them, or 93 million Americans, are obese. That number is predicted to increase to 120 million in 5 years. Obesity is associated with premature death and, after smoking, is the second leading cause of preventable death in the United States today. Approximately 300,000 deaths in the United States each year are associated with obesity.

It has been determined that as the BMI increases to greater than 25, there is an increased risk of developing certain diseases associated with overweight and obesity, including:

- Hypertension
- Cardiovascular disease
- Dyslipidemia (high blood cholesterol levels, high blood triglyceride levels, or both)
- Type 2 diabetes
- Colon cancer
- Gallbladder disease
- Breast and endometrial cancer
- Sleep apnea and respiratory problems
- Osteoarthritis

Obesity is considered a chronic condition that requires a multiple treatment approach including a behavioral therapy program, low-calorie diet, and suitable aerobic exercise program. Primary care physicians often manage individuals with mild and moderate obesity, but morbidly obese patients are usually referred to a bariatric specialist. **Bariatrics** is the branch of medicine that deals with the treatment and control of obesity and diseases associated with obesity. ∎

PROCEDURE 20-1   Measuring Weight and Height

Outcome Measure weight and height.

Equipment Supplies

- Upright balance scale

Weight

1. **Procedural Step.** Sanitize your hands.
2. **Procedural Step.** Check the scale to ensure it is balanced as follows:

   a. Make sure the upper and lower weights are on zero. When the weights are on zero, they are all the way to the left of the calibration bars.

   b. Look at the indicator point. If the scale is balanced, the indicator point is resting in the center of the balance area.

   c. If the indicator point rests below the center, adjust the screw on the balance knob by turning it clockwise (to the right) until the indicator point rests in the center of the balance area.

   d. If the indicator point rests above the center, adjust the screw on the balance knob by turning it counterclockwise (to the left) until the indicator point rests in the center of the balance area.

Ensure that the upper and lower weights are on zero. (From Bonewit-West K: *Clinical procedures for medical assistants,* ed 7, St. Louis, 2008, Saunders.)

Correct the balance by adjusting the screw on the balance knob. (From Bonewit-West K: *Clinical procedures for medical assistants,* ed 7, St. Louis, 2008, Saunders.)

Principle. If the scale is not balanced, the weight measurement will be inaccurate.

3. **Procedural Step.** Greet the patient and introduce yourself.
4. **Procedural Step.** Identify the patient and explain to the patient that you will be measuring his or her height and weight.
5. **Procedural Step.** Instruct the patient to remove shoes and outer clothing such as a jacket or sweater. A good medical aseptic practice is to place a paper towel on the platform of the scale to protect the patient's feet.
   Principle. Removing heavy clothing and shoes allows a more accurate measurement of the patient's weight.
6. **Procedural Step.** Assist the patient onto the scale, and instruct the patient not to move.
   Principle. It is not possible to balance the scale if the patient is moving.
7. **Procedural Step.** Balance the scale as follows:

   a. Move the lower weight to the notched groove that does not cause the indicator point to drop to the bottom of the calibration area. Ensure that the lower weight is seated firmly in its groove.

   b. Slide the upper weight slowly along its calibration bar by tapping it gently until the indicator point comes to a rest at the center of the balance area.

   Principle. Not seating the lower weight firmly in its groove results in an inaccurate reading.

Slide the upper weight by tapping it gently. (From Bonewit-West K: *Clinical procedures for medical assistants,* ed 7, St. Louis, 2008, Saunders.)

8. **Procedural Step.** Read the results to the nearest quarter pound by adding the measurement on the lower scale to the measurement on the upper scale. Jot down this value or make a mental note of it.
9. **Procedural Step.** Ask the patient to step off of the scale platform. Provide assistance if needed.

Height

1. Procedural Step. Slide the movable calibration rod upward until the measuring bar is well above the patient's apparent height. Open the measuring bar to its horizontal position.

Slide the bar upward until it is well above the patient's height. (From Bonewit-West K: *Clinical procedures for medical assistants,* ed 7, St. Louis, 2008, Saunders.)

2. Procedural Step. Instruct the patient to step onto the scale platform with his or her back to the scale. Provide assistance if needed. Instruct the patient to stand erect and look straight ahead.
Principle. Looking straight ahead helps the patient to stand erect and balanced, which ensures an accurate measurement.

3. Procedural Step. Carefully lower the measuring bar (keeping it horizontal) until it rests gently on top of the patient's head with the hair compressed. The measuring bar should form a 90-degree angle with the calibration rod.
Principle. The measuring bar must be at a 90-degree angle to ensure an accurate height measurement.

4. Procedural Step. Keeping the measuring bar in a horizontal position, instruct the patient to step down and put on his or her shoes. Hold the bar in a horizontal position until the patient has stepped off the scale.

5. Procedural Step. Read the height measurement from the top down to the nearest quarter-inch marking at the junction of the stationary calibration rod and the movable calibration rod. (*Note:* If the patient's height is less than the top value of the stationary rod, read the measurement from the bottom up directly on the stationary calibration rod.) Jot down this value or make a mental note of it.

6. Procedural Step. Return the measuring bar to its vertical (resting) position, and slide the movable calibration rod to its lowest position. Return the weights to zero.

Lower the bar until it rests on top of the patient's head. (From Bonewit-West K: *Clinical procedures for medical assistants,* ed 7, St. Louis, 2008, Saunders.)

Read the measurement to the nearest quarter-inch marking. (From Bonewit-West K: *Clinical procedures for medical assistants,* ed 7, St. Louis, 2008, Saunders.)

7. Procedural Step. Sanitize your hands, and chart the results. Include the date and time and the patient's weight and height measurements. The weight should be charted in pounds to the nearest quarter pound, and the height should be charted in feet and inches to the nearest quarter inch.

CHARTING EXAMPLE

Date	
11/5/10	10:15 a.m. Wt: 155. Ht: 5' 6¹/₄" _____
	_____ Hope Fauber, CMA (AAMA)

PROCEDURE 20-1

PROCEDURE 20-2

POSITIONING AND DRAPING

Correct positioning of the patient facilitates the examination by permitting better access to the part being examined or treated. The basic positions used in the medical office are sitting, supine, prone, dorsal recumbent, lithotomy, Sims, knee-chest, and Fowler's.

The position used depends on the type of examination or procedure to be performed. More than one position may be used to examine the same body part during the physical examination. The sitting and supine positions are both used to examine the chest. It is important to know the correct position for each examination or treatment. When positioning a patient, the medical assistant should explain the position to the patient and assist the patient in attaining it.

It is important to take the patient's endurance and degree of wellness into consideration when positioning a patient. Patients who are weak or ill may be unable to assume a position or may require special assistance in attaining it. Some positions, such as the lithotomy and knee-chest positions, are embarrassing and uncomfortable. A patient should not be kept in these positions any longer than necessary. Some patients (especially elderly ones) become dizzy after a time in certain positions, such as the knee-chest position. These patients should be allowed to rest before they get off the examining table. The medical assistant should also assist patients off the examining table to prevent falls.

The patient is draped during positioning to provide for modesty, comfort, and warmth. Only the part to be examined should be exposed. Patient gowns and drapes used in the medical office are usually made of paper but also may be made of cloth. Procedures 20-2 through 20-9 present proper positioning and draping of the patient.

Text continued on p. 397

Memories *from* Externship

Hope Fauber: During my externship at a student health center at a 4-year college, I was responsible for working up patients for gynecologic examinations. The two-piece drapes had the top opening in the front and the bottom opening in the back. After explaining this to an Asian student who spoke very little English, I noticed that she had the openings opposite of what I had explained. I explained again, with words and gestures, that she needed to reverse the openings. To my surprise, she stood up, turned around in a circle, and sat down! ■

Prepare for Success

 PROCEDURE 20-2   Sitting Position

Outcome Position and drape a patient in the sitting position. The sitting position is used to examine the head, neck, chest, and upper extremities and to measure vital signs.

Equipment/Supplies

- Examining table
- Disposable patient gown
- Disposable patient drape

1. **Procedural Step.** Sanitize your hands. Greet the patient and introduce yourself.
2. **Procedural Step.** Identify the patient and explain the type of examination or procedure that will be performed.
3. **Procedural Step.** Provide the patient with a patient gown. Instruct the patient to remove clothing as appropriate for the type of examination being performed and to put on the patient gown with the opening in front. The disrobing facility should provide privacy, a place to sit, and a place to hang clothing.
4. **Procedural Step.** Pull out the footrest of the examining table, and assist the patient into a sitting position. The patient's buttocks and thighs should be firmly supported on the edge of the table.

Sitting position. (From Bonewit-West K: *Clinical procedures for medical assistants,* ed 7, St. Louis, 2008, Saunders.)

5. Procedural Step. Place a drape over the patient's thighs and legs to provide warmth and modesty.

6. Procedural Step. After completion of the examination, assist the patient down from the table. Return the footrest to its normal position. Instruct the patient to get dressed. Discard the gown and drape in a waste container.

Place the drape over the patient's thighs and legs. (From Bonewit-West K: *Clinical procedures for medical assistants,* ed 7, St. Louis, 2008, Saunders.)

PROCEDURE 20-3   Supine Position

Outcome Position and drape a patient in the supine position. The supine position is used to examine the head, chest, abdomen, and extremities.

Equipment/Supplies

- Examining table
- Disposable patient gown
- Disposable patient drape

1. Procedural Step. Sanitize your hands. Greet the patient and introduce yourself.

2. Procedural Step. Identify the patient and explain the type of examination or procedure that will be performed.

3. Procedural Step. Provide the patient with a patient gown. Instruct the patient to remove clothing as appropriate for the type of examination being performed and to put on the patient gown with the opening in front. The disrobing facility should provide privacy, a place to sit, and a place to hang clothing.

4. Procedural Step. Pull out the footrest of the examining table, and assist the patient into a sitting position. Place a drape over the patient's thighs and legs.

5. Procedural Step. Ask the patient to move back on the table. As the patient is doing this, pull out the table extension while supporting the patient's lower legs.

Pull out the table extension while supporting the patient's legs. (From Bonewit-West K: *Clinical procedures for medical assistants,* ed 7, St. Louis, 2008, Saunders.)

Continued

PROCEDURE 20-3

PROCEDURE 20-3   Supine Position—cont'd

6. Procedural Step. Ask the patient to lie on his or her back with the legs together. Provide assistance if needed. The patient's arms may be placed above the head or alongside the body.

Position the patient on the back with the legs together. (From Bonewit-West K: *Clinical procedures for medical assistants,* ed 7, St. Louis, 2008, Saunders.)

7. Procedural Step. Position the drape lengthwise over the patient to provide warmth and modesty. As the physician examines the patient, move the drape according to the body parts being examined.

Place a drape lengthwise over the patient. (From Bonewit-West K: *Clinical procedures for medical assistants,* ed 7, St. Louis, 2008, Saunders.)

8. Procedural Step. After completion of the examination, assist the patient into a sitting position. Slide the table extension back into place while supporting the patient's lower legs.

9. Procedural Step. Assist the patient down from the table. Instruct the patient to get dressed. Return the footrest to its normal position. Discard the gown and drape in a waste container.

PROCEDURE 20-4   Prone Position

Outcome Position and drape a patient in the prone position. The prone position is used to examine the back and assess extension of the hip joint.

Equipment/Supplies

- Examining table
- Disposable patient gown
- Disposable patient drape

1. Procedural Step. Sanitize your hands. Greet the patient and introduce yourself.

2. Procedural Step. Identify the patient and explain the type of examination or procedure that will be performed.

3. Procedural Step. Provide the patient with a patient gown. Instruct the patient to remove clothing as

appropriate for the type of examination being performed and to put on the patient gown with the opening in back. The disrobing facility should provide privacy, a place to sit, and a place to hang clothing.

4. Procedural Step. Pull out the footrest of the examining table, and assist the patient into a sitting position. Place a drape over the patient's thighs and legs.

5. Procedural Step. Ask the patient to move back on the table. As the patient is doing this, pull out the table extension while supporting the patient's lower legs.

6. Procedural Step. Ask the patient to lie on his or her back. Provide assistance if needed. Position the drape lengthwise over the patient.

7. Procedural Step. Ask the patient to turn onto his or her stomach by rolling toward you. Provide assistance for this step by helping her turn and adjusting the drape to provide modesty.

Principle. This step prevents the patient from accidentally rolling off the table.

8. Procedural Step. Position the patient with the legs together and the head turned to one side. The arms can be placed above the head or alongside the body.

Position the patient's legs together with the head turned to one side. (From Bonewit-West K: *Clinical procedures for medical assistants,* ed 7, St. Louis, 2008, Saunders.)

9. Procedural Step. Adjust the drape as needed so that it is positioned lengthwise over the patient to provide warmth and modesty. As the physician examines the patient, move the drape according to the body parts being examined.

Place a drape lengthwise over the patient. (From Bonewit-West K: *Clinical procedures for medical assistants,* ed 7, St. Louis, 2008, Saunders.)

10. Procedural Step. After completion of the examination, ask the patient to turn back over by rolling toward you. Assist the patient into a supine position and then into a sitting position. Slide the table extension back into place while supporting the patient's lower legs.

11. Procedural Step. Assist the patient down from the table. Return the footrest to its normal position. Instruct the patient to get dressed. Discard the gown and drape in a waste container.

PROCEDURE 20-5   Dorsal Recumbent Position

Outcome Position and drape a patient in the dorsal recumbent position. The dorsal recumbent position is used to perform vaginal and rectal examinations, insert a urinary catheter, and examine the head, neck, chest, and extremities of patients who have difficulty maintaining the supine position. The supine position is an uncomfortable position for patients with respiratory problems, back injury, or lower back pain. Bending the legs (rather than lying flat) is more comfortable for these patients and is easier to maintain.

Equipment/Supplies

- Examining table
- Disposable patient gown
- Disposable patient drape

1. Procedural Step. Sanitize your hands. Greet the patient and introduce yourself.

2. Procedural Step. Identify the patient and explain the type of examination or procedure that will be performed.

3. Procedural Step. Provide the patient with a patient gown. Instruct the patient to remove clothing as

appropriate for the type of examination being performed and to put on the patient gown with the opening in front. The disrobing facility should provide privacy, a place to sit, and a place to hang clothing.

4. Procedural Step. Pull out the footrest of the examining table, and assist the patient into a sitting position. Place a drape over the patient's thighs and legs.

Continued

PROCEDURE 20-5   Dorsal Recumbent Position—cont'd

5. Procedural Step. Ask the patient to move back on the table. As the patient is doing this, pull out the table extension while supporting the patient's lower legs.

6. Procedural Step. Ask the patient to lie on her back. Provide assistance if needed. The arms can be placed above the head or alongside the body. Position the drape diagonally over the patient.

7. Procedural Step. Ask the patient to bend the knees and place each foot at the edge of the examining table with the soles of the feet flat on the table. Provide assistance during this step. Push in the table extension and the footrest.

Ask the patient to bend the knees and place each foot at the edge of the examining table. (From Bonewit-West K: *Clinical procedures for medical assistants*, ed 7, St. Louis, 2008, Saunders.)

8. Procedural Step. Adjust the drape as needed to provide the patient with warmth and modesty. The drape should be positioned diagonally, with one corner over the patient's chest and the opposite corner falling between the patient's legs and completely covering the pubic area.

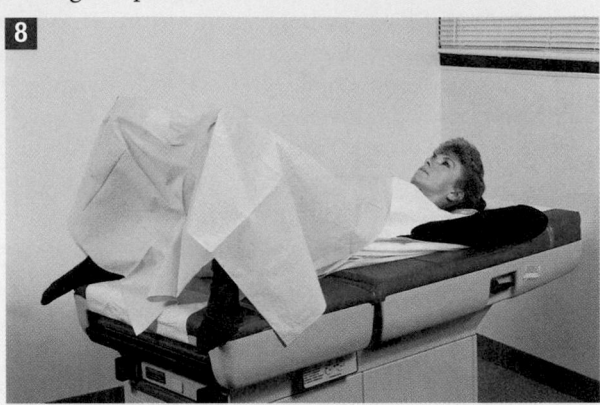

Place a drape diagonally over the patient. (From Bonewit-West K: *Clinical procedures for medical assistants*, ed 7, St. Louis, 2008, Saunders.)

9. Procedural Step. When the physician is ready to examine the genital area, the center corner of the drape is folded back over the abdomen.

10. Procedural Step. After completion of the examination, pull out the footrest and the table extension. Assist the patient into a supine position and then into a sitting position. Slide the table extension back into place while supporting the patient's lower legs.

11. Procedural Step. Assist the patient down from the table. Return the footrest to its normal position. Instruct the patient to get dressed. Discard the gown and drape in a waste container.

PROCEDURE 20-6   Lithotomy Position

Outcome Position and drape a patient in the lithotomy position. The lithotomy position is used for vaginal, pelvic, and rectal examinations. The lithotomy position is the same as the dorsal recumbent position except that the patient's feet are placed in stirrups. The lithotomy position provides maximal exposure to the genital area and facilitates insertion of a vaginal **speculum.** Because this is an uncomfortable position for the patient to maintain, the patient should not be put into this position until just before the examination.

Equipment/Supplies

- Examining table
- Disposable patient gown
- Disposable patient drape

1. Procedural Step. Sanitize your hands. Greet the patient and introduce yourself.

2. Procedural Step. Identify the patient and explain the type of examination or procedure that will be performed.

3. Procedural Step. Provide the patient with a patient gown. Instruct the patient to remove clothing as appropriate for the type of examination being performed and put on the patient gown with the opening in front. If the patient is wearing socks, tell her that she may keep them on during the procedure. The disrobing facility should provide privacy, a place to sit, and a place to hang clothing.

Principle. Socks help to keep the patient's feet warm after they are placed in the metal stirrups.

4. **Procedural Step.** Some medical offices use disposable stirrup covers. If this is the case, apply a cover to each stirrup. Pull out the footrest of the examining table, and assist the patient into a sitting position. Place a drape over the patient's thighs and legs.

Principle. Stirrup covers provide a soft, warm, nonslip surface for the patient's feet.

5. **Procedural Step.** When the physician is ready to examine the patient, ask the patient to move back on the table. As the patient is doing this, pull out the table extension while supporting the patient's lower legs.

6. **Procedural Step.** Ask the patient to lie on the back. Provide assistance if needed. The arms can be placed above the head or alongside the body.

7. **Procedural Step.** Position the drape over the patient to provide warmth and modesty. The drape should be positioned diagonally with one corner over the patient's chest and the opposite corner between the patient's feet.

8. **Procedural Step.** Pull out the stirrups and position them at an angle. Position the stirrups so that they are level with the examining table and pulled out approximately 1 foot from the edge of the table. Check to make sure the stirrups are not too far apart or too close together. Lock the stirrups into place.

Principle. If the stirrups are too far apart, it is uncomfortable for the patient. If the stirrups are too close together, the patient will be unable to move her buttocks to the edge of the table as needed for the examination.

9. **Procedural Step.** Ask the patient to bend the knees and place each foot, one at a time, into a stirrup. Provide assistance during this step. Push in the table extension and the footrest.

10. **Procedural Step.** Instruct the patient to slide the buttocks all the way down to the edge of the examining table and let her legs fall apart as far as is comfortable.

11. **Procedural Step.** Reposition the drape as needed so that one corner is over the patient's chest and the opposite corner falls between the patient's legs and completely covers the perineal area. When the physician is ready to examine the genital area, the center corner of the drape is pulled up and folded back over the knees.

Ask the patient to slide the buttocks to the edge of the table and to rotate the thighs outward. (From Bonewit-West K: *Clinical procedures for medical assistants,* ed 7, St. Louis, 2008, Saunders.)

Position the drape diagonally. (From Bonewit-West K: *Clinical procedures for medical assistants,* ed 7, St. Louis, 2008, Saunders.)

12. **Procedural Step.** After completion of the examination, pull out the footrest and table extension. Ask the patient to slide the buttocks back from the end of the table. Lift the patient's legs out of the stirrups at the same time, and place them on the table extension (supine position). Remove the stirrup covers and discard them in a waste container. Return the stirrups to their normal position. Assist the patient into a sitting position. Slide the table extension back into place while supporting the patient's lower legs.

Principle. Lifting both the patient's legs out of the stirrups at the same time avoids strain on the back and abdominal muscles.

13. **Procedural Step.** Assist the patient down from the table. Return the footrest to its normal position. Instruct the patient to get dressed. Discard the gown and drape in a waste container.

PROCEDURE 20-6

PROCEDURE **20-7**   Sims Position

Outcome Position and drape a patient in the Sims position. This position, also known as the *left lateral position*, is used to examine the vagina and rectum, measure rectal temperature, perform a flexible sigmoidoscopy, and administer an enema.

Equipment/Supplies

- Examining table
- Disposable patient gown
- Disposable patient drape

1. **Procedural Step.** Sanitize your hands. Greet the patient and introduce yourself.
2. **Procedural Step.** Identify the patient and explain the type of examination or procedure that will be performed.
3. **Procedural Step.** Provide the patient with a patient gown. Instruct the patient to remove clothing from the waist down and put on the patient gown with the opening in back. The disrobing facility should provide privacy, a place to sit, and a place to hang clothing.
4. **Procedural Step.** Pull out the footrest of the examining table, and assist the patient into a sitting position. Place a drape over the patient's thighs and legs.
5. **Procedural Step.** Ask the patient to move back on the table. As the patient is doing this, pull out the table extension while supporting the patient's lower legs.
6. **Procedural Step.** Ask the patient to lie on his or her back. Provide assistance if needed.
7. **Procedural Step.** Position the drape lengthwise over the patient to provide warmth and modesty.
8. **Procedural Step.** Ask the patient to turn onto the left side. Provide assistance during this step to prevent the

patient from accidentally rolling off the table and adjust the drape to provide modesty. The patient's left arm should be positioned behind the body and the right arm forward with the elbow bent. Assist the patient in flexing the legs. The right leg is flexed sharply, and the left leg is flexed slightly.

9. **Procedural Step.** Adjust the drape as needed. When the physician is ready to examine the patient, a small portion of the drape is folded back to expose the anal area.

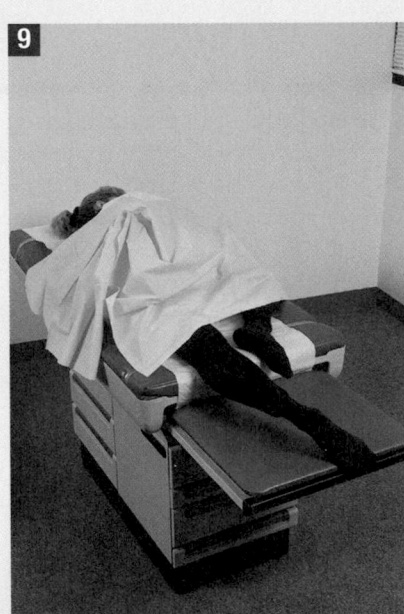

Adjust the drape as needed. (From Bonewit-West K: *Clinical procedures for medical assistants,* ed 7, St. Louis, 2008, Saunders.)

10. **Procedural Step.** After completion of the examination, assist the patient into a supine position and into a sitting position. Slide the table extension back into place while supporting the patient's lower legs.
11. **Procedural Step.** Assist the patient down from the table. Return the footrest to its normal position. Instruct the patient to get dressed. Discard the gown and drape in a waste container.

The right leg is flexed sharply, and the left leg is flexed slightly. (From Bonewit-West K: *Clinical procedures for medical assistants,* ed 7, St. Louis, 2008, Saunders.)

PROCEDURE 20-8   Knee-Chest Position

Outcome Position and drape a patient in the knee-chest position. The knee-chest position is used to examine the rectum and perform a proctoscopic examination because it provides maximal exposure to the rectal area. This is a difficult position to maintain; the patient should not be put into this position until just before the examination.

Equipment/Supplies

- Examining table
- Disposable patient gown
- Disposable patient drape

1. **Procedural Step.** Sanitize your hands. Greet the patient and introduce yourself.
2. **Procedural Step.** Identify the patient and explain the type of examination or procedure that will be performed.
3. **Procedural Step.** Provide the patient with a patient gown. Instruct the patient to remove clothing from the waist down and put on the gown with the opening in back. The disrobing facility should provide privacy, a place to sit, and a place to hang clothing.
4. **Procedural Step.** Pull out the footrest of the examining table, and assist the patient into a sitting position. Place a drape over the patient's thighs and legs.
5. **Procedural Step.** Ask the patient to move back on the table. As the patient is doing this, pull out the table extension while supporting the patient's lower legs.
6. **Procedural Step.** Assist the patient into the supine position and then into the prone position, making sure to have the patient roll toward you. Position the drape diagonally over the patient to provide warmth and modesty.
7. **Procedural Step.** Ask the patient to bend the arms at the elbows and rest them alongside the head. Ask the patient to elevate the buttocks while keeping the back straight. The patient's head should be turned to one side, and the weight of the body should be supported by the chest. A pillow under the chest can give

The buttocks are elevated, and the head is turned to one side. (From Bonewit-West K: *Clinical procedures for medical assistants,* ed 7, St. Louis, 2008, Saunders.)

additional support and aid relaxation. The knees and lower legs are separated approximately 12 inches.
8. **Procedural Step.** Adjust the drape diagonally as needed with one corner over the patient's back and the opposite corner over the buttocks and falling between the patient's legs. When the physician is ready to examine the patient, a small portion of the drape is folded back to expose the anal area.

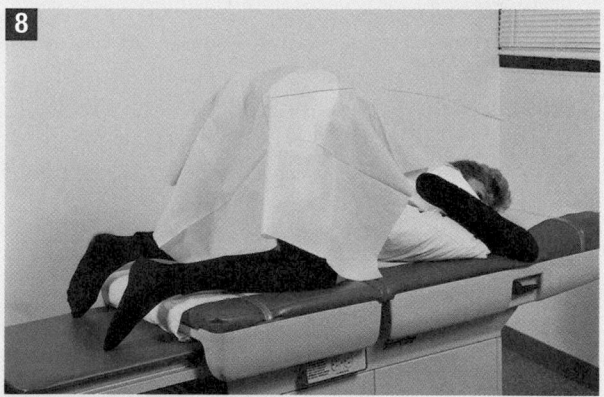

Position the drape diagonally. (From Bonewit-West K: *Clinical procedures for medical assistants,* ed 7, St. Louis, 2008, Saunders.)

9. **Procedural Step.** After completion of the examination, assist the patient into a prone position and then into a supine position. Allow the patient to rest in the supine position before he or she sits up.
   Principle. Patients (especially elderly ones) frequently become dizzy after being in the knee-chest position and should be allowed to rest before they sit up.
10. **Procedural Step.** Assist the patient into a sitting position. Slide the table extension back into place while supporting the patient's lower legs.
11. **Procedural Step.** Assist the patient down from the table. Return the footrest to its normal position. Instruct the patient to get dressed. Discard the gown and drape in a waste container.

PROCEDURE 20-8

PROCEDURE 20-9 Fowler's Position

Outcome Position and drape a patient in the Fowler's position. Fowler's position is used to examine the upper body of patients with cardiovascular and respiratory problems, such as congestive heart failure, emphysema, and asthma. These patients find it easier to breathe in this position than in a sitting or supine position. This position is also used to draw blood from patients who are likely to faint.

Equipment/Supplies

- Examining table
- Disposable patient gown
- Disposable patient drape

1. **Procedural Step.** Sanitize your hands. Greet the patient and introduce yourself.
2. **Procedural Step.** Identify the patient and explain the type of examination or procedure that will be performed.
3. **Procedural Step.** Provide the patient with a patient gown. Instruct the patient to remove clothing as appropriate for the type of examination being performed and to put on the patient gown with the opening in front. The disrobing facility should provide privacy, a place to sit, and a place to hang clothing.
4. **Procedural Step.** Position the head of the table as follows:
   a. For a semi-Fowler's position, the table should be positioned at a 45-degree angle.
   b. For a full Fowler's position, the table should be positioned at a 90-degree angle.

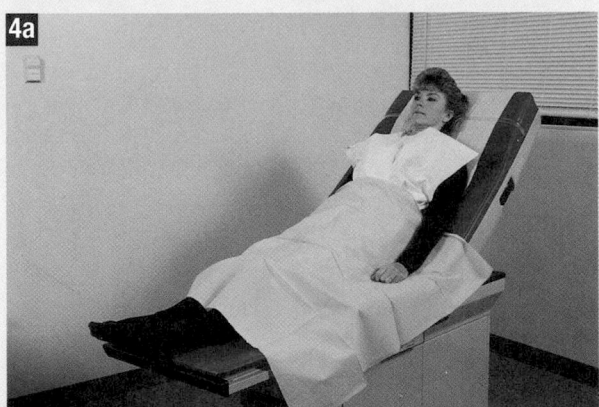

Position the table at a 45-degree angle for a semi-Fowler's position. (From Bonewit-West K: *Clinical procedures for medical assistants,* ed 7, St. Louis, 2008, Saunders.)

5. **Procedural Step.** Pull out the footrest of the examining table, and assist the patient into a sitting position. Place a drape over the patient's thighs and legs.

6. **Procedural Step.** Pull out the table extension while supporting the patient's lower legs. Ask the patient to lean back against the table head. Provide assistance during this step.

Ask the patient to lean back against the table head. (From Bonewit-West K: *Clinical procedures for medical assistants,* ed 7, St. Louis, 2008, Saunders.)

7. **Procedural Step.** Position the drape lengthwise over the patient to provide warmth and modesty. As the physician examines the patient, move the drape according to the body parts being examined.
8. **Procedural Step.** After completion of the examination, assist the patient into a sitting position. Slide the table extension back into place while supporting the patient's lower legs.
9. **Procedural Step.** Assist the patient down from the table. Instruct the patient to get dressed. Return the head of the table and the footrest to their normal positions. Discard the gown and drape in a waste container.

PROCEDURE 20-9

ASSESSMENT OF THE PATIENT

The extent of patient assessment during the physical examination depends on the purpose of the examination and the patient's condition. A complete physical examination involves a thorough assessment of all the body systems. Table 20-2 outlines the specific assessments included in a complete physical examination. The physician uses an organized and systematic approach in performing a physical examination, starting with the patient's head and proceeding toward the feet. Using this type of approach facilitates the examination process and requires the fewest position changes by the patient. The physician notes the results of the physical examination in the patient's medical record. Figure 20-6 is an example of a preprinted form for this purpose.

Patients who exhibit symptoms of illness usually require only selected portions of the physical examination. A patient who comes to the medical office with the symptoms of bronchitis usually does not require a complete physical examination; rather, the physician examines the body system that is most likely to be associated with the symptoms. Four assessment techniques are used to obtain information during the physical examination: inspection, palpation, percussion, and auscultation.

Inspection

Inspection involves observation of the patient for any signs of disease, and of the four assessment techniques, it is the one most frequently used. Good lighting, either natural or artificial, is important for effective observation. The patient's color, speech, deformities, skin condition (e.g., rashes, scars, warts), body contour and symmetry, orientation to the surroundings, body movements, and anxiety level are assessed through inspection. The medical assistant should develop a high level of detailed observational skills to assist the physician in assessing physical characteristics.

Palpation

Palpation is the examination of the body using the sense of touch (Figure 20-7). The physician uses palpation to determine the placement and size of organs, the presence of lumps, and the existence of pain, swelling, or tenderness. Examining the breasts and taking the pulse are performed by palpation. Palpation often helps verify data obtained by inspection. The patient's verbal and facial expressions are also observed during palpation to assist in the detection of abnormalities.

The two types of palpation, light and deep, are categorized by the amount of pressure applied. *Light palpation* of structures is performed to determine areas of tenderness. The fingertips are placed on the part to be examined and are gently depressed approximately one-half inch. *Deep palpation* is used to examine the condition of organs such as those in the abdomen. Two hands are used for deep palpation. One hand is used to support the body from below, and the other hand is used to press over the area to be palpated. Deep palpation is used by the physician to perform a bimanual pelvic examination.

Text continued on p. 402

Table 20-2 Physician Assessment during the Physical Examination			
Body Structure	**Assessment**	**Normal Findings**	**Abnormal Findings**
General appearance	Observation of body build, posture, gait	Good posture and balance Steady gait	Poor posture or balance Unsteady, irregular, or staggering gait
	Determination of weight and height	Weight within ideal range	Patient is overweight or underweight
	Observation of hygiene and grooming	Good hygiene and grooming	Poor hygiene and grooming
	Observation for signs of illness	No signs of illness	Obvious signs of illness
	Observation of attitude, emotional state, mood	Patient speaks clearly and is cooperative	Patient is uncooperative, withdrawn, incoherent, negative, or hostile
Skin	Inspection of skin for color, vascularity, lesions	Smooth, supple, free of blemishes No unusual color	Blisters, wounds, lesions, rashes, swelling Unusual skin color (e.g., flushing, cyanosis, jaundice, pallor)
	Palpation of temperature, moisture, turgor, texture	Warm to touch	Rough, dry, flaky skin Poor skin turgor

Continued

Table 20-2 Physician Assessment during the Physical Examination—cont'd

Body Structure	Assessment	Normal Findings	Abnormal Findings
Head and neck	Inspection of size, shape, contour of head	Round head with prominences in front and back	Head is asymmetric or of unusual size
	Inspection of hair and scalp	Hair is resilient, evenly distributed, and not excessively dry or oily	Loss of hair Scaliness or dryness of scalp Presence of lice or other parasites
	Palpation of head and neck	No lumps, swelling, tenderness, or lesions of head or neck	Lumps, swelling, tenderness, or lesions of head or neck
Eyes	Evaluation of visual acuity and color vision	Good visual ability with or without glasses or contact lenses Appropriate color perception	Poor visual acuity or blindness Color blindness
	Evaluation of visual field	No visual field loss	Gaps in field of vision
	Inspection of eyelids and eyeballs	Eyes are bright	Dull or glossy eyes
	Inspection of conjunctiva	Pink mucous membranes	Inflamed mucous membranes Excessive tearing Drainage from eyes
	Inspection of eye movements	Eyes move equally in all directions	Drooping eyelids Uncoordinated eye movements
	Tests for pupillary reaction using penlight	Pupils are black, are equal in size, react appropriately to light	Dilated, constricted, or unequal pupils
	Inspection of internal eye structures using ophthalmoscope	Reddish-pink retina, even caliber, intact retinal blood vessels	Cloudy lens or narrowed blood vessels
Ears	Test for hearing using tuning fork or **audiometer**	Good hearing ability	Limited hearing or deafness
	Inspection of size, shape, symmetry of ears	Ears are symmetric and proportionate to head	Ears are asymmetric and not proportionate to the head
	Inspection of external ear canal and tympanic membrane using an otoscope	Cerumen is soft and easily removed No drainage or discomfort Skin of ear canal is intact, pink, warm, and slightly moist Tympanic membrane is pearly gray and semitransparent	Lesions, redness, or swelling of external ear canal Drainage from ear Pain when ear is moved Impacted cerumen Tympanic membrane is red, bulging, or perforated
Nose	Inspection of size, shape, symmetry of nose	Nose is symmetric, straight, not tender	Nose is asymmetric, deformed, flaring, or tender
	Inspection of nostrils using nasal speculum	Septum is intact and midline Nasal mucosa is moist and pink	Deviation or perforation of septum Redness, swelling, polyps, or discharge Nostrils are obstructed
	Test for sense of smell	Correct or very few incorrect responses to odors	Absent, decreased, exaggerated, or unequal responses to test substances
Mouth and pharynx	Inspection of lips for contour, color, texture	Pink, moist, soft, smooth lips	Pallor, cyanosis, blisters, swelling, cracking, excessive dryness of lips
	Inspection of mucosa	Pink, moist mucous membranes	Pale or dry mucosa with ulcers or abrasions

Table 20-2 Physician Assessment during the Physical Examination—cont'd

Body Structure	Assessment	Normal Findings	Abnormal Findings
Mouth and pharynx—cont'd	Inspection of gums and palate	Smooth, pink, moist, firm gums Hard palate is firm and white Soft palate is pink and cushiony	Gums are red, bleeding, swollen, tender, spongy, or receding
	Inspection of teeth	Smooth, white enamel; regularly spaced teeth or well-fitting dentures	Missing or loose teeth, dental caries, poor-fitting dentures
	Inspection of tongue	Moist, pink, slightly rough-surfaced tongue	Tongue is dry, furry, smooth, red, or ulcerated
	Inspection of pharynx	Pink and smooth pharynx Tonsils are pink and normal in size Gag reflex is present	Pharynx is red, swollen, or ulcerated Tonsils are red or swollen Absent gag reflex
Arms and hands	Inspection of hands and arms for general appearance	Firm, strong muscles Normal range of motion in joints	Muscle weakness, lack of control or coordination Restricted range of motion
	Palpation of arm muscles	Good muscle control and coordination	
	Palpation for tenderness or lumps	No tenderness or lumps	Tenderness or lumps of hands or arms
	Inspection of fingernails	Colorless nail plate with a convex curve Smooth nail texture	Indentation, infection, brittleness, thickening, or angulation of nails Cyanosis or pallor of nails
Chest and lungs	Inspection of size and shape of chest	Chest is symmetric	Abnormal chest contour
	Assessment of respiratory rate, rhythm, depth	Normal respiratory rate, rhythm, depth	Labored, slow, rapid, or irregular respirations
	Percussion of chest		
	Auscultation of breath sounds	Normal breath sounds No cough	Flat or dull lung sounds Noisy breath sounds Productive or nonproductive cough
	Palpation of ribs	No tenderness of ribs	Tenderness of ribs
Heart	Auscultation of heart sounds	Normal heart sounds	Irregular heartbeats or murmur
	Auscultation of apical pulse, rate, rhythm, volume	Regular, strong heartbeats	Rates slower or more rapid than normal
	Palpation of peripheral pulses	Palpable peripheral pulses	Weak or absent peripheral pulses
	Auscultation of blood pressure	Blood pressure within normal range for age	Low or high blood pressure
	Assessment of peripheral vascular perfusion	Skin is pink, resilient, moist Immediate return of color to nail beds	Cyanosis, pallor, edema Poor capillary filling in nail beds
	Electrocardiogram to assess heart function	Normal heart function	Abnormal electrocardiogram
Breasts	Inspection of size, symmetry, contour	Breasts are round, smooth, symmetric	Retraction, dimpling, redness, or swelling of breasts
	Inspection of nipple	Nipples are round and equal in size, are similar in color, appear soft and smooth Areola is round and pink	Bleeding, cracking, discharge, or inversion of nipples

Continued

Table 20-2 Physician Assessment during the Physical Examination—cont'd

Body Structure	Assessment	Normal Findings	Abnormal Findings
Breasts—cont'd	Palpation of breasts and axillary lymph nodes	No lumps or tenderness of breasts or axillary lymph nodes	Lumps or tenderness of breasts or axillary lymph nodes
Abdomen	Inspection of contour, symmetry, skin condition, integrity	Symmetric contour Unblemished skin Soft abdomen	Asymmetric contour Rash or other skin lesions Abdominal distention
	Auscultation of bowel sounds	Active bowel sounds	Increased, diminished, or absent bowel sounds
	Percussion to assess underlying organs Palpation of underlying organs, tenderness, lumps	Normal position and size of liver and spleen	Tenderness or lumps Enlarged liver or spleen
Genitalia and rectum	*Male* Inspection of penis and urethra	Penis is smooth	Ulceration or discharge from penis
	Inspection of scrotum and palpation of testes	Testicles are smooth, firm, and movable within scrotal sac Scrotum is symmetric	Lumps or tenderness of scrotum, testes, or prostate gland
	Palpation of rectum and prostate gland	Increased pigmentation in anal area Good anal sphincter tone	Enlarged prostate gland Hemorrhoids or relaxed anal sphincter
	Stool specimen to test for occult blood	Absence of occult blood in stool	Occult blood in stool
	Female Inspection of external genitalia	External genitalia are smooth and without lesions	Ulceration or redness or swelling of external genitalia
	Inspection of vagina and cervix using vaginal speculum	Vaginal mucosa is pink and moist Cervix is pink and smooth	Lacerations, tenderness, redness, or discharge from vagina or cervix
	Specimen collection from vagina and cervix for Pap test	Pap test is normal	Pap test is abnormal
	Bimanual pelvic examination	No tenderness or lumps of uterus and ovaries	Tenderness or lumps of uterus and ovaries
	Palpation of rectum	Good anal sphincter tone	Hemorrhoids or relaxed anal sphincter
	Stool specimen to test for occult blood	Increased pigmentation in anal area	Occult blood in stool
Lower extremities	Inspection of legs for general appearance and palpation of legs	Firm, strong muscles Normal range of motion in joints	Muscle weakness, lack of control or coordination Restricted range of motion Tenderness or lumps Limp or foot dragging during walking
	Inspection of toenails	Smooth nail texture	Indentation, infection, brittleness, thickening, or angulation of nails
Neurologic	Determination of mental status and level of consciousness	Alert and responds appropriately Oriented to person, place, and time	Responds inappropriately Disoriented
	Determination of sense of pain and touch	Normal response to pain and touch	Diminished or absent response to stimuli
	Use of percussion hammer to test reflexes	Normal reflexes	Abnormal or absent reflexes

From Bonewit-West K: *Clinical procedures for medical assistants*, ed 7, St. Louis, 2008, Saunders.

PHYSICAL EXAMINATION

INSTRUCTIONS:
(WNL) Within Normal Limits
(POS) Positive findings (X) Omitted

1. GENERAL

a. Posture _____
b. Gait _____
c. Speech _____
d. Appearance _____
e. Emotion _____

2. HEAD

a. Hair _____
b. Masses _____
c. Shape _____
d. Bruits _____
e. Tenderness _____
f. Sinus _____
g. Articulations _____

3. EYES

a. Lids R ___ L ___
b. Sclera R ___ L ___
c. Conjunctiva R ___ L ___
d. Muscles R ___ L ___
e. Cornea R ___ L ___
f. Pupils R ___ L ___
g. Fundi R ___ L ___
h. Light R ___ L ___
i. Bruits R ___ L ___
j. Accommodation R ___ L ___

4. EARS

a. Pinna R ___ L ___
b. Canal R ___ L ___
c. Drum R ___ L ___
d. Weber _____
e. Rinne _____

5. NOSE

a. Septum _____
b. Mucosa R ___ L ___
c. Obstruction ___

6. MOUTH/THROAT

a. Lips _____
b. Breath _____
c. Tongue _____
d. Pharynx _____
e. Tonsils _____
f. Teeth _____
g. Dentures _____
h. Caries _____
i. Larynx _____
j. Floor _____

7. NECK

a. Thyroid _____
b. Trachea _____
c. Veins _____
d. Nodes R ___ L ___
e. Bruits R ___ L ___
f. Carotid R ___ L ___

8. LUNGS

a. Chest _____
b. Symmetry _____
c. Diaphragm _____
d. Rubs _____
e. Bruits _____
f. Sounds _____
g. Fremitus _____

9. HEART

a. PMI _____
b. Rate _____
c. Rhythm _____
d. Thrill ___
e. Rub _____
f. Murmur _____
g. Palpation _____

10. BREASTS

a. Nodes R ___ L ___
b. Nipple R ___ L ___
c. Areolae R ___ L ___
d. Symmetry _____
e. Discharge _____

11. ABDOMEN

a. Sounds _____
b. Masses _____
c. Tenderness _____
d. Organs _____
e. Hernia R ___ L ___
f. Bruits R ___ L ___
g. Femoral R ___ L ___
h. Ing. nodes R ___ L ___

12. MUSCULOSKELETAL

a. Cervical _____
b. Thoracic _____
c. Lumbar _____
d. Sacral _____
e. Pelvic _____
f. Rib cage _____

13. FEMALE GENITALS

a. Labia _____
b. Bartholin gland _____
c. Urethra _____
d. Vagina _____
e. Cervix _____
f. Uterus _____
g. Adnexa _____
   R ___ L ___
h. Pap smear done _____

14. MALE GENITALS

a. Penis _____
b. Scrotum _____
c. Testicles _____
d. Discharge _____
e. Scars _____
f. Meatus _____
g. Epididymis _____

15. RECTAL

a. Masses _____
b. Anus _____
c. Sphincter _____
d. Prostate _____
e. Pilonidal _____
f. Fissure _____
g. Hemorrhoids _____
h. Sigmoid _____
   _____cm.
i. Mucosa _____
j. Other _____

16. SKIN

a. Scars _____
b. Marks _____
c. Texture _____
d. Sweat _____
e. Color _____
f. Ulcers _____

17. NEUROLOGICAL

	Strength*	Reflex**
a. Biceps	R ___ L ___	R ___ L ___
b. Triceps	R ___ L ___	R ___ L ___
c. Knee	R ___ L ___	R ___ L ___
d. Ankle	R ___ L ___	R ___ L ___

e. Romberg _____
f. Babinsky _____
g. Cranial N _____
h. Sensory _____
i. Coordination _____
j. Tremor _____
k. Vibratory _____

*When testing strength use grades:
Weak (W); Normal (N); Strong (S)

**When testing reflexes use:
Absent (A); Present (P); Brisk (B)

18. EXTREMITIES

a. Range of Motion
   Shoulder _____   Knee _____
   Elbow _____   Ankle _____
   Wrist _____   Hand _____
   Hip _____   Foot _____
      Phalanges _____

b. General UR ___ UL ___ LR ___ LL ___
c. Muscular UR ___ UL ___ LR ___ LL ___
d. Bruits UR ___ UL ___ LR ___ LL ___
e. Edema UR ___ UL ___ LR ___ LL ___
f. Varicosities UR ___ UL ___ LR ___ LL ___

Signature _____

Figure 20-6. A preprinted form for recording the results of the physical examination. (From Bonewit-West K: *Clinical procedures for medical assistants,* ed 7, St. Louis, 2008, Saunders.)

What Would You Do? What Would You *Not* Do?

Case Study 3

Ben-Yi Sun has brought his father, Chang-Yi Sun, to the medical office. Chang-Yi Sun is 76 years old and lives with Ben-Yi and his family. Because there is a large Asian population in the community, the medical office personnel have learned two things about the Asian culture: (1) They are brought up to respect elders, and elders are always considered first, and (2) Asians have a great respect for harmony. If they do not understand something, they may not admit it to avoid disrupting harmony. Ben-Yi Sun speaks very good English, but his father understands only a few words of English. Chang-Yi Sun has been diagnosed with hypertension, and he needs education about going on a low-sodium diet. He also needs instructions on taking his blood pressure at home and recording the results. ■

Figure 20-7. Palpation is the examination of the body using the sense of touch. (From Bonewit-West K: *Clinical procedures for medical assistants,* ed 7, St. Louis, 2008, Saunders.)

Percussion

Percussion involves tapping the patient with the fingers and listening to the sounds produced to determine the size, density, and location of organs. This technique is often used to examine the lungs and abdomen.

The fingertips are used to produce a sound vibration similar to that of tapping a drumstick on a drum. The non-dominant hand is placed directly on the area to be assessed, with the fingers slightly separated. The dominant hand is used to strike the joint of the middle finger placed on the patient to produce the sound vibration (Figure 20-8). Structures that are dense, such as the liver, spleen, and heart, produce a dull sound. Empty or air-filled structures, such as the lungs, produce a hollow sound. Any condition that changes the density of an organ or tissue, such as fluid in the lungs, would change the quality of the sound.

Auscultation

Auscultation is an examination technique that involves listening with a stethoscope to the sounds produced within the body. This technique is used to listen to the heart and lungs or to measure blood pressure. Environmental noise interferes with effective auscultation of body sounds and should be minimized. The diaphragm of the stethoscope chest piece is used to assess high-pitched sounds, such as lung and bowel sounds; the bell of the stethoscope chest piece is used to assess low-pitched sounds, such as those produced by the heart and vascular system. The chest piece should be cleaned with an antiseptic wipe and warmed with the hands before being placed on the patient.

ASSISTING THE PHYSICIAN

During the patient assessment, the medical assistant should assist the physician as required. This includes helping the patient change positions for the physician's examination of the different parts of the body, handing the physician instruments and supplies, and reassuring the patient to reduce apprehension. When the examination is completed, the medical assistant should assist the patient off the examining table and provide additional information if needed, such as scheduling a return visit or patient education to promote wellness. Procedure 20-10 describes the procedure for assisting with the physical examination.

Figure 20-8. Percussion involves tapping the patient with the fingers. **A,** The nondominant hand is placed directly on the area to be assessed, with the fingers slightly separated. **B,** The fingers of the dominant hand are used to strike the joint of the middle finger to produce a sound vibration. (From Bonewit-West K: *Clinical procedures for medical assistants,* ed 7, St. Louis, 2008, Saunders.)

PROCEDURE **20-10**   Assisting with the Physical Examination

Outcome Prepare the patient and assist with a physical examination.

Equipment/Supplies

- Examining table
- Equipment for the type of examination to be performed

1. **Procedural Step.** Prepare the examining room. Ensure that the room is clean, free of clutter, and well lit and that the room temperature is comfortable for the patient.
2. **Procedural Step.** Sanitize your hands.
3. **Procedural Step.** Assemble the equipment according to the type of examination to be performed and the physician's preference. Arrange the instruments and supplies in a neat and orderly manner on a table or tray. Do not allow one item to lie on top of another.
4. **Procedural Step.** Obtain the patient's medical record. Go to the waiting room and ask the patient to come back to the examining room.
5. **Procedural Step.** Escort the patient to the examining room.

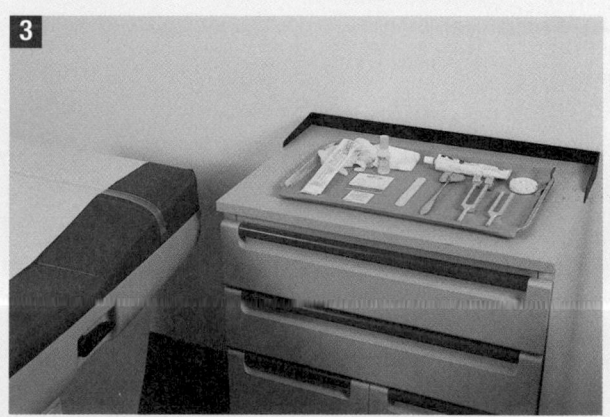

Assemble the equipment. (From Bonewit-West K: *Clinical procedures for medical assistants,* ed 7, St. Louis, 2008, Saunders.)

Continued

PROCEDURE 20-10   Assisting with the Physical Examination—cont'd

6. Procedural Step. Ask the patient to be seated. Greet the patient and introduce yourself using a calm and friendly manner. Identify the patient by his or her full name and date of birth.

Principle. Identifying the patient correctly avoids mistaking one patient for another. Using a calm and friendly manner helps to put the patient at ease.

Greet and identify the patient by name and date of birth. (From Bonewit-West K: *Clinical procedures for medical assistants,* ed 7, St. Louis, 2008, Saunders.)

7. Procedural Step. Seat yourself so that you face the patient at a distance of 3 to 4 feet.

8. Procedural Step. Obtain and record the patient's symptoms following the procedure outlined in Procedure 36-4 in Chapter 36.

9. Procedural Step. Measure the patient's vital signs, and chart the results.

10. Procedural Step. Measure the weight and height of the patient, and chart the results.

11. Procedural Step. Instruct and prepare the patient for the examination as follows:

a. Ask the patient whether he or she needs to empty the bladder before the examination. If a urine specimen is needed, the patient will be required to void into a urine container.

b. Provide the patient with a patient gown. Instruct the patient to remove all clothing and put on the patient gown. Offer assistance if you sense the patient may have trouble undressing.

c. Tell the patient to have a seat on the examining table after putting on the patient gown. Inform the patient that the physician will be with him or her soon and leave the room to provide the patient with privacy.

Instruct the patient for the examination. (From Bonewit-West K: *Clinical procedures for medical assistants,* ed 7, St. Louis, 2008, Saunders.)

Principle. An empty bladder makes the examination easier and is more comfortable for the patient.

12. Procedural Step. Make the medical record available to the physician. The medical office has a designated location where the record is placed, such as a small shelf mounted on the wall next to the outside of the examining room door or in a chart holder on the outside of the examining room door. Position the medical record so that patient-identifiable information is not visible. Check to make sure that the patient is ready to be seen by the physician. Before entering a patient's room, knock lightly on the door to let the patient know that you are getting ready to enter the room. If a patient is ready to be seen, inform the physician. This may be done using a color-coded flagging system mounted on the wall next to the examining room.

Principle. HIPAA requires protection of a patient's health information.

13. Procedural Step. Assist the physician with the examination of the body systems as follows:

a. Ensure that the patient is positioned correctly in a sitting position on the examining table. This allows the physician to examine the patient's head, eyes, ears, nose, mouth and pharynx, neck, chest, lungs, and heart.

b. Hand the physician the **ophthalmoscope, otoscope,** and tongue depressor.

c. Dim the light when the physician is ready to use the ophthalmoscope. The dim light helps dilate the patient's pupils, providing the physician better visualization of the interior of the eye.

d. After use, the tongue depressor should be transferred by holding it at the center to prevent contact

Transfer the tongue depressor by holding it at the center. (From Bonewit-West K: *Clinical procedures for medical assistants,* ed 7, St. Louis, 2008, Saunders.)

with the patient's secretions, which may contain pathogens. Dispose of the tongue depressor in a regular waste container.

e. Offer reassurance to the patient to reduce apprehension.

14. Procedural Step. Position the patient as required for examination of the remaining body systems. Place and drape the patient in the proper position for examination of a particular part of the body.

15. Procedural Step. Assist and instruct the patient as follows:

a. Allow the patient to rest in a sitting position on the examining table before he or she gets off it. Some patients become dizzy after being positioned on the examining table.

b. Assist the patient off the examining table to prevent falls.

c. Instruct the patient to get dressed. Provide assistance if needed.

d. Provide the patient with any necessary instructions, such as patient education and scheduling a return visit. Give instructions involving medical

care in terms the patient can understand; do not use medical terms.

e. Sanitize the hands, and chart any instructions given to the patient in his or her medical record.

f. Escort the patient to the reception area.

16. Procedural Step. Clean the examining room in preparation for the next patient as follows:

a. Discard the paper on the examining table. If body secretions have gotten on the examining table, apply gloves, and clean and disinfect the table. Unroll a fresh length of paper on the table.

b. Discard all disposable supplies into an appropriate waste container.

c. Ensure that there are an ample number of clean gowns and drapes and other supplies.

d. Remove reusable equipment to a work area for sanitization, sterilization, or disinfection as required by the medical office policy.

Unroll a fresh length of paper. (From Bonewit-West K: *Clinical procedures for medical assistants,* ed 7, St. Louis, 2008, Saunders.)

PROCEDURE 20-10

MEDICAL PRACTICE *and the* LAW

Activities involved in the physical examination can be sensitive for the patient. Information obtained while taking the patient history is confidential; revealing this information to anyone is unethical and illegal. A good rapport is essential for obtaining complete information, especially when asking sensitive questions. Complete information is necessary for accurate diagnosis and treatment.

Preparing the patient for a physical examination can be embarrassing for the patient. Keep in mind your duty to "do good" and "do no harm" to the patient. This involves proper knowledge and techniques and a professional, caring, and helpful attitude. Draping the patient correctly allows only minimal exposure. Incorrect

draping or positioning that is unnecessarily uncomfortable could become a legal issue. Patients who are young, very old, or weak should never be left alone on an examining table. A fall from a table often results in harm and potential for a lawsuit.

Finally, while assisting the physician, be supportive of the patient as much as you are able. While the physician concentrates on the examination, you should continually assess the patient and provide for any needs, including assistance, encouragement, and physical comfort. Be patient, polite, and professional in all directions given to the patient. You may have done this many times, but this could be the first time for a frightened, ill patient. ∎

What Would You Do? What Would You *Not* Do? **RESPONSES**

Case Study 1
Page 380

What Did Hope Do?

❑ Empathized with Abbey and told her that a lot of patients feel just like she does about having their weight taken. Explained that the information in her medical record is strictly confidential.

❑ Told Abbey that weight is important so that the physician can properly diagnose and treat her condition, and that medication dosage is often based on a person's weight.

❑ Told Abbey that she could stand on the scale backward while her weight is being measured so that she would not see the reading on the scale.

❑ Returned the weights to zero before Abbey got off the scale.

❑ Recorded Abbey's weight in her chart without telling her the results.

❑ Encouraged Abbey to see the physician when she needs to so that she stays as healthy as possible.

What Did Hope Not *Do?*

❑ Did not make any comments about Abbey's body or weight after weighing her.

❑ Did not criticize Abbey for letting her weight stand in the way of coming in when she needed health care.

What Would You Do/What Would You *Not* Do? Review Hope's response and place a checkmark next to the information you included in your response. List the additional information you included in your response.

_____

_____

_____

_____

Case Study 2
Page 382

What Did Hope Do?

❑ Listened carefully to Mikayla and showed concern verbally and nonverbally.

❑ Carefully charted the information relayed by Mikayla so that the physician would be aware of all aspects of Mikayla's problem.

❑ Told Mikayla that she needs to talk to the physician about wanting some medicine for heartburn.

❑ Encouraged Mikayla to talk to her parents about what's been going on with her.

What Did Hope Not *Do?*

❑ Did not agree with Mikayla that she needs to lose more weight.

❑ Did not make comments about Mikayla being too thin.

What Would You Do/What Would You *Not* Do? Review Hope's response and place a checkmark next to the information you included in your response. List the additional information you included in your response.

_____

_____

_____

_____

Case Study 3
Page 402

What Did Hope Do?

❑ Greeted Chang-Yi first before greeting his son.

❑ Spoke clearly and slowly to Ben-Yi in a normal tone of voice.

❑ Gave them a brochure on low-sodium diets and went over the foods that are low in sodium.

❑ Asked Chang-Yi (via Ben-Yi's translating) to indicate the foods he likes that he thinks would be low in sodium. Determined whether these foods are low in sodium.

❑ Showed Ben-Yi how to take his father's blood pressure. Had Ben-Yi practice taking his father's blood pressure.

❑ Made sure that Chang-Yi and Ben-Yi understood all of the information before they left the office.

What Did Hope Not *Do?*

❑ Was careful not to ignore Chang-Yi.

What Would You Do/What Would You *Not* Do? Review Hope's response and place a checkmark next to the information you included in your response. List the additional information you included in your response.

_____

_____

_____

_____

TERMINOLOGY REVIEW

Audiometer An instrument used to measure hearing.

Auscultation The process of listening to the sounds produced within the body to detect signs of disease.

Bariatrics The branch of medicine that deals with the treatment and control of obesity and diseases associated with obesity.

Clinical diagnosis A tentative diagnosis of a patient's condition obtained through the evaluation of the health history and the physical examination, without the benefit of laboratory or diagnostic tests.

Diagnosis The scientific method of determining and identifying a patient's condition.

Differential diagnosis A determination of which of two or more diseases with similar symptoms is producing a patient's symptoms.

Inspection The process of observing a patient to detect signs of disease.

Mensuration The process of measuring a patient.

Ophthalmoscope An instrument for examining the interior of the eye.

Otoscope An instrument for examining the external ear canal and tympanic membrane.

Palpation The process of feeling with the hands to detect signs of disease.

Percussion The process of tapping the body to detect signs of disease.

Percussion hammer An instrument with a rubber head, used for testing reflexes.

Prognosis The probable course and outcome of a patient's condition and the patient's prospects for recovery.

Speculum An instrument for opening a body orifice or cavity for viewing.

Symptom Any change in the body or its functioning that indicates a disease might be present.

ON THE WEB

For Information on Nutrition:

American Dietetic Association: www.eatright.org

Ask the Dietitian: www.dietitian.com

For Information on Weight Control and Fitness:

American Obesity Association: www.obesity.org

Obesity Action Coalition: www.obesityaction.org

Weight Watchers: www.weightwatchers.com

E-Diets: www.ediets.com

Calorie Control Council: www.caloriecontrol.org

Cyber Diet: www.cyberdiet.com

For Information on Accessing Health Information:

InteliHealth: www.intelihealth.com

Mayo Clinic: www.mayoclinic.com

U.S. Department of Health and Human Services: www.os.dhhs.gov

American Academy of Family Physicians: Family Doctor: www.familydoctor.org

Healthfinder: www.health.gov

WebMD: www.webmd.com

Medline Plus: www.nlm.nih.gov/medlineplus

 PREPARE FOR CERTIFICATION Visit the Evolve site at http://evolve.elsevier.com/Bonewit/today/ to actively Prepare for your Certification.

 *Check out the **Companion CD** bound with the book to access additional interactive activities.*

21

Eye and Ear Assessment and Procedures

LEARNING OBJECTIVES

The Eye
1. Define visual acuity.
2. State the cause and visual difficulty of the following:
   - Myopia
   - Hyperopia
   - Presbyopia
3. Explain the differences among an ophthalmologist, optometrist, and optician.
4. Explain the significance of the top and bottom numbers next to each line of letters on the Snellen eye chart.
5. Explain the difference between congenital and acquired color vision defects.
6. List the reasons to perform an eye irrigation and an eye instillation.

The Ear
1. Identify conditions that may cause conductive and sensorineural hearing loss.
2. List and describe the ways in which hearing acuity can be tested.
3. List the reasons to perform an ear irrigation and an ear instillation.

PROCEDURES

Assess distance visual acuity.
Assess near visual acuity.
Assess color vision.
Perform an eye irrigation.
Perform an eye instillation.

Perform an ear irrigation.
Perform an ear instillation.

CHAPTER OUTLINE

Introduction to the Eye
Visual Acuity
    Assessment of Distance Visual Acuity
    Assessment of Near Visual Acuity
Assessment of Color Vision
    Ishihara Test
Eye Irrigation
Eye Instillation

Introduction to the Ear
Assessment of Hearing Acuity
    Types of Hearing Loss
    Hearing Acuity Tests
Ear Irrigation
Ear Instillation

CAAHEP COMPETENCIES

Clinical Competencies
Patient Care
- Prepare patient for and assist with routine and specialty examinations.
- Prepare patient for and assist with procedures, treatments, and minor office surgery.

General Competencies
Patient Instruction
- Instruct individuals according to their needs.
- Provide instruction for health maintenance and disease prevention.

ABHES COMPETENCIES

Clinical Duties
- Prepare patients for procedures.
- Prepare patients for and assist physician with routine and specialty examinations and treatments and minor office surgeries.

Instruction
- Instruct patients with special needs.
- Teach patients methods of health promotion and disease prevention.

KEY TERMS

audiometer (aw-dee-OM-eh-ter)
canthus (KAN-thus)
cerumen
hyperopia (HYE-per-OP-ee-uh)
impacted
instillation (IN-still-AY-shun)

irrigation (EAR-ih-GAY-shun)
myopia (mye-OH-pee-uh)
otoscope (AH-toe-skope)
presbyopia (PRESS-bee-OH-pee-uh)
refraction (ree-FRAK-shun)
tympanic membrane (tim-PAN-ik MEM-brane)

Introduction to the Eye

The medical assistant is responsible for performing a variety of assessments and procedures that involve the eye. An understanding of the structure and function of the eye is essential to mastering skill in these areas. Refer to Chapter 10 to review the structure and function of the eye.

A visual acuity test is usually part of the routine physical examination. This test is a screening test to detect deficiencies in vision. The medical assistant may also be responsible for assessing color vision with the use of specially prepared colored plates. As a result of this testing, color blindness can be detected. Color blindness is an inability to distinguish certain colors; the most common problem is with the colors red and green. Color blindness is particularly significant if the patient is involved in an activity that relies on the ability to distinguish colors, such as electronics and interior decorating.

The medical assistant is responsible for performing or teaching the patient to perform eye irrigations and instillations. **Irrigation** is washing a body canal with a flowing solution. **Instillation** is dropping a liquid into a body cavity. Eye irrigations and instillations should be performed using the important principles of medical asepsis outlined in Chapter 17.

VISUAL ACUITY

Visual acuity refers to acuteness or sharpness of vision. A person with normal visual acuity can see clearly and is able to distinguish fine details close up and at some distance.

Errors of refraction are the most common causes of defects in visual acuity (Figure 21-1). **Refraction** refers to the ability of the eye to bend the parallel light rays coming into it so that they can be focused on the retina. An *error of*

refraction means that the light rays are not being refracted or bent properly and are not adequately focused on the retina. A defect in the shape of the eyeball can cause a refractive error. Errors of refraction can be improved with corrective lenses.

A person who is nearsighted has a condition termed **myopia.** The eyeball is too long from front to back, causing the light rays to be brought to a focus in front of the retina. A myopic person has difficulty seeing objects at a distance and may squint and have headaches as a result of eyestrain. A corrective lens (e.g., eyeglasses, contact lenses) or laser eye surgery can correct this condition, which then allows the light rays to come to a focus on the retina.

A person who is farsighted has a condition known as **hyperopia.** The eyeball is too short from front to back, resulting in a different type of refractive error, in which the light rays are brought to a focus behind the retina. The individual has difficulty viewing objects at a reading or working distance. An individual with hyperopia may experience blurring, headaches, and eyestrain while performing up-close tasks. A corrective lens can improve this condition by causing the light rays to come to a focus on the retina.

In most people, a decrease in the elasticity of the lens of the eye begins to occur after age 40 years. This condition, **presbyopia,** results in a decreased ability to focus clearly on close objects.

If a defect in visual acuity is detected, the patient is referred to an eye specialist for further evaluation. Several types of specialists are involved in the care of the eyes. An *ophthalmologist* is a physician who specializes in diagnosing and treating diseases and disorders of the eye. An ophthalmologist is qualified to prescribe ophthalmic and systemic medications and to perform eye surgery. An *optometrist* is a licensed primary health care provider who has expertise in measuring visual acuity and prescribing corrective lenses for the treatment of refractive errors. An optometrist is also

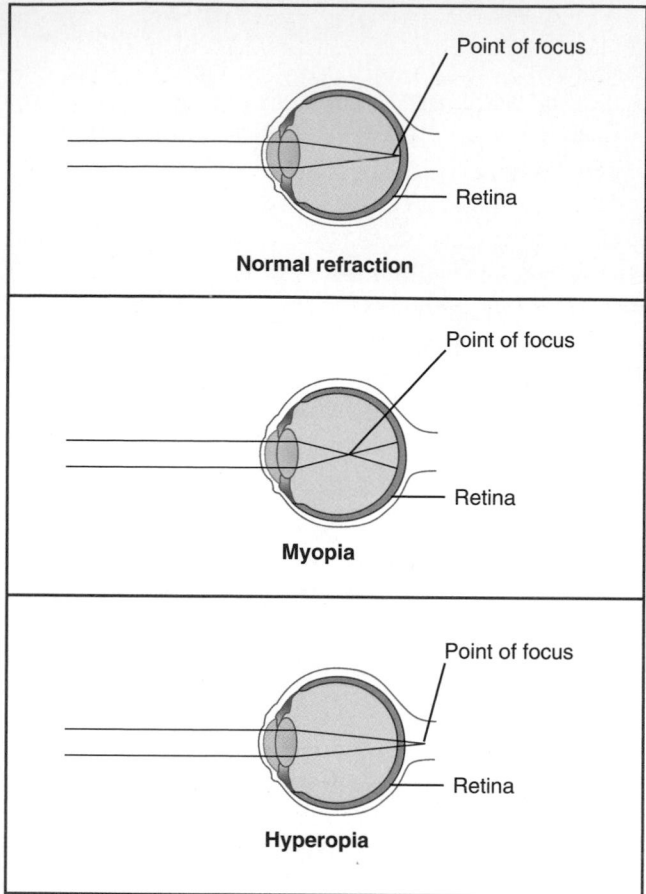

Errors of Refraction

Figure 21-1. Diagram of normal refraction compared with myopia (nearsightedness) and hyperopia (farsightedness), which are errors of refraction that cause visual defects. (From Bonewit-West K: *Clinical procedures for medical assistants,* ed 7, St. Louis, 2008, Saunders.)

qualified to diagnose and treat disorders and diseases of the eye and to prescribe ophthalmic medications. An optometrist is not a physician and is not permitted to prescribe systemic medications or to perform eye surgery. An *optician* is a professional who interprets and fills prescriptions for eyeglasses and contact lenses.

Assessment of Distance Visual Acuity

Myopia can be diagnosed (in combination with other tests) by a distance visual acuity (DVA) test. In the medical office, the Snellen eye chart is most often used. Two types of charts are commonly used. One type is used for school-age children and adults and consists of a chart of letters in decreasing sizes (Figure 21-2). The other type is used for preschool children, non–English-speaking people, and nonreaders; it is composed of the capital letter E in decreasing sizes and arranged in different directions (Figure 21-3). Visual acuity charts with pictures of familiar objects are also available for use with preschool children. Testing with these charts tends to be less accurate than with the Snellen charts. Some children are unable to identify the objects because of lack of recognition, not because of a defect in visual acuity. It is

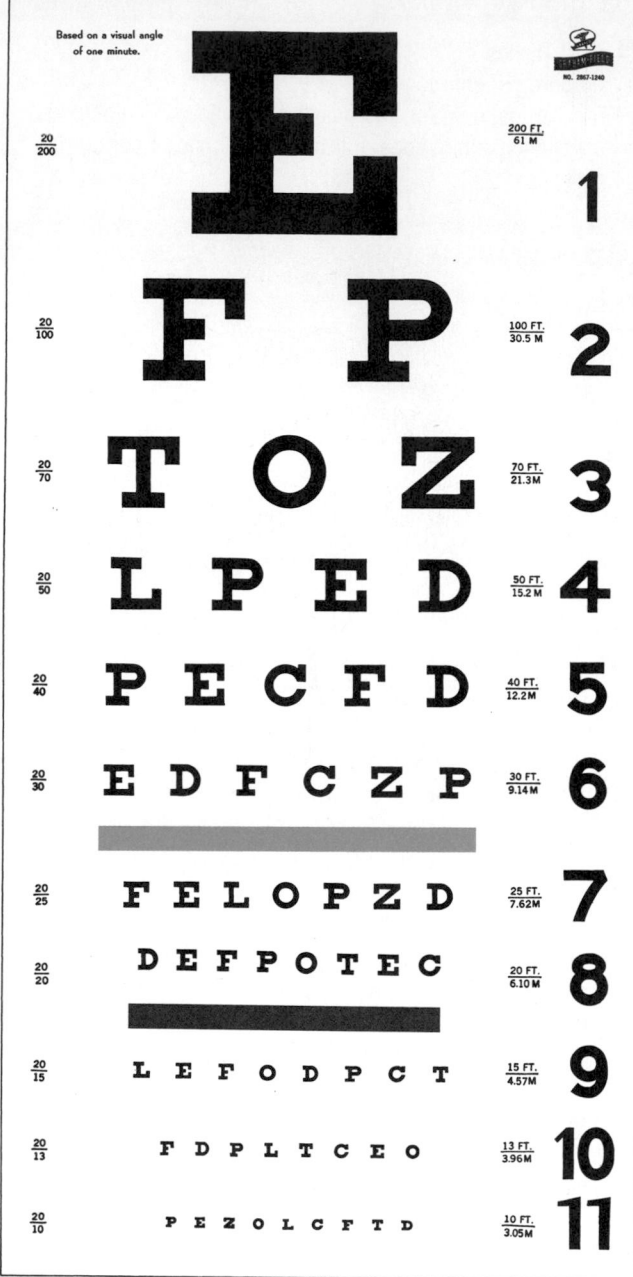

Figure 21-2. Snellen eye chart consisting of letters in decreasing sizes; this chart is used to measure distance visual acuity. (From Bonewit-West K: *Clinical procedures for medical assistants,* ed 7, St. Louis, 2008, Saunders.)

suggested that the Snellen Big E chart be used with preschool children.

Conducting a Snellen Test

The visual acuity test should be performed in a well-lit room that is free of distractions. The test is usually performed at a distance of 20 feet; this can be conveniently marked off in the medical office with paint or a piece of tape so that it does not have to be remeasured every time the test is performed.

A visual acuity reading of 20/15 means this was the smallest line that the individual could read at a distance of 20 feet. It indicates above-average acuity for distance vision. People with normal acuity would be able to read this line at 15 feet.

The acuity of each eye should be measured separately, traditionally beginning with the right eye. Most physicians prefer that the patient wear his or her contact lenses or glasses, except reading glasses, during the test; the medical assistant should record in the patient's chart that corrective lenses were worn by the patient during the test. An eye occluder should be held over the eye not being tested. The patient's hand should not be used to cover the eye because this may encourage peeking through the fingers, especially in the case of children. The patient should be instructed to leave open the eye not being tested because closing it causes squinting of the eye that is being tested. The procedure for measuring DVA is outlined in Procedure 21-1.

Assessing Distance Visual Acuity in Preschool Children

With minor variations, Procedure 21-1 can be used to test DVA in preschool children. The Snellen Big E chart is used for this purpose.

A child needs a complete and thorough explanation of what is expected of him or her before beginning the test. Tell the child you will be playing a pointing game. Do not force the child to play the game because the results would then tend to be inaccurate. Draw the capital letter E on an index card, and teach the child to point in the direction of the open part of the E by turning the card in different directions (up, down, to the right, and to the left). Using such phrases as "fingers" or the "legs of the table" to describe the open part of the E helps the child understand what is expected (Figure 21-4). Allow the child to practice the pointing game with the index card until you are sure this level of skill has been mastered. Be sure to praise the child when the correct response is given.

The child might need help holding the eye occluder in place. The aid of another person such as the parent would then be required.

Assessment of Near Visual Acuity

Near visual acuity (NVA) testing assesses the patient's ability to read close objects (i.e., at a reading or working distance); the test results are used to detect hyperopia and presbyopia.

The test is conducted with a card similar to the Snellen eye chart; however, the size of the type ranges from the size of newspaper headlines down to considerably smaller print, such as would be found in a telephone directory (Figure 21-5). The test card is available in a variety of forms, such as printed paragraphs, printed words, and pictures.

The test should be performed in a well-lit room free of distractions. It is conducted with the patient holding the test card at a distance between 14 and 16 inches. If the patient wears reading glasses, they should be worn during

20/200	200 FT. / 61 M 1
20/100	100 FT. / 30.5 M 2
20/70	70 FT. / 21.7 M 3
20/50	50 FT. / 15.2 M 4
20/30	30 FT. / 9.1 M 5
20/20	20 FT. / 6.1 M 6
20/15	15 FT. / 4.6 M 7
20/10	10 FT. / 3.05 M 8

Figure 21-3. Snellen Big E eye chart consisting of the capital letter E in decreasing sizes and arranged in different directions; this chart is used to measure distance visual acuity. (From Bonewit-West K: *Clinical procedures for medical assistants,* ed 7, St. Louis, 2008, Saunders.)

Two numbers, separated by a line, appear at the side of each row of letters on the chart. The number above the line represents the distance (in feet) at which the test is conducted. It is usually 20 feet because most eye tests are conducted at this distance. The number below the line represents the distance from which a person with normal visual acuity can read the row of letters. The line marked 20/20 indicates normal DVA, or 20/20 vision. This means a person could read what he or she was supposed to read at a distance of 20 feet.

A visual acuity reading of 20/30 means this was the smallest line that the individual could read at a distance of 20 feet. People with normal acuity would be able to read this line at a distance of 30 feet.

Figure 21-4. A, Cammie teaches a preschool child to point in the direction of the open part of the capital letter E. **B,** Cammie performs the Snellen Big E visual acuity test. (From Bonewit-West K: *Clinical procedures for medical assistants,* ed 7, St. Louis, 2008, Saunders.)

Highlight on Eye Assessment

Vision disorders are the fourth most common disability in the United States. Studies show that vision disorders are the most prevalent disabling condition in children. Because of this, it is recommended that children have a complete eye examination starting at age 3. Children and adults should have an eye examination every 2 to 3 years up to 60 years of age. Individuals older than 60 years should have yearly eye examinations.

Individuals who have risk factors for eye disorders should have an eye examination every year. Examples of risk factors are diabetes and hypertension.

Visual acuity is considered normal for the various age groups if it falls within the following values:

Newborn	20/500
Infant 1-6 mo	20/200 to 20/90
Infant 6-12 mo	20/60
Child 12-18 mo	20/40
Child 2-3 yr	20/30
Child 3-18 yr	20/20
Adult 18 yr or older	20/20

Legal blindness is defined as a visual acuity measurement of 20/200 or less in both eyes with the use of corrective lenses.

The term *color blind* is not an accurate term to describe an individual with abnormal color vision because the inability to distinguish any colors at all is extremely rare. Most individuals with a color vision abnormality are unable to distinguish certain hues of color, such as red and green. A better term is *color vision defect.*

Defective color vision is usually congenital. It is found in 8% of men and 5% of women.

Studies show that there is no significant correlation between defective color vision and increased automobile accidents. Most drivers who have a color vision defect are able to distinguish traffic lights by the different light intensities and by the position of the light on the traffic signal. ∎

the test. The acuity should be measured in each eye separately, traditionally beginning with the right eye. An eye occluder should be held over the eye not being tested. The patient should be instructed to keep the covered eye open because closing it may cause squinting of the eye that is being tested. The patient is asked to read or identify orally each line or paragraph of type. During the test, the patient should be observed for unusual symptoms, such as squinting, tilting the head, or watering of the eyes, which may indicate that the patient is having difficulty reading the card. The patient continues until reaching the smallest type that can be read.

The results are recorded as the smallest type that the patient could comfortably read with each eye at the distance at which the card is held (i.e., 14 to 16 inches). The recording is based on the type of test card used to conduct the test. One type of card uses a recording method similar to that used with the Snellen eye test. For this type of NVA

No. 1.
.37M

In the second century of the Christian era, the empire of Rome comprehended the fairest part of the earth, and the most civilized portion of mankind. The frontiers of that extensive monarchy were guarded by ancient renown and disciplined valor. The gentle but powerful influence of laws and manners had gradually cemented the union of the provinces. Their peaceful inhabitants enjoyed and abused the advantages of wealth.

No. 2.
.50M

fourscore years, the public administration was conducted by the virtue and abilities of Nerva, Trajan, Hadrian, and the two Antonines. It is the design of this, and of the two succeeding chapters, to describe the prosperous condition of their empire; and afterwards, from the death of Marcus Antoninus, to deduce the most important circumstances of its decline and fall; a revolution which will ever be remembered, and is still felt by

No. 3.
.62M

the nations of the earth. The principal conquests of the Romans were achieved under the republic; and the emperors, for the most part, were satisfied with preserving those dominions which had been acquired by the policy of the senate, the active emulations of the consuls, and the martial enthusiasm of the people. The seven first centuries were filled with a rapid succession of triumphs; but it was

No. 4.
.75M

reserved for Augustus to relinquish the ambitious design of subduing the whole earth, and to introduce a spirit of moderation into the public councils. Inclined to peace by his temper and situation, it was very easy for him to discover that Rome, in her present exalted situation, had much less to hope than to fear from the chance of arms; and that, in the prosecution of

No. 5.
1.00M

the undertaking became every day more difficult, the event more doubtful, and the possession more precarious, and less beneficial. The experience of Augustus added weight to these salutary reflections, and effectually convinced him that, by the prudent vigor of

No. 6.
1.25M

his counsels, it would be easy to secure every concession which the safety or the dignity of Rome might require from the most formidable barbarians. Instead of exposing his person or his legions to the arrows of the Parthinians, he obtained, by an honor-

No. 7.
1.50M

able treaty, the restitution of the standards and prisoners which had been taken in the defeat of Crassus. His generals, in the early part of his reign, attempted the reduction of Ethiopia and Arabia Felix. They marched near a thou-

No. 8.
1.75M

sand miles to the south of the tropic; but the heat of the climate soon repelled the invaders, and protected the unwarlike natives of those sequestered regions

No. 9.
2.00M

The northern countries of Europe scarcely deserved the expense and labor of conquest. The forests and morasses of Germany were

No. 10.
2.25M

filled with a hardy race of barbarians who despised life when it was separated from freedom; and though, on the first

No. 11.
2.50M

attack, they seemed to yield to the weight of the Roman power, they soon, by a signal

Figure 21-5. Example of a near visual acuity card. (From Bonewit-West K: *Clinical procedures for medical assistants*, ed 7, St. Louis, 2008, Saunders.)

card, the results would be recorded as 14/14 for a patient with normal NVA. This means the patient read what was supposed to be read at a distance of 14 inches. Also included in the recording should be the date and time, corrective lenses worn, and any unusual symptoms exhibited by the patient.

ASSESSMENT OF COLOR VISION

Defects in color vision may be classified as congenital or acquired. *Congenital defects* are more common and refer to a color vision deficiency that is inherited and present at birth. Congenital color vision deficiencies most often affect males. *Acquired defects* refer to a color vision deficiency that is acquired after birth, resulting from such factors as an eye injury, disease, and certain drugs. Color vision tests, such as the Ishihara test (Figure 21-6), detect congenital color vision disturbances and are commonly performed in the medical office. A basic screening for color vision can be performed by asking the patient to identify the red and green lines on the Snellen eye chart.

What Would You Do? What Would You *Not* Do?

Case Study 1

Nicole Neason brings her daughter, Haley, to the office for a camp physical. Haley just completed the fourth grade and is going to summer camp for 2 weeks with Tess, her best friend. Tess wears glasses, and Haley thinks they are really cool. She often asks to try on Tess's glasses and wishes she could wear glasses just like her best friend. When Haley is measured for visual acuity, she misses a few letters on the 20/70 line, the 20/50 line, the 20/40 line, and the 20/20 line. She is unable to read any of the letters on the 20/15 line. After the examination, Haley wants to know if she's missed enough letters to be able to get glasses. ∎

Ishihara Test

The Ishihara test for color blindness is a convenient and accurate method to detect total congenital color blindness and red-green color blindness by assessing an individual's ability to perceive primary colors and shades of color. The

Figure 21-6. Ishihara color plates. Polychromatic plates. In the upper figure, a person with normal color vision reads 74, but a person with red-green color blindness reads 21. In the lower figure, a red-blind person (protanope) reads 2, but a green-blind person (deuteranope) reads 4. A normal-vision person reads 42. Reproduced plates are not good for testing for color deficiency. (From Ishihara J: *Tests for color blindness,* Tokyo, 1920, Kanehara.)

Ishihara book contains a series of polychromatic plates of primary-colored dots arranged to form a numeral against a background of similar dots of contrasting colors (see Figure 21-6). Patients with normal color vision are able to read the appropriate numeral; however, patients with color vision defects read the dots either as not forming a number at all or as forming a number different from the one identified by the individual with normal color vision. The first plate in the Ishihara book is designed to be read correctly by all individuals (with normal vision and exhibiting color vision deficiencies) and should be used to explain the procedure to the patient.

The book includes plates with winding colored lines for patients who are unable to identify the numbers by name, such as preschool children and non–English-speaking people. The patient should be asked to trace the line formed by the colored dots using a cotton swab or the eraser end of a pencil. The patient's finger should not be used to do the tracing because soiled fingers over time can degrade the polychromatic plates.

The Ishihara test should be conducted in a quiet room illuminated by natural daylight. If this is not feasible, a room lit with electric light may be used; however, the light should be adjusted to resemble the effect of natural daylight as much as possible. Using light other than just described, such as bright sunlight, may change the appearance of shades of color on the plates, leading to inaccurate test results.

The medical assistant is responsible for performing the color vision test and recording results in the patient's chart.

Putting It All into Practice

My name is Cammie Lindner, and I work for an ear, nose, and throat (ENT) surgeon. There are administrative responsibilities in my job; however, the focus is on the clinical aspects, including vital signs measurement, allergy testing, immunotherapy, and assisting with minor office surgeries, such as excision of skin lesions and tympanostomy tube insertions. Over the past years in an ENT practice, there have been many challenging and rewarding situations. A recent incident was one that certainly falls into the rewards category.

A young girl came into the office from the emergency department for repair of a facial laceration. It had been quite a day for her, so it was understandable that she was a bit nervous and upset. As the suturing was performed, she grasped her mother's hand as I tried to discuss interests and school with her. She did fine and was very relieved when the last suture was done.

On her return visit for the suture removal, her mother could not accompany her. As I was showing her to the examination room, she quietly asked if I would be in the room. I said, "If you would like, I certainly will." She anxiously nodded yes. As the sutures were removed, she squeezed my hand tighter and tighter. After all of them were out, she first checked her appearance in the mirror, then turned before going out the door and gave me a big hug and a "thank you." Days like this one are truly great rewards and make you feel you really can make a difference in someone's care. ■

Prepare for Success

The physician assesses the results to determine whether the patient has a deficiency in color vision.

The Ishihara test consists of 14 color plates. Plates 1 through 11 are used to conduct the basic test, and plates 12, 13, and 14 are used to assess further patients who exhibit a red-green color deficiency. It is unnecessary to include these plates (12, 13, and 14) in the test of patients who exhibit normal color vision. In interpreting the results, if 10 or more plates are read correctly, the patient's color vision is considered normal. If 7 or fewer of the 11 Ishihara plates are read correctly, the patient is identified as having a color vision deficiency. It would be unusual for the medical assistant to obtain results in which the patient read 8 or 9 plates correctly. The test is structured so that a patient with a color vision defect generally does not read 8 or 9 plates correctly and the rest incorrectly.

If a defect in color vision is detected, the patient is referred for additional assessment of color vision to an ophthalmologist or optometrist, who would use more precise color vision tests. The procedure for assessing color vision using the Ishihara color plates is outlined in Procedure 21-2.

PROCEDURE 21-1 Assessing Distance Visual Acuity—Snellen Chart

Outcome Assess DVA.

Equipment/Supplies

- Snellen eye chart
- Eye occluder
- Antiseptic wipe

1. Procedural Step. Sanitize your hands.

2. Procedural Step. Assemble the equipment. Perform the test in a well-lit room that is free of distractions. Wipe the eye occluder with an antiseptic wipe, and allow it to dry completely.
Principle. The eye occluder should be disinfected before use.

3. Procedural Step. Greet the patient and introduce yourself. Identify the patient and explain the procedure. Tell the patient that he or she will be asked to read several lines of letters. The patient should not have an opportunity to study or memorize the letters before beginning the test.

4. Procedural Step. Determine whether the patient wears contact lenses or glasses (other than reading glasses). If the patient wears such aids, he or she should be told to keep them on during the test.

5. Procedural Step. Ask the patient to stand on the marked line located 20 feet from the chart.

6. Procedural Step. Position the center of the Snellen chart at the patient's eye level. Stand next to the chart during the test to indicate to the patient the line to be identified.
Principle. Ensure that the chart is at the patient's eye level rather than your eye level, to provide the most accurate results.

7. Procedural Step. Test the acuity of each eye separately. Measure the visual acuity of the right eye first.
Principle. The medical assistant should establish a pattern of beginning with the same eye (traditionally the right eye) every time the test is performed. This helps to reduce errors during the recording of results.

8. Procedural Step. Ask the patient to cover the left eye with the eye occluder. If the patient wears eyeglasses, tell him or her to place the occluder in front of the glasses gently to prevent the glasses from being moved out of their normal position. Instruct the patient to keep the left eye open. During the test, the medical assistant should check to make sure the patient is keeping the left eye open.
Principle. Eyeglasses moved out of normal position may lead to inaccurate test results. Keeping the left eye open prevents squinting of the right eye, which temporarily improves vision, leading to inaccurate test results.

9. Procedural Step. Instruct the patient not to squint during the test because squinting temporarily improves vision. Ask the patient to identify orally one line at a time on the Snellen chart, starting with the 20/70 line (or a line that is several lines above the 20/20 line).
Principle. It is best to start at a line above the 20/20 line to give the patient a chance to gain confidence and to become familiar with the test procedure.

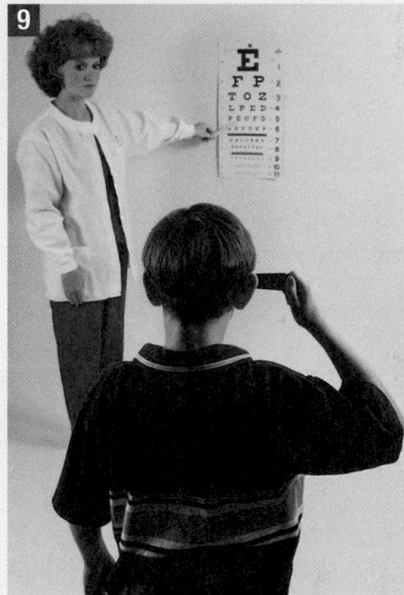

Ask the patient to identify one line at a time. (From Bonewit-West K: *Clinical procedures for medical assistants,* ed 7, St. Louis, 2008, Saunders.)

10. Procedural Step. If the patient is able to read the 20/70 line, proceed down the chart until reaching the smallest line of letters the patient can read. If the patient is unable to read the 20/70 line, proceed up the chart until the smallest line of letters the patient can read is reached.

11. Procedural Step. While the patient is reading the letters, observe him or her for unusual symptoms, such as squinting, tilting of the head, or watering of the eyes.
Principle. These symptoms may indicate that the patient is having difficulty identifying the letters.

12. Procedural Step. Jot down the numbers next to the smallest line of letters that the patient is able to read. If one or two letters are missed, record the visual

Continued

PROCEDURE 21-1

PROCEDURE 21-1   Assessing Distance Visual Acuity—Snellen Chart—cont'd

acuity with a minus sign next to the bottom number, along with the number of letters missed. If more than two letters are missed, the previous line is recorded.

13. Procedural Step. Ask the patient to cover the right eye with the eye occluder and keep the right eye open. Measure the visual acuity in the left eye as described in steps 8 through 10. During the test, check to make sure the patient is keeping the right eye open.

Ask the patient to cover the right eye and keep the right eye open. (From Bonewit-West K: *Clinical procedures for medical assistants,* ed 7, St. Louis, 2008, Saunders.)

Principle. Keeping the right eye open prevents squinting of the left eye.

14. Procedural Step. Chart the procedure. Include the date and time, the name of the test (Snellen test), the visual acuity results, and any unusual symptoms the patient exhibited during the test. Also chart whether the patient was wearing corrective lenses during the test. Use the following abbreviations: s̄c without correction or c̄c with correction.

Latin abbreviations are used to record visual acuity. The abbreviation for the right eye is OD *(oculus dexter),* the abbreviation for the left eye is OS *(oculus sinister),* and the abbreviation for both eyes is OU *(oculus uterque).*

15. Procedural Step. Disinfect the eye occluder with an antiseptic wipe, and sanitize your hands.

CHARTING EXAMPLE	
Date	
11/5/10	3:30 p.m. Snellen test, s̄c: OD 20/20-1.
	OS 20/25. Exhibited squinting, OD. ————
	—————————— C. Lindner, CMA (AAMA)

see DVD

PROCEDURE 21-2   Assessing Color Vision—Ishihara Test

Outcome Assess color vision.

Equipment/Supplies

- Ishihara book
- Cotton swab

1. **Procedural Step.** Sanitize your hands. Assemble the equipment.
2. **Procedural Step.** Conduct the test in a quiet room illuminated by natural daylight.
   Principle. Using unnatural light may change the appearance of the shades of color on the plates, leading to inaccurate test results.
3. **Procedural Step.** Greet the patient and introduce yourself. Identify the patient and explain the procedure. Using the first (practice) plate as an example, instruct the patient to identify orally numbers formed by colored dots. Tell the patient that 3 seconds will be given to identify each plate.
   Principle. The first plate is designed to be read correctly by all individuals and is used to explain the procedure to the patient.

4. Procedural Step. Hold the first color plate 30 inches (75 cm) from the patient, at a right angle to the patient's line of vision. The patient should keep both eyes open during the test.

5. **Procedural Step.** Ask the patient to identify the number on the plate. If the plate consists of a traceable winding colored line, ask the patient to trace the line using a cotton swab or the eraser end of a pencil. The patient's finger should not be used to make the tracing.
   Principle. The patient's finger should not be used to trace the line because soiled fingers can degrade the plate over time.

Hold the color plate 30 inches from the patient. (From Bonewit-West K: *Clinical procedures for medical assistants,* ed 7, St. Louis, 2008, Saunders.)

6. Procedural Step. Record results after each plate. Continue until the patient has viewed all the plates. To record the color vision results, use the plate identification number and the number given by the patient. If the patient is unable to identify a number, the mark "X" should be recorded to indicate that the patient could not read the plate. Examples:

Plate 5: 21 This means the patient read the number 21 on plate 5.

Plate 6: X This means the patient could not identify a number on plate 6.

Plate 11: Traceable This means that the patient correctly traced a winding line on plate 11.

7. Procedural Step. Complete the charting entry. Include the date and time, the name of the test (Ishihara test), and any unusual symptoms the patient exhibited during the test, such as squinting or rubbing the eyes.

8. Procedural Step. Return the Ishihara book to its proper place. The book of color plates must be stored in a closed position to protect it from light.

Principle. Exposing the plates to excessive and unnecessary light results in fading of the color.

CHARTING EXAMPLE

Plate No.	Normal Person	Results
1	12	12
2	8	8
3	5	5
4	29	29
5	74	21
6	7	X
7	45	45
8	2	2
9	X	X
10	16	16
11	Traceable	Traceable
11/6/10	10:00 a.m.	
	C. Lindner, CMA (AAMA)	

EYE IRRIGATION

An eye irrigation involves washing the eye with a flowing solution. Eye irrigations are performed for the following purposes: to cleanse the eye by washing away foreign particles, ocular discharges, or harmful chemicals; to relieve inflammation through the application of heat; and to apply an antiseptic solution. Procedure 21-3 shows how to perform an eye irrigation.

EYE INSTILLATION

An eye instillation involves the dropping of a liquid into the lower conjunctival sac of the eye. Eye instillations are performed to treat eye infections (with medication), soothe an irritated eye, dilate the pupil, and anesthetize the eye during an eye examination or treatment. Medication to be instilled in the eye may come in the form of a liquid, as ophthalmic drops, or as an ophthalmic ointment. The eye drops are usually dispensed in a flexible plastic container with an attached dropper. Eye ointment is dispensed in a small metal tube with a small tip for applying the medication. Procedure 21-4 shows how to perform an eye instillation.

What Would You Do? What Would You *Not* Do?

Case Study 2

Peter Mitchell comes in with his 5-year-old son, Clive. Clive is diagnosed with conjunctivitis, and the physician prescribes Poly-trim ophthalmic suspension. Mr. Mitchell says that Clive does not cooperate very well when having drops put in his eyes and asks for any ideas that might make it less of an ordeal. Mr. Mitchell has 7-year-old twin girls at home and wants to know what can be done so they do not get pink eye. He asks if it would be all right to instill the drops in the twins' eyes as a preventive measure. ■

PATIENT TEACHING Conjunctivitis

Answer questions patients have about conjunctivitis.

What is conjunctivitis?

Conjunctivitis, often referred to as *pink eye,* is an inflammation of the conjunctiva. The conjunctiva is a thin, transparent membrane that covers the white of the eye. Conjunctivitis occurs when the conjunctiva becomes infected with a bacterium or virus. Other causes of conjunctivitis include allergies, the prolonged use of contact lenses, and irritation from wind, dust, and smoke. Conjunctivitis is almost always harmless and clears up by itself within 2 weeks. If it is caused by a bacterium, the physician may prescribe antibiotic eye drops or ointment.

What are the symptoms of conjunctivitis?

Most types of conjunctivitis are relatively painless. The eye is red or pink because of irritation, and there is a feeling of sandiness or grittiness in the eye. A discharge is usually present, which dries at night when the eyes are closed. This may cause the eyelids to be stuck together in the morning. Other symptoms include tearing, itching, and sensitivity of the eye to light.

Is conjunctivitis contagious?

Conjunctivitis caused by a virus or bacterium is highly contagious. It can be spread easily from one eye to another and throughout a family or classroom in a matter of days.

How can we avoid spreading conjunctivitis?

The following measures help prevent the spread of conjunctivitis:

- Avoid touching or rubbing the infected eye, which can spread the infection to the other eye or other people.
- Sanitize your hands frequently with soap, particularly after touching the eyes or face.
- Do not share washcloths, towels, or pillows with anyone.
- Do not wear contact lenses or eye makeup until the conjunctivitis is completely gone.
- Discard eye makeup that is used while you are infected to prevent reinfection.
- Encourage the patient to practice techniques that prevent the spread of conjunctivitis.
- If the physician has prescribed eye medication, teach the patient (or parent) the proper procedure for performing an eye instillation.
- Give the patient educational materials on conjunctivitis. ∎

PROCEDURE 21-3   Performing an Eye Irrigation

Outcome Perform an eye irrigation.

Equipment/Supplies

- Disposable gloves (nonpowdered)
- Irrigating solution
- Solution basin
- Bath thermometer
- Disposable rubber bulb syringe
- Basin
- Moisture-resistant towel
- Gauze pads

1. **Procedural Step.** Sanitize your hands.
2. **Procedural Step.** Assemble the equipment. If both eyes are to be irrigated, two sets of equipment must be used to prevent cross-infection from one eye to the other. Normal saline is generally used to irrigate the eye. Perform the following:
   a. Carefully check the label of the irrigating solution three times to make sure you have the correct solution. The first time is after you remove the solution container from the shelf. Compare the label of the solution container with the physician's instructions. Normal saline is generally used to irrigate the eye.
   b. Check the expiration date of the solution.
   c. Warm the irrigating solution to body temperature (98.6°F [37°C]) by placing the solution container in a basin of warm water. Use a bath thermometer to make sure the temperature of the water used to warm the solution does not exceed body temperature.

   d. Check the solution label a second time before pouring the solution.
   e. Pour the solution as follows:
      Palm the label of the container and remove the cap. Place the cap on a flat surface with the open end up. Pour the solution into the basin and replace the cap without contaminating it. Cover the basin to keep the solution warm.
   f. Check the solution label a third time before returning the container to its storage area.
   Principle. The solution label should be carefully checked three times to prevent an error. Outdated solutions may produce undesirable effects and should be discarded. If the solution is too cold or too warm, it will be uncomfortable for the patient. Palming the label prevents solution from dripping on the label and obscuring it or loosening the label. Placing the cap open end up prevents contamination.
3. **Procedural Step.** Greet the patient and introduce yourself. Identify the patient and explain the proce-

dure and purpose of the irrigation. If the patient wears glasses or contact lenses, ask him or her to remove them.

4. **Procedural Step.** Position the patient. The patient may be placed in a sitting or lying position. Place a moisture-resistant towel on the patient's shoulder to protect the patient's clothing. Position a basin tightly against the patient's cheek under the affected eye to catch the irrigating solution, and ask the patient to hold it in place. Ask the patient to tilt the head in the direction of the affected eye.

   Principle. The patient is positioned so that the solution flows away from the unaffected eye to prevent cross-infection.

5. **Procedural Step.** Apply nonpowdered gloves. Cleanse the eyelids from inner to outer **canthus** with a moistened gauze pad to remove any discharge or debris on

(From Bonewit-West K: *Clinical procedures for medical assistants,* ed 7, St. Louis, 2008, Saunders.)

Cleanse the eyelids from inner to outer canthus. (From Bonewit-West K: *Clinical procedures for medical assistants,* ed 7, St. Louis, 2008, Saunders.)

the lids. The inner canthus is the inner junction of the eyelids next to the nose. The outer canthus is the junction of the eyelids farthest from the nose. Normal saline or the solution ordered for the irrigation may be used. Discard the gauze pad after each wipe.

Principle. Nonpowdered gloves avoid irritation of the patient's eye with powder that may have gotten on the outside of the glove. The eyelids should be clean to prevent foreign particles from entering the eye during the irrigation. Cleansing from inner to outer canthus prevents cross-infection.

6. **Procedural Step.** Fill the irrigating syringe with the solution by squeezing the bulb and slowly releasing it until the desired amount of solution enters the bulb. Instruct the patient to keep both eyes open and find a focal point in the room and focus on it.

   Principle. Looking at a focal point helps the patient keep the irrigated eye open during the procedure.

7. **Procedural Step.** Separate the eyelids with the index finger and thumb to expose the lower conjunctiva and to hold the upper eyelid open.

   Principle. The medical assistant must hold the eye open during the procedure because the patient will have a tendency to close it.

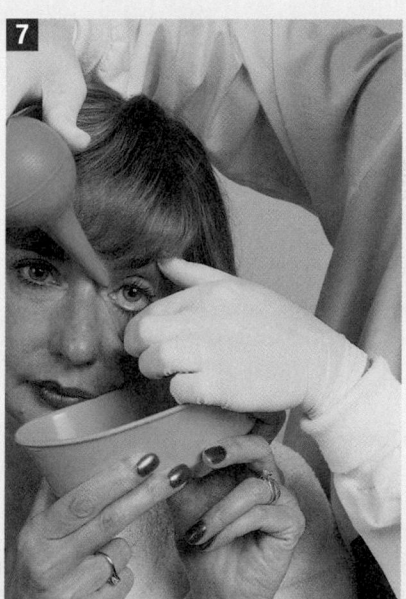

Separate the eyelids, and hold the tip of the syringe 1 inch above the eye. (From Bonewit-West K: *Clinical procedures for medical assistants,* ed 7, St. Louis, 2008, Saunders.)

8. **Procedural Step.** Hold the tip of the syringe approximately 1 inch above the eye. Gently release the solution onto the eye at the inner canthus. This allows the solution to flow over the eye at a moderate rate from the inner to outer canthus. Direct the solution to the lower conjunctiva. To prevent injury, do not allow the tip of the syringe to touch the eye.

Continued

PROCEDURE 21-3   Performing an Eye Irrigation—cont'd

Principle. The solution flows away from the unaffected eye to prevent cross-infection. The cornea is sensitive and can be harmed easily. The irrigating solution must be directed to the lower conjunctiva to prevent injury to the cornea.

9. **Procedural Step.** Refill the syringe, and continue irrigating until the desired results have been obtained or all the solution is used, depending on the purpose of the irrigation.

10. **Procedural Step.** Dry the eyelids from inner to outer canthus with a gauze pad.

11. **Procedural Step.** Remove the gloves, and sanitize your hands.

12. **Procedural Step.** Chart the procedure. Include the following: the date and time; which eye was irrigated; the type, strength, and amount of solution used; and any significant observations and patient reactions. Use

one of these abbreviations to indicate which eye was irrigated:

OU—Both eyes
OD—Right eye
OS—Left eye

13. **Procedural Step.** Remove reusable equipment to a work area for sanitization, sterilization, or disinfection as required by the medical office policy.

CHARTING EXAMPLE

Date	
11/5/10	10:30 a.m. Irrigated OS c̄ sterile saline @ 98.6° F. No complaints of discomfort.
	———————————— C. Lindner, CMA (AAMA)

PROCEDURE 21-4   Performing an Eye Instillation

Outcome Perform an eye instillation.

Equipment/Supplies

- Disposable gloves (nonpowdered)
- Ophthalmic drops or ophthalmic ointment as ordered by the physician
- Tissues
- Gauze pads

1. **Procedural Step.** Sanitize your hands.
2. **Procedural Step.** Assemble the equipment, and perform the following:
   a. Check the drug label three times to make sure you have the correct medication. The first time should be when you remove the medication from the shelf. The medication label must bear the word *ophthalmic.*
   b. Check the medication label a second time against the physician's instructions. Also check the dosage ordered by the physician.
   c. Check the expiration date.
   d. Check the medication label a third time before the cap is removed to instill the medication.
   Principle. The drug label should be carefully checked three times to prevent a medication error. Medication not bearing the word *ophthalmic* must never be placed in the eye because it could injure the eye. An outdated medication may produce undesirable effects and should be discarded.
3. **Procedural Step.** Greet the patient and introduce yourself. Identify the patient and explain the proce-

dure and purpose of the instillation. If the patient wears glasses or contact lenses, ask him or her to remove them.

4. **Procedural Step.** Help the patient into a sitting or supine position.

5. **Procedural Step.** Apply nonpowdered gloves. Prepare the medication. **Eye drops:** If the medication requires mixing, shake the container well. Check the medication label for the third time, and remove the cap from the container. **Eye ointment:** Check the medication label for the third time, and remove the cap from the tip of the tube.
   Principle. Nonpowdered gloves avoid irritation of the patient's eyes with powder that may have gotten on the outside of the gloves.

6. **Procedural Step.** Ask the patient to look up at the ceiling, and expose the lower conjunctival sac by using the fingers of the nondominant hand placed over a tissue. The fingers should be placed on the patient's cheekbone just below the eye, and the skin of the cheek should be drawn gently downward.

Principle. Looking up helps keep the patient from blinking when the drops are instilled.

7. Procedural Step. Insert the medication. **Eye drops:** Invert the container and hold the tip of the dropper approximately ½ inch above the eye sac. Do not allow the dropper to touch the eye or any other surface. Gently squeeze the container and place the correct number of eye drops in the center of the lower conjunctival sac. Never place the drops directly on the eyeball. Replace the cap on the container. **Eye ointment:** Gently squeeze the tube and place a thin ribbon of ointment along the length of the lower conjunctival sac from inner to outer canthus. Be careful not to touch the tip of the ointment tube to the eye or any other surface. Discontinue the ribbon by twisting the tube. Replace the cap on the tube.

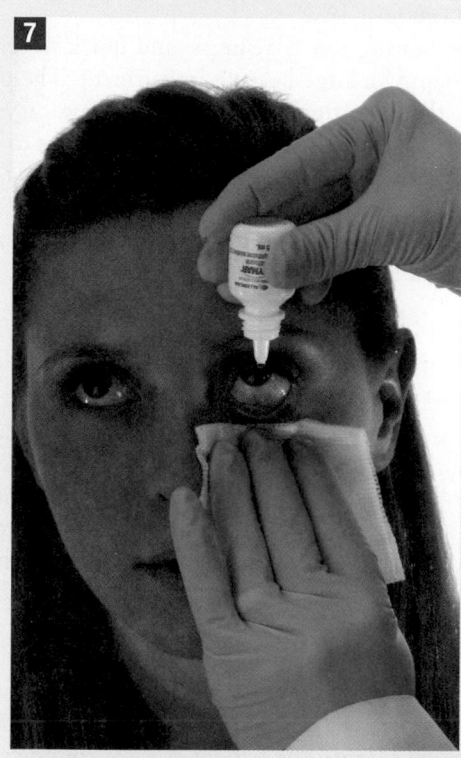

7

Ask the patient to look up, and insert the medication. (From Bonewit-West K: *Clinical procedures for medical assistants,* ed 7, St. Louis, 2008, Saunders.)

Principle. Touching the dropper or tip of the tube to the eye (or other surfaces) could injure the eye and contaminate the medication. Placing the medication in the conjunctival sac, rather than directly on the eyeball, is more comfortable for the patient.

8. Procedural Step. Ask the patient to close his or her eyes gently and move the eyeballs. Instruct the patient not to shut the eyes tight or to blink and to keep the eyes closed for 1 to 2 minutes. Tell the patient that the instillation may blur the vision temporarily.

Principle. Moving the eyeballs helps distribute the medication over the entire eye. Keeping the eyes closed allows the medication to be absorbed. If the eyes are shut tightly or if the patient blinks, the drops or ointment may be pushed out of the eye.

9. Procedural Step. Dry the eyelid from inner to outer canthus with a gauze pad to remove excess medication.

10. Procedural Step. Remove the gloves, and sanitize your hands.

11. Procedural Step. Chart the procedure. The medication dosage for eye drops is recorded in the number of drops instilled. The abbreviation for drop is *gtt;* for drops, *gtts.* The number of drops must be recorded in Roman numerals (i.e., i, ii) following the *gtt* abbreviation. The recording should include the date and time, the name and strength of the medication, the number of drops or amount of ointment, which eye received the instillation, your observations, and the patient's reaction.

12. Procedural Step. Return the medication to its proper storage area.

CHARTING EXAMPLE	
Date	
11/5/10	2:30 p.m. Atropine sulfate, 1% gtts ii OU.
	Pt states a temporary blurring of vision. ——
	———————————— C. Lindner, CMA (AAMA)

Introduction to the Ear

The medical assistant is responsible for performing a variety of procedures that involve the ear. An understanding of the structure and function of the ear is essential to mastering skill in these areas. Refer to Chapter 10 to review the structure and function of the ear.

Hearing tests may be part of a routine physical examination. When interacting with the patient, the medical assistant should be alert to signs that indicate the patient might be having difficulty hearing what is being said. A whispered voice next to the patient's ear can be a screening test for hearing acuity. The use of tuning forks or an audiometer provides a more accurate determination of hearing acuity. An **audiometer** is an instrument that emits sound waves at various frequencies. The patient is instructed to indicate when a sound at a given frequency can be heard.

The medical assistant is responsible for performing or teaching the patient to perform ear irrigations and instillations. Ear irrigations and instillations should be performed using the important principles of medical asepsis outlined in Chapter 17.

PROCEDURE 21-4

ASSESSMENT OF HEARING ACUITY

The assessment of hearing acuity is an integral part of a complete physical examination. It is possible for an individual to have a hearing loss and not be aware of it. Early detection and treatment of hearing problems help prevent permanent hearing loss.

An individual with normal hearing should be able to hear the frequencies of normal speech, which range from 300 to 4000 Hz (hertz, or cycles per second) at a normal sound intensity. Patients who exhibit hearing loss are referred to an otolaryngologist or an audiologist for further evaluation.

Types of Hearing Loss

Hearing loss is of three types: conductive, sensorineural, and mixed. *Conductive hearing loss* is the most common and results when there is a physical interference with the normal conduction of sound waves through the external and middle ear. Because of the interference, the amount of sound reaching the inner ear is less than normal, resulting in hearing impairment. Conductive loss in the external ear may be caused by an obstruction in the external ear canal, such as **impacted cerumen,** swelling from external otitis (swimmer's ear), foreign bodies, and benign growths such as polyps. Conductive loss in the middle ear may be caused by serous otitis media (fluid in the middle ear) or acute otitis media (infection in the middle ear), a perforated **tympanic membrane,** or otosclerosis. The cause of conductive hearing loss often can be detected by examining the external ear canal with an **otoscope.** Hearing is frequently restored by removing the obstruction (e.g., impacted cerumen) or treating the disorder (e.g., serous otitis media).

Sensorineural hearing loss results from damage to the inner ear or auditory nerve. With this type of hearing loss, the sound is conducted normally through the outer and middle ear structures, but because of a problem with the perception of sound waves, a hearing deficit occurs. Specific causes of sensorineural loss include hereditary factors, intense noise exposure over time, tumors, degenerative changes from the normal aging process, ototoxicity caused by certain medications and infectious diseases, such as measles, mumps, and meningitis. *Mixed hearing loss* is a combination of conductive and sensorineural loss.

Hearing Acuity Tests

Numerous tests can be used to assess hearing acuity. Tests range from the simple gross screening test to qualitative tests using a tuning fork to highly specific quantitative tests using an audiometer. It is important to test only one ear at a time because a hearing deficit can exist in one ear only. The ear not being tested should be blocked by an earplug or masked. *Masking* involves the presentation of sound (usually noise) to the ear not being tested so that the patient's response is based only on hearing in the ear being tested.

Gross Screening Test

The gross hearing test is a simple and quick screening test used to identify a large hearing impairment. The physician performs the screening test during the physical examination. Hearing is assessed by asking the patient to repeat a simple word or series of numbers whispered from a distance of 1 to 2 feet from the ear. When a hearing loss is discovered, a tuning fork or audiometer is used for a more precise assessment of hearing.

Tuning Fork Tests

Tuning fork tests provide a general assessment of hearing acuity and may be part of the physical examination. A tuning fork with a frequency of 512 Hz or 1024 Hz is generally used because these frequencies fall within the range of normal speech. The Weber and Rinne tests are the tuning fork tests most commonly performed by the physician; they are used to identify conductive and sensorineural hearing loss.

The *Weber test* is a useful assessment of hearing loss when one ear hears better than the other. The tuning fork is set in vibration, and the base of the fork is placed on the center of the patient's head. The patient is asked to indicate where the sound is heard best. A patient with normal hearing would hear the sound equally in both ears or in the center of the head. Figure 21-7 illustrates the Weber test and describes the interpretation of results.

The *Rinne test* compares the duration of sound perception by air conduction with that of bone conduction. The tuning fork is set in vibration, and the base of the fork is placed against the bone of the mastoid process. The patient is instructed to indicate when the sound is no longer heard. The prongs of the fork (still vibrating) are placed in the air about 1 inch from the opening of the patient's ear canal, and the patient indicates when the sound is no longer heard. An individual with normal hearing is able to hear the sound at least twice as long through air conduction as through bone conduction. Figure 21-8 illustrates the Rinne test and describes the interpretation of results.

What Would You Do? What Would You *Not* Do?

Case Study 3

Willow Basil brings in her 6-year-old daughter, Jade. For the past 3 days, Jade has been running a fever and has had persistent pain and hearing loss in her left ear. Mrs. Basil practices alternative medicine and uses prescription medications as little as possible. She says that she has been trying herbal therapy and aromatherapy to make Jade better, but it does not seem to be helping. Jade is diagnosed with acute otitis media, and the physician prescribes amoxicillin for 10 days. Mrs. Basil wants to know if she has to give Jade the amoxicillin for the entire 10 days. She asks if she can stop using it when Jade starts feeling better. Mrs. Basil also wants to know if the ear infection will cause a permanent problem with Jade's hearing. ■

Normal Hearing
The patient hears the sound equally in both ears or in the center of the head.

Conductive Hearing Loss
The patient hears the sound better in the problem ear.

Sensorineural Hearing Loss
The patient does not hear the sound as well in the problem ear.

Figure 21-7. Weber test. (From Bonewit-West K: *Clinical procedures for medical assistants*, ed 7, St. Louis, 2008, Saunders.)

Bone conduction

Normal Hearing
The patient hears the sound at least twice as long through air conduction as through bone conduction.

Conductive Hearing Loss
The patient hears the sound longer by bone conduction than by air conduction.

Sensorineural Hearing Loss
The sound is reduced. The patient will also hear the sound longer through air conduction than through bone conduction but not twice as long.

Air conduction

Figure 21-8. Rinne test. (From Bonewit-West K: *Clinical procedures for medical assistants,* ed 7, St. Louis, 2008, Saunders.)

Figure 21-9. A, Audiometer. **B,** The patient signals when he hears a sound. (Courtesy GSI [Grason-Stadler, Inc.], Milford, NH.)

Memories *from* Externship

Cammie Lindner: There is one characteristic that is shared by all patients. I first noticed this during my externships, and it does not seem to matter what type of practice it is. Patients like to feel special and to be treated that way. They like consistency in their physician and in the office staff, in seeing familiar faces. This is especially hard during externship. The time spent is too short to truly get to know the patients, but it is a great learning experience.

It is important to observe the staff and patient communication and interaction skills. By doing this, you can decide which ones you admire and those that you do not wish to copy. The following are just a few of the guidelines that have helped me: (1) Call patients by name, and be sure that they know your name. (2) Follow through with what you have told patients you will do, and keep them updated if circumstances change. (3) Smile and do not let one patient's negative attitude interfere with your care of others. (4) Take time to listen.

When you do begin your career, it does not take long to get into a routine and start knowing your patients. When patients see a familiar face, they are more willing to share information that can contribute to improved communication and good health care. ■

Prepare for Success

Audiometry

Audiometry is the measurement of hearing acuity using a special instrument called an **audiometer.** An audiometer quantitatively measures hearing for the various frequencies of sound waves. Audiometry is a more specific hearing acuity test because it provides information on how extensive a hearing loss is and which frequencies are involved. It is important that the test be conducted in a quiet room because outside noise may affect the results, especially in the lower frequencies. The patient wears headphones placed snugly over the ears (Figure 21-9). The audiometer delivers a single frequency at a time at specific intensities, starting with low-frequency tones of 250 to 500 Hz and going to very high frequencies of 6000 to 8000 Hz. The patient is asked to signal when he or she hears a sound so that the patient's hearing threshold for each frequency can be determined. The hearing acuity in each ear is assessed separately, and the results are plotted on a graph known as an *audiogram.* The medical assistant may be responsible for performing audiometry in the medical office. Before operating an audiometer, however, the medical assistant must receive extensive on-site training by an audiologist to ensure that proper technique is used to conduct the test.

Tympanometry

Tympanometry is not a hearing test, but it does help determine the cause of hearing loss, so it is presented in this section. The tympanometer consists of an earpiece attached to an electronic device (Figure 21-10). The earpiece is placed snugly in the patient's ear, and low-frequency sound waves are directed against the eardrum while pressure is applied in the ear canal. With a normal ear, the eardrum exhibits mobility in response to the pressure, as indicated on a graphic readout known as a *tympanogram.* If there is fluid in the middle ear, the eardrum does not move, but remains stiff, as indicated on the tympanogram. Tympanometry is useful in diagnosing serous otitis media (fluid in the middle ear), which is a common cause of temporary hearing loss in children.

PATIENT TEACHING Acute Otitis Media

Answer questions patients have about otitis media.

What is a middle ear infection?
An infection of the middle ear is medically referred to as *acute otitis media*. It is an inflammation of the middle ear caused by an infection and can occur in one or both ears. It is common in young children 3 months to 3 years old, but is unusual in adults. A middle ear infection is not serious if treated promptly and effectively. If not treated, however, middle ear infections can lead to serious complications, such as acute mastoiditis, meningitis, and permanent hearing loss.

What causes a middle ear infection?
It is believed that a middle ear infection as a result of a blocked eustachian tube may be caused by an upper respiratory infection or allergy. The blockage causes fluid to build up in the middle ear. This fluid is an ideal place for bacteria to grow. If this occurs, the result is acute otitis media.

What are the symptoms of a middle ear infection?
The most common symptoms are intense pain, fever, and temporary hearing loss. Other symptoms may include dizziness, nausea and vomiting, and (if the eardrum ruptures) drainage from the ear.

How does the physician know whether a middle ear infection is present?
The physician examines the ears with an otoscope. If a middle ear infection is present, the eardrum is red and swollen, as a result of irritation from the infection, and there is pus and mucus behind the eardrum.

How is the infection treated?
A middle ear infection is usually treated with an oral antibiotic for 10 to 14 days. It is important to take all of the antibiotic prescribed; otherwise, the ear infection may recur. The physician may also recommend a decongestant to help open the blocked eustachian tube. After the acute infection is over, fluid may remain trapped in the middle ear. This condition is known as *serous otitis media* and, if not treated, may last for days, weeks, months, or even a year. Although fluid in the middle ear is painless, it may result in a feeling of fullness or pressure in the ears and temporary hearing loss.

Why are middle ear infections so common in children?
In children, the eustachian tube is positioned horizontally and is shorter and narrower than in adults. When a child has an upper respiratory infection, bacteria can travel easily to the middle ear. In addition, swelling from the respiratory infection can block this narrow tube, which causes fluid to build up in the middle ear.
- Encourage the patient to complete the entire prescribed course of antibiotics.
- If the physician has prescribed ear drops, teach the patient (or parent) the proper procedure for performing an ear instillation.
- Encourage early treatment of upper respiratory infections.
- Give the patient educational materials on otitis media. ■

Highlight on Hearing Impairment

The number of individuals with a hearing impairment has gradually increased over the past 20 years. Factors that contribute to this increase include an aging population and a noisier environment.

It is estimated that approximately 28 million people in the United States have a hearing loss severe enough to interfere with their daily activities, whereas another 2 million individuals are profoundly deaf.

Precise screening of preschool children for hearing loss is difficult. This is because tuning fork tests and audiometry require the ability to signal in response to sound, and children up to age 4 or 5 years have trouble mastering this skill.

Most state, county, and local school systems require hearing screening as a prerequisite for entrance to school and again at periodic intervals, usually during the first, third, fifth, and seventh grades.

Risk factors for hearing impairment in children include family history of deafness, premature birth, low birth weight, measles, mumps, high fevers, meningitis, recurrent or chronic ear infections, and the maternal rubella infection during pregnancy.

Signs of hearing impairment in children are poor attentiveness, delayed speech development, and persistent problems with articulation. Signs of hearing impairment in adults include frequent requests for words or statements to be repeated, leaning toward the speaker, turning the head, cupping the ears, and speaking in a loud or unvaried tone of voice.

The most common cause of conductive hearing loss in children is fluid in the middle ear, which prevents the tympanic membrane from vibrating freely. In adults, the most common cause of conductive loss is otosclerosis, a condition in which the stapes becomes

Continued

Highlight on Hearing Impairment—cont'd

fixed because of calcium deposits and less able to pass on vibrations when sound enters the ear.

The loudness of sound is measured in units called *decibels* (dB). Sounds of less than 75 dB, even after long exposure, are unlikely to cause hearing loss. Normal conversation is approximately 60 dB, and a whisper in a quiet library is 30 to 40 dB.

Permanent sensorineural hearing loss can result when the ear is repeatedly bombarded with loud sound over time. Standards set by OSHA indicate that continued exposure to noise louder than 85 dB eventually harms an individual's hearing by damaging the tiny hair cells in the organ of Corti. The organ of Corti is a structure in the cochlea (inner ear) that converts sound waves into nerve impulses for transmission to the brain. This type of sensorineural hearing loss is known as *noise-induced hearing loss.* It is most often seen in individuals who frequently listen to loud music, fire guns without wearing ear protection, or are exposed to loud noise as part of their jobs. The following are examples of common noises and the decibel level of each:

Noise	Decibels
Normal breathing	10
Humming of a refrigerator	40
Television	70
Vacuum cleaner	60-85
Motorcycle	95-100
Personal stereo system with earphones (on high)	115
Rock concert	120
Chain saw	120
Auto stereo on high	125
Jet taking off	140
Firecracker	150
Firearms	140-170

Many hearing impairments can be helped with the use of a hearing aid. Individuals who benefit most from a hearing aid have mild-to-moderate conductive hearing loss. Individuals with sensorineural or mixed hearing loss have more trouble finding a suitable hearing aid and often get less satisfactory results. ■

EAR IRRIGATION

An ear irrigation is the washing of the external auditory canal with a flowing solution. Ear irrigations are performed for the following purposes: to cleanse the external auditory canal to remove cerumen, discharge, or a foreign body; to relieve inflammation by applying an antiseptic solution; and to apply heat to the ear. Before irrigating, impacted cerumen must be softened by instilling warm mineral oil or hydrogen peroxide for 10 to 15 minutes. Procedure 21-5 shows how to perform an ear irrigation. An ear irrigation should not be performed if the tympanic membrane is perforated because it could result in a severe irritation or infection of the middle ear.

EAR INSTILLATION

An ear instillation involves the dropping of a liquid into the external auditory canal. Ear instillations are performed to soften impacted cerumen, combat infection with the use of antibiotic ear drops, and relieve pain. The ear drops are usually dispensed in a flexible plastic container with an attached dropper. Procedure 21-6 shows how to perform an ear instillation.

Figure 21-10. A, Tympanometer. **B,** The earpiece is placed snugly in the patient's ear. (Courtesy GSI [Grason-Stadler, Inc.], Milford, NH.)

PROCEDURE 21-5 Performing an Ear Irrigation

Outcome Perform an ear irrigation.

Equipment/Supplies

- Disposable gloves
- Irrigating solution
- Solution basin
- Bath thermometer
- Irrigating syringe

- Ear basin
- Moisture-resistant towel
- Gauze pads
- Ear wick

1. Procedural Step. Sanitize your hands.

2. Procedural Step. Assemble the equipment. If both ears are to be irrigated, two sets of equipment must be used to prevent cross-infection from one ear to the other. Perform the following:

a. Carefully check the label of the irrigating solution three times to make sure you have the correct solution. The first time is after you remove the solution container from the shelf. Compare the label of the solution container with the physician's instructions.

b. Check the expiration date of the solution.

c. Warm the irrigating solution to body temperature (98.6°F [37°C]) by placing the solution container in a basin of warm water. Use a bath thermometer to make sure the temperature of the water used to warm the solution does not exceed body temperature.

d. Check the solution label a second time before pouring the solution.

e. Pour the solution as follows:
Palm the label of the container and remove the cap. Place the cap on a flat surface with the open end up. Pour the solution into the basin and replace the cap without contaminating it. Cover the basin to keep the solution warm.

f. Check the solution label a third time before returning the container to its storage area.

Assemble the equipment. (From Bonewit-West K: *Clinical procedures for medical assistants,* ed 7, St. Louis, 2008, Saunders.)

Principle. The solution label should be carefully checked three times to prevent an error. An outdated solution may produce undesirable effects. If the solution is too cold or too warm, it might stimulate the inner ear and the patient will become dizzy. Palming the label prevents the solution from dripping on the label and obscuring it or loosening the label. Placing the cap open end up prevents contamination.

3. Procedural Step. Greet the patient and introduce yourself. Identify the patient and explain the procedure. Explain the purpose of performing the irrigation—for example, to remove cerumen. Tell the patient the procedure is not painful; however, he or she may feel a minimal amount of discomfort and occasional dizziness, fullness, and warmth as the ear solution comes in contact with the tympanic membrane.

4. Procedural Step. Help the patient into a sitting position with the head tilted toward the affected ear. Place a moisture-resistant towel on the patient's shoulder under the ear to be irrigated to protect clothing and to prevent water from running down the neck. Instruct the patient to hold the ear basin tightly against the neck under the affected ear to catch the irrigating solution.

Principle. The patient is positioned so that gravity aids the flow of the solution out of the ear and into the basin.

5. Procedural Step. Apply gloves. Cleanse the outer ear with a moistened gauze pad to remove any discharge or debris present. Normal saline or the solution ordered for the irrigation may be used.

Principle. The outer ear should be clean to prevent foreign particles from entering the ear canal during the irrigation.

6. Procedural Step. Fill the syringe with the irrigating solution (approximately 50 ml). Expel air from the syringe.

Principle. Air forced into the ear is uncomfortable for the patient.

7. Procedural Step. Straighten the external ear canal. The canal is straightened by gently pulling the ear upward and backward for adults and children older than 3 years old and downward and backward for children 3 years old and younger.

Continued

PROCEDURE **21-5**   Performing an Ear Irrigation—cont'd

Principle. Straightening the canal permits the irrigating solution to reach all areas of the canal.

8. **Procedural Step.** Insert the syringe tip into the ear, but not too deeply. Make sure that the tip of the syringe does not obstruct the canal opening so that the solution can flow freely out of the canal.
   Principle. Inserting the tip of the syringe too deeply causes discomfort for the patient.

   Obstruction of the canal causes pressure to build up in the canal, resulting in patient discomfort and possible injury to the tympanic membrane.

9. **Procedural Step.** Inject the irrigating solution toward the roof of the ear canal. It is important that the solution be injected toward the roof of the canal to prevent it from being injected directly onto the tympanic membrane.
   Principle. The tip of the syringe should be directed at the roof of the canal to prevent injury to the tympanic membrane and to aid in the removal of foreign particles by allowing the solution to flow down the length of the canal and out the bottom. In addition, severe patient discomfort and dizziness may occur if the solution is injected directly onto the tympanic membrane.

Inject the irrigating solution toward the roof of the ear canal. (From Bonewit-West K: *Clinical procedures for medical assistants,* ed 7, St. Louis, 2008, Saunders.)

10. **Procedural Step.** Refill the syringe, and continue irrigating until the desired results have been obtained or all the solution is used, depending on the purpose of

the irrigation. Observe the returning solution to note the material present (e.g., cerumen, discharge, a foreign object) and the amount (small, moderate, or large).

11. **Procedural Step.** Dry the outside of the ear with a gauze pad. Have the patient lie on the affected side on the treatment table. Tell the patient that the ear will feel sensitive for a short time. Place a cotton wick loosely in the ear canal for 15 minutes if instructed to do so by the physician.
    Principle. Any solution remaining in the ear canal should be allowed to drain out. A cotton wick makes the patient's ear feel less sensitive after the irrigation.

12. **Procedural Step.** Remove the gloves, and sanitize your hands.

13. **Procedural Step.** Chart the procedure. Include the following: the date and time; which ear was irrigated; the type, strength, and amount of solution used; the amount and type of material returned in the irrigating solution; any significant observations; and patient reactions. Use one of these abbreviations to indicate which ear was irrigated:
    AU—Both ears
    AD—Right ear
    AS—Left ear

14. **Procedural Step.** Remove reusable equipment to a work area for sanitization, sterilization, or disinfection as required by the medical office policy.

CHARTING EXAMPLE	
Date	
11/15/10	2:15 p.m. Irrigated AD c̄ saline, 200 ml @ 98.6° F. Mod amt of cerumen present in returned solution. Cotton wick placed in ear canal × 15 min. No complaints of discomfort.
	—————————— C. Lindner, CMA (AAMA)

PROCEDURE 21-6 **Performing an Ear Instillation**

Outcome Perform an ear instillation.

Equipment/Supplies

* Disposable gloves
* Otic drops
* Gauze pad

1. **Procedural Step.** Sanitize your hands.
2. **Procedural Step.** Assemble the equipment, and perform the following:
   a. Check the drug label three times to make sure you have the correct medication. The first time should be when you remove the medication from the shelf. The medication label must bear the word *otic*.
   b. Check the medication label a second time against the physician's instructions. Also check the dosage ordered by the physician.
   c. Check the expiration date.
   d. Check the medication label a third time before the cap is removed to instill the medication.
   Principle. The drug label should be carefully checked three times to prevent a medication error. Medication not bearing the word *otic* must not be placed in the ear because it could injure the ear. An outdated medication may produce undesirable effects.
3. **Procedural Step.** Greet the patient and introduce yourself. Identify the patient and explain the procedure and purpose of the instillation.
4. **Procedural Step.** Position the patient in a sitting position.
5. **Procedural Step.** Warm the drops to body temperature by holding the medication container in the palms of your hands for a few minutes. Do not warm the drops by placing them in hot water.
   Principle. If the drops are too cold or too warm, they might stimulate the inner ear, causing the patient to become dizzy.
6. **Procedural Step.** Apply gloves. If the medication requires mixing, shake the container well. Check the medication label for the third time, and remove the cap from the container.
   Principle. Gravity aids in the flow of the medication into the ear canal.
7. **Procedural Step.** Ask the patient to tilt his or her head in the direction of the unaffected ear. Straighten the external auditory canal. The canal is straightened by pulling the ear upward and backward for adults and children older than 3 years old and downward and backward for children 3 years old and younger.
   Principle. Straightening the canal permits the medication to reach all areas of the canal.
8. **Procedural Step.** Invert the container and place the tip of the dropper at the opening of the ear canal.

Gently squeeze the container and instill the correct number of drops along the side of the canal. Replace the cap on the container.

Instill the medication along the side of the ear canal. (From Bonewit-West K: *Clinical procedures for medical assistants,* ed 7, St. Louis, 2008, Saunders.)

9. **Procedural Step.** Instruct the patient to lie on the unaffected side for 2 to 3 minutes.
   Principle. Lying on the unaffected side prevents the medication from running out and allows complete distribution of the medication.
10. **Procedural Step.** Place a moistened cotton wick loosely in the ear canal for 15 minutes if instructed to do so by the physician.
    Principle. The cotton wick prevents the medication from running out when the patient sits up. Moistening the wick prevents the medication from being absorbed by the cotton.

Continued

PROCEDURE 21-6   Performing an Ear Instillation—cont'd

11. **Procedural Step.** Remove the gloves, and sanitize your hands.
12. **Procedural Step.** Chart the procedure. Include the date and time, the name and strength of the medication, the number of drops, which ear received the instillation, any significant observations, and the patient's reaction.
13. **Procedural Step.** Return the medication to its storage area.

CHARTING EXAMPLE

Date	
11/20/10	9:30 a.m. Auralgan gtts ii, AD. No discharge present. Pt states a relief of pain. —————— —————————— C. Lindner, CMA (AAMA)

MEDICAL PRACTICE and the LAW

Legal issues concerning eye and ear assessment are similar to the legal issues that concern any assessment. Accurate assessments done properly are necessary for accurate diagnoses and treatment and to prevent injuries to these structures.

Patient Rights

Patients entering the office have six major rights, which are enforceable by law, as follows:

1. The right to have the physician and medical assistant *do good for them.* Failure results in malpractice.
2. The right to *be treated fairly.* This is enforced by discrimination and employment laws.
3. The right to *be free.* This is exercised by giving informed consent and advance directives.
4. The right *not to be harmed.* Licensure protects patients by ensuring a minimal level of skill.
5. The right of fidelity, or *being true.* This includes confidentiality, telling the truth, and loyalty to the patient.
6. The right to *life.* This concerns cases of abortion, assisted suicide, and euthanasia.

If any of these rights is violated, the patient has the right to sue. ■

What Would You Do? What Would You *Not* Do?   RESPONSES

Case Study 1
Page 413

What Did Cammie Do?
❑ Talked with Haley (on her level) about why someone needs to wear glasses.
❑ Retested Haley with the Snellen chart to see if she missed the same letters.
❑ Tested Haley with the Big E chart to give the physician an additional measurement to make an interpretation of Haley's visual acuity.

What Did Cammie **Not** *Do?*
❑ Did not tell Haley that she needs glasses.
❑ Did not scold Haley for trying to miss letters on the test.

What Would You Do/What Would You *Not* Do? Review Cammie's response and place a checkmark next to the information you included in your response. List the additional information you included in your response.

_____
_____
_____
_____

Case Study 2
Page 417

What Did Cammie Do?
❑ Gave Mr. Mitchell some suggestions on how to put drops in Clive's eyes so that it is less scary. One idea is to have Clive lie down flat and close his eyes. Place the drops in the inner corner of his eye next to the bridge of his nose, letting them make a little lake there. When Clive relaxes and opens his eye, the drops will gently flow into his eye.
❑ Talked with Clive (on his level) about why he needs eye drops.
❑ Told Mr. Mitchell that the eye drops were prescribed for Clive, and they should be used only for Clive. Told him that if the twins developed conjunctivitis, he should call the office.

What Would You Do? What Would You *Not* Do?   RESPONSES—cont'd

❑ Gave Mr. Mitchell suggestions for preventing the twins from getting conjunctivitis (not touching the infected eye, frequent handwashing, not sharing toys or towels).

What Did Cammie Not *Do?*

❑ Did not tell Mr. Mitchell to hold Clive down or force drops in his eyes.

❑ Did not tell Mr. Mitchell that he should know better than to think about giving the twins a medication not prescribed for them.

What Would You Do/What Would You *Not* Do? Review Cammie's response and place a checkmark next to the information you included in your response. List the additional information you included in your response.

_____

_____

_____

_____

Case Study 3
Page 422

What Did Cammie Do?

❑ Explained to Mrs. Basil that Jade may begin to feel better after several days of antibiotics, but not all of the germs causing her ear infection will have been killed by then. If she does not give

Jade the full course of antibiotics, the infection could come back.

❑ Documented all the medications that Mrs. Basil has administered to Jade.

❑ Gave Mrs. Basil a patient information brochure on acute otitis media.

❑ Told Mrs. Basil that she needs to talk to the physician about her concern regarding hearing loss because he is most qualified to answer that question.

❑ Encouraged Mrs. Basil to bring Jade in sooner when she develops fever and ear pain.

What Did Cammie Not *Do?*

❑ Did not criticize Mrs. Basil for waiting so long to bring Jade in.

❑ Did not offer a personal opinion about alternative medicine.

What Would You Do/What Would You *Not* Do? Review Cammie's response and place a checkmark next to the information you included in your response. List the additional information you included in your response.

_____

_____

_____

⟳ TERMINOLOGY REVIEW

Audiometer An instrument used to measure hearing acuity quantitatively for the various frequencies of sound waves.

Canthus The junction of the eyelids at either corner of the eye.

Cerumen Ear wax.

Hyperopia Farsightedness.

Impacted Wedged firmly together so as to be immovable.

Instillation The dropping of a liquid into a body cavity.

Irrigation The washing of a body canal with a flowing solution.

Myopia Nearsightedness.

Otoscope An instrument used to examine the external ear canal and tympanic membrane.

Presbyopia A decrease in the elasticity of the lens that occurs with aging, resulting in a decreased ability to focus on close objects.

Refraction The deflection or bending of light rays by a lens.

Tympanic membrane A thin, semitransparent membrane between the external ear canal and the middle ear that receives and transmits sound waves. Also known as the *eardrum.*

ON THE WEB

For Information on the Eye:

American Optometric Association: www.aoa.org

American Academy of Ophthalmology: www.aao.org

National Eye Institute: www.nei.nih.gov

All About Vision: www.allaboutvision.com

Sight and Hearing Association: www.sightandhearing.org

American Academy of Optometry: www.aaopt.org

American Association for Pediatric Ophthalmology and Strabismus: www.aapos.org

For Information on the Ear:

American Academy of Audiology: www.audiology.org

National Institute on Deafness and Other Communication Disorders: www.nidcd.nih.gov

Healthy Hearing: www.healthyhearing.com

Hear It: www.hear-it.org

League for the Hard of Hearing: www.lhh.org

 PREPARE FOR CERTIFICATION   Visit the Evolve site at http://evolve.elsevier.com/Bonewit/today/ to actively Prepare for your Certification.

 *Check out the **Companion CD** bound with the book to access additional interactive activities.*

22

Physical Agents to Promote Tissue Healing

LEARNING OBJECTIVES

Local Application of Heat and Cold

1. Give examples of moist and dry applications of heat and cold.
2. State the factors to consider when applying heat and cold.
3. List the effects of local application of heat, and state reasons for applying heat.
4. List the effects of local application of cold, and state reasons for applying cold.

Ambulatory Aids

1. List factors that are taken into consideration when ambulatory aids are prescribed.
2. Explain the difference between an axillary crutch and a forearm crutch.
3. State conditions that may result when axillary crutches are not fitted properly.
4. List the guidelines that should be followed by the patient to ensure safe use of crutches.
5. State the use of each of the following crutch gaits: four-point gait, two-point gait, three-point gait, swing-to gait, and swing-through gait.
6. List and describe the three types of canes.
7. Identify the patient conditions that warrant the use of a cane or walker.

PROCEDURES

Apply each of the following heat treatments:
  Heating pad
  Hot soak
  Hot compress
  Chemical hot pack
Apply each of the following cold treatments:
  Ice bag
  Cold compress
  Chemical cold pack

Measure a patient for axillary crutches.
Instruct a patient in the proper use of crutches.
Instruct a patient in the proper procedure for each of the following crutch gaits:
  Four-point
  Two-point
  Three-point
  Swing-to
  Swing-through
Instruct a patient in the use of a cane.
Instruct a patient in the proper use of a walker.

CHAPTER OUTLINE

Introduction to Tissue Healing
Local Application of Heat and Cold
  Factors Affecting the Application of Heat and Cold
  Heat
  Cold

Ambulatory Aids
  Crutches
  Canes
  Walkers

CAAHEP COMPETENCIES

Clinical Competencies
Patient Care

- Prepare and maintain examination and treatment areas.
- Prepare patient for and assist with procedures, treatments, and minor office surgeries.

General Competencies
Patient Instructions

- Instruct individuals according to their needs.
- Provide instruction for health maintenance and disease prevention.

ABHES COMPETENCIES

Communication
- Adaptation for individualized needs

Clinical Duties
- Prepare and maintain examination and treatment area.
- Prepare patient for and assist physician with routine and specialty examinations and treatments and minor office surgeries.

Instruction
- Teach patients methods of health promotion and disease prevention.

KEY TERMS

ambulation (AM-byoo-LAY-shun)
ambulatory
compress (KOM-press)
edema (uh-DEE-muh)
erythema (err-uh-THEE-muh)

exudate (EKS-oo-date)
soak
sprain
strain
suppuration (SUP-er-AY-shun)

Introduction to Tissue Healing

Physical agents are often employed in the medical office to promote tissue healing for individuals who experience a disability as a result of injury, disease, or loss of a body part. Physical agents are used therapeutically to improve circulation, provide support, and promote the return of motion so that the individual can perform the activities of daily living. Physical agents frequently used in the medical office include the local application of heat and cold and ambulatory aids, such as crutches, canes, and walkers.

LOCAL APPLICATION OF HEAT AND COLD

The application of heat and cold is used therapeutically to treat conditions such as infection and trauma. The medical assistant may be responsible for applying various forms of heat and cold at the medical office or for instructing patients in the proper procedure for applying heat or cold at home. The medical assistant should have a basic understanding of the physiologic effects of heat and cold on the body and possible adverse reactions if they are not administered correctly.

Heat and cold can be applied in moist or dry forms. The common applications of dry and moist heat and cold are as follows:
1. *Dry heat:* heating pad, chemical hot pack
2. *Moist heat:* hot soak, hot compress
3. *Dry cold:* ice bag, chemical cold pack
4. *Moist cold:* cold compress

Heat and cold are applied for short periods (generally 15 to 30 minutes) to produce the desired therapeutic results. The application may be repeated at time intervals specified by the physician. Prolonged application of heat or cold is not recommended because it can result in adverse secondary effects. The type of heat or cold application used for a particular condition depends on the purpose of the application, the location and condition of the affected area, and the age and general health of the patient. The physician instructs the medical assistant to apply a heat or cold treatment based on these factors.

Heat and cold receptors in the skin readily adapt to changes in temperature, eventually resulting in diminished heat or cold sensations. The temperature actually remains the same and is providing the intended therapeutic effects. The patient, not perceiving the same degree of temperature, may want to increase the intensity of the application, however, without realizing the inherent dangers. Excessive heat or cold could result in tissue damage. A common example of this situation is a patient who turns up the setting of a heating pad from medium to high when the heating pad no longer feels warm. The medical assistant should fully explain to the patient the necessity of maintaining a safe temperature range during the application.

Factors Affecting the Application of Heat and Cold

Before applying heat or cold, certain factors must be taken into consideration to prevent unfavorable reactions, such as tissue necrosis. The temperature may need to be adjusted based on the following conditions:
1. **The age of the patient.** Young children and elderly patients tend to be more sensitive to the application of heat or cold.
2. **Location of the application.** Certain areas of the body are more sensitive to the application of heat or cold, especially thin areas of the skin and areas that are usually covered by clothing, such as the chest, back, and abdomen. The skin on the hands and face is not as sensitive and is better able to tolerate temperature change.

Putting It All into Practice

My name is Marlyne Cooper, and I am a certified medical assistant. I work in a community health center. My primary responsibilities are to take patients back to the examination rooms and to prepare them for procedures and treatments. I take the patient's chief complaint and the health history. I greet each patient in a kind and calm way. This helps put the patient at ease before the physician goes into the examining room.

I once worked in a private office with a small waiting room and narrow hall. One of my regular patients was a healthy young 20-year-old man who was confined to a wheelchair by a spinal injury from an automobile accident. He had great difficulty maneuvering his motorized chair in tight spaces, and he felt embarrassed and conspicuous sitting in the middle of the waiting room. I began bringing him through the larger back door into the physician's office, directly into an examination room. Talking about things we had in common, such as an interest in sports and movies, made him feel more at ease. By making the situation as easy as possible for him, he was able to keep his dignity and not draw attention to his special needs. ∎

Prepare for Success

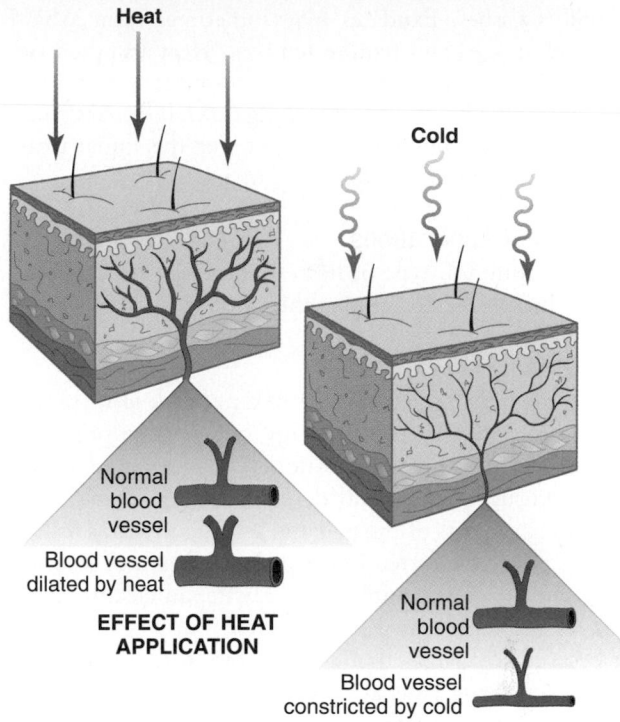

Figure 22-1. Effects of the local application of heat and cold. (From Wood LA, Rambo BJ: *Nursing skills for allied health services,* vol 2, Philadelphia, 1980, Saunders.)

Broken skin, such as is found with an open wound, is more sensitive to heat and cold and is more prone to tissue damage.

3. **Impaired circulation.** Patients with impaired circulation tend to be more sensitive to heat and cold. This impairment may be at the site of the application or may be a systemic problem involving the entire body that is a result of certain conditions, such as peripheral vascular disease, diabetes mellitus, or congestive heart failure.

4. **Impaired sensation.** Patients with impaired sensation, such as diabetic patients, must be watched carefully because tissue damage may occur from the application of heat or cold without the patient's awareness.

5. **Individual tolerance to change in temperature.** Some individuals cannot tolerate temperature change as easily as others.

The medical assistant should observe the area to which the heat or cold has been applied before, during, and after the treatment for signs indicating that a modification of temperature is necessary. Prolonged erythema or paleness, pain, swelling, and blisters should be reported to the physician. The medical assistant also should ask the patient whether the application feels comfortable or is too hot or too cold.

Heat

Local Effects of Heat

The application of moderate heat to a localized area of the body for a short time (approximately 15 to 30 minutes) produces *dilation,* or an increase in diameter, of the blood vessels in the area as the body tries to rid itself of excess heat (Figure 22-1). This results in an increased blood supply to the area, and tissue metabolism increases. Nutrients and oxygen are provided to the cells at a faster rate, and wastes and toxins are carried away faster. The skin in the area becomes warm and exhibits erythema. **Erythema** is the reddening of the skin caused by dilation of superficial blood vessels in the skin.

These physiologic effects of moderate heat applied to a localized area promote healing. Prolonged application of heat (more than 1 hour) produces secondary effects, however, that reverse this healing process. Blood vessels constrict, and blood supply to the area decreases. The medical assistant must be careful to apply heat for the length of time specified by the physician.

Purpose of Applying Heat

Heat functions in relieving pain, congestion, muscle spasms, and inflammation. Conditions for which the local application of heat is often prescribed are low back pain, arthritis, menstrual cramping, and localized abscesses.

Heat promotes muscle relaxation and is often used for the relief of pain caused by excessive contraction of muscle fibers. **Edema,** or swelling, in the tissues can be reduced through the application of heat because the increased blood supply functions to increase the absorption of fluid from the tissues through the lymphatic system.

Heat, usually in the form of a hot **compress,** can be used to soften exudates. An **exudate** is a discharge produced by the body's tissues. Exudates may sometimes form a hard crust over an area and require removal. Heat also increases **suppuration,** or the process of pus formation, to help in the relief of inflammation by breaking down infected tissues. Heat is not recommended, however, for the initial treatment of acute inflammation or trauma.

Type of Heat Applications

The most common type of heat applications are described next, including the conditions they are often used to treat.

Heating Pad

The electric heating pad consists of a network of wires that function to convert electric energy into heat to provide a constant and even heat application. The wires must not be bent or crushed. This could damage the pad, resulting in overheating of parts of the pad and leading to burns or fire. Pins must not be inserted in the pad as a means of securing it; if a pin comes in contact with a wire, an electric shock could result. To prevent electric hazards, heating pads should not be used over areas that contain moisture, such as wet dressings. Heating pads are often used to relieve pain and muscle spasms.

Hot Soak

A **soak** is the direct immersion of a body part in water or a medicated solution. A soak can be applied to an extremity or a part of the torso. Hot soaks are used to cleanse open wounds, increase suppuration, increase the blood supply to an area to hasten the healing process, and apply a medicated solution to an area.

Hot Compress

A hot compress is a soft, moist, absorbent cloth, such as a washcloth, that is immersed in a warm solution and applied to a body part. Hot compresses are used to increase suppuration, improve circulation to a body part to aid in healing, promote drainage from infection, and soften exudates. Applying a hot compress to an open wound requires the use of sterile technique.

Chemical Hot Pack

Chemical hot packs are available in a variety of sizes and shapes. When activated, they provide a specific degree of heat for a specific period of time (usually 30 to 60 minutes), as indicated on the package label. A chemical hot pack consists of a vinyl bag containing calcium chloride crystals and a smaller bag (encased in the vinyl bag) containing water. Pressure is applied with the hands to break the inner bag. The water in the inner bag combines with the calcium chloride crystals to produce heat. After using the pack, it should be discarded in an appropriate receptacle. Chemical hot packs should be stored at room temperature and are used as an alternative to a heating pad to relieve pain and muscle spasms.

Procedures 22-1, 22-2, 22-3, and 22-6 (see later) present proper application of heat with a heating pad, hot soak, hot compress, and chemical hot pack.

Cold

Local Effects of Cold

The application of moderate cold to a localized area produces *constriction,* or a decrease in diameter, of blood vessels in the area as the body attempts to prevent heat loss (see Figure 22-1). This constriction leads to decreased blood supply to the area. Tissue metabolism decreases, less oxygen is used, and fewer wastes accumulate. The skin becomes cool and pale. Prolonged application of cold (more than 1 hour) has a reverse secondary effect. Blood vessels dilate, and there is an increase in tissue metabolism. To prevent secondary effects, the medical assistant must apply cold for the recommended length of time only.

Purpose of Applying Cold

The application of moderate cold for a short time is used to prevent edema. Cold may be applied immediately after an individual has suffered direct trauma, such as a bruise, minor burn, **sprain, strain,** joint injury, or fracture. The cold limits the accumulation of fluid in the body tissues by constricting blood vessels and reducing the leakage of fluid into the tissues. Through the constriction of peripheral blood vessels, cold can be used to control bleeding. Cold temporarily relieves pain because of its anesthetic, or numbing, effect, which reduces stimulation of the pain receptors. Cold also slows the movement of blood and tissue fluids in the affected area, resulting in less pressure against pain receptors and therefore less pain. In the early stages of an infection, the local application of cold inhibits the activity of microorganisms. In this way, suppuration is decreased and inflammation is reduced. Cold applications should always be placed in a protective covering because applying cold directly to the skin could result in a skin burn.

Types of Cold Applications

Ice Bag

An ice bag consists of a waterproof bag with a screw-on cap. Before use, it must be filled with small pieces of ice and placed in a protective covering. Ice bags are used to prevent swelling, control bleeding, and relieve pain and inflammation.

Cold Compress

A cold compress is a soft, moist, absorbent cloth, such as a washcloth, that is immersed in a cold solution and applied

---

What Would You Do? What Would You *Not* Do?

Case Study 1

Aaron Collins is at the office. Aaron recently helped a friend move, and the next day he developed intense pain in his lower back. To alleviate the pain, he slept on a heating pad, but when he woke up, his back was red and blistered. Aaron says he turned the setting on the heating pad to high because his back was hurting so much and he thought that it would help his back feel better sooner. Aaron wants to know the best way to apply heat using a heating pad. He also wants to know what he can do to prevent low back pain in the future. ∎

to a body part. Cold compresses are used to relieve pain and inflammation and to treat conditions such as headaches, injury to the eyes, and pain after tooth extraction.

Chemical Cold Pack

Chemical cold packs are available in a variety of sizes and shapes. When activated, they provide a specific degree of coldness for a specific period of time (usually 30 to 60 minutes), as indicated on the package label. Most cold packs consist of a vinyl bag of ammonium nitrate crystals. Enclosed in this bag is a smaller vinyl bag of water. The cold pack is activated by applying pressure until the inner bag ruptures.

This releases the water into the larger bag, and a chemical reaction occurs between the crystals and water, producing coldness. These packs are disposable, and when the coldness diminishes, they should be discarded in an appropriate receptacle. Chemical cold packs should be stored at room temperature. They are used as an alternative to ice bags for the local application of cold to prevent swelling, control bleeding, and relieve pain and inflammation.

Procedures 22-4, 22-5, and 22-6 present proper application of cold with an ice bag, a cold compress, and a chemical cold pack.

Text continued on p. 443

PROCEDURE 22-1　Applying a Heating Pad

Outcome Apply a heating pad.

Equipment/Supplies

- Heating pad with a protective covering

1. **Procedural Step.** Sanitize your hands.
2. **Procedural Step.** Assemble the equipment.
3. **Procedural Step.** Greet the patient and introduce yourself. Identify the patient and explain the procedure. Explain the purpose of the application (e.g., to relieve pain).
4. **Procedural Step.** Place the heating pad in the protective covering.
   Principle. The protective covering provides more comfort for the patient and absorbs perspiration.

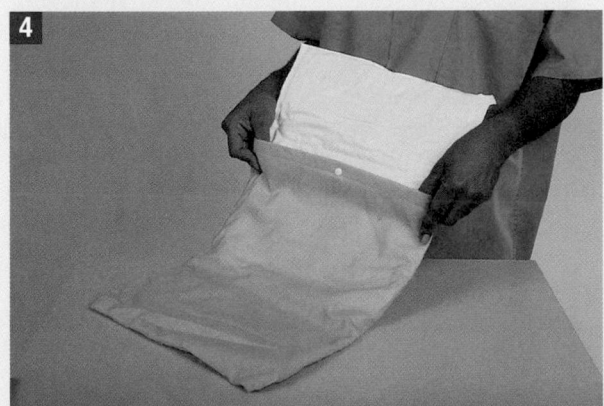

Place the heating pad in a protective covering. (From Bonewit-West K: *Clinical procedures for medical assistants,* ed 7, St. Louis, 2008, Saunders.)

5. **Procedural Step.** Connect the plug to an electric outlet. Set the selector switch at the proper setting, as designated by the physician (usually low or medium).
6. **Procedural Step.** Place the heating pad on the patient's affected body area. Ask the patient how the temperature feels. The heating pad should feel warm but not uncomfortable.

7. **Procedural Step.** Instruct the patient not to lie on the pad or turn the control higher to prevent burns.
   Principle. Lying on the pad causes heat to accumulate and burn the patient. The patient's heat receptors eventually become adjusted to the temperature change, resulting in a decreased heat sensation, and the patient may be tempted to increase the temperature. Turning the control higher results in excessive heat on the patient's skin, which could burn the patient.
8. **Procedural Step.** Check the patient periodically for signs of an increase or decrease in redness or swelling, and ask the patient whether the site is painful. Administer the treatment for the proper length of time as designated by the physician.
9. **Procedural Step.** Sanitize your hands, and chart the procedure. Include the date and time, method of heat application (heating pad), temperature setting of the pad, location and duration of the application, appearance of the application site, and patient's reaction. Also, chart any instructions provided to the patient on applying a heating pad at home.
10. **Procedural Step.** Properly care for equipment, and return it to its storage location.

CHARTING EXAMPLE

Date	
12/10/10	10:15 a.m. Heating pad on medium setting applied to lower back x 20 min. Area appears pink following application. Pt states a relief of pain and better mobility. Provided instructions on the application of a heating pad at home. —— M. Cooper, CMA (AAMA)

PROCEDURE 22-2   Applying a Hot Soak

Outcome Apply a hot soak.

Equipment/Supplies

- Soaking solution ordered by the physician
- Bath thermometer
- Basin
- Bath towels

1. **Procedural Step.** Sanitize your hands.
2. **Procedural Step.** Assemble the equipment. Check the label on the solution container to make sure you have the correct solution as ordered by the physician. Place the solution containers in a basin of warm water. Warm the soaking solution to a temperature between 105°F and 110°F (41°C and 44°C).
3. **Procedural Step.** Greet the patient and introduce yourself. Identify the patient and explain the procedure. Explain the purpose of the application (e.g., to apply a medicated solution).
4. **Procedural Step.** Fill the basin one-third to two-thirds full with the warmed soaking solution.
5. **Procedural Step.** Check the temperature of the solution with a bath thermometer. The temperature for an adult should be 105°F to 110°F (41°C to 44°C).
6. **Procedural Step.** Assist the patient into a comfortable position to avoid fatigue and muscle strain. Pad the side of the basin with a towel for the patient's comfort.
7. **Procedural Step.** Slowly and gradually immerse the patient's affected body part in the solution. Ask the patient how the temperature feels.
   Principle. The affected body part should become accustomed to the change in temperature gradually.
8. **Procedural Step.** Test the temperature of the solution frequently. To keep the solution at a constant temperature, remove cooler fluid every 5 minutes and replace it with hot solution. Pour the hot solution in near the edge of the basin by placing your hand between the patient and the solution. Stir the solution as you pour.
   Principle. The solution should be added away from the patient's body part to prevent splashing hot fluid on the patient. Stirring in the solution helps distribute the heat and keep the temperature constant.
9. **Procedural Step.** Check the patient's skin periodically for signs of an increase or decrease in redness or swelling, and ask the patient whether the site is painful. Apply the hot soak for the proper length of time as designated by the physician (usually 15 to 20 minutes).

Replace cooler solution with hot solution. (From Bonewit-West K: *Clinical procedures for medical assistants,* ed 7, St. Louis, 2008, Saunders.)

10. **Procedural Step.** Dry the affected part completely and gently.
11. **Procedural Step.** Sanitize your hands, and chart the procedure. Include the date and time, method of heat application (hot soak), name and strength of the solution, temperature of the soak, location and duration of the application, appearance of the application site, and patient's reaction.
12. **Procedural Step.** Properly care for equipment, and return it to its storage location.

CHARTING EXAMPLE	
Date	
12/12/10	1:15 p.m. Normal saline hot soak @ 105° F applied to ®ankle x 20 min. Area appears pink following application. Pt states less stiffness in ankle. — M. Cooper, CMA (AAMA)

PROCEDURE 22-3   Applying a Hot Compress

Outcome Apply a hot compress.

Equipment/Supplies

- Solution ordered by the physician
- Bath thermometer
- Basin
- Washcloths
- Waterproof covering
- Towel

1. **Procedural Step.** Sanitize your hands.
2. **Procedural Step.** Assemble the equipment. Check the label on the solution container to make sure you have the correct solution as ordered by the physician. Place the solution containers in a basin of warm water. Warm the soaking solution to a temperature between 105°F and 110°F (41°C and 44°C).
3. **Procedural Step.** Greet the patient and introduce yourself. Identify the patient and explain the procedure. Explain the purpose of the application (e.g., to soften an exudate).
4. **Procedural Step.** Fill the basin half full with warmed solution. Check the temperature of the solution with the bath thermometer. The temperature for an adult should be 105°F to 110°F (41°C to 44°C).
5. **Procedural Step.** Completely immerse the compress in the solution. Wring the compress to remove excess moisture. The compress should be wet but not dripping. Apply it lightly at first to the affected site to allow the patient to become used to the heat gradually. You may want to cover the compress with a waterproof cover to help hold in the heat. Ask the patient how the temperature feels. The compress should be as hot as the patient can comfortably tolerate.

   Principle. The waterproof cover prevents cool air currents from coming into contact with the compress and reduces the number of times the compress needs to be changed.

Apply the compress to the affected site. (From Bonewit-West K: *Clinical procedures for medical assistants,* ed 7, St. Louis, 2008, Saunders.)

6. **Procedural Step.** Place additional compresses in the solution so that they are ready for use.
7. **Procedural Step.** Repeat the application of the compress every 2 to 3 minutes for the duration of time specified by the physician (usually 15 to 20 minutes). Check the patient's skin periodically for signs of an increase or decrease in redness or swelling, and ask the patient whether the site is painful.
8. **Procedural Step.** Check the temperature of the solution periodically. Remove cooler fluid and replace it with hot solution if needed. Administer the treatment for the proper length of time as designated by the physician.
9. **Procedural Step.** Dry the affected part thoroughly and gently.
10. **Procedural Step.** Sanitize your hands, and chart the procedure. Include the date and time, method of heat application (hot compress), name and strength of the solution, temperature of the solution, location and duration of the application, appearance of the application site, and patient's reaction.
11. **Procedural Step.** Properly care for equipment, and return it to its storage location.

Wring out the compress. (From Bonewit-West K: *Clinical procedures for medical assistants,* ed 7, St. Louis, 2008, Saunders.)

CHARTING EXAMPLE

Date	
12/20/10	10:30 a.m. Normal saline hot compress @ 110° F applied to Ⓡ forearm x 20 min. No complaints of discomfort. ————————— M. Cooper, CMA (AAMA)

PROCEDURE 22-3

PROCEDURE 22-4 Applying an Ice Bag

Outcome Apply an ice bag.

Equipment/Supplies

- Ice bag with a protective covering
- Small pieces of ice (ice chips or crushed ice)

1. **Procedural Step.** Sanitize your hands.
2. **Procedural Step.** Assemble the equipment.
3. **Procedural Step.** Greet the patient and introduce yourself. Identify the patient and explain the procedure. Explain the purpose of applying the ice bag (e.g., to prevent swelling).
4. **Procedural Step.** Check the ice bag for leakage.
   Principle. A leaking bag would get the patient wet and cause chilling.
5. **Procedural Step.** Fill the bag one half to two thirds full with small pieces of ice.
   Principle. Small pieces of ice work better than large pieces because they reduce the air spaces in the bag, resulting in better conduction of cold. In addition, small pieces of ice allow the bag to mold better to the body area.
6. **Procedural Step.** Expel air from the bag by squeezing the empty top half of the bag together and screwing on the stopper.
   Principle. Air is a poor conductor of cold and makes it difficult to mold the ice bag to the body area.

Expel air from the bag. (From Bonewit-West K: *Clinical procedures for medical assistants*, ed 7, St. Louis, 2008, Saunders.)

7. **Procedural Step.** Place the bag in the protective covering.
   Principle. The protective covering provides for patient comfort and absorbs the moisture that condenses on the outside of the bag.
8. **Procedural Step.** Place the bag on the patient's affected body area. Ask the patient how the temperature feels.

The application of ice is usually uncomfortable, but most patients tolerate it when they know how much benefit may be derived from it.
Principle. Individuals vary in their ability to tolerate cold.

9. **Procedural Step.** Check the patient's skin periodically for signs of an increase or decrease in redness or swelling, and ask the patient whether the site is painful. If extreme paleness and numbness or a mottled blue appearance occurs at the application site, remove the bag and notify the physician.
10. **Procedural Step.** Refill the bag with ice as needed, and change the protective covering if needed. Administer the treatment for the proper length of time, as designated by the physician (usually until the area feels numb, approximately 15 to 30 minutes).
11. **Procedural Step.** Sanitize your hands, and chart the procedure. Include the date and time, method of cold application (ice bag), location and duration of the application, appearance of the application site, and patient's reaction. Also, chart any instructions provided to the patient on applying an ice bag at home.
12. **Procedural Step.** Properly care for the ice bag. Dispose of or launder the protective covering as required. Cleanse the ice bag with a warm detergent solution, rinse thoroughly, and dry by hanging the bag upside down with the top removed. Store the bag by screwing on the stopper, leaving air inside to prevent the sides from sticking together.

CHARTING EXAMPLE

Date	
12/22/10	11:30 a.m. Ice bag applied to Ⓡ knee x 20
	min. Pt complained of slight discomfort
	during the application. Area appears less
	swollen following application. Provided
	instructions on the application of an ice bag
	at home. _____ M. Cooper, CMA (AAMA)

PROCEDURE 22-5   Applying a Cold Compress

Outcome Apply a cold compress.

Equipment/Supplies

- Ice cubes
- Basin
- Washcloths

- Towel
- Ice bag

1. **Procedural Step.** Sanitize your hands.
2. **Procedural Step.** Assemble the equipment. Check the label on the solution container to make sure you have the correct solution as ordered by the physician.
3. **Procedural Step.** Greet the patient and introduce yourself. Identify the patient and explain the procedure. Explain the purpose of the application (e.g., to treat an eye injury).
4. **Procedural Step.** Place large ice cubes in the basin. Add the solution until the basin is half full.
   Principle. Using larger pieces of ice prevents them from sticking to the compress and slows the rate at which they melt in the solution.

Place large ice cubes in the basin. (From Bonewit-West K: *Clinical procedures for medical assistants,* ed 7, St. Louis, 2008, Saunders.)

5. **Procedural Step.** Completely immerse the compress in the solution. Wring the compress to rid it of excess moisture. The compress should be wet but not dripping. Apply it lightly at first to the affected site to allow the patient to become used to the cold gradually.

The compress can be covered with an ice bag to help keep it cold and to reduce the number of times it needs to be changed. Ask the patient how the temperature feels.

6. **Procedural Step.** Place additional compresses in the solution to be ready for use.
7. **Procedural Step.** Repeat the application of the compress every 2 to 3 minutes for the duration of time specified by the physician (usually 15 to 20 minutes). Check the patient's skin periodically for signs of an increase or decrease in redness or swelling, and ask the patient whether the site is painful.
8. **Procedural Step.** Add ice if needed to keep the solution cold. Administer the treatment for the proper length of time designated by the physician.
9. **Procedural Step.** Thoroughly dry the affected part.
10. **Procedural Step.** Sanitize your hands, and chart the procedure. Include the date and time, method of cold application (cold compress), location and duration of the application, appearance of the application site, and patient's reaction.
11. **Procedural Step.** Properly care for equipment, and return it to its storage location.

CHARTING EXAMPLE

Date	
12/27/10	9:15 a.m. Normal saline cold compress
	applied to bridge of nose x 15 min. Nose
	appears less swollen following application.
	Tolerated application well. ——————
	—————— M. Cooper, CMA (AAMA)

PROCEDURE 22-5

PROCEDURE 22-6   Applying a Chemical Pack

Outcome Apply a chemical cold pack and a chemical hot pack.

The procedure for applying a chemical cold or hot pack is as follows:

1. **Procedural Step.** Shake the crystals to the bottom of the bag.
2. **Procedural Step.** Squeeze the bag firmly with your hands to break the inner water bag.
3. **Procedural Step.** Shake the bag vigorously to mix the contents.
4. **Procedural Step.** Cover the bag with a protective covering.
5. **Procedural Step.** Apply the bag to the affected area. Check the patient's skin periodically.
6. **Procedural Step.** Administer the treatment for the proper length of time.
7. **Procedural Step.** Discard the bag in an appropriate receptacle.
8. **Procedural Step.** Sanitize your hands and chart the procedure. Include the date and time, method of application (chemical cold or hot pack), location and dura-tion of the application, appearance of the application site, and the patient's reaction.

Chemical packs. **A,** Chemical cold pack. **B,** Chemical hot pack. (From Bonewit-West K: *Clinical procedures for medical assistants,* ed 7, St. Louis, 2008, Saunders.)

PATIENT TEACHING   Low Back Pain

Answer questions patients have about low back pain.

What causes low back pain?
Low back pain is one of the most common health problems in the United States. Approximately 80% of Americans are affected by low back pain at some time during their life. The most frequent cause of low back pain is poor posture and poor body mechanics, which strain the muscles and ligaments that support the back. Other causes include physical inactivity, excessive body weight, disc damage, osteoarthritis, and congenital deformities.

How might the physician treat low back pain?
To treat low back pain caused by strain, the physician might pre-scribe bed rest, local application of heat or cold, massage, medica-tions, back manipulation, use of back-supporting devices, deep-heating treatments such as ultrasound, and exercises to strengthen the supporting structures of the back and prevent the back pain from recurring or becoming chronic.

What can be done to prevent low back pain?
Most cases of low back pain can be prevented by practicing good posture and body mechanics.
- Encourage patients to follow practices that prevent strain to the lower back.
- Teach the patient the procedure for the local application of heat or cold as prescribed by the physician.
- Provide the patient with a sheet that describes and illustrates the correct way to perform back exercises prescribed by the physician.
- Provide the patient with educational materials on low back pain. ∎

PATIENT TEACHING   Body Mechanics

Teach patients the essentials of good posture and body mechanics as follows:

Standing and walking
Stand and walk with the chin tucked in, head up, back flattened, and pelvis held straight. Wear comfortable low-heeled shoes that offer good support.

Lifting
To lift an object, always bend the body at the knees and hips. Never bend from the waist. Lift the object with the leg muscles and hold it close to the body at waist level. Never lift anything heavier than you can easily manage or higher than waist level.

PATIENT TEACHING Body Mechanics—cont'd

Sitting

Sit in a chair with a firm back. The feet should be flat on the floor, and the knees should be level with the hips. Sit firmly against the back of the chair; avoid slumping. Using a pillow in the small of the back or a footstool to raise the knees also reduces strain on the back.

Driving

Ensure that the car seat is not too far back. Stretching for the pedals strains the back. The car seat should be positioned so that the driver's back is straight and the knees are raised.

Sleeping

Sleep on a firm, comfortable mattress that supports the back and does not allow it to sag. Sleep on your side with knees bent or on your back with a pillow under the knees. Do not sleep on your stomach because this causes the body to sag into the mattress, which results in strain to the back, neck, and shoulders. ■

Memories *from* Externship

Marlyne Cooper: At my first externship site, I was scared to death about having to give injections to small children. I didn't want to hurt them. A 6-month-old infant was brought to the office for her immunizations. My externship supervisor wanted me to give the injections. The infant was so small, and she was crying before I even gave her the first injection. I knew that when I gave the injection, she was going to cry even more, and that made me feel bad. My supervisor was there with me, and she talked me through it. It turned out that it wasn't as bad as I had thought it would be. My supervisor was very helpful in keeping me calm. After that first experience, I felt much more comfortable when I had to give an injection to a small child. ■

Prepare for Success

AMBULATORY AIDS

Mechanical assistive devices are used by individuals who require aid in ambulation. The word **ambulation** means "walking"; patients who are **ambulatory** are able to walk as opposed to being confined to a wheelchair or a bed. Ambulatory aids include crutches, canes, and walkers. The device used depends on factors such as the type and severity of the disability, the amount of support required, and the patient's age and degree of muscular coordination. The ambulatory aid may be prescribed for a temporary condition, such as a fracture, a sprain to a lower extremity, and disability after orthopedic surgery. It may also be prescribed for a long-term condition, such as paralysis, deformity, and permanent weakness of the lower extremities.

Crutches

Crutches are artificial supports that consist of wood or tubular aluminum. They are used for patients who require assistance in walking as a result of disease, injury, or birth defects of the lower extremities. Crutches function by removing weight from the legs and transferring it to the arms. The two main crutch types are the axillary crutch and the forearm crutch (Figure 22-2). The axillary and the

Highlight on Ambulatory Aids

Many people who could benefit from ambulatory aids are not using them. The primary reason is that they do not know how to use them correctly, become discouraged, and quit using them.

Other types of aids available to assist individuals with physical disabilities include raised toilet seats, handle bars, carrying devices, tub seats, overbed tables, and swivel cushions for assistance in getting into and out of cars.

If an individual needs help in learning to drive with a physical disability, the local bureau of vocational rehabilitation or the state motor vehicle department can provide information on qualified instruction available in the community.

Walking with an ambulatory aid is a physiologic stressor to the body because it requires more energy than normal walking does. Because of this, individuals need to rest frequently when using an ambulatory aid.

Many people need to have their crutches lengthened after they have had them for awhile. This is because their posture improves as they gain confidence in walking with them. Children and teenagers who use crutches for a long time also need frequent adjustments as they grow.

A cane can provide security to the individual using it; however, it can be more trouble than it is worth if it is the incorrect size. It is estimated that two thirds of people who buy canes select one that is too long.

Some walkers are designed to fit over chairs and toilets, allowing the user additional support when rising or sitting. Folding walkers are available, and they are easy to store and transport. ■

forearm crutch require rubber tips, which increase the surface tension to prevent the crutches from slipping on the floor.

The *axillary crutch* is used most frequently and is made of wood or tubular aluminum. This type of crutch has a shoulder rest and handgrips and extends from the ground almost to the patient's axilla.

The *forearm crutch,* also known as a *Lofstrand crutch,* consists of a single adjustable tube of aluminum that extends

- Teach patients the guidelines for the proper use of crutches.
- Provide the patient with an exercise sheet that illustrates exercises to strengthen arm muscles before beginning crutch walking.
- Teach the patient the crutch gaits prescribed by the physician, and have the patient demonstrate the gaits before leaving the office.

- Provide the patient with a list of local vendors who provide crutch services, such as repairs and supplies (e.g., rubber tips, crutch pads).
- Provide the patient with printed educational materials on the use of crutches and crutch gaits. ∎

AXILLARY CRUTCH   FOREARM CRUTCH

Figure 22-2. Types of crutches. (From Bonewit-West K: *Clinical procedures for medical assistants,* ed 7, St. Louis, 2008, Saunders.)

to the forearm. A metal cuff attached to the crutch fits securely around the patient's forearm, and a handgrip covered with rubber extends from the crutch for weight bearing. The metal cuff and the handgrip stabilize the patient's wrists to make walking safer and easier. One advantage of the forearm crutch is that the individual can release the handgrip, enabling use of the hand, while the metal cuff holds the crutch in place. Individuals who are paraplegic or have cerebral palsy use the forearm crutch most often.

Axillary Crutch Measurement

The patient must be measured for axillary crutches to ensure the correct crutch length and the proper placement of the handgrip. Incorrectly fitted crutches increase the patient's risk of developing back pain, nerve damage, and injuries to the axillae and palms of the hands. Procedure 22-7 presents the correct way to measure a patient for axillary crutches.

If the crutches are too long, the shoulder rests exert pressure on the patient's axillae. This can injure the radial nerve in the brachial plexus, which eventually may lead to *crutch palsy,* a condition of muscular weakness in the forearm, wrist, and hand. In addition, crutches that are too long force

the patient's shoulders forward, preventing the patient from pushing his or her body off the ground. Crutches that are too short force the patient to be bent over and uncomfortable, also making them awkward to use. If the handgrips are too low, pressure is put on the patient's axillae, whereas handgrips that are too high are awkward.

Wooden crutches are made with bolts and wing nuts, which allow proper adjustment of the length and handgrip level. Aluminum crutches consist of aluminum tubes. Spring-loaded pushbuttons on an inner tube "pop out" into holes on an outer tube to allow proper adjustment of the crutch length.

Crutch Guidelines

It is important that the patient receive specific guidelines to ensure safety while using crutches, to prevent injuries and falls. The medical assistant is responsible for instructing the patient in the following guidelines:

1. Wear well-fitting flat shoes with firm, nonskid soles to provide good traction and stability.
2. Use correct posture to prevent strain on muscles and joints and to maintain proper body balance.
3. Support your weight with your hands on the handgrips and the axillary pads pressing against the sides of the rib cage. The body weight should not be supported by the axillae because pressure on the axillae may cause crutch palsy.
4. Look ahead when walking, rather than down at your feet.
5. Be aware of the surface on which you are walking. It should be clean, flat, dry, and well lighted. Throw rugs and objects serving as obstacles should temporarily be removed from your environment to prevent falls.
6. Keep the crutches about 4 to 6 inches out from the side of your feet when walking to prevent obstruction of the pathway for the feet.
7. Take steps by moving the crutches forward a safe and comfortable distance, preferably 6 inches. When first learning to use the crutches, take small steps rather than large ones. Do not move forward more than 12 to 15 inches with each step. A greater distance might cause the crutches to slide forward and you to lose your balance.
8. Report tingling or numbness in the upper body to the physician. You might be using the crutches incorrectly, or they might be the wrong size for you.
9. Extra padding can be added to the shoulder rests of your crutches to make them more comfortable. If you

do this, ensure that the extra padding does not press against your axillae, but rather against your lateral rib cage. The handgrips can also be padded for increased comfort.

10. To prevent slipping, keep the crutch tips dry to maintain their surface friction. If they become wet, dry them completely before use.

11. Inspect the crutch tips regularly. They should be securely attached. If the crutch tips are worn down, they should be replaced with tips of the proper size.

12. For wooden crutches, periodically check the wing nuts holding the central strut and handgrips in place to ensure that they are tight.

Crutch Gaits

The type of crutch gait used depends on the amount of weight the patient is able to support with one or both legs and the patient's physical condition and muscular coordination. The patient should learn a fast and a slow gait. The faster gait is used for making speed in open areas, and the slower one is used in crowded places. In addition, learning more than one gait reduces patient fatigue because a different combination of muscles is used for each gait. Procedure 22-8 provides guidelines and charts for use in instructing the patient on how to walk with crutches.

Canes

A cane is a lightweight, easily movable device made of wood or aluminum with a rubber tip and is used to help provide balance and support. Canes are generally used by patients who have weakness on one side of the body, such as patients with hemiparesis, joint disabilities, or defects of the neuromuscular system. The three main types of canes are the *standard cane, tripod cane,* and *quad cane* (Figure 22-3). The standard cane provides the least amount of support and is used by patients who require only slight assistance in walking. The tripod and quad canes have three and four legs, respectively, a bent shaft, and a T-shaped handle with grips. They are easier to hold and provide greater stability than a standard cane because of the wider base of support. In addition, multilegged canes are able to stand alone, which frees the arms when the patient is getting up from a chair. The disadvantage of a multilegged cane is that it is bulkier and more difficult to move.

A cane is held on the side of the body that is opposite to the side that needs support. The cane length must be properly adjusted to ensure optimal stability. The cane handle should be approximately level with the greater trochanter, and the elbow should be flexed at a 25- to 30-degree angle. The patient should be instructed to stand erect and not lean on the cane to ensure good balance. Procedure 22-9 presents guidelines on instructing the patient on how to walk with a cane.

Walkers

A walker is an ambulatory aid consisting of an aluminum frame with handgrips and four widely placed legs with rubber suction tips and one open side (Figure 22-4). A

Figure 22-3. Examples of a quad cane *(left)* and a standard cane *(right)*. (From Bonewit-West K: *Clinical procedures for medical assistants,* ed 7, St. Louis, 2008, Saunders.)

Figure 22-4. A walker. (From Bonewit-West K: *Clinical procedures for medical assistants,* ed 7, St. Louis, 2008, Saunders.)

walker is light and easily movable. Walkers are available with wheels that facilitate movement of the walker. They are also available with a fold-up feature that allows them to be easily transported in a vehicle. For proper ambulation, the walker should extend from the ground to approximately the level of the patient's hip joint. Procedure 22-10 presents guidelines on instructing the patient on how to walk with a walker.

Walkers are used most often by geriatric patients with weakness or balance problems. Walkers are also used during the healing process for patients who have had knee or hip joint replacement surgery. These patients need more help with balance and walking than can be provided by crutches or a cane. Because of its wide base, a walker provides the patient with a great amount of stability and security. Disadvantages of a walker include a slow pace and difficulty in maneuvering the walker in a small room.

PROCEDURE 22-7

What Would You Do? What Would You *Not* Do?

Case Study 2

Thaddeus Bernard calls the office. Thaddeus fractured the femur of his left leg in a skiing accident 2 weeks ago. The physician applied a long leg fiberglass cast, and Thaddeus was properly fitted with aluminum crutches. Thaddeus says that he is having some problems with his crutches. He is complaining of weakness in his forearms and hands and some tingling and numbness in his fingers. He also says that he has bruises under his arms. Thaddeus says that after he got home, his crutches didn't seem to fit right, so he readjusted them. Thaddeus is getting ready to return to college and wants to know the best way to carry his books while using crutches. ■

PROCEDURE 22-7 Measuring for Axillary Crutches

Outcome Measure an individual for axillary crutches.

Determining Crutch Length

For you to determine crutch length correctly, the patient must wear shoes while being measured. The measurement can be taken while the patient is standing.

1. **Procedural Step.** Ask the patient to stand erect.
2. **Procedural Step.** Position the crutches with the crutch tips at a distance of 2 inches (5 cm) in front of and 4 to 6 inches (15 cm) to the side of each foot. (The large dots in the figure represent crutch tips.)
3. **Procedural Step.** Adjust the crutch length so that the shoulder rests are approximately 1½ to 2 inches (about 2 finger-widths) below the axilla.
   Wooden Crutches. The length of the crutch is adjusted by removing the bolt and wing nut and sliding the central strut (support piece) at the bottom upward or downward as needed to attain the proper length. The strut is secured by replacing the bolt and securely fastening the wing nut.

Position for measuring for crutches. (From Bonewit-West K: *Clinical procedures for medical assistants,* ed 7, St. Louis, 2008, Saunders.)

Tubular Aluminum Crutches. The length of the crutch is adjusted by pressing the spring-loaded push-button with your thumb and sliding the outer tube upward or downward as needed to attain the proper length. The spring-loaded button on the inner tube

should be allowed to "pop out" into the appropriate hole on the outer tube.

Handgrip Positioning

When the crutch length has been adjusted, the correct placement of the handgrips must be determined.

1. **Procedural Step.** Ask the patient to stand erect with a crutch under each arm and to support his or her weight by the handgrips.
2. **Procedural Step.** Adjust the handgrips on the crutches so that the patient's elbow is flexed to an angle of approximately 30 degrees. The handgrip level is adjusted by removing the bolt and wing nut and sliding the handgrip upward or downward, as required. The handgrip is secured by replacing the bolt and tightly fastening the wing nut. The angle of elbow flexion can be verified using a measuring device known as a *goniometer.* A goniometer is an instrument that measures the angle of a joint.
3. **Procedural Step.** Check the fit of the crutches. If the crutches are measured correctly, the medical assistant should be able to insert two fingers between the top of the crutch and the axilla when the patient is standing erect with the crutches under the arms.

Insert two fingers between the top of the crutch and the axilla. (From Bonewit-West K: *Clinical procedures for medical assistants,* ed 7, St. Louis, 2008, Saunders.)

PROCEDURE 22-8   Instructing a Patient in Crutch Gaits

Outcome Instruct a patient in the following crutch gaits: four-point, two-point, three-point, swing-to, and swing-through.

Tripod Position

The tripod position is the basic crutch stance used before crutch walking. It provides a wide base of support and enhances stability and balance.

Instruct the patient in the tripod position as follows:
1. **Procedural Step.** Stand erect, and face straight ahead.
2. **Procedural Step.** Place the tips of the crutches 4 to 6 inches (15 cm) in front of the feet and 4 to 6 inches (10 to 15 cm) to the side of each foot. (The large dots in the figure represent crutch tips.)

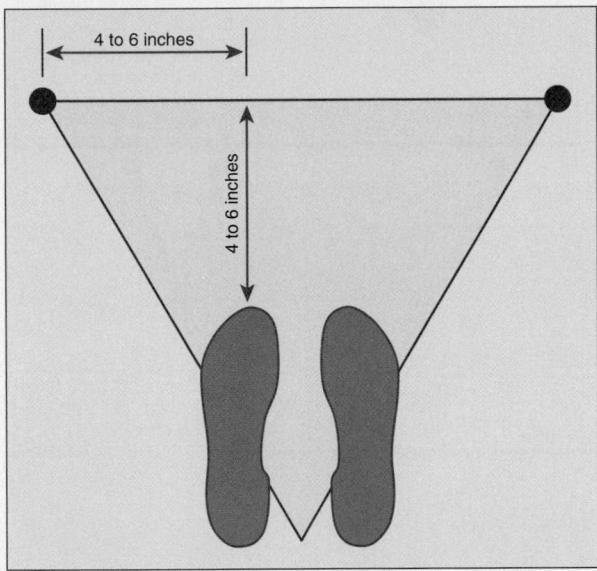

Tripod position. (From Bonewit-West K: *Clinical procedures for medical assistants,* ed 7, St. Louis, 2008, Saunders.)

Four-Point Gait

The four-point gait is a basic and slow gait. To use this gait, the patient must be able to bear considerable weight on both legs. The four-point gait is the most stable and safest of the crutch gaits because it provides at least three points of support at all times. It is used most often by patients who have leg muscle weakness or spasticity, poor muscular coordination or balance, or degenerative leg joint disease. Instruct the patient in the procedure for the four-point gait following the steps in the accompanying figure.

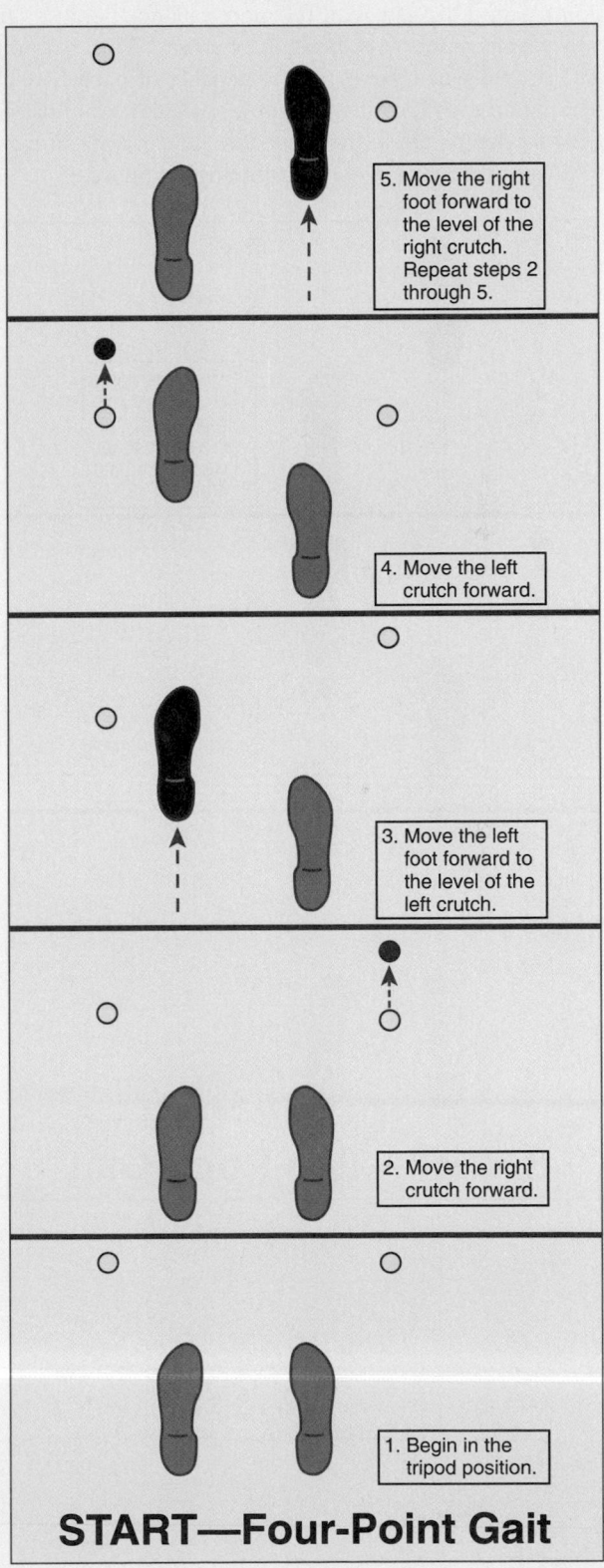

5. Move the right foot forward to the level of the right crutch. Repeat steps 2 through 5.

4. Move the left crutch forward.

3. Move the left foot forward to the level of the left crutch.

2. Move the right crutch forward.

1. Begin in the tripod position.

START—Four-Point Gait

PROCEDURE 22-8

Continued

Two-Point Gait

The two-point gait is similar to, but faster than, the four-point gait. This gait requires more balance because only two points support the body at one time. The two-point gait is used when the patient is capable of partial weight bearing on each foot and has good muscular coordination. Instruct the patient in the procedure for the two-point gait following the steps in the accompanying figure.

Three-Point Gait

The three-point gait is used by patients who cannot bear weight on one leg. The patient must be able to support his or her full weight on the unaffected leg. With this gait, the crutches and the unaffected leg alternately bear the patient's weight. This gait is used most often by amputees without a prosthesis, patients with musculoskeletal or soft tissue trauma to a lower extremity (e.g., fracture, sprain),

3. Move the right crutch and left foot forward at the same time. Repeat steps 2 and 3.

2. Move the left crutch and right foot forward at the same time.

1. Begin in the tripod position.

START—Two-Point Gait

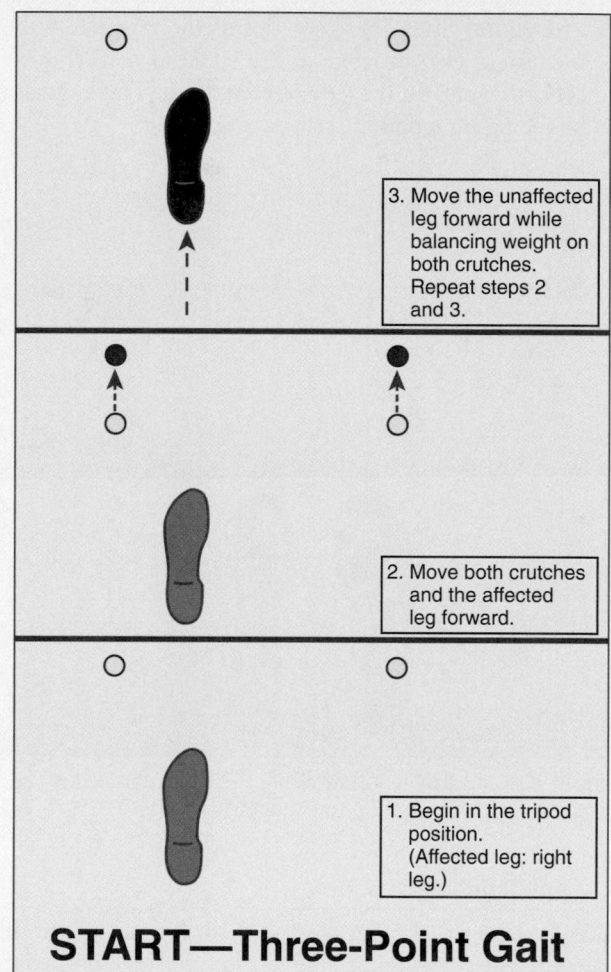

3. Move the unaffected leg forward while balancing weight on both crutches. Repeat steps 2 and 3.

2. Move both crutches and the affected leg forward.

1. Begin in the tripod position. (Affected leg: right leg.)

START—Three-Point Gait

patients with acute leg inflammation, and patients who have had recent leg surgery. To use this gait, the patient must have good muscular coordination and arm strength. Instruct the patient in the procedure for the three-point gait, following the steps in the accompanying figure.

extremity disabilities, such as paralysis, and by patients who wear supporting braces on their legs.

Instruct the patient in the procedure for the swing-to and the swing-through crutch gaits, following the steps in the accompanying figures.

Swing Gaits

The swing gaits include the swing-to gait and the swing-through gait and are used by patients with severe lower

3. Lift and swing the body to the crutches. Repeat steps 2 and 3.

2. Move both crutches forward together.

1. Begin in the tripod position.

START—Swing-To Gait

3. Lift and swing the body past (or through) the crutches. Repeat steps 2 and 3.

2. Move both crutches forward together.

1. Begin in the tripod position.

START—Swing-Through Gait

PROCEDURE 22-9

see DVD

PROCEDURE **22-9**   Instructing a Patient in the Use of a Cane

Outcome Instruct the patient in the use of a cane.

1. **Procedural Step.** Hold the cane on the strong side of the body (i.e., in the hand opposite the affected extremity).
2. **Procedural Step.** Place the tip of the cane 4 to 6 inches to the side of the foot.
3. **Procedural Step.** Move the cane forward approximately 12 inches (1 foot).
4. **Procedural Step.** Move the affected leg forward to the level of the cane.

5. **Procedural Step.** Move the strong leg forward and ahead of the cane and weak leg.
6. **Procedural Step.** Repeat steps 3 through 5.
   Note: The cane and affected leg can be moved forward simultaneously (steps 3 and 4); however, the patient has less support with this method.

PROCEDURE 22-10 Instructing a Patient in the Use of a Walker

Outcome Instruct the patient in the use of a walker.

1. Procedural Step. Pick up the walker, and move it forward approximately 6 inches.

2. Procedural Step. Move the right foot and then the left foot up to the walker.

3. Procedural Step. Repeat steps 1 and 2.

PROCEDURE 29-10

MEDICAL PRACTICE and the LAW

The procedures described in this chapter deal with the goal of returning full function to an injured area. Sometimes, despite correct treatment, full function does not return. This problem can become a legal issue if the patient believes he or she should have healed fully or cannot return to work. To protect yourself, follow each procedure to the letter and record the patient's progress (or lack of progress) carefully in the medical record. Sometimes the patient is involved in insurance fraud and falsely complains of pain or impaired function to continue receiving disability benefits. If you suspect this is the case, objectively document the functions you have seen the patient perform.

The application of heat and cold must be performed precisely to maximize effectiveness of the treatment without injury to the patient. Failure to follow procedures correctly or to obtain the correct temperature could leave you legally liable.

The ultrasound machine, if used incorrectly, can burn the patient. To protect yourself and benefit the patient, keep the applicator head moving at all times and keep adequate coupling agent on the skin at all times.

Ambulatory aids used correctly can help the patient regain mobility. If crutches are used improperly, the patient could fall or develop nerve or other injuries. When instructing about ambulation aid use, allow enough time for the patient to give a return demonstration and send home written instructions in case the patient forgets what was taught. ■

What Would You Do? What Would You Not Do? RESPONSES

Case Study 1
Page 436

What Did Marlyne Do?

❑ Empathized with Aaron for being in so much pain.

❑ Explained to Aaron that he should never sleep on a heating pad because the heat builds up and causes the type of burn he experienced.

❑ Explained to Aaron that it is best to apply heat for 15 to 30 minutes at a time with the pad set no higher than the medium setting. Told him the pad may not feel warm after his body gets used to it, but that it is still helping him. Told Aaron that the high setting could burn his skin.

❑ Told Aaron how to prevent low back pain by using good body mechanics, especially during lifting.

What Did Marlyne Not Do?

❑ Did not criticize Aaron for sleeping on the heating pad or turning the pad to the high setting.

What Would You Do?/What Would You Not Do? Review Marlyne's response and place a checkmark next to the information you included in your response. List the additional information you included in your response.

_____

_____

_____

_____

Case Study 2
Page 446

What Did Marlyne Do?

❑ Listened carefully and empathetically to Thaddeus' problems and concerns with his crutches.

❑ Explained to Thaddeus that the crutches were adjusted to fit him properly at the office and that he may have caused some problems by readjusting them.

❑ Scheduled an appointment for Thaddeus to come in that day so the physician can examine him and his crutches can be checked for proper length.

❑ Went over crutch guidelines and crutch gaits with Thaddeus again when he came to the office for his appointment.

❑ Told Thaddeus that he should use a backpack to carry his books to keep his hands free to move on his crutches. Stressed that he should keep his backpack as light as possible and keep the weight evenly distributed on his back (i.e., use both straps).

What Did Marlyne Not Do?

❑ Did not tell Thaddeus to readjust the crutches himself.

❑ Did not tell Thaddeus that he should have paid more attention when he was being instructed in crutch guidelines.

What Would You Do/What Would You Not Do? Review Marlyne's response and place a checkmark next to the information you included in your response. List the additional information you included in your response.

_____

_____

_____

TERMINOLOGY REVIEW

Ambulation Walking or moving from one place to another.

Ambulatory Able to walk as opposed to being confined to bed or a wheelchair.

Compress A soft, moist, absorbent cloth that is folded in several layers and applied to a part of the body in the local application of heat or cold.

Edema The retention of fluid in the tissues, resulting in swelling.

Erythema Reddening of the skin caused by dilation of superficial blood vessels in the skin.

Exudate A discharge produced by the body's tissues.

Soak The direct immersion of a body part in water or a medicated solution.

Sprain Trauma to a joint that causes injury to the ligaments.

Strain An overstretching of a muscle caused by trauma.

Suppuration The process of pus formation.

ON THE WEB

For Information on Rehabilitation and Disability:

National Rehabilitation Information Center (NARIC): www.naric.com

American Academy of Orthopaedic Surgeons: www.aaos.org

About.Com—Orthopedics: orthopedics.about.com

American Physical Therapy Association: www.apta.org

American Chiropractic Association: www.amerchiro.org

American Occupational Therapy Association: www.aota.org

National Stroke Association (NSA): www.stroke.org

Arthritis Foundation: www.arthritis.org

National Institute of Arthritis and Musculoskeletal and Skin Diseases: www.niams.nih.gov

American Academy of Physical Medicine and Rehabilitation: www.aapmr.org

PREPARE FOR CERTIFICATION Visit the Evolve site at http://evolve.elsevier.com/Bonewit/today/ to actively Prepare for your Certification.

CD *Check out the* **Companion CD** *bound with the book to access additional interactive activities.*

23

The Gynecologic Examination and Prenatal Care

LEARNING OBJECTIVES

PROCEDURES

Gynecologic Examination
1. State the purpose of the gynecologic examination.
2. Identify the components of the gynecologic examination.

Breast Examination
1. Explain the purpose of a breast examination.

Instruct a woman in the procedure for a breast self-examination.

Pelvic Examination
1. Explain the purpose of a pelvic examination.
2. List and describe the four parts of the pelvic examination.
3. State the purpose of a Pap test.
4. List advantages and disadvantages of the liquid-based Pap test.
5. List and describe each category on a cytology request for a Pap test.

Prepare a woman for a gynecologic examination.
Assist the physician with a gynecologic examination.
Complete a cytology requisition form.

Vaginal Infections
1. Identify the symptoms of the following:
   Trichomoniasis
   Candidiasis
   Chlamydia
   Gonorrhea
2. Explain how each of the above-listed infections is diagnosed and treated.

Assist in the collection of a vaginal microbiologic specimen.

Prenatal Visits
1. Explain the purpose of each part of the prenatal record.
2. List and explain the purpose of each procedure included in the initial prenatal examination.
3. List and explain the purpose of each prenatal laboratory test.
4. Explain the purpose of return prenatal visits.
5. Explain the purpose of each of the following:
   Triple screen test
   Ultrasound scan
   Amniocentesis
   Fetal heart rate monitoring

Calculate the expected date of delivery.

Complete a prenatal health history.
Assist with an initial prenatal examination.
Assist with a return prenatal examination.

Six Weeks–Postpartum Visit
1. Explain the purpose of the 6 weeks–postpartum visit.
2. State the procedures included in the postpartum examination.

Assist with a 6 weeks–postpartum examination.

CHAPTER OUTLINE

CAAHEP COMPETENCIES

Clinical Competencies
Patient Care
- Obtain and record patient history.
- Prepare and maintain examination and treatment areas.
- Prepare patient for and assist with routine and specialty examinations.

General Competencies
Professional Communications
- Respond to and initiate written communications.
- Recognize and respond to verbal communications.
- Recognize and respond to nonverbal communications.

Patient Instruction
- Instruct individuals according to their needs.
- Provide instruction for health maintenance and disease prevention.

ABHES COMPETENCIES

Communication
- Recognize and respond to verbal and nonverbal communication.
- Adaptation for individualized needs.

Clinical Duties
- Interview and record patient history.
- Prepare patients for procedures.
- Prepare and maintain examination and treatment area.
- Prepare patient for and assist physician with routine and specialty examinations and treatments and minor office surgeries.

Instruction
- Teach patients methods of health promotion and disease prevention.

KEY TERMS

Gynecology
adnexal (ad-NEKS-al)
amenorrhea (AY-men-ah-REE-ah)
atypical (ay-TIP-ih-kul)
cervix (SER-viks)
colposcopy (kol-POS-koe-pee)
cytology (sy-TOL-oh-jee)
dysmenorrhea (DIS-men-ah-REE-ah)
dyspareunia (DIS-pah-ROO-nee-ah)
dysplasia (dis-PLAY-shah)
ectocervix (EK-toe-SER-viks)
endocervix (EN-doe-SER-viks)
external os (eks-TER-nal AHS)
gynecology (gie-nuh-KOL-oh-jee)
menopause (MEN-oh-paws)

menorrhagia (men-uh-RAY-jee-ah)
metrorrhagia (met-ro-RAY-jee-ah)
perimenopause (PEAR-ee-MEN-oh-paws)
perineum (pear-ih-NEE-um)
risk factor
vulva (VUL-va)
Obstetrics
abortion (ah-BOR-shun)
Braxton Hicks contractions (BRAK-stun HIKS con-TRAK-shuns)
dilation (of the cervix) (die-LAY-shun)
effacement (eh-FAYS-ment)
embryo (EM-bree-oh)
engagement
expected date of delivery (EDD)
fetal heart rate

fetal heart tones
fetus (FEE-tus)
fundus (FUN-dus)
gestation (jess-TAY-shun)
gestational age (jess-TAY-shun-al)
infant
lochia (LOE-kee-uh)
multigravida (MUL-tee-GRAV-ih-duh)
multipara (mul-TIH-pear-uh)
nullipara (nul-IH-pear-uh)
obstetrics (ob-STEH-triks)

position
postpartum (poest-PAR-tum)
preeclampsia (PREE-ih-KLAMP-see-ah)
prenatal (pree-NAY-tul)
presentation
primigravida (PRIH-mih-GRAV-ih-duh)
primipara (prih-MIH-pear-uh)
puerperium (PYOO-ur-PEER-ee-um)
quickening
toxemia (tok-SEE-mee-uh)
trimester (try-MES-ter)

Introduction to the Gynecologic Examination and Prenatal Care

The medical assistant should have knowledge of gynecology and obstetrics to assist in examinations and treatments in these specialties. Gynecologic examinations are frequently and routinely performed in the medical office. Prenatal care consists of a series of scheduled medical office visits for the promotion of the health of the mother and fetus during the pregnancy. Obtaining the patient's cooperation makes the gynecologic or prenatal examination proceed more smoothly and, as a result, makes the patient feel more comfortable. The medical assistant can help by explaining the purpose of the procedure to the patient. If the patient understands the beneficial results to be derived from the examination, she is more likely to participate as required. This chapter discusses the gynecologic examination and prenatal care and the procedures involved with both.

GYNECOLOGIC EXAMINATION

GYNECOLOGY

Gynecology is the branch of medicine that deals with diseases of the reproductive organs of women. The gynecologic examination is frequently and routinely performed in the medical office and generally includes a *breast examination* and a *pelvic examination.*

The purpose of the gynecologic examination is to assess the health of the female reproductive organs to detect early signs of disease, leading to early diagnosis and treatment. This examination may be part of a general physical examination, or it may be performed by itself. Although assisting with the gynecologic examination is a routine procedure for the medical assistant, the patient may not consider it a routine examination. To reduce apprehension or embarrassment, the medical assistant should fully explain the procedure to the patient and offer to answer any questions.

Terms Related to Gynecology

The medical assistant should have a thorough knowledge of the female reproductive system (refer to Chapter 16) and the following terms associated with the female reproductive system:

Amenorrhea The absence or cessation of the menstrual period. Amenorrhea occurs normally before puberty, during pregnancy, and after menopause.

Cervix The lower narrow end of the uterus that opens into the vagina.

Colposcopy Examination of the cervix using a colposcope (a lighted instrument with a magnifying lens).

Dysmenorrhea Pain associated with the menstrual period.

Dyspareunia Pain in the vagina or pelvis experienced by a woman during sexual intercourse.

Dysplasia The growth of abnormal cells. Dysplasia is a precancerous condition that may or may not develop into cancer.

Menopause The permanent cessation of menstruation, which usually occurs between the ages of 45 and 55 with an average age of 51.

Menorrhagia Excessive bleeding during a menstrual period, in the number of days, the amount of blood, or both. Also called *dysfunctional uterine bleeding.*

Metrorrhagia Bleeding between menstrual periods.

Perimenopause Before the onset of menopause, the phase during which a woman with regular periods changes to irregular cycles and increased periods of amenorrhea.

Perineum The external region between the vaginal orifice and the anus in a female and between the scrotum and the anus in a male.

Risk factor Anything that increases an individual's chance of developing a disease. Some risk factors (e.g., smoking) can be avoided, but others cannot (e.g., age, family history).

BREAST EXAMINATION

The physician usually begins the gynecologic examination with the breast examination. The medical assistant is responsible for assisting the patient into the supine position. The physician inspects the breasts and nipples for swelling, dimpling, puckering, and change in skin texture. The nipples are checked for abnormalities such as bleeding and discharge. The breasts and axillary lymph nodes are palpated for lumps, hard knots, and thickening.

The patient should know how to examine her breasts at home for the presence of lumps and other changes with a breast self-examination (BSE). Most breast cancers are first discovered by women themselves. The American Cancer Society (ACS) recommends that women 20 years old and older examine their breasts once every month. The medical assistant may be responsible for instructing the patient in this procedure at the medical office (Procedure 23-1). If a lump or other change is discovered, the woman should schedule an appointment with her physician as soon as possible. Most breast lumps are not cancerous, but the physician must make that diagnosis.

PELVIC EXAMINATION

The purpose of the pelvic examination is to assess the size, shape, and location of the reproductive organs and to detect the presence of disease. The pelvic examination consists of the following components:

1. Inspection of the external genitalia, vagina, and cervix
2. Collection of a specimen for a Pap test
3. Bimanual pelvic examination
4. Rectal-vaginal examination

For the pelvic examination, the patient is positioned in the lithotomy position. The patient lies on the table on her back, with her feet in the stirrups and her buttocks at the bottom edge of the table. The stirrups should be level with the examining table and pulled out approximately 1 foot from the edge of the table. The patient's knees should be bent and relaxed, and her thighs should be rotated outward as far as is comfortable. This position helps relax the vulva and perineum and facilitates insertion of the vaginal speculum. The patient should be properly draped to reduce exposure and to provide warmth. The lithotomy position is difficult to maintain, and the patient should not be placed in this position until the physician is ready to begin the examination.

The medical assistant can help the patient relax during the examination by telling her to breathe deeply, slowly, and evenly through the mouth. If the patient is relaxed, it is easier for the physician to insert the vaginal speculum and to perform the bimanual pelvic examination; it is also more comfortable for the patient. It is recommended that the medical assistant remain in the room during the pelvic examination to provide legal protection for the physician, reassure the patient, and assist the physician. Procedure 23-2 outlines the medical assistant's role in assisting the physician with a gynecologic examination.

Inspection of External Genitalia, Vagina, and Cervix

The physician begins the pelvic examination with inspection of the external genitalia. The **vulva** is inspected for swelling, ulceration, and redness.

Next, the physician inserts a vaginal speculum into the vagina. Specula are available in two forms—metal and plastic. Metal specula are reusable and must be sanitized and sterilized after each use. Plastic specula are disposable and are designed to be used only once. Vaginal specula come

Putting It All into Practice

My name is Yin-Ling Wu, and I am a registered medical assistant. I work with 10 physicians in a large clinic. My primary job responsibilities include documenting patient histories and complaints, taking vital signs, and assisting physicians with patient examinations and procedures.

One experience that has probably affected me more than any other occurred while I was working in obstetrics and gynecology. A full-term prenatal patient came in for a routine weekly appointment late one afternoon. By this stage of the pregnancy, you have seen the patients often enough to develop a more personal relationship. I was obtaining her vital signs and asking the routine questions when she said, "I haven't felt the baby move for 2 days." This immediately sent up a red flag, but I was careful to hide my concern until I was out of her room. The physician was unable to pick up any fetal heart tones, so she immediately did an ultrasound. It showed that the fetus had died. The patient was alone and extremely upset. I stayed with her until her family came.

Although there was little medical treatment given during this time, I do believe that my medical assisting training and experience made a difference in knowing what to do and say to help comfort the patient through this crisis. ■

Prepare for Success

What Would You Do? What Would You *Not* Do?

Case Study 1

Carol Wooster, 42 years old, has come to the office for a gynecologic examination. She has not had a gynecologic examination in 10 years. Mrs. Wooster picked up a BSE brochure at a local health fair and performed a breast examination at home. She is now concerned because she found some unusual things. Her right breast is slightly larger than her left breast, her left nipple is pulled in, and she found some freckles on her right breast. Mrs. Wooster explains that she has not had a gynecologic examination in such a long time because her periods have been normal and regular. She also says that the physician will probably want her to have a mammogram, and she has heard that it hurts to have one. Mrs. Wooster is afraid that the physician will be annoyed with her for not having had a gynecologic examination sooner. ■

PATIENT TEACHING   Breast Self-Examination

Answer questions patients have about breast self-examination (BSE).

When should I examine my breasts?

Beginning at age 20, you should examine your breasts once a month according to your reproductive status as follows:

- **Regular periods:** Approximately 2 to 3 days after your menstrual period has ended. At this time, your breasts are least likely to be tender or swollen, and it will be easier to perform the examination.
- **No periods (because of menopause or hysterectomy):** Any day of the month is fine; however, it helps to choose a particular day, such as the first day of the month or an easy-to-remember date such as the date of your birthday.
- **Hormone therapy:** If you are taking hormones, talk to the physician about when to examine your breasts.

Why is it important to examine my breasts every month?

The purpose of a BSE is not just to find lumps, but also to notice when there are changes in your breasts. The best way to do this is to become as familiar as possible with your breasts. By examining your breasts once every month, you will learn what is normal for you, and it will be easier to notice changes.

What is considered normal?

Breast tissue normally feels a little lumpy and uneven. The left and right breast may not be the same size; most women's breasts are slightly different in size. Many women have a normal thickening or ridge of firm tissue under the lower curve of the breast where it attaches to the chest wall. Throughout your life, changes also can occur in the size, shape, and feel of your breasts because of aging, weight changes, the menstrual cycle, pregnancy, breastfeeding, and use of birth control pills or other hormones.

What should be reported to the physician?

Early breast cancer does not usually cause pain. When breast cancer first develops, there may be no symptoms at all. As the cancer grows, it can cause changes that should be reported to the physician. Contact your physician immediately if any of the following changes occurs:

- Any new lump, hard knot, or thickening in the breast or underarm area
- A change in the size or shape of the breast
- A puckering or dimpling of the skin of the breast or nipple
- A change in skin texture of the breast or nipple
- A nipple that becomes retracted (pulled in)
- A discharge or bleeding from the nipple ∎

---

in three sizes—small, medium, and large. The physician determines the size required based on the physical and sexual maturity of the patient. The function of the speculum is to hold the walls of the vagina apart to allow visual inspection of the vagina and cervix (Figure 23-1).

A metal vaginal speculum is cold and should be warmed before use by placing it on a heating pad or by storing it in a warming drawer. A warmed speculum is more comfortable for the patient. It is important not to overheat the speculum, however; one that is too hot is just as uncomfortable as one that is too cold. A disposable plastic speculum does not hold the cold and does not need to be warmed.

If a specimen needs to be obtained for a Pap smear or a microbiologic test, the speculum should not be lubricated because this would interfere with the test results. In these situations, the speculum can be moistened with warm water, which helps to lubricate it and facilitates insertion.

The physician inspects the vagina and cervix for color, lacerations, ulcerations, tenderness, nodules, and discharge. If an abnormal discharge is present, the physician obtains a specimen for microbiologic examination. Examples of pathologic conditions that produce a discharge include vaginal infections such as *trichomoniasis, candidiasis, chlamydia,* and *gonorrhea,* which are discussed in detail later.

Pap Test

A Pap test is usually part of the pelvic examination. It is a simple and painless **cytology** evaluation named after its

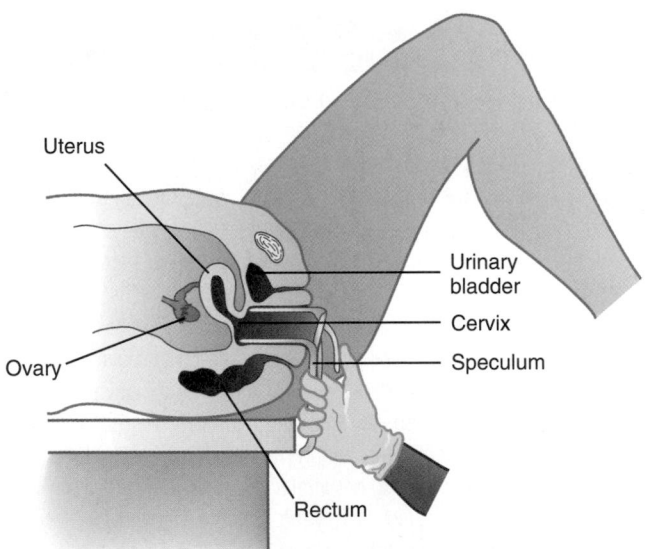

Figure 23-1. Insertion of the vaginal speculum for visualization of the vagina and cervix. (From Bonewit-West K: *Clinical procedures for medical assistants,* ed 7, St. Louis, 2008, Saunders.)

developer, Dr. George Papanicolaou (1883-1962). It is used for the early detection of cervical cancer. Almost all cancers of the cervix can be cured if detected early enough. The Pap test is also used to detect abnormal (**atypical**) cells of the cervix that might develop into cancer if not treated. In some

Highlight on Breast Cancer

Breast cancer is one of the most common types of cancer among American women. The American Cancer Society (ACS) estimates that one of every nine women in the United States develops breast cancer at some point in her lifetime. Every year, more than 200,000 women learn they have breast cancer, and about 40,000 of them die from the disease. Most women (82%) diagnosed with breast cancer are older than 50 years old, but breast cancer does occur in younger women.

Survival Rate

The 5-year survival rate for breast cancer that has spread to a distant site in the body (metastasized) is only 21%. The 5-year survival rate for small, localized tumors is 94%. If the cancer has spread to lymph nodes in the region of the breast, the 5-year survival rate is 73%. These encouraging statistics are the result of advances in early detection of breast cancer and better treatment, including improved surgical procedures, radiation therapy, chemotherapy, hormonal therapy, and biologic therapy.

Recommendations for Early Detection

The ACS and the National Cancer Institute recommend a three-point program for the early detection of breast cancer: (1) monthly breast self-examination, (2) periodic clinical breast examination by a physician, and (3) screening mammography.

Risk Factors

Breast cancer results from the abnormal growth of cells in breast tissue. It occurs more often in the left breast than in the right, and more often in the upper outer quadrant of the breast. The cause of abnormal growths in the breasts is unknown; therefore every woman should consider herself at risk for breast cancer. Certain factors seem to place a woman at higher than normal risk for breast cancer, however, including the following:

- **Age.** The risk of breast cancer increases as women get older. Most women diagnosed with breast cancer are older than age 50.
- **Personal history.** Women with cancer in one breast have a greater chance of developing a new cancer in the other breast or in another part of the same breast.
- **Family history.** A woman's risk of developing breast cancer increases if her mother, sister, or daughter had breast cancer, especially at a young age.
- **Breast biopsy.** Women who have had a breast biopsy that indicated certain types of benign breast disease (characterized by atypical hyperplasia) have an increased risk of developing breast cancer.
- **Breast cancer genes.** A woman who has inherited mutations in breast cancer genes (mutations of the *BRCA1* and *BRCA2* genes) from either parent is more likely to develop breast cancer.
- **Reproductive history.** Women who began menstruating at an early age (before age 12) or who went through menopause at a late age (after age 55) have a slightly increased risk of breast cancer.
- **Childbearing.** Women who have never had a child or women who had their first child late (after age 30) have a slightly increased risk of developing breast cancer.
- **Hormone replacement therapy (HRT).** Studies indicate that long-term use of HRT for relief of menopausal symptoms increases the risk of breast cancer.
- **Radiation treatment.** Women who have had radiation of the chest before age 30 as a treatment for another type of cancer (e.g., Hodgkin's disease) have a significantly increased risk of developing breast cancer.
- **Lifestyle factors.** Studies suggest that the use of alcohol (more than two drinks per day) increases the risk of breast cancer. Obesity, especially for women after menopause, may also increase the risk of breast cancer.

Warning Signs

The warning signs of possible breast cancer include a lump, hard knot, or thickening in the breast or armpit; a change in breast color or texture; dimpling or puckering; nipple discharge; changes in the size or shape of the breast; and an enlargement of the lymph nodes.

Diagnosis

A biopsy is the only conclusive method of determining whether a breast lump or suspicious area seen on a mammogram is benign or malignant. A biopsy involves the surgical removal and analysis of all or part of the lump. Biopsy methods include needle biopsy, incisional biopsy (removal of a portion of the lump), excisional biopsy (removal of the entire lump), and mammographic localization with biopsy. The physician may recommend one or more of these procedures to evaluate a lump or other change in the breast.

Eighty percent of breast lumps are benign. A lump or suspicious area is often the result of a benign breast condition, such as normal hormonal changes, fibrocystic breast disease, or a fibroadenoma. ∎

---

cases, the Pap test can detect cancer of the endometrium; however, it is less reliable in doing so.

The ACS recommends a woman have her first Pap test beginning within 3 years of having vaginal intercourse or at 21 years of age, whichever is earlier. Screening should be performed every year with the direct smear Pap test or every 2 years with the liquid-based Pap test. The ACS guidelines further state that beginning at age 30, women who have tested negative for three or more consecutive Pap tests may be screened every 2 to 3 years. Women who are at high risk for cervical cancer or who have had abnormal Pap test results should continue to be screened annually. Factors that place a woman at a higher risk for cervical cancer include diethylstilbestrol (DES) exposure before birth, human immunodeficiency virus (HIV) infection, or a weakened immune system due to organ transplantation, chemotherapy, or chronic steroid use.

Patient Instructions

A Pap specimen must not be collected from a woman during her menstrual period because the red blood cells obscure the specimen and interfere with an accurate evaluation. The patient should be instructed to schedule her Pap test 10 to 20 days after the first day of her last menstrual period (LMP). The patient should be told not to douche or insert tampons, medications, or contraceptive spermicides into the vagina for 2 days before having a Pap test. Douching and tampon insertion reduce the number of cells available for analysis, and vaginal medications and spermicides change the pH of the vagina, making the specimen nonrepresentative or invalid. The patient should also be told to abstain from sexual intercourse for 2 days before the Pap test. Recent sexual intercourse can produce inflammatory changes that can interfere with visualization of abnormal cells that may be present.

Specimen Collection

The outermost layer of the cervix consists of a thin, flat layer of cells, approximately 10 layers thick, known as *squamous epithelial cells.* With the speculum in place, the physician collects a sampling of these cells for evaluation by the laboratory. A scraping of epithelial cells is taken from the **ectocervix** and the **endocervix.** A scraping of cells can also be collected from the vagina; however, this is not usually done unless the physician has observed a lesion on the vaginal wall or the maturation index is to be determined. The technique used by the physician to collect the epithelial cells is described next.

Vaginal Specimen

If a vaginal specimen is necessary, it is collected first, before the cervical and endocervical specimens. The rounded end of the plastic spatula is used to collect the specimen. If a routine vaginal specimen is being obtained, it is collected from the vaginal pool in the posterior fornix of the vagina, which is located just below the cervix (Figure 23-2A). If the physician is collecting a specimen from a lesion on the

Vaginal Specimen

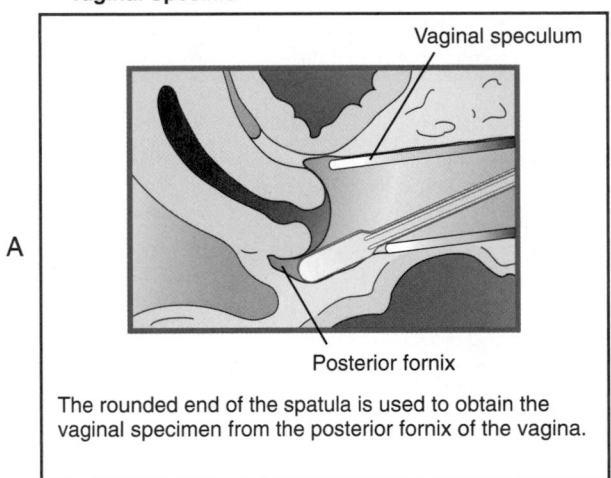

A

The rounded end of the spatula is used to obtain the vaginal specimen from the posterior fornix of the vagina.

Cervical Specimen

B

The S-shaped end of the spatula is placed inside the cervical canal and rotated 360 degrees over the surface of the cervix.

Endocervical Specimen

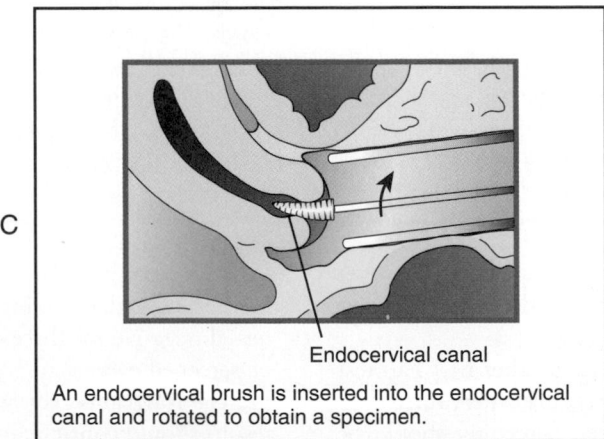

C

An endocervical brush is inserted into the endocervical canal and rotated to obtain a specimen.

Figure 23-2. Obtaining the Pap specimen. (From Bonewit-West K: *Clinical procedures for medical assistants,* ed 7, St. Louis, 2008, Saunders.)

vaginal wall, a scraping of cells is taken from the area of the lesion. To obtain a specimen for a determination of the maturation index (discussed later), the physician obtains the vaginal specimen from the upper third of the lateral vaginal wall.

Cervical Specimen

The physician obtains the cervical specimen by placing the S-shaped end of the plastic spatula just inside the cervical canal at the **external os** and rotating the blade 360 degrees over the surface of the ectocervix at the squamocolumnar junction, where cervical cancer is most often found (Figure 23-2B). The ectocervix is the part of the cervix that projects into the vagina and is lined with stratified squamous epithelium.

Endocervical Specimen

The physician collects this specimen from the endocervix. The endocervix consists of the mucous membrane lining the endocervical canal. This is accomplished by inserting an endocervical brush into the endocervical canal and rotating the brush (Figure 23-2C). The endocervical brush is made up of soft bristles designed to be inserted into the canal without causing damage to it.

Preparation Methods

Two methods are used to prepare a specimen for a Pap test. The traditional method is the *direct smear* (Pap smear), and the newer method is the *liquid-based preparation*.

Direct Smear

With the direct smear method, a thin smear of each specimen is spread on a glass slide that has a frosted edge. The medical assistant must label each slide on its frosted edge with a lead pencil according to the source of the specimen as follows: *V (vaginal), C (cervical),* or *E (endocervical).* Slides on which all three specimens can be placed are also available. These slides are divided into thirds and prelabeled with *V, C,* and *E.*

The smears must be fixed immediately by flooding the slides with 95% ethyl alcohol or by lightly spraying the slides with a commercial cytology spray fixative. The slides must be fixed before they dry to avoid inaccurate results. The purpose of the fixative is to maintain the normal appearance of the cells; to protect the slides from contaminants in the air, such as dust and bacteria; and to attach the smear firmly to the slide. The cytology fixative must be allowed to dry thoroughly; the slides are then ready for transport to a laboratory for evaluation. To protect the slides during transport, they must be placed in a slide container designed especially for this purpose.

Liquid-Based Preparation

A newer method to prepare the specimen for evaluation is the liquid-based preparation. Brand names include Thin-Prep, AutoCyte, and SurePath. Although more expensive than the direct smear method, the liquid-based method is growing in popularity. Using this method improves the quality of the specimen, resulting in fewer slides that are unsatisfactory for evaluation. A better quality specimen also reduces the occurrence of false-negative test results.

The specimen for a liquid-based preparation can be obtained using the specimen collection technique described earlier. A plastic spatula (S-shaped end) is used to collect the ectocervical specimen, and an endocervical brush is used to collect the endocervical specimen. If a vaginal specimen is necessary, it is collected first using the rounded end of the spatula as previously described.

The Pap specimen can also be collected using a broom, a newer collection device made of flexible plastic. The physician inserts the central bristles of the broom into the endocervical canal deep enough to allow the shorter bristles to contact the outside of the cervix fully. The broom is gently pushed and rotated in a clockwise direction (Figure 23-3). In this way, a specimen from the ectocervix and the endocervix can be collected at the same time.

When the Pap specimen has been collected, the medical assistant is responsible for performing one of the following depending on the brand of liquid-based preparation being used:

1. Rinse the collection device in the vial of liquid preservative, and discard the collection device (performed with ThinPrep).
2. Remove the tip of the collection device, and deposit it in the vial of preservative. Discard the handle (performed with SurePath).

The preservative maintains the specimen and prevents it from drying out during transport to the laboratory. After being received by the laboratory, the vial is placed in an automated slide preparation processor. The automated processor performs several important functions. First, it separates the cells from debris present in the specimen, and then it disperses a representative cell sample onto a slide in

The bristles of the broom are inserted into the endocervical canal and then gently pushed and rotated in a clockwise direction so that both an ectocervical and endocervical specimen can be collected at the same time.

Figure 23-3. Collecting a Pap specimen using a broom. (From Bonewit-West K: *Clinical procedures for medical assistants,* ed 7, St. Louis, 2008, Saunders.)

a thin, uniform layer. The slide is next immersed in a fixative to maintain the normal appearance of the cells.

The ways in which the liquid-based method provides a better-quality specimen than the direct smear method are as follows:

- With the direct smear method, only a small portion of the specimen is smeared on the slide; most of it is thrown away with the collection device. With the liquid-based method, the collection device is rinsed or the tip is deposited in a vial of liquid that preserves all or most of the specimen. Having more of the specimen available allows the laboratory to evaluate it better.
- When a Pap specimen is collected, it includes unnecessary debris, such as blood, mucus, and inflammatory cells. With the direct smear method, the debris is smeared on the slide along with the cells. This debris may obscure the cells in the specimen, making it difficult to evaluate them. With the liquid-based method, the automated processor removes a large portion of the debris from the specimen and transfers the cells to a glass slide. This provides the cytotechnologist with a clear, unobstructed view of the epithelial cells.
- With the direct smear method, the cells have a tendency to clump together when they are smeared on the slide, making them more difficult to evaluate. With the liquid-based method, the automated processor disperses the cells onto the slide in a thin, even layer. In this way, the cells are spread out, making it easier for the cytotechnologist to evaluate them.

Cytology Request

A cytology request must accompany all Pap specimens. Figure 23-4 is an example of a cytology request form. The medical assistant is responsible for completing the request, which includes the following categories.

General Information

General information includes the physician's name, address, and phone number and the patient's name, address, identification number, date of birth, and date of LMP. Insurance information is also required in this section for third-party billing.

Date and Time of Collection

The date and time of collection indicates to the laboratory the number of days that have passed since the collection, providing the laboratory with information regarding the freshness of the specimen.

Collection Method

Under the collection method category, the medical assistant must indicate whether the specimen is a direct smear (Pap smear) or a liquid-based preparation.

Source of the Specimen

The purpose of this category is to identify the origin of the specimen because it is impossible for the laboratory to obtain this information by looking at the specimen.

The medical assistant checks one or more of the following boxes on the form: cervical, endocervical, or vaginal.

Collection Technique

The collection device or devices used to obtain the specimen must be indicated. The medical assistant checks one or more of the following boxes on the form: spatula, brush, or broom.

Patient History

Information on the present and past health status of the patient is specified under the patient history category. The medical assistant must check the following boxes that apply to the patient: pregnant, lactating, oral contraceptives, postmenopausal, hormone replacement therapy, postmenopausal bleeding, postpartum, intrauterine death (IUD), postcoital bleeding, DES exposure, and previous abnormal smear. This information assists the laboratory in evaluating the specimen.

Previous Treatment

Any previous treatment for a precancerous or cancerous condition of the cervix is indicated under this category. The medical assistant checks the appropriate box on the form if any of the following procedures have been performed on the patient: colposcopy and biopsy, cryosurgery, loop electrocautery excision procedure (LEEP), laser vaporization, conization, hysterectomy, radiation, and chemotherapy.

Evaluation of the Pap Specimen

Before a Pap slide can be evaluated, it must be stained by a laboratory technician. Staining is performed on slides prepared by the direct smear method and the liquid-based method. The purpose of staining is to allow better viewing of the morphology of the epithelial cells. The slide is studied under a microscope for evidence of abnormalities by a specially trained technician, known as a *cytotechnologist*. When an abnormality is detected, it is reviewed by a *cytopathologist* (a physician specializing in pathology), who makes a final evaluation. The findings are recorded on a cytology report and returned to the medical office.

A more recent development in the evaluation of Pap slides is the use of automated cytology computer-imaging devices. An abnormal slide may contain only a few abnormal cells among thousands of normal cells. Because of this, these abnormal cells may be missed during the evaluation by the cytotechnologist. A cytology computer-imaging device is able to examine every cell on the slide and select and display cells that appear "most abnormal." The cytotechnologist can evaluate these cells further under a microscope. In this way, the cytotechnologist is able to focus his or her expertise and decision making on preselected areas of the slide.

Maturation Index

The maturation index must be performed on a sampling of cells taken from the upper third of the lateral vaginal wall. The *maturation index* refers to the percentage of parabasal,

GYN CYTOLOGY REQUISITION

THOMAS WOODSIDE, MD
501 MAIN ST
ST. LOUIS, MO 63146
(314) 555–0093

PATIENT INFO

Patient's Name (Last)	(First)	(MI)	Date of Birth MO	DAY	YR	Collection Time : AM PM	Collection Date MO	DAY	YR	Patient's ID #

Patient's Address   Phone

City   State   ZIP

RESP. PARTY

Name of Responsible Party (if different from patient)

Address of Responsible Party   APT #

City   State   ZIP

INSURANCE

Patient's Relationship to Responsible Party   ☐ 1. Self   ☐ 2. Spouse   ☐ 3. Child   ☐ 4. Other

Insurance Comany Name	Plan	Carrier Code
Subscriber/Member #	Location	Group #

Insurance Address   Physician's Provider #

City   State   ZIP

Employer's Name or Number   Insured SSN

Diagnosis/Signs/Symptoms in ICD-9 Format (Highest Specificity)

R E Q U I R E D

ICD-9 codes are the internationally accepted method of describing the clinical picture of the patient. All diagnoses should be provided by the ordering physician or his or her authorized designee. The following is a partial list of of common diagnoses in ICD-9 format. Most third party payers require an ICD-9 code to indicate the medical necessity of the test(s) and or profile(s) ordered. For a complete list of all ICD-9 codes, please refer to a current ICD-9 manual.

V76.2 Routine Cervical Pap Smear	616.0 Cervicitis	626.8 Abnormal Bleeding
V15.89 High Risk Cervical Screening	616.10 Vaginitis	627.1 Postmenopausal Bleeding
V22.2 Pregnancy	617.0 Endometriosis, Uterus	627.3 Atrophic Vaginitis
079.4 Human Papillomavirus	622.1 Dysplasia, Cervix	795.0 Abnormal Cervical Pap Smear
180.0 Malignant Neoplasm, Cervix	623.0 Dysplasia, Vagina	

COLLECTION METHOD

Liquid-Based Prep
192055 ☐ ThinPrep Pap Test

192039 ☐ ThinPrep Pap Test w/reflex to HPV
        Hybrid Capture when ASC-US or SIL

192047 ☐ ThinPrep Pap Test w/reflex to high-risk only
        HPV Hybrid Capture when ASC-US

Pap Smear
009100 ☐ 1 Slide   009191 ☐ 2 Slides

Pap Smear and Maturation Index
009209 ☐ 1 Slide   190074 ☐ 2 Slides

SOURCE OF SPECIMEN

☐ Cervical
☐ Endocervical
☐ Vaginal

Date LMP

___/___/___
Mo   Day   Year

COLLECTION TECHNIQUE

☐ Spatula
☐ Brush
☐ Broom
☐ Other
_____

PATIENT HISTORY

☐ Pregnant
☐ Lactating
☐ Oral Contraceptives
☐ Postmenopausal
☐ Hormone Replacement
   Therapy

☐ PMP Bleeding
☐ Postpartum
☐ IUD
☐ Postcoital Bleeding
☐ DES Exposure
☐ Previous Abnormal
   Pap Test

☐ Other _____

PREVIOUS TREATMENT   Date/Results

☐ None
☐ Colposcopy and Bx   _____
☐ Cryosurgery   _____
☐ LEEP   _____
☐ Laser Vaporization   _____
☐ Conization   _____
☐ Hysterectomy   _____
☐ Radiation   _____
☐ Chemotherapy   _____

Figure 23-4. Cytology request form. (From Bonewit-West K: *Clinical procedures for medical assistants,* ed 7, St. Louis, 2008, Saunders.)

intermediate, and superficial cells present in the specimen. The maturation index provides the physician with an endocrine evaluation of the patient, which can assist in evaluating the cause of infertility, menopausal or postmenopausal bleeding, or amenorrhea and can help assess the results of treatment with hormones. If the physician orders a maturation index along with the Pap test, the medical assistant must indicate this on the cytology request by checking the box labeled *Maturation Index* (see Figure 23-4). Numerous factors affect the results of the maturation index; it is impor-

tant to indicate on the cytology request the presence of abnormal bleeding, hormone treatment, or treatment with digitalis, corticosteroids, or thyroid medication.

Cytology Report

The Bethesda System (TBS) is the standard for reporting the results of a Pap test on the cytology report (Figure 23-5). The National Cancer Institute in Bethesda, Maryland, developed this system. It provides a detailed cytologic description (Table 23-1), rather than a numerical result (as

GYN CYTOLOGY REPORT

| RIVERVIEW MEDICAL LABORATORY
DEPARTMENT OF PATHOLOGY
2501 GRANT AVENUE
ST. LOUIS, MO 63146
(314) 555–3443 | PATIENT: Heather Jones
PATIENT NO: 45876
DOB: 10/20/65
SUBMITTING: T. Woodside, MD |

Date of Specimen: 7/01/10	SPECIMEN TYPE
Date Received: 7/02/10	☒ ThinPrep ☐ Conventional Pap Smear
Date Reported: 7/06/10	

Performed By: Richard McVay, Cytotechnologist   **Checked By:** Melissa Wagner, Pathologist

SPECIMEN ADEQUACY	GENERAL CATEGORIZATION
☒ Satisfactory for Evaluation ☐ Unsatisfactory for Evaluation	☐ Negative for Intraepithelial Lesion or Malignancy (*see Interpretation/Result*) ☒ Epithelial Cell Abnormality (*see Interpretation/Result*) ☐ Other (*see Interpretation/Result*)

INTERPRETATION/RESULT

A. BENIGN CELLULAR CHANGES

☐ Infection:
  ☐ Trichomonas vaginalis
  ☐ Fungal organisms morphologically compatible w/ Candida species
  ☐ Cellular changes associated with herpes simplex virus
  ☐ Bacterial infection morphologically compatible with gardnerella
  ☐ Cytoplasmic inclusions suggestive of chlamydia

☐ Reactive changes
  ☐ Without inflammation
  ☐ With inflammation
  ☐ Atrophy with inflammation (atrophic vaginitis)
  ☐ Radiation effect
  ☐ Repair
  ☐ Hyperkeratosis
  ☐ Parakeratosis

B. EPITHELIAL CELL ABNORMALITIES

☒ Squamous Cell
  ☒ Atypical Squamous Cells of Undetermined Significance (ASC-US)
  ☐ Atypical Squamous Cells of Higher Risk (ASC-H)
  ☐ Low-Grade Squamous Intraepithelial Lesion (LSIL)
  ☐ High-Grade Squamous Intraepithelial Lesion (HSIL)
  ☐ Squamous Cell Carcinoma
☐ Glandular Cell
  ☐ Atypical Glandular Cells of Undetermined Significance (AGUS)
  ☐ Adenocarcinoma

Figure 23-5. Cytology report form (The Bethesda System). (From Bonewit-West K: *Clinical procedures for medical assistants*, ed 7, St. Louis, 2008, Saunders.)

Table 23-1 Pap Test Results

Test Result	Interpretation
Negative for intraepithelial lesion or malignancy	Epithelial cells were normal, and there were no precancerous or cancerous findings
Atypical squamous cells of undetermined significance (ASC-US)	Cells are only slightly abnormal. Nature and cause of abnormality cannot be determined. These slightly altered cells usually return to normal on their own, resulting in negative results on subsequent Pap tests
Atypical squamous cells of higher risk (ASC-H)	Minor abnormal changes in cells with unknown causes, but at risk of progressing to HSIL. Further testing is required to determine whether this is a minor condition or one that may progress to HSIL
Low-grade squamous intraepithelial lesion (LSIL)	Abnormal cells that show definite minor changes, but are unlikely to progress to cancer (general term for this is *mild dysplasia*). LSIL may be caused by HPV infection, but of a type that is not likely to lead to cervical cancer
High-grade squamous intraepithelial lesion (HSIL)	Abnormal cell changes that have higher likelihood of progressing to cancer. Although not cancerous yet, abnormal cells may become cancerous if treatment is not obtained (general term for this is *moderate-to-severe dysplasia*). HSIL is often caused by HPV infection of a type associated with cervical cancer
Carcinoma	Usually means patient has cervical cancer. Most women with cervical cancer also test positive for HPV infection

From Bonewit-West K: *Clinical procedures for medical assistants,* ed 7, St. Louis, 2008, Saunders.
HPV, Human papillomavirus.

with the previous class I through V system). For this reason, TBS is a more effective means of communicating the results of the Pap test to the physician.

Bimanual Pelvic Examination

After obtaining the smear for the Pap test, the physician withdraws the speculum and performs a bimanual pelvic examination. The physician inserts the index and middle fingers of a lubricated gloved hand into the vagina. The fingers of the other hand are placed on the woman's lower abdomen. Between the two hands, the physician can palpate the size, shape, and position of the uterus and ovaries and detect tenderness or lumps (Figure 23-6).

Rectal-Vaginal Examination

The last part of the pelvic examination is a rectal-vaginal examination. The physician inserts one gloved finger into the vagina and another gloved finger into the rectum to obtain information about the tone and alignment of the pelvic organs and the **adnexal** region (ovaries, fallopian tubes, and ligaments of the uterus). The presence of hemorrhoids, fistulas, and fissures also can be noted. During this examination, the physician may want to obtain some fecal material from the rectum to test for occult blood in the stool, which requires a guaiac slide test (e.g., Hemoccult). This is typically performed on women beginning at 40 years of age. The medical assistant is responsible for assisting with the collection and testing the specimen for occult blood. This procedure (fecal occult blood testing) is presented in detail in Chapter 28.

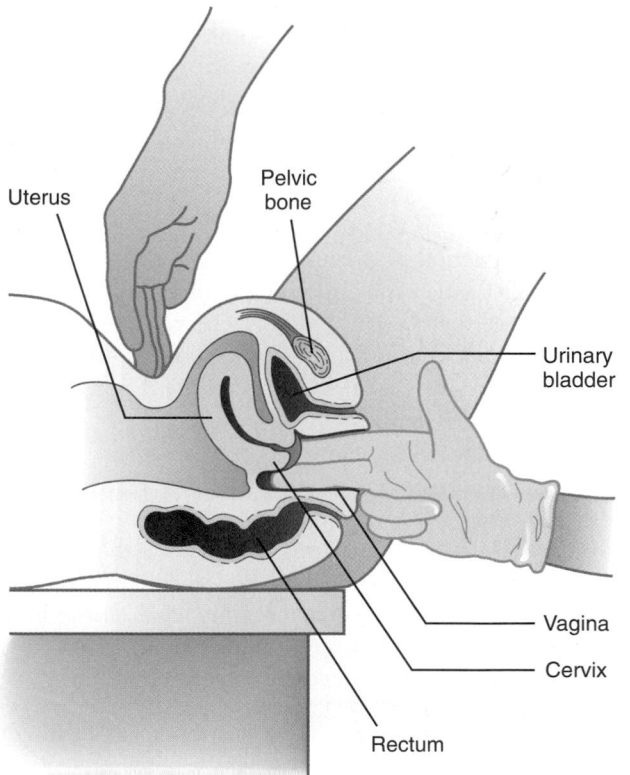

Figure 23-6. The bimanual pelvic examination. (From Bonewit-West K: *Clinical procedures for medical assistants,* ed 7, St. Louis, 2008, Saunders.)

Text continued on p. 470

PROCEDURE 23-1   Breast Self-Examination Instructions

Outcome Instruct a patient in the procedure for performing a BSE.

Equipment/Supplies

- Small pillow

1. Procedural Step. Greet the patient and introduce yourself. Identify the patient and inform her that you will be showing her how to perform a BSE. Discuss with her the purpose of a BSE and when to examine the breasts (see the box *Patient Teaching: Breast Self-Examination*).

2. Procedural Step. Explain to the patient that a complete BSE should be performed in three ways—before a mirror, lying down, and in the shower.
Principle. Using three methods results in a thorough examination, making it more likely that breast changes will be detected.

Instruct the patient in the procedure for performing a BSE as follows:

Before a Mirror

3. Procedural Step. Remove clothing from the waist up. Stand in front of a large mirror with your arms relaxed at your sides. Observe each breast for the following:
  a. Change in size or shape
  b. Swelling, puckering, or dimpling of the skin
  c. Change in skin texture
  d. Retraction of the nipple
  e. Changes in size or position of one nipple compared with the other
Principle. Puckering and dimpling of the skin or retraction of the nipple may mean that a tumor is pulling the skin inward.

4. Procedural Step. Slowly raise your arms over your head, and repeat the same inspection listed in procedural step 3.
Principle. When the arms are moved at the same time into the same positions, both breasts and nipples should react to the movement in the same way. A change in one breast (e.g., dimpling or puckering of the skin) and not the other should be reported to your physician.

Raise your arms over your head. (From Bonewit-West K: *Clinical procedures for medical assistants,* ed 7, St. Louis, 2008, Saunders.)

5. Procedural Step. Rest your palms on your hips and press down firmly to flex your chest muscles. Repeat the inspection in procedural step 3.
Principle. Flexing the chest muscles allows abnormalities to become more apparent.

Press down firmly to flex the chest muscles. (From Bonewit-West K: *Clinical procedures for medical assistants,* ed 7, St. Louis 2008, Saunders.)

6. Procedural Step. Gently squeeze the nipple of each breast with your fingertips and look for a discharge.

Lying Down

7. Procedural Step. To examine the right breast, lie on your back and place a small pillow (or folded towel) under your right shoulder. Place your right hand behind your head.
Principle. The purpose of this step is to flatten the breast and distribute the breast tissue more evenly on the chest, making it easier to palpate the breast tissue.

8. Procedural Step. Extend your left hand with the fingers held flat. The pads of the middle three fingers of the left hand are used to perform the examination. The finger pads include the top third of each finger. Do not use the tips of the fingers. Use small rotating motions (about the size of a dime) and continuous firm pressure with the finger pads.
Principle. The finger pads are more sensitive than the fingertips, making it easier to detect an abnormality.

Use the pads of the middle three fingers. (From Bonewit-West K: *Clinical procedures for medical assistants,* ed 7, St. Louis, 2008, Saunders.)

9. Procedural Step. Use one of the following patterns to move around the breast: circular, vertical strip, or wedge. Choose the pattern that is easiest for you. When you have chosen a pattern, use the same pattern each time you examine your breasts.

Use one of three patterns to examine the breasts. (From Bonewit-West K: *Clinical procedures for medical assistants,* ed 7, St. Louis, 2008, Saunders.)

Circular
  a. Visualize the breast as a clock face.
  b. Start at the outside top edge of the breast.
  c. Proceed clockwise around the entire outer rim of the breast until your fingers return to the starting point.
  d. Move in about 1 inch toward the nipple, and make the same circling motion again.
  e. Move around the breast in smaller and smaller circles until you reach the nipple.

Vertical Strip
  a. Mentally divide the breast into strips.
  b. Start in the underarm area and slowly move your fingers downward until they are below the breast.
  c. Move your fingers about 1 inch toward the middle, and slowly move back up.
  d. Repeat until the entire breast has been examined.

Wedge
  a. Mentally divide your breast into wedges similar to the pieces of a pie.
  b. Starting at the outer edge of the breast, move your fingers toward the nipple and back to the edge of the breast.
  c. Check your entire breast, covering one small wedge-shaped section at a time.

  Principle. Using a specific pattern ensures that the entire breast is examined.

10. Procedural Step. Holding the middle three fingers of your hand together with the thumb extended, use your finger pads and the pattern you selected to examine the right breast thoroughly. Press firmly enough to feel the different breast tissues. The breast should be palpated for lumps, hard knots, and thickening. Breast tissue normally feels a little lumpy and uneven.

Examine the right breast. (From Bonewit-West K: *Clinical procedures for medical assistants,* ed 7, St. Louis, 2008, Saunders.)

11. Procedural Step. Examine the entire chest area from your collarbone to the base of a properly fitted bra and from the breastbone to the underarm. Pay special attention to the area between the breast and underarm, including the underarm itself. A ridge of firm tissue in the lower curve of the breast is normal. Continue the examination until every part of the breast has been examined, including the nipple.
  Principle. An enlarged node in the armpit can also be a sign of breast cancer even if nothing can be felt in the breast.

12. Procedural Step. Repeat this procedure on the left breast. Place a small pillow (or folded towel) under the left shoulder, and place your left hand behind your head. Use the finger pads of the right hand to examine the left breast.

In the Shower

13. Procedural Step. Gently lather each breast.
  Principle. Fingers glide easily over wet, soapy skin, making it easier to detect changes in the breast.

14. Procedural Step. Place your right hand behind your head. Extend your left hand with the fingers held flat. With the finger pads of the middle three fingers, use small rotating motions (about the size of a dime) and continuous firm pressure with the finger pads to examine the right breast. Use your preferred pattern (circular, vertical strip, or wedge) to palpate for lumps, hard knots, and thickening. Examine the area between the breast and underarm, including the underarm itself.
  Principle. The upright position makes it easier to examine the upper and outer portions of the breast.

15. Procedural Step. Repeat the procedure on the left breast. Place the left arm behind the head, and use the right fingers to examine the left breast.

Continued

PROCEDURE 23-1

PROCEDURE 23-2

PROCEDURE **23-1** Breast Self-Examination Instructions—cont'd

Examine the breasts in the shower. (From Bonewit-West K: *Clinical procedures for medical assistants,* ed 7, St. Louis, 2008, Saunders.)

16. Procedural Step. Instruct the patient to report lumps and other changes to the physician immediately. Reassure the patient that most breast lumps are not cancerous, but the only way to know for sure is to see the physician as soon as possible.

17. Procedural Step. Chart the procedure. Include the date and time and the type of instructions given to the patient. If you gave a printed instruction sheet or educational brochure to the patient, document this as well.

CHARTING EXAMPLE

Date	
9/7/10	11:00 a.m. Instructions provided for a BSE. Pt given a BSE educational brochure. ———————————— Y. Wu, RMA

PROCEDURE **23-2** Assisting with a Gynecologic Examination

Outcome Assist with a gynecologic examination. The following procedure describes the medical assistant's role in assisting with a gynecologic examination consisting of breast and pelvic examinations, including a Pap test and a fecal occult blood test.

Equipment/Supplies

- Disposable gloves
- Examining gown and drape
- Disposable vaginal speculum
- Water-based lubricant
- Gauze pads

- Hemoccult slide and developing solution
- Tissues
- Cytology request form
- Biohazard specimen transport bag

Direct Smear Method

- Glass slides with frosted edge
- Cytology fixative
- Plastic spatula
- Endocervical brush
- Slide container

Liquid-Prep Method

- Vial with preservative (ThinPrep, SurePath)
- Plastic spatula and endocervical brush or cytology broom

1. Procedural Step. Sanitize your hands.

2. Procedural Step. Assemble the equipment. Complete as much of the cytology request form as possible. Some information on the form requires input from the patient, such as the LMP, and must be completed later. Prepare the collection materials as follows:

Pap Smear Method. Using a lead pencil, identify the slides on the frosted edge with the patient's name, date, and source of the specimen using the following abbreviations: *V (vaginal), C (cervical),* and *E (endocervical).*

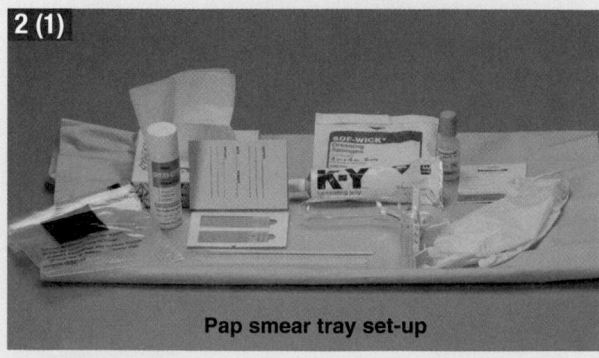

Pap smear tray set-up

Assemble equipment. (From Bonewit-West K: *Clinical procedures for medical assistants,* ed 7, St. Louis, 2008, Saunders.)

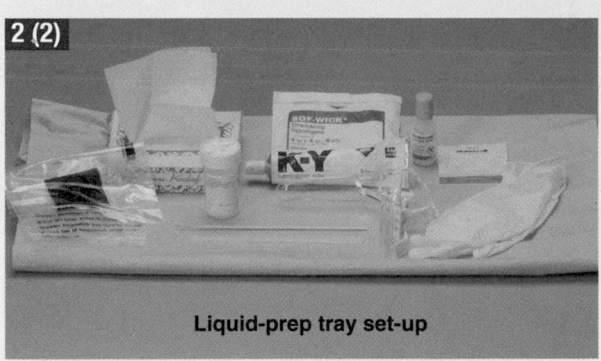

Liquid-prep tray set-up

Assemble equipment. (From Bonewit-West K: *Clinical procedures for medical assistants,* ed 7, St. Louis, 2008, Saunders.)

Liquid-Prep Method. Check the expiration date on the vial. Label the vial with the date and the patient's name and identification number. The identification number is located on the cytology request form.

Principle. If the vial is outdated, it should be discarded because it may lead to inaccurate test results.

3. **Procedural Step.** Greet the patient and introduce yourself. Identify the patient and explain the procedure.

4. **Procedural Step.** Escort the patient to the examining room and ask her to be seated. Seat yourself so that you are facing the patient. Ask the patient whether she has any problems or concerns, and record the information in the patient's chart. Ask the patient the necessary questions to complete the rest of the cytology request form.

5. **Procedural Step.** Measure the patient's vital signs, height, and weight, and chart the results.

6. **Procedural Step.** Instruct and prepare the patient for the examination as follows:

   a. Ask the patient whether she needs to empty the bladder before the examination. If a urine specimen is necessary, instruct the patient in the proper collection of the specimen.

   b. Provide the patient with a patient gown. Instruct the patient to remove all clothing and to put on the patient gown with the opening in front. If the patient is wearing socks, tell her she can keep them on. Offer assistance if you sense the patient may have trouble undressing.

   c. Tell the patient to have a seat on the examining table after she has put on the examining gown.

   d. Inform the patient that the physician will be with her soon, and leave the room to give her privacy.

Principle. An empty bladder makes the examination easier and is more comfortable for the patient. Wearing socks helps keep the patient's feet warm during the examination.

Provide the patient with a gown (From Bonewit-West K: *Clinical procedures for medical assistants,* ed 7, St. Louis, 2008, Saunders.)

7. **Procedural Step.** Make the medical record available for review by the physician. The medical office has a designated location where the record is placed, such as a small shelf mounted on the wall next to the outside of the examining room door or in a chart holder on the outside of the examining room door. Position the medical record so that patient-identifiable information is not visible.

Principle. Before going into the room, the physician will want to review the patient's measurements and urine test results documented by the medical assistant. HIPAA requires protection of a patient's health information.

8. **Procedural Step.** Check to make sure the patient is ready to be seen by the physician. Before entering a patient's room, always knock lightly on the door to let the patient know you are getting ready to enter the room. Inform the physician that the patient is ready. This may be done using a color-coded flagging system mounted on the wall next to the examining room.

9. **Procedural Step.** Assist the patient into a supine position, and properly drape her for the breast examination.

10. **Procedural Step.** Assist the patient into the lithotomy position for the pelvic examination.

11. **Procedural Step.** Prepare the vaginal speculum by removing it from the warming drawer and performing one of the following:

Pap Smear Method. Moisten the blades of the speculum with warm water.

Liquid Prep Method. Thinly lubricate the blades of the speculum with a water-based lubricant.

Principle. Preparing the vaginal speculum facilitates its insertion into the vagina.

Continued

12. **Procedural Step.** Prepare the light for the physician as follows:
    a. *Overhead examination lamp:* Adjust and focus the light for the physician.
    b. *Speculum-illumination system:* Snap the light source device into the light holder on the vaginal speculum and turn it on. The lighting system produces a beam of light that shines through the blades of the speculum for visualization of the vagina and cervix.
       Principle. Visualization of the vagina and cervix requires direct light.

13. **Procedural Step.** Hand the vaginal speculum to the physician. Reassure the patient, and help her relax the abdominal muscles during the examination by telling her to breathe deeply, slowly, and evenly through the mouth.
    Principle. If the patient is relaxed, the examination proceeds more smoothly and is more comfortable for her.

14. Procedural Step. Apply gloves, and assist with the collection of the Pap specimen as follows:
    a. **Direct Smear Method**
       (1) Hold each slide so that the physician can smear the specimen on it.
       (2) Fix each slide immediately after collection by flooding it with 95% ethyl alcohol or by spraying it with a cytology fixative. The slide should be sprayed lightly with a continuous motion from a distance of 5 to 6 inches.
       (3) Allow the slides to air dry for 5 to 10 minutes, and place them in a protective slide container.
    b. **Liquid-Prep Method (ThinPrep)**
    Spatula and Brush Method
       (1) Remove the cap from the ThinPrep vial, and hold it so that the physician can insert the spatula into the vial.
       (2) Rinse the plastic spatula in the liquid preservative by vigorously swirling it around in the solution 10 times.
       (3) Discard the spatula in a biohazard waste container.
       (4) Hold the vial so that the physician can insert the endocervical brush into the vial.
       (5) Rinse the brush in the liquid preservative by vigorously rotating it in the solution 10 times while pushing the brush against the vial wall. Swirl the brush in the solution to further release cellular material.
       Discard the brush in a biohazard waste container. Securely tighten the cap so that the torque line on the cap passes the torque line on the vial.

14a (2)

Spray lightly from a distance of 5 to 6 inches. (From Bonewit-West K: *Clinical procedures for medical assistants,* ed 7, St. Louis, 2008, Saunders.)

14b (2)

Vigorously swirl the spatula in the preservative. (From Bonewit-West K: *Clinical procedures for medical assistants,* ed 7, St. Louis, 2008, Saunders.)

Broom Method
(1) Remove the cap from the ThinPrep vial, and hold it so that the physician can insert the broom into the vial.
(2) Rinse the broom in the liquid preservative by pushing the broom vigorously into the bottom of the vial 10 times. This motion forces the

Rotate the brush in the preservative. (From Bonewit-West K: *Clinical procedures for medical assistants,* ed 7, St. Louis, 2008, Saunders.)

Push the broom vigorously into the bottom of the vial. (From Bonewit-West K: *Clinical procedures for medical assistants,* ed 7, St. Louis, 2008, Saunders.)

broom bristles apart, releasing cervical cells into the solution. Swirl the broom vigorously in the liquid preservative to further release cellular material.

(3) Discard the broom in a biohazard waste container. Tighten the cap so that the torque line on the cap passes the torque line on the vial.

c. **Liquid-Prep Method (SurePath)**

(1) Remove the cap from the SurePath vial, and hold it so that the physician can insert the collection device into the vial.

(2) Break off or disconnect the tip of the collection device from the handle.

(3) Discard the handle of the collection device in a waste container.

(4) Repeat the previous steps until the physician has collected all of the specimens needed for the Pap test.

(5) Securely tighten the cap on the vial.

15. **Procedural Step.** Turn off the examining lamp or disconnect the light source from the vaginal speculum. Discard the disposable vaginal speculum in a biohazard waste container. Apply lubricant to a gauze square. Hold it out so that the physician can apply lubricant to his or her gloves to perform the bimanual and rectal-vaginal examinations. Assist with the collection of the fecal specimen for the fecal occult blood test.

Principle. Applying lubricant to a gauze square (rather than directly to the physician's gloved fingers) prevents the opening of the tube of lubricant from touching the physician's gloves and contaminating the contents of the tube.

Hold the gauze with the lubricant for the physician. (From Bonewit-West K: *Clinical procedures for medical assistants,* ed 7, St. Louis, 2008, Saunders.)

Continued

PROCEDURE 23-2

PROCEDURE 23-2   Assisting with a Gynecologic Examination—cont'd

16. **Procedural Step.** After the examination, assist the patient into a sitting position, and allow her the opportunity to rest for a moment. Offer the patient tissues to remove excess lubricant from the perineum. Assist the patient off the examining table.
    Principle. Some patients (especially geriatric) become dizzy after being on the examining table and should be allowed to rest before sitting up.

17. **Procedural Step.** Instruct the patient to get dressed. Tell the patient how and when she will be notified of Pap test results.

18. **Procedural Step.** Test the fecal occult blood specimen, and chart the results.

19. **Procedural Step.** Prepare the Pap specimen for transport to the laboratory. Place the specimen (slide container or vial) in a biohazard specimen transport bag, and seal the bag. Insert the cytology requisition into the outside pocket of the bag, and tuck the top of the requisition under the flap. Place the bag in the appropriate location for pickup by the laboratory.

20. **Procedural Step.** Chart the transport of the Pap specimen to an outside laboratory.

21. **Procedural Step.** Clean the examining room.

Insert the laboratory request into the outside pocket. (From Bonewit-West K: *Clinical procedures for medical assistants,* ed 7, St. Louis, 2008, Saunders.)

CHARTING EXAMPLE

Date	
9/7/10	10:00 a.m. Hemoccult: negative.
	Instructions provided for BSE. ThinPrep
	Pap specimen to Medical Center Laboratory
	for cytology. —————————— Y. Wu, RMA

VAGINAL INFECTIONS

The vagina provides a warm, moist environment, which tends to encourage the growth of various organisms that can result in a vaginal infection, or *vaginitis.* If an unusual vaginal discharge is present, suggesting a vaginal infection, a specimen is obtained to identify the invading organism. A specimen of the discharge is collected at the medical office and is evaluated there or placed in a transport medium that is picked up by a laboratory courier and transported to an outside medical laboratory for evaluation. The patient should be instructed not to douche before coming to the medical office because the physician would be unable to observe the discharge or obtain a specimen for microbiologic analysis.

The medical assistant is responsible for assembling the appropriate supplies for the collection and evaluation of the suspected invading organism. The medical assistant must label all specimens with the patient's name, the date, and the source of the specimen. If the specimen is to be transported to an outside medical laboratory for evaluation, a laboratory request form must be completed. The request form indicates the source of the specimen, the physician's clinical diagnosis, the microbiologic examination requested, and other pertinent information, such as medications the patient is taking. The physician's clinical assessment of the patient's signs and symptoms, along with the results of the laboratory evaluation of the specimen, are used to diagnose the presence of a vaginal infection.

Medical assistants should protect themselves from infection with a pathogen while assisting with the collection and evaluation of the specimen by practicing good techniques of medical asepsis. Methods used to identify the invading organism and the supplies required for the collection and evaluation of organisms that cause common vaginal infections are presented next.

Figure 23-7. *Trichomonas vaginalis* under a microscope. (Modified from Mahon C, Manuselis G: *Textbook of diagnostic microbiology*, ed 2, Philadelphia, 2000, Saunders.)

Trichomoniasis

Trichomonas vaginalis, the causative agent of trichomoniasis (trich), is a pear-shaped protozoan with four flagella, which allow for the motility of the organism (Figure 23-7). Trichomoniasis is usually, but not always, spread through sexual intercourse. Symptoms of this infection include a profuse, frothy vaginal discharge that is usually yellowish green and has an unpleasant odor; itching and irritation of the vulva and vagina; dyspareunia; and dysuria. The cervix may exhibit small red spots, a condition known as "strawberry cervix."

Trichomonas may be identified at the medical office by a wet preparation, which involves placing a small amount of the discharge on a microscope slide using a sterile swab, adding a drop of isotonic saline to it, and placing a coverslip over the mixture to protect it (Figure 23-8). The slide is examined under the microscope and observed for the presence of the lashing movements of the flagella and the motility of the organism.

If the physician prefers to have an outside laboratory evaluate the specimen, it must be placed in a tube containing a transport medium. The specimen must be transported as soon as possible (within 24 hours) to prevent it from dying, which would impede visualization of the motility of the organism.

Trichomoniasis is treated with the oral administration of metronidazole (Flagyl). The woman and her sexual partner must be treated at the same time to prevent reinfection because her partner may harbor the organism without displaying noticeable symptoms.

Candidiasis

Candida albicans is a yeastlike fungus normally found in the intestinal tract and is a frequent contaminant of the vagina; however, it usually does not produce symptoms indicating a vaginal infection. Conditions such as pregnancy, diabetes mellitus, and prolonged antibiotic therapy produce changes

Wet Preparation

A small amount of the vaginal discharge is placed on the slide.

A drop of normal saline is added to the specimen.

A coverslip is placed over the specimen to protect it during examination under the microscope.

Figure 23-8. Preparing a wet preparation for the identification of *Trichomonas vaginalis*. (From Bonewit-West K: *Clinical procedures for medical assistants*, ed 7, St. Louis, 2008, Saunders.)

in the vagina that may precipitate a candidal infection of the vagina, commonly referred to as a "yeast infection." Symptoms of candidiasis include white patches on the mucous membrane of the vagina; a thick, odorless, cottage cheese–like discharge; vulval irritation; and dysuria. The discharge is extremely irritating and usually results in burning and intense itching.

Candida may be identified microscopically in the medical office by placing a specimen of the vaginal discharge on a slide using a sterile swab and adding a drop of a 10% solution of potassium hydroxide (KOH). The KOH dissolves cellular debris present in the smear and allows better visualization of yeast buds, spores, or hyphae (fungus filaments), indicating the presence of *C. albicans* (Figure 23-9). If the specimen is to be transported to a medical laboratory for identification, it must be placed in a transport medium to prevent drying and death of the organism.

Candidiasis is treated with the application of vaginal ointments or suppositories, such as miconazole (Monistat), clotrimazole (Gyne-Lotrimin), and nystatin (Mycostatin), or the oral administration of fluconazole (Diflucan). Candidiasis tends to recur; the woman should be instructed to contact the medical office if the symptoms of the yeast infection reappear.

Figure 23-9. *Candida albicans* under a microscope. (Modified from Mahon C, Manuselis G: *Textbook of diagnostic microbiology*, ed 2, Philadelphia, 2000, Saunders.)

Chlamydia

Chlamydia is caused by the bacterium *Chlamydia trachomatis.* It is a gram-negative intracellular bacterium; it grows and multiplies in the cytoplasm of the host cell. Chlamydia is the most frequently reported and fastest-spreading sexually transmitted disease in the United States, particularly among adolescent girls and young women.

Most women with chlamydia have no symptoms and are not aware of having the condition. Because of this, many women do not seek medical care until serious complications have occurred. After infection, chlamydia first attacks the cervix, resulting in cervicitis. If symptoms do occur, they may include one or more of the following: dysuria, itching and irritation of the genital area, and a yellowish, odorless vaginal discharge. These symptoms usually appear 1 to 3 weeks after the patient has been infected.

If not treated, chlamydia can spread further into the female reproductive tract and cause *pelvic inflammatory disease* (PID). The symptoms of PID include lower abdominal pain, fever, nausea and vomiting, dyspareunia, vaginal discharge, and bleeding between periods. Complications of PID are serious and include chronic pelvic pain, scarring of the fallopian tubes, ectopic pregnancy, and infertility.

Symptoms of a chlamydial infection in men include mild dysuria and a thin, watery discharge from the penis. Men are more likely to have symptoms than women; however, the symptoms may appear only early in the day and be so mild that they are ignored. If the infection is not treated, it can cause *epididymitis,* a painful condition of the testicles that could result in infertility.

When diagnosed early, chlamydia can be treated successfully with antibiotics. The antibiotics most often used are azithromycin (Zithromax) and doxycycline. The patient's partner should also be tested for chlamydia so that if treatment is necessary, it can be administered as soon as possible.

Chlamydia is most frequently diagnosed using a DNA-based detection test known as the *DNA-probe test.* This test is able to detect the presence of the genes of chlamydia

bacteria. The physician collects a specimen using a sterile swab. The specimen is collected from the endocervical canal of a female patient and from the urethra of a male patient. Male patients should be instructed not to void for 1 hour before the collection of the specimen to prevent chlamydia organisms from being washed out of the urethra. After collection, the specimen is placed in a tube containing a transport medium to preserve the specimen until it reaches the laboratory. See the box *Chlamydia and Gonorrhea Specimen Collection* for detailed instructions on how to collect a chlamydia specimen.

Gonorrhea

Gonorrhea is caused by the bacterium *Neisseria gonorrhoeae,* which is a gram-negative diplococcus. Gonorrhea is an infection of the genitourinary tract that is transmitted through sexual intercourse. Chlamydia often occurs in association with gonorrhea; approximately 25% to 40% of patients infected with gonorrhea also have chlamydia.

Women who have contracted gonorrhea may have no symptoms or may exhibit dysuria and a yellow vaginal discharge. The symptoms of gonorrhea (if they occur) appear 2 to 10 days after infection and may be so mild that they are ignored. As the disease progresses, it can spread farther into the reproductive tract, resulting in PID. As mentioned previously, PID can lead to serious complications such as infertility.

Men who have contracted gonorrhea exhibit more symptoms than do women, including dysuria and a whitish discharge from the penis, which may progress to a thick and creamy discharge. The burning and pain experienced during urination is often severe, which usually prompts an infected man to seek early treatment. If not treated, gonorrhea may cause epididymitis, which could lead to infertility.

Gonorrhea can be treated effectively with antibiotics. In recent years, gonorrhea bacteria have become resistant to the antibiotics typically used to treat the disease. Because of this, newer types of antibiotics have been developed. One of the most effective antibiotics used to treat gonorrhea is ceftriaxone, which is administered in one dose through an injection.

The medical office most frequently uses a DNA-probe test to diagnose gonorrhea. This test detects the presence of the genes of the gonorrhea bacterium. Before the development of the DNA-probe test, a culture test was most often used to diagnose gonorrhea. Although occasionally still used, the disadvantage of this method is that gonorrhea is difficult to culture. Special procedures must be performed after the collection of the specimen to ensure the organism remains alive during transport to the laboratory. This includes an atmosphere of carbon dioxide and a specially enriched Thayer-Martin culture medium. Most offices now prefer the DNA-probe test, which is just as accurate as the culture test but much easier when preparing the specimen for transport to the laboratory. The procedure for obtaining a specimen for the DNA-probe test is outlined in the box *Chlamydia and Gonorrhea Specimen Collection.*

Highlight on Sexually Transmitted Diseases

Sexually transmitted diseases (STDs) are among the most common infectious diseases in the United States today. Each year, more than 15 million new cases of STDs are reported in the United States. If this trend continues, at least one in four Americans will contract an STD at some time in his or her life. STDs are most prevalent among teenagers and young adults; nearly two thirds of STDs are contracted by individuals 15 to 25 years old.

Transmission
STDs are spread most often by sexual contact (vaginal, anal, or oral) with an infected person. They are less commonly spread by skin-to-skin contact and by the use of contaminated needles among drug users. More than 20 STDs have been identified. The most common STDs are chlamydia, gonorrhea, herpes, HPV, hepatitis B, HIV, and syphilis. Currently, a preventive vaccine is available for HPV and hepatitis B.

Symptoms
An STD sometimes causes no symptoms at all, particularly in women. If symptoms do occur, they include one or more of the following: an unusual discharge from the penis or vagina; itching, redness, or soreness of the genitals; sores or blisters on or around the genitals, anus, or both; and pain or burning during urination.

With or without symptoms, an STD can be spread to someone else. If symptoms develop, they may be so mild that they go unnoticed, or they may be confused with symptoms of other diseases. Because of this, STDs may go undetected and untreated. If not treated, many STDs result in serious complications, such as infertility. In addition, some STDs can be passed from an infected mother to her infant before or during birth.

Treatment
When diagnosed early, most STDs can be treated effectively, and many can be cured. Antibiotics can cure STDs caused by bacteria, such as chlamydia, gonorrhea, and syphilis. Medications have been developed to control the symptoms of STDs caused by viruses, such as herpes and HPV; however, they cannot eliminate the virus from the body.

Prevention and Control
All STDs can be prevented. The best way to prevent STDs is to practice abstinence or to have a mutually monogamous sexual relationship with an uninfected partner. If an individual's lifestyle does not follow one of these patterns, the following can be done to reduce the risk of contracting an STD:
- Before having a sexual relationship, partners should discuss their sexual histories with each other and get tested for STDs.
- Use a condom during sexual intercourse. If the condom is not used correctly, however, an individual still could contract an STD.
- Limit the number of sexual partners. The risk of an STD increases with each new partner, particularly if it is unknown how many previous partners that person has had.

Plan of Action
Sexually active individuals who are not in a monogamous relationship should have regular health checkups and ask to be tested for STDs. These individuals should also learn to recognize the symptoms of STDs and check themselves for signs of STD infection once a month.

If an individual thinks he or she has an STD, a physician should be consulted as soon as possible. If an individual has been treated for an STD and still has symptoms, he or she should return to the physician for further evaluation. It is possible to have more than one STD at a time and to become reinfected with the same STD.

An individual diagnosed with an STD should inform his or her partner immediately so that the partner can be tested. It is also important for an infected person to take all prescribed medication and to abstain from intercourse until a physician has determined that he or she is no longer contagious. ■

What Would You Do? What Would You *Not* Do?

Case Study 2
Dagny Fairchild comes to the office. She is 16 years old, and her father is a lawyer and her mother is a chemical engineer. Her boyfriend was diagnosed 2 weeks ago with chlamydia. Dagny was hesitant to come in because she does not have any symptoms, and her boyfriend always uses a condom. She is worried about her parents finding out that she is sexually active and what they will think if she has one of "those diseases." Dagny is also afraid and extremely embarrassed about what will be "done to her" to determine whether she has chlamydia. She tells Yin-Ling that she is thinking of leaving the office and not seeing the physician at all. (*Note:* Dagny lives in a state that allows minors to receive health care services without parental consent.) ■

PRENATAL CARE

OBSTETRICS

Obstetrics is the branch of medicine that deals with the supervision of women's health during pregnancy, childbirth, and the puerperium. **Prenatal** refers to the care of a preg-

nant woman before delivery of the infant. Prenatal care consists of a series of scheduled medical office visits for the promotion of the health of the mother and fetus through prevention of disease and early detection, diagnosis, and treatment of problems common to pregnancy (e.g., anemia, urinary tract infection, preeclampsia). Early detection of

Chlamydia and Gonorrhea Specimen Collection

DNA-Based Detection Test

The procedure for collecting a specimen for the DNA test is outlined below. The chlamydia and gonorrhea tests can be performed on the same specimen.

1. The medical assistant assembles supplies needed to collect the specimen, including a vaginal speculum, clean disposable gloves, and the DNA-probe collection kit. The collection kit includes cotton-tipped swabs and a tube of transport medium.
2. The transport tube must be labeled with the following information: patient's name and identification number, date and time of collection, and physician's name and phone number.

**DNA-probe set-up
(Female patient)**

(From Bonewit-West K: *Clinical procedures for medical assistants*, ed 7, St. Louis, 2008, Saunders.)

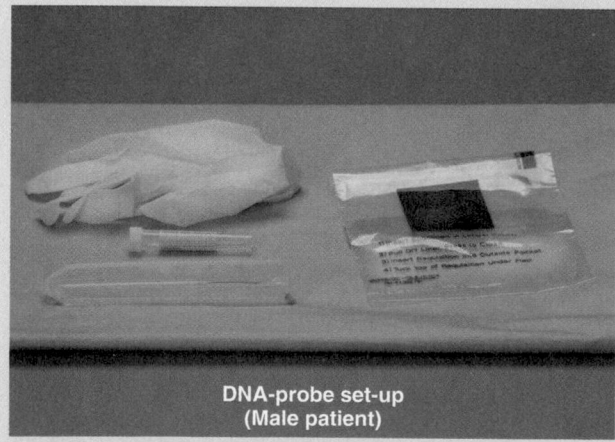

**DNA-probe set-up
(Male patient)**

(From Bonewit-West K: *Clinical procedures for medical assistants*, ed 7, St. Louis, 2008, Saunders.)

3. The physician collects the specimen as follows:
   - **Female Patient:** The physician inserts a vaginal speculum into the vagina. Using a cotton-tipped swab, the physician first removes excess mucus or discharge from the cervix. Next, the physician collects the specimen by inserting another cotton-tipped swab into the endocervical canal and rotating it for 5 to 10 seconds. This ensures a good sampling of the specimen.
   - **Male Patient:** The patient must not urinate for 1 hour before the collection to prevent any urethral discharge from being washed away. The physician inserts a small-tipped cotton swab 2 to 4 cm into the penis. The swab is gently rotated for 3 to 5 seconds to dislodge cells and to ensure contact with all urethral surfaces.
4. The physician withdraws the swab.
5. The medical assistant should ensure that the transport medium is at the bottom of the tube. The medical assistant unscrews the cap and holds the tube for the physician.

The physician inserts the swab into the transport tube and breaks off the shaft of the swab at the score line. (From Bonewit-West K: *Clinical procedures for medical assistants*, ed 7, St. Louis, 2008, Saunders.)

6. The physician inserts the swab into the transport tube and breaks off the shaft of the swab at the score line.
7. The medical assistant places the cap on the tube and twists it until it clicks into place. The tube is placed in a biohazard specimen transport bag along with the laboratory requisition for pickup by the laboratory.

---

medical problems helps prevent serious complications in the mother and fetus.

Obstetric Terminology

The medical assistant should know the common terms related to obstetrics, as follows:

Braxton Hicks contractions   Intermittent and irregular painless uterine contractions that occur throughout pregnancy. They occur more frequently toward the end of pregnancy and are sometimes mistaken for true labor pains.

Dilation   The stretching of the external os (of the cervix) from an opening of a few millimeters to an opening large enough to allow the passage of an infant (approximately 10 cm).

Effacement The thinning and shortening of the cervical canal from its normal length of 1 to 2 cm to a structure with paper-thin edges in which there is no canal at all. Effacement occurs late in pregnancy, during labor, or both. The purpose of effacement, along with dilation, is to permit the passage of the infant into the birth canal.

Embryo The child in utero from the time of conception to the beginning of the first trimester (i.e., the first 2 months of development).

Engagement The entrance of the fetal head or the presenting part into the pelvic inlet.

Fetus The child in utero, from the third month after conception to birth; during the first 2 months of development, it is called an *embryo*.

Fundus The dome-shaped upper portion of the uterus between the fallopian tubes.

Gestation The period of intrauterine development from conception to birth; the period of pregnancy. The average pregnancy lasts about 280 days, or 40 weeks, from the date of conception to childbirth.

Gestational age The age of the fetus between conception and birth.

Infant A child from birth to 12 months old.

Multigravida A woman who has been pregnant more than once.

Multipara A woman who has completed two or more pregnancies to the age of viability regardless of whether they ended in live infants or stillbirths.

Nullipara A woman who has not carried a pregnancy to the point of fetal viability (20 weeks of gestation).

Position The relation of the presenting part of the fetus to the maternal pelvis.

Postpartum Occurring after childbirth.

Preeclampsia A major complication of pregnancy, the cause of which is unknown, characterized by increasing hypertension, albuminuria, and edema. If the condition is neglected or not treated properly, preeclampsia may develop into eclampsia, which could cause maternal convulsions and coma. Preeclampsia generally occurs between the 20th week of pregnancy and the end of the first week postpartum.

Presentation Indication of the part of the fetus that is closest to the cervix and is delivered first. A cephalic presentation is a delivery in which the fetal head is presenting against the cervix. A breech presentation is a delivery in which the buttocks or feet are presented instead of the head.

Primigravida A woman who is pregnant for the first time.

Primipara A woman who has carried a pregnancy to fetal viability (20 weeks of gestation) for the first time, regardless of whether the infant was stillborn or alive at birth.

Puerperium The period of time (usually 4 to 6 weeks) after delivery in which the uterus and body systems are returning to normal.

Memories *from* Externship

Yin-Ling Wu: During my externship, I was assigned to an OB/GYN clinic. They had an ultrasound technician working there who ran all the scans on prenatal patients. She would always bring the pictures out so we could all look at them. They always looked like a big blob to me—I could never see anything.

One day, a patient whom one of the medical assistants knew really well came into the office. The patient agreed to let us all come in for her ultrasound. It was her first time getting an ultrasound. When the technician put the ultrasound probe on her abdomen, we could see the outline of the whole baby. You could even see a tiny arm and fingers, and it looked like the baby was waving. The look of joy and amazement on the mom's face was unforgettable. After that, I knew I was in the right profession. ■

Prepare for Success

Quickening The first movements of the fetus in utero as felt by the mother, which usually occurs between 16 and 20 weeks of gestation and is felt consistently thereafter.

Toxemia A condition that can occur in pregnant women that includes preeclampsia and eclampsia. If preeclampsia goes undiagnosed or is not satisfactorily controlled, it could develop into eclampsia, which is characterized by convulsions and coma.

Trimester Three months, or one third, of the gestational period. The 9 months of pregnancy are divided into three trimesters, each consisting of 3 months. From conception to 3 months is the first trimester, from 4 to 6 months is the second trimester, and from 7 to 9 months is the third trimester.

PRENATAL VISITS

The medical office visits for prenatal and postpartum care of the pregnant woman can be grouped into three major categories as follows:
1. First prenatal visit
2. Return prenatal visits
3. Six weeks–postpartum visit

First Prenatal Visit

The first prenatal visit generally occurs after the woman has missed her second menstrual period; if problems exist, the woman is seen after missing her first menstrual period. Regardless of whether or not the patient is happy and excited about the pregnancy, the first visit is often a stressful experience for the patient. The medical assistant plays an important role in relaxing the patient and relieving her anxiety.

The first prenatal visit requires more time than subsequent prenatal visits; sufficient time should be scheduled to allow a complete and accurate initial assessment of the pregnant woman. The components of the first prenatal visit vary depending on the medical office, but they generally include the following:

1. Completion of a prenatal record form.
2. Initial prenatal examination, consisting of a complete physical examination. Of particular importance are the breast, abdominal, and pelvic examinations. Pelvic measurements may be taken at this time or during a return prenatal visit.
3. Prenatal patient education.
4. Laboratory tests.

Prenatal Record

The prenatal record provides information regarding the past and present health of the patient and serves as a database and flow sheet for subsequent prenatal visits. The prenatal record is essential in helping identify high-risk patients. The medical assistant is usually responsible for collecting a portion of the information required for the prenatal record. Many types of printed prenatal record forms are available (Figure 23-10). The specific form used in the medical office is based on the physician's preference and the method used for conducting the prenatal examination.

PRENATAL HEALTH HISTORY

PATIENT INFORMATION

Date: _____   EDD: _____   Referred By: _____

Name: _____   Phone (home): _____
       LAST   FIRST   MIDDLE   Phone (work): _____

Address: _____   Emergency Contact: _____

_____   Phone: _____
       CITY   STATE   ZIP

Date of Birth: ____/____/____   Age: ____   Marital Status: _____
Occupation: _____
Education: ☐ High School   ☐ College   ☐ Post-graduate

PAST MEDICAL HISTORY

	O Neg / + Pos	DETAIL POSITIVE REMARKS INCLUDE DATE AND TREATMENT		O Neg / + Pos	DETAIL POSITIVE REMARKS INCLUDE DATE AND TREATMENT
1. DIABETES			16. D (Rh) SENSITIZED		
2. HYPERTENSION			17. PULMONARY (TB, ASTHMA)		
3. HEART DISEASE			18. RHEUMATIC FEVER		
4. AUTOIMMUNE DISORDER			19. BLEEDING TENDENCY		
5. KIDNEY DISEASE/UTI			20. GYN SURGERY		
6. NEUROLOGIC/EPILEPSY			21. OPERATIONS/HOSPITALIZATIONS (YEAR AND REASON)		
7. PSYCHIATRIC					
8. HEPATITIS/LIVER DISEASE					
9. VARICOSITIES/PHLEBITIS			22. ANESTHETIC COMPLICATIONS		
10. THYROID DYSFUNCTION			23. HISTORY OF ABNORMAL PAP		
11. TRAUMA/DOMESTIC VIOLENCE			24. UTERINE ANOMALY/DES		
12. BLOOD TRANSFUSION			25. INFERTILITY		

	AMT/DAY PREPREG.	AMT/DAY PREG.	# YEARS USE			
				25. INFERTILITY		
				26. SEXUALLY TRANSMITTED DISEASE		
13. TOBACCO						
14. ALCOHOL						
15. STREET DRUGS				27. OTHER		

IMMUNIZATIONS:

Mark an X next to those you have had.

☐ Influenza   ☐ Chickenpox
☐ Hepatitis B ☐ Pneumococcal
☐ Hib   ☐ Tuberculin Test
☐ Polio   ☐ Tetanus Booster
☐ MMR

ALLERGIES:

List all allergies (foods, drugs, environment).   ☐ None

_____
_____
_____
_____
_____

MENSTRUAL HISTORY

Menarche: Age of Onset _____   GYN Disorders (List): _____
Frequency: Q ____ Days   _____
Duration: ____ Days
Amount of Flow: ☐ Small   ☐ Moderate ☐ Large   On contraceptive at conception? ☐ Yes ☐ No

Figure 23-10. Example of a prenatal record form. (From Bonewit-West K: *Clinical procedures for medical assistants,* ed 7, St. Louis, 2008, Saunders.)

Obtaining and recording information in the prenatal record from one visit to the next provides an opportunity for the medical assistant to develop a rapport with the patient. It is also an excellent time to relay information to her regarding various aspects of the prenatal and postnatal period, such as an explanation of the changes occurring in her body, the signs and symptoms of labor, nutrition of the infant (breastfeeding and bottle feeding), and care of the newborn infant. The prenatal record form should be completed in a quiet setting that is free from distractions. This gives the patient the confidence to discuss areas of concern openly, which helps ensure a complete and accurate prenatal history.

Past Medical History

The past medical history focuses on conditions that could affect the health of the mother and fetus, such as kidney disease, liver disease, heart disease, hypertension, sexually transmitted diseases, phlebitis, diabetes, tuberculosis, thyroid disorders, drug allergies, alcohol and tobacco intake, drug addiction, previous abnormal Pap tests, infertility problems, and surgeries. In addition, the medical assistant

OBSTETRIC HISTORY

G _____ (Total Pregnancies) T _____ (Term) P _____ (Preterm) A _____ (Abortions)? L _____ (Living Children)

PREVIOUS PREGNANCIES:

DATE MONTH/ YEAR	WEEKS GEST.	LENGTH OF LABOR	BIRTH WEIGHT	SEX M/F	TYPE DELIVERY	ANES.	MATERNAL COMPLICATIONS	INFANT COMPLICATIONS

PRESENT PREGNANCY HISTORY

NAUSEA			ABDOMINAL PAIN		
VOMITING			URINARY COMPLAINTS		
FATIGUE			VAGINAL BLEEDING		
BREAST CHANGES			VAGINAL DISCHARGE		
INDIGESTION			PRURITIS		
CONSTIPATION			ACCIDENTS		
PERSISTENT HEADACHES			SURGERY		
DIZZINESS			X-RAYS		
VISUAL DISTURBANCE			RUBELLA EXPOSURE		
EDEMA (SPECIFY AREA)			OTHER VIRAL INFECTIONS		

LMP ____/____/____ Mo Day Year   Amount of Flow: ☐ Small   ☐ Moderate ☐ Large

CURRENT MEDICATIONS: (Include prescription, OTC, herbal, and vitamins). ☐ None

Medication _____   Frequency _____

INITIAL PHYSICAL EXAMINATION

DATE ____/____/____

1. HEENT	☐ NORMAL	☐ ABNORMAL	12. VULVA	☐ NORMAL	☐ CONDYLOMA	☐ LESIONS
2. FUNDI	☐ NORMAL	☐ ABNORMAL	13. VAGINA	☐ NORMAL	☐ INFLAMMATION	☐ DISCHARGE
3. TEETH	☐ NORMAL	☐ ABNORMAL	14. CERVIX	☐ NORMAL	☐ INFLAMMATION	☐ LESIONS
4. THYROID	☐ NORMAL	☐ ABNORMAL	15. UTERUS SIZE	_____ WEEKS		☐ FIBROIDS
5. BREASTS	☐ NORMAL	☐ ABNORMAL	16. ADNEXA	☐ NORMAL	☐ MASS	
6. LUNGS	☐ NORMAL	☐ ABNORMAL	17. RECTUM	☐ NORMAL	☐ ABNORMAL	
7. HEART	☐ NORMAL	☐ ABNORMAL	18. DIAGONAL CONJUGATE	☐ REACHED	☐ NO	_____ CM
8. ABDOMEN	☐ NORMAL	☐ ABNORMAL	19. SPINES	☐ AVERAGE	☐ PROMINENT	☐ BLUNT
9. EXTREMITIES	☐ NORMAL	☐ ABNORMAL	20. SACRUM	☐ CONCAVE	☐ STRAIGHT	☐ ANTERIOR
10. SKIN	☐ NORMAL	☐ ABNORMAL	21. SUBPUBIC ARCH	☐ NORMAL	☐ WIDE	☐ NARROW
11. LYMPH NODES	☐ NORMAL	☐ ABNORMAL	22. GYNECOID PELVIC TYPE	☐ YES	☐ NO	

COMMENTS (Number and explain abnormals): _____

_____

_____

_____ **EXAM BY** _____

Figure 23-10, cont'd.

Continued

PATIENT'S NAME _____

INTERVAL PRENATAL HISTORY

Date 20__	Weeks Gestation	Height of Fundus (cm)	Weight	B/P	Urine Glucose	Urine Protein	FHT	Vaginal Examination	Presentation	Edema	Discharge	Bleeding	Contractions	Fetal Activity	NST	Next Appt.	Initials

PLANS/EDUCATION   (COUNSELED ☑)

☐ ANESTHESIA PLANS _____

☐ TOXOPLASMOSIS PRECAUTIONS (CATS/RAW MEAT) _____

☐ CHILDBIRTH CLASSES _____

☐ PHYSICAL/SEXUAL ACTIVITY _____

☐ LABOR SIGNS _____

☐ NUTRITION COUNSELING _____

☐ BREAST OR BOTTLE FEEDING _____

☐ NEWBORN CAR SEAT _____

☐ POSTPARTUM BIRTH CONTROL _____

☐ ENVIRONMENTAL/WORK HAZARDS _____

☐ TUBAL STERILIZATION _____

☐ VBAC COUNSELING _____

☐ CIRCUMCISION _____

☐ TRAVEL _____

☐ LIFESTYLE, TOBACCO, ALCOHOL _____

REQUESTS _____

_____

_____

TUBAL STERILIZATION   DATE   INITIALS

CONSENT SIGNED   ___/___/___   _____

Figure 23-10, cont'd.

solicits information from the patient regarding immunizations and childhood diseases to provide the physician with the information needed to assess her antibody protection against such diseases.

Menstrual History

A menstrual history is obtained from the patient. It includes the date of the onset of menstruation, menstrual interval cycle, duration, amount of flow (recorded as small, moderate, or large), and any gynecologic disorders. The form also includes a space for the patient to indicate whether or not she was using a method of contraception when she became pregnant.

Obstetric History

A thorough obstetric history is a component of the prenatal record and provides the opportunity to obtain information from the patient related to previous pregnancies. If a woman is a multigravida, information about each pregnancy is obtained, including the length of the pregnancy, hours of labor, type of delivery (vaginal or cesarean section), type of anesthesia, sex and weight of the newborn, and maternal or infant complications. The obstetric history assists in identifying areas that may need to be investigated further or monitored during the prenatal period. Women with previous complications, such as premature labor, gestational diabetes, or postpartum hemorrhaging, are at risk for having these problems again.

Present Pregnancy History

The present pregnancy history establishes a baseline for the present health status of the prenatal patient. In addition, the patient is queried regarding any warning signs that may be present and may place the mother or fetus in jeopardy,

LABORATORY		PATIENT'S NAME _____		
INITIAL LABS	**DATE**	**RESULTS**	**REVIEWED**	**COMMENTS**
BLOOD TYPE	/ /	A B AB O		
Rh FACTOR	/ /	☐ Pos ☐ Neg		
Rh ANTIBODY SCREEN	/ /	☐ Pos ☐ Neg		
HCT/HGB	/ /	_____% _____ g/dL		
RUBELLA ANTIBODY TITER	/ /	Immune Nonimmune		
VDRL	/ /	☐ NR ☐ R		
HBsAg (HEPATITIS B)	/ /	☐ Pos ☐ Neg		
HIV	/ /	☐ Pos ☐ Neg ☐ Declined		
URINE CULTURE/SCREEN	/ /			
PAP TEST	/ /	☐ Normal ☐ Abnormal		
CHLAMYDIA (DNA PROBE)	/ /	☐ Pos ☐ Neg		
GONORRHEA (DNA PROBE)	/ /	☐ Pos ☐ Neg		
7–20 WEEK LABS (WHEN INDICATED/ELECTED)	**DATE**	**RESULTS**	**REVIEWED**	**COMMENTS**
ULTRASOUND #1 (7–12 WEEKS)	/ /	EDD:		
ULTRASOUND #2 (18–20 WEEKS)	/ /	EFW:		
TRIPLE SCREEN (15–20 WEEKS)	/ /			
CVS	/ /			
AMNIOCENTESIS	/ /			
24–28 WEEK LABS (WHEN INDICATED)	**DATE**	**RESULTS**	**REVIEWED**	**COMMENTS**
HCT/HGB	/ /	_____ % _____ g/dL		
GCT (24–28 WKS)	/ /	1 Hour _____		
GTT (IF SCREEN ABNORMAL)	/ /	_____ FBS _____ 1 Hour _____ 2 Hour _____ 3 Hour		
D (Rh) ANTIBODY SCREEN	/ /			
D IMMUNE GLOBULIN (RhIG) GIVEN (28 WKS)	/ /	SIGNATURE		
32–36 WEEK LABS	**DATE**	**RESULTS**	**REVIEWED**	**COMMENTS**
HCT/HGB (32 WKS)	/ /	_____ % _____ g/dL		
ULTRASOUND #3 (34 WKS)	/ /	EFW:		
GROUP B STREP (35–37 WKS)	/ /	☐ Pos ☐ Neg		
ADDITIONAL LAB TESTS	**DATE**	**RESULTS**	**REVIEWED**	**COMMENTS**
	/ /			
	/ /			
	/ /			
	/ /			
	/ /			

Figure 23-10, cont'd.

such as persistent headaches, visual disturbances, abdominal pain, vaginal bleeding, or discharge. The patient is also asked whether she has experienced any of the early signs of pregnancy, such as nausea, vomiting, fatigue, and breast changes.

All prescribed or over-the-counter medications (including vitamin supplements and herbal products) the patient is taking must be recorded. Certain medications cross the placental barrier and could be harmful to the developing fetus. The patient should be instructed not to take any medications without first checking with the physician.

In the space provided under the present pregnancy history, the medical assistant needs to record the first day of the patient's LMP. The LMP is used to calculate due date, or **expected date of delivery (EDD),** by using Nägele's rule: Add 7 days to the first day of the LMP, subtract 3 months, and add 1 year (EDD = LMP + 7 days − 3 months + 1 year). For example, if the first day of the patient's LMP was June 10, 2009, the EDD is March 17, 2010. The problem is set up as follows:

6	10	2009	(LMP)
−3	+ 7	+ 1	(Applying Nägele's rule)
3	17	2010	(Delivery date)

Using Nägele's rule, approximately 4% of patients deliver spontaneously on the EDD; most patients deliver during the period extending from 7 days before to 7 days after the EDD.

Gestation calculators are commercially available that can be used to determine the delivery date by lining up an arrow and the date of the LMP, using a movable inner cardboard wheel (Figure 23-11). These calculators require less time to determine the EDD than using Nägele's

Figure 23-11. Gestation calculator. The last menstrual period is July 20, and the estimated date of delivery is April 25. (From Bonewit-West K: *Clinical procedures for medical assistants,* ed 7, St. Louis, 2008, Saunders.)

rule, and they provide information on the probable size (length and weight) of the fetus on any given date. The accuracy of gestation calculators is comparable to that of Nägele's rule. If the patient is unsure of the date of her LMP, the physician estimates the length of gestation by other methods, such as fundal height measurement and sonography.

Interval Prenatal History

The interval prenatal history is also included in the prenatal record form; its purpose is to update the record. During every return visit, essential data are collected and recorded in this section, including weight, blood pressure, urine testing results, fundal height measurement, and fetal heart rate. A general inquiry is made regarding the occurrence of additional signs of pregnancy, such as fetal movement or Braxton Hicks contractions, and how the patient is feeling and any concerns or symptoms since the last prenatal visit.

This information is recorded and assists the medical staff in planning, implementing, and evaluating individual needs. Particular attention is focused on risk factors, such as hypertension, thrombophlebitis, and uterine bleeding, which could influence the course of the pregnancy.

Initial Prenatal Examination

Purpose

The initial prenatal examination is of particular importance because it results in confirmation of the pregnancy and establishes a baseline for the woman's state of health. It includes a thorough gynecologic examination (breast and pelvic examinations) and a general physical examination of the other body systems, although the latter may be performed during a subsequent prenatal visit, depending on the medical office routine.

Women often have little or no medical supervision during their childbearing years; the physical examination is of particular importance in establishing a baseline for the woman's general state of health and in identifying high-risk prenatal patients. Conditions such as obesity, hypertension, severe varicosities, and uterine size inappropriate for the due date can be diagnosed by the physician, and necessary treatment or monitoring can be instituted to help prevent complications.

Preparation of the Patient

When the patient arrives at the medical office and the prenatal record form has been completed, the medical assistant is responsible for taking and recording the patient's vital signs, height, and weight to provide a database for subsequent prenatal visits. The patient is asked to disrobe completely and put on an examining gown with the opening in front. The medical assistant must give complete and thorough instructions so the patient knows exactly what is expected. The patient should be asked whether she needs to empty her bladder because an empty bladder facilitates the examination and is more comfortable for her. If the office policy is such that a specimen is necessary for urine testing at the initial prenatal visit, the patient will be required to void.

Special precautions should be taken in assisting the prenatal patient. The medical assistant should support the patient as she gets onto and off the scale and examining table to ensure her safety and comfort. This is especially important as the pregnancy progresses and the patient becomes more awkward and off balance.

The medical assistant is responsible for setting up the tray required for the examination. The setup includes the equipment and supplies required for the procedures to be performed. During the prenatal examination, the medical assistant is responsible for positioning the patient as required for each aspect of the examination and assisting the physician as needed.

Patient Education

At the conclusion of the initial prenatal examination and after the patient is dressed, the physician talks with her regarding instructions on diet, weight gain, rest, sleep, employment, exercise, travel, sexual intercourse, dental care, smoking, alcohol, and drugs. Many offices have a prenatal guidebook designed especially for this purpose that is given to each patient to use as a reference. Some offices also use a series of teaching films that the patient views during the return prenatal visit while waiting to see the physician. The physician also prescribes a daily vitamin supplement to be taken during the prenatal period to ensure that the mother and fetus obtain an adequate supply of vitamins and minerals.

When the physician is finished talking with the patient, the medical assistant is responsible for scheduling the next prenatal visit and for ensuring that the patient understands the instructions for maintaining health and preventing disease during the pregnancy. The medical assistant should tell the patient to report the occurrence of any warning signs during the pregnancy (see the *Warning Signs during Pregnancy* box) and not to take any medications without first checking with the physician. The patient should also be encouraged to contact the medical office should any questions or problems arise.

Laboratory Tests

The physician orders many laboratory tests to assist in the assessment of the patient's state of health and to detect problems that may put the pregnancy at risk. Several tests, such as the Pap test and the chlamydia and gonorrhea tests, require the physician to collect the specimens at the medical

---

Warning Signs during Pregnancy

Signs of Infection
- Fever
- Vaginal discharge
- Dysuria
- Increased frequency of urination
- Marked decrease in urinary output

Signs of Spontaneous Abortion
- Vaginal bleeding
- Persistent low back pain
- Abdominal pain and cramping

Signs of Preeclampsia
- Severe, persistent headache
- Dizziness
- Blurred vision
- Sudden swelling of hands, feet, or face
- Sudden, rapid weight gain
- Abdominal pain

Signs of Placental or Fetal Problems
- Vaginal spotting or bleeding
- Abdominal pain and cramping
- Back pain
- Noticeable decrease in fetal activity
- No fetal movement

Signs of Preterm Labor
- Regular or frequent contractions (more than four to six per hour)
- Recurring low, dull backache
- Menstrual-like cramping
- Unusual pressure in the pelvis, low back, abdomen, or thighs

---

office and have them transported by laboratory courier to an outside laboratory for evaluation. The specimen required for the prenatal blood tests must be obtained through a venipuncture to provide a sufficient quantity of blood for the number of tests ordered. The blood specimen is collected at the medical office or at an outside laboratory.

It is important to have these initial tests completed as soon as possible to provide the physician with the test results by the time of the next scheduled prenatal visit. Based on the results of the prenatal examination and the laboratory tests, the physician may order additional tests to assess the patient's condition. Certain tests and procedures are scheduled later in the pregnancy, such as the glucose challenge test (GCT) and the group B streptococcus (GBS) test. The prenatal laboratory tests that are usually performed on a pregnant woman are described next.

Urine Tests
Urinalysis
A complete urinalysis is performed, including physical, chemical, and microscopic analyses of the urine; a clean-catch midstream urine specimen is generally required for the test. If bacteria are found in the urine specimen, the physician usually requests a urine culture and sensitivity test to determine the possible presence of a urinary tract infection. A pregnancy test also may be performed on the urine specimen, if ordered by the physician.

Swab Tests
Pap Test
A Pap test is done for the detection of abnormalities of cell growth to diagnose precancerous or cancerous conditions of the cervix. This test can also be used for hormonal assessment (maturation index) and to assist in the detection of vaginal infections.

Chlamydia and Gonorrhea
Specimens are taken from the endocervical canal and sent to the laboratory to rule out chlamydia and gonorrhea. Chlamydia can be passed from an infected woman to her infant during childbirth, resulting in conjunctivitis and pneumonia in the newborn. If a gonorrheal infection is present at the time of delivery, the *N. gonorrhoeae* organism could infect the infant's eyes during passage through the birth canal. This results in *ophthalmia neonatorum,* which, if not treated, could lead to blindness. For this reason, most states require that pregnant women be tested for gonorrhea and that the eyes of newborns be treated with antibiotic or silver nitrate drops immediately after birth to kill any gonococcal bacteria that may be present. A patient who is diagnosed with chlamydia or gonorrhea requires immediate treatment with an appropriate antibiotic to prevent problems for herself and her child.

Trichomoniasis and Candidiasis
If an excessive irritating vaginal discharge is present, the physician obtains a specimen to rule out trichomoniasis and candidiasis. It is important to control candidiasis before delivery to prevent the development of thrush, a yeastlike

infection of the infant's mucous membrane of the mouth or throat.

Group B Streptococcus

GBS is a common bacterium often found in the vagina and rectum of healthy women. Normally, one of four pregnant women carries GBS. GBS is not harmful to a pregnant woman, but it can cause life-threatening infections in the newborn. While passing through the birth canal, a newborn can become infected with the bacteria carried by the mother. When infected, the infant may develop an infection of the blood (septicemia), pneumonia, or meningitis.

To prevent GBS infection of the newborn, a pregnant woman is tested for the bacteria between 35 and 37 weeks' gestation. Using two swabs, the physician collects specimens from the vagina and the rectum. The specimen swabs are placed in a transport tube and sent to the laboratory to be cultured for GBS. If GBS is found, intravenous antibiotics are administered to the woman every 4 hours during labor until delivery. In most cases, this antibiotic administration prevents the newborn from becoming infected with GBS. In situations in which the newborn does become infected with GBS, antibiotics are administered immediately and the infant is closely monitored.

Blood Tests

Complete Blood Count

The complete blood count (CBC) is a basic screening test used to assist in assessing the patient's state of health. It includes a hemoglobin, hematocrit, white blood cell count, red blood cell count, differential white blood cell count, platelet count, and red blood cell indices. Of particular importance with respect to the prenatal patient are the hemoglobin and hematocrit evaluations, which are described here.

Hemoglobin and Hematocrit

Low hemoglobin or hematocrit values are seen in cases of anemia. Prenatal patients tend to develop anemia because there is an increased demand for and correlating increased production of red blood cells during pregnancy; the physician carefully reviews the results of these tests. If the hemoglobin or hematocrit value is low, further hematologic evaluation is usually required. If necessary, therapy is instituted, which usually consists of an iron supplement and nutritional counseling. The hemoglobin and hematocrit values are checked again at approximately 32 weeks of gestation as a precaution against anemia before delivery.

Rh Factor and ABO Blood Type

Tests are performed to anticipate ABO blood type and Rh factor incompatibilities. If the patient is Rh-negative, the father's blood type must also be evaluated. If the father's blood type is Rh-positive, the possibility of an Rh incompatibility exists. This situation warrants the performance of an Rh antibody titer test and repeat antibody titers throughout the pregnancy to determine whether the mother's antibody level is increasing. An increased Rh antibody level could be dangerous to the developing fetus. It can result in severe anemia, jaundice, brain damage, heart failure, and sometimes death of the fetus.

Glucose Challenge Test

A GCT is performed between 24 and 28 weeks of gestation to screen for gestational diabetes mellitus (GDM). This test works by assessing the body's response to a measured glucose solution. The patient does not need to fast for this test, and there is no preparation required other than arriving at the laboratory at the scheduled time. To perform the GCT, the patient is asked to drink 50 g of a glucose solution, and her glucose level is measured 1 hour later. A woman with a glucose level of less than 140 mg/dL does not have GDM and requires no further testing. If the glucose level is greater than 140 mg/dL, the test is abnormal. Not all women with elevated results have diabetes, however, and further testing using the 3-hour glucose tolerance test (GTT) must be performed before a final diagnosis can be made.

Serology Test for Syphilis

The microorganism that causes syphilis, *Treponema pallidum,* can cross the placental barrier and infect the fetus; this could result in IUD or cause the fetus to be born with congenital syphilis. Infants with congenital syphilis are often born with deformities and may become blind, deaf, paralyzed, or insane. The tests most commonly employed to screen for the presence of syphilis are the Venereal Disease Research Laboratory (VDRL) test and the rapid plasma reagin (RPR) test. The test results are reported as nonreactive, weakly reactive, or reactive. Because these tests are screening tests, a weakly reactive or reactive test result warrants more specific testing to arrive at a diagnosis for syphilis. Examples of these tests are the fluorescent treponemal antibody absorption (FTA-ABS) test and the *Treponema pallidum* particle agglutination assay (TPPA) test.

A prenatal serology test for syphilis is mandated by most states and should be performed early in the pregnancy, before fetal damage occurs. A patient who has contracted syphilis requires treatment with an appropriate antibiotic.

What Would You Do? What Would You *Not* Do?

Case Study 3

Johanna Kruger is 24 years old and pregnant with her first child. She is at the office for her first prenatal visit. She is quite upset. Her best friend just had her first baby and the baby died 24 hours later from a GBS infection. Johanna is afraid that the same thing will happen to her baby. She wants to be tested for GBS as soon as possible. She has some antibiotics at home and is thinking of taking them. Johanna is worried because she has been experiencing some problems with her pregnancy. She is sick all day, her breasts hurt, and yesterday she had some spotting. Johanna is hesitant to tell all of this to the physician because he might think she worries too much. ■

Rubella Antibody Titer

The rubella antibody titer assesses the level of antibody against rubella (German measles) in the patient's blood and is used to determine whether the woman is immune to rubella. If the mother contracts rubella during pregnancy, serious congenital abnormalities can occur in the fetus. Patients who lack immunity should be immunized against rubella within 6 weeks of delivery.

Rh Antibody Titer (on Rh-Negative Blood Specimens)

An Rh antibody titer detects the amount of circulating Rh antibodies against red blood cells. These antibodies can occur in a pregnant woman who is Rh-negative and is carrying an Rh-positive fetus; an Rh antibody titer is performed on all Rh-negative blood specimens. Repeat antibody titer levels are also performed during the pregnancy to determine whether the woman's antibody level is increasing. As previously indicated, an increased Rh antibody level could be dangerous to the developing fetus. As a preventive measure, Rh-negative women with the potential of having an Rh-positive infant and who test negative for Rh antibodies are given two injections of Rh immune globulin (RhoGAM). The Rh immune globulin prevents the formation of the Rh antibodies in the mother, which avoids Rh incompatibility complications during the next pregnancy. The first injection is given at 28 weeks of gestation, and the second injection is administered within 72 hours of delivery.

Hepatitis B and Human Immunodeficiency Virus

The Centers for Disease Control and Prevention recommends that pregnant women have a blood test, the HBsAg test, to screen for hepatitis B virus. Women who have positive HBsAg test results have an increased risk of spontaneous **abortion** or preterm labor. In addition, the mother may transmit hepatitis B to the infant, particularly during delivery or in the first few days of life. This risk can be greatly reduced by administering hepatitis B immune globulin (HBIG) and the hepatitis B vaccine within 12 hours of birth to the newborns of women who have tested positive for hepatitis B. It is also recommended that testing for HIV, the virus that causes AIDS, be offered to all pregnant women, particularly women at risk for contracting HIV. Infants born to women who are HIV positive are at risk of developing the disease.

Return Prenatal Visits

Return prenatal visits provide the opportunity for a continuous assessment of the health of the mother and the fetus. During each visit, essential data are collected and recorded in the prenatal record, resulting in an updated record at each visit, as discussed in this section. If signs or symptoms of a pathologic condition are present, the physician performs selected aspects of the physical examination as needed to diagnose and treat the condition. In addition, diagnostic and laboratory tests may be ordered to assist in diagnosis and treatment. The usual schedule of visits for prenatal care is listed as follows. A patient who exhibits complications is seen more frequently for closer monitoring.

- Every 4 weeks for the first 28 weeks
- Every 2 weeks until 36 weeks
- Weekly thereafter until delivery

The return prenatal visit also provides the opportunity for the physician and the medical assistant to lend support to the mother, provide her with ongoing prenatal education to reduce apprehension and anxiety, and ensure that the mother is well informed and prepared during her pregnancy, childbirth, and the postpartum period. The medical assistant plays an important role in prenatal education and should take the necessary time with each patient to provide appropriate information and allow the patient to ask questions. Procedure 23-3 outlines the medical assistant's role in the return prenatal visit.

The patient is asked to obtain a urine specimen during each return prenatal visit. The medical assistant is responsible for testing the specimen for glucose and protein using a reagent strip and for recording results in the prenatal record. A positive reaction to glucose may indicate the development of GDM or a prediabetic condition, and a positive reaction to protein may indicate a urinary tract infection or preeclampsia. Further testing is usually necessary to arrive at a final diagnosis and institute treatment.

During the return visit, the physician performs one or more of the following procedures, depending on the stage of the pregnancy: (1) palpation of the woman's abdomen to measure fundal height, (2) measurement of the fetal heart rate, and (3) a vaginal examination. These procedures are discussed in detail next.

Fundal Height Measurement

The pregnant uterus rises gradually into the abdominal cavity, and the fundus is palpable between 8 and 13 weeks of gestation. The first fundal height measurement, which is usually performed during the first prenatal visit, is used as a guideline for all subsequent measurements. The physician measures the fundal height by placing one end of a flexible, nonstretchable centimeter tape measure on the superior aspect of the symphysis pubis and measuring to the crest or top of the uterine fundus (Figure 23-12). The measurement is recorded on a flow chart in the patient's prenatal record. By 20 weeks, the fundus reaches the lower border of the umbilicus, and between 36 and 37 weeks, it reaches the tip of the sternum. During the first and second trimesters, measuring the fundal height provides a rough estimate of the duration of the pregnancy (Figure 23-13). Because fetal weights vary considerably during the third trimester, it is difficult to use fundal height measurements as an estimate of the duration of the pregnancy in the last trimester.

In addition to assessing the duration of the pregnancy, the fundal height measurements permit variations from normal to become apparent and are used to assess whether fetal development is progressing normally. Growth that is too rapid or too slow must be evaluated further by the

Figure 23-12. Measurement of fundal height. The physician places one end of a centimeter tape measure on the superior aspect of the symphysis pubis and measures to the top of the uterine fundus. (From Bonewit-West K: *Clinical procedures for medical assistants,* ed 7, St. Louis, 2008, Saunders.)

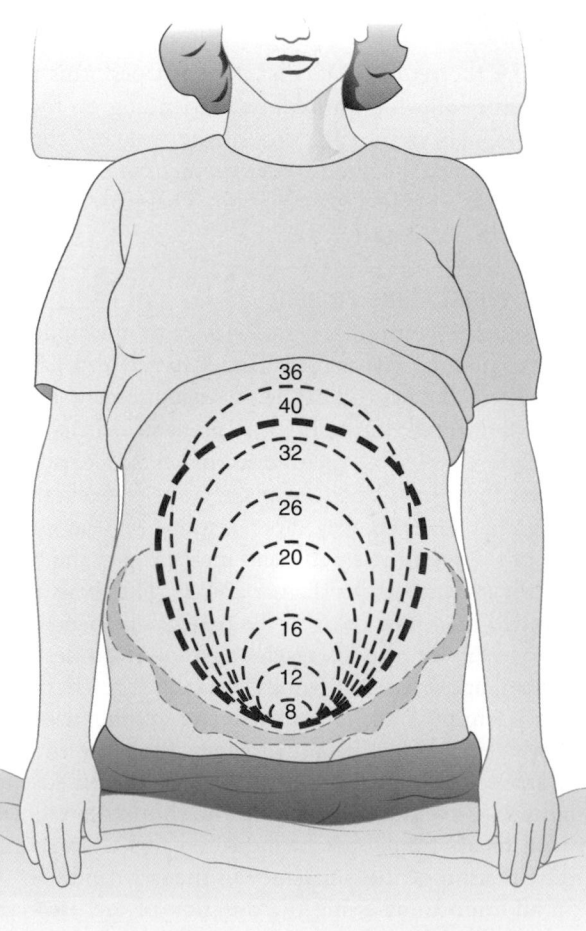

Figure 23-13. Fundal height showing gestational age in weeks. (From Bonewit-West K: *Clinical procedures for medical assistants,* ed 7, St. Louis, 2008, Saunders.)

physician as a possible indication of high-risk conditions, such as multiple pregnancies, polyhydramnios, ovarian tumor, and intrauterine growth retardation, IUD, or an error in estimating the fetal progress.

Fetal Heart Tones

The normal **fetal heart rate** is between 120 and 160 beats per minute with a regular rhythm. A very slow or rapid fetal heart rate usually indicates fetal distress. The term **fetal heart tones** refers to the heartbeat of the fetus as heard through the mother's abdominal wall. The fetal heart tones can be heard with a Doppler fetal pulse detector between 10 and 12 weeks of gestation. The Doppler fetal pulse detector converts ultrasonic waves into audible sounds of the fetal pulse.

The Doppler device consists of a main control unit and a probe (Figure 23-14A). The probe head contains a transducer and electronic components, which generate the sound waves. The probe head is delicate and must be handled carefully, making sure not to drop or knock the head to prevent damaging it.

Because air is a poor conductor of sound, an ultrasound coupling gel must first be spread on the mother's abdomen in the area to be examined. The gel is usually applied by the medical assistant, and its purpose is to increase conductivity of the sound waves between the abdomen and the transducer.

The physician places the head of the probe into the gel on the mother's abdomen and slowly moves it until the fetal heart tones are located. The Doppler device amplifies the fetal heart tones, and they are broadcast through a built-in loudspeaker in the main unit. A volume control provides

Figure 23-14. **A,** Parts of a Doppler device. **B,** The probe of the Doppler device is moved across the abdomen to detect the fetal pulse. (From Bonewit-West K: *Clinical procedures for medical assistants,* ed 7, St. Louis, 2008, Saunders.)

| Before labor | Early effacement | Complete effacement | Complete dilation |

Figure 23-15. Effacement and dilation occur to permit the passage of the infant into the birth canal. The cervical canal shortens from its normal length of 1 to 2 cm to a structure with paper-thin edges in which there is no canal at all. The cervix dilates from an opening a few millimeters wide to an opening large enough to allow the passage of the infant (approximately 10 cm). (From Bonewit-West K: *Clinical procedures for medical assistants,* ed 7, St. Louis, 2008, Saunders.)

adjustment of the sound level as required. (Fetal heart tones sound like the hoofbeats of a galloping horse, and when the probe is over the placenta, a windlike sound is heard.) The Doppler device may also have an LCD screen, which provides a digital display of the fetal pulse rate. Stereo headphones come with the Doppler device to allow private listening. The loudspeaker is muted when the headphones are connected (Figure 23-14B).

After the procedure, the medical assistant should remove excess gel from the mother's abdomen with a paper towel. The probe head is cleaned using a damp cloth or a paper towel. The Doppler device should be properly stored in its carrying case to prevent it from becoming damaged.

Vaginal Examination

In the absence of vaginal bleeding, vaginal examinations may be performed at any time during the pregnancy; however, in a normal pregnancy, there is usually no need to perform a vaginal examination until the patient nears term. The vaginal examination is usually begun approximately 2 to 3 weeks from the EDD and is performed to confirm the presenting part and to determine the degree, if any, of cervical dilation and effacement. The purpose of dilation and effacement is to permit the passage of the infant from the uterus into the birth canal (Figure 23-15).

Special Tests and Procedures

The pregnancy can be evaluated with one or more of the following special tests and procedures: triple screen test, obstetric ultrasound scan, amniocentesis, and fetal heart rate monitoring. These are not considered routine procedures; however, they involve little or no risk to the mother or the fetus. Because some of these tests may be performed in the obstetric medical office, the medical assistant should have a general knowledge of these procedures.

Obstetric Ultrasound Scan

An obstetric ultrasound scan is a diagnostic imaging technique, similar to sonar, used to view the fetus in utero. It allows continuous viewing of the fetus and shows fetal movement. The physician or an ultrasound technologist performs the procedure. The primary purposes of an ultrasound scan are to evaluate the health of the fetus and determine gestational age. This is accomplished by viewing the image of the fetus and by taking various measurements of the image, such as the crown-rump length; biparietal diameter, which is a side-to-side measurement of the fetal head; femur length; and abdominal circumference.

Obstetric ultrasound scanning uses high-frequency sound waves that are directed into the uterus through a transducer. When the sound waves reach the uterus, they "bounce" back to the transducer, similar to an echo. These reflected sound waves are converted into an image, or *sonogram* (Figure 23-16), which is displayed on a monitor screen. The monitor is usually positioned so the mother can observe the image on the screen if she wishes.

Although an obstetric ultrasound scan can be performed at any time during the pregnancy, it is often performed between 7 and 12 weeks of gestation and again between 18 and 20 weeks. A third scan is sometimes done around 34 weeks of gestation. Box 23-1 outlines this schedule and what can be assessed at these times.

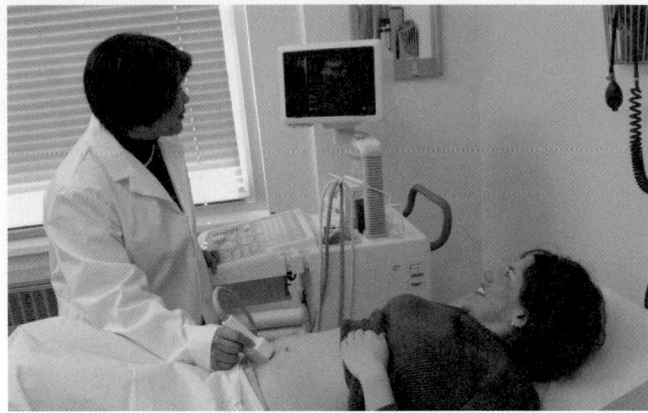

Figure 23-16. Obstetric ultrasound scan. (From Bonewit-West K: *Clinical procedures for medical assistants,* ed 7, St. Louis, 2008, Saunders.)

BOX 23-1 Purpose of Obstetric Ultrasound Scanning

Between 7 and 12 Weeks
- To confirm pregnancy by detecting fetal heart motion
- To determine gestational age by taking measurements of the embryo and embryonic sac
- To detect an ectopic pregnancy

Erect fetal penis. *1,* Urethra; *2,* corpus cavernosum; *3,* shaft; *4,* glans; *5,* foreskin. (From Callen P: *Ultrasonography in obstetrics and gynecology,* ed 4, Philadelphia, 2000, Saunders.)

Embryo at approximately 9 weeks' gestation. (From Greer I, Cameron I, Kitchener H, Prentice A: *Mosby's color atlas and text of obstetrics and gynecology,* St. Louis, 2001, Mosby.)

Between 18 and 20 Weeks
- To determine fetal growth, size, and weight by taking measurements of the fetus
- To detect the presence of multiple fetuses
- To examine the brain, spinal cord, heart, lungs, gastrointestinal tract, reproductive organs, kidneys, bladder, bowel, and extremities of the fetus
- To detect congenital abnormalities
- To determine the location of the placenta
- To determine the cause of bleeding or spotting

Twins. (From Bonewit-West K: *Clinical procedures for medical assistants,* ed 7, St. Louis, 2008, Saunders.)

BOX 23-1　Purpose of Obstetric Ultrasound Scanning—cont'd

External female genitalia. *1,* Major labium; *2,* minor labium; *3,* vaginal cleft; *4,* thighs. (From Callen P: *Ultrasonography in obstetrics and gynecology,* ed 4, Philadelphia, 2000, Saunders.)

At 34 Weeks
- To evaluate fetal growth, size, and weight by taking measurements of the fetus

- To verify location of the placenta
- To confirm fetal presentation in uncertain cases

Other Purposes
- To diagnose uterine and pelvic abnormalities during pregnancy
- To view the fetus, placenta, and amniotic fluid during tests such as amniocentesis and chorionic villus sampling
- To confirm intrauterine death

Amniocentesis being performed under ultrasound guidance. (From Greer I, Cameron I, Kitchener H, Prentice A: *Mosby's color atlas and text of obstetrics and gynecology,* St. Louis, 2001, Mosby.)

From Bonewit-West K: *Clinical procedures for medical assistants,* ed 7, St. Louis, 2008, Saunders.

PATIENT TEACHING　Obstetric Ultrasound Scan

1. Emphasize the importance of preparing properly for the examination.
2. Provide the patient with educational materials on obstetric ultrasound.
3. Answer questions patients have about an obstetric ultrasound scan.

What is an ultrasound scan?
An ultrasound scan is performed to look at the fetus in the uterus with the use of sound waves. During the examination, a gel is spread over your abdomen, and a scanning device is moved lightly over the area. The baby's image is displayed on a monitor similar to a television screen. During the examination, pictures of your baby will be taken and you will be given a copy for your baby album. If you choose, you may bring a standard VHS tape for the ultrasonographer to record your baby on videotape. The ultrasound examination usually takes about 30 minutes.

Why is an ultrasound scan performed?
Ultrasound scanning is used to determine the age and position of the fetus, the location of the placenta, and the number of babies present, and overall to help the physician monitor and manage the pregnancy.

What preparation is necessary?
To prepare for an abdominal ultrasound, you will need to drink 32 oz of fluid 1 hour before the examination. Drink all the water within 15 to 20 minutes, and do not void until the examination has been completed. You should wear comfortable clothing. A two-piece outfit is recommended so that you do not have to undress completely.

Is an ultrasound scan safe?
No known side effects or risks to either mother or fetus during an ultrasound examination exist. Ultrasound does not use x-rays. No long-term risks have been detected. The procedure is painless, and the only discomfort is from a full bladder, which will make you want to go to the bathroom. When the examination is completed, you will have the opportunity to do so.

Can I learn the sex of my baby through an ultrasound scan?
Although an ultrasound scan is not performed only to determine the sex of the baby, it is sometimes possible (usually by 20 weeks) to tell whether the baby is a boy or girl, depending on the position of the baby in the uterus. Because not all parents want to know their baby's sex in advance, you will not automatically be told the baby's sex if it is determined, but you will be given the opportunity to make the choice of knowing or not knowing. ■

Amniocentesis

Amniocentesis is a diagnostic procedure that can be performed between 15 and 18 weeks' gestation. Amniocentesis aids in prenatal diagnosis of certain genetically transmitted errors of metabolism, congenital abnormalities, and chromosomal disorders such as Down syndrome. It is also used to detect fetal jeopardy or distress and, later in the pregnancy, to assess fetal lung maturity. Amniocentesis can also determine whether the infant is a boy or girl.

To perform the procedure, the physician inserts a long, thin needle through the mother's abdomen and into the amniotic sac surrounding the fetus (Figure 23-17). An obstetric ultrasound scan is always performed in conjunction with amniocentesis so that the physician can view the position of the fetus, placenta, and amniotic fluid. This allows the physician to know the exact place to insert the needle. The physician withdraws a sample (about 1 tablespoon) of fluid, which contains fetal cells. The fluid is sent to a laboratory for study. It usually takes 1 to 3 weeks to evaluate the amniotic fluid and report the results.

Although the complication rate for an amniocentesis is extremely low, it is not risk free. There is a slight risk of bleeding, leakage of fluid, and infection of the amniotic fluid. There is also a slight possibility of miscarriage. Because of these risks, amniocentesis is offered only to women whose pregnancies are at risk for fetal abnormalities. This includes women who are 35 years old or older, women who have a child with a genetic or neural tube defect, women who have abnormal triple screen test results, women who have or whose partner has a chromosomal abnormality, and women who are or whose partner is a carrier for a metabolic disease.

Fetal Heart Rate Monitoring

Fetal heart rate monitoring is performed later in the pregnancy to obtain information on the physical condition of the fetus. Specific conditions that may warrant this procedure are fetal growth that is not progressing well, decreased amniotic fluid, decreased fetal activity, elevation of the mother's blood pressure, gestational diabetes, and an overdue infant.

To perform the procedure, an electronic microphone is strapped to the mother's abdomen to amplify the fetal heartbeat. A gel is usually applied under the microphone to make the sounds clearer. The fetal heartbeat is heard and displayed on a screen and printed on special paper.

Medical Assisting Responsibilities

The medical assistant has many important responsibilities in the return prenatal examination, which are outlined in Procedure 23-3. The medical assistant is responsible for assembling the equipment and supplies required for the examination, for obtaining information to update the prenatal record, for preparing the patient for the examination, and for assisting the physician during the examination. The physician depends on the medical assistant to have the urine test results and certain measurements, such as blood pressure and weight, completed and recorded in advance to allow him or her the opportunity to review these measurements before examining the patient.

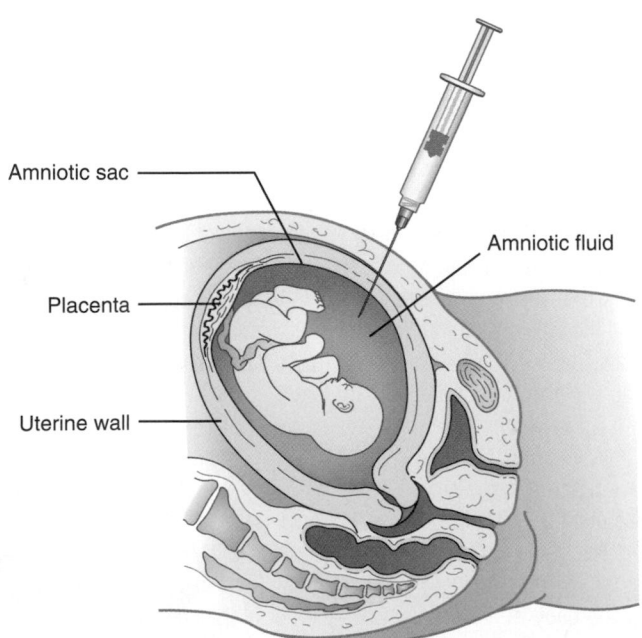

Amniotic sac

Placenta

Uterine wall

Amniotic fluid

Figure 23-17. Amniocentesis. (From Bonewit-West K: *Clinical procedures for medical assistants,* ed 7, St. Louis, 2008, Saunders.)

What Would You Do? What Would You *Not* Do?

Case Study 4

Wynita Lopez is at the office with her husband. She is 32 years old and 18 weeks pregnant. It took Wynita a long time, almost 6 years, to get pregnant. She is excited and happy about being pregnant but, at the same time, sad and confused. Her test results on her triple screen test came back indicating the possibility that her baby has Down syndrome. A repeat test was done with the same results. Wynita just finished having an ultrasound that showed a normal baby, but Wynita and her husband understand that the only way to know for sure is to have an amniocentesis. Wynita does not know what to do. She is afraid of having an amniocentesis because of the chance of miscarriage. She also knows her triple screen test could be a false-positive. Wynita is unsure what her decision would be if the baby did have Down syndrome. Her husband is visibly distressed and wants Wynita to make all the decisions, saying he will be supportive of whatever she decides. Right now she wants as much information as she can get about all of this before she makes a decision. She feels "safer" being at the medical office and does not want to go home just yet. ■

PROCEDURE 23-3 Assisting with a Return Prenatal Examination

Outcome Assist with a return prenatal examination.

Equipment/Supplies

- Urine specimen container
- Centimeter tape measure
- Doppler fetal pulse detector
- Ultrasound coupling gel
- Paper towels

- Disposable vaginal speculum
- Disposable gloves
- Water-based lubricant
- Gauze pads
- Examining gown and drape

1. **Procedural Step.** Sanitize your hands.
2. **Procedural Step.** Set up the tray for the prenatal examination. The equipment and supplies depend on the procedures to be included in the examination, which may include one or more of the following:
   a. Fundal height measurement
   b. Measurement of fetal heart tones
   c. Examination of the legs, feet, and face for edema and development of varicosities
   d. Taking a specimen for the diagnosis of a vaginal infection
   e. Vaginal examination

Set up the prenatal tray. (From Bonewit-West K: *Clinical procedures for medical assistants,* ed 7, St. Louis, 2008, Saunders.)

3. **Procedural Step.** Greet the patient and introduce yourself. Identify the patient and explain the procedure. Provide the patient with a urine specimen container, and ask her to obtain a urine specimen.
   Principle. A urine specimen is necessary to test for glucose and protein at each prenatal visit. In addition, an empty bladder makes the examination easier and is more comfortable for the patient.
4. **Procedural Step.** Escort the patient to the examining room, and ask her to be seated. Seat yourself so that you are facing the patient. Ask the patient whether she has experienced any problems since the last prenatal visit, and record information in the appropriate section in her prenatal record.

Principle. The physician investigates any unusual or abnormal signs or symptoms relayed by the patient.

5. **Procedural Step.** Measure the patient's blood pressure, and chart the results in the prenatal record. If the blood pressure is elevated, allow the patient to relax, and then measure the blood pressure again.
   Principle. Taking the blood pressure again gives the opportunity to determine whether the elevation was due to emotional excitement.

Measure the patient's blood pressure. (From Bonewit-West K: *Clinical procedures for medical assistants,* ed 7, St. Louis, 2008, Saunders.)

6. **Procedural Step.** Weigh the patient, and chart the results in the prenatal record.
   Principle. Maternal weight gain or loss assists in assessing fetal development, as well as the mother's nutrition and state of health.
7. **Procedural Step.** Instruct and prepare the patient for the examination. Have her remove or pull up her outer clothing to expose the abdominal area. If the physician will be performing a vaginal examination, the patient also must remove her underpants; otherwise, she may leave them on. Tell the patient to have a seat on the examining table when she is finished getting ready for the examination. Inform the patient that the physician will be with her soon and leave the room to give her privacy.

Continued

PROCEDURE **23-3** **Assisting with a Return Prenatal Examination—cont'd**

Weigh the patient. (From Bonewit-West K: *Clinical procedures for medical assistants,* ed 7, St. Louis, 2008, Saunders.)
Apply a liberal amount of coupling gel. (From Bonewit-West K:

8. **Procedural Step.** Using a reagent strip, test the urine specimen for glucose and protein, and chart the results. *Note:* The urine specimen may be tested at any time before the physician examines the patient; however, a convenient time to test the specimen is while the patient is disrobing.
   Principle. The prenatal patient's urine must be tested at every visit to assist in the early detection and prevention of disease.

9. **Procedural Step.** Make the medical record available for review by the physician. The medical office has a designated location where the record is placed, such as a small shelf mounted on the wall next to the outside of the examining room door or in a chart holder on the outside of the examining room door. Position the medical record so that patient-identifiable information is not visible.
   Principle: Before going into the room, the physician will want to review the patient's chart and information documented by the medical assistant. HIPAA requires protection of a patient's health information.

10. **Procedural Step.** Check to make sure the patient is ready to be seen by the physician. Before entering a patient's room, always knock lightly on the door to let the patient know you are getting ready to enter the room. Inform the physician. This may be done using a color-coded flagging system mounted on the wall next to the examining room.

11. **Procedural Step.** Assist the patient into a supine position, and properly drape her. Provide support and reassurance to the patient to help her relax during the examination.
    Principle. The patient should be properly draped so that she is warm and comfortable.

12. **Procedural Step.** Assist the physician as required for the prenatal examination, as follows:
    a. **Fundal Height Measurement:** Hand the physician the tape measure for the determination of the fundal measurement.
    b. **Fetal Heart Tones:** Apply a liberal amount of coupling gel to the patient's abdomen. Turn on the Doppler fetal pulse detector and hand it to the physician. When the physician is finished, remove excess gel from the patient with a paper towel. Clean the probe head of the Doppler device with a damp cloth or a paper towel. Place the probe head back in its holder.
    c. **Vaginal Specimen:** Assist the patient into the lithotomy position if a specimen is to be taken for the detection of a vaginal infection. Assist with the collection of the specimen as required.
    d. **Vaginal Examination:** Assist the patient into the lithotomy position if a vaginal examination is to be performed.

Clinical procedures for medical assistants, ed 7, St. Louis, 2008, Saunders.)

13. Procedural Step. After the examination, assist the patient into a sitting position, and allow her the opportunity to rest for a moment. If a vaginal examination was performed, offer the patient tissues to remove excess lubricating jelly from the perineum. Assist her off the examining table to prevent falls. Instruct the patient to get dressed. Leave the room to provide the patient with privacy.

Principle. The patient may become dizzy after being on the examining table and should be allowed to rest before getting off the table. The medical assistant must provide for the safety of the prenatal patient while she is getting off the examining table.

14. Procedural Step. Provide prenatal patient teaching and further explanation of the physician's instructions as required to meet individual patient needs. Escort the patient to the reception area.

15. Procedural Step. Clean the examining room in preparation for the next patient, and, if necessary, prepare specimens for transport to an outside medical laboratory.

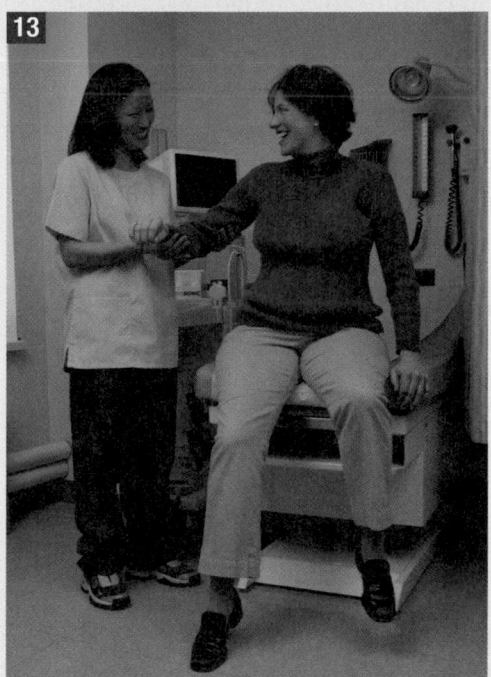

Assist the patient off the examining table. (From Bonewit-West K: *Clinical procedures for medical assistants,* ed 7, St. Louis, 2008, Saunders.)

SIX WEEKS–POSTPARTUM VISIT

The **puerperium** includes the period of time in which the body systems are returning to their prepregnant or nearly prepregnant state, which is usually 4 to 6 weeks after delivery. During this time, numerous changes occur in the woman's body. The *involution of the uterus* (i.e., the process by which it returns to its normal size and state) occurs; this includes healing of any injuries sustained to the birth canal during delivery.

During the puerperium, the patient experiences a vaginal discharge shed from the lining of the uterus, known as **lochia.** Lochia consists of blood, tissue, white blood cells, mucus, and some bacteria. The color of the lochia is an indication of the progress of the healing of the uterus. For the first 3 days after delivery, the lochia consists almost entirely of blood and, because of its red color, is termed *lochia rubra.* By approximately 4 days postpartum, the amount of blood decreases and the discharge becomes pink or brownish and is known as *lochia serosa.* By 10 days postpartum, the flow should decrease and the lochia should become yellowish white; this is known as *lochia alba.* Lochia usually continues in consistently decreasing amounts (from moderate to scant to occasional spotting) and becomes paler in color until the third week after delivery, when it usually disappears altogether. It would not be considered unusual for the discharge to last the entire 6 weeks, however.

The patient should be instructed to contact the medical office under the following circumstances: if the amount of discharge increases rather than decreases; if the discharge is absent within the first 2 weeks after delivery; if it changes to red after having been yellowish white, which indicates bleeding; or if it takes on a foul odor, which indicates infection. Menstruation usually begins approximately 2 months after delivery in a nonnursing mother and 3 to 6 months after delivery in a nursing mother.

During the puerperium, the patient should be encouraged to avoid fatigue, avoid lifting heavy objects, and consume a nutritious, well-balanced diet that helps maintain health and promote healing. The physician will want to see the patient at the medical office at the end of the 6-week period. The purpose of the 6 weeks–postpartum visit is to evaluate the general physical condition of the patient, to ensure there are no residual problems from childbearing, and to provide the patient with education regarding methods of contraception and infant care. During this visit the patient is queried about problems or abnormalities related to vaginal discharge, urinary or bowel function, and breastfeeding if she is nursing. This information is recorded in the patient's chart. The postpartum visit provides an excellent opportunity for the medical assistant to instruct the patient in the technique for performing a BSE and to educate her in the importance of returning to the medical office annually for a Pap test.

During the postpartum examination, the physician evaluates the patient's general appearance, performs breast and pelvic examinations, and checks to determine whether the muscle tone has returned to the muscles of the abdominal wall. During the puerperium, atypical cells may be sloughed off into the cervical and vaginal mucus as part of the normal healing process. Because of this, the Pap test is not included in the postpartum visit. If the patient has problems with hemorrhoids or varicosities, the physician discusses any further treatment required. If the patient does not have

antibody protection to rubella, as has been evidenced through the prenatal laboratory tests, she receives rubella immunization at this time (if it was not administered in the hospital). In addition, hemoglobin and hematocrit determinations are usually performed on the postpartum patient to screen for anemia caused by blood loss during delivery and the puerperium.

MEDICAL PRACTICE and the LAW

Mature Minor

A difficult and complex issue facing policy makers today involves whether a minor should be able to obtain health care services without a parent's consent. A minor is an individual who has not reached the age of majority; in most states, minors reach majority at 18 years old (at that time, individuals are legally able to make their own decisions regarding health care).

Over the past 3 decades, many states have passed legislation permitting minors to receive some health care services without parental consent. These include contraceptive services, testing and treatment for sexually transmitted diseases, prenatal care and delivery services, treatment for alcohol and drug abuse, and outpatient mental health care. States that have passed such legislation reason that some minors might avoid seeking the care that they need for certain conditions if they had to have parental consent. The one major exception to this is abortion. Most states have laws that require the involvement of at least one parent in a minor's decision to have an abortion.

In recent years, some states have given minors even greater authority to make health care decisions for themselves by adopting what is known as the *mature minor rule.* This allows an individual in the middle to late teens who exhibits the intelligence and maturity to understand the nature and consequences of a medical treatment to consent to such treatment without parental consent.

It is important for the medical assistant to become familiar with the laws in his or her state regarding a minor's right to consent to health care to help the medical assistant in making appropriate decisions with respect to minors. For example, if a state does not allow a minor to obtain prenatal care without parental consent, the medical assistant would not be permitted to make an appointment for a minor who is pregnant; rather, it would have to be scheduled by the minor's parent. Consent by minors to health care services will continue to be a complex issue; the medical assistant must keep up to date with changes in his or her state. ■

What Would You Do? What Would You *Not* Do? RESPONSES

Case Study 1
Page 455

What Did Yin-Ling Do?

❑ Reassured Mrs. Wooster that the physician is there to help her and stressed that he will be pleased that she has come to the office for an examination.

❑ Commended Mrs. Wooster on performing a BSE at home and encouraged her to continue performing a BSE each month. Asked her whether she had any questions on how to perform a BSE.

❑ Told Mrs. Wooster that some breast changes are normal and others are not normal, and the only way to know for sure is to be examined by the physician.

❑ Told Mrs. Wooster that it is important to have a periodic gynecologic examination even if her periods are normal. Explained to her that some conditions can be present without symptoms. Took plenty of time with her so that she would feel comfortable coming back again in the future for a gynecologic examination. Gave Mrs. Wooster a patient information brochure on gynecologic examinations.

❑ Gave Mrs. Wooster a patient information brochure on mammograms, and explained the mammogram procedure to reduce her apprehension. Explained that the procedure is not painful, but there may be some minor discomfort. Provided her with some tips on reducing discomfort that may occur, such as avoiding caffeine several days before the procedure and having the office schedule the mammogram a week after her menstrual period.

What Did Yin-Ling Not Do?

❑ Did not criticize Mrs. Wooster for waiting so long to schedule a gynecologic examination.

❑ Did not tell Mrs. Wooster that there is no discomfort involved with a mammogram.

What Would You Do?/What Would You *Not* Do? Review Yin-Ling's response and place a checkmark next to the information you included in your response. List additional information you included in your response.

_____
_____
_____
_____

Case Study 2
Page 473

What Did Yin-Ling Do?

❑ Stressed to Dagny how important it is that she be seen by the physician. Explained that she could be infected with chlamydia and not know it because chlamydia often has no symptoms, especially in women.

❑ Explained to Dagny that state law allows her to be treated for a sexually transmitted disease without permission from her parents. Told her the law was created to encourage minors to seek treatment for sexually transmitted diseases.

❑ Commended Dagny on practicing safe sex. Relayed to her that if a condom is not used correctly, or if it tears, she might not be protected from getting a sexually transmitted disease. That is another reason she should be tested.

❑ Explained to Dagny what will occur during the examination and what the physician will be doing. Relayed techniques that Dagney could use to relax during the procedure.

What Did Yin-Ling Not *Do?*

❑ Did not tell Dagny everything would be all right and that she probably does not have chlamydia.

❑ Did not ask Dagny whether she knew how her boyfriend got chlamydia.

❑ If Dagny still insisted on leaving, did not try to prevent her from doing so.

What Would You Do?/What Would You *Not* Do? Review Yin-Ling's response and place a checkmark next to the information you included in your response. List additional information you included in your response.

_____
_____
_____
_____

Case Study 3
Page 482

What Did Yin-Ling Do?

❑ Tried to calm Johanna by telling her that it is normal for her to be worried and concerned. Explained that the purpose of her prenatal visits are so that the physician can keep a close watch on her and detect any problems that might occur.

❑ Reassured Johanna that she does not need to be afraid to tell the physician any of her concerns because he is there to help her and her baby.

❑ Told Johanna that it is important not to take any medications during her pregnancy without first checking with the physician because some medications could be harmful to her baby.

❑ Told Johanna that her problems and concerns would be relayed to the physician and that he would want to talk to her about them. Explained that the physician would also talk with her about being tested for GBS.

What Did Yin-Ling Not *Do?*

❑ Did not tell Johanna that it was all right to take the antibiotics.

What Would You Do?/What Would You *Not* Do? Review Yin-Ling's response and place a checkmark next to the information you included in your response. List additional information you included in your response.

_____
_____
_____
_____

Case Study 4
Page 488

What Did Yin-Ling Do?

❑ Escorted Mr. and Mrs. Lopez to a private room in the office. Tried to relax them and told them that whatever they choose to do will be the right decision for them. Reassured them that they could stay at the office for as long as they wanted.

❑ Gave Mrs. Lopez the information she requested that was available at the office and provided her with a list of resources approved by the physician that she could contact for further information.

❑ Asked Mr. and Mrs. Lopez whether they had any more questions they wanted to ask the physician.

What Did Yin-Ling Not *Do?*

❑ Did not give Mr. and Mrs. Lopez advice on what they should do.

What Would You Do?/What Would You *Not* Do? Review Yin-Ling's response and place a checkmark next to the information you included in your response. List additional information you included in your response.

_____
_____
_____
_____

TERMINOLOGY REVIEW

Abortion The termination of the pregnancy before the fetus reached the age of viability (20 weeks).

Adnexal Adjacent.

Amenorrhea The absence or cessation of the menstrual period. Amenorrhea occurs normally before puberty, during pregnancy, and after menopause.

Atypical Deviation from the normal.

Braxton Hicks contractions Intermittent and irregular painless uterine contractions that occur throughout pregnancy. They occur more frequently toward the end of pregnancy and are sometimes mistaken for true labor pains.

Cervix The lower narrow end of the uterus that opens into the vagina.

Colposcopy Examination of the cervix using a colposcope (a lighted instrument with a magnifying lens).

Cytology The science that deals with the study of cells, including their origin, structure, function, and pathology.

Dilation (of the cervix) The stretching of the external os from an opening a few millimeters wide to an opening large enough to allow the passage of an infant (approximately 10 cm).

Dysmenorrhea Pain associated with the menstrual period.

Dyspareunia Pain in the vagina or pelvis experienced by a woman during sexual intercourse.

Dysplasia The growth of abnormal cells. Dysplasia is a precancerous condition that may or may not develop into cancer.

Ectocervix The part of the cervix that projects into the vagina and is lined with stratified squamous epithelium.

EDD Expected date of delivery, or due date.

Effacement The thinning and shortening of the cervical canal from its normal length of 1 to 2 cm to a structure with paper-thin edges in which there is no canal at all. Effacement occurs late in pregnancy, during labor, or both. The purpose of effacement along with dilation is to permit the passage of the infant into the birth canal.

Embryo The child in utero from the time of conception to the beginning of the first trimester.

Endocervix The mucous membrane lining the cervical canal.

Engagement The entrance of the fetal head or the presenting part into the pelvic inlet.

Expected date of delivery (EDD) Projected birth date of the infant.

External os The opening of the cervical canal of the uterus into the vagina.

Fetal heart rate The number of times per minute the fetal heart beats.

Fetal heart tones The sounds of the heartbeat of the fetus heard through the mother's abdominal wall.

Fetus The child in utero from the third month after conception to birth; during the first 2 months of development, it is called an *embryo*.

Fundus The dome-shaped upper portion of the uterus between the fallopian tubes.

Gestation The period of intrauterine development from conception to birth; the period of pregnancy. The average pregnancy lasts about 280 days, or 40 weeks, from the date of conception to childbirth.

Gestational age The age of the fetus between conception and birth.

Gynecology The branch of medicine that deals with the diseases of reproductive organs of women.

Infant A child from birth to 12 months of age.

Lochia A discharge from the uterus after delivery that consists of blood, tissue, white blood cells, and some bacteria.

Menopause The permanent cessation of menstruation, which usually occurs between the ages of 45 and 55.

Menorrhagia Excessive bleeding during a menstrual period, in the number of days or the amount of blood or both. Also called *dysfunctional uterine bleeding* (DUB).

Metrorrhagia Bleeding between menstrual periods.

Multigravida A woman who has been pregnant more than once.

Multipara A woman who has completed two or more pregnancies to the age of fetal viability regardless of whether they ended in live infants or stillbirths.

Nullipara A woman who has not carried a pregnancy to the point of fetal viability (20 weeks of gestation).

Obstetrics The branch of medicine concerned with the care of the woman during pregnancy, childbirth, and the postpartal period.

Perimenopause Before the onset of menopause, the phase during which the woman with regular periods changes to irregular cycles and increased periods of amenorrhea.

Perineum The external region between the vaginal orifice and the anus in a female and between the scrotum and the anus in a male.

Position The relation of the presenting part of the fetus to the maternal pelvis.

Postpartum Occurring after childbirth.

Preeclampsia A major complication of pregnancy, the cause of which is unknown, characterized by increasing hypertension, albuminuria, and edema. If this condition is neglected or not treated properly, it may develop into eclampsia, which could cause maternal convulsions and coma. Preeclampsia generally occurs between the 20th week of pregnancy and the end of the first week postpartum.

Prenatal Before birth.

TERMINOLOGY REVIEW—cont'd

Presentation Indication of the part of the fetus that is closest to the cervix and is delivered first. A cephalic presentation is a delivery in which the fetal head is presenting against the cervix. A breech presentation is a delivery in which the buttocks or feet are presented instead of the head.

Primigravida A woman who is pregnant for the first time.

Primipara A woman who has carried a pregnancy to fetal viability (20 weeks of gestation) for the first time, regardless of whether the infant was stillborn or alive at birth.

Puerperium The period of time, usually 4 to 6 weeks after delivery, in which the uterus and the body systems are returning to normal.

Quickening The first movements of the fetus in utero as felt by the mother, which usually occurs between 16 and 20 weeks of gestation and is felt consistently thereafter.

Risk factor Anything that increases an individual's chance of developing a disease. Some risk factors (e.g., smoking) can be avoided, but others cannot (e.g., age, family history).

Toxemia A condition that can occur in pregnant women that includes preeclampsia and eclampsia. If preeclampsia goes undiagnosed or is not satisfactorily controlled, it could develop into eclampsia, characterized by convulsions and coma.

Trimester Three months, or one third, of the gestational period of pregnancy.

Vulva The region of the external female genital organs.

ON THE WEB

For Information on Sexually Transmitted Diseases:

National Institute of Allergy and Infectious Diseases: www.niaid.nih.gov

Centers for Disease Control Division of Sexually Transmitted Diseases (located under "Disease Facts and Information"): www.cdc.gov/std

Planned Parenthood: www.plannedparenthood.org

American Social Health Association: www.ashastd.org

Herpes Information: www.gotherpes.com

HPV Information: www.gothpv.com

For Information on Women's Health:

The National Women's Health Information Center: www.4women.gov

The Universe of Women's Health: www.obgyn.net

For Information on Contraceptives:

Planned Parenthood: www.plannedparenthood.org

Ultimate Birth Control Links: www.ultimatebirthcontrol. com

Reproductive Health Online: www.reproline.jhu.edu

For Information on Menopause:

North American Menopause Society: www.menopause. org

Menopause Online: www.menopause-online.com

For Information on Pregnancy and Childbirth:

Childbirth: www.childbirth.org

StorkNet's Pregnancy Guide: www.pregnancyguideonline. com

What to Expect: www.whattoexpect.com

The American College of Obstetricians and Gynecologists: www.acog.com

American Baby: www.americanbaby.com

Baby Zone: www.babyzone.com

Lamaze International: www.lamaze.org

LaLeche League: www.laleche.org

 PREPARE FOR CERTIFICATION   Visit the Evolve site at http://evolve.elsevier.com/Bonewit/today/ to actively Prepare for your Certification.

 *Check out the **Companion CD** bound with the book to access additional interactive activities.*

24

The Pediatric Examination

LEARNING OBJECTIVES

Pediatric Office Visits
1. List the components of the well-child visit.
2. State the usual schedule for well-child visits.
3. Explain the purpose of the sick-child visit.
4. List the procedures performed by the medical assistant during pediatric office visits.
5. Explain why it is important to develop a rapport with the pediatric patient.

Growth Measurements
1. State the importance of measuring the child's weight, height (or length), and head circumference during each office visit.
2. State the functions served by a growth chart.

Pediatric Blood Pressure Measurement
1. State the importance of measuring a child's blood pressure.
2. List the three factors that determine whether a child has hypertension.

Collection of a Urine Specimen
1. List the reasons for collecting a urine specimen from a child.

Pediatric Injections
1. State the range for the gauge and length of needles used for intramuscular and subcutaneous pediatric injections.
2. Explain the use of each of the following pediatric injection sites: dorsogluteal, vastus lateralis, and deltoid.

Immunizations
1. Describe the schedule for immunization of infants and children recommended by the American Academy of Pediatrics.
2. State the information that must be provided to parents as required by the National Childhood Vaccine Injury Act.
3. List the information that must be recorded in the medical record after administering an immunization.

Newborn Screening Test
1. Explain the purpose of a newborn screening test.
2. List the symptoms of phenylketonuria (PKU).
3. State what occurs if PKU is left untreated.

PROCEDURES

Carry an infant using the following positions:
Cradle
Upright

Plot pediatric growth values on a growth chart.
Measure the weight and length of an infant.
Measure the head and chest circumference of an infant.

Measure the blood pressure of a child.

Collect a urine specimen using a pediatric urine collector.

Locate the following pediatric intramuscular injection sites:
Dorsogluteal
Vastus lateralis
Deltoid
Administer an intramuscular injection to an infant.
Administer a subcutaneous injection to an infant.

Read and interpret a vaccine information statement.
Record information on a pediatric vaccine administration record.

CHAPTER OUTLINE

Introduction to the Pediatric Examination
Pediatric Office Visits
Developing a Rapport
Carrying the Infant
  Cradle Position
  Upright Position
Growth Measurements
  Weight
  Length and Height
  Head and Chest Circumference
  Growth Charts
Pediatric Blood Pressure Measurement
  Special Guidelines for Children
  Correct Cuff Size

  Cooperation of the Child
  Blood Pressure Classifications
Collection of a Urine Specimen
Pediatric Injections
  Types of Needles
  Intramuscular Injection Sites
Immunizations
  National Childhood Vaccine Injury Act
Newborn Screening Test

CAAHEP COMPETENCIES

Clinical Competencies
Patient Care
- Prepare and maintain examination and treatment areas.
- Prepare patient for and assist with routine and specialty examinations.
- Prepare patient for and assist with procedures, treatments, and minor office surgeries.
- Maintain medication and immunization records.

General Competencies
Patient Instruction
- Instruct individuals according to their needs.
- Provide instruction for health maintenance and disease prevention.

ABHES COMPETENCIES

Clinical Duties
- Prepare and maintain examination and treatment areas.
- Prepare patient for and assist physician with routine and specialty examinations and treatments and minor office surgeries.
- Maintain medication and immunization records.

Instruction
- Teach patients methods of health promotion and disease prevention.

KEY TERMS

adolescent
immunity (ih-MYOO-nih-tee)
immunization (IM-yoo-nih-ZAY-shun)
infant
length
pediatrician (PEE-dee-uh-TRIH-shun)
pediatrics (pee-dee-AT-riks)

preschool (PREE-skool) child
school-age child
toddler (TOD-ler)
toxoid (TOKS-oid)
vaccine (vak-SEEN)
vertex (VER-teks)

Introduction to the Pediatric Examination

Pediatrics is the branch of medicine that deals with the care and development of children and the diagnosis and treatment of diseases in children. A **pediatrician** is a physician who specializes in pediatrics. Many physicians in general practice accept pediatric patients. It is essential that the medical assistant develop the skills needed to assist the physician in the care and treatment of children.

PEDIATRIC OFFICE VISITS

Pediatric patient office visits fall into two broad categories. The first is the *well-child visit* (also termed *health maintenance visit*), in which the physician progressively evaluates the growth and development of the child. A physical examination is performed during each well-child visit and is directed toward discovering any abnormal conditions commonly associated with the stage of development reached by the child. Table 24-1 provides an outline of normal development during infancy. The child also receives necessary immunizations during these visits.

Another important component of the well-child visit is *anticipatory guidance.* Anticipatory guidance is the process of providing parents with information to prepare them for anticipated developmental events and to assist them in promoting their children's well-being. Topics that are commonly included are safety, nutrition, sleep, play, exercise, development, and discipline.

The interval between well-child visits depends on the medical office, but it frequently follows this schedule after birth: 1 month, 2 months, 4 months, 6 months, 9 months, 12 months, 15 months, 18 months, 24 months, and yearly thereafter.

The second category of pediatric patient office visits is the *sick-child visit.* The child is exhibiting the signs and symptoms of disease, and the physician evaluates the patient's condition to arrive at a diagnosis and prescribe treatment.

During well-child and sick-child visits, the medical assistant performs many of the same procedures that have been presented in previous chapters (e.g., measurement of temperature, pulse, respiration, and blood pressure; measurement of weight and height; measurement of visual acuity; assisting with the physical examination). This chapter discusses procedures specifically related to the pediatric patient and variations in procedures previously presented.

DEVELOPING A RAPPORT

The medical assistant must establish a rapport with the pediatric patient. If the medical assistant gains the child's

What Would You Do? What Would You *Not* Do?

Case Study 1

My-Lai Chang comes into the office with Christopher Chang, her 2-month-old son. Christopher is here for his 2-month well-child visit. Mrs. Chang is very distraught. She says that Christopher has episodes of nonstop crying every day that last 2 to 3 hours at a time. She is breastfeeding Christopher and says that the crying is worse after he nurses. Although Mrs. Chang realizes that Christopher has colic, she feels guilty because it seems "her milk" is making it worse. She is also having problems with sore nipples and engorgement. She really wanted to breastfeed Christopher, but she is thinking of stopping because it just seems too hard to do. Christopher measures in the 50th percentile for weight and length. Mrs. Chang is worried that he is not growing enough and thinks it is because she is not producing enough milk. ■

Table 24-1 Milestones of Gross and Fine Motor Development in Infancy		
Average Age (mo)	**Gross Motor**	**Fine Motor**
1	Turns head from side to side	Grasping reflex present
2	Holds head at 45-degree angle when prone	Holds rattle briefly
3	Begins rolling over	Grasps rattle or dangling objects
4	Slight head lag when pulled to sitting position	Brings objects to mouth
5	No head wobble when held in sitting position	Transfers objects from hand to hand
6	Sits without support	Manipulates and examines large objects with hands
7	Stands while holding on	Reaches for, grabs, and retains object
8	Pulls self to stand	Grasps objects with thumb and finger
9	Crawls backwards	Begins to show hand preference
10	Creeps on hands and knees	Hits cup with spoon
11	Walks using furniture for support	Picks up small objects with thumb and forefinger (pincer grasp)
12	Stands alone easily	Puts three or more objects into container
12-16	Walks alone easily	Turns two or three pages in large cardboard book

From Leahy JM, Kizilay PE: *Foundations of nursing practice,* Philadelphia, 1998, Saunders.

trust and confidence, the child is likely to cooperate during an examination or procedure. Interacting with children requires special techniques. The techniques employed depend on the age of the child. **Toddlers** and **preschool children** often respond well to making a game of the procedure. Explaining the purpose of an instrument (e.g., the stethoscope) to a **school-age child** and allowing him or her to hold the instrument or even to help during the procedure may overcome fears in that age group (Figure 24-1).

The medical assistant should always explain the procedure to children who are able to understand. Each child must be approached at his or her level of understanding. To do this, the medical assistant should know what to expect from a child at a particular age, in terms of motor and social development. Each child has his or her own individual rate of development; the descriptions of normal development based on age are meant to serve as a guide only and may have to be modified to meet individual needs. In addition, it is normal for an ill child to regress to an earlier level of behavior. Table 24-2 outlines techniques that can be used with various age groups to gain their cooperation during an examination or procedure.

CARRYING THE INFANT

The medical assistant needs to lift and carry the **infant** to perform various procedures, such as measurement of length and weight. The infant should be lifted and carried in a manner that is safe and comfortable. Proper positions include the cradle and upright positions.

Cradle Position

The medical assistant slides the left hand and arm under the infant's back and grasps the infant's arm from behind. The thumb and fingers should encircle the infant's forearm. The infant's head, shoulders, and back are supported by the medical assistant's arm. Next the medical assistant slips the right arm up and under the infant's buttocks. The infant is cradled in the arm with his or her body resting against the medical assistant's chest (Figure 24-2).

Upright Position

The medical assistant slips the right hand under the infant's head and shoulders. The fingers should be spread apart to support the infant's head and neck. The left forearm is slipped under the infant's buttocks to help support the infant's weight. The infant should be allowed to rest against the medical assistant's chest with the cheek resting on the medical assistant's shoulder (Figure 24-3).

GROWTH MEASUREMENTS

One of the best methods to evaluate the progress of a child is to measure his or her growth. The weight, height (or length), and head circumference (up to age 3 years) of a child should be measured during each office visit and plotted on a growth chart.

Weight

A child's weight is often used to determine nutritional needs and the proper dosage of a medication to administer to the

exce

Figure 24-1. The medical assistant should develop a rapport with children to gain their trust and cooperation. Making a game of the procedure **(A)** and explaining the purpose of the stethoscope and allowing the child to hold it **(B)** help the child overcome fears. (From Bonewit-West K: *Clinical procedures for medical assistants,* ed 7, St. Louis, 2008, Saunders.)

Table 24-2 Techniques for Interacting with Children

Technique	Infant (Birth-1 yr)	Toddler (1-3 yr)	Preschool (3-6 yr)	School Age (6-12 yr)	Adolescent (12-18 yr)
Avoid sudden motion and loud or abrupt noises	♥				
Limit number of strangers in room	♥				
Use distractions, bright objects, rattles, and talking to gain cooperation	♥				
Physically restrain child if necessary to ensure safety	♥	♥	♥		
Allow physical contact with parent during procedure	♥	♥	♥		
Encourage parent to comfort child after procedure	♥	♥	♥		
Use play to explain procedure (e.g., dolls, puppets)		♥	♥		
Perform procedures quickly, if possible		♥	♥		
Use concrete terms, rather than abstract terms		♥	♥		
Avoid words that have more than one meaning (e.g., shot)		♥	♥		
Give child permission to cry, yell, or otherwise express pain verbally		♥	♥		
Praise child for cooperative behavior		♥	♥	♥	
Allow child to handle equipment, if possible			♥	♥	
Make sure child understands body part to be involved			♥	♥	
Try to describe how procedure will feel			♥	♥	
Tell child about any discomfort that may be felt, but don't dwell on it			♥	♥	
Stress benefits of anything child may find pleasurable afterward (e.g., stickers, feeling better)			♥	♥	
Give child choices when possible (e.g., arm to use)			♥	♥	
Suggest ways to maintain control (e.g., counting, deep breathing, relaxation)			♥	♥	
Use drawing and diagrams to illustrate parts of body that will be involved			♥	♥	
Encourage participation such as holding instrument during procedure			♥	♥	
Include child in decision-making process				♥	♥
Discuss risks of procedure					♥
Provide information about appearance changes that might result					♥
Give child educational brochures or have him or her view videos about procedure					♥
Ask parent to step out if child does not want parent in examining room					♥

From Bonewit-West K: *Clinical procedures for medical assistants,* ed 7, St. Louis, 2008, Saunders.

child. The medical assistant should exercise care in measuring weight. Infants are weighed in a recumbent position, as outlined in Procedure 24-1. Older children are weighed in a standing position, as presented in Chapter 20.

Length and Height

Another measure of a child's growth is **length,** or height (stature). Length is measured in children younger than 24 months. The recumbent length is a measurement from the **vertex** of the head to the heel of the infant in a supine position, as outlined in Procedure 24-1. Two people are often needed to determine the length of an infant accurately. The parent's help can be requested; the medical assistant must provide the parent with thorough instructions on what is to be done. Older children have their height measured in a standing position (Figure 24-4), as presented in Chapter 20.

Head and Chest Circumference

Infancy is a period of rapid brain growth. Because of this, the head circumference is an important measurement. The head circumference for a newborn ranges from 32 to 38 cm, or 12½ to 15 inches. A 10-cm (4-inch) increase in head circumference occurs within the first year of life.

The head circumference of children younger than 3 years old should be routinely measured and plotted on a head circumference growth chart. Measurement of head circumference is an important screening measure for microencephaly and macroencephaly.

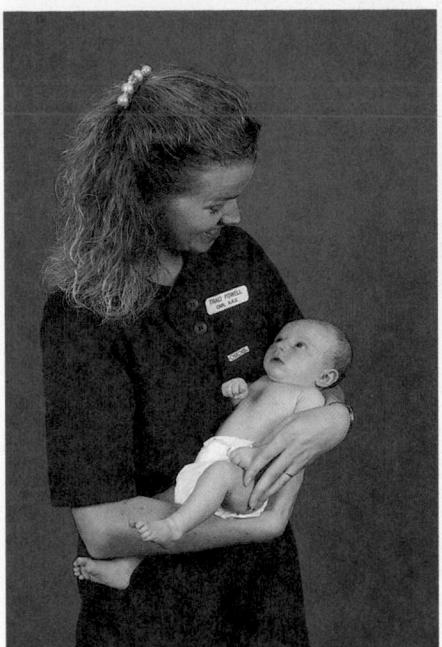

Figure 24-2. Traci holds the infant in the cradle position. (From Bonewit-West K: *Clinical procedures for medical assistants*, ed 7, St. Louis, 2008, Saunders.)

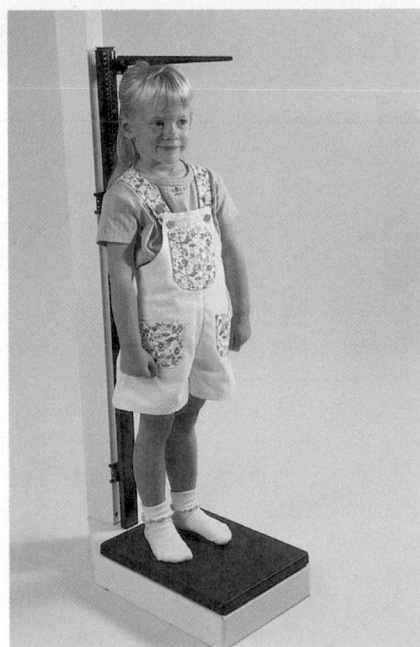

Figure 24-4. Measuring the height of a child. (From Bonewit-West K: *Clinical procedures for medical assistants*, ed 7, St. Louis, 2008, Saunders.)

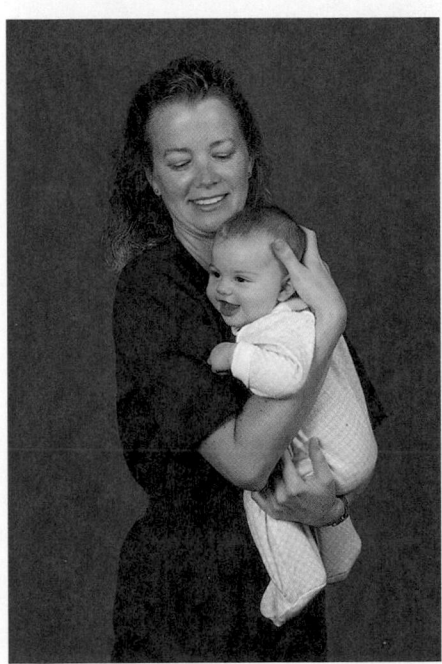

Figure 24-3. Traci holds the infant in the upright position. (From Bonewit-West K; *Clinical procedures for medical assistants*, ed 7, St. Louis, 2008, Saunders.)

At birth, a newborn's head circumference is about 2 cm larger than his or her chest circumference. The chest grows at a faster rate than the cranium, and between 6 months and 2 years of age, the measurements are about the same. After age 2 years, the chest circumference is greater than the

head circumference. The measurement of the chest circumference is valuable in a comparison with the head circumference, but not by itself. The chest circumference is not typically measured on a routine basis; this measurement is done only when a heart or lung abnormality is suspected. Procedure 24-2 outlines the procedure for measuring the head and chest circumference of an infant.

Growth Charts

Growth charts should be part of every child's permanent record. The National Center for Health Statistics developed growth charts to assist physicians in determining whether the growth of a child is normal. The charts can be used to identify children with growth or nutritional abnormalities. The medical assistant is usually responsible for plotting the child's measurements on the growth chart (Procedure 24-3).

Growth charts provide a means of comparing a child's weight and length (or height) with that of other children of the same age. For example, the medical assistant calculates the growth percentile of an 18-month-old boy and finds that he is in the 25th percentile for weight and the 80th percentile for length. This means that 75% of 18-month-old boys weigh more than he does, and 25% weigh less than he does. It also means that 20% of 18-month-old boys are taller, and 80% are shorter. Although comparing a child with other children of the same age is one use of growth charts (particularly by parents), it is not the most important use.

The primary use of growth charts is to look at the child's growth pattern. If a child has always hovered around a

Putting It All into Practice

My name is Traci Powell, and I am a certified medical assistant. I work in the pediatrics department of a large multispecialty clinic. My job responsibilities are mostly clinical; however, I do assist in the front office when needed. I love working with the children and have enjoyed watching them grow over the years.

A coworker and I recently organized a local AAMA (American Association of Medical Assistants) chapter. Our chapter provides AAMA continuing education units (CEUs). Our members attend state and national conventions every year, and they hold state and national leadership positions. It is my goal to see the medical assisting profession continue to grow and advance in the health care field. With advanced training for CMAs (AAMA) being developed by the AAMA and the great increase in managed care, opportunities for CMAs (AAMA) are growing tremendously.

It is interesting how your education, training, and experience all come together, especially in a crisis. Early one morning when I arrived at work, a mother was waiting with a small child who was approximately 2 years old. The child was dusky in color, panicky, and having trouble breathing. Apparently the child had gotten into some dry beans the previous night and had inhaled one into her lung. None of the physicians were in the building yet, and this child was in respiratory distress. We immediately called a Code Blue, put her on oxygen, and made arrangements for a squad car to take her to Children's Hospital, where a surgeon was waiting. All went well, and she is a healthy little girl today.

Looking back, I am grateful for a good, solid medical assisting education; a PALS (Pediatric Advance Life Support) certification; and experience in working with children so that I was able to help that child through a life-threatening experience. I firmly believe that no matter how long a person has been in the medical field or what his or her profession is, continuing education is essential to stay current in the ever-changing health care field. ■

Prepare for Success

Highlight on Childhood Obesity

Statistics

An epidemic of childhood obesity is occurring in the United States; the incidence of obesity in children has doubled over the past 20 years. Approximately 25% of Americans younger than age 19 are overweight or obese, which equates to one of every four children. A child is considered overweight if his or her weight falls in the 85th to 95th percentile for age, gender, and height on the National Center for Health Statistics growth charts. When a child's weight exceeds the 95th percentile for age, gender, and height, he or she is considered obese.

Causes

The primary causes of childhood obesity are overeating and inadequate exercise. Other causes include hormonal and genetic problems, but these are much less likely, occurring in only 5% of obese children. The risk of obesity tends to be greater among children who have obese parents. After age 3, the likelihood that obesity will persist into adulthood increases as an obese child gets older. When an obese child reaches age 6, the probability is more than 50% that obesity will persist into adulthood. Of obese **adolescents,** 70% to 80% remain obese as adults.

Related Problems

Problems associated with childhood obesity include high blood pressure, type 2 diabetes, orthopedic problems caused by increased stress on weight-bearing joints, skin disorders such as dermatitis, sleep apnea, low self-esteem, social isolation, and feelings of rejection and depression. Some authorities believe that the social and psychological problems are the most significant consequences of childhood obesity.

Prevention

It is much easier to prevent childhood obesity than to treat it after it has occurred. Authorities believe that the primary focus should be on educating parents about the problems associated with childhood obesity and helping them employ preventive measures. Guidelines for preventing childhood obesity include the following:

- Provide a healthy diet, with 30% or fewer calories coming from fat.
- Encourage active play.
- Do not use food for reward, comfort, or bribes.
- Limit television, video, and computer time.
- Limit the amount of "junk" food kept in the home.
- Do not make the child eat when he or she is not hungry.
- Do not offer dessert as a reward for finishing a meal.
- Encourage the child to drink water instead of sweet beverages.
- Do not frequently eat at fast-food restaurants.

Treatment

The treatment of childhood obesity is difficult, and the success rate is not particularly high. Children seem to be most successful at losing weight and keeping it off when the entire family is involved. Parents should eat healthy meals and snacks with their children. The most successful diets are those that use ordinary foods in controlled portions, rather than diets that require the avoidance of specific foods. Parents also should spend time being active with their children. Activities should stress self-improvement rather than competition. ■

certain percentile in height and weight, there is no need for concern. If a child is in the 20th percentile for weight but has always been in this percentile, he is likely growing normally. It would be more concerning if the child had been

in the 75th percentile and dropped to the 20th percentile. The physician investigates any significant change or rapid increase or decrease in a child's growth pattern.

Text continued on p. 508

PROCEDURE 24-1   Measuring the Weight and Length of an Infant

Outcome Measure the weight and length of an infant.

Equipment/Supplies

- Pediatric balance scale (table model)

1. **Procedural Step.** Sanitize your hands.
2. **Procedural Step.** Greet the infant's parent and introduce yourself. Identify the infant and explain the procedure to the parent. The weight of the infant is usually measured first. Depending on the medical office policy, ask the parent to perform one of the following:
   a. Remove the infant's clothing and put a dry diaper on the infant.
   b. Remove the infant's clothing, including the diaper.
   Principle. The infant should not be weighed with a wet diaper because it could increase the infant's weight considerably. Also, growth charts for infants and young children base their percentiles on the weight of the child without clothing.
3. **Procedural Step.** Unlock the pediatric scale, and place a clean paper protector on it. Check the balance scale for accuracy, making sure to compensate for the weight of the paper.
   Principle. The paper protector prevents cross-contamination and reduces the spread of disease from one patient to another.
4. **Procedural Step.** Gently place the infant on his or her back on the table of the scale. Place one hand slightly above the infant as a safety precaution.
5. **Procedural Step.** Balance the scale as follows:
   a. Move the lower weight to the notched groove that does not cause the indicator point to drop to the bottom of the calibration area. Ensure that the lower weight is seated firmly in its groove.
   b. Slowly slide the upper weight along its calibration bar by tapping it gently until the indicator point comes to a rest at the center of the balance area.
   Principle. Not seating the lower weight firmly in its groove results in an inaccurate reading.
6. **Procedural Step.** Read the results in pounds and ounces while the infant is lying still. Jot down this value or make a mental note of it. (*Note:* The result on the pictured scale is 15 lb and 2 oz.)
7. **Procedural Step.** Return the balance to its resting position, and lock the scale.

Balance the scale. (From Bonewit-West K: *Clinical procedures for medical assistants,* ed 7, St. Louis, 2008, Saunders.)

Read the results in pounds and ounces. (From Bonewit-West K: *Clinical procedures for medical assistants,* ed 7, St. Louis, 2008, Saunders.)

8. **Procedural Step.** Place the vertex (top) of the infant's head against the headboard at the zero mark. Ask the parent to hold the infant's head in this position.
9. **Procedural Step.** Straighten the infant's knees, and place the soles of his or her feet firmly against the upright footboard (to create a right angle).
10. **Procedural Step.** Read the infant's length in inches (to the nearest ⅛ inch) from the measure. Jot down this value or make a mental note of it. (*Note:* The result on this scale is 25½ inches.)

Continued

PROCEDURE 24-1

PROCEDURE 24-2

PROCEDURE 24-1   Measuring the Weight and Length of an Infant—cont'd

Properly position the infant. (From Bonewit-West K: *Clinical procedures for medical assistants,* ed 7, St. Louis, 2008, Saunders.)

11. **Procedural Step.** Gently remove the infant from the table, and hand him or her to the parent. Return the headboard and footboard to their resting positions.
12. **Procedural Step.** Sanitize your hands, and chart the results.

Read the length in inches. (From Bonewit-West K: *Clinical procedures for medical assistants,* ed 7, St. Louis, 2008, Saunders.)

CHARTING EXAMPLE

Date	
8/10/10	9:30 a.m. Wt. 15 lb 2 oz. Length 25 ½ in. _____
	_____ T. Powell, CMA (AAMA)

PROCEDURE 24-2   Measuring Head and Chest Circumference of an Infant

Outcome Measure the head and chest circumference of an infant.

Equipment/Supplies

• Flexible nonstretch tape measure

Measurement of Head Circumference

1. **Procedural Step.** Sanitize your hands, and assemble the equipment.
2. **Procedural Step.** Position the infant. The infant should be placed on his or her back on the examining table. An alternative position is to have the parent hold the infant.
3. **Procedural Step.** Position the tape measure around the infant's head at the greatest circumference. This is usually accomplished by placing the tape slightly above the eyebrows and pinna of the ears and around the occipital prominence at the back of the skull.
4. **Procedural Step.** Read the results in centimeters (or inches) to the nearest 0.5 cm (or ¼ inch). Jot down this value or make a mental note of it. Sanitize your hands, and chart the results.

Position the tape measure around the infant's head. (From Bonewit-West K: *Clinical procedures for medical assistants,* ed 7, St. Louis, 2008, Saunders.)

CHARTING EXAMPLE

Date	
8/10/10	10:00 a.m. Head circumference: 42 ½ cm. _____
	_____ T. Powell, CMA (AAMA)

Measurement of Chest Circumference

1. **Procedural Step.** Position the infant on his or her back on the examining table.
2. **Procedural Step.** Encircle the tape around the infant's chest at the nipple line. It should be snug, but not so tight that it leaves a mark.
3. **Procedural Step.** Read the results in centimeters (or inches) to the nearest 0.5 cm (or ¼ inch). Jot down this value or make a mental note of it. Sanitize your hands, and chart the results.

CHARTING EXAMPLE

Date	
8/15/10	10:00 a.m. Chest circumference: 42 cm. — ———————— T. Powell, CMA (AAMA)

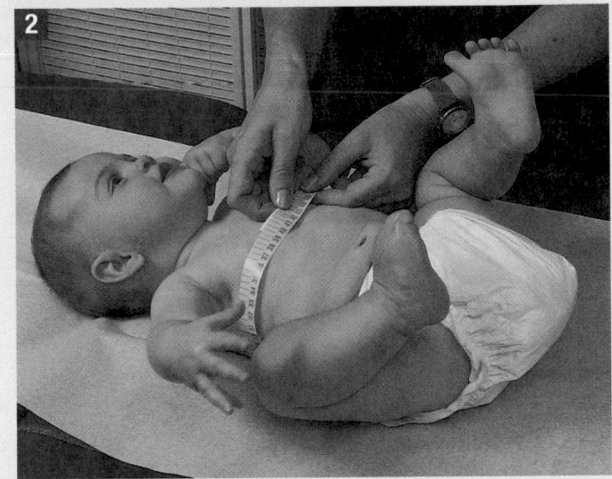

Encircle the tape around the infant's chest. (From Bonewit-West K: *Clinical procedures for medical assistants,* ed 7, St. Louis, 2008, Saunders.)

PROCEDURE 24-3   Calculating Growth Percentiles

Outcome Plot a pediatric growth value on a growth chart.

Equipment/Supplies

- Pediatric growth chart

1. **Procedural Step.** Select the proper growth chart.
2. **Procedural Step.** Locate the child's age in the horizontal column at the bottom of the chart.
3. **Procedural Step.** Locate the growth value in the vertical column under the appropriate category (weight, length or stature, and head circumference).
4. **Procedural Step.** Draw an imaginary vertical line from the child's age mark and an imaginary horizontal line from the child's growth mark. Find the site at which the two lines intersect on the graph, and place a dot on this site.
5. **Procedural Step.** To determine the percentile in which the child falls, follow the curved percentile line upward to read the value located on the right side of the chart. Interpolation is necessary if the value does not fall exactly on a percentile line. (*Interpolation* means that you must estimate a percentile that falls between a larger and smaller known percentile.)
6. **Procedural Step.** Chart the results. Include the date and time and each growth percentile.
   Note: The weight (15 lb, 2 oz), length (25½ inches), and head circumference (42.5 cm) of the child in Procedures 24-1 and 24-2 have been plotted on a growth chart. This child is 5 months old. Locate these values on the appropriate growth chart to ensure you obtain the same percentiles.

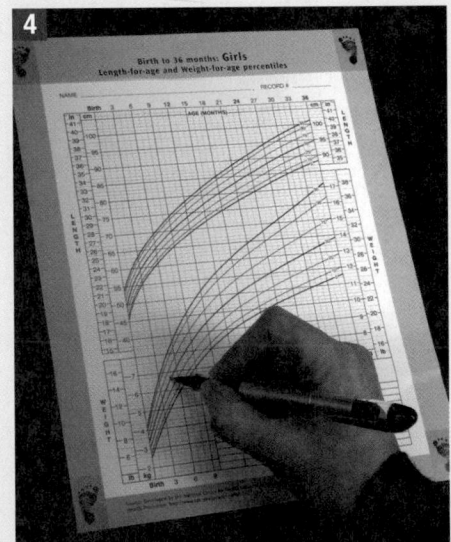

(From Bonewit-West K: *Clinical procedures for medical assistants,* ed 7, St. Louis, 2008, Saunders.)

CHARTING EXAMPLE

Date	
10/22/10	10:30 a.m. Weight: 55%. Length: 70%. ——— Head Circum: 67% —— T. Powell, CMA (AAMA)

Continued

PROCEDURE 24-3

Birth to 36 months: Girls
Length-for-age and Weight-for-age percentiles

NAME _____

RECORD # _____

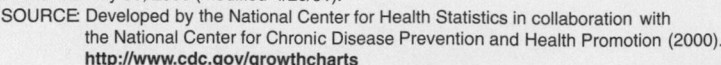

Published May 30, 2000 (modified 4/20/01).
SOURCE: Developed by the National Center for Health Statistics in collaboration with
the National Center for Chronic Disease Prevention and Health Promotion (2000).
http://www.cdc.gov/growthcharts

CDC

SAFER · HEALTHIER · PEOPLE™

Birth to 36 months: Boys
Length-for-age and Weight-for-age percentiles

NAME _____

RECORD # _____

Published May 30, 2000 (modified 4/20/01).
SOURCE: Developed by the National Center for Health Statistics in collaboration with
the National Center for Chronic Disease Prevention and Health Promotion (2000).
http://www.cdc.gov/growthcharts

AGE (MONTHS)

LENGTH

WEIGHT

95
90
75
50
25
10
5

Mother's Stature _____   Gestational
Father's Stature _____   Age: _____ Weeks   Comment

Date	Age	Weight	Length	Head Circ.	
	Birth				

PROCEDURE 24-3

SAFER · HEALTHIER · PEOPLE™

PEDIATRIC BLOOD PRESSURE MEASUREMENT

The American Academy of Pediatrics recommends that all children 3 years old and older have their blood pressure measured annually. Measuring pediatric blood pressure helps to identify children at risk for developing hypertension as adults. High blood pressure in children can be caused by kidney disease and, to a lesser degree, by heart disease. When the condition is treated, the blood pressure usually returns to normal. Overweight children usually have higher blood pressure than children of normal weight. Losing weight through a prescribed diet and regular physical activity often reduces blood pressure in these children.

Special Guidelines for Children

The procedure for measuring blood pressure in children is the same as that for adults and is presented in Chapter 19. Some special pediatric guidelines must be taken into consideration.

Correct Cuff Size

The most important criterion in obtaining an accurate pediatric blood pressure measurement is selecting the correct cuff size. If the cuff is too small, the reading may be falsely high. If the cuff is too large, the reading may be falsely low. Blood pressure cuffs come in a variety of sizes and are measured in centimeters (cm). The size of a cuff refers to its inner inflatable bladder, rather than its cloth cover. Table 24-3 lists the range of cuff sizes commercially available. The name of the cuff (e.g., child, adult) does not imply it is appropriate for that age. An 8-year-old overweight child may need an adult-sized cuff.

For an accurate blood pressure measurement, the bladder of the cuff should encircle 80% to 100% of the arm. The child's arm circumference should be assessed midpoint between the acromion process (shoulder) and the olecranon process (elbow). Figure 24-5 shows how to determine the correct pediatric cuff size.

Cooperation of the Child

Another important factor to consider when taking pediatric blood pressure is preparing the child for the procedure. It is important to gain the child's cooperation and to ensure that the child is relaxed. Apprehension can cause the blood pressure to be falsely high. To reduce a child's anxiety level, carefully explain the procedure to the child, and, if appro-

Table 24-3 Acceptable Bladder Dimensions for Arms of Different Sizes		
Cuff	Bladder Length (cm)	Arm Circumference Range at Midpoint (cm)
Newborn	6	Less than 6
Infant	15	6-15
Child	21	16-21
Small adult	24	22-26
Adult	30	27-34
Large adult	38	35-44
Adult thigh	42	45-52

From Bonewit-West K: *Clinical procedures for medical assistants,* ed 7, St. Louis, 2008, Saunders.

 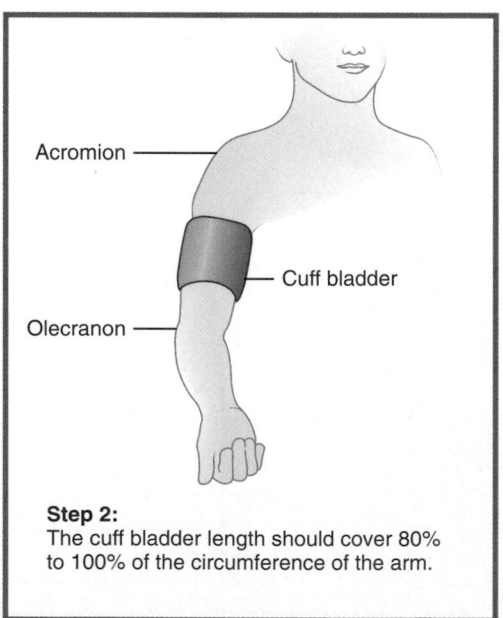

Figure 24-5. Determination of proper blood pressure cuff size. (From Bonewit-West K: *Clinical procedures for medical assistants,* ed 7, St. Louis, 2008, Saunders.)

priate, allow him or her to handle the equipment before measuring blood pressure. The blood pressure should be measured after the child has been sitting quietly for 3 to 5 minutes (Figure 24-6).

Blood Pressure Classifications

Blood pressure varies depending on the age of the child and his or her height and gender. The National High Blood Pressure Education Program (NHBPEP) prepared a set of tables that physicians use to determine whether a child's blood pressure is higher than the average among children of the same age and height. If a child has a blood pressure that is higher than 90% to 95% of most other children of the same age, height, and gender, the child may have high blood pressure.

The NHBPEP tables (one for boys and one for girls) allow precise classification of blood pressure according to body size, which avoids misclassifying children at the extreme ends of normal growth. A very tall child would not be mistakenly diagnosed as having hypertension, and hypertension would not be missed in a very short child. The NHBPEP tables used by physicians to assist in the diagnosis of hypertension in children can be found at the National Heart, Lung, and Blood Institute website (http://www.nhlbi.nih.gov/guidelines/hypertension/child_tbl.pdf).

Blood pressure varies throughout the day in children as a result of normal fluctuations in physical activity and emotional stress. If a child's blood pressure is elevated, two more readings must be taken at different visits before the physician can make a diagnosis of hypertension.

COLLECTION OF A URINE SPECIMEN

A urinalysis may be performed on a pediatric patient for the following reasons: to screen for the presence of disease as part

Figure 24-6. Traci measures the blood pressure of a pediatric patient. (From Bonewit-West K: *Clinical procedures for medical assistants*, ed 7, St. Louis, 2008, Saunders.)

What Would You Do? What Would You *Not* Do?

Case Study 2

Wanda Tilley comes to the office with her 10-year-old daughter, Courtney. Courtney has a skin condition on her legs that needs to be evaluated by the physician. Courtney has been obese since she was 4 years old. Mrs. Tilley is also obese and is not too concerned about Courtney's weight. She says that Courtney must have inherited her "fat gene," and there's not much that can be done about it. Courtney's favorite activities are playing video games and reading. She would like to join the community swim team, but she's too embarrassed for anyone to see her in a bathing suit. Courtney says the other kids are always making fun of her at school. She says that they call her "two-ton Tilley" and "double-roll," and they don't want to sit with her at lunch. Courtney wants her mom to home-school her because she's getting to the point where she can't take it anymore. She doesn't want the doctor to examine her because he'll see how fat she is and say bad things about it. ∎

Memories *from* Externship

Traci Powell: I still remember how difficult it was at times as a student. I had been out of high school for more than a year, so I had to get back into the routine of studying. I worried about whether I would do well, whether I would be able to find a good job, and whether I would like medical assisting. Adding to these concerns was the financial burden of putting myself through school. I took advantage of grants and a student loan. Throughout the last 6 months of my education, I also worked full-time as an aide on the midnight shift at a nursing home while attending school full-time during the day. As if that were not enough, my first child was well on her way into this world as I was finishing up the last quarter of my degree. There were so many times that I was tired, frustrated, and broke, but I kept pushing myself to do my best because I knew this was going to be my lifetime career, and I wanted to excel in my profession. My determination paid off. Today I have a great medical assisting position that I love, with an institution that is one of the best employers in the area. ∎

Prepare for Success

of a general physical examination, to assist in the diagnosis of a pathologic condition, or to evaluate the effectiveness of therapy. The collection of a urine specimen from a child who exhibits bladder control is performed using the technique outlined in Chapter 30. Collecting a urine specimen from an infant or young child who cannot urinate voluntarily involves the use of a pediatric urine collector.

Pediatric urine collectors are designed to be used with both sexes. The urine collector consists of a clear plastic disposable bag containing a hypoallergenic pressure-sensitive adhesive around the opening of the bag. The adhesive firmly attaches the urine collector to the genitalia. Procedure 24-4 outlines the procedure for applying a pediatric urine collector.

PROCEDURE 24-4 Applying a Pediatric Urine Collector

Outcome Apply a pediatric urine collector.

Equipment/Supplies

- Disposable gloves
- Personal antiseptic wipes
- Pediatric urine collector bag

- Urine specimen container and label
- Regular waste container

---

1. **Procedural Step.** Sanitize your hands.
2. **Procedural Step.** Assemble the equipment.
3. **Procedural Step.** Greet the infant's parent and introduce yourself. Identify the infant and explain the procedure to the parent.
4. **Procedural Step.** Apply gloves. Position the child. The child should be placed on his or her back with the legs spread apart. The medical assistant may need another individual to hold the child's legs apart.
   Principle. This position facilitates cleansing of the genitalia and permits proper application of the urine collector bag.
5. **Procedural Step.** Cleanse the child's genitalia.
   Female: Using a front-to-back motion (pubis to anus), cleanse each side of the meatus with a separate wipe. With a third wipe, cleanse directly down the middle (directly over the urinary meatus). Discard each wipe after cleansing. Allow the area to dry completely.
   Male: If the child is not circumcised, retract the foreskin of the penis. Cleanse the area around the meatus and the urethral opening (meatal orifice) in a manner similar to that used to cleanse the female patient. Use a separate wipe for each swipe. Cleanse the scrotum last, using a fresh wipe. Discard each wipe after cleansing. Allow the area to dry completely.
   Principle. The urinary meatus and surrounding area must be cleansed to prevent contaminants, such as baby powder, fecal material, and microorganisms, from entering the urine specimen, which could affect the test results. A front-to-back motion must be used to prevent drawing microorganisms from the anal area into the area being cleansed. The area must be completely dry to ensure an airtight adhesion of the collection bag to prevent leakage of urine.
6. **Procedural Step.** Remove the paper backing from the urine collector bag. This exposes the hypoallergenic

6 (1)

Remove the paper backing from the urine collector bag. (From Bonewit-West K: *Clinical procedures for medical assistants,* ed 7, St. Louis, 2008, Saunders.)

6 (2)

Firmly press the adhesive surface to the skin surrounding the external genitalia. (From Bonewit-West K: *Clinical procedures for medical assistants,* ed 7, St. Louis, 2008, Saunders.)

6 (3)

Female: The opening of the bag should be directly over the urinary meatus. (From Bonewit-West K: *Clinical procedures for medical assistants,* ed 7, St. Louis, 2008, Saunders.)

Male: The penis and scrotum are projected through the opening of the bag. (From Bonewit-West K: *Clinical procedures for medical assistants,* ed 7, St. Louis, 2008, Saunders.)

adhesive surface around the opening of the bag. Firmly attach the bag in the following manner:

Female: Stretch the perineum taut, and firmly place the bottom of the adhesive surface on the infant's perineum. Starting at the perineum and working upward, firmly press the adhesive surface to the skin surrounding the external genitalia, ensuring there is no puckering. The opening of the bag should be directly over the urinary meatus. The excess of the bag should be positioned toward the child's feet.

Male: Position the bag so that the child's penis and scrotum are projected through the opening of the bag. Starting at the perineum and working upward, firmly press the adhesive surface to the skin surrounding the penis and scrotum, ensuring there is no puckering. The excess of the bag should be positioned toward the child's feet.

Principle. The adhesive surface of the bag must be attached securely with no puckering to prevent leakage.

7. **Procedural Step.** Loosely diaper the child. Check the urine collector bag every 15 minutes until a urine specimen is obtained.
   Principle. The diaper helps hold the urine collector bag in place. The bag must be checked frequently. Once the infant has urinated, moisture from the urine may cause the adhesive surface to become loose and leak, especially with an active infant.
8. **Procedural Step.** When the child has voided, gently remove the urine collector bag by holding the bottom of the adhesive surface against the infant's skin and carefully peeling the bag off from the top to the bottom.
   Principle. The bag must be removed gently because pulling the adhesive away too quickly may cause discomfort and irritation of the child's skin.
9. **Procedural Step.** Clean the genital area with a personal antiseptic wipe. Rediaper the child.
10. **Procedural Step.** Transfer the urine specimen into a urine specimen container, and tightly apply the lid. Label the container with the child's name, the date, the time of collection, and the type of specimen (i.e., urine). Dispose of the collector bag in a regular waste container. (*Note:* The urine collector bag can be used as a urine container to transport the specimen to the laboratory. This is accomplished by folding the adhesive sponge ring in half along its vertical axis and pressing the adhesive surfaces firmly together to ensure a tight seal.)
11. **Procedural Step.** Based on the medical office routine, test the urine specimen, or prepare it for transfer to an outside laboratory; be sure to include a completed laboratory request form. If the specimen cannot be tested or transferred immediately, preserve it by placing it in the refrigerator.
    Principle. Changes occur in a urine specimen that is left sitting out at room temperature, which can lead to inaccurate test results.
12. **Procedural Step.** Remove the gloves, and sanitize your hands.
13. **Procedural Step.** Chart the procedure. Include the date, the time of collection, and the type of specimen (i.e., urine). If the specimen is to be transported to an outside laboratory, indicate this information, including the laboratory tests ordered.

PROCEDURE 24-4

CHARTING EXAMPLE

Date	
8/12/10	10:15 a.m. Urine specimen collected for culture. Picked up by Medical Center Lab on 8/12/10. —————— T. Powell, CMA (AAMA)

PEDIATRIC INJECTIONS

Administering an injection to a child is an important responsibility. The experience a child has with early injections influences the child's attitude toward later ones. If the child is old enough to understand, the procedure should be explained. The medical assistant should be honest and attempt to gain the child's trust and cooperation. The child should be told the truth about the injection—that it will hurt, but only for a short time. Explaining that the medicine will help him or her get better is also advisable. Another person should be present to assist. The assistant can help position the child and can divert or restrain him or her if necessary. If the child struggles and fights excessively, the medical assistant should delay the injection and consult the physician.

The administration of injections is presented in Chapter 26. Before undertaking the study of pediatric injections, the medical assistant should review this chapter thoroughly, concentrating on the location of injection sites and the procedures for preparing and administering injections. The same basic technique is used to administer an injection to an adult and a child. Variations in procedure are explained in the following section.

Types of Needles

The gauge and length of the needle used for intramuscular injections vary, depending on the consistency of the medication to be administered and the size of the child. Thick or oily preparations require a larger-needle lumen, and the needle must be long enough to reach muscle tissue. A needle length ranging from ⅝ inch to 1 inch is generally used to administer an intramuscular injection to a child, and the gauge of the needle generally ranges between 22 and 25 depending on the viscosity of the medication. The length of the needle used to administer a pediatric subcutaneous injection ranges from ⅜ inch to ½ inch, and the gauge of the needle ranges from 23 to 25.

Intramuscular Injection Sites

Pediatric injection sites vary based on the age of the child. The specific site to be injected is stated in the package insert accompanying the medication. Until the child is walking, the gluteus muscle is small, not well developed, and covered with a thick layer of fat. An injection in the dorsogluteal site may come dangerously close to the sciatic nerve. The danger is increased if the child is squirming or fighting. Because serious trauma can result from incorrect administration of an injection in this area, it is recommended that the dorsogluteal site not be used until the child has been walking for at least 1 year (Figure 24-7).

The vastus lateralis muscle site is recommended for injections of infants and young children. It is located on the anterior surface of the midlateral thigh, away from major nerves and blood vessels, and it is large enough to accommodate the injected medication (Figure 24-8). The length of the needle used depends on the overall size of the thigh.

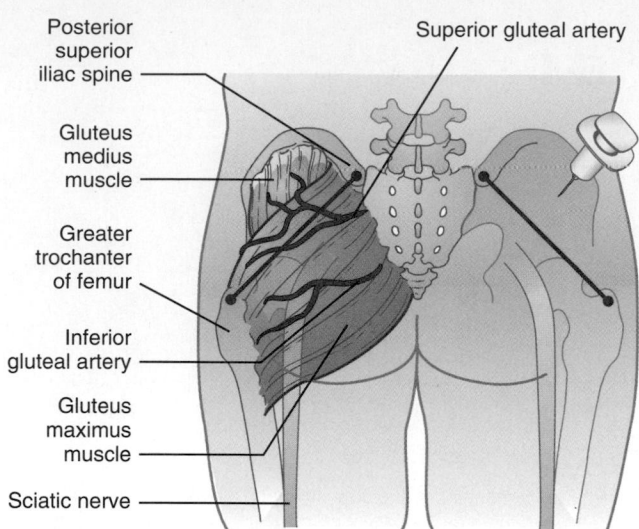

Figure 24-7. Dorsogluteal intramuscular injection site. (Courtesy Wyeth Laboratories, Madison, NJ.)

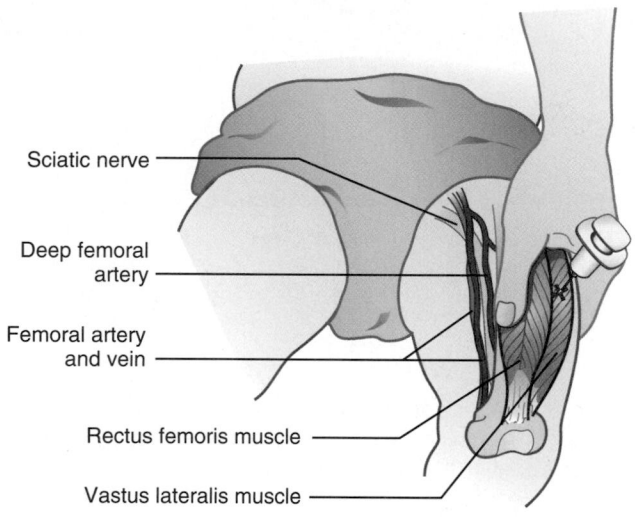

Figure 24-8. Vastus lateralis intramuscular injection site. (Courtesy Wyeth Laboratories, Madison, NJ.)

It should be long enough to penetrate the muscle belly for proper absorption to occur. A 1-inch needle is often used. To administer the injection, the infant is placed on his or her back. The thigh is grasped to compress the muscle tissue and stabilize the extremity. The injection is administered following the procedure outlined in Chapter 26.

The deltoid muscle is shallow and can accommodate only a small amount of medication. In addition, repeated injections to this site are painful. To administer the injection, the deltoid muscle mass should be grasped at the injection site and compressed between the thumb and fingers. The needle should be inserted pointing slightly upward toward the shoulder (Figure 24-9).

After giving the injection, the medical assistant or the child's parent should hold the infant and provide comfort and show approval so that the child associates something other than pain with this procedure.

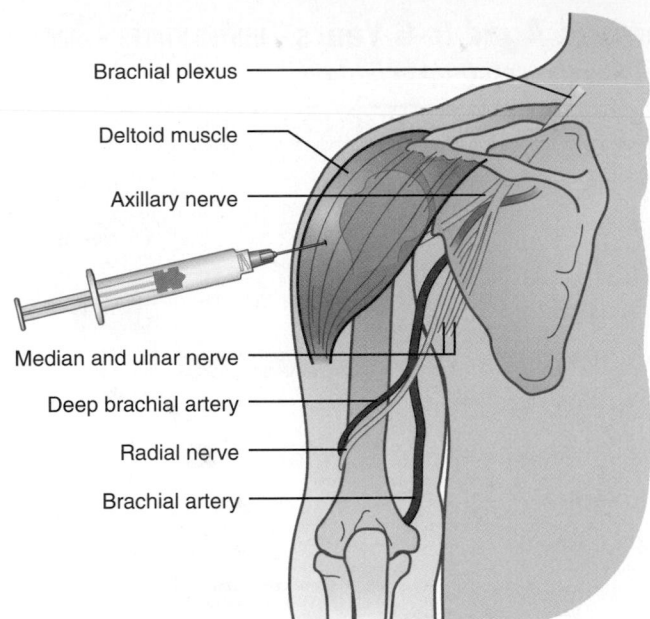

Brachial plexus

Deltoid muscle

Axillary nerve

Median and ulnar nerve

Deep brachial artery

Radial nerve

Brachial artery

Figure 24-9. Deltoid intramuscular injection site. (Courtesy Wyeth Laboratories, Madison, NJ.)

IMMUNIZATIONS

Immunity is the resistance of the body to the effects of harmful agents, such as pathogenic microorganisms and their toxins. The process of becoming immune or rendering an individual immune through the use of a **vaccine** or **toxoid** is known as active, artificial **immunization.** Immunizations build the body's defenses and protect an individual from attack by certain infectious diseases.

Immunizations should be administered to infants and young children during well-child visits according to an immunization schedule (Figure 24-10). The American Academy of Pediatrics recommends following the schedule outlined in Figure 24-10. This schedule is intended as a guide to be used with any modifications needed to meet the requirements of an individual or group.

The medical assistant should be familiar with every immunization that is given, including its use, common side effects, route of administration, dosage, and method of storage. The drug manufacturer includes a package insert with each vaccine and toxoid that contains valuable information about the drug. Drug references, such as the *Physician's Desk Reference,* can also be used to locate information on immunizations. Immunizations administered to infants and children, along with the routes of administration and common minor problems, are listed in Table 24-4.

Parents should be provided with an immunization record card (Figure 24-11) at their infant's first well-child visit. They should be instructed to bring this card to every visit so that their child's immunizations can be recorded. Parents should be informed of the possible normal side effects of each immunization and given instructions on how to respond if they occur.

National Childhood Vaccine Injury Act

The National Childhood Vaccine Injury Act (NCVIA), which became effective in 1988, requires that parents be provided with information about the benefits and risks of childhood immunizations. To help medical offices comply with these regulations, the Centers for Disease Control and Prevention developed a set of vaccine information statements (VISs). A VIS explains, in lay terminology, the benefits and risks of a vaccine. See Figure 24-12 for a DTaP VIS.

The NCVIA requires that the appropriate VIS be given to the child's parent or guardian before the child receives a dose of any immunization listed in Table 24-4. The medical assistant must give the parent or guardian enough time to read the VIS before the immunization is administered. In addition, the medical assistant must chart the following information in the patient's medical record: the name and publication date of each VIS provided to the parent and the date the VIS was given to the parent. The publication date of the VIS is located at the bottom of the VIS. VISs are also available for pneumococcal polysaccharide, meningococcal, rabies, yellow fever, typhoid, Japanese encephalitis, anthrax, and smallpox. Their use is strongly encouraged by the NCVIA, but not required, because these vaccines are not administered to children on a routine basis.

The NCVIA also requires that the following information be recorded in each patient's medical record after the administration of the vaccine: the date of administration of the vaccine, the manufacturer and lot number of the vaccine, the signature and title of the health care provider who administered the vaccine, and the address of the medical office where the vaccine was administered. Figure 24-13 shows an example of a pediatric vaccine administrative record.

What Would You Do? What Would You *Not* Do?

Case Study 3

Stacy Jones, a legal secretary, brings her 5-year-old son, Matthew, in for a kindergarten physical. Stacy has read the VISs for the DTaP, IPV, and MMR immunizations that Matthew will be getting at this visit and has some questions. She wants to know why polio is not given orally anymore. She also wants to know why children are immunized against chickenpox because it is such a harmless disease. She is annoyed because she thinks that children are receiving too many unnecessary injections these days. Matthew is extremely afraid of "shots" and says that no one with a needle is getting anywhere near him. Stacy is protective of Matthew and knows that he will be hard to handle. She wants to know whether this set of immunizations could just be skipped. She says that most of these diseases do not even exist anymore and that she noticed, from reading the vaccine sheets, that there are a lot of possible side effects. ■

Recommended Immunization Schedule for Persons Aged 0–6 Years—UNITED STATES • 2008
For those who fall behind or start late, see the catch-up schedule

Vaccine ▼ Age ▶	Birth	1 month	2 months	4 months	6 months	12 months	15 months	18 months	19–23 months	2–3 years	4–6 years	
Hepatitis B[1]	HepB	HepB		see footnote 1		HepB						**Range of recommended ages**
Rotavirus[2]			Rota	Rota	Rota							
Diphtheria, Tetanus, Pertussis[3]			DTaP	DTaP	DTaP	see footnote 3	DTaP				DTaP	
Haemophilus influenzae type b[4]			Hib	Hib	*Hib*[4]	Hib						**Certain high-risk groups**
Pneumococcal[5]			PCV	PCV	PCV	PCV				PPV		
Inactivated Poliovirus			IPV	IPV		IPV					IPV	
Influenza[6]						Influenza (Yearly)						
Measles, Mumps, Rubella[7]						MMR					MMR	
Varicella[8]						Varicella					Varicella	
Hepatitis A[9]						HepA (2 doses)				HepA Series		
Meningococcal[10]										MCV4		

This schedule indicates the recommended ages for routine administration of currently licensed childhood vaccines, as of December 1, 2007, for children aged 0 through 6 years. Additional information is available at www.cdc.gov/vaccines/recs/schedules. Any dose not administered at the recommended age should be administered at any subsequent visit, when indicated and feasible. Additional vaccines may be licensed and recommended during the year. Licensed combination vaccines may be used whenever any components of the combination are indicated and other components of the vaccine are not contraindicated and if approved by the Food and Drug Administration for that dose of the series. **Providers should consult the respective Advisory Committee on Immunization Practices statement for detailed recommendations, including for high risk conditions:** http://www.cdc.gov/vaccines/pubs/ACIP-list.htm. Clinically significant adverse events that follow immunization should be reported to the Vaccine Adverse Event Reporting System (VAERS). Guidance about how to obtain and complete VAERS form is available at www.vaers.hhs.gov or by telephone, 800-822-7967.

1. Hepatitis B vaccine (HepB). *(Minimum age: birth)*
At birth:
- Administer monovalent HepB to all newborns prior to hospital discharge.
- If mother is hepatitis B surface antigen (HBsAg)-positive, administer HepB and 0.5 mL of hepatitis B immune globulin (HBIG) within 12 hours of birth.
- If mother's HBsAg status is unknown, administer HepB within 12 hours of birth. Determine the HBsAg status as soon as possible and if HBsAg-positive, administer HBIG (no later than age 1 week).
- If mother is HBsAg-negative, the birth dose can be delayed, **in rare cases,** with a provider's order and a **copy of the mother's** negative HBsAg laboratory report in the infant's medical record.

After the birth dose:
- The HepB series should be completed with either monovalent HepB or a combination vaccine containing HepB. The second dose should be administered at age 1–2 months. The final dose should be administered no earlier than age 24 months. Infants born to HBsAg-positive mothers should be tested for HBsAg and antibody to HBsAg after completion of at least 3 doses of a licensed HepB series, at age 9–18 months (generally at the next well-child visit).

4-month dose:
- It is permissible to administer 4 doses of HepB when combination vaccines are administered after the birth dose. If monovalent HepB is used for doses after the birth dose, a dose at age 4 months is not needed.

2. Rotavirus vaccine (Rota). *(Minimum age: 6 weeks)*
- Administer the first dose at age 6–12 weeks.
- Do not start the series later than age 12 weeks.
- Administer the final dose in the series by age 32 weeks. Do not administer any dose later than age 32 weeks.
- Data on safety and efficacy outside of these age ranges are insufficient.

3. Diphtheria and tetanus toxoids and acellular pertussis vaccine (DTaP). *(Minimum age: 6 weeks)*
- The fourth dose of DTaP may be administered as early as age 12 months, provided 6 months have elapsed since the third dose.
- Administer the final dose in the series at age 4–6 years.

4. *Haemophilus influenzae* type b conjugate vaccine (Hib). *(Minimum age: 6 weeks)*
- If PRP-OMP (PedvaxHIB® or ComVax® [Merck]) is administered at ages 2 and 4 months, a dose at age 6 months is not required.
- TriHIBit® (DTaP/Hib) combination products should not be used for primary immunization but can be used as boosters following any Hib vaccine in children age 12 months or older.

5. Pneumococcal vaccine. *(Minimum age: 6 weeks for pneumococcal conjugate vaccine [PCV]; 2 years for pneumococcal polysaccharide vaccine [PPV])*
- Administer one dose of PCV to all healthy children aged 24–59 months having any incomplete schedule.
- Administer PPV to children aged 2 years and older with underlying medical conditions.

6. Influenza vaccine. *(Minimum age: 6 months for trivalent inactivated influenza vaccine [TIV]; 2 years for live, attenuated influenza vaccine [LAIV])*
- Administer annually to children aged 6–59 months and to all close contacts of children aged 0–59 months.
- Administer annually to children 5 years of age and older with certain risk factors, to other persons (including household members) in close contact with persons in groups at higher risk, and to any child whose parents request vaccination.
- For healthy nonpregnant persons (those who do not have underlying medical conditions that predispose them to influenza complications) ages 2–49 years, either LAIV or TIV may be used.
- Children receiving TIV should receive 0.25 mL if age 6-35 mos or 0.5 mL if age 3 years or older.
- Administer 2 doses (separated by 4 weeks or longer) to children younger than 9 years who are receiving influenza vaccine for the first time or who were vaccinated for the first time last season, but only received one dose.

7. Measles, mumps, and rubella vaccine (MMR). *(Minimum age: 12 months)*
- Administer the second dose of MMR at age 4–6 years. MMR may be administered before age 4–6 years, provided 4 weeks or more have elapsed since the first dose.

8. Varicella vaccine. *(Minimum age: 12 months)*
- Administer second dose at age 4–6 years; may be administered 3 months or more after first dose.
- Don't repeat second dose if administered 28 days or more after first dose.

9. Hepatitis A vaccine (HepA). *(Minimum age: 12 months)*
- HepA is recommended for all children aged 1 yr (i.e., aged 12–23 months). The 2 doses in the series should be administered at least 6 months apart.
- Children not fully vaccinated by age 2 years can be vaccinated at subsequent visits.
- HepA is recommended for certain other groups of children, including in areas where vaccination programs target older children.

10. Meningococcal vaccine. *(Minimum age: 2 years for meningococcal conjugate vaccine (MCV4) and for meningococcal polysaccharide vaccine (MPSV4))*
- MCV4 is recommended for children aged 2–10 years with terminal complement deficiencies or anatomic or functional asplenia and certain other high-risk groups. Use of MPSV4 is also acceptable.
- Persons who received MPSV4 3 or more years prior and remain at increased risk for meningococcal disease should be vaccinated with MCV4.

The Recommended Immunization Schedules for Persons Aged 0–18 Years are approved by the Advisory Committee on Immunization Practices (www.cdc.gov/vaccines/recs/acip), the American Academy of Pediatrics (http://www.aap.org), and the American Academy of Family Physicians (http://www.aafp.org).

DEPARTMENT OF HEALTH AND HUMAN SERVICES • CENTERS FOR DISEASE CONTROL AND PREVENTION • SAFER • HEATHIER • PEOPLE™

CS103164

Figure 24-10. Immunization schedule. (From Department of Health and Human Services, Centers for Disease Control and Prevention, United States, 2008.)

Table 24-4 Childhood and Adolescent Immunizations

Immunization	Route of Administration	Common Minor Problems after Administration
Hep B (hepatitis B vaccine)	IM	Mild fever Soreness at injection site
DTaP (diphtheria and tetanus toxoids and acellular pertussis vaccine)	IM	Fever, irritability, tiredness, and poor appetite Redness or swelling at injection site Soreness or tenderness at injection site (occurs 1-3 days after injection)
Hib (*Haemophilus influenzae* type B conjugate vaccine)	IM	Redness, swelling and warmth at injection site; fever greater than 101°F (38.3°C) Redness, warmth, or swelling at injection site (occurs within 1 day after injection; lasts 2-3 days)
IPV (inactivated polio vaccine)	IM or SC	Soreness and redness at injection site
MMR (measles, mumps, and rubella vaccine)	SC	Fever, mild rash (1-2 weeks after administration; lasts 1-3 days)
Varicella (chickenpox vaccine)	SC	Fever, mild rash Soreness, redness, or swelling at injection site
PCV (pneumococcal conjugate vaccine)	IM	Tenderness at the injection site; mild fever Irritability and drowsiness Loss of appetite
MCV4 (meningococcal vaccine)	IM	Pain and redness at injection site
Influenza vaccine	IM	Soreness or redness at the injection site, fever and malaise for 1-2 days
Hep A (hepatitis A vaccine)	IM	Pain and swelling at the injection site

From Bonewit-West K: *Clinical procedures for medical assistants,* ed 7, St. Louis, 2008, Saunders.
IM, Intramuscular; *SC,* subcutaneous.

PATIENT TEACHING   Childhood Immunizations

- Encourage parents to have their children immunized.
- Emphasize to parents the importance of maintaining an immunization record card that documents all of their children's immunizations.
- Provide parents with educational materials on the importance of immunizations.
- Answer questions patients have about childhood immunizations.

What is immunity?

Immunity is the resistance of the body to microorganisms that cause disease. When an individual has an infection, the body responds by producing disease-fighting substances known as *antibodies.* Antibodies usually remain in the body even after the individual has recovered from the disease. This protects the individual from getting that disease again.

How do immunizations prevent disease?

The microorganisms that cause disease or their toxins are weakened or killed and made into vaccines. These vaccines are injected into the body. The body reacts to these vaccines the same way that it responds to the disease itself, by producing antibodies. These antibodies last for a long time, often for life, to defend the body against disease.

What childhood diseases can be prevented through immunization?

The reduction of childhood disease by immunization during the past 40 years has been dramatic. Thirteen diseases can be prevented by routine immunization: hepatitis B, diphtheria, tetanus, pertussis (whooping cough), *Haemophilus influenzae* type B infections, polio, measles, mumps, rubella (German measles), chickenpox (varicella), pneumococcal infections (meningitis and blood infections), hepatitis A, and influenza (flu). Except for tetanus, all these diseases are contagious. They can be spread from child to child and from one community to another. When children are not protected against them, serious outbreaks of disease can still occur.

Haven't most of these diseases been eliminated in the United States?

Although most of the vaccine-preventable diseases have been reduced to very low levels in the United States, this is not true worldwide. Some of these diseases are quite prevalent in other countries. An infected traveler can bring these diseases into the United States without knowing it. If Americans were not immunized, these diseases could quickly spread throughout the population and cause an epidemic. Only when a disease has been eradicated worldwide is it safe to stop vaccinating for that particular disease.

Continued

PATIENT TEACHING Childhood Immunizations—cont'd

Do immunizations have side effects?

Vaccines are among the safest and most reliable medications available. Minor side effects may occur, however, after administration of an immunization. They do not last long and may include a slight fever and irritability; redness, swelling, and soreness at the injection site; and a mild rash. Rarely, the effects can be more serious; if any unusual symptoms occur after immunization, it is important to contact the physician immediately. Overall, the benefits of vaccines to prevent childhood diseases are greater than the possible risks for almost all children.

Are immunizations required by law?

Every state has laws requiring immunization against some or all of these diseases before children enter school. Children who get their immunizations not only benefit from the protection these immunizations provide, but also they contribute to the well-being of everyone by reducing the chance for disease to spread. ∎

IMMUNIZATION RECORD

Name _____

Birthdate _____

Immunization	DATE	DATE	DATE	DATE	DATE
Heb B (Hepatitis B)					
DTaP (Diphtheria, Tetanus, and Pertussis)					
Hib (Haemophilius Influenzae Type b)					
IPV (Inactivated Polio Vaccine)					
MMR (Measles, Mumps, Rubella)					
Varicella (Chickenpox)					
PCV (Pneumococcal Conjugate Vaccine)					
MCV4 (Meningococcal Vaccine)					
Tuberculin (Mantoux) **RESULT**					
Tetanus Booster					
Other					

Figure 24-11. Immunization record card. (From Bonewit-West K: *Clinical procedures for medical assistants,* ed 7, St. Louis, 2008, Saunders.)

NEWBORN SCREENING TEST

A newborn screening test is performed on an infant to screen for the presence of certain metabolic and endocrine diseases. These diseases that are screened vary by state but typically include phenylketonuria (PKU), biotinidase deficiency, congenital adrenal hyperplasia, maple sugar urine disease, congenital hypothyroidism, galactosemia, homocystinuria, and sickle cell anemia. The most important of these is PKU, which is discussed in more detail in the following paragraphs.

PKU is a congenital hereditary disease caused by a lack of the enzyme *phenylalanine hydroxylase.* This enzyme is necessary to convert phenylalanine, an amino acid, into tyrosine, which is an amino acid necessary for normal metabolic functioning. Without this enzyme, phenylalanine accumulates in the blood and, if the accumulation is left untreated, causes mental retardation and other abnormalities, such as tremors and poor muscle coordination. In most cases, on early detection, a special low-phenylalanine diet and close periodic monitoring can prevent adverse effects. Normal development usually occurs if treatment is started before the child reaches 3 to 4 weeks of age. To promote the best development of cognitive abilities, most authorities recommend lifelong dietary restriction of phenylalanine. Although PKU is not a common condition (affecting 1 in every 12,000 births), early diagnosis and treatment lead to a better prognosis.

Phenylalanine can be detected in the blood of an affected infant only after the infant has been receiving breast or formula milk. Infants taking formula can be tested earlier than breastfed infants because formula contains phenylalanine, whereas the "first breast milk," or colostrum, does not. The test results of breastfed infants are usually invalid until the mother begins producing milk.

All states require by law that infants undergo newborn screening. The best time to perform the test is between 1 and 7 days after birth. In most states, the newborn screening test is performed before the infant leaves the hospital. If the test results come back indicating abnormal or invalid results, the infant needs to be retested. Most repeat tests are required because of invalid test results due to the collection of an

DIPHTHERIA TETANUS & PERTUSSIS VACCINES

W H A T Y O U N E E D T O K N O W

1 | Why get vaccinated?

Diphtheria, tetanus, and pertussis are serious diseases caused by bacteria. Diphtheria and pertussis are spread from person to person. Tetanus enters the body through cuts or wounds.

DIPHTHERIA causes a thick covering in the back of the throat.
• It can lead to breathing problems, paralysis, heart failure, and even death.

TETANUS (Lockjaw) causes painful tightening of the muscles, usually all over the body.
• It can lead to "locking" of the jaw so the victim cannot open his mouth or swallow. Tetanus leads to death in up to 2 out of 10 cases.

PERTUSSIS (Whooping Cough) causes coughing spells so bad that it is hard for infants to eat, drink, or breathe. These spells can last for weeks.
• It can lead to pneumonia, seizures (jerking and staring spells), brain damage, and death.

Diphtheria, tetanus, and pertussis vaccine (DTaP) can help prevent these diseases. Most children who are vaccinated with DTaP will be protected throughout childhood. Many more children would get these diseases if we stopped vaccinating.

DTaP is a safer version of an older vaccine called DTP. DTP is no longer used in the United States.

2 | Who should get DTaP vaccine and when?

Children should get 5 doses of DTaP vaccine, one dose at each of the following ages:

✓ 2 months   ✓ 4 months   ✓ 6 months
   ✓15-18 months   ✓ 4-6 years

DTaP may be given at the same time as other vaccines.

3 | Some children should not get DTaP vaccine or should wait

• Children with minor illnesses, such as a cold, may be vaccinated. But children who are moderately or severely ill should usually wait until they recover before getting DTaP vaccine.

• Any child who had a life-threatening allergic reaction after a dose of DTaP should not get another dose.

• Any child who suffered a brain or nervous system disease within 7 days after a dose of DTaP should not get another dose.

• Talk with your doctor if your child:
  - had a seizure or collapsed after a dose of DTaP,
  - cried non-stop for 3 hours or more after a dose of DTaP,
  - had a fever over 105°F after a dose of DTaP.

Ask your health care provider for more information. Some of these children should not get another dose of pertussis vaccine, but may get a vaccine without pertussis, called **DT**.

4 | Older children and adults

DTaP is not licensed for adolescents, adults, or children 7 years of age and older.

But older people still need protection. A vaccine called **Tdap** is similar to DTaP. A single dose of Tdap is recommended for people 11 through 64 years of age. Another vaccine, called **Td**, protects against tetanus and diphtheria, but not pertussis. It is recommended every 10 years. There are separate Vaccine Information Statements for these vaccines.

| Diphtheria/Tetanus/Pertussis | 5/17/2007 |

Figure 24-12. Vaccine information statement for DTaP. (Courtesy Centers for Disease Control and Prevention, Atlanta.)

Continued

5 | What are the risks from DTaP vaccine?

Getting diphtheria, tetanus, or pertussis disease is much riskier than getting DTaP vaccine.

However, a vaccine, like any medicine, is capable of causing serious problems, such as severe allergic reactions. The risk of DTaP vaccine causing serious harm, or death, is extremely small.

Mild Problems (Common)
- Fever (up to about 1 child in 4)
- Redness or swelling where the shot was given (up to about 1 child in 4)
- Soreness or tenderness where the shot was given (up to about 1 child in 4)

These problems occur more often after the 4th and 5th doses of the DTaP series than after earlier doses. Sometimes the 4th or 5th dose of DTaP vaccine is followed by swelling of the entire arm or leg in which the shot was given, lasting 1-7 days (up to about 1 child in 30).

Other mild problems include:
- Fussiness (up to about 1 child in 3)
- Tiredness or poor appetite (up to about 1 child in 10)
- Vomiting (up to about 1 child in 50)

These problems generally occur 1-3 days after the shot.

Moderate Problems (Uncommon)
- Seizure (jerking or staring) (about 1 child out of 14,000)
- Non-stop crying, for 3 hours or more (up to about 1 child out of 1,000)
- High fever, over 105°F (about 1 child out of 16,000)

Severe Problems (Very Rare)
- Serious allergic reaction (less than 1 out of a million doses)
- Several other severe problems have been reported after DTaP vaccine. These include:
  - Long-term seizures, coma, or lowered consciousness
  - Permanent brain damage.

  These are so rare it is hard to tell if they are caused by the vaccine.

Controlling fever is especially important for children who have had seizures, for any reason. It is also important if another family member has had seizures. You can reduce fever and pain by giving your child an *aspirin-free* pain reliever when the shot is given, and for the next 24 hours, following the package instructions.

6 | What if there is a moderate or severe reaction?

What should I look for?

Any unusual conditions, such as a serious allergic reaction, high fever or unusual behavior. Serious allergic reactions are extremely rare with any vaccine. If one were to occur, it would most likely be within a few minutes to a few hours after the shot. Signs can include difficulty breathing, hoarseness or wheezing, hives, paleness, weakness, a fast heart beat or dizziness. If a high fever or seizure were to occur, it would usually be within a week after the shot.

What should I do?

- **Call** a doctor, or get the person to a doctor right away.
- **Tell** your doctor what happened, the date and time it happened, and when the vaccination was given.
- **Ask** your doctor, nurse, or health department to report the reaction by filing a Vaccine Adverse Event Reporting System (VAERS) form.

Or you can file this report through the VAERS web site at **www.vaers.hhs.gov**, or by calling **1-800-822-7967**. *VAERS does not provide medical advice*

7 | The National Vaccine Injury Compensation Program

In the rare event that you or your child has a serious reaction to a vaccine, a federal program has been created to help pay for the care of those who have been harmed.

For details about the National Vaccine Injury Compensation Program, call **1-800-338-2382** or visit the program's website at **www.hrsa.gov/vaccinecompensation.**

8 | How can I learn more?

- Ask your health care provider. They can give you the vaccine package insert or suggest other sources of information.

- Call your local or state health department's immunization program.

- Contact the Centers for Disease Control and Prevention (CDC):
  - Call **1-800-232-4636 (1-800-CDC-INFO)**
  - Visit the National Immunization Program's website at **www.cdc.gov/nip**

U.S. DEPARTMENT OF HEALTH & HUMAN SERVICES
Centers for Disease Control and Prevention

Vaccine Information Statement	
DTaP (5/17/07)	42 U.S.C. § 300aa-26

Figure 24-12, cont'd.

PEDIATRIC VACCINE ADMINISTRATION RECORD

Name _____
     (first)   (MI)   (last)

DOB _____

Physician _____

Address _____
     _____

SITE ABBREVIATIONS:

RVL: Right vastus lateralis

LVL: Left vastus lateralis

RD: Right deltoid

LD: Left deltoid

Vaccine	Type of Vaccine[1] (generic abbreviation)	Date Given (mo/day/yr)	Dose	Site	Vaccine		Vaccine Information Statement		Signature of Vaccinator
					Lot #	Mfr.	Date on VIS	Date Given	
Hepatitis B[2] (e.g., HepB, Hib-HepB, DTaP-HepB-IPV) Give IM.									
Diphtheria, Tetanus, Pertussis[2] (e.g., DTaP, DTaP-Hib, DTaP-HepB-IPV, DT, Tdap, Td) Give IM.									
Haemophilus influenzae **type b**[2] (e.g., Hib, Hib-HepB, DTaP-Hib) Give IM.									
Polio[2] (e.g., IPV, DTaP-HepB-IPV) Give IPV SC or IM. Give DTaP-HepB-IPV IM.									
Pneumococcal (e.g., PCV, conjugate; PPV, polysaccharide) Give PCV IM. Give PPV SC or IM.									
Measles, Mumps, Rubella[5] (e.g., MMR, MMRV) Give SC.									
Varicella[5] (e.g., Var, MMRV) Give SC.									
Meningococcal (e.g., MCV4, conjugate; MPSV4, polysaccharide) Give MCV4 IM and MPSV4 SC.									
Influenza[5] (e.g., TIV, inactivated; LAIV, live attenuated) Give TIV IM. Give LAIV IN.									
Other									

1. Record the generic abbreviation for the type of vaccine given (e.g., DTaP-Hib, PCV), *not* the trade name.
2. For combination vaccines, fill in a row for each separate antigen in the combination.

Figure 24-13. Pediatric vaccine administration record. (Modified from Immunization Action Coalition, St. Paul, Minn.)

inadequate amount of the blood specimen. Newborn screening retesting is usually performed at a hospital laboratory but may sometimes be performed in the medical office.

The newborn screening test card (Figure 24-14) includes an information section that must be completed before the test is performed. The newborn screening test is performed on capillary blood obtained from the fleshy part of the lateral or medial posterior curve of the plantar surface of the infant's heel (Figure 24-15A and B). The blood specimen is placed on a special filter paper attached to the newborn screening test card (Figure 24-16) and mailed to an outside laboratory for analysis. The results are ready in a few days. If one of the newborn screening test results is positive, further testing is performed.

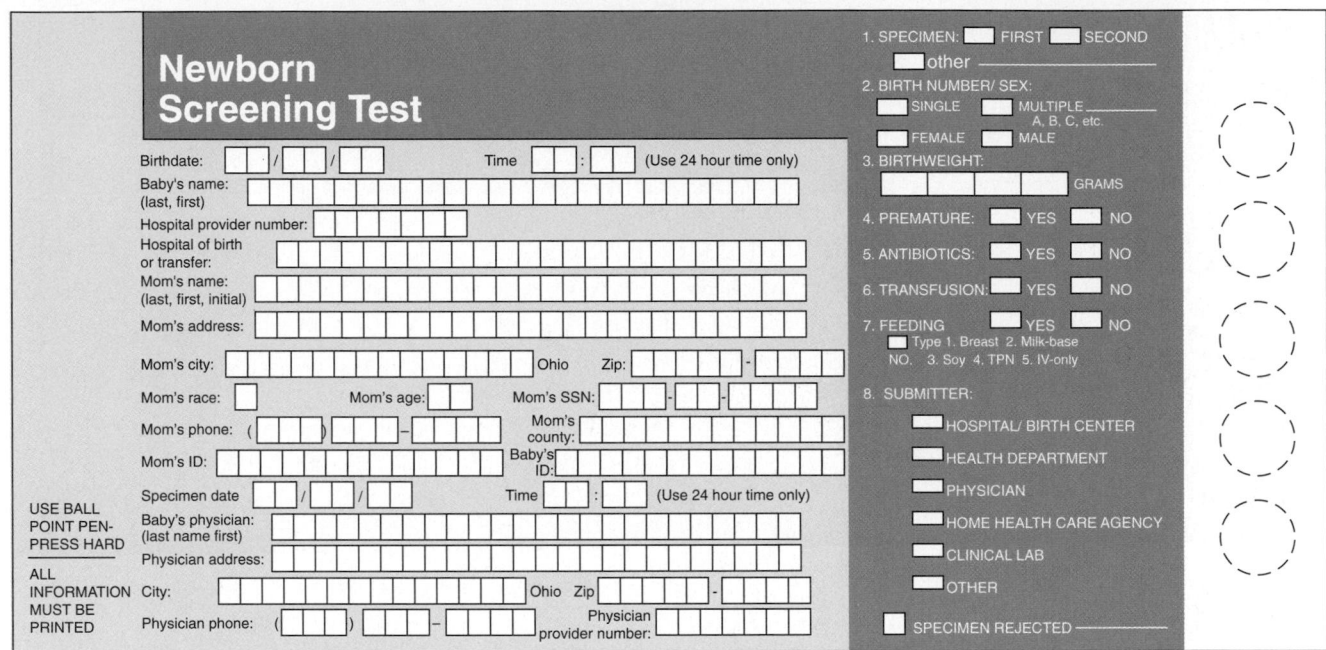

Figure 24-14. Newborn screening test card. (From Bonewit-West K: *Clinical procedures for medical assistants,* ed 7, St. Louis, 2008, Saunders.)

Figure 24-15. **A,** Heel puncture sites for a pediatric patient. **B,** Puncture of the medial posterior curve of the plantar surface of an infant's heel. (From Bonewit-West K: *Clinical procedures for medical assistants,* ed 7, St. Louis, 2008, Saunders.)

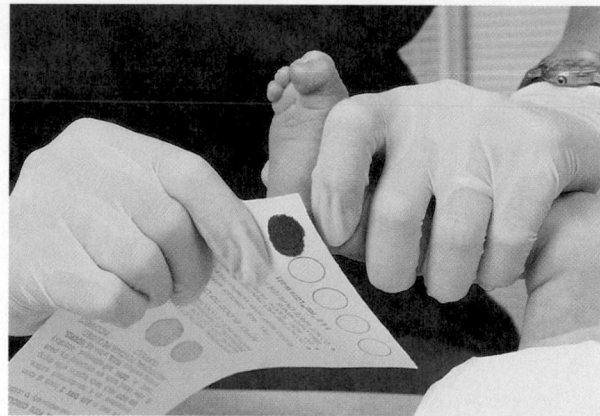

Figure 24-16. Applying a drop of blood to the first circle on the filter paper on the newborn screening test card. (From Bonewit-West K: *Clinical procedures for medical assistants,* ed 7, St. Louis, 2008, Saunders.)

MEDICAL PRACTICE *and the* LAW

Children are not small adults. They must be treated as individuals, according to their developmental level. Pediatric patients (except for emancipated minors) cannot give written or verbal consents. Make sure a parent or legal guardian is available for consent. A babysitter or grandparent cannot give consent for treatment without written permission from a parent or legal guardian. Similarly, patient information can be given only to a parent or legal guardian.

If your office sees pediatric patients, you have a responsibility to be aware of developmental needs and milestones of children at various ages. This is necessary for accurate developmental assessment. ■

What Would You Do? What Would You *Not* Do?   RESPONSES

Case Study 1
Page 498

What Did Traci Do?
❑ Listened patiently to Mrs. Chang and allowed her to vent her frustrations.
❑ Reassured Mrs. Chang that her milk is very nutritious for Christopher. Gave her a brochure on breastfeeding that included information on what to do for sore nipples and engorgement.
❑ Gave Mrs. Chang the names and phone numbers of community resources for nursing mothers.
❑ Told Mrs. Chang that Christopher's weight and length do not fall in the underweight category on his growth chart. Showed her Christopher's growth chart so that she could see that Christopher is progressing normally.

What Did Traci Not Do?
❑ Did not tell Mrs. Chang to cheer up because the colic would eventually go away on its own.
❑ Did not give a personal opinion on whether Mrs. Chang should breastfeed or bottle-feed her infant.

What Would You Do?/What Would You *Not* Do? Review Traci's response and place a checkmark next to the information you included in your response. List additional information included in your response.

_____

_____

_____

_____

Case Study 2
Page 509

What Did Traci Do?
❑ Explained to Mrs. Tilly that childhood obesity has doubled in the past 20 years and has become a serious health concern.
❑ Told Mrs. Tilly that she could have a big impact on Courtney's life by preparing healthy meals and eating them with her and by becoming involved in activities with Courtney, such as taking walks.
❑ Spent some time talking with Courtney about her interests and complimented Courtney on her achievements.

Continued

What Would You Do? What Would You *Not* Do? RESPONSES—cont'd

❏ Encouraged Courtney to join the swim team. Told her that lots of people do not like to be seen in a bathing suit and encouraged her not to let that stand in her way of doing something she wants to do.

❏ Reassured Courtney that the doctor wants to help her and that he would never say anything bad about her weight.

What Did Traci Not Do?

❏ Did not agree with Mrs. Tilly that there is nothing that can be done about Courtney's weight problem.

❏ Did not tell Courtney that she needs to lose weight or she might develop serious health problems such as diabetes.

What Would You Do?/What Would You *Not* Do? Review Traci's response and place a checkmark next to the information you included in your response. List additional information included in your response.

_____

_____

_____

_____

Case Study 3
Page 513

What Did Traci Do?

❏ Explained to Stacy that it is rare, but sometimes a child develops polio from getting the oral polio vaccine. Told her that this does not occur with the injectable polio vaccine.

❏ Explained to Stacy that chickenpox is usually a mild disease, but it can be serious, especially in young infants and adults.

❏ Explained to Stacy that most side effects from vaccines are mild, and the complications from the diseases far outweigh the possible side effects.

❏ Told Stacy that these diseases have been reduced to very low levels in the United States, but they still occur in other countries.

Explained that infected travelers can bring these diseases to the United States and infect individuals who are not immunized.

❏ Reminded Stacy that these immunizations are required for Matthew to start kindergarten.

❏ Talked with Matthew on his level about why he needs to be immunized.

❏ Told Matthew that they would play a game so that it would not hurt as much. Taught him to hold up his finger and pretend that it was a birthday candle; when the injection was given, told him to keep blowing out the candle until he was told to stop.

❏ Told Matthew that he could choose a prize from the treasure chest after he had his immunizations.

What Did Traci Not Do?

❏ Did not ignore or minimize Stacy's concerns.

❏ Did not tell Stacy that the answers to all her questions are in the vaccine information sheets that she was just given.

❏ Did not tell Stacy it would be all right to skip Matthew's immunizations.

❏ Did not refer to the immunizations as "shots" when talking with Matthew.

❏ Did not tell Matthew that it would not hurt when he gets his immunizations.

What Would You Do?/What Would You *Not* Do? Review Traci's response and place a checkmark next to the information you included in your response. List additional information included in your response.

_____

_____

_____

_____

⟲ TERMINOLOGY REVIEW

Adolescent An individual 12 to 18 years old.

Immunity The resistance of the body to the effects of a harmful agent, such as a pathogenic microorganism and its toxins.

Immunization (active, artificial) The process of becoming immune or of rendering an individual immune through the use of a vaccine or toxoid.

Infant A child from birth to 12 months old.

Length (recumbent) The measurement from the vertex of the head to the heel of the foot in a supine position.

Pediatrician A physician who specializes in the care and development of children and the diagnosis and treatment of children's diseases.

Pediatrics The branch of medicine that deals with the care and development of children and the diagnosis and treatment of children's diseases.

Preschool child A child 3 to 6 years old.

School-age child A child 6 to 12 years old.

Toddler A child 1 to 3 years old.

Toxoid A toxin (a poisonous substance produced by a bacterium) that has been treated by heat or chemicals to destroy its harmful properties. It is administered to an individual to prevent an infectious disease by stimulating the production of antibodies in that individual.

Vaccine A suspension of attenuated (weakened) or killed microorganisms administered to an individual to prevent an infectious disease by stimulating the production of antibodies in that individual.

Vertex The top of the head.

ON THE WEB

For Information on Child Health:

KidsHealth: www.kidshealth.com

Healthy Kids: www.healthykids.com

ParentCenter: parentcenter.babycenter.com

Pediatric on Call: www.pediatriconcall.com

Kids Source Online: www.kidsource.com

American Academy of Pediatrics: www.aap.org

For Information on Childhood Conditions:

Attention Deficit Hyperactivity Disorder: www.add-adhd.org

Attention Deficit Disorder Association: www.add.org

Cerebral Palsy: www.about-cerebral-palsy.org

American Academy for Cerebral Palsy and Developmental Medicine: www.aacpdm.org

Child Abuse: www.preventchildabuse.org

American Professional Society on the Abuse of Children: www.apsac.org

Cystic Fibrosis: www.cysticfibrosis.com

Cystic Fibrosis Foundation: www.cff.org

Dental Health: Colgate World of Care: www.colgate.com

American Dentistry Association: www.ada.org

The Tooth Fairy Online: www.asis.com/toothfairy

Diabetes: American Diabetes Association: www.diabetes.org

Children with Diabetes: www.childrenwithdiabetes.com

Down Syndrome: www.downsyndrome.com

Spina Bifida Association of America: www.sbaa.org

National SIDS/Infant Death Resource Center: www.sidscenter.org

Influenza Information: www.cdc.gov/flu

SIDS Alliance: www.sidsalliance.org

For Information on Immunizations:

Centers for Disease Control and Prevention: Vaccine Information Statements: www.cdc.gov/vaccines

American Academy of Pediatrics Childhood Immunization Support Program: www.cispimmunize.org

American Academy of Family Physicians: Recommendations for Immunizations: www.aafp.org

The Children's Hospital of Philadelphia Vaccine Education Center: www.chop.edu

Every Child by Two: www.ecbt.org

National Network for Immunization Information: www.immunizationinfo.org

---

PREPARE FOR CERTIFICATION   Visit the Evolve site at http://evolve.elsevier.com/Bonewit/today/ to actively Prepare for your Certification.

 Check out the **Companion CD** bound with the book to access additional interactive activities.

Conception: fertilize egg

14 days (gygot) 14 th day

embrio

Embryo; The child in utero from the time of conception to the beginning of the first trimester (first 2 months of development)

fetus: 3 month of first trimester (3 month after conception to birth;

Infant: birth to 1 year

Toddler: 1 to 3

Preschool: 3 to 6

School: 6 to 12

Adolescent: 12 to 18

25

Minor Office Surgery

LEARNING OBJECTIVES

Surgical Asepsis
1. Identify procedures that require the use of surgical asepsis.
2. Describe the medical assistant's responsibilities during a minor surgical procedure.
3. List the guidelines to follow to maintain surgical asepsis during a sterile procedure.
4. Identify and explain the use and care of instruments commonly used for minor office surgery.

Wound Healing
1. Explain the difference between a closed wound and an open wound, and give examples of each.
2. List and explain the three phases of the healing process.
3. List and describe the different types of wound drainage.
4. List the functions of a dressing.

Sutures
1. Explain the method used to measure the diameter of suturing material.
2. Describe the two types of sutures (absorbable and nonabsorbable), and give examples of their uses.
3. Categorize suturing needles according to type of point and shape.

Medical Office Surgical Procedures
1. Explain the purpose of and procedure for each of the following minor surgical operations: sebaceous cyst removal, incision and drainage of a localized infection, needle biopsy, ingrown toenail removal, colposcopy, cervical punch biopsy, and cryosurgery.
2. Explain the principles underlying each step in the minor office surgery procedures.

PROCEDURES

Apply and remove sterile gloves.
Open a sterile package.
Add an article to a sterile field.
Pour a sterile solution.

Change a sterile dressing.

Remove sutures.
Remove surgical staples.
Apply and remove adhesive skin closures.
Set up a tray for each of the following surgical procedures:
> Suture insertion
> Sebaceous cyst removal
> Incision and drainage of a localized infection
> Needle biopsy
> Ingrown toenail removal
> Colposcopy
> Cervical punch biopsy
> Cryosurgery

Assist the physician with minor office surgery.

CAAHEP COMPETENCIES

Clinical Competencies
Patient Care
- Prepare patient and assist with procedures, treatments, and minor office surgeries.

General Competencies
Legal Concepts
- Identify and respond to issues of confidentiality.
- Perform within legal and ethical boundaries.

Patient Instruction
- Provide instruction for health maintenance and disease prevention.

ABHES COMPETENCIES

Clinical Duties
- Prepare patient for procedures.
- Prepare patient for and assist physician with routine and specialty examinations and treatments and minor office surgeries.

Instruction
- Teach patients methods of health promotion and disease prevention.

Legal Concepts
- Determine needs for documentation and reporting.

abrasion (ah-BRAY-shun)
abscess (AB-sess)
absorbable suture (ab-SOR-ba-bul SOO-chur)
approximation (ah-PROKS-lh-MAY-shun)
bandage
biopsy (BYE-op-see)
capillary action (KAP-ill-air-ee AK-shun)
colposcope (KOL-poe-skope)
colposcopy (kol-POS-koe-pee)
contaminate (kon-TAM-in-ate)
contusion (kon-TOO-shun)
cryosurgery (KRY-oh-SURJ-er-ee)
exudate (EKS-oo-date)
fibroblast (FYE-broh-blast)
forceps (FORE-seps)
furuncle (FYOOR-un-kul)
hemostasis (hee-moe-STAY-sis)
incision (in-SIH-shun)
infection (in-FEK-shun)
infiltration (in-fill-TRAY-shun)

inflammation (in-flah-MAY-shun)
laceration (lass-ur-AY-shun)
ligate (LIH-gate)
local anesthetic (LOE-kul an-es-STET-ik)
Mayo (MAY-oe) tray
needle biopsy (NEE-dul BYE-op-see)
nonabsorbable suture (non-ab-SOR-ba-bul SOO-chur)
postoperative (post-OP-er-uh-tiv)
preoperative (pree-OP-er-uh-tiv)
puncture (PUNK-shur)
scalpel (SKAL-pul)
scissors
sebaceous cyst (suh-BAY-shus SIST)
serum (SEER-um)
sterile (STARE-ul)
surgical asepsis (SUR-jih-kul ay-SEP-sis)
sutures (SOO-churz)
swaged (SWAYJD) needle
wound

Introduction to Minor Office Surgery

Various types of minor surgical operations are performed in the medical office, such as insertion of sutures, sebaceous cyst removal, mole removal, incision and drainage of infections, needle biopsies, cervical biopsies, and ingrown toenail removal. The physician explains the nature of the surgical procedure and any risks to the patient and offers to answer questions. The medical assistant is responsible for explaining the patient preparation required for the procedure and for obtaining the patient's signature on a written consent to treatment form, which grants the physician permission to perform the surgery (Figure 25-1).

Additional responsibilities of the medical assistant include preparing the treatment room, preparing the patient, preparing the minor surgery tray, assisting the physician during the procedure, administering postoperative care to the patient, and cleaning the treatment room after the procedure.

The treatment room must be spotlessly clean, and the medical assistant should ensure that the physician has adequate lighting for the procedure. The patient is positioned and draped according to the procedure to be performed. The skin is prepared as specified by the physician. Hair around the operative site is a contaminant and may need to be removed by shaving. The skin is cleansed, and an appropriate antiseptic is applied to the area to reduce the number of microorganisms present.

The medical assistant prepares the minor surgery tray using **sterile** technique. The specific instruments and sup-

plies included in each setup vary, depending on the type of surgery to be performed and the physician's preference. The medical assistant must become familiar with the instruments and supplies required for each surgical procedure performed in the medical office.

During the minor surgery, the medical assistant is present to assist the physician as needed and to lend support to the patient. The medical assistant should become completely familiar with the assisting techniques (e.g., swabbing blood from the operative site) required for each surgical procedure performed in the medical office and learn to anticipate the physician's needs to help the procedure go quickly and smoothly.

After the minor surgery, the medical assistant should remain with the patient as a safety precaution to prevent accidental falls and other injuries and to make sure the patient understands the postoperative instructions. The medical assistant removes and properly cares for all used instruments and supplies and cleans the treatment room in preparation for the next patient.

SURGICAL ASEPSIS

Surgical asepsis, also known as *sterile technique,* refers to practices that keep objects and areas sterile, or free from all living microorganisms and spores. Surgical asepsis protects the patient from pathogenic microorganisms that may enter the body and cause disease. It is always employed under the following circumstances: when caring for broken skin, such as open wounds and suture punctures; when a skin surface

---

(attach label or complete blanks)

First name: _____ Last name: _____

Date of Birth: _____ Month _____ Day _____ Year

Account Number: _____

Procedure Consent Form

I, _____, hereby consent to have

Dr. _____ perform _____.

I have been fully informed of the following by my physician:

1. The nature of my condition.
2. The nature and purpose of the procedure.
3. An explanation of risks involved with the procedure.
4. Alternative treatments or procedures available.
5. The likely results of the procedure.
6. The risks involved with declining or delaying the procedure.

My physician has offered to answer all questions concerning the proposed procedure.

I am aware that the practice of medicine and surgery is not an exact science, and I acknowledge that no guarantees have been made to me about the results of the procedure.

Patient _____   Date _____
        (or guardian and relationship)

Witnessed _____   Date _____

Figure 25-1. Consent to treatment form. (From Bonewit-West K: *Clinical procedures for medical assistants,* ed 7, St. Louis, 2008, Saunders.)

is being penetrated, as by a surgical incision for a mole removal or the administration of an injection (the needle must remain sterile); and when a body cavity is entered that is normally sterile, such as during the insertion of a urinary catheter. Sterility of instruments and supplies is achieved through the use of disposable sterile items or by sterilizing reusable articles.

A sterile object that touches any unsterile object is automatically considered contaminated and must not be used. If the medical assistant is in doubt or has a question concerning the sterility of an article, he or she should consider it contaminated and replace it with a sterile article.

Sterility of the hands cannot be attained. Sanitizing the hands renders them medically aseptic and must be performed before and after every surgical procedure using proper technique (see Chapter 17). To prevent contamination of sterile articles, sterile gloves must be worn while picking up or transferring articles during a sterile procedure. Procedure 25-1 describes the procedure for applying and removing sterile gloves.

Specific guidelines must be observed during a sterile procedure to maintain surgical asepsis. See the accompanying box on *Guidelines for Surgical Asepsis.*

INSTRUMENTS USED IN MINOR OFFICE SURGERY

A variety of surgical instruments are used for minor office surgery. Most instruments are made of stainless steel and have either a bright, highly polished finish or a dull finish. The medical assistant should become familiar with the name, use, and proper care of all instruments used in the medical office. Some common instruments are described here and are illustrated in Figure 25-2.

Scalpels

A **scalpel** is a small, straight surgical knife consisting of a handle and a thin, sharp blade that has a convex edge. It is used to make surgical incisions and can divide tissue with the least possible trauma to the surrounding structures. Both reusable and disposable scalpels are available; scalpels that have a reusable handle and a disposable blade are used most frequently.

Scissors

Scissors are cutting instruments that have straight (str) or curved (cvd) blades. Both blade tips may be sharp (s/s), both may be blunt (b/b), or one tip may be blunt and the other sharp (b/s). The two parts of a pair of scissors come together

Guidelines for Surgical Asepsis

1. Take precautions to prevent sterile packages from becoming wet. Wet packages draw microorganisms into the package owing to the **capillary action** of the liquid, resulting in contamination of the sterile package. If a sterile package that has been prepared at the medical office becomes wet, it must be rewrapped and resterilized; if a disposable sterile package becomes wet, it must be discarded.
2. A 1-inch border around the sterile field is considered contaminated or unsterile because this area may have become contaminated while the sterile field was being set up.
3. Always face the sterile field. If you must turn your back to it or leave the room, a sterile towel must be placed over the sterile field.
4. Hold all sterile articles above waist level. Anything out of sight might become contaminated. The sterile articles also should be held in front of you and should not touch your uniform.
5. To avoid contamination, place all sterile items in the center, not around the edges, of the sterile field.
6. Be careful not to spill water or solutions on the sterile field. The area beneath the field is contaminated, and microorganisms are drawn up onto the field by the capillary action of the liquid, resulting in contamination of the field.
7. Do not talk, cough, or sneeze over a sterile field. Water vapor from the nose, mouth, and lungs is carried outward by the air and contaminates the sterile field.
8. Do not reach over a sterile field. Dust or lint from your clothing may fall onto it, or your unsterile clothing may accidentally touch it.
9. Do not pass soiled dressings over the sterile field.
10. Always acknowledge if you have contaminated the sterile field so that proper steps can be taken to regain sterility.

at a hinge joint known as a *box lock.* The type of scissors employed depends on the intended use. The various types of scissors are listed and described next.

- *Operating scissors* have straight, delicate blades with sharp cutting edges and are used to cut through tissue. They are available with sharp/sharp, blunt/blunt, or blunt/sharp tips.
- *Suture scissors* are used to remove sutures. The hook on the tip aids in getting under a suture, and the blunt end prevents puncturing of the tissues.
- *Bandage scissors* are inserted beneath a dressing or bandage to cut it for removal. The flat blunt prow can be inserted beneath a dressing without puncturing the skin.
- *Dissecting scissors* have thick blades with a fine cutting edge used to divide tissue and are available with straight or curved blades. Both blade tips of dissecting scissors are blunt.

Forceps

Forceps are two-pronged instruments for grasping and squeezing. Some forceps have a spring handle (e.g., thumb, tissue, splinter, and dressing forceps) that provides the proper tension for grasping tissue. As shown in Figure 25-2, some varieties have toothed clasps on the handle, known as *ratchets,* to hold the tips securely together (e.g., Allis tissue forceps, hemostatic forceps, sponge forceps). The ratchets are designed to allow closure of the instrument at three or more positions. The various types of forceps are listed and described next.

- *Thumb forceps* have serrated tips and are used to pick up tissue or to hold tissue between adjacent surfaces. Serrations are sawlike teeth that grasp tissue and prevent it from slipping out of the jaws of the instrument.
- *Tissue forceps* have teeth to prevent them from slipping and are used to grasp tissue. Tissue forceps are identified by the number of apposing teeth on each jaw (e.g., 1 × 2,

2 × 3, 3 × 4). The teeth should approximate tightly when the instrument is closed.
- *Splinter forceps* have sharp points that are useful in removing foreign objects, such as splinters, from the tissues.
- *Dressing forceps* are used in the application and removal of dressings. They have blunt ends that contain coarse cross-striations used for grasping.
- **Hemostatic forceps** have serrated tips, ratchets, and box locks and are available with straight or curved blades. Hemostats are used to clamp off blood vessels and to establish **hemostasis** until the vessels can be closed with sutures. The ratchets keep the hemostat tightly shut when it is closed. They should mesh together smoothly when the instrument is closed; if they spring back open, the instrument is in need of repair. The serrations on a hemostat prevent the blood vessel from slipping out of the jaws of the instrument.
- *Sponge forceps,* as the name implies, have large serrated rings on the tips for holding sponges. A *sponge* is a porous, absorbent pad, such as a 4-inch gauze pad, used to absorb fluids, apply medication, or cleanse an area.

Miscellaneous Instruments

Various miscellaneous instruments used in the medical office are listed and described next.

- *Needle holders* have serrated tips, ratchets, and box locks; they are used to grasp a curved needle firmly to insert it through the skin flaps of an incision.
- *Retractors* are used to hold tissues aside to improve the exposure of the operative area.

Care of Surgical Instruments

Surgical instruments are expensive, are delicate yet durable, and last for many years if handled and maintained properly. The care an instrument receives depends to a large degree

Figure 25-2. Instruments used in minor office surgery. (Courtesy Elmed, Addison, Ill.)

Continued

on the parts making up the instrument (e.g., box lock, ratchet, cutting edge, serrations). The medical assistant works with instruments while setting up a sterile tray, performing certain procedures such as suture removal and sterile dressing change, and cleaning up after minor office surgery and during the sanitization and sterilization process. During each of these procedures, guidelines must be followed to prolong the life span of each instrument and to ensure its proper functioning:

1. Always handle instruments carefully. Dropping an instrument on the floor or throwing an instrument into a basin could damage it.
2. Do not pile instruments in a heap because they become entangled and might be damaged when separated.
3. Keep sharp instruments separate from the rest of the instruments to prevent damaging or dulling the cutting edge. Also, keep delicate instruments, such as lensed instruments, separate to protect them from damage.
4. To prolong the proper functioning of the ratchet, keep instruments with a ratchet in an open position when not in use.

5. Rinse blood and body secretions off an instrument as soon as possible to prevent them from drying and hardening on the instrument.
6. When performing procedures that require surgical instruments, always use the instrument for the purpose for which it was designed. Substituting one type of instrument for another could damage it.
7. Sanitize and sterilize instruments using proper technique.

COMMERCIALLY PREPARED STERILE PACKAGES

Commercially prepared disposable packages are used frequently and may contain one particular article (e.g., sterile dressing) or a complete sterile setup (e.g., one for the removal of sutures). The directions for opening the package are stated on the outside of the package; they should be followed carefully to prevent contamination of the sterile contents. Procedure 25-2 describes opening a sterile package.

Figure 25-2, cont'd.

Putting It All into Practice

My name is Trudy Browning, and I have worked as the office manager of an internal medicine office for the past 7 years. My job includes front and back office duties, including scheduling appointments, transcription, patient calls, patient workups, injections, electrocardiograms, and venipuncture. The most interesting part of my job is dealing with the many different personalities of the patients that I come in contact with daily.

A patient who had not been to the clinic for a while came in one day. His graduation from college had been delayed because he had developed a pilonidal cyst that needed to be surgically removed. At onset, these cysts can be very painful and usually require daily cleaning and packing. From my experience with pilonidal cyst care, I knew that 1 to 2 months of treatment is usually required before full recovery is achieved.

The physician and I prepared for the initial treatment and noticed the surgical site was very large and deep. We knew this treatment would take much longer than usual. Treatment was provided daily for 3 months. Subsequent treatments continued every other day for 2 months. Through our continuous contact, we became good friends with the patient.

Our patient graduated at the end of the spring quarter and moved out of state. He stays in contact with us and is still undergoing treatment. He made a difference in our lives because he always maintained a positive attitude and was very pleasant, making our job easier. We made a difference in his life through the good health care we provided and our continuing friendship. ■

One type of commercially prepared package is the peel-apart package (commonly referred to as a *peel-pack*). This type of sterile package has an edge with two flaps that can be pulled apart in the following manner: Grasp each unsterile flap between your bent index finger and extended thumb and, rolling your hands outward, pull the package apart (Figure 25-3A). The inside of the wrapper and the contents are sterile, and to prevent contamination, they must not be touched with bare hands. The medical assistant can place the contents of the peel-pack directly on the sterile field by step-

Halsted Mosquito
Hemostatic Forceps
Straight or Curved

Kelly Hemostatic
Forceps
Straight or Curved

Foerster
Sponge Forceps

Rochester-Pean
Hemostatic Forceps
Straight or Curved

Ochsner-Kocher Hemostatic
Forceps Straight or Curved
1 × 2 Teeth

Crile-Wood
Needle Holder

Volkmann Rake Retractor

Sharp   Blunt

Senn-Mueller Retractor

Figure 25-2, cont'd.

ping back slightly from the field and gently ejecting or "flipping" the contents onto the center of the sterile field (Figure 25-3B). Stepping back prevents the unsterile outer wrapper and the medical assistant's hands from crossing over the sterile field, which would result in contamination.

The contents of the package can also be removed with a sterile gloved hand. This technique is useful during minor office surgery when the physician needs additional supplies, such as gauze pads and sutures. The medical assistant opens the sterile package, and the physician removes the sterile contents from the package using a gloved hand (Figure 25-3C). The inside of the package can be used as a sterile field by opening the peel-apart package completely and laying it flat on a clean, dry surface (Figure 25-3D).

Once a sterile package has been opened and set up, the medical assistant may need to pour a sterile solution, such as an antiseptic, into a container located on the field. To do so, the steps of surgical asepsis outlined in Procedure 25-3 should be followed.

Text continued on p. 537

Figure 25-3. Methods for removing the sterile contents of a peel-apart package so that sterility is maintained. **A,** Grasp each flap between a bent index finger and an extended thumb and roll hands outward to pull apart. **B,** Step back and eject the contents onto the field. **C,** The medical assistant opens the pack, and the physician removes the sterile contents with a gloved hand. **D,** The inside of the peel-apart package can be used as a sterile field. (From Bonewit-West K: *Clinical procedures for medical assistants,* ed 7, St. Louis, 2008, Saunders.)

PROCEDURE 25-1   Applying and Removing Sterile Gloves

Outcome Apply and remove sterile gloves.

The medical assistant must wear sterile gloves to perform a sterile procedure, such as a dressing change, or to assist the physician during minor office surgery. The medical assistant must learn to put on the gloves using the principles of surgical asepsis so as not to contaminate them.

Gloves must be removed in a manner that protects the medical assistant from contaminating the clean hands with pathogens that might be on the outside of the gloves. This is accomplished by not allowing the bare hands to come in contact with the outside of the gloves.

Equipment/Supplies

- Sterile gloves

Applying Sterile Gloves

1. **Procedural Step.** Remove all rings and put them in a safe place. Wash your hands with an antimicrobial soap.

   Principle. Rings may cause the gloves to tear. The warm, moist environment inside gloves provides ideal growing conditions for the multiplication of transient microorganisms on the hands. Washing the hands with an antimicrobial removes these microorganisms and also deposits an antibacterial film on your hands to discourage the growth of bacteria. This prevents the transmission of pathogens.

2. **Procedural Step.** Choose the appropriate-sized gloves; they should not be too small or too large. The gloves should fit snugly but not be too tight.

   Principle. If your gloves are too small, they may rip as you apply them or become uncomfortable to wear. If they are too large, you may find it difficult to perform your tasks.

3. **Procedural Step.** Place the glove package on a clean, flat surface. Open the glove package without touching the inside of the wrapper. The tops of the gloves are turned down to form a cuff.

   Principle. The hands are not sterile, and the inside of the wrapper is sterile.

4. **Procedural Step.** Pick up the first glove on the inside of the cuff with the fingers of the opposite hand, being sure not to touch the outside of the glove with your ungloved hand.

   Principle. After applying the gloves, the inside of the cuff lies next to your skin and does not remain sterile; therefore it is permissible to pick up the glove by the cuff. The outside of the glove is sterile, and touching it would contaminate it. If a glove becomes contaminated, you must obtain a new pair of gloves and repeat the procedure.

Pick up the first glove on the inside of the cuff. (From Bonewit-West K: *Clinical procedures for medical assistants,* ed 7, St. Louis, 2008, Saunders.)

5. **Procedural Step.** Step back and pull the glove on. Allow the cuff to remain turned back on itself.

   Principle. Stepping back prevents your unsterile hand from passing over the glove still in the glove package, which would contaminate it.

6. **Procedural Step.** Pick up the second glove by slipping your sterile gloved fingers under its cuff and grasping the opposite side the cuff with your thumb.

   Principle. The cuff is sterile and may be touched by the sterile gloved hand.

Pick up the second glove. (From Bonewit-West K: *Clinical procedures for medical assistants,* ed 7, St. Louis, 2008, Saunders.)

7. **Procedural Step.** Remove your thumb from the cuff and pull the glove on. Turn back the cuff.

Turn back the cuff. (From Bonewit-West K: *Clinical procedures for medical assistants,* ed 7, St. Louis, 2008, Saunders.)

8. **Procedural Step.** Turn back the cuff of the first glove by reaching under the cuff with the other gloved hand. Do not allow the sterile glove to come in contact with the inside of the cuff. Adjust the gloves to a comfortable position. Inspect the gloves for tears.

Continued

PROCEDURE **25-1**   Applying and Removing Sterile Gloves—cont'd

Principle. The area under the folded cuff is sterile and may be touched by the sterile gloved hand. The inside of the cuff has previously been touched by your clean hands and is not sterile. If a tear is present, a new pair of gloves must be applied.

Removing Sterile Gloves

1. Procedural Step. With your gloved left hand, grasp the outside of the right glove 1 to 2 inches from the top. (*Note:* It does not matter which glove is removed first—you may start with the left glove if you prefer.)

Grasp the outside of the glove. (From Bonewit-West K: *Clinical procedures for medical assistants,* ed 7, St. Louis, 2008, Saunders.)

2. Procedural Step. Slowly pull the right glove off the hand. It turns inside out as it is removed from your hand.

3. Procedural Step. Pull the right glove free, and scrunch it into a ball with your gloved left hand.

Scrunch the glove into a ball. (From Bonewit-West K: *Clinical procedures for medical assistants,* ed 7, St. Louis, 2008, Saunders.)

4. Procedural Step. Place the index and middle fingers of the right hand on the inside of the left glove. Do not allow your clean hand to touch the outside of the glove.

Place the fingers on the inside of the glove. (From Bonewit-West K: *Clinical procedures for medical assistants,* ed 7, St. Louis, 2008, Saunders.)

5. Procedural Step. Pull the second glove off the left hand. It turns inside out as it is removed from your hand, enclosing the balled-up right glove. Discard both gloves in an appropriate waste container. If your gloves are visibly contaminated with blood or other potentially infectious materials, discard them in a biohazard waste container; otherwise, they can be discarded in a regular waste container.

Pull the glove off the hand. (From Bonewit-West K: *Clinical procedures for medical assistants,* ed 7, St. Louis, 2008, Saunders.)

6. Procedural Step. Sanitize your hands thoroughly to remove any microorganisms that may have come in contact with your hands.

PROCEDURE 25-2 · Opening a Sterile Package

Outcome Open a sterile package. A sterile package that has been wrapped after the procedure for wrapping presented in Chapter 18 is opened using the procedure outlined here. The sterile package may be in the form of a commercially prepared disposable package (e.g., sterile dressing change) or a pack that has been assembled and sterilized at the medical office (e.g., sebaceous cyst removal pack); in both cases, the inside of the sterile wrapper serves as the sterile field.

Equipment/Supplies

- Sterile package

1. **Procedural Step.** Sanitize your hands.
2. **Procedural Step.** Assemble the equipment.
3. **Procedural Step.** Check the pack to make sure it is not wet, torn, or opened. These factors cause contamination of the sterile contents and the pack must not be used. If autoclave tape has been used to close the pack, check to make sure the tape has changed color.
   Principle. Autoclave tape indicates the pack has been through the sterilization process, but it does not verify that the contents of the pack are sterile.

Check the sterilization indicator. (From Bonewit-West K: *Clinical procedures for medical assistants,* ed 7, St. Louis, 2008, Saunders.)

4. **Procedural Step.** Place the wrapped package on the table so that the top flap of the wrapper opens away from you. Always face the sterile field and do not talk, laugh, cough, or sneeze over the field. These actions contaminate the sterile field.
5. **Procedural Step.** Loosen and remove the fastener on the wrapped package, and discard it in a waste container.

6. **Procedural Step.** Open the first flap away from the body. Handle only the outside of the wrapper.
   Principle. The medical assistant should open the sterile package so as not to reach over the sterile contents. Otherwise, dust or lint from unsterile clothing may fall on the contents of the package and cause contamination.

Open the first flap away from the body. (From Bonewit-West K: *Clinical procedures for medical assistants,* ed 7, St. Louis, 2008, Saunders.)

7. **Procedural Step.** Without crossing over the sterile field, open the left and right flaps.
8. **Procedural Step.** Open the flap closest to the body by lifting it toward you. Touch only the outside of the wrapper.
9. **Procedural Step.** Adjust the sterile wrapper by the corners as needed to make sure it lies in proper position on the tray or table.
10. **Procedural Step.** Check the sterilization indicator on the inside of the pack to make sure it has changed appropriately. This indicates the contents of the pack are sterile.

Continued

PROCEDURE 25-2

Open the left and right flaps. (From Bonewit-West K: *Clinical procedures for medical assistants,* ed 7, St. Louis, 2008, Saunders.)

Open the flap closest to the body. (From Bonewit-West K: *Clinical procedures for medical assistants,* ed 7, St. Louis, 2008, Saunders.)

PROCEDURE 25-3   Pouring a Sterile Solution

Outcome Pour a sterile solution.

Equipment/Supplies

- Sterile solution
- Sterile container
- Sterile towel

1. **Procedural Step.** Read the label of the solution to ensure that you have the correct solution.
2. **Procedural Step.** Check the expiration date on the solution. Do not use an outdated solution.
   Principle. Outdated solutions may produce undesirable effects and should be discarded.
3. **Procedural Step.** Check the solution label a second time to make sure you have the correct solution.
4. **Procedural Step.** Place the palm of your hand over the label. Remove the cap by touching only the outside and place the cap on a flat surface with the open end up. Do not place the cap on the sterile field, as the outside of the cap is contaminated.
   Principle. Palming the label prevents the solution from dripping on the label and obscuring it. Handling the cap by the outside prevents contamination of the inside. Placing the cap with the open end up prevents contamination of the inside of the cap by an unsterile surface.
5. **Procedural Step.** Rinse the lip of the bottle (if it has been previously used) by pouring a small amount of solution into a separate container.
   Principle. Rinsing the lip washes away any microorganisms that may be on it.
6. **Procedural Step.** Pour the proper amount of solution into the sterile container at a height of approximately

6 inches. Do not allow the neck of the bottle to come in contact with the sterile container, and be careful not to splash solution onto the sterile field.
Principle. Pouring from a height of approximately 6 inches reduces splashing and prevents contamination of the sterile container with the outside of the (unsterile) bottle.

Pour the proper amount of solution. (From Bonewit-West K: *Clinical procedures for medical assistants,* ed 7, St. Louis, 2008, Saunders.)

7. **Procedural Step.** Replace the cap on the container without contaminating it. Check the label a third time to ensure that you have poured the correct solution.

WOUNDS

A **wound** is a break in the continuity of an external or internal surface caused by physical means. Wounds can be accidental or intentional (as when the physician makes an incision during a surgical operation). The two basic types of wounds are closed and open.

A *closed wound* involves an injury to the underlying tissues of the body without a break in the skin surface or mucous membrane; an example is a contusion, or bruise. A **contusion** results when the tissues under the skin are injured and is often caused by a blunt object. Blood vessels rupture, allowing blood to seep into the tissues, which results in a bluish discoloration of the skin. After several days, the color of the contusion turns greenish yellow as a result of oxidation of blood pigments. Bruising commonly occurs with injuries such as fractures, sprains, strains, and black eyes. *Open wounds* involve a break in the skin surface or mucous membrane that exposes the underlying tissues; examples include incisions, lacerations, punctures, and abrasions. Figure 25-4 illustrates specific wounds.

- An **incision** is a clean, smooth cut caused by a sharp instrument, such as a knife, razor, or piece of glass. Deep incisions are accompanied by profuse bleeding; in addition, damage to muscles, tendons, and nerves may occur.
- A **laceration** is a wound in which the tissues are torn apart, rather than cut, leaving ragged and irregular edges. Lacerations are caused by dull knives, large objects that have been driven into the skin, and heavy machinery. Deep lacerations result in profuse bleeding, and a scar often results from the jagged tearing of the tissues.

- A **puncture** is a wound made by a sharp-pointed object piercing the skin layers—for example, a nail, splinter, needle, wire, knife, bullet, or animal bite. A puncture wound has a very small external skin opening, and for this reason bleeding is usually minor. A tetanus booster may be administered with this type of wound because the tetanus bacteria grow best in a warm anaerobic environment, such as the one in a puncture.
- An **abrasion** or scrape is a wound in which the outer layers of the skin are scraped or rubbed off, resulting in an oozing of blood from ruptured capillaries. Abrasions are often caused by falling on gravel and floors (floor burn). These falls can result in skinned knees and elbows.

Wound Healing

The skin is a protective barrier for the body and is considered its first line of defense. When the surface of the skin has been broken, it is easy for microorganisms to enter and cause **infection.** The body has a natural healing process that works to destroy invading microorganisms and to restore the structure and function of the damaged tissues, as is described next.

Phases of Wound Healing

Wound healing occurs in three phases, which are described here and illustrated in Figure 25-5.

Phase 1

Phase 1, also called the *inflammatory phase,* begins as soon as the body is injured. This phase lasts approximately 3 to 4 days. During this phase, a fibrin network forms, resulting

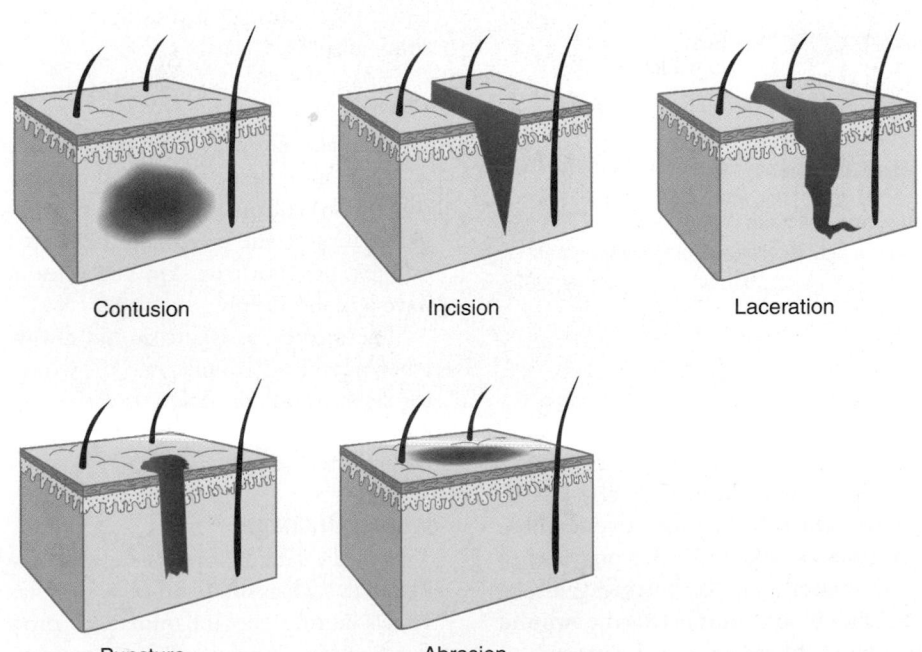

Contusion   Incision   Laceration

Puncture   Abrasion

Figure 25-4. Types of wounds. (From Bonewit-West K: *Clinical procedures for medical assistants,* ed 7, St. Louis, 2008, Saunders.)

PATIENT TEACHING | **Wound Care**

Explain the following to the patient regarding wounds:
- The type of wound that the patient has: incision, laceration, puncture, or abrasion.
- The purpose of suturing the wound: to close the skin and protect against further contamination, to facilitate healing, and to leave a smaller scar.
- If a tetanus toxoid has been administered, explain the purpose of this immunization: to protect against tetanus (lockjaw).
- Teach the patient how to care for the wound, as follows:
  - Keep the dressing clean and dry. If it becomes wet, contact the medical office to schedule a sterile dressing change.
  - Apply an ice bag for swelling (if prescribed by the physician).

- Report immediately any signs that the wound is infected. These signs include:
  a. Fever
  b. Persistent or increased pain, swelling, or drainage
  c. Red streaks radiating away from the wound
  d. Increased redness or warmth
- Notify the office if the sutures become loose or break.
- Return as instructed by the physician for the removal of sutures.
- Teach the patient how to apply an ice bag (if prescribed by the physician).
- Give the patient written instructions on wound care to refer to at home. ■

Phase 1: Inflammatory Phase

Phase 2: Granulation Phase

Phase 3: Maturation Phase

Figure 25-5. Phases of wound healing. (From Bonewit-West K: *Clinical procedures for medical assistants,* ed 7, St. Louis, 2008, Saunders.)

in a blood clot that "plugs" up the opening of the wound and stops the flow of blood. The blood clot eventually becomes the scab. The inflammatory process also occurs during this phase. **Inflammation** is the protective response of the body to trauma, such as cuts and abrasions, and to the entrance of foreign matter, such as microorganisms. During inflammation, the blood supply to the wound increases, which brings white blood cells and nutrients to the site to assist in the healing process. The four local signs of inflammation are redness, swelling, pain, and warmth.

The purpose of inflammation is to destroy invading microorganisms and to remove damaged tissue debris from the area so that proper healing can occur.

Phase 2

Phase 2 is also called the *granulation phase* and typically lasts 4 to 20 days. During this phase, **fibroblasts** migrate to the wound and begin to synthesize collagen. Collagen is a white protein that provides strength to the wound. As the amount of collagen increases, the wound becomes stronger, and the chance that the wound will open decreases. There also is a growth of new capillaries during this phase to provide the damaged tissue with an abundant supply of blood. As the capillary network develops, the tissue becomes a translucent red color. This tissue is known as *granulation tissue*. Granulation tissue consists primarily of collagen and is fragile and shiny and bleeds easily.

Phase 3

Phase 3, also known as the *maturation phase,* begins as soon as granulation tissue forms and can last for 2 years. During this phase, collagen continues to be synthesized, and the granulation tissue eventually hardens to white scar tissue. Scar tissue is not true skin and does not contain nerves or have a blood supply.

The medical assistant should always inspect the wound when providing wound care. The wound should be observed for signs of inflammation and the amount of healing that has occurred. This information should be charted in the patient's record.

Wound Drainage

The medical term for drainage is **exudate.** An exudate is material, such as fluid and cells, that has escaped from blood vessels during the inflammatory process. The exudate is deposited in tissue or on tissue surfaces and is often present in a wound. When providing wound care, the medical assistant should always inspect the wound for drainage and chart this information in the patient's record. There are three major types of exudates: serous, sanguineous, and purulent.

- **Serous exudate.** A serous exudate consists chiefly of **serum,** which is the clear portion of the blood. Serous drainage is clear and watery. An example of a serous exudate is the fluid in a blister from a burn.
- **Sanguineous exudate.** A sanguineous exudate is red and consists of red blood cells. This type of drainage results when capillaries are damaged, allowing the escape of red blood cells, and is frequently seen in open wounds. A bright-red sanguineous exudate indicates fresh bleeding, and a dark exudate indicates older bleeding.
- **Purulent exudate.** A purulent exudate contains pus, which consists of leukocytes, dead liquefied tissue debris, and dead and living bacteria. Purulent drainage is usually thick and has an unpleasant odor. It is white in color but may acquire tinges of pink, green, or yellow depending on the type of infecting organism. The process of pus formation is *suppuration.*

In addition to the exudates just described, mixed types of exudates are often observed in a wound. A *serosanguineous exudate* consists of clear and blood-tinged drainage and is commonly seen in surgical incisions. A *purosanguineous exudate* consists of pus and blood and is often seen in a new wound that is infected.

STERILE DRESSING CHANGE

Surgical asepsis must be maintained when one is caring for and applying a dry sterile dressing (abbreviated as *DSD*) to an open wound. The medical assistant must take care to prevent infection in clean wounds and to decrease infection in wounds already infected. The function of a sterile dressing is to protect the wound from contamination and trauma, to absorb drainage, and to restrict motion, which may interfere with proper wound healing. The size, type, and amount of dressing material used during a sterile dressing change depend on the size and location of the wound and the amount of drainage.

Sterile folded *gauze pads* are used in the medical office for a sterile dressing change. This type of dressing absorbs drainage, but the gauze has a tendency to stick to the wound when the drainage dries. Gauze pads come in a variety of sizes, including 4×4, 3×3, and 2×2; the 4×4 size is used most frequently.

Nonadherent pads are also used as a sterile dressing; they have one surface impregnated with agents that prevent the dressing from sticking to the wound. One brand of this type of material is Telfa pads. The nonadherent side, which is shiny, is placed next to the wound. Telfa dressings are often used to cover burned skin. Procedure 25-4 presents the procedure for changing a sterile dressing.

Petrolium jelly

 PROCEDURE 25-4   Changing a Sterile Dressing

Outcome Change a sterile dressing.

Equipment/Supplies

- Mayo stand
- Biohazard waste container

Side Table

- Clean disposable gloves
- Antiseptic swabs
- Sterile gloves
- Plastic waste bag
- Hypoallergenic adhesive tape
- Scissors

Sterile Field

- Sterile dressing
- Sterile thumb forceps

1. **Procedural Step.** Wash your hands with an antimicrobial soap.
2. **Procedural Step.** Assemble the equipment. Set up the nonsterile items on a side table or counter. Position the waterproof waste bag in a location convenient for disposal of contaminated items.

Prepare the side table. (From Bonewit-West K: *Clinical procedures for medical assistants,* ed 7, St. Louis, 2008, Saunders.)

Continued

PROCEDURE 25-4 Changing a Sterile Dressing—cont'd

3. Procedural Step. Greet the patient and introduce yourself. Identify the patient and explain the procedure. Instruct the patient not to move during the procedure. Adjust the light so that it is focused on the dressing.

4. Procedural Step. Apply clean gloves. Loosen the tape on the dressing, and pull it toward the wound. Carefully and gently remove the soiled dressing by pulling it upward. Do not touch the inside of the dressing that was next to the open wound. If the dressing is stuck to the wound, it can be loosened by moistening it with a normal saline solution. Place the soiled dressing in the waste bag without allowing the dressing to touch the outside of the bag.

Principle. Gentle dressing removal avoids unnecessary stress on the wound. Touching the inside of the dressing can transfer an infected discharge to your gloves.

Remove the soiled dressing. (From Bonewit-West K: *Clinical procedures for medical assistants,* ed 7, St. Louis, 2008, Saunders.)

5. Procedural Step. Inspect the wound, and observe for the following: amount of healing; presence of inflammation; and presence of drainage, including the amount (scant, moderate, or profuse) and type of drainage.

Principle. Drainage is classified as serous (containing serum), sanguineous (red and composed of blood), serosanguineous (containing serum and blood), or purulent (containing pus and appearing white with tinges of yellow, pink, or green, depending on the type of infecting microorganism). Purulent drainage is usually thick and has an unpleasant odor.

6. Procedural Step. Open the pouch containing the sterile antiseptic swabs, and place it in a convenient location or hold it in your nondominant hand.

7. Procedural Step. Using the antiseptic swabs, apply the antiseptic to the wound. Apply the antiseptic from the top to the bottom of the wound, working from the center to the outside of the wound. Use a new swab for each motion. Discard each contaminated swab in the waste bag after use.

Principle. The purpose of the antiseptic is to decrease the number of microorganisms in the wound.

Apply an antiseptic to the wound. (From Bonewit-West K: *Clinical procedures for medical assistants,* ed 7, St. Louis, 2008, Saunders.)

8. Procedural Step. Remove the clean disposable gloves, and discard them in the waste bag without contaminating yourself. Sanitize your hands and prepare the sterile field using surgical asepsis. Items are either placed onto a sterile field or contained in a prepackaged set-up. Instruct the patient not to talk, laugh, sneeze, or cough over the sterile field.

Principle. Microorganisms are carried in water vapor from the mouth, nose, and lungs and can be transferred onto the sterile field.

Prepare the sterile field. (From Bonewit-West K: *Clinical procedures for medical assistants,* ed 7, St. Louis, 2008, Saunders.)

9. Procedural Step. Open a package of sterile gloves, and apply them.

10. Procedural Step. Pick up the sterile dressing with your gloved hand or sterile forceps. Place the sterile dressing over the wound by lightly dropping it in place. Do not move the dressing once you have dropped it into place. Discard the gloves or forceps in the waste bag.

Principle. Dropping the dressing over the wound and not moving it prevents the transfer of microorganisms from the skin to the center of the wound.

11. **Procedural Step.** Apply hypoallergenic adhesive tape to hold the dressing in place. The tape must be long enough to adhere to the skin, but not so long that it loosens when the patient moves. The strips of tape should be evenly spaced, with strips at each end of the dressing.

12. **Procedural Step.** Instruct the patient in wound care as follows:

a. Provide the patient with written wound care instructions (see the patient teaching box on wound care in this chapter).

b. Explain the wound care instructions, and ask the patient whether he or she has any questions. Tell the patient to keep the wound clean and dry and to contact the office if signs of infection occur, such as excessive swelling, pain, or discharge.

c. Ask the patient to sign the instruction sheet on the appropriate line.

d. Witness the patient's signature by signing your name in the appropriate space on the form. Include today's date.

e. Before the patient leaves the medical office, make a copy of the instruction sheet. Give a signed copy of the wound care instructions to the patient, and file the original in the patient's medical record.

Principle. The filed copy protects the physician legally in the event that the patient fails to follow the instructions and causes further harm or damage to the wound.

13. **Procedural Step.** Return the equipment. Tightly secure the bag containing the soiled dressing and contaminated articles, and dispose of it in a biohazard waste container.

Principle. Contaminated items must be disposed of properly to prevent the spread of infection.

14. **Procedural Step.** Sanitize your hands.

15. **Procedural Step.** Chart the procedure. Include the date and time, location of the dressing, condition of the wound, type and amount of drainage, care of the wound, and any problems the patient experienced with the wound. Also chart the instructions given to the patient on wound care.

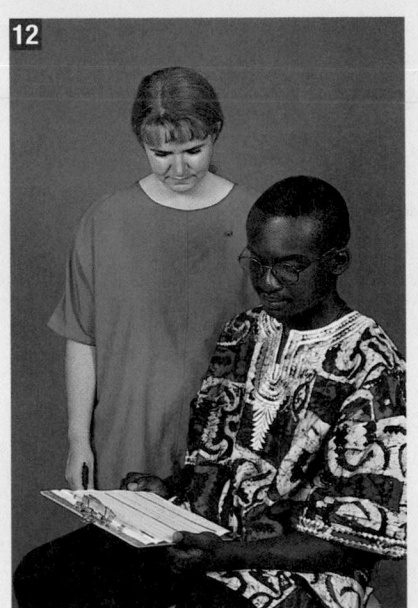

Instruct the patient in wound care. (From Bonewit-West K: *Clinical procedures for medical assistants,* ed 7, St. Louis, 2008, Saunders.)

CHARTING EXAMPLE	
Date	
9/20/10	10:30 a.m. Dressing changed Ⓛ ant forearm. Scant amt of serous drainage noted. Sl redness around incision line. Sutures intact and suture line in good approximation. Incision cleaned c̄ Betadine and DSD applied. No complaints of pain or discomfort. Explained wound care. Written instructions provided. Signed copy filed in chart. To return in 2 days for suture removal. —————————— T. Browning, CMA (AAMA)

SUTURES

The insertion and removal of **sutures** are commonly performed in the medical office. Sutures may be required to close a surgical incision or to repair an accidental wound. They **approximate,** or bring together, the edges of the wound with surgical stitches and hold them in place until proper healing can occur. Sutures also protect the wound from further contamination and minimize the amount of scar formation. A **local anesthetic** is necessary to numb the area before the sutures are inserted.

Types of Sutures

Sutures are available in two types: absorbable and nonabsorbable. **Absorbable sutures** consist of surgical gut or synthetic materials, such as polyglycolic acid (Dexon), polyglactin 910 (Vicryl), polydioxanone (PS II), polyglyconate (Maxon), and poliglecaprone (Monocryl) (Figure 25-6A). Surgical gut is made from sheep or cow intestine. This type of suturing material is gradually digested by tissue enzymes and absorbed by the body's tissues 5 to 20 days after insertion, depending on the kind of surgical gut employed. Plain

Figure 25-6. Swaged suture packets. **A,** Absorbable sutures. **B,** Nonabsorbable sutures. (From Bonewit-West K: *Clinical procedures for medical assistants,* ed 7, St. Louis, 2008 Saunders.)

Memories *from* Externship

Trudy Browing: I remember observing my first minor office surgery during my externship. It was a sebaceous cyst removal. The cyst was located on the calf of the patient's left leg. I helped in setting up the surgical tray and prepared and draped the site. I tried to explain to the patient what was going on to prepare her for the procedure. I think the patient was calmer than I was. The physician entered the room with a medical assistant on hand. Although I was in the room primarily to observe, I helped the physician with his surgical gloves and in numbing the site. I watched the physician make the incision and cut out and remove a large cyst.

Everything was going smoothly until the physician started to suture the wound. I felt like someone had turned the heat up really high; the room seemed to get really hot. I started to feel dizzy. I smiled at the physician and excused myself. He just smiled back at me, and I left the room. I went outside the room and caught my breath. I regained my composure and reentered the room. The physician was still suturing the wound. As I watched him run the needle through the skin and pull the suture tight, it really got to me. I smiled and told the physician that I would wait outside until they were done. After the physician left the room, I went back to help clean up. I felt so stupid. Later that day, the physician looked at me and said: "Got a little warm in there, didn't it?" He just laughed and said that what I did was normal and not to worry about it. He made me feel better about myself. After that incident, I went in alone and helped him with cyst removals, and it didn't bother me at all. ■

Prepare for Success

surgical gut has a rapid absorption time, whereas chromic surgical gut is treated to slow down its rate of absorption in the tissues. Absorbable sutures are frequently used to suture subcutaneous tissue, fascia, intestines, bladder, and peritoneum and to **ligate,** or tie off, vessels. Because the suturing of this type of tissue is generally done during surgery performed by the physician in the hospital with the patient under a general anesthetic, the medical office may not stock absorbable suture material.

Nonabsorbable sutures (Figure 25-6B) are not absorbed by the body and either remain permanently in the body tissues and become encapsulated by fibrous tissue or are removed (e.g., skin sutures). Nonabsorbable sutures are used to suture skin; this type of suture is used frequently in the medical office. Nonabsorbable sutures are made from materials that are not affected by tissue enzymes. These materials include silk, cotton, nylon (Ethilon), braided polyester (Ti-Cron), polypropylene (Prolene), stainless steel, and surgical skin staples.

Suture Size and Packaging

Sutures are measured by their gauge, which refers to the diameter of the suturing material. The size ranges from numbers below 0 (pronounced "aught") to numbers above 0. The diameter of the suture material increases with each number above 0 and decreases with each number below 0. If the size of a particular suture material ranges from 6-0 to 4, the available sizes include 6-0, 5-0, 4-0, 3-0, 2-0, 0, 1, 2, 3, and 4. Size 6-0 are very fine sutures, and size 4 are very heavy sutures. Size 2-0 (00) sutures have a smaller diameter than size 0 sutures.

Nonabsorbable sutures with a smaller gauge (5-0 to 6-0) are used for suturing incisions in delicate tissue, such as the face and neck, whereas nonabsorbable heavy sutures are used for firmer tissue, such as the chest and abdomen. Finer sutures also leave less scar formation and are used when cosmetic results are desired.

Sutures come in individual packages that consist of an outer peel-apart package and a sterile inner packet. They are labeled according to the type of suture material (e.g., surgical silk), the size (e.g., 4-0), and the length of the suturing material (e.g., 18 inches). The type and size of material used are based on the nature and location of the tissue being sutured and the physician's preference. To repair a laceration of the arm, the physician might use a 4-0 surgical silk suture. The physician informs the medical assistant of the type and size of sutures needed.

Suture Needles

Needles used for suturing are categorized according to their type of point and their shape. A needle with a sharp point is a *cutting needle,* and one with a round point is a *noncutting needle.* Cutting needles (Figure 25-7A) are used for firm tissues, such as skin; the sharp point helps push the needle through the tissue. Noncutting or blunt needles are used to penetrate tissues that offer a small amount of resistance, such as the fascia, intestine, liver, spleen, kidney, subcutaneous tissue, and muscle.

A suture needle is either curved or straight (see Figure 25-7A). *Curved needles* permit the physician to dip in and out of the tissue. A needle holder must be used with a curved needle. A *straight needle* is used when the tissue can be displaced sufficiently to permit the needle to be pushed and pulled through the tissue. Straight needles do not require the use of a needle holder.

Some needles have an eye through which the suture material is inserted, and some needles are **swaged** (Figure 25-7B). *Swaged* means that the suture and needle are one continuous unit; the needle is permanently attached to the end of the suture. Swaged needles are used frequently because they offer several advantages over eyed needles. One advantage is that the suture material does not slip off the needle, as might occur with suture material threaded through the eye of a needle. Another advantage is that tissue trauma is reduced because a swaged needle has only a single strand of suture that must be pulled through the tissue compared with a double strand in an eyed needle. The swaged needle can be pulled through the tissue with less resulting trauma. Swaged suture packets are labeled to specify the gauge, type, and length of suture material; the type of needle point (cutting or noncutting); and the needle shape (curved or straight) (see Figure 25-6).

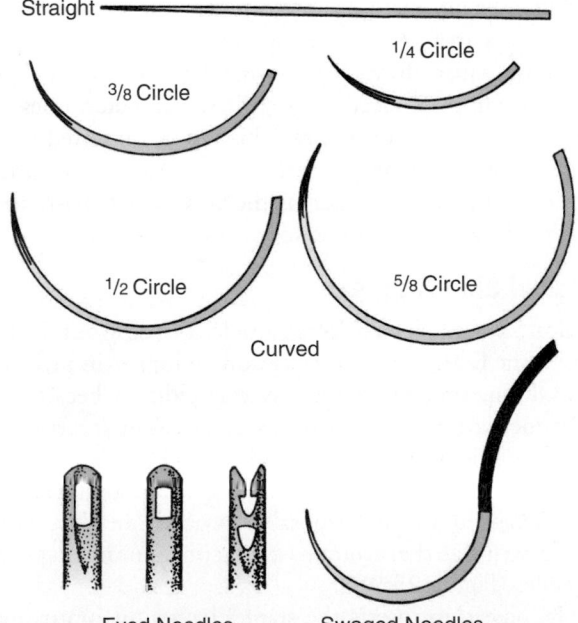

Figure 25-7. Common suture needles. **A,** Needles with a cutting point. **B,** Eyed needles and a swaged needle. (**A** modified from *Perspectives on sutures,* copyright © 2007, Covidien. All rights reserved. Reprinted with the permission of Covidien. **B** modified from Nealon TF Jr: *Fundamental skills in surgery,* ed 4, Philadelphia, 1994, Saunders.)

Insertion of Sutures

The medical assistant may be responsible for preparing the suture tray and for assisting the physician during the insertion of the sutures. The physician designates the size and type of suture material and needle required. Because sutures, needles, and suture-needle combinations (swaged needles) are contained in peel-apart packages, they can be added to the sterile field by flipping them onto the sterile field or by placing them there with a sterile gloved hand (Figure 25-8).

Suture Insertion Setup

The items required for a suture insertion setup are listed next.

Items Placed to the Side of the Sterile Field
- Clean disposable gloves
- Antiseptic solution
- Surgical scrub brush
- Antiseptic swabs
- Sterile gloves
- Local anesthetic
- Antiseptic wipe to cleanse the vial
- Tetanus toxoid with needle and syringe

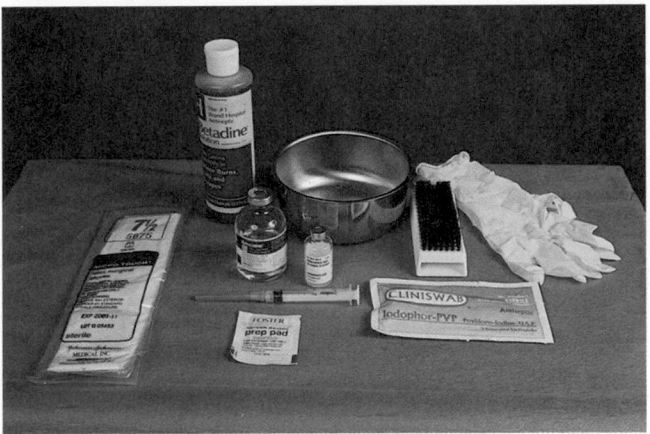

Suture insertion side table. (From Bonewit-West K: *Clinical procedures for medical assistants,* ed 7, St. Louis, 2008, Saunders.)

Items Included on the Sterile Field
- Fenestrated drape
- Syringe and needle for drawing up the local anesthetic
- Hemostatic forceps
- Thumb forceps
- Tissue forceps
- Dissecting scissors
- Operating scissors
- Needle holder
- Suture
- Sterile 4 × 4 gauze

Flipping sutures onto the sterile field.

Figure 25-8. Adding sutures to a sterile field. (From Bonewit-West K: *Clinical procedures for medical assistants,* ed 7, St. Louis, 2008, Saunders.)

The physician removing the sutures with a sterile gloved hand.

Suture insertion sterile field. (From Bonewit-West K: *Clinical procedures for medical assistants,* ed 7, St. Louis, 2008, Saunders.)

Suture Removal

When the wound has healed such that it no longer needs the support of nonabsorbable suture material, the sutures must be removed. The length of time the sutures remain in place depends on their location and the amount of healing that must occur. Some areas of the body, such as the head and neck, have a good blood supply; the sutures do not need to remain there as long as they do in other areas because this area heals more rapidly.

Sutures must always be left in place long enough for proper healing to occur. The physician determines the length of time, but in general, skin sutures inserted in the face and neck are removed in 3 to 5 days, and sutures inserted in other areas, such as the skin of the chest, arms, legs, hands, and feet, are removed in 7 to 10 days.

Surgical Skin Staples

Surgical skin staples are often used to close wounds. Stapling is the fastest method of closure of long skin incisions. In addition, trauma to the tissue is reduced because the tissue does not have to be handled much when inserting the staples. Surgical staples are stainless steel and are inserted into the skin using a special skin stapler. Skin staplers are available as reusable or disposable devices. The skin stapler holds a cartridge that contains a prescribed number and size of staples (Figure 25-9).

The physician inserts the staples by gently approximating the tissues with tissue forceps. The skin stapler is held over the site, and the staple is inserted into the skin. Skin stapling produces excellent cosmetic results, and the staples are easy to remove with a specially designed staple remover.

Figure 25-9. Disposable skin stapler. (From Bonewit-West K: *Clinical procedures for medical assistants,* ed 7, St. Louis, 2008, Saunders.)

The medical assistant is frequently responsible for removing sutures and staples. This procedure should be done only after the physician has given a written or verbal order to the medical assistant. Procedure 25-5 presents the method used to remove sutures and skin staples.

What Would You Do? What Would You *Not* Do?

Case Study 1

Kerry Ventura brings her 6-year-old son Cory to the medical office. Cory got a new bike for his birthday and just learned how to ride it without training wheels. While going around a corner, he lost his balance and fell and cut his left knee. The incision is about 1½ inches long. Cory is going to need sutures to approximate the wound. Mrs. Ventura is very upset and blames herself. She says that she should have been watching him more closely. Mrs. Ventura wants to know why Steri-Strips cannot be used to close the incision. She says that it would be a lot less painful for Cory than having stitches. When asked to sign the consent to treatment form for Cory, Mrs. Ventura says she does not want to sign the form until her husband has a chance to read it. She says that right now he is in Japan for 2 weeks on a business trip. ■

PROCEDURE 25-5

PROCEDURE **25-5** Removing Sutures and Staples

Outcome Remove sutures and staples.

Equipment/Supplies

- Antiseptic swabs
- Clean disposable gloves
- Sterile 4 × 4 gauze
- Surgical tape
- Mayo stand
- Biohazard waste container

For Suture Removal

- Suture removal kit, which includes:
  - Suture scissors
  - Thumb forceps
  - Sterile 4 × 4 gauze

For Staple Removal

- Staple removal kit, which includes:
  - Staple remover
  - Sterile 4 × 4 gauze

1. Procedural Step. Wash your hands with an antimicrobial soap. Assemble the equipment.

Principle. Washing the hands with an antimicrobial soap removes microorganisms from the hands and also deposits an antimicrobial film on your hands to discourage the growth of bacteria.

Suture removal setup. (From Bonewit-West K: *Clinical procedures for medical assistants,* ed 7, St. Louis, 2008, Saunders.)

Continued

PROCEDURE 25-5   Removing Sutures and Staples—cont'd

1 (2)

Staple removal setup. (From Bonewit-West K: *Clinical procedures for medical assistants,* ed 7, St. Louis, 2008, Saunders.)

2. Procedural Step. Greet the patient and introduce yourself. Identify the patient and explain the procedure.

3. Procedural Step. Position the patient as required to provide good access to the site. Adjust the light so that it is focused on the wound. Verify that the sutures (or staples) are intact and that the incision line is approximated and not gaping. Check that the incision line is not infected. If the incision line is not approximated or if redness, swelling, or a discharge is present, do not remove the sutures; notify the physician.
Principle. The sutures (or staples) should not be removed unless the incision line is approximated and free from infection.

4. Procedural Step. Open the suture or staple removal kit, keeping the contents of the kit sterile. Most kits are opened by peeling back a top cover, which exposes a plastic tray that holds the necessary instruments and supplies.

4

Open the suture removal kit. (From Bonewit-West K: *Clinical procedures for medical assistants,* ed 7, St. Louis, 2008, Saunders.)

5. Procedural Step. Apply clean gloves. Cleanse the incision line with an antiseptic swab to destroy microorganisms and to remove any dried exudate encrusted around the sutures or staples. Clean the wound from the top to the bottom, working from the center to the outside of the wound. Use a new swab for each cleansing motion. Allow the skin to dry.
Principle. Dried exudate must be removed to allow unimpeded removal of the sutures or staples.

6. Procedural Step. Remove the sutures or staples. Tell the patient that he or she will feel a pulling or tugging sensation as each suture (or staple) is removed, but that it will not be painful. Count the number of sutures or staples removed. Check the patient's chart to make sure the same number are removed as were inserted by the physician.

6 (1)

Cut the suture below the knot on the side closest to the skin. (From Nealon TF Jr: *Fundamental skills in surgery,* ed 4, Philadelphia, 1994, Saunders.)

6 (2)

Gently pull the suture out. (From Nealon TF Jr: *Fundamental skills in surgery,* ed 4, Philadelphia, 1994, Saunders.)

PROCEDURE 25-5

PROCEDURE 25-5

To remove sutures:

a. Using the sterile thumb forceps provided in the kit, pick up the knot of the first suture.

b. Place the curved tip of the suture scissors under the suture. Using the sterile suture scissors, cut the suture below the knot on the side of the suture closest to the skin. Cut the suture as close to the skin as possible.

c. Using a smooth, continuous motion, gently pull the suture out of the skin. Remove the suture without allowing any portion that was previously outside to be pulled back through the tissue lying beneath the incision line. Place the suture on the 4 × 4 gauze included in the suture kit.

6 (3)

Place the bottom jaws of the staple remover under the staple. (From Bonewit-West K: *Clinical procedures for medical assistants*, ed 7, St. Louis, 2008, Saunders.)

(Reformed staple)

Firmly squeeze the staple handles until they are fully closed. (From Bonewit-West K: *Clinical procedures for medical assistants*, ed 7, St. Louis, 2008, Saunders.)

d. Continue in this manner until all the sutures have been removed.

Principle. To prevent infection, the suture must be removed without pulling any portion that has been outside the skin back through the tissue lying beneath the incision line.

To remove staples:

a. Gently place the bottom jaws of the staple remover under the staple to be removed.

b. Firmly squeeze the staple handles until they are fully closed.

c. Carefully lift the staple remover upward to remove the staple from the incision line. Place the staple on the 4 × 4 gauze included in the staple kit.

d. Continue in this manner until all the staples have been removed.

7. **Procedural Step.** Cleanse the site with an antiseptic swab. Some physicians want the medical assistant to apply adhesive skin closures after removing the sutures or staples to provide additional support to the wound as it continues to heal.

8. **Procedural Step.** Apply a dry sterile dressing if indicated by the physician.

9. **Procedural Step.** Dispose of the sutures (or staples) and the gauze in a biohazard waste container.

10. **Procedural Step.** Remove the gloves, and sanitize your hands.

11. **Procedural Step.** Chart the procedure. Include the date and time, the status of the sutures (or staples) and incision line, the number of sutures (or staples) removed, the location of the site, care of the wound (i.e., application of an antiseptic or dressing), and the patient's reaction. Chart any instructions given to the patient.

CHARTING EXAMPLE	
Date	
9/20/10	10:30 a.m. Sutures intact and incision line in good approximation. No signs of infection. Sutures x6 removed from Ⓡ ant forearm. Incision line cleaned c̄ Betadine and DSD applied. Instructions provided on dressing care. ———— T. Browning, CMA (AAMA)

Adhesive Skin Closures

Adhesive skin closures may be used for wound repair to approximate the edges of a laceration or incision. Skin closures consist of sterile, hypoallergenic tape that is commercially available in a variety of widths and lengths and is strong enough to approximate a wound until healing occurs.

Brand names for adhesive skin closures are Steri-Strip (3M Corporation) and Proxi-Strip (Johnson & Johnson) (Figure 25-10).

Adhesive skin closures may be used when not much tension exists on the skin edges. The strips of tape are applied transversely across the line of incision to approxi-

Figure 25-10. Adhesive skin closures in different sizes. (From Bonewit-West K: *Clinical procedures for medical assistants,* ed 7, St. Louis, 2008, Saunders.)

mate the skin edges. The advantages of adhesive skin closures are that they eliminate the need for sutures and a local anesthetic, they are easy to apply and remove, they have a lower incidence of wound infection compared with sutures, and they result in less scarring than sutures. The disadvantage of this method is that there is less precision in bringing the wound edges together compared with suturing the wound. In addition, adhesive skin closures cannot be used on certain areas of the body where the adhesive has difficulty adhering to the skin. This includes areas that harbor moisture (e.g., palms of the hands, soles of the feet, axilla) and hairy areas of the body (e.g., scalp, a man's chest).

The medical assistant is frequently responsible for applying adhesive skin closures. Procedure 25-6 outlines this procedure. Approximately 5 to 10 days after application, the skin closures usually loosen and fall off on their own. If they require removal by the medical assistant, the method presented at the end of Procedure 25-6 should be followed.

 PROCEDURE 25-6   Applying and Removing Adhesive Skin Closures

Outcome Apply and remove adhesive skin closures.

Equipment/Supplies

- Clean disposable gloves
- Sterile gloves
- Antiseptic solution
- Surgical scrub brush
- Antiseptic swabs

- Tincture of benzoin
- Sterile cotton-tipped applicator
- Adhesive skin closure strips
- Sterile 4 × 4 gauze pads
- Surgical tape

Application of Adhesive Skin Closures

1. Procedural Step. Wash your hands with an antimicrobial soap and assemble the equipment.

Assemble the equipment. (From Bonewit-West K: *Clinical procedures for medical assistants,* ed 7, St. Louis, 2008, Saunders.)

2. Procedural Step. Greet the patient and introduce yourself.

3. Procedural Step. Identify the patient and explain the procedure.

4. Procedural Step. Position the patient as required for application of the strips. Adjust the light so that it is focused on the wound. Apply clean gloves. Inspect the wound for signs of redness, swelling, and drainage. (*Note:* Chart this information in the patient's record after completing the procedure.)

5. Procedural Step. Gently scrub the wound using an antiseptic solution (e.g., Betadine solution) and a sterile gauze pad or a surgical scrub brush. Clean at least 3 inches around the wound, removing all debris, skin oil, and exudates. Allow the skin to dry or pat dry with gauze squares. (*Note:* Change gloves as needed to maintain cleanliness.)

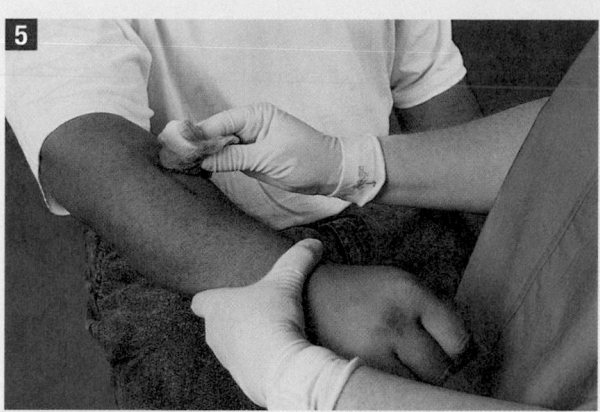

Clean the wound. (From Bonewit-West K: *Clinical procedures for medical assistants,* ed 7, St. Louis, 2008, Saunders.)

6. Procedural Step. Apply an antiseptic to the site using antiseptic swabs such as Betadine swabs. Apply the antiseptic from the top to the bottom of the wound, working from the center to the outside of the wound. Use a new swab for each motion. Allow the skin to dry completely.
Principle. The antiseptic decreases the number of microorganisms in the wound. The skin must be completely dry to ensure adhesion of the skin closures to the skin.

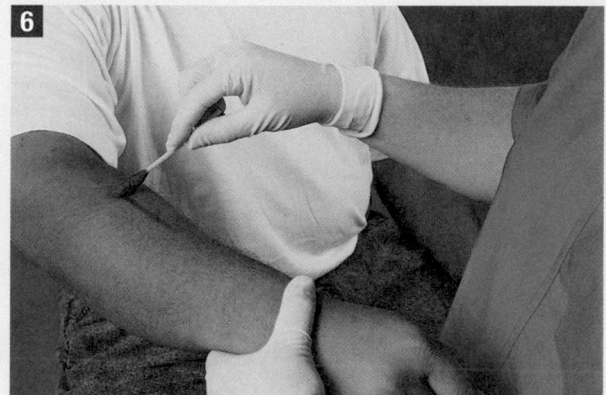

Apply an antiseptic to the wound. (From Bonewit-West K: *Clinical procedures for medical assistants,* ed 7, St. Louis, 2008, Saunders.)

7. Procedural Step. If dictated by the medical office policy, apply a thin coat of tincture of benzoin to the skin parallel to each side of the wound with a sterile cotton-tipped applicator. Do not allow the tincture of benzoin to touch the wound. Allow the skin to dry. Remove the gloves, and wash your hands with an antimicrobial soap.
Principle. Tincture of benzoin facilitates adhesion of the strips to the skin.

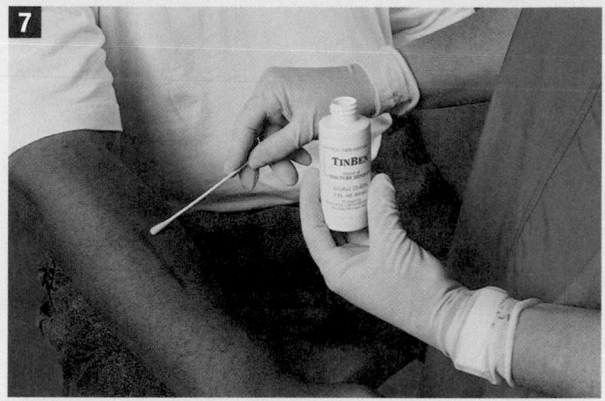

Apply tincture of benzoin. (From Bonewit-West K: *Clinical procedures for medical assistants,* ed 7, St. Louis, 2008, Saunders.)

8. Procedural Step. Open the plastic peel-apart package of strips using sterile technique as follows:
a. Grasp each flap of the package between the thumbs and bent index fingers. Pull the package apart.
b. Peel back the package until it is completely open.
c. Lay the opened package flat on a clean dry surface. The inside of the package serves as the sterile field.

9. Procedural Step. Apply sterile gloves. Fold the card of strips along its perforated tab, and tear off the tab, which exposes the ends of the strips, making them easier to grasp. Peel a strip of tape off the card at a 45-degree angle to the card.

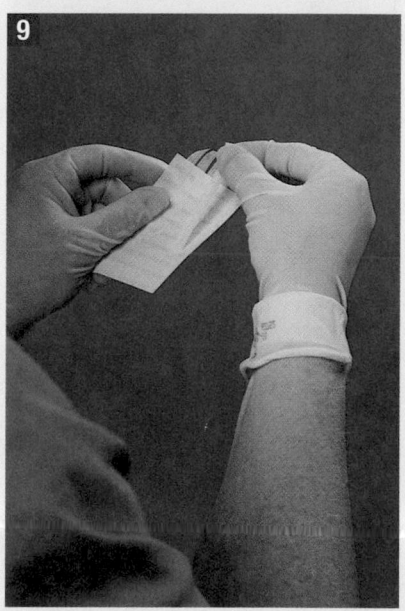

Peel a strip of tape off the card. (From Bonewit-West K: *Clinical procedures for medical assistants,* ed 7, St. Louis, 2008, Saunders.)

PROCEDURE 25-6

Continued

PROCEDURE 25-6 **Applying and Removing Adhesive Skin Closures—cont'd**

10. Procedural Step. Check that the skin surface is dry. Position the first strip over the center of the wound as follows:

a. Secure one end of the strip of tape to the skin on one side of the wound by pressing down firmly on the tape.

b. Stretch the strip transversely across the line of the incision until the edges of the wound are approximated exactly. If necessary, use your gloved hand to assist in bringing the edges of the wound together.

c. Secure the strip on the skin on the other side of the wound by pressing down firmly on the tape.

Principle. Approximating the wound exactly facilitates good healing and minimizes scar formation.

Position the first strip over the center of the wound. (From Bonewit-West K: *Clinical procedures for medical assistants,* ed 7, St. Louis, 2008, Saunders.)

11. Procedural Step. Apply the second strip perpendicular to the wound on one side of the center strip. The space between the strips should be approximately 1/8 inch. Apply a third strip on the other side of the center strip at a 1/8-inch interval. Continue applying the strips at 1/8-inch intervals until the edges of the wound are approximated. If at any time the skin surfaces become moist with perspiration, blood, or serum, wipe the area dry with a sterile gauze pad before applying the next strip.

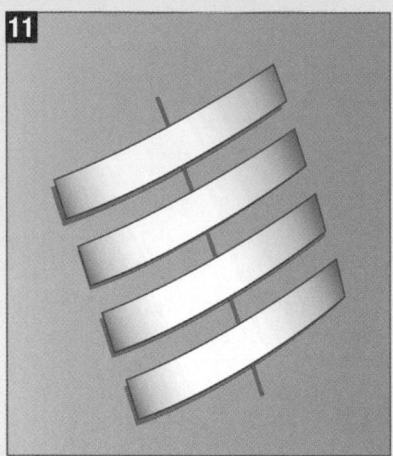

Apply the strips until the edges of the wound are approximated. (From Bonewit-West K: *Clinical procedures for medical assistants,* ed 7, St. Louis, 2008, Saunders.)

Principle. Applying the strips in this manner facilitates good **approximation** of the wound. Spacing the strips at 1/8-inch intervals allows proper drainage of the wound.

12. Procedural Step. Apply two closures approximately 1/2 inch from the ends of the strips and parallel to the wound (ladder fashion).

Principle. Applying a strip along each edge redistributes the tension and assists in holding the strips firmly in place.

Apply a strip along each edge. (From Bonewit-West K: *Clinical procedures for medical assistants,* ed 7, St. Louis, 2008, Saunders.)

13. Procedural Step. Apply a dry sterile dressing over the strips if indicated by the physician (see Procedure 25-4).

14. Procedural Step. Remove the gloves, and sanitize your hands.

15. Procedural Step. Instruct the patient in wound care as follows:

a. Provide the patient with written wound care instructions (see the patient teaching box on wound care in this chapter).

b. Explain the wound care instructions, and ask the patient whether he or she has any questions.

c. Ask the patient to sign the instruction sheet on the appropriate line.

d. Witness the patient's signature by signing your name in the appropriate space on the form. Include today's date.

e. Before the patient leaves the medical office, make a copy of the instruction sheet. Give a signed copy of the wound care instructions to the patient, and file the original in the patient's medical record.

Principle. An instruction sheet signed by the patient provides legal documentation that wound care instructions were provided to the patient in the event that the patient fails to follow the instructions and causes further harm or damage to the wound.

Ask the patient to sign the instruction sheet. (From Bonewit-West K: *Clinical procedures for medical assistants,* ed 7, St. Louis, 2008, Saunders.)

16. Procedural Step. Chart the procedure. Include the date and time, the appearance of the wound, wound preparation, the number of strips applied, the location of the wound, the care of the wound, and the patient's reaction. Chart verbal and written instructions given to the patient concerning wound care.

CHARTING EXAMPLE

Date	
9/20/10	10:30 a.m. Incision approx 5 cm long located
	on (R) post forearm. Redness noted on edge
	of wound. Sl amt of serous drainage noted.
	Wound scrubbed c̄ Betadine sol and Betadine
	antiseptic applied. Applied Steri-Strips x4.
	Incision in good approximation. Applied DSD.
	Explained wound care. Written instructions
	provided. Signed copy filed in chart. To return
	in 5 days for removal of strips. _____
	_____ T. Browning, CMA (AAMA)

Removal of Adhesive Skin Closures

Adhesive skin closures usually loosen and fall off on their own approximately 5 to 10 days following application. If they require removal, the procedure outlined below should be followed by the medical assistant.

1. Procedural Step. Sanitize your hands. Greet the patient and introduce yourself. Identify the patient and explain the procedure.

2. Procedural Step. Position the patient as required. Adjust the light so that it is focused on the wound. Check that the skin closures are intact and that the incision line is approximated and not gaping. Check that incision line is not infected. If the incision line is not approximated or if redness, swelling, or a discharge is present, do not remove the skin closures; notify the physician.

3. Procedural Step. Position a 4 × 4 gauze pad in a convenient location. Apply clean gloves.

4. Procedural Step. Remove the skin closures as follows:

a. Gently grasp one end of a strip of tape with the dominant hand.

b. Stabilize the skin with one finger of the nondominant hand.

c. Slowly loosen and peel off one half of the strip of tape from the outside to the wound margin, keeping the peeled-off section of the strip close to the skin surface and pulled back over itself. As you remove the strip from the skin, continue moving the finger as needed to support the newly exposed skin. Always pull the strip toward the wound. Never pull the strip away from the wound because tension on the wound site could disrupt the healing process.

Continued

PROCEDURE 25-6

PROCEDURE 25-6 Applying and Removing Adhesive Skin Closures—cont'd

d. Remove the other half of the strip of tape from the outside to the wound margin in the manner just described.

e. When both halves of the strip are completely loosened, gently lift the strip up and away from the wound surface. Place the strip on a 4 × 4 gauze pad.

f. Continue in this manner until all the skin closures have been removed.

5. **Procedural Step.** Cleanse the site with an antiseptic swab. Apply a dry sterile dressing if indicated by the physician (see Procedure 25-4).

6. **Procedural Step.** Dispose of the strips and gauze in a biohazard waste container. Remove the gloves, and sanitize your hands.

7. **Procedural Step.** Chart the procedure. Include the date and time, the status of the skin closures, the number of skin closures removed, the location of the site, the care of the wound, and the patient's reaction. Chart any instructions given to the patient.

CHARTING EXAMPLE	
Date	
9/25/10	10:30 a.m. Skin closures intact and in good approximation. No signs of infection. Strips x 4 removed from Ⓡ post forearm. Incision line cleaned c̄ Betadine and DSD applied. Instructions provided on dressing care.
	——————— T. Browning, CMA (AAMA)

ASSISTING WITH MINOR OFFICE SURGERY

Tray Setup

Assisting with minor office surgery requires a thorough knowledge of the instruments and supplies for each tray setup and the type of assistance required by the physician during the surgery. The medical assistant must be able to work quickly and efficiently and to anticipate the physician's needs.

The instruments and supplies for the surgery must be set on a sterile field. Many offices maintain index cards indicating the appropriate instruments and supplies for each minor office surgery tray setup. The card may also include information regarding the type of skin preparation, the position of the patient, the physician's glove size, the type of suture material, **preoperative** instructions, and **postoperative** instructions. The index cards are generally kept in a file box and are filed alphabetically by the type of surgery. The medical assistant should pull the card before setting up for the minor office surgery and use it as a guide to ensure that all the required articles are placed on the sterile field. The medical assistant may set up the sterile tray either before or after preparing the patient's skin. The sterile tray setup must not become contaminated. If the medical assistant must turn away from the sterile tray or leave the room after setting up, a sterile towel must be placed over the tray to maintain sterility.

Methods Used to Set Up a Sterile Tray

A common method used to set up a sterile tray is to use prepackaged sterile setups wrapped in disposable sterilization paper or muslin that are prepared by the medical office through autoclave sterilization (see Procedure 25-2). These setups are labeled according to use (e.g., suture pack, cyst removal pack) and contain most of the instruments and supplies required for the minor office surgery indicated on the label. The medical assistant opens the wrapped package on a flat surface, such as a **Mayo tray.** A Mayo tray is a broad, flat metal tray placed on a stand that can be used to hold sterile instruments and supplies; the inside of the wrapped package is sterile and serves as the sterile field. Several additional articles not contained in the prepackaged setup (e.g., an antiseptic, sterile 4 × 4 gauze pads, disposable syringes and needles, sutures) may need to be added to the sterile field when the package is opened. If an antiseptic solution is poured into a basin on the sterile field, it is performed according to Procedure 25-3. Items in peel-apart packages are added by flipping them onto the sterile field or by placing them on the field using a sterile gloved hand.

Another method used to set up a sterile tray is to place all the necessary articles on the sterile field by flipping them onto the sterile field from peel-apart packages. With this method, the sterile field is prepared by placing a sterile towel over a tray, such as a Mayo tray or other flat surface. The sterile towel must be handled by the corners only so as not to **contaminate** it. It must not be fanned through the air, but instead must be laid down gently and slowly to prevent airborne contamination.

Side Table

Some articles required for minor office surgery are not placed on the sterile field, but are set on an adjacent table or counter. These articles, such as a surgical scrub brush, are not sterile and must not be placed on the sterile field. The local anesthetic, which is a sterile solution, is in a vial that is not sterile and must *not* be placed on the sterile field. The physician needs to apply gloves to perform the surgery.

PROCEDURE 25-6

Although the gloves are sterile, the outside wrapper is not; the package of gloves must not be placed on the sterile field. In addition, it is easier for the physician to apply gloves from a side table or counter. To facilitate applying the gloves, the medical assistant opens the outside wrapper for the physician.

Skin Preparation

The patient's skin must be prepared before the minor office surgery because the skin contains an abundance of microorganisms. If these microorganisms were to enter the body through the operative site, a wound infection could develop. It is impossible to sterilize skin because chemical agents required to kill all living microorganisms are too strong to be placed on the skin surfaces. The operative site and an area surrounding it must be cleaned and prepared in such a way as to remove as many microorganisms as possible to reduce the risk of surgical wound contamination.

Shaving the Site

Hair supports the growth of microorganisms, and the physician may want the medical assistant to shave the skin at and around the operative site. Shave preparation trays are commercially available and include several gauze sponges, a measured amount of antiseptic soap, a container for soapy water, and a disposable safety razor. The skin should be pulled taut as it is shaved, and the medical assistant must be careful to prevent nicks. When all the hair has been removed, the shaved area should be rinsed and dried thoroughly.

Cleansing the Site

The operative site must be cleaned with an antiseptic solution such as povidone-iodine (Betadine Surgical Scrub) or chlorhexidine gluconate (Hibiclens) (Figure 25-11). The medical assistant should scrub the operative area with a surgical scrub brush using a firm circular motion, moving from the inside outward. The area is rinsed using gauze pads saturated with water and is blotted dry with sterile gauze.

Antiseptic Application

When the patient's skin has been shaved (if required) and cleansed, an antiseptic is applied to the operative area, followed by the application of a sterile drape. The antiseptic decreases the number of microorganisms on the patient's skin; a common antiseptic is Betadine. A disposable sterile fenestrated drape (Figure 25-12) is the type of drape most commonly used. It has an opening that is placed directly over the operative site. A fenestrated drape covers a wide area of skin around the operative area, leaving only the operative site exposed. This provides a sterile area around the operative site and decreases contamination of the patient's surgical wound.

Local Anesthetic

Minor office surgeries often require the use of a local anesthetic; local anesthetics frequently used in the medical office

Figure 25-11. Cleansing solutions. (From Bonewit-West K: *Clinical procedures for medical assistants,* ed 7, St. Louis, 2008, Saunders.)

Figure 25-12. Fenestrated drape. (From Bonewit-West K: *Clinical procedures for medical assistants,* ed 7, St. Louis, 2008, Saunders.)

include lidocaine hydrochloride (Xylocaine) and procaine hydrochloride (Novocaine). The physician injects the local anesthetic into the tissue surrounding the operative site, a process termed **infiltration,** to produce a loss of sensation in that area and prevent the patient from feeling pain during the surgery. Local anesthetics begin working in 5 to 15 minutes and have a duration of action of 1 to 3 hours, depending on the type of anesthetic.

Some physicians prefer to use a local anesthetic containing *epinephrine.* Epinephrine is a vasoconstrictor that prolongs the local effect of the anesthetic and decreases the rate of systemic absorption of the local anesthetic. It accomplishes this by constricting the blood vessels at the operative site. The physician informs the medical assistant what type, strength, and amount of the local anesthetic are necessary for the minor office surgery. Xylocaine is available in 0.5%, 1%, 1.5%, and 2% solutions. The physician may order 1 ml of Xylocaine 2% with epinephrine to suture a laceration of the forearm.

Preparing the Anesthetic

The local anesthetic is drawn up into the syringe according to the procedure presented in Chapter 26. The vial must first be cleansed using an antiseptic wipe. The correct amount of anesthetic solution is withdrawn into the syringe. This may be performed by the medical assistant or the physician. The medical assistant withdraws the anesthetic into the syringe and hands it to the physician, who has not yet applied sterile gloves. The physician injects the anesthetic into the patient's tissues and then applies sterile gloves to begin the surgery.

The physician may prefer to draw the anesthetic solution into the syringe after he or she has applied sterile gloves. The medical assistant should first show the label of the vial to the physician and then hold the vial securely while the physician withdraws the medication (Figure 25-13). The

medical assistant must hold the vial because the outside of the vial is medically aseptic and cannot be touched by the physician's sterile gloved hand.

If the medical assistant prepares the anesthetic injection, the needle and syringe are not placed on the sterile field, but are assembled off to the side. If the physician withdraws the anesthetic, the needle and syringe are placed on the sterile field.

Assisting the Physician

The type of assistance required by the physician during minor office surgery is based on the type of surgery and physician's preference. Some physicians want the medical assistant to apply sterile gloves and assist directly by handing instruments and supplies from the sterile field. An instrument should be handed to the physician in a firm, confident manner so that the instrument does not slip out of the physician's hand and drop on the floor. The instrument should be placed in the physician's hand in its functional position; that is, the position in which it is to be used (Figure 25-14). If the instrument is handed correctly, the physician should not have to reposition the instrument to use it.

The medical assistant is responsible for adding any instruments or supplies to the sterile field that the physician requires after the surgery has begun, such as another hemostat, additional 4 × 4 gauze pads, and sutures. This is generally accomplished using peel-apart packages and either flipping the contents onto the sterile field or holding the package open and allowing the physician to remove the contents with a gloved hand. In assisting with minor office surgery, it is essential to know all steps in the procedure so that the physician's needs are anticipated and the surgery proceeds smoothly and efficiently.

The physician may obtain a tissue specimen that is sent to the laboratory for histologic examination. The specimen must be placed in an appropriate-sized container with a preservative. The medical assistant is responsible for label-

Figure 25-13. Drawing up the local anesthetic. **A,** Trudy holds up the vial so that the physician can verify the name and strength of the local anesthetic. **B,** Trudy holds the vial securely while the physician withdraws the medication. (From Bonewit-West K: *Clinical procedures for medical assistants,* ed 7, St. Louis, 2008, Saunders.)

Figure 25-14. Trudy hands a hemostat to the physician in its functional position. (From Bonewit-West K: *Clinical procedures for medical assistants,* ed 7, St. Louis, 2008, Saunders.)

ing the specimen container with the patient's name, date, and type of specimen. The medical assistant must also complete a laboratory requisition to accompany the specimen; this is known as a *biopsy requisition* (Figure 25-15).

When the minor office surgery is completed, the physician may want the medical assistant to place a dry sterile dressing over the surgical wound to protect it from contamination or injury or to absorb drainage. The medical assistant is also responsible for assisting the patient and cleaning the examining room.

Procedure 25-7 describes the medical assistant's responsibilities while assisting with minor office surgery. Specific instruments and supplies required for the minor office surgery depend on the type of surgery being performed and the physician's preference. Knowing the name and function of the surgical instruments shown in Figure 25-2 enables the medical assistant to set up for each type of minor surgery performed in the medical office. If the medical office uses prepackaged sterile setups, the medical assistant should have already assembled the instruments and supplies in the package during the sanitization and sterilization process; however, the instruments and supplies should be checked after the pack is opened to ensure that all the sterile articles are included.

Text continued on p. 560

What Would You Do? What Would You *Not* Do?

Case Study 2

Abbey Mendy is having a sebaceous cyst removed from her neck. She wants to know why the antiseptic applied to her neck is orange and whether it is going to stain her skin permanently. During the procedure Abbey reaches her hand up to adjust her hair and accidentally touches the physician's gloved hand. After the procedure, a sterile dressing is applied to her neck, and she is given an appointment to return to have her sutures removed. Abbey becomes alarmed when she is told that the cyst will be sent to the laboratory for a biopsy. She wants to know whether the physician is not telling her everything about her condition and that maybe he thinks she has cancer. Abbey asks if her neighbor can take out her sutures. She says that he has worked as a veterinary assistant for the past 8 years and has lots of experience in removing stitches. ■

DIAGNOSTIC PATHOLOGY ASSOCIATES, INC

HISTOPATHOLOGY/CYTOPATHOLOGY REQUISITION

BILL TO: ☐ ACCOUNT ☐ MEDICARE ☐ BLUE SHIELD ☐ PATIENT ☐ MEDICAID ☐ OTHER	PATIENT NAME (LAST, FIRST, MIDDLE INITIAL)		PATIENT ID	ROOM NO.
SEX	BIRTHDATE / /	DATE COLLECTED	TIME COLLECTED A.M. P.M.	REQUESTING PHYSICIAN	SPECIAL INSTRUCTIONS
RESPONSIBLE PARTY NAME		RESPONSIBLE PARTY ADDRESS		CITY, STATE, ZIP
PHONE	MEDICAID ID NUMBER	MEDICARE HIC NUMBER		INSURANCE COMPANY NAME
INSURANCE COMPANY ADDRESS		GROUP NUMBER	CONTRACT NUMBER	COVERAGE CODE	PATIENT/INSURED RELATIONSHIP ☐ SELF ☐ SPOUSE ☐ DEPEND.

PATIENT AUTHORIZATION: I AUTHORIZE THE RELEASE OF ANY MEDICAL INFORMATION NECESSARY TO PROCESS A CLAIM. I PERMIT A COPY OF THIS AUTHORIZATION TO BE USED IN PLACE OF THE ORIGINAL AND REQUEST PAYMENT OF ANY MEDICAL INSURANCE BENEFITS EITHER TO ME OR TO THE PARTY WHO ACCEPTS ASSIGNMENT. SIGNED X_____ DATE _____

TISSUE EXAM: ☐ GROSS & MICROSCOPIC ☐ GROSS ONLY	SOURCE OF SPECIMEN:	CLINICAL DIAGNOSIS:
SPECIMEN TYPE: ☐ BIOPSY ☐ SCRAPING ☐ BRUSHING ☐ WASHING ☐ FLUIDS ☐ FINE NEEDLE ☐ OTHER _____	☐ PHONE REPORT (NEXT WORKING DAY) COPIES TO: _____	PATIENT HISTORY:

Figure 25-15. Biopsy requisition. (Courtesy Diagnostic Pathology Associates, Westerville, Ohio.)

PROCEDURE 25-7

Highlight on the History of Surgery

Primitive Surgery

Surgery evolved from very primitive beginnings. The first record of a surgical operation dates back to 350,000 BC. Primitive humans believed that headaches were caused by demons that had gained entrance to the head and were unable to get out. To release the demons, a hole was chiseled through the patient's skull with a sharp flint. Early operating instruments consisted of sharpened flints and crude hammers. Sharpened animal teeth were used for bloodletting and drainage of abscesses. Ancient records show that suturing materials consisted of dried gut, dried tendon, strips of hide, horsehair, and fibers from tree bark. To help form a clot, bleeding wounds were covered with materials such as rabbit fur, shredded tree bark, egg yolk, and cobwebs.

Early 1800s

In the early 1800s, surgical instruments were still almost nonexistent. Kitchen knives and penknives doubled as scalpels, and table forks were used as retractors. Physicians would use household pincushions to hold their suturing needles. The same sponges were used for every patient to wipe away blood and other secretions. Because of these conditions, the most trivial operations were likely to be followed by infection, and death occurred in half of all surgical operations. Joseph Lister, an English surgeon, was one of the first individuals to advocate the use of antiseptics during surgery. Lister insisted on the use of antiseptics on the hands of his surgical team, instruments, wounds, and dressings. Many surgeons ridiculed Lister's ideas, but in 1879 his antiseptic principles were, at long last, formally adopted by the medical profession. Today, Lister is known as the father of modern surgery.

Mid-1800s

Anesthetic agents, such as ether and chloroform, were discovered in the mid-1800s. Before this time, various methods were used to subdue and restrain patients during surgery, such as having the patient consume alcohol before the operation and strapping the patient to the operating table. With the advent of anesthetics, new surgical procedures never before considered possible came into existence. This resulted in new demands for surgical instruments and the necessity for smaller and more delicate instruments.

Late 1800s and Early 1900s

The late 1800s and early 1900s saw dramatic advances in surgical operations and techniques. The most notable include the invention of the steam sterilizer, which permitted sterilization of surgical instruments and supplies; the use of surgical gowns, caps, masks, and gloves during surgery; the monitoring of a patient's condition while under anesthesia; the development of stainless steel, which provided a superior material for manufacturing surgical instruments; and the establishment of standards for manufacturing and packaging sutures. Other discoveries important to surgery during this time included the discovery of x-rays by Wilhelm Roentgen; the discovery of penicillin by Alexander Fleming; the discovery that cocaine could be used as a local anesthetic by William Halsted; and the development of endoscopic instruments, such as the laryngoscope, bronchoscope, and sigmoidoscope, for viewing internal structures of the body.

The breakthroughs in surgical technology established through the ages laid the foundation for present-day complex surgical procedures, such as laser surgery, open-heart surgery, and microsurgery. It is incredible to think that it all started with a sharpened flint! ∎

PROCEDURE 25-7   Assisting with Minor Office Surgery

Outcome Set up a surgical tray, and assist with minor office surgery.

Equipment/Supplies

- Mayo stand
- Instruments and supplies for the type of surgery to be performed
- Biohazard waste container

Preparing the Tray

1. **Procedural Step.** Determine the type of minor office surgery to be performed. The physician instructs the medical assistant as to the type of surgery and provides any additional information needed to set up for the surgery, such as the type of local anesthetic and sutures to be used. If the medical office maintains a minor office surgery filing system, pull the file card that indicates the instruments and supplies required for the type of surgery to be performed.

2. **Procedural Step.** Prepare the examining room. Make sure the room is clean and well lighted.

3. **Procedural Step.** Sanitize your hands.
4. **Procedural Step.** Set up nonsterile articles on a side table or counter. If a specimen container is included in the setup, label the container with the patient's name, date, and type of specimen.

   Principle. Articles that are not sterile cannot be placed on the sterile field because they would contaminate it.

5. **Procedural Step.** Wash your hands with an antimicrobial soap and set up the minor office surgery tray on a clean, dry, flat surface, using the principles of surgical asepsis. The sterile tray can be set up as follows:

   Prepackaged setup:
   a. Select the appropriate package from the supply shelf, and place it on a Mayo tray or other flat surface.
   b. Open the prepackaged setup using the inside of the wrapper as the sterile field. Check the sterilization indicator to make sure the contents of the pack are sterile.
   c. Add other articles to the sterile field that are necessary for the surgery but not contained in the sterile package, such as 4 × 4 gauze, sutures, and a fenestrated drape.

Open the sterile pack using the inside of the wrapper as the sterile field. (From Bonewit-West K: *Clinical procedures for medical assistants,* ed 7, St. Louis, 2008, Saunders.)

Transferring articles to a sterile field:
a. Pick up the folded sterile towel by two corner ends and allow it to unfold; make sure it does not touch an unsterile surface.
b. Lay the sterile towel down gently and slowly over the Mayo tray, making sure it does not brush against an unsterile surface, such as your uniform. Do not allow your arms to pass over the towel as

you lay it down because this would result in contamination of the sterile field.

Lay the sterile towel down gently and slowly. (From Bonewit-West K: *Clinical procedures for medical assistants,* ed 7, St. Louis, 2008, Saunders.)

c. Transfer instruments and supplies to the sterile field from wrapped or peel-apart packages.

   Principle. The principles of surgical asepsis must be followed to prevent contamination of the sterile field.

6. **Procedural Step.** Apply a sterile glove, and arrange the articles neatly on the sterile field. Do not allow one article to lie on top of another. Check that all the instruments and supplies required for the surgery are available on the sterile field.

   Principle. Instruments and supplies can be located quickly and efficiently on a neat and orderly sterile field. Sterile gloves must be used to prevent contamination of the sterile articles.

Arrange the articles neatly on the sterile field. (From Bonewit-West K: *Clinical procedures for medical assistants,* ed 7, St. Louis, 2008, Saunders.)

Continued

PROCEDURE 25-7

PROCEDURE 25-7   Assisting with Minor Office Surgery—cont'd

7. Procedural Step. Cover the tray setup with a sterile towel by picking up the towel by two corner ends and placing it gently and slowly over the setup. Do not allow your arms to pass over the sterile field as you lay it down.

Principle. The towel prevents the sterile tray from becoming contaminated. The towel must be picked up by the corner ends to prevent contaminating it and should be moved slowly and not fanned through the air to prevent airborne contamination. Passing the arms over the sterile field results in contamination of the field.

Cover the tray setup with a sterile towel. (From Bonewit-West K: *Clinical procedures for medical assistants,* ed 7, St. Louis, 2008, Saunders.)

Preparing the Patient

8. Procedural Step. Greet the patient and introduce yourself. Identify the patient by full name and date of birth. Explain the procedure, and prepare the patient for the minor office surgery as follows:
a. Try to allay the patient's fear or anxiety.
b. Ask the patient whether he or she needs to void before the surgery.
c. Provide instructions to the patient about any clothing that must be removed and putting on an examination gown, if required. Enough clothing must be removed to expose the operative area completely and to avoid getting the antiseptic or blood on the patient's clothing.
d. Instruct the patient not to move during the procedure and not to talk, laugh, sneeze, or cough over the sterile field.

Principle. Minor office surgery is often a frightening experience for the patient, and reassurance should be offered to reduce apprehension. The amount of clothing that must be removed depends on the type of minor office surgery being performed. By moving, the patient may accidentally contaminate the sterile field or touch the operative site. Microorganisms are carried in water vapor from the mouth, nose, and lungs and can be transferred onto the sterile field.

9. Procedural Step. Position the patient. The position is determined by the type of minor office surgery to be performed. The patient is positioned in such a way as to provide the best possible exposure and accessibility to the operative site. *Note:* If a difficult position must be maintained, such as the knee-chest position, the patient should not be positioned until the physician is ready to begin the minor office surgery.

10. Procedural Step. Adjust the light so that it is focused on the operative site.

11. Procedural Step. Prepare the patient's skin by performing the following:
a. Apply clean disposable gloves.
b. If hair is present, the skin at and around the operative site may need to be shaved. The skin should be pulled taut as it is shaved. The area is rinsed and dried thoroughly.
c. Cleanse the patient's skin with an antiseptic solution and a surgical scrub brush using a firm, circular motion and moving from the inside outward. Do not return to an area just cleansed. The area is rinsed using gauze pads saturated with water and blotted dry with a sterile gauze pad.
d. Apply an antiseptic to the site using antiseptic swabs such as Betadine. Allow the skin to dry. Alternatively, the physician may place a fenestrated drape over the operative site and then apply the antiseptic.
e. Remove the gloves, and sanitize your hands.

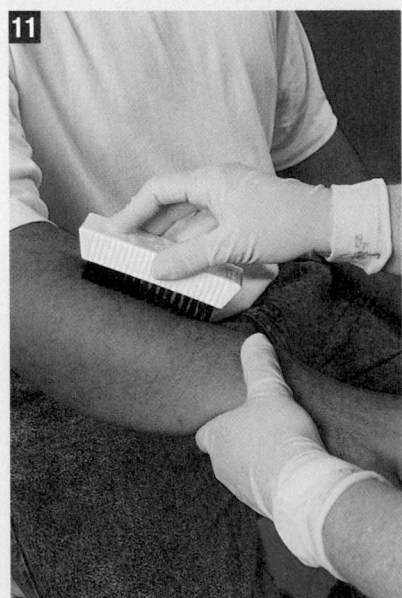

Cleanse the patient's skin with an antiseptic solution. (From Bonewit-West K: *Clinical procedures for medical assistants,* ed 7, St. Louis, 2008, Saunders.)

12. Procedural Step. Verify that everything is prepared for the minor office surgery, and inform the physician that the patient is ready.

Assisting the Physician

13. Procedural Step. Assist the physician as required during the minor office surgery, following the principles of surgical asepsis. The physician drapes the patient, injects the local anesthetic, and performs the surgery. The responsibilities of the medical assistant may include the following:

a. Uncover the sterile tray setup by picking up the sterile towel covering it. The towel should be picked up by two corner ends and removed slowly and gently without allowing the arms to pass over the sterile field.

b. Open the outer glove wrapper for the physician to facilitate the application of sterile gloves.

c. Withdraw the local anesthetic into a syringe and hand it to the physician, or hold the vial while the physician withdraws the local anesthetic.

d. Adjust the light as needed by the physician for good visualization of the operative site.

e. Restrain patients such as children.

f. Relax and reassure the patient during the minor office surgery.

g. Hand instruments and supplies to the physician. (Sterile gloves are required.)

h. Keep the sterile field neat and orderly. (Sterile gloves are required.)

i. Hold a basin in which the physician can deposit soiled instruments and supplies, such as hemostats and gauze sponges. (Clean gloves are required.)

Hold a basin for the physician to deposit soiled instruments. (From Bonewit-West K: *Clinical procedures for medical assistants,* ed 7, St. Louis, 2008, Saunders.)

j. Retract tissue from an area to allow the physician the best access to and visibility of the operative site. (Sterile gloves are required.)

k. Sponge blood from the operative site. (Sterile gloves are required.)

l. Add instruments and supplies to the sterile field as required by the physician.

m. Hold the specimen container to accept a tissue specimen received from the physician. (Clean gloves are required.) Do not touch the inside of the container because it is sterile.

Hold the container to accept a tissue specimen. (From Bonewit-West K: *Clinical procedures for medical assistants,* ed 7, St. Louis, 2008, Saunders.)

n. After the physician has inserted a suture, cut the ends of the suture material approximately $\frac{1}{8}$ inch above the knot of the suture (sterile gloves are required).

14. Procedural Step. Apply a sterile dressing to the surgical wound, if ordered by the physician (see Procedure 25-4).
Principle. The sterile dressing protects the wound from contamination and injury and absorbs drainage.

15. Procedural Step. After the surgery, perform the following:

a. Stay with the patient as a safety precaution and to assist and instruct the patient.

b. Ensure that postoperative instructions regarding any type of medical care to be administered at home are understood. If the patient has a wound or if sutures have been inserted, he or she should be told to keep the area clean and dry and to report any signs of infection, such as excessive redness, swelling, discharge, or increase in pain. Provide the patient with written wound care instructions (see the patient teaching box on wound care in this chapter). Ask the patient if he or she has any questions. Have the patient sign the instruction sheet. Witness the patient's signature. Before the patient leaves the office, make a copy of the instruction sheet. Give a copy to the patient and file the original in the patient's chart.

c. Relay information regarding the return visit for postoperative care, such as the removal of sutures or a dressing change.

d. Help the patient off the table to prevent falls.

Continued

PROCEDURE 25-7   Assisting with Minor Office Surgery—cont'd

e. Instruct the patient to get dressed, offering assistance if needed.

f. Any instructions or information given must be charted in the patient's medical record.

Principle. The patient (especially an elderly one) may become dizzy after the minor office surgery and may fall when getting off the examining table. The filed copy protects the physician legally, in the event that the patient fails to follow instructions and causes harm or damage to the operative site.

16. **Procedural Step.** If a specimen was collected, it must be transferred to the laboratory in a tightly closed, properly labeled specimen container. Prepare the specimen for transport. Complete a biopsy request form to accompany the specimen. Place the specimen container in a biohazard specimen bag and seal it. Place the biopsy request in the outer pocket of the bag. Record information in the patient's chart, including the date the specimen was picked up or sent to the laboratory and the name of the laboratory.

Principle. Recording information regarding transport of the specimen documents that the specimen was sent to the laboratory.

17. **Procedural Step.** Clean the examining room. Handle the instruments carefully so as not to damage them. Be especially careful with sharp instruments to prevent cutting yourself. Blood and body secretions should be rinsed off the instruments immediately to prevent them from drying and hardening. The instruments must be sanitized and sterilized when it is convenient to do so; follow the procedures presented in Chapter 18. Discard disposable articles contaminated with blood or other potentially infectious materials in a biohazard waste container.

Principle. Surgical instruments are expensive and must be handled carefully to prolong their life span. Hardened blood and secretions on an instrument are difficult to remove. Disposable articles must be discarded in an appropriate manner to prevent the spread of infection.

CHARTING EXAMPLE

Date	
9/25/10	2:00 p.m. Applied DSD to Ⓡ post forearm.
	Instructed patient on suture care. Written
	instructions provided. Signed copy filed in
	chart. To return in 5 days for removal of
	sutures. Sebaceous cyst specimen sent to
	Medical Center Laboratory for biopsy on
	9/25/10. ——— T. Browning, CMA (AAMA)

MEDICAL OFFICE SURGICAL PROCEDURES

The most common surgical procedures performed in the medical office are presented on the following pages. A discussion of the procedure is also presented.

Sebaceous Cyst Removal

A **sebaceous cyst** is a thin, closed sac or capsule that contains secretions from a sebaceous, or oil, gland. It forms when the outlet of the gland becomes obstructed. The built-up secretion of sebum from the gland causes swelling, and the lining of the cyst consists of the stretched sebaceous gland. Sebaceous cysts are soft to firm in consistency and are generally elevated and filled with an odorous cheesy material. This type of cyst can occur anywhere on the body except on the palms of the hands and the soles of the feet—these areas do not contain sebaceous glands. Sebaceous cysts tend to occur most frequently on the scalp, face, ears, neck, and back.

A sebaceous cyst is usually painless and nontender, although it may become infected; to avoid this, the cyst should be excised by the physician. If it is already infected, the physician does not excise the cyst, but drains it and performs the removal at a later time.

Procedure

A sebaceous cyst is removed as follows:

1. A local anesthetic is used to numb the area.
2. The physician makes an incision, removes the cyst, and sutures the surgical incision (Figure 25-16).
3. The cyst is placed in a specimen container with a preservative and sent to the laboratory for examination by a pathologist.
4. A sterile dressing is applied to the operative site.

Surgical Incision and Drainage of Localized Infections

An **abscess** is a collection of pus in a cavity surrounded by inflamed tissue (Figure 25-17). It is caused by a pathogen that invades the tissues, usually via a break in the skin. An abscess serves as a defense mechanism of the body to keep an infection localized by walling off the microorganisms, preventing them from spreading through the body. A **furuncle,** also known as a *boil,* is a localized staphylococcal infection that originates deep within a hair follicle. Furuncles produce pain and itching. The skin initially becomes red and then turns white and necrotic over the top of the furuncle. Erythema and induration usually surround it.

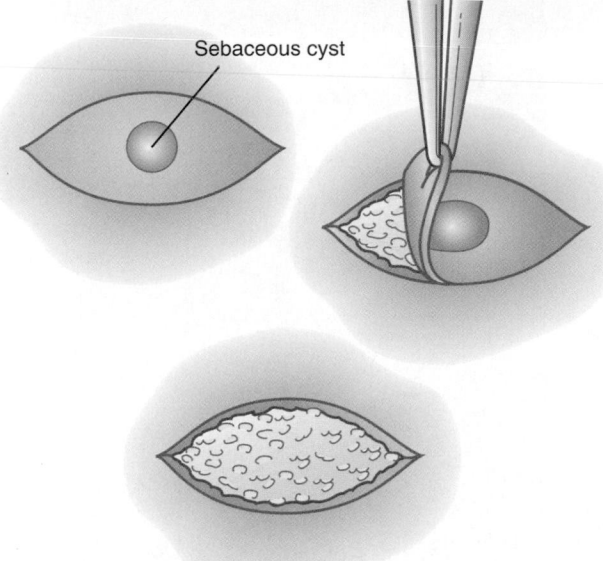

Figure 25-16. Sebaceous cyst removal. The physician makes an incision, removes the cyst, and sutures the surgical incision. (From Nealon TF Jr: *Fundamental skills in surgery,* ed 4, Philadelphia, 1994, Saunders.)

Figure 25-17. An abscess is a collection of pus in a cavity surrounded by inflamed tissue. (From Nealon TF Jr: *Fundamental skills in surgery,* ed 4, Philadelphia, 1994, Saunders.)

Procedure

Localized infections, such as abscesses, furuncles, and infected sebaceous cysts, that do not rupture and drain naturally may need to be incised and drained by the physician as follows:

1. A local anesthetic is generally used for the procedure.
2. A scalpel is used to make the incision. Either a rubber Penrose drain or a gauze wick is inserted into the wound to keep the edges of the tissues apart, which facilitates drainage of the exudate. The exudate contains pathogenic microorganisms; the medical assistant should be careful to avoid contact with the exudate while assisting with the minor surgery.
3. A sterile dressing of several thicknesses is applied over the operative site to absorb the drainage.

Postoperative Instructions

The physician may prescribe the application of warm compresses to be applied by the patient at home. Applying heat to the operative site helps to promote healing. If the physician orders this treatment, the medical assistant should instruct the patient in this procedure properly according to the information outlined in Chapter 22 (see Procedure 22-3).

Needle Biopsy

A **biopsy** is the removal and examination of tissue from the living body. The tissue is usually examined under a microscope. Biopsies are most often performed to determine whether a tumor is malignant or benign; however, a biopsy may also be used as a diagnostic aid for other conditions, such as infections. A **needle biopsy** is a type of biopsy in which tissue from deep within the body is obtained by the insertion of a biopsy needle through the skin. The advantage of a needle biopsy is that a sample of tissue can be obtained that might otherwise require a major surgical operation.

Procedure

1. The procedure is performed under a local anesthetic, and because an incision is not required, the patient does not have to undergo the discomfort and inconvenience of an operative recovery.
2. The tissue specimen is placed in a container with a preservative and sent to the laboratory for examination by a pathologist.
3. A small dressing, placed over the needle puncture site, is usually sufficient to protect the operative site and promote healing.
4. After the procedure, the patient should be observed for any evidence of complications related to the procedure.

Ingrown Toenail Removal

An ingrown toenail occurs when the edge of the toenail grows deeply into the nail groove and penetrates the surrounding skin, resulting in pain and discomfort to the patient (Figure 25-18A). Ingrown toenails are caused by external pressure, such as from tight shoes, or from trauma, improper nail trimming, or infection. The protruding nail acts as a foreign body, usually resulting in secondary infection and inflammation. In mild cases, this condition is treated by inserting a small piece of cotton packing under the toenail to raise the nail edge away from the tissue of the nail groove (Figure 25-18B). In severe and recurring cases, part of the nail must be surgically removed, which relieves pain by decreasing the nail pressure on the soft tissues.

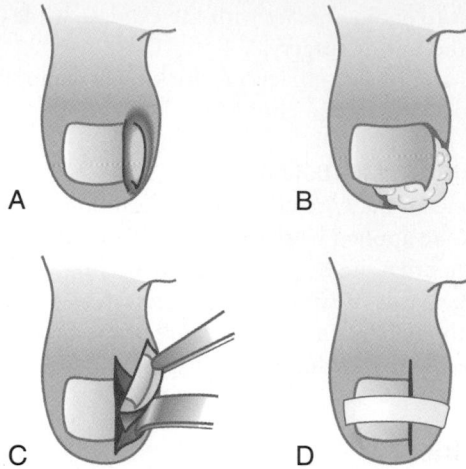

Figure 25-18. Ingrown toenail. **A,** The edge of the toenail grows deeply into the nail groove. **B,** In mild cases, treatment consists of inserting a small piece of cotton packing under the toenail. **C,** In severe and recurring cases, a wedge of the nail is surgically removed. **D,** A strip of surgical tape is applied over the area. (From Nealon TF Jr: *Fundamental skills in surgery,* ed 4, Philadelphia, 1994, Saunders.)

Procedure

An ingrown toenail is removed as follows:

1. Before the surgical procedure is performed, the affected foot must be soaked in tepid water containing an antibacterial skin solution for 10 to 15 minutes to soften the nail plate and decrease the possibility of bacterial infection.
2. The patient is placed in a reclining position with the foot adequately supported, and the toe is shaved to remove hair, which would act as a contaminant.
3. An antiseptic is applied to the affected toe, which is numbed using a local anesthetic.
4. Using surgical toenail scissors, the physician surgically removes a wedge of the nail (Figure 25-18C).
5. A sterile gauze dressing or a strip of surgical tape is applied over the area to protect the operative site and to promote healing (Figure 25-18D).

Colposcopy

Colposcopy is the visual examination of the vagina and cervix by means of a lighted instrument with a binocular magnifying lens, known as a **colposcope** (Figure 25-19). The purpose of colposcopy is to examine the vagina and cervix to determine areas of abnormal tissue growth. Colposcopy is performed following abnormal Pap test results, to evaluate a vaginal or cervical lesion observed during a pelvic examination, or after treatment for cancer of the cervix. To prepare for the procedure, the patient should be instructed not to insert anything (e.g., tampons, vaginal medications, spermicides) into the vagina for 24 to 48 hours before the procedure. The lens of the colposcope is positioned approximately 12 inches (30 cm) from the opening of the vagina. The lens magnifies tissue, facilitating the inspection of cervical cells and the obtaining of a biopsy specimen. For a routine colposcopic examination, a magnification ranging

Figure 25-19. A colposcope. (From Apgar BS, Brotzman GL, Spitzer M: *Colposcopy: principles and practice—an integrated textbook and atlas,* Philadelphia, 2002, Saunders.)

from 6× to 15× is generally used. The colposcope may be placed on an adjustable stand or attached to the side of the examining table and swung out before use.

Procedure

Colposcopy is performed as follows:

1. The patient is assisted into a lithotomy position and prepared as for a pelvic examination.
2. The physician inserts a vaginal speculum into the vagina.
3. A long, cotton-tipped applicator moistened with saline is used to wipe the cervix to remove the mucous film that normally covers it. The saline also provides better visualization of the cervical epithelium because dry cervical epithelium is not transparent and does not allow satisfactory viewing of the vascular pattern of the cervix.
4. The colposcope is focused on the cervix, and the physician inspects the saline-moistened cervix.
5. The cervix is swabbed with acetic acid, using a long, cotton-tipped applicator. The acetic acid dissolves cervical mucus and other secretions; the acetic acid provides the best contrast between normal and abnormal tissue, allowing easier visualization of dysplastic and neoplastic epithelium.
6. The cervical epithelium may also be stained with Lugol's iodine solution using a long, cotton-tipped applicator.

This provides another means to identify unhealthy epithelium. The healthy epithelium of the cervix contains glycogen, which can absorb the iodine, causing the epithelium to stain a dark brown color. Conversely, abnormal epithelium, such as would constitute a malignancy, does not contain glycogen and is unable to absorb the iodine.

7. If an abnormal area is observed, the physician obtains a cervical biopsy specimen using punch biopsy forceps, which is described next.

Cervical Punch Biopsy

A cervical biopsy is performed in combination with colposcopy to remove a cervical tissue specimen for examination

What Would You Do? What Would You *Not* Do?

Case Study 3

Sadira Wisal has been referred to the office for a colposcopy by her family physician. Her last Pap test came back as abnormal, and a repeat Pap test 3 months later was also abnormal. While having her vital signs taken, Sadira bursts into tears. She tearfully explains that she's afraid that she has cancer, and that no one at her regular physician's office told her what to expect from this procedure. Sadira does not understand why she has to have this procedure done, and she does not know what the physician will be doing during the procedure. She says that she feels stupid, but she does not even know what a cervix is. Sadira also worries that the procedure will affect her ability to have children. ■

by a pathologist. The purpose of the biopsy is to determine whether the specimen is benign or malignant. Cervical biopsies are often performed following abnormal Pap test results. The procedure is usually performed 1 week after the end of the menstrual period, when the cervix is the least vascular. To prepare for the procedure, the patient should be told not to douche; use tampons, vaginal medications, or spermicides; or have intercourse for 2 days before the examination.

Procedure

A cervical biopsy is performed as follows:

1. The patient is positioned and draped in a lithotomy position. An anesthetic is not necessary; because the cervix has few pain receptors, the patient experiences little discomfort from the procedure. Some patients experience mild cramping and pinching when the specimen is being removed from the cervix.
2. The physician inserts a vaginal speculum into the vagina for proper visualization of the cervix.
3. To assist in obtaining the specimen, the physician may stain the cervix with Lugol's solution.
4. The colposcope is focused on the cervix, and the physician inspects the cervix.
5. Using cervical biopsy punch forceps, the physician obtains several tissue specimens (Figure 25-20A) from the abnormal cervical epithelium (Figure 25-20B).

Cervix

Punch forceps

A

Kevorkian punch tip

Wittner punch tip

Universal handle

B

Figure 25-20. Cervical punch biopsy. **A,** Obtaining a tissue specimen from the cervix using cervical biopsy punch forceps. **B,** Cervical biopsy punch forceps. (Courtesy Elmed, Addison, Ill.)

6. The specimen is placed in a container with a preservative and is sent to the laboratory for examination by a pathologist.
7. If bleeding occurs, the physician controls it with gauze packing, a hemostatic solution (e.g., Monsel's solution), or electrocautery.
8. The patient is given a sanitary pad at the office after the procedure to absorb any discharge.

Postoperative Instructions

Postoperative instructions include the following:
1. The patient should be informed that a minimum amount of bleeding may follow the procedure.
2. The patient should be instructed to contact the physician if bleeding is heavier than normal menstrual bleeding.
3. A foul-smelling, gray-green vaginal discharge may occur several days after the procedure and continue for 3 weeks. The patient should be informed that this discharge results from normal healing of cervical tissue and gradually diminishes as the healing progresses.
4. An appointment is scheduled approximately 1 week following the procedure to make sure that healing is taking place and to discuss the biopsy results.

Cryosurgery

Cervical

Cervical **cryosurgery,** also known as *cryotherapy,* is often used to treat chronic cervicitis and cervical erosion through the use of freezing temperatures. The procedure can be performed without an anesthetic, although occasionally a mild analgesic is necessary immediately afterward. The cryosurgery unit consists of a long metal probe attached to a cooling-agent tank (Figure 25-21). The principal cooling agents are liquid nitrogen, nitrous oxide, and carbon dioxide gas; of these, liquid nitrogen is used most often. The probe

Figure 25-21. Cryosurgery unit. (From Zakus S: *Clinical skills for medical assistants,* ed 4, Philadelphia, 2001, Saunders.)

is placed in contact with the infected area, and the cooling agent flows through the probe, freezing the cervical tissue to 40°C to 80°C. This causes the cells to die and slough off so that the cervical covering can eventually be replaced with new, healthy epithelial tissue. The regeneration of cervical tissue occurs within approximately 4 to 6 weeks after the procedure.

Procedure

Cryosurgery is performed as follows:
1. The patient is draped and assisted into the lithotomy position.
2. The physician inserts a vaginal speculum for proper visualization of the cervix.
3. The cervix is swabbed with an acid-saline solution to remove mucus and other contaminants.
4. The metal probe is placed in contact with the affected area, and the cryosurgery unit is turned on.
5. The cooling agent is permitted to flow over the cervical area for approximately 3 minutes. During the procedure, the patient may experience some pain resembling menstrual cramping, which usually lasts about 30 minutes.
6. When the procedure has been completed, the medical assistant should assist the patient as needed and observe her for signs of discomfort or vertigo.
7. The patient is given a sanitary pad at the office after the procedure to absorb any discharge.

Postoperative Instructions

Postoperative instructions include the following:
1. The patient should be informed of the type of discharge that normally occurs after the cryosurgery. On the first postoperative day, the patient will develop a heavy, clear, watery vaginal discharge, which usually reaches its maximum by the sixth day.
2. The patient should be told to use sanitary pads, rather than tampons, at home. In addition, a vaginal cream may be prescribed to promote healing and the formation of new epithelial tissue.
3. The patient should be told that continuation of the discharge for approximately 4 weeks is normal, but that the development of a foul odor should be reported to the physician.
4. The patient should be informed that the next menstrual period will be heavier than normal and may involve some cramping.
5. The patient is usually instructed to abstain from intercourse for 4 weeks after the procedure and to douche with a solution of dilute vinegar and water.
6. The patient must schedule a return visit 6 weeks after the procedure to ensure that proper healing has occurred.

Skin Lesions

In the medical office, cryosurgery may also be used to remove benign skin lesions, such as common warts. Only a small amount of cooling agent is required for skin lesions, so the cryosurgery unit is considerably smaller than the one described for cervical cryosurgery. Most physicians use liquid nitrogen contained in a small, pressurized, stainless steel canister with an attached probe. The physician applies the liquid nitrogen to the skin lesion until it turns white, which indicates that freezing of the tissue has occurred. During the procedure, the patient feels a slight burning or stinging sensation as the cooling agent is applied. After cryosurgery, a blister develops and dries to a scab in 1 week to 10 days and eventually sloughs off. The patient should be told to keep the area clean and dry until the scab has sloughed off. In some cases, the treatment may not result in complete destruction of the lesion; two or more treatments may be required to remove the lesion.

BANDAGING

A **bandage** is a strip of woven material used to wrap or cover a part of the body. The function of the bandage may be to apply pressure to control bleeding, to protect a wound from contamination, to hold a dressing in place, or to protect, support, or immobilize an injured part of the body.

Guidelines for Application

The bandage should be applied so that it feels comfortable to the patient, and it must be fastened securely with metal clips or adhesive tape. Guidelines for applying a bandage are as follows:

1. Observe the principles of medical asepsis during the application of a bandage.
2. Ensure that the area to which a bandage is applied is clean and dry.
3. Do not apply a bandage directly over an open wound. To prevent contamination of the wound, apply first a sterile dressing and then the bandage. The bandage should extend at least 2 inches (5 cm) beyond the edge of the dressing.
4. To prevent irritation, do not allow the skin surfaces of two body parts (e.g., two fingers) to touch. In addition, the patient's perspiration provides a moist environment that encourages the growth of microorganisms. A piece of gauze should be inserted between the two body parts.
5. Ensure that joints and prominent parts of bones are padded to prevent the bandage from rubbing the skin and causing irritation.
6. Bandage the body part in its normal position with joints slightly flexed to avoid muscle strain.
7. Apply the bandage from the distal to the proximal part of the body to aid the venous return of blood to the heart.
8. As you apply the bandage, ask the patient whether it feels comfortable. The bandage should fit snugly enough that it does not fall off, but not so tightly that it impedes circulation.
9. If possible, leave the fingers and toes exposed when bandaging an extremity. This provides the opportunity to check them for signs of impairment in circulation. Signs indicating that the bandage is too tight include coldness, pallor, numbness, cyanosis of the nailbeds, swelling, pain, and tingling sensations. If any of these signs occurs, loosen the bandage immediately.
10. If a bandage roll is dropped during the procedure, obtain a new bandage and begin again.

Types of Bandages

Three basic types of bandages are used in the medical office. A *roller bandage* is a long strip of soft material wound on itself to form a roll. It ranges from 0.5 to 6 inches (1.3 to 15.2 cm) wide and from 2 to 5 yards (1.83 to 4.57 m) long. The width used depends on the part being bandaged. Roller bandages are usually made of sterilized gauze. Gauze is porous and lightweight, molds easily to a body part, and is relatively inexpensive and disposable. Because it is made of loosely woven cotton, however, it may slip and fray easily. *Kling gauze* is a special type of gauze that stretches; this allows it to cling, and, as a result, it molds and conforms better to the body part than does regular gauze.

Elastic bandages are made of woven cotton that contains elastic fibers. One brand name of elastic bandages is the Ace bandage. Although elastic bandages are expensive, they can be washed and used again. The medical assistant must be extremely careful when applying an elastic bandage because it is easy to apply it too tightly and impede circulation. Elastic adhesive bandages may also be used; these have an adhesive backing to provide a secure fit.

Bandage Turns

Five basic bandage turns are used, alone or in combination. The type of turn used depends on which body part is to be bandaged, and whether the bandage is used for support or immobilization or for holding a dressing in place.

The *circular turn* is applied to a part of uniform width, such as toes, fingers, or the head. Each turn completely overlaps the previous turn. Two circular turns are used to anchor a bandage at the beginning and end of a spiral, spiral-reverse, figure-eight, or recurrent turn (Figure 25-22).

The *spiral turn* is applied to a part of uniform circumference, such as the fingers, arms, legs, chest, or abdomen. Each spiral turn is carried upward at a slight angle and should overlap the previous turn by one half to two thirds the width of the bandage (Figure 25-23).

The *spiral-reverse turn* is useful for bandaging a part that varies in width, such as the forearm or lower leg. Reversing each spiral turn allows for a smoother fit and prevents gaping caused by the variation in the contour of the limb. The thumb is used to make the reverse halfway through each spiral turn. The bandage is directed downward and folded on itself while it is kept parallel to the lower edge of the previous turn. Each turn should overlap the previous one by two thirds the width of the bandage. The reverse turn is used as often as needed to provide a uniform fit (Figure 25-24).

1. Place the end of the roller bandage on a slant.

2. Encircle the part while allowing the corner of the bandage to extend.

3. Turn down the corner of the bandage.

4. Make another circular turn around the part.

Figure 25-22. Procedure for anchoring a bandage. (From Bonewit-West K: *Clinical procedures for medical assistants,* ed 7, St. Louis, 2008, Saunders.)

Figure 25-23. Procedure for making the spiral turn. (From Bonewit-West K: *Clinical procedures for medical assistants,* ed 7, St. Louis, 2008, Saunders.)

A

B

C

Figure 25-24. Procedure for making the spiral-reverse turn. **A,** Encircle the part while keeping the bandage at a slant. **B,** Reverse the spiral turn using the thumb or index finger, and direct the bandage downward and fold it on itself. **C,** Keep the bandage parallel to the lower edge of the previous turn. (From Bonewit-West K: *Clinical procedures for medical assistants,* ed 7, St. Louis, 2008, Saunders.)

Figure 25-25. Procedure for applying an elastic bandage around the ankle using a figure-eight turn. (From Leake MJ: *A manual of simple nursing procedures,* Philadelphia, 1971, Saunders.)

Figure 25-26. Procedure for using the recurrent turn to bandage the end of a stump. (From Bonewit-West K: *Clinical procedures for medical assistants,* ed 7, St. Louis, 2008, Saunders.)

The *figure-eight turn* is generally used to hold a dressing in place or to support and immobilize an injured joint, such as the ankle, knee, elbow, or wrist. The figure-eight turn consists of slanting turns that alternately ascend and descend around the part and cross over one another in the middle, resembling the figure 8. Each turn overlaps the previous one by two thirds the width of the bandage (Figure 25-25).

The *recurrent turn* is a series of back-and-forth turns used to bandage the tips of fingers or toes, the stump of an amputated extremity, or the head. The bandage is anchored by using two circular turns and is passed back and forth over the tip of the part to be bandaged, first on one side and then on the other side of the first center turn. Each turn should overlap the previous turn by two thirds the width of the bandage (Figure 25-26).

MEDICAL PRACTICE *and the* LAW

Surgical procedures are invasive and painful, and they have the potential for harmful complications and subsequent lawsuits. Before having a surgical procedure performed, the patient must sign a consent to treatment form. It is the medical assistant's responsibility to witness the patient's signature, but it is the physician's responsibility to inform the patient of the procedure to be performed and its risks, alternative procedures, and benefits. The physician may delegate some or all of these tasks to the medical assistant, but *do not* accept this responsibility. Patients cannot sign for themselves if they are minors or if they are impaired by drugs or disease, such as Alzheimer's disease. In these cases, consent must be obtained from the legal guardian or next of kin. Before asking a patient to sign a consent to treatment form, ask whether he or she has any questions. If so, make sure the information is given before the consent is signed. Make sure you know what procedures require informed consent in your office.

During the procedure, your duty is to assist the physician and maintain surgical asepsis. If this is broken, you must inform the physician and remedy the situation. There is no such thing as "almost sterile."

After the surgical procedure, the medical assistant must give the patient home care instructions. Home care must be performed exactly to ensure proper healing. Instructions should be given verbally, demonstrated, and given in writing. Written instructions must be in the correct language and at the patient's reading level. Pictures included with the written instructions can clarify difficult points. Many offices purchase preprinted instructions for common surgical procedures. Make sure the signs of infection are listed on these sheets, along with instructions to call the physician if they occur, or if any other problems or questions arise. ∎

What Would You Do? What Would You *Not* Do? RESPONSES

Case Study 1
Page 545

What Did Trudy Do?
❏ Tried to calm and reassure Mrs. Ventura. Told her that children at this age are prone to accidents and that she should not blame herself.
❏ Told Mrs. Ventura that Cory's wound could not be held together effectively with Steri-Strips. Explained that sutures would help the wound heal better.
❏ Told Mrs. Ventura that the doctor could not perform the procedure unless she signs the consent form. Explained that Cory's wound should be sutured as soon as possible to prevent infection and to minimize scarring.
❏ Asked Mrs. Ventura whether she would like to talk with the doctor again about any questions she has about the procedure before signing the form.

What Did Trudy Not *Do?*
❏ Did not prepare Cory for the suture insertion procedure until Mrs. Ventura signed the consent to treatment form.

What Would You Do?/What Would You *Not* Do? Review Trudy's response and place a checkmark next to the information you included in your response. List additional information you included in your response.

_____
_____
_____
_____

Case Study 2
Page 555

What Did Trudy Do?
❏ Explained to Abbey that the antiseptic contains iodine, which appears orange when it is applied to the skin. Assured her that the iodine would not stain her skin permanently and that it would wear off in a few days.
❏ Calmly and discreetly opened a new pair of sterile gloves so that the physician could reapply sterile gloves. Reminded Abbey not to move during the procedure.

What Would You Do? What Would You *Not* Do? RESPONSES—cont'd

- ❏ Told Abbey that all tissues removed from patients are routinely sent to the laboratory for a biopsy. Reassured her that the doctor has told her everything he knows about her condition.
- ❏ Made it clear to Abbey that her neighbor is not permitted to remove her sutures. Stressed to her that the doctor needs to check her incision before the sutures are removed to ensure that proper healing has occurred.

What Did Trudy Not Do?

- ❏ Did not scold Abbey for contaminating the physician's sterile gloved hand.

What Would You Do?/What Would You *Not* Do? Review Trudy's response and place a checkmark next to the information you included in your response. List additional information you included in your response.

_____

_____

_____

_____

Case Study 3
Page 563

What Did Trudy Do?

- ❏ Listened empathetically to Sadira, and tried to calm and reassure her.

- ❏ Spent some time going over the colposcopy procedure and what to expect.
- ❏ Answered as many of Sadira's questions as possible. Reassured her that a lot of people do not know what a cervix is and that she was asking some very good questions.
- ❏ Asked the physician to spend some time talking with Sadira before the procedure to answer the questions that Trudy was not qualified to answer.
- ❏ Ensured that Sadira understood all of the information about the procedure before asking her to sign a consent to treatment form.

What Did Trudy Not Do?

- ❏ Did not tell Sadira that her family physician and staff should have spent some time explaining the procedure to her so that she did not have to worry so much.
- ❏ Did not tell Sadira that she does not have cancer.

What Would You Do?/What Would You *Not* Do? Review Trudy's response and place a checkmark next to the information you included in your response. List additional information you included in your response.

_____

_____

_____

_____

TERMINOLOGY REVIEW

Abrasion A wound in which the outer layers of the skin are damaged; a scrape.

Abscess A collection of pus in a cavity surrounded by inflamed tissue.

Absorbable suture Suture material that is gradually digested by tissue enzymes and absorbed by the body.

Approximation The process of bringing two parts, such as tissue, together through the use of sutures or other means.

Bandage A strip of woven material used to wrap or cover a part of the body.

Biopsy The surgical removal and examination of tissue from the living body. Biopsies are generally performed to determine whether a tumor is benign or malignant.

Capillary action The action that causes liquid to rise along a wick, tube, or gauze dressing.

Colposcope A lighted instrument with a binocular magnifying lens used to examine the vagina and cervix.

Colposcopy The visual examination of the vagina and cervix using a colposcope.

Contaminate As it relates to sterile technique, to cause a sterile object or surface to become unsterile.

Contusion An injury to the tissues under the skin that causes blood vessels to rupture, allowing blood to seep into the tissues; a bruise.

Cryosurgery The therapeutic use of freezing temperatures to destroy abnormal tissue.

Exudate A discharge produced by the body's tissues.

Fibroblast An immature cell from which connective tissue can develop.

Forceps A two-pronged instrument for grasping and squeezing.

Furuncle A localized staphylococcal infection that originates deep within a hair follicle. Also known as a *boil.*

Hemostasis The arrest of bleeding by natural or artificial means.

Continued

TERMINOLOGY REVIEW—cont'd

Incision A clean cut caused by a cutting instrument.

Infection The condition in which the body, or part of it, is invaded by a pathogen.

Infiltration The process by which a substance passes into and is deposited within the substance of a cell, tissue, or organ.

Inflammation A protective response of the body to trauma and the entrance of foreign matter. The purpose of inflammation is to destroy invading microorganisms and to repair injured tissue.

Laceration A wound in which the tissues are torn apart, leaving ragged and irregular edges.

Ligate To tie off and close a structure, such as a severed blood vessel.

Local anesthetic A drug that produces a loss of feeling and an inability to perceive pain in only a specific part of the body.

Mayo tray A broad, flat metal tray placed on a stand and used to hold sterile instruments and supplies when it has been covered with a sterile towel.

Needle biopsy A type of biopsy in which tissue from deep within the body is obtained by the insertion of a biopsy needle through the skin.

Nonabsorbable suture Suture material that is not absorbed by the body and either remains permanently in the body tissue and becomes encapsulated by fibrous tissue or is removed.

Postoperative After a surgical operation.

Preoperative Preceding a surgical operation.

Puncture A wound made by a sharp pointed object piercing the skin.

Scalpel A surgical knife used to divide tissues.

Scissors A cutting instrument.

Sebaceous cyst A thin, closed sac or capsule that contains fatty secretions from a sebaceous gland.

Serum The clear, straw-colored part of the blood that remains after the solid elements have been separated out of it.

Sterile Free of all living microorganisms and bacterial spores.

Surgical asepsis Practices that keep objects and areas sterile or free from microorganisms.

Sutures Material used to approximate tissues with surgical stitches.

Swaged needle A needle with suturing material permanently attached to its end.

Wound A break in the continuity of an external or internal surface caused by physical means.

ON THE WEB

For Information on Surgery and Emergency Medicine:

The American College of Surgeons: www.facs.org

American Red Cross: www.redcross.org

Ethicon Incorporated: www.ethicon.com

Federal Emergency Management Agency: www.fema.gov

PREPARE FOR CERTIFICATION   Visit the Evolve site at http://evolve.elsevier.com/Bonewit/today/ to actively Prepare for your Certification.

CD   *Check out the Companion CD bound with the book to access additional interactive activities.*

26

Administration of Medication and Intravenous Therapy

LEARNING OBJECTIVES

Introduction to the Administration of Medication

1. Explain the difference between administering, prescribing, and dispensing medication.
2. State the common routes for administering medication.
3. List and describe the six sections of the PDR.
4. List and describe the categories of information in a drug package insert.
5. Describe the Food and Drug Administration's responsibilities with respect to drugs.
6. List and define the four names of drugs.
7. Classify drugs according to preparation.
8. Classify drugs according to the action they have on the body.
9. List the guidelines for writing metric and apothecary notations.
10. List and describe the five schedules for controlled drugs.
11. List and explain the parts of a prescription.
12. Explain the purpose of a medication record.
13. Describe the factors that affect the action of drugs in the body.
14. List and describe the possible adverse effects of medication.
15. List the guidelines for preparing and administering medication.

Oral Administration

1. Explain why the oral route is most frequently used to administer medication.
2. State where the absorption of most oral medications occurs.

Parenteral Administration

1. State the advantages and disadvantages of the parenteral route of administration.
2. Identify the parts of a needle and syringe, and explain their functions.
3. State the ranges of gauge and length of needles for the following injections: intradermal, subcutaneous (SC), and intramuscular (IM).
4. State the purpose of safety-engineered syringes.
5. Describe the dispensing units available for injectable medications.
6. State which tissue layers of the body are used for intradermal, SC, and IM injections.
7. List the medications commonly administered through the following routes: SC and IM.
8. Explain the reason for administering medication with the Z-track method.

PROCEDURES

Research a drug using the *Physician's Desk Reference* (PDR).
Interpret a drug package insert.
Calculate drug dosage.
Complete a prescription form.
Complete a medication record form.

Prepare and administer oral medications.

Reconstitute a powdered drug for parenteral administration.
Withdraw medication from a vial.
Withdraw medication from an ampule.
Locate appropriate SC injection sites.
Administer an SC injection.
Locate each of the following IM injection sites: dorsogluteal, deltoid, vastus lateralis, and ventrogluteal.
Administer an IM injection.
Administer an injection using the Z-track method.
Administer an intradermal injection.

Tuberculin Testing

1. List the symptoms of active tuberculosis (TB).
2. Explain the purpose of tuberculin testing.
3. Explain the significance of a positive reaction to a tuberculin test.
4. List the diagnostic procedures that might be performed after a positive tuberculin test.

Administer a Mantoux test, and read the test results.
Administer a tine test, and read the test results.
Complete a TB test record card.

Allergy Testing

1. Define an allergy, and name common allergens.
2. Explain what occurs during an allergic reaction.
3. List the guidelines for direct skin allergy testing.
4. State the purpose of the following types of allergy tests: patch testing, skin-prick testing, intradermal skin testing, and radioallergosorbent assay testing.

Perform allergy skin testing.

Intravenous Therapy

1. Explain the advantages of outpatient intravenous (IV) therapy.
2. Identify the role of the entry-level medical assistant in IV therapy.
3. State the indications for outpatient IV therapy.
4. Describe how medication is administered through the following methods: direct IV injection, intermittent IV administration, and continuous IV administration.
5. Identify when the following medications may be administered intravenously in an outpatient setting: antibiotics, chemotherapy, monoclonal antibodies, and analgesics.
6. State when each of the following may be administered intravenously in an outpatient setting: fluids and electrolytes, nutritional supplements, and blood products.

CHAPTER OUTLINE

Introduction to the Administration of Medication
Administering, Prescribing, and Dispensing Medication
Legal Aspects
Routes of Administration
Drug References
Food and Drug Administration
Drug Nomenclature
Classification of Drugs Based on Preparation
  Liquid Preparations
  Solid Preparations
Classification of Drugs Based on Action
Systems of Measurement for Medication
  Metric System
  Apothecary System
  Household System
Converting Units of Measurement
Controlled Drugs
Prescription
  Parts of a Prescription
  Generic Prescribing
  Completing a Prescription Form
Medication Record
Factors Affecting Drug Action
  Therapeutic Effect
  Undesirable Effects of Drugs

Guidelines for Preparation and Administration of Medication
Oral Administration
Parenteral Administration
  Parts of a Needle and Syringe
  Safety-Engineered Syringes
  Preparation of Parenteral Medication
  Storage
  Reconstitution of Powdered Drugs
  Subcutaneous Injections
  Intramuscular Injections
  Intradermal Injections
Tuberculin Testing
  Tuberculosis
  Purpose of Tuberculin Testing
  Tuberculin Test Reactions
  Tuberculin Testing Methods
  Mantoux Test
Allergy Testing
  Allergy
  Allergic Reaction
  Diagnosis and Treatment
  Types of Allergy Tests
Intravenous Therapy
  Advantages of Outpatient Intravenous Therapy
  Medical Office–Based Intravenous Therapy

CAAHEP COMPETENCIES

Clinical Competencies
Patient Care
- Apply pharmacology principles to prepare and administer oral and parenteral medications.
- Maintain medication and immunization records.

General Competencies
Legal Concepts
- Document appropriately.
- Demonstrate knowledge of federal and state health care legislation and regulations.

ABHES COMPETENCIES

Clinical Duties
- Prepare and administer oral and parenteral medications as directed by physician.
- Maintain medication and immunization records.

Legal Concepts
- Document accurately.
- Dispose of controlled substances in compliance with government regulations.
- Monitor legislation related to current health care issues and practices.

KEY TERMS

adverse reaction (AD-vers ree-AK-shun)
allergen (AL-er-jen)
allergy (AL-er-jee)
ampule (AM-pyool)
anaphylactic reaction (an-uh-ful-AK-tik ree-AK-shun)
autoimmune disease
chemotherapy
controlled drug
conversion (kon-VER-shun)
cubic centimeter (KYOO-bik SEN-tih-mee-ter) (cc)
DEA number
dose
drug
enteral nutrition
gauge (GAYJ)
hemophilia
immune globulin
induration (in-dur-AY-shun)
infusion

inhalation (in-hal-AY-shun)
inscription (in-SKRIP-shun)
intradermal injection (in-tra-DER-mal in-JEK-shun)
intramuscular (in-tra-MUS-kyoo-lar) (IM) injection
intravenous (in-tra-VEE-nus) (IV) therapy
oral (OR-ul) administration
parenteral (par-EN-ter-al)
pharmacology (far-ma-KOL-oh-jee)
prescription
signatura (sig-na-CHUR-ah)
subcutaneous (sub-kyoo-TAY-nee-us) (SC) injection
sublingual (sub-LIN-gwal) administration
subscription (sub-SKRIP-shun)
superscription (soo-per-SKRIP-shun)
topical (TOP-ih-kul) administration
transfusion
vial (VIE-ul)
wheal (WEE-ul)

Introduction to the Administration of Medication

Pharmacology is the study of drugs and includes the preparation, use, and action of drugs in the body. A **drug** is a chemical that is used for the treatment, prevention, or diagnosis of disease. Most drugs are produced synthetically, but they also can be obtained from other sources, such as animals, plants, and minerals.

ADMINISTERING, PRESCRIBING, AND DISPENSING MEDICATION

Medication may be administered, prescribed, or dispensed in the medical office. Medication that is administered is actually given to a patient at the office. Medication is prescribed when a physician provides a patient with a handwritten or computer-generated prescription for a drug to be filled at a pharmacy. Prescriptions can also be telephoned or faxed to the pharmacy by the physician, depending on the preference of the patient. Dispensed medication is given to a patient at the office to be taken at home; for example, the physician gives a patient drug samples to take home.

LEGAL ASPECTS

An important responsibility of the medical assistant is the administration of medication. (One should check the laws of the state to ensure that it is legally permissible for the medical assistant to administer medication.) The medical assistant should administer medication only under the direction of the physician. In all states, it is unlawful to administer medication in the medical office without the consent of the physician.

ROUTES OF ADMINISTRATION

Common routes of administration of medication are oral, **sublingual, inhalation,** rectal, vaginal, **topical,** intradermal, subcutaneous (SC), intramuscular (IM), and intravenous (IV). The route of administration depends on the type of drug being given, the dosage form, the intended action, and the rapidity of response desired. The route by which medication is most commonly administered in the medical office is the parenteral route. **Parenteral** refers to sites outside the gastrointestinal tract; this term is most commonly used to refer to the administration of medication by injection.

DRUG REFERENCES

The medical assistant is obligated to become familiar with the drugs that are most frequently used in his or her office. It is essential to know their indications, adverse reactions, route of administration, dosage, and storage. With each drug (including drug samples and injectable medications), the manufacturer includes a *package insert,* which contains valuable information regarding the drug. In addition, many drug references are available. The *Physician's Desk Reference* (PDR) is frequently used in the medical office. The PDR contains information on most major prescription pharmaceutical products available in the United States. The drug information in the PDR consists of the actual drug package insert. Figure 26-1 provides guidelines for using the PDR. These guidelines not only assist in learning how to use the PDR, but they also provide the necessary information for understanding how to interpret drug package inserts. Drug information is also available on the Internet on certain recognized websites; many of these sites are listed at the end of the chapter in the box titled *On the Web: For Information on Pharmacology.*

FOOD AND DRUG ADMINISTRATION

The U.S. Food and Drug Administration (FDA) is a federal agency in the Department of Health and Human Services. The FDA is responsible for determining whether new food products, drugs, vaccines, medical devices, cosmetics, and other products are safe before they are released for human use.

The FDA determines the safety and effectiveness of prescription and nonprescription (over-the-counter [OTC]) drugs. Pharmaceutical manufacturers are required to submit new drug applications to the FDA for review and approval before products can be released for human use.

The FDA is also responsible for determining whether a medication will be available with or without a prescription. Medications that require a prescription have been determined by the FDA to be safe and effective when used under the guidance of a physician. Prescription medication labels must bear the following statement: *Caution: Federal law prohibits dispensing without a prescription.*

Nonprescription medications are drugs that the FDA determines to be safe and effective for use without physician supervision. Nonprescription medications have a low incidence of adverse reactions when the consumer follows the directions and warnings on the label. Examples of nonprescription medications include mild pain relievers, topical antibiotics, topical corticosteroids, cold medications, and laxatives.

DRUG NOMENCLATURE

Each drug has four names: the chemical, generic, official, and brand, or trade, name.
1. **Chemical name.** The chemical name provides a precise description of the drug's chemical composition; pharmaceutical manufacturers and pharmacists are most concerned with the chemical makeup of a drug.
2. **Generic name.** The generic name is assigned by the pharmaceutical manufacturer who develops the drug, before it receives official approval by the FDA. The generic name is often a shortened derivative of the chemical name.
3. **Official name.** The official name is the name under which the drug is listed in official publications, such as the *United States Pharmacopeia* and the *National Formulary.* Official publications set specific standards to regulate the strength, purity, packaging, safety, labeling, and dosage form of each drug. The generic name is frequently used for the official name.
4. **Brand name.** The brand name is the name under which a pharmaceutical manufacturer markets a drug. Because a drug may be manufactured by more than one pharmaceutical company, it may have several brand names. The generic name of a common analgesic is acetaminophen; brand names for this drug include Tylenol, Tempra, Datril, Exdol, Panadol, and Liquiprim.

GUIDELINES FOR USING THE PHYSICIAN'S DESK REFERENCE

The *Physician's Desk Reference* (PDR) is published annually by the Medical Economics Company with the cooperation of the pharmaceutical manufacturers whose products are included in it. This reference includes essential information on most major prescription pharmaceutical products available in the United States. The PDR is divided into color-coded sections, which are described below.

SECTION 1: MANUFACTURER'S INDEX
(Color Code: White)

The Manufacturer's Index lists pharmaceutical manufacturers in alphabetical order along with a list of drugs that are manufactured by each company. This index provides all of the necessary information, should the manufacturer need to be contacted regarding a particular drug.

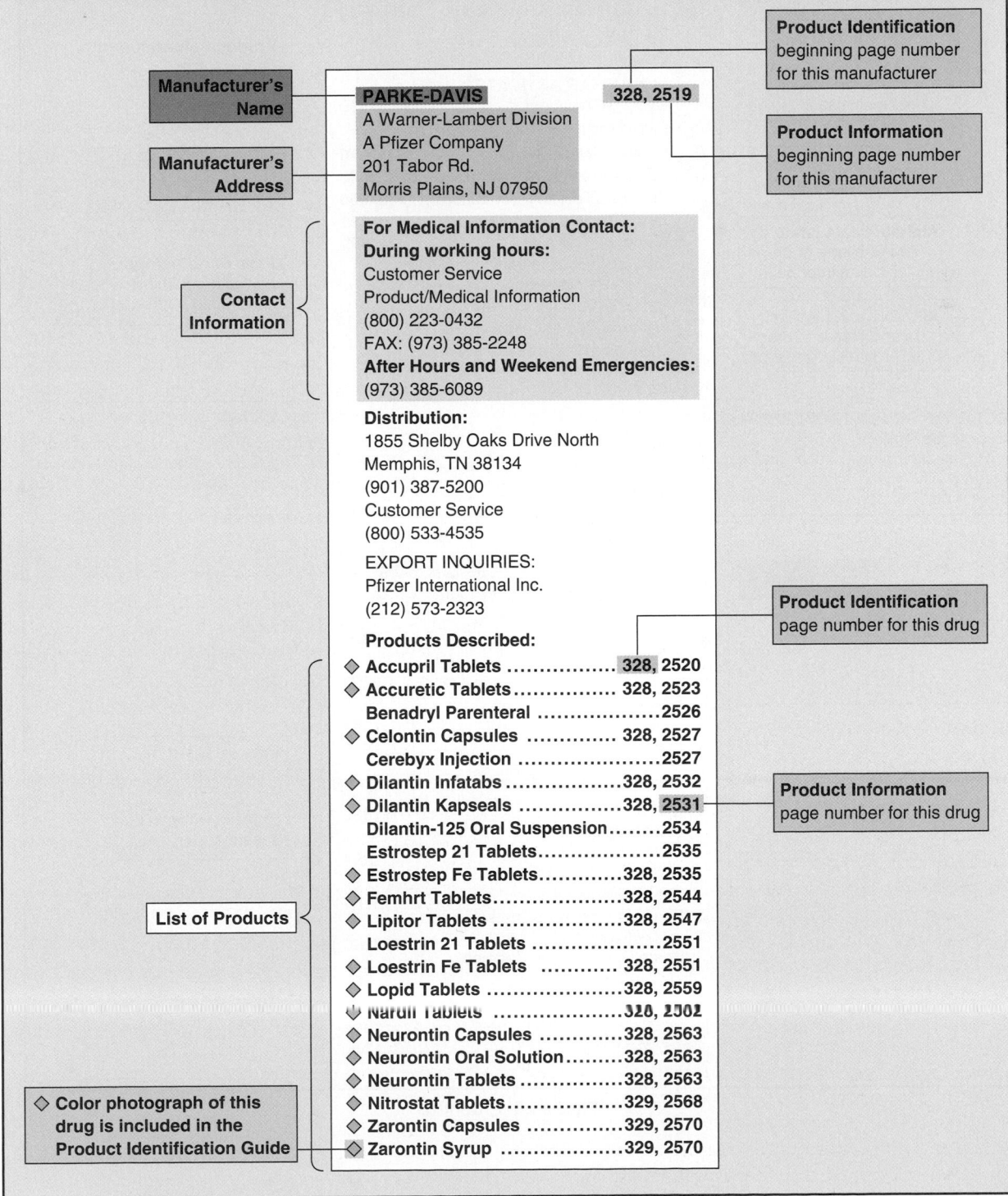

Manufacturer's Name

PARKE-DAVIS   328, 2519

Manufacturer's Address

A Warner-Lambert Division
A Pfizer Company
201 Tabor Rd.
Morris Plains, NJ 07950

Product Identification beginning page number for this manufacturer

Product Information beginning page number for this manufacturer

Contact Information

For Medical Information Contact:
During working hours:
Customer Service
Product/Medical Information
(800) 223-0432
FAX: (973) 385-2248
After Hours and Weekend Emergencies:
(973) 385-6089

Distribution:
1855 Shelby Oaks Drive North
Memphis, TN 38134
(901) 387-5200
Customer Service
(800) 533-4535

EXPORT INQUIRIES:
Pfizer International Inc.
(212) 573-2323

Product Identification page number for this drug

Products Described:

Product	Pages
◇ Accupril Tablets	328, 2520
◇ Accuretic Tablets	328, 2523
Benadryl Parenteral	2526
◇ Celontin Capsules	328, 2527
Cerebyx Injection	2527
◇ Dilantin Infatabs	328, 2532
◇ Dilantin Kapseals	328, 2531
Dilantin-125 Oral Suspension	2534
Estrostep 21 Tablets	2535
◇ Estrostep Fe Tablets	328, 2535
◇ Femhrt Tablets	328, 2544
◇ Lipitor Tablets	328, 2547
Loestrin 21 Tablets	2551
◇ Loestrin Fe Tablets	328, 2551
◇ Lopid Tablets	328, 2559
◇ Nardil Tablets	328, 2502
◇ Neurontin Capsules	328, 2563
◇ Neurontin Oral Solution	328, 2563
◇ Neurontin Tablets	328, 2563
◇ Nitrostat Tablets	329, 2568
◇ Zarontin Capsules	329, 2570
◇ Zarontin Syrup	329, 2570

Product Information page number for this drug

List of Products

◇ **Color photograph of this drug is included in the Product Identification Guide**

Figure 26-1. Guidelines for using the *Physician's Desk Reference.* (From Bonewit-West K: *Clinical procedures for medical assistants,* ed 7, St. Louis, 2008, Saunders.)

Continued

SECTION 2: BRAND AND GENERIC NAME INDEX
(Color Code: Pink)
   This section consists of an alphabetical listing of the drugs included in the PDR by both generic and brand names. This section allows for the quick and easy location of drug information.

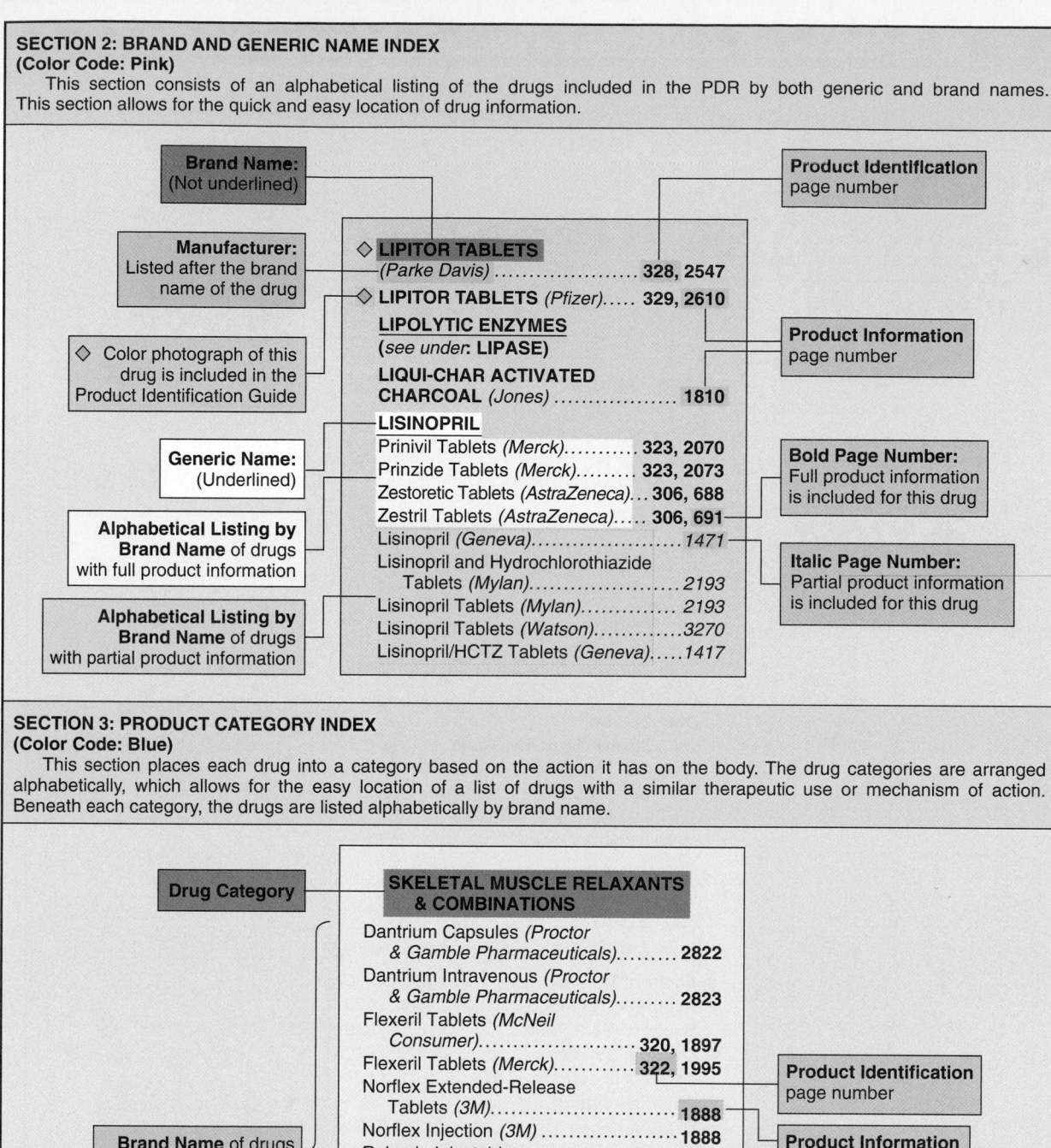

SECTION 3: PRODUCT CATEGORY INDEX
(Color Code: Blue)
   This section places each drug into a category based on the action it has on the body. The drug categories are arranged alphabetically, which allows for the easy location of a list of drugs with a similar therapeutic use or mechanism of action. Beneath each category, the drugs are listed alphabetically by brand name.

Figure 26-1, cont'd.

**SECTION 4: PRODUCT IDENTIFICATION GUIDE
(Color Code: Gray)**

This section provides a full-color (actual size) photograph of the tablets and capsules included in the PDR. The drugs are arranged alphabetically by manufacturer. A variety of other dosage forms are also illustrated, but are shown in less than actual size (e.g., inhalers, injectable drugs in vials). This section provides valuable assistance in identifying a drug.

**SECTION 5: PRODUCT INFORMATION
(Color Code: White)**

This index makes up the main section of the PDR and contains product information on approximately 3000 drug products. The drugs are arranged alphabetically by manufacturer; under the manufacturer, the drugs are listed alphabetically by brand name. The information included in this section consists of the actual drug package inserts. The following information is included for each medication:

DESCRIPTION: This category consists of a general description of the drug and includes the following information: brand name (with pronunciation), generic name, drug category, dosage form (e.g., tablets, capsules), route of administration, chemical name and structural formula, and the inactive ingredients contained in the drug. This category also indicates if the product requires a prescription (Rx) or if it is available over-the-counter (OTC). The symbol C and a Roman numeral appearing next to the drug it indicates that it is a scheduled drug and that a prescription written for this drug requires the physician's DEA number.

CLINICAL PHARMACOLOGY: This category describes how the drug functions in the body to produce its therapeutic effect. Also included is an analysis of the absorption, distribution, metabolism, and excretion of the drug after it enters the body.

INDICATIONS AND USAGE: This category presents a list of the conditions that the drug has been formally approved to treat by the Food and Drug Administration (FDA).

CONTRAINDICATIONS: This category includes situations in which the drug should not be used because the risk of using the drug in these situations outweighs any possible benefit. Contraindications include administration of the drug to patients known to have a hypersensitivity (allergy) to it and use of the drug in patients who have a substantial risk of being harmed by it because of their particular age, sex, concurrent use of another drug, disease state, or condition (e.g., pregnancy).

WARNINGS: This category describes serious adverse reactions and potential safety hazards that may occasionally occur with the use of the drug and what should be done if they occur.

PRECAUTIONS: This category includes information regarding any special care that needs to be taken by the physician for the safe and effective use of the drug. Information typically presented in this category includes:

- **General Precautions:** Lists any disease states or situations may require special consideration when the drug is being taken.
- **Information for Patients:** Includes information that should be relayed to the patient to ensure safe and effective use of the drug.
- **Laboratory Tests:** Indicates the laboratory tests that may be helpful in following the patient's response to the drug or in identifying possible adverse reactions to the drug.
- **Drug Interactions:** Lists any known interactions of this drug with other drugs that can affect the proper functioning of the drug.
- **Laboratory Test Interactions:** Includes any laboratory tests that may be affected when taking the medication.
- **Pregnancy:** Indicates the pregnancy category of the drug.

ADVERSE REACTIONS: This category describes the unintended and undesirable effects that may occur with the use of the drug. Some adverse reactions are harmless and therefore often tolerated by the patient in order to obtain the therapeutic effect of the drug. Other adverse reactions may be harmful to the patient and warrant discontinuing the medication.

OVERDOSAGE: This category describes symptoms associated with an overdosage of the drug, as well as the complications that can occur and the treatment to institute for an overdosage.

DOSAGE AND ADMINISTRATION: This category lists the recommended adult dosage, the usual dosage range of the drug, and the route of administration (e.g., by mouth, sublingual, IM). Also included is information about the intervals recommended between doses, the usual duration of treatment, and any modification of dosage needed for special groups such as children, the elderly, and patients with renal or hepatic disease.

HOW SUPPLIED: This category indicates the dosage forms that are available (e.g., 20-mg tablets), the units in which the dosage form is available (e.g., bottles of 100; 5-ml multiple-dose vial), information to help identify the dosage form (shape and color), and the handling and storage conditions for the drug.

SECTION 6: DIAGNOSTIC PRODUCT INFORMATION

This section includes product information on diagnostic products. They are listed alphabetically by manufacturer and provide information on the use of these products. An example of diagnostic product included in this section is Tubersol, which is used to perform tuberculin testing.

Additional information included in the PDR is listed below:

- **FDA Drug Information Centers**
- **Key to Controlled Substances Categories**
- **Key to FDA Use-In-Pregnancy Ratings**

Figure 26-1, cont'd.

What Would You Do? What Would You *Not* Do?

Case Study 1

Carol Okasinski, 56 years old, is a new patient. She was a patient of another physician in the community; however, his receptionist was often rude to her, and she decided not to go there anymore. Mrs. Okasinski is obese and has hypertension, type 2 diabetes, osteoarthritis in her hands and knees, and problems with depression. While filling in the health history form, she says she cannot fill in the names of the medications she is taking. She is on a lot of medications prescribed by her previous physician. She says she could not get the childproof pill containers open because of the arthritis in her hands, so she had her husband throw away the childproof containers and transfer each medication into an easy-to-open plastic container. She knows when to take her medications, but she does not know the names of them or why she is taking them. She has brought in a bag with all her medications in their plastic containers. ■

The medical assistant should be familiar with the generic and the brand names of the medications commonly prescribed and administered in the medical office.

CLASSIFICATION OF DRUGS BASED ON PREPARATION

Drugs are available in two basic forms: liquid and solid. A medication may be available in both these forms (liquid and solid), which permits it to be administered to different types of patients. A liquid preparation of an antibiotic is administered to young children, and the solid preparation (e.g., tablets) of the same medication is administered to older children and adults. The following list includes the common categories of drugs based on preparation.

Liquid Preparations

Elixir   A drug that is dissolved in a solution of alcohol and water. Elixirs are sweetened and flavored and are taken orally. *Example:* Dimetapp Elixir.

Emulsion   A mixture of fats or oils in water. *Example:* Soyacol Emulsion.

Liniment   A drug combined with oil, soap, alcohol, or water. Liniments are applied externally, using friction, to produce a feeling of heat or warmth. *Example:* Heet Liniment.

Lotion   An aqueous preparation that contains suspended ingredients. Lotions are used to treat external skin conditions. They work to soothe, protect, and moisten the skin and to destroy harmful bacteria. *Example:* Caladryl Lotion.

Solution   A liquid preparation that contains one or more completely dissolved substances. The dissolved substance is known as the *solute,* and the liquid in which it is dissolved is known as the *solvent. Example:* Polysporin Ophthalmic Solution.

Spirit   A drug combined with an alcoholic solution that is volatile (a substance that is volatile evaporates readily). *Example:* aromatic spirit of ammonia.

Spray   A fine stream of medicated vapor, usually used to treat nose and throat conditions. *Example:* Dristan Nasal Spray.

Suspension   A drug that contains solid insoluble drug particles in a liquid; the preparation must be shaken before administration. *Example:* Amoxicillin Oral Suspension.

Suspension   A pressurized form in which solid aerosol or liquid drug particles are suspended in a gas to be dispensed in a cloud or mist. *Example:* Proventil Inhalation Aerosol.

Syrup   A drug dissolved in a solution of sugar, water, and sometimes a flavoring to disguise an unpleasant taste. *Example:* Robitussin Cough Syrup.

Tincture   A drug dissolved in a solution of alcohol or alcohol and water. *Example:* tincture of iodine.

Solid Preparations

Tablet   A powdered drug that has been pressed into discs. Some tablets are scored; that is, they are marked with an indentation so that they can be broken into halves or quarters for proper dosage. *Example:* Tylenol Tablets.

Chewable tablet   A powdered drug that has been flavored and pressed into a disc. Chewable tablets are often used for antacids, antiflatulents, and children's medication. *Example:* Pepto-Bismol Chewable Tablets.

Sublingual tablet   A powdered drug that has been pressed into a disc and is designed to dissolve under the tongue, which permits its rapid absorption into the bloodstream. *Example:* nitroglycerin sublingual tablets (Nitrostat).

Enteric-coated tablet   A tablet coated with a substance that prevents it from dissolving until it reaches the intestines. The coating protects the drug from being destroyed by gastric juices and prevents it from irritating the stomach lining. To prevent the active ingredients from being released prematurely in the stomach, enteric-coated tablets must not be crushed or chewed. *Example:* Ecotrin Enteric-Coated Aspirin.

Capsule   A drug contained in a gelatin capsule that is water-soluble and functions to prevent the patient from tasting the drug. *Example:* Benadryl Capsules.

Sustained-release capsule   A capsule containing granules that dissolve at different rates to provide a gradual and continuous release of medication. This reduces the number of doses that must be administered. (Sustained-release medication also comes in other preparations, such as tablets and caplets.) *Example:* Contac 12-Hour Sustained-Release Capsules.

Caplet   A drug contained in an oblong tablet with a smooth coating to make swallowing easier. *Example:* Advil Caplets.

Lozenge   A drug contained in a candylike base. Lozenges are circular and are designed to dissolve on the tongue. *Example:* Chloraseptic Throat Lozenges.

Cream A drug combined in a base that is generally non-greasy, resulting in a semisolid preparation. Creams are applied externally to the skin. *Example:* Hydrocortisone Topical Cream.

Ointment A drug with an oil base, resulting in a semi-solid preparation. Ointments are applied externally to the skin and are usually greasy. *Example:* Cortisporin Topical Ointment.

Suppository A drug mixed with a firm base, such as cocoa butter, that is designed to melt at body temperature. A suppository is shaped into a cylinder or a cone for easy insertion into a body cavity, such as the rectum or vagina. *Example:* Preparation H Suppositories.

Transdermal patch A patch with an adhesive backing, which contains a drug, that is applied to the skin.

The drug enters the circulation after being absorbed through the skin. *Example:* nitroglycerin patches (Nitro-Dur).

CLASSIFICATION OF DRUGS BASED ON ACTION

Drugs can also be classified according to the action they have on the body. The medical assistant should know in which category a particular drug belongs and its primary use and major therapeutic effects. Table 26-1 contains classifications based on action and examples of drugs that are commonly administered and prescribed in the medical office.

Text continued on p. 585

Table 26-1 Classification of Drugs Based on Action

Drug Category	Primary Use and Major Therapeutic Effects	COMMONLY PRESCRIBED DRUGS Generic	Brand
Analgesics (Opioid)	*Used* to manage moderate to severe pain *Work* by altering perception of and response to painful stimuli	codeine/APAP hydrocodone/APAP meperidine oxycodone oxycodone/APAP propoxyphene N/APAP tramadol	▶ Tylenol w/ Codeine (III) ▶ Vicodin (III) Demerol (II) ▶ Oxycontin (II) ▶ Percocet (II) ▶ Darvocet-N (IV), ▶ Ultram
Analgesics/ Antipyretics	*Used* to manage mild to moderate pain and to reduce fever *Work* by relieving pain and reducing fever	acetaminophen aspirin **NSAID** ibuprofen naproxen	Tylenol* Bayer,* Ecotrin* Advil,* Motrin* Aleve,* Naprosyn
Anesthetics (Local)	*Used* to produce local anesthesia through loss of feeling to a body part *Work* by preventing initiation and conduction of normal nerve impulses in body part	lidocaine dibucaine	Xylocaine Nupercainal ointment*
Antacids	*Used* to treat heartburn, hyperacidity, indigestion, and gastroesophageal reflux disease, and to promote healing of ulcers *Work* by neutralizing gastric acid to relieve gastric pain and irritation	aluminum hydroxide/ magnesium hydroxide calcium carbonate	Maalox,* Mylanta* Tums*
Anti-Alzheimer's Agents	*Used* to treat mild to moderate dementia associated with Alzheimer's disease *Work* by elevating acetylcholine concentration in cerebral cortex	donepezil	Aricept
Antianemics	**Iron Supplements** *Used* to prevent or cure iron-deficiency anemia *Work* by increasing amount of iron in body **Vitamin B$_{12}$ Injections** *Used* to treat pernicious anemia *Work* by increasing amount of vitamin B$_{12}$ in body **Folic Acid Supplements** *Used* to promote normal fetal development *Work* by stimulating production of red blood cells, white blood cells, and platelets	ferrous sulfate iron dextran cyanocobalamin folic acid	Feosol* DexFerrum, InFed Cobex, Cyanoject ▶ Folvite
Antianginals	*Used* to relieve or prevent angina attacks *Work* by increasing blood supply to myocardial tissue	**Nitrate** nitroglycerin	Nitro-Bid, Nitrostat

Continued

Table 26-1 Classification of Drugs Based on Action—cont'd

Drug Category	Primary Use and Major Therapeutic Effects	COMMONLY PRESCRIBED DRUGS	
		Generic	Brand
Antianxiety Agents	**Used** to treat anxiety **Work** at many levels in central nervous system to produce anxiolytic (anxiety-relieving) effect	alprazolam diazepam	▶ Xanax (IV) Valium (IV)
Anticholinergics	**Used** to decrease preoperatively oral and respiratory secretions **Work** by blocking effects of acetylcholine in autonomic nervous system	atropine	Atro-Pen
Anticoagulants	**Used** to prevent and treat venous thrombosis, pulmonary embolism, and myocardial infarction by preventing clot extension and formation **Work** by delaying or preventing blood coagulation	warfarin enoxaparin	▶ Coumadin Lovenox
Anticonvulsants	**Used** to prevent or relieve seizures **Work** by decreasing incidence and severity of seizures	clonazepam divalproex phenytoin	▶ Klonopin (IV) ▶ Depakote ▶ Dilantin
Antidepressants	**Used** to prevent, cure, or alleviate depression, and to treat anxiety disorders (panic attacks) and obsessive-convulsive disorder **Work** by inhibiting reuptake of neurotransmitters in central nervous system	**Selective Serotonin Reuptake Inhibitors (SSRIs)** fluoxetine paroxetine sertraline **Miscellaneous** bupropion venlafaxine	 ▶ Prozac ▶ Paxil ▶ Zoloft ▶ Wellbutrin-SR ▶ Effexor XR

Antidiabetics	**Oral Hypoglycemics**
	Used to manage non–insulin-dependent type 2 diabetes mellitus
	Work by stimulating release of insulin from pancreas and increasing sensitivity to insulin
	Insulins
	Used to manage diabetes mellitus
	Work by reducing blood glucose levels
		glipizide
		glyburide
		metformin
		
		regular insulin
		
		NPH insulin
		
		insulin glargine
		insulin lispro
			▶ Glucotrol XL
			▶ Micronase
			▶ Glucophage
			
			Humulin R,*
			  Novolin R*
			▶ Humulin N,*
			  Novolin N*
			Lantus
			Humalog

Antidiarrheals	**Used** to control and relieve diarrhea **Work** by inhibiting peristalsis, reducing fecal volume, and preventing loss of fluids and electrolytes	bismuth subsalicylate diphenoxylate/atropine kaolin/pectin loperamide	Pepto-Bismol* Lomotil (V) Kaopectate* Imodium*
Antidysrhythmics	**Used** to control or prevent cardiac dysrhythmias **Work** by decreasing myocardial excitability and slowing conduction velocity	procainamide propranolol	Pronestyl Inderal
Antiemetics	**Used** to prevent or relieve nausea and vomiting **Work** by depressing chemoreceptor trigger zone in central nervous system to inhibit nausea and vomiting	ondansetron prochlorperazine promethazine	Zofran Compazine ▶ Phenergan
Antiflatulents	**Used** to relieve discomfort of excess gas and bloating in gastrointestinal tract **Work** by causing coalescence of gas bubbles in intestinal tract	simethicone	Gas-X,* Mylanta Gas*
Antifungals	**Used** to treat fungal infections **Work** by killing or inhibiting growth of susceptible fungi	amphotericin B fluconazole miconazole nystatin	Fungizone ▶ Diflucan Monistat* Mycostatin*
Antigout Agents	**Used** to prevent attacks of gout **Work** by inhibiting production of uric acid	allopurinol colchicine	▶ Zyloprim Colchicine tablets
Antihelmintics	**Used** to treat worm infections (pinworms, roundworms, hookworms) **Work** by destroying worms	mebendazole	Vermox

Table 26-1 Classification of Drugs Based on Action—cont'd

Drug Category	Primary Use and Major Therapeutic Effects	COMMONLY PRESCRIBED DRUGS	
		Generic	**Brand**
Antihistamines	*Used* to relieve symptoms associated with allergies (increased sneezing; rhinorrhea; itchy eyes, nose, and throat) *Work* by blocking effects of histamine at histamine receptor sites	cetirizine chlorpheniramine desloratadine diphenhydramine fexofenadine hydroxyzine loratadine	►Zyrtec Chlor-Trimetron* ►Clarinex Benadryl* ►Allegra ►Atarax, Vistaril ►Claritin*
Antihypertensives	*Used* to manage hypertension *Work* by causing systemic vasodilation to reduce blood pressure	**Angiotensin-Converting Enzyme Inhibitors** lisinopril quinapril **Peripherally Acting Adrenergic Blockers** clonidine doxazosin **Angiotensin II Receptor Antagonists** losartan valsartan **Beta Blockers** atenolol metoprolol propranolol **Calcium Channel Blockers** amlodipine diltiazem **Vasodilators** hydralazine **Miscellaneous** amlodipine/benazepril losartan/hydrochlorothiazide	 ►Prinivil ►Accupril ►Catapres ►Cardura ►Cozaar ►Diovan ►Tenormin ►Toprol XL ►Inderal ►Norvasc ►Cardizem Apresoline ►Lotrel ►Hyzaar
Antiimpotence Agents	*Used* to treat erectile dysfunction *Work* by promoting increased blood flow to penis	sildenafil	►Viagra
Antiinfectives	*Used* to treat infections *Work* by killing or inhibiting growth of bacteria	**Penicillins** amoxicillin amoxicillin/clavulanate benzathine penicillin penicillin V procaine penicillin **Macrolides** azithromycin clarithromycin erythromycin **Cephalosporins** cefprozil ceftriaxone cephalexin **Fluoroquinolones** ciprofloxacin levofloxacin **Tetracycline** tetracycline	 ►Amoxil ►Augmentin Bicillin Veetids Wycillin ►Zithromax ►Biaxin Ery-Tab, Pediazole ►Cefzil Rocephin ►Keflex ►Cipro ►Levaquin Achromycin

Continued

Table 26-1 Classification of Drugs Based on Action—cont'd

Drug Category	Primary Use and Major Therapeutic Effects	COMMONLY PRESCRIBED DRUGS Generic	COMMONLY PRESCRIBED DRUGS Brand
Antiinfectives—cont'd		**Aminoglycosides**	
		kanamycin	Kantrex
		neomycin	Neobiotic
		tobramycin	Tobrax
		Sulfonamides	
		trimethoprim/ sulfamethoxazole	Bactrim
		Miscellaneous	
		mupirocin	▶ Bactroban
		nitrofurantoin	▶ Macrobid
Antiinflammatory Agents	*Used* to relieve signs and symptoms of osteoarthritis and rheumatoid arthritis in adults *Work* by decreasing pain and inflammation	aspirin celecoxib ibuprofen indomethacin naproxen valdecoxib	Bayer,* Ecotrin* ▶ Celebrex Advil,* Motrin* Indocin Aleve,* Naprosyn ▶ Bextra
Antimanics	*Used* to treat bipolar affective disorders *Work* by altering cation transport in nerves and muscles	lithium	Eskalith, Eskalith CR
Antimigraines	*Used* in acute treatment of migraine attacks *Work* by causing vasoconstriction in large intracranial arteries	sumatriptan	▶ Imitrex
Antineoplastics	*Used* to treat tumors *Work* by preventing development, growth, or proliferation of malignant cells	cyclophosphamide methotrexate	Cytoxan Mexate
Anti-Parkinson's Agents	*Used* to treat symptoms of Parkinson's disease *Work* by restoring balance between acetylcholine and dopamine in central nervous system	carbidopa/levodopa	Sinemet
Antiprotozoals	*Used* to treat protozoal infections *Work* by destroying protozoa	metronidazole	Flagyl
Antipsychotics	*Used* to treat psychotic disorders *Work* by blocking dopamine and serotonin receptors in central nervous system	olanzapine risperidone quetiapine	▶ Zyprexa Risperdal ▶ Seroquel
Antiretrovirals	*Used* to manage HIV infections and to reduce maternal-fetal transmission of HIV *Work* by inhibiting replication of retroviruses	zidovudine	Retrovir
Antispasmodics	*Used* to control hypermotility in irritable bowel syndrome, spastic colitis, spastic bladder, and pylorospasm *Work* by preventing or relieving spasms of gastrointestinal or genitourinary tracts	dicyclomine hyoscyamine	Bentyl Levsin
Antituberculars	*Used* to treat tuberculosis *Work* by killing or inhibiting growth of mycobacteria	pyrazinamide	PMS-Pyrazinamide
Antitussives	*Used* in prevention or relief of coughs caused by minor viral upper respiratory infections or inhaled irritants *Work* by suppressing cough reflex by direct effect on cough center in central nervous system	benzonatate dextromethorphan guaifenesin/codeine	Tessalon Robitussin DM* Robitussin A-C (V)
Antiulcers	*Used* to manage ulcers, gastroesophageal reflux disease, heartburn, indigestion, and gastric hyperacidity *Work* by preventing accumulation of acid in stomach	**Gastric Pump Inhibitors** esomeprazole lansoprazole omeprazole **H$_2$-Receptor Antagonists** famotidine ranitidine	Nexium ▶ Prevacid Prilosec* Pepcid AC* ▶ Zantac*

Table 26-1 Classification of Drugs Based on Action—cont'd

Drug Category	Primary Use and Major Therapeutic Effects	COMMONLY PRESCRIBED DRUGS Generic	Brand
Antivirals	*Used* to manage herpes infections *Work* by inhibiting viral replication	acyclovir valacyclovir	▶ Zovirax Valtrex
Bone Resorption Inhibitors	*Used* to treat and prevent osteoporosis *Work* by inhibiting resorption of bone	alendronate raloxifene risedronate	▶ Fosamax ▶ Evista ▶ Actonel
Bronchodilators	*Used* to manage reversible airway obstruction caused by asthma or chronic obstructive pulmonary disease *Work* by relaxing smooth muscle of respiratory tract, resulting in bronchodilation	albuterol fluticasone/salmeterol ipratropium/albuterol montelukast	▶ Proventil ▶ Advair Diskus ▶ Combivent ▶ Singulair
Cardiac Glycosides	*Used* to treat congestive heart failure and cardiac arrhythmias *Work* by increasing strength and force of myocardial contractions and slowing heart rate	digoxin	Lanoxicaps, ▶ Lanoxin
Central Nervous System Stimulants	*Used* to treat narcolepsy and manage attention-deficit/hyperactivity disorder *Work* by increasing level of catecholamines in central nervous system	atomoxetine dextroamphetamine saccharate and sulfate methylphenidate	▶ Strattera ▶ Adderall (II) Ritalin (II), ▶ Concerta (II)
Contraceptives (Hormonal)	*Used* to prevent pregnancy and to regulate menstrual cycle *Work* by inhibiting ovulation	**Oral Contraceptives** ethinyl estradiol/norethindrone **Injectable Contraceptives** medroxyprogesterone **Transdermal Contraceptives** ethinyl estradiol/norelgestromin **Vaginal Ring Contraceptives** ethinyl estradiol/etonogestrel	 ▶ Kariva, ▶ Ortho-Novum ▶ Depo-Provera Ortho Evra NuvaRing
Corticosteroids	**Systemic Corticosteroids** *Used* to treat inflammation, allergies, asthma, and autoimmune disorders and as replacement therapy in adrenal insufficiency *Work* by suppressing inflammation and modifying normal immune response **Nasal Corticosteroids** *Used* to treat chronic nasal inflammatory conditions (e.g., allergic rhinitis) *Work* by suppressing inflammation and reducing hypersecretions of respiratory tract	cortisone fluticasone hydrocortisone methylprednisolone fluticasone mometasone prednisone triamcinolone	Cortone ▶ Flovent Cortef Depo-Medrol ▶ Flonase Nasonex Deltasnoe ▶ Nasacort
Decongestants	*Used* to decrease nasal congestion *Work* by producing vasoconstriction in respiratory tract mucosa	oxymetazoline phenylephrine pseudoephedrine	Afrin,* Dristan* Neo-Synephrine* Sudafed*
Diuretics	*Used* to manage hypertension, edema in congestive heart failure, and renal disease *Work* by removing excess fluid from the body by increasing urine output	**Loop Diuretic** furosemide **Thiazide Diuretics** chlorthalidone hydrochlorothiazide **Potassium-Sparing Diuretics** spironolactone triamterene	 ▶ Lasix Hygroton Esidrix, HydroDiuril Aldactone ▶ Dyrenium

Continued

Table 26-1 Classification of Drugs Based on Action—cont'd

Drug Category	Primary Use and Major Therapeutic Effects	COMMONLY PRESCRIBED DRUGS Generic	Brand
Electrolyte Replacements	*Used* to treat or prevent electrolyte depletion *Work* by replacing electrolytes in body	**Potassium Supplements** potassium chloride	▶ K-Dur, ▶ Klor-Con
Emetics	*Used* to treat poisoning *Work* by inducing vomiting	syrup of ipecac	—
Expectorants	*Used* to manage coughs by expelling mucus *Work* by decreasing viscosity of bronchial secretions to promote clearance of mucus from respiratory tract	guaifenesin	Robitussin,* Naldecon*
Hormone Replacements	*Used* to treat moderate to severe vasomotor symptoms of menopause *Work* by restoring hormonal balance	conjugated estrogens conjugated estrogen/ progesterone estradiol/norethindrone	▶ Premarin ▶ Prempro Activella
Immunizations	*Used* to prevent (vaccine-preventable) diseases *Work* by stimulating body to produce antibodies	diphtheria, tetanus toxoids, and acellular pertussis vaccine *Haemophilus* b conjugate vaccine hepatitis A vaccine hepatitis B vaccine inactivated polio vaccine influenza virus vaccine types A and B measles, mumps, and rubella vaccine meningococcal conjugate vaccine pneumococcal 7-valent conjugate vaccine rubella vaccine varicella vaccine	Daptacel, Infanrix, Tripedia ActHIB, HibTITER Havrix, Vaqta Engerix-B, Recombivax HB IPOL Fluogen, Fluzone M-R-Vax II, M-M-R II Menactra Pneumovax II, Prevnar Meruvax II Varivax
Immunosuppressants	*Used* to treat severe rheumatoid arthritis and to prevent and treat rejection of transplanted organs *Work* by inhibiting body's normal immune response	methotrexate	Rheumatrex
Laxatives	*Used* to relieve constipation *Work* by promoting defecation of normal, soft stool	bisacodyl docusate psyllium	Dulcolax* Colace* Metamucil*
Lipid-Lowering Agents	*Used* to lower cholesterol to reduce risk of myocardial infarction and stroke *Work* by inhibiting enzyme needed to synthesize cholesterol in body	atorvastatin ezetimibe pravastatin rosuvastat simvastatin	▶ Lipitor ▶ Zetia ▶ Pravachol ▶ Crestor ▶ Zocor
Muscle Relaxants (Skeletal)	*Used* to treat acute painful musculoskeletal conditions *Work* by relaxing skeletal muscles	carisoprodol cyclobenzaprine	▶ Soma ▶ Flexeril
Ophthalmic Antiinfectives	*Used* to treat eye infections *Work* by destroying bacteria	dexamethasone/tobramycin polymyxin/neomycin tobramycin	TobraDex Neosporin Tobrex
Otic Preparations	*Used* to treat ear conditions **Antiinfectives** *Work* by relieving ear pain **Antiinfectives** *Work* by treating otitis externa **Cerumenolytics** *Work* by softening cerumen	benzocaine neomycin/polymyxin/ hydrocortisone carbamide peroxide	Auralgan Cortisporin Otic Debrox*

Table 26-1 Classification of Drugs Based on Action—cont'd

Drug Category	Primary Use and Major Therapeutic Effects	COMMONLY PRESCRIBED DRUGS Generic	COMMONLY PRESCRIBED DRUGS Brand
Platelet Inhibitors	*Used* to reduce incidence of myocardial infarction and stroke *Work* by interfering with ability of platelets to adhere to each other	clopidogrel salicylates	▶ Plavix Aspirin*
Sedatives and Hypnotics	*Used* for short-term treatment of insomnia *Work* by promoting sleep by central nervous system depression	eszopiclone phenobarbital temazepam zolpidem	Lunesta (IV) Luminal (IV) Restoril (IV) ▶ Ambien (IV)
Smoking Deterrents	*Used* to manage nicotine withdrawal to cease cigarette smoking *Work* by providing nicotine during controlled withdrawal from cigarette smoking	nicotine	Nicorette Gum,* Nicotrol Inhaler, Nicoderm Patch,* Commit Lozenges*
Thrombolytic Agents	*Used* for acute management of coronary thrombosis (myocardial infarction) *Work* by dissolving existing clots	alteplase reteplase streptokinase	Activase Retavase Streptase
Thyroid Preparations	**Thyroid Hormones** *Used* as replacement or substitute therapy for diminished or absent thyroid functioning of many causes *Work* by increasing basal metabolic rate **Antithyroid Agents** *Used* to treat hyperthyroidism *Work* by inhibiting thyroid hormone synthesis, reducing basal metabolic rate	levothyroxine methimazole	▶ Levoxyl, ▶ Synthroid Tapazole
Urinary Tract Antispasmodics	*Used* to treat overactive bladder function *Work* by inhibiting bladder contractions	oxybutynin tolterodine	Ditropan Detrol
Vasopressors	*Used* to treat severe allergic reactions and cardiac arrest *Work* by increasing blood pressure and cardiac output and by dilating bronchi	epinephrine	Adrenalin, EpiPen
Weight Control Agents	*Used* to manage obesity **Appetite Suppressants** *Work* by suppressing appetite center in central nervous system **Lipase Inhibitors** *Work* by inhibiting action of lipase to decrease absorption of dietary fats	 diethylpropion phentermine orlistat	 Tenuate (IV) Fastin (IV) Xenical

Modified from Bonewit-West K: *Clinical procedures for medical assistants,* ed 7, St. Louis, 2008, Saunders.
(II), Schedule II drug; *(III),* schedule III drug; *(IV),* schedule IV drug.
*Available over-the-counter.
▶ Top-200 most prescribed drugs.

SYSTEMS OF MEASUREMENT FOR MEDICATION

Three systems of measurement are used in the United States for prescribing, administering, and dispensing medication: the metric system, apothecary system, and household system. The metric system is the most common system used to measure medication because it provides a more exact measurement and is easier to use. Some physicians occasionally use the apothecary system; the medical assistant should be familiar with this system. The third system of measurement, the household system, is the least accurate and is generally used only when a patient takes liquid medication at home.

Systems of measurement have units of weight, volume, and length. *Weight* refers to the heaviness of an item, and *volume* refers to the amount of space occupied by a substance. *Length* is a unit of linear measurement of the distance from one point to another. Although length is not used to administer medication, it is used in other aspects of the medical office. The head circumference of infants is measured in centimeters (cm), a metric unit of linear measurement.

To prepare and administer medication properly and to avoid medication errors, the medical assistant must have a thorough knowledge of the specific units of measurement for these three systems and must be able to convert within each and from one system to another. A basic discussion of the metric, apothecary, and household systems is presented next. A more thorough study of these systems, including conversion of units and dose calculation, is included in Chapter 26 of the Study Guide.

Metric System

The metric system was developed in France in the latter part of the eighteenth century in an effort to simplify measurement. Most European countries are required by law to use this system for the measurement of weight, volume, and length. Overall, the metric system is used for most scientific and medical measurements. Pharmaceutical companies use the metric system to measure and label medications.

The metric system employs a uniform decimal scale based on units of 10, making it very flexible and logical. The basic metric units of measurement are the gram, liter, and meter. The *gram* is a unit of weight used to measure solids, the *liter* is a unit of volume used to measure liquids, and the *meter* is a linear unit used to measure length or distance. The metric units used most often in the administration of medication in the medical office are the milligram, gram, milliliter, and cubic centimeter. Because a **cubic centimeter (cc)** is the amount of space occupied by 1 milliliter (ml), these two units can be used interchangeably (i.e., 1 ml = 1 cc).

Prefixes added to the words *gram, liter,* and *meter* designate smaller or larger units of measurement in the metric system. The same prefixes are used with all three units. For example, *milli* is used as follows: *milli*gram, *milli*liter, and *milli*meter. A prefix changes the value of the basic unit of measurement by the same amount. The prefix *milli* describes a unit that is $1/1000$ of the basic unit: 1 gram is equal to 1000 milligrams, 1 liter is equal to 1000 milliliters, and 1 meter is equal to 1000 millimeters. The box *Metric Notation Guidelines* lists the metric units of measurement and equivalent values in different units. Specific guidelines are used in the medical notation of metric units and doses, which also are presented in the box. To read prescriptions and medication orders, to record medication administration, and, most importantly, to avoid medication errors, the medical assistant must be familiar with and be able to follow these guidelines.

Metric Notation Guidelines

Follow these guidelines when using the metric notation of measurement and dosage.

1. The units of metric measurement are written using the following abbreviations:

   Weight
   microgram: mcg or μg
   milligram: mg
   gram: g
   kilogram: kg

   Volume
   milliliter: ml
   cubic centimeter: cc
   liter: L

2. Do not use a period with the abbreviation of metric units because it might be mistaken for another letter or symbol.
   Correct: mg
               ml
   Incorrect: mg.
               ml.

3. Use Arabic numerals (e.g., 1, 2, 3, 4) to express the quantity of the dose.
   Correct: 4 mg
   Incorrect: iv mg

4. Place the numeral that expresses the quantity of the dose in front of the abbreviation. To make it easier to read, leave a (single) space between the quantity and the abbreviation.
   Correct: 5 ml
   Incorrect: ml 5
               5ml

5. Write a fraction of a dose as a decimal.
   Correct: 0.5 g
   Incorrect: ½ g

6. If the dose is a fraction of a unit, place a zero before the decimal point as a means of focusing on the fractional dose. This reduces the possibility of misreading the dose as a whole number.
   Correct: 0.5 g (this reduces the possibility of not seeing the decimal point and reading the dose as 5 grams)
   Incorrect: .5 g

7. Do not place a decimal point and a zero after a whole number. The decimal point may be overlooked, resulting in a 10-fold overdose error.
   Correct: 1 ml (this reduces the possibility of not seeing the decimal point and reading the dose as 10 ml)
   Incorrect: 1.0 ml

Metric System: Conversion of Equivalent Values
Weight
   1000 micrograms = 1 milligram
   1000 milligrams = 1 gram
   1000 grams = 1 kilogram
Volume
   1000 milliliters = 1 liter
   1000 liters = 1 kiloliter
   1 milliliter = 1 cubic centimeter

Apothecary System

The apothecary system is older and less accurate than the metric system. It was brought to the United States from England during the eighteenth century. Pharmacists used this system during the colonial period to compound and measure medications. This system is gradually being phased out for measurement of medication in favor of the metric system. Until that process is completed, however, the medical assistant must be familiar with this system and be able to use it to administer medication.

The basic unit of weight in the apothecary system is the *grain,* derived from the weight of a large grain of wheat, which was used to balance the material being weighed. The next largest unit of measurement is the *scruple;* however, this unit is not used to administer medication. The remaining units, in order of increasing weight, are *dram, ounce,* and *pound.* The pound is not generally used in the administration of medication. The medical assistant should note, however, that in the apothecary system the pound is equal to 12 ounces, in contrast to the more familiar *avoirdupois* pound used to measure body weight, which is equal to 16 ounces.

Measures of liquid volume in the apothecary system correlate closely with measures of dry weight in the same system. The smallest unit of measurement is the *minim,* meaning "the least." A minim is approximately equivalent to a volume of water that weighs 1 grain. A minim glass or a syringe calibrated in minims must be used to measure with this unit. The remaining units of liquid volume in the apothecary system, in order of increasing volume, are *fluid dram, fluid ounce, pint, quart,* and *gallon.* The basic unit of linear measurement is the *inch,* followed by *foot, yard,* and *mile.* Most Americans are familiar with apothecary units of measurement because of their use in everyday life. For example, milk is available in pints, quarts, and gallons, and height is measured in feet and inches.

The box *Apothecary Notation Guidelines* lists the units of measurement in the apothecary system and equivalent values in different units. It also includes guidelines for the medical notation of apothecary units.

Apothecary Notation Guidelines

Follow these guidelines when using the medical notation of apothecary units and dosage.

1. The units of apothecary measurement are usually written with abbreviations and symbols as follows:

   Weight
   grain: gr
   dram: dr or ℥
   ounce: oz or ℥

   Volume
   minim: ℳ
   fluid dram: f℥; fluid ounce: f℥
   pint: pt
   quart: qt
   gallon: gal

2. When writing symbols and abbreviations to express apothecary units, use lowercase Roman numerals to express the dose quantity.
   Correct: ℥ vi (6 ounces)
   Incorrect: 6 ℥
   ℥6

3. Place the Roman numeral expressing dose quantity after the symbol or abbreviation.
   Correct: ℥ ii (2 drams)
   gr v (5 grains)
   Incorrect: ii ℥
   v gr

4. A line may be placed over the roman numerals. Dots are placed above the line for emphasis as a safeguard against error.
   Correct: f ℥ iii (3 fluid drams)
   Incorrect: f ℥ III

5. Write "ss" to designate one half of a dose, and place it after the apothecary symbol or abbreviation.
   Correct: gr ss
   Incorrect: gr ½

6. Write fractions (other than ½) in Arabic numerals, and place them after the apothecary symbol or abbreviation.
   Correct: gr ¼
   Incorrect: gr 0.25; ¼ gr

   Note: If abbreviations and symbols are not used to express apothecary units of measurement, Arabic numerals must be used to express dose quantity and are placed before the unit of measurement. Example: ¼ grain.

Apothecary System: Conversion of Equivalent Values

Weight
60 grains = 1 dram
8 drams = 1 ounce
12 ounces = 1 pound

Volume
60 minims = 1 fluid dram
8 fluid drams = 1 fluid ounce
16 fluid ounces = 1 pint
2 pints = 1 quart
4 quarts = 1 gallon

Table 26-2 Household System: Conversion of Common Values	
Abbreviations	
drop:	gtt
teaspoon:	tsp
tablespoon:	T
ounce:	oz
cup:	c
Volume	
60 gtt =	1 tsp
3 tsp =	1 T
6 tsp =	1 oz
2 T =	1 oz
6 oz =	1 teacup
8 oz =	1 glass

From Bonewit-West K: *Clinical procedures for medical assistants,* ed 7, St. Louis, 2008, Saunders.

Household System

The household system is more complicated and less accurate for administering liquid medication than either the metric or apothecary system. Nevertheless, most individuals are familiar with this system because of its frequent use in the United States. This system of measurement may be the only one the patient can understand and safely use to take liquid medication at home. Most patients are more comfortable measuring medication in drops and teaspoons than in minims and milliliters. In addition, the patient is more likely to have household measuring devices on hand than to have metric measuring devices. If a precise measurement is necessary, however, the metric system must be used, and the medical assistant should instruct the patient in the use of the metric measuring device.

Volume is the only household unit of measurement used to administer medication. The basic unit of liquid volume in the household system is the *drop (gtt),* which is approximately equal to 0.6 ml in the metric system and 1 minim in the apothecary system. These units cannot be considered exact equivalents because the size of the drop varies based on temperature, the viscosity of the liquid, and the size of the dropper. The remaining units, in order of increasing volume, are *teaspoon, tablespoon, ounce (fluid ounce), cup,* and *glass.* Table 26-2 lists the units of liquid volume measurement in the household system and equivalent values in different units.

CONVERTING UNITS OF MEASUREMENT

Changing from one unit of measurement to another is known as **conversion.** Conversion is required when medication is ordered in a unit of measurement that differs from

the medication's label. The dose quantity must be mathematically translated or converted to the unit of measurement of the medication on hand. If the physician orders 5 grams of an oral solid medication, and the medication label expresses the drug strength in milligrams, the medical assistant would need to convert the grams into milligrams to know how much medication to administer. Converting units of measurement can be classified into the following categories: (1) conversion of units within a measurement system and (2) conversion of units from one measurement system to another.

Converting units within a measurement system allows a quantity to be expressed in two different but equal units of measurement within *one* system. An example of converting units of weight within the metric system is as follows: 1 gram is equal to 1000 milligrams. Converting from one measurement system to another allows a quantity written in one measurement system to be expressed in an equivalent unit of measurement in *another* system. An example of a conversion from the apothecary system to the metric system is as follows: 1 grain (apothecary system) is equivalent to 60 milligrams (metric system).

Conversion requires the use of a conversion table to indicate the equivalent values of various units of measurement. Conversion tables of equivalent values in these three measurement systems are included in this chapter:

Metric conversion—Metric Notation Guidelines box
Apothecary conversion—Apothecary Notation Guidelines box
Household conversion—Table 26-2

Tables used to convert from one system to another consist of approximate rather than exact equivalents, and a 10% error usually occurs in making these conversions. Conversion tables used to convert from one system to another are presented in Table 26-3.

The medical assistant must be careful when using conversion tables to avoid errors in interpolation. The numbers on conversion tables are small and close together; it is easy to misread the chart from one column to the other. To reduce this possibility, a straightedge should be used when reading a conversion table.

CONTROLLED DRUGS

By means of federal and state legislation, restrictions are placed on drugs that have potential for abuse. These drugs are known as **controlled drugs.** They are classified into five categories, called *schedules,* which are based on their abuse potential. Table 26-4 lists, describes, and provides examples of the schedules for controlled drugs.

To administer, prescribe, or dispense controlled drugs, the physician must register every year with the Drug Enforcement Administration (DEA). The physician is assigned a registration number known as the **DEA number.** Every time a prescription for a controlled drug is written, the physician must put his or her DEA number in the appropriate space on the prescription blank.

Table 26-3 Conversion Charts for Systems of Measurement

CONVERSION CHART FOR METRIC AND APOTHECARY SYSTEMS (COMMON APPROXIMATE EQUIVALENTS)

Metric System to Apothecary System			Apothecary System to Metric System		
Weight			**Weight**		
60 mg	=	1 gr	15 gr	=	1000 mg (1 g)
1 g	=	15 gr	10 gr	=	600 mg
29 g	=	1 dr	7½ gr	=	500 mg
30 g	=	1 oz	5 gr	=	300 mg
1 kg	=	2.2 lb	3 gr	=	200 mg
Volume			1½ gr	=	100 mg
0.06 ml	=	1 ℥	1 gr	=	60 mg *to 65mg*
1 ml (cc)	=	15 ℥	¾ gr	=	50 mg
4 ml	=	1 f℥	½ gr	=	30 mg
30 ml	=	1 f℥	¼ gr	=	15 mg
500 ml	=	1 pt	⅙ gr	=	10 mg
1000 ml (1 L)	=	1 qt	⅛ gr	=	8 mg
			$\frac{1}{12}$ gr	=	5 mg
			$\frac{1}{15}$ gr	=	4 mg
			$\frac{1}{20}$ gr	=	3 mg
			$\frac{1}{30}$ gr	=	2 mg
			$\frac{1}{40}$ gr	=	1.5 mg
			$\frac{1}{50}$ gr	=	1.2 mg
			$\frac{1}{60}$ gr	=	1 mg
			$\frac{1}{100}$ gr	=	0.6 mg
			$\frac{1}{120}$ gr	=	0.5 mg
			$\frac{1}{150}$ gr	=	0.4 mg
			$\frac{1}{200}$ gr	=	0.3 mg
			$\frac{1}{300}$ gr	=	0.2 mg
			$\frac{1}{600}$ gr	=	0.1 mg

EQUIVALENCES IN HOUSEHOLD, APOTHECARY, AND METRIC UNITS (VOLUME)

Household	Apothecary	Metric
1 gtt	= 1 ℥	= 0.06 ml
15 gtt	= 15 ℥	= 1 ml (1 cc)
1 tsp	= ⅙ f℥	= 5 (4) ml*
1 T	= ½ f℥	= 15 ml
2 T	= 1 f℥	= 30 ml
1 oz	= 1 f℥	= 30 ml
1 teacup	= 6 f℥	= 180 ml
1 glass	= 8 f℥	= 240 ml

From Bonewit-West K: *Clinical procedures for medical assistants,* ed 7, St. Louis, 2008, Saunders.
*The American standard teaspoon is accepted as 5 ml; however, 4 ml can be used as the equivalent to provide a more accurate conversion.

PRESCRIPTION

A **prescription** is a physician's order authorizing the dispensing of a drug by a pharmacist. Prescriptions can be authorized in different forms, including handwritten, computer-generated, and telephoned or faxed to a pharmacy.

Abbreviations and symbols are usually used to write a prescription. They are also used to record medication infor-

mation in the patient's chart. Common abbreviations used in the medical office for writing prescriptions are included in Table 26-5.

The medical assistant should ensure that all prescription pads are kept in a safe place and out of reach of individuals who may want to obtain drugs illegally. The stock supply of prescription pads should be locked in a drawer.

Table 26-4 Classification of Controlled Drugs

Classification	Description	Examples	
		Generic	**Brand**
Schedule I	High potential for abuse No accepted medical use Use may lead to severe physical or psychological dependence Not available for prescribing May be used for research with appropriate limitations	GHB Heroin LSD Marijuana MDMA (Ectasy) Mescaline Methaqualone (Quaalude) Phencyclidine (PCP) Psilocybin	— — — — — — — — —
Schedule II	High potential for abuse Accepted medical use in United States Abuse may lead to severe psychological or physical dependence Prescription must be in writing in indelible ink or typed Emergency telephone order permitted only for immediate amount needed to treat patient; written prescription must be provided to pharmacist within 7 days No refills allowed Manufacturer's label marked C-II	**Analgesics** Cocaine Codeine Fentanyl Hydrocodone Hydromorphone Meperidine Methadone Morphine Oxycodone Oxycodone/APAP Oxycodone/ASA **Central Nervous System Stimulants** Dextroamphetamine Methylphenidate Methamphetamine **Sedatives/Hypnotics** Amobarbital Glutethimide Pentobarbital Secobarbital	 — — Sublimaze Hycodan Dilaudid Demerol Dolophine Roxanol OxyContin Percocet Percodan Dexedrine, Adderall Ritalin Desoxyn — Amytal Doriden Nembutal, Seconal
Schedule III	Intermediate potential for abuse Accepted medical use in United States Abuse may lead to low to moderate physical dependence and moderate to high psychological dependence Telephone and fax orders permitted If authorized by physician, prescription can be refilled five times within 6 mo from issue date Prescription expires 6 mo from issue date Manufacturer's label marked C-III	**Anabolic Steroids** Oxandrolone Oxymetholone **Analgesics** Buprenorphine Butalbital compound Codeine combined with nonopioid analgesic Hydrocodone combined with nonopioid analgesic **Central Nervous System Stimulant** Benzphetamine **Male Hormone** Testosterone **Sedative/Hypnotic** Butabarbital	 Anavar Oranabol Buprenex Fiorinal Tylenol w/ codeine, Soma w/ codeine, Empirin w/ codeine Vicodin, Lortab, Lorcet, Tussionex Didrex Androderm, Delatestryl Butisol

Table 26-4 Classification of Controlled Drugs—cont'd

Classification	Description	Examples	
		Generic	**Brand**
Schedule IV	Low potential for abuse Accepted medical use in United States Abuse may lead to limited physical or psychological dependence Telephone and fax orders permitted If authorized by physician, prescription can be refilled five times within 6 mo of issue date Prescription expires 6 mo from issue date Manufacturer's label marked C-IV	**Analgesics**	
		Butorphanol	Stadol
		Pentazocine	Talwin
		Propoxyphene	Darvon, Darvocet-N
		Antianxiety Agents	
		Alprazolam	Xanax
		Buspirone	BuSpar
		Chlordiazepoxide	Librium
		Clorazepate	Tranxene
		Diazepam	Valium
		Halazepam	Paxipam
		Lorazepam	Ativan
		Meprobamate	Equanil
		Oxazepam	Serax
		Anticonvulsant	
		Clonazepam	Klonopin
		Central Nervous System Stimulants	
		Modafinil	Provigil
		Pemoline	Cylert
		Sedatives/Hypnotics	
		Chloral hydrate	Noctec
		Eszopiclone	Lunesta
		Ethchlorvynol	Placidyl
		Flurazepam	Dalmane
		Midazolam	Versed
		Phenobarbital	Luminal
		Temazepam	Restoril
		Triazolam	Halcion
		Zaleplon	Sonata
		Zolpidem	Ambien
		Weight Control Agents	
		Diethylpropion	Tenuate
		Phentermine	Fastin
		Sibutramine	Meridia
Schedule V	Very low potential for abuse Accepted medical use in United States Abuse may lead to low physical or psychological dependence Telephone and fax orders permitted Prescribing polices determined by state and local regulations. In most states: Number of refills determined by physician Prescription expires 1 yr from issue date Some are available without prescription to patients older than 18 yr Manufacturer's label marked C-V	Cough suppressants with small amounts of codeine	Robitussin A-C, Cheracol syrup
		Antidiarrheals containing paregoric	Parepectolin, Kapectolin PG
		Diphenoxylate/atropine	Lomotil

From Bonewit-West K: *Clinical procedures for medical assistants,* ed 7, St. Louis, 2008, Saunders.

My name is Theresa Cline, and I work for four physicians in a family practice medical office. I have worked there ever since I graduated from college with an associate's degree in medical assisting. One experience that I will never forget taught our entire office staff a valuable lesson. It involved a woman who came to our office because she had lacerated her wrist while using a butcher knife. After the wound was sutured, I gave her a tetanus injection because she was past due for one. Shortly thereafter, she became very nauseated and dizzy, and I made her lie down on the examining table. She asked me to get her a cold drink of water and I left the room to do so. Apparently, while I was gone she must have tried to sit up or turn over because she rolled off the table and struck the back of her head on the floor. She sustained a laceration to her scalp, which also had to be sutured. Owing to her persistent symptoms of severe nausea, vomiting, and headache, it was decided that she should be admitted to the hospital for neurologic observation and x-ray studies.

The vital lesson that this experience taught everyone in our office was that you must never leave a patient alone, not even for a minute to get something, if there is the slightest indication that he or she is not feeling perfectly fine. Another staff member should be called to obtain whatever is necessary. From that point on, this has been our office policy and procedure. ■

Prepare for Success

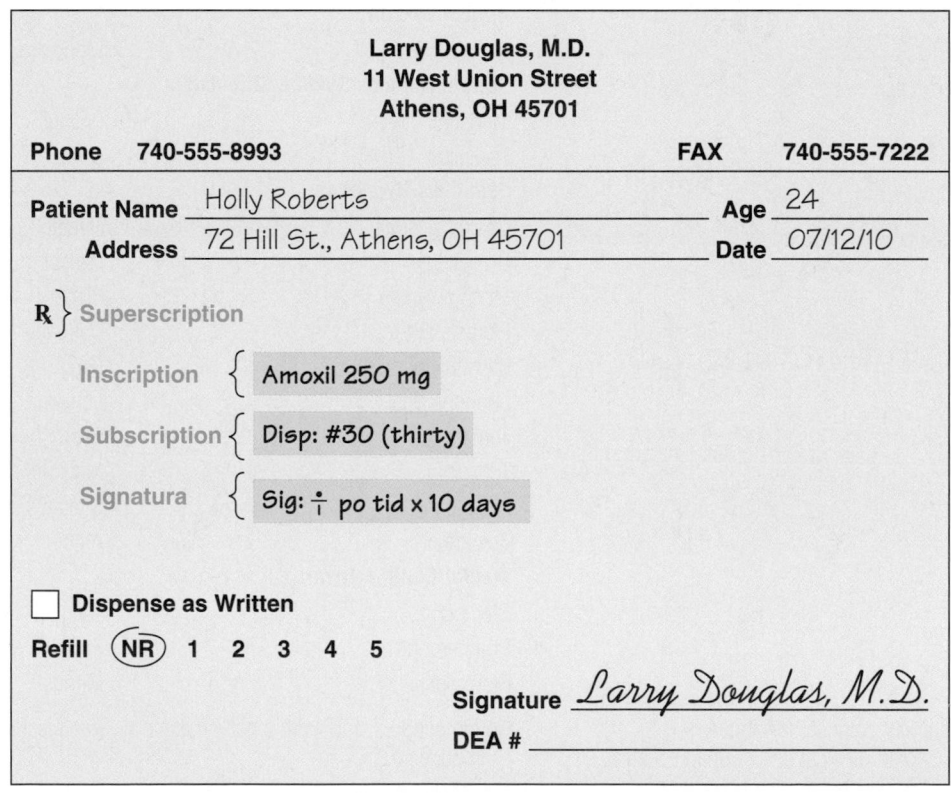

Figure 26-2. Example of a prescription. (From Bonewit-West K: *Clinical procedures for medical assistants,* ed 7, St. Louis, 2008, Saunders.)

Parts of a Prescription

A prescription is written on a specially designed form. It includes directions to the pharmacist for filling the prescription and instructions to the patient for taking the medication (Figure 26-2). The specific information that the prescription must include follows:

- **Date.** A pharmacist cannot fill a prescription unless the date the prescription was issued is indicated on the form. The reason for this is that a prescription expires after a

certain length of time. In most states, a prescription for a drug (with the exception of controlled drugs) expires 1 year from the date of issue. After this time, the prescription (or any refills left on the prescription) cannot be filled.

- **Physician's name, address, telephone number, and fax number.** This information is preprinted on the prescription form. It identifies the physician issuing the prescription and provides the necessary information should the

Table 26-5 Common Abbreviations and Symbols Used in Medication Documentation

Abbreviation or Symbol	Meaning	Abbreviation or Symbol	Meaning
a̅a̅	of each	OS	left eye
ac	before meals	OTC	over-the-counter
AD	right ear	OU	in each eye
ad lib	as desired	℥ or oz	ounce
aq	water	p̄	after
admin	administer, administration	pc	after meals
AM or a.m.	morning	Pt or pt	patient
APAP	acetaminophen	per	by
AS	left ear	PM or p.m.	evening
ASA	aspirin	po or PO	by mouth
AU	in each ear	prn	as needed
bid	twice a day	qAM	every morning
c̄	with	qd	every day
cap(s)	capsule(s)	qh	every hour
cc	cubic centimeter	q (2, 3, 4) h	every (2, 3, 4) hours
DAW	dispense as written	qid	four times a day
dil	dilute	qod	every other day
ℨ or dr	dram	qs	of sufficient quantity
elix	elixir	Rx	take
g	gram	s̄	without
gr	grain	SC or SQ	subcutaneous
gtt(s)	drop(s)	SL	sublingual
h or hr	hour	sol	solution
hs	at bedtime	ss	one half
ID	intradermal	STAT	immediately
IM	intramuscular	T	tablespoon
INH	inhalation	tab(s)	tablet(s)
IV	intravenous	tid	three times a day
kg	kilogram	tsp	teaspoon
L	liter	#	number
liq	liquid	×	times
ℳ	minim	Ø	no, none
med(s)	medication(s)	ī	one
mg	milligram	ī̄ī	two
min	minute	ī̄ī̄ī	three
ml	milliliter	ī̄v	four
NPO	nothing by mouth	v̄	five
OD	right eye		

From Bonewit-West K: *Clinical procedures for medical assistants,* ed 7, St. Louis, 2008, Saunders.

pharmacist have a question and need to contact the medical office.

- **Patient's name and address.** This information is important for insurance billing and in properly dispensing the medication.
- **Patient's age.** The patient's age is important to the pharmacist when he or she double-checks the physician's order to ensure the proper dose is being dispensed. The most common errors in dosage occur among children and the elderly, who may not require the standard dose of a drug because these age groups metabolize drugs differently. The patient's age also allows the pharmacist to double-check that the drug is age appropriate for the patient. For example, *ciprofloxacin* (e.g., Cipro) should not be taken by children and adolescents because this antibiotic can damage cartilage in individuals younger than 18 years old.
- **Superscription.** The superscription consists of the symbol *Rx.* This symbol comes from the Latin word *recipe* and means "take."

- **Inscription.** The inscription states the name of the drug and the dose (e.g., Amoxil 250 mg). Most drugs are available in various doses; it is important that the correct dose be prescribed. For example, Amoxil comes in the following doses: 125 mg, 250 mg, and 500 mg.
- **Subscription.** The subscription gives directions to the pharmacist. At present, it is generally used to designate the number of doses to be dispensed. To prevent a prescription from being altered illegally, it is recommended that numbers and letters be used to indicate the quantity to be dispensed (e.g., #30 [thirty]).
- **Signatura.** The signatura (abbreviated *Sig.*) is a Latin term that means "write" or "label" and indicates the information to be included on the medication label. It consists of directions to the patient for taking the medication. The name of the medication is also included on the label so that the patient can identify the medication.
- **Refill.** This part of the prescription indicates the number of times the prescription may be refilled.

- **Physician's signature.** A prescription cannot be filled unless it is signed by the physician.
- **DEA number.** The number assigned to the physician by the DEA must appear on the prescription for a controlled drug. See Table 26-4 for examples of controlled drugs.

Generic Prescribing

Generic prescribing means that the physician writes the prescription using the generic rather than the brand name of the drug. Because many pharmaceutical manufacturers may produce the same generic drug and sell it under different brand names, price competition often results. If the physician prescribes a drug using its generic name, the pharmacist is permitted to fill it with the drug that offers the best savings to the patient. In addition, most states allow the pharmacist the option of filling the prescription with a chemically equivalent generic drug, even if the drug has been prescribed by brand name. If the physician wants the prescription to be filled with a specific brand of drug,

---

PATIENT TEACHING | **Prescription Medications**

To avoid adverse reactions, teach patients the proper guidelines for taking prescription medication. These guidelines are as follows:

Know the names of all your prescription and nonprescription medications. Nonprescription drugs are known as *over-the-counter* (OTC) drugs; they are drugs that can be purchased without a prescription. Vitamin supplements and herbal products are considered OTC drugs.

Know why you are taking each medication. It is important to know the desired therapeutic outcome and the common side effects of each medication and guidelines ("do's and don'ts") to follow when taking the medication.

Take your medication exactly as prescribed, at the right times and in the right amounts. The medication may not work properly if it is not taken as directed. If the dose is too small, the drug may not produce its intended therapeutic effect; exceeding the recommended dosage could result in a toxic effect.

Inform the physician if new symptoms or adverse effects develop when you are taking the medication. The physician may need to change your dosage or prescribe a different medication. Alternative medications that the physician can prescribe to treat your condition are usually available.

Take the medication for the prescribed duration of time, even after you begin to feel better. If you do not complete the entire course of drug therapy, your condition may recur. Not taking all of a prescribed antibiotic may cause an infection to return, and it may be worse than the first infection.

Tell the physician if you decide not to take your medication. Otherwise, the physician may think your medication is not working. Not taking a medication prescribed by the physician

could be serious because it may allow your condition to worsen.

Do not take additional medications, including OTC medications, without checking with the physician. All drugs, including OTC medications, are designed to have an effect on the body. Some combinations of drugs cause serious reactions. In some cases, one drug cancels the effects of another and prevents it from working.

Never take a medication that was prescribed for someone else. Physicians prescribe medication based on an individual's age, weight, sex, and condition. Taking a medication prescribed for someone else can have serious results.

Keep all medications in their original containers to avoid taking the wrong medication by mistake. Store your medications in their original containers from the pharmacy. Basic information about your medication is on the original container. Medications that are not clearly marked may be taken inadvertently by the wrong person.

Store your medications in a safe place, away from the reach of children. Ask for child-resistant safety closures, and ensure that the caps of the bottles are closed tightly. Accidental drug poisoning in children is a common and preventable problem. Also, do not take your medication in front of young children because they may want to mimic your behavior.

Store medications in a cool, dry place or as stated on the label. Do not store capsules or tablets in the bathroom or kitchen because heat or moisture may cause the medication to break down.

Discard unused portions of prescription medications and outdated OTC medications. Medications should be discarded by flushing them down the toilet. Medications that are past their expiration date may produce adverse effects in the body. ■

instructions must be indicated on the prescription form, such as "Dispense as Written (DAW)," or words of a similar meaning (see Figure 26-2).

Completing a Prescription Form

The physician is responsible for having accurate and pertinent information on the prescription form. If delegated by the physician, a prescription form can be completed by the medical assistant and signed by the physician. The physician must review the prescription thoroughly before signing it to ensure all of the information is correct. If the medical assistant is delegated this responsibility, he or she must carefully follow the important guidelines presented in the box *Guidelines for Completing a Prescription Form.*

Guidelines for Completing a Prescription Form

- Work in a quiet, well-lit area that is free of distractions.
- Use an indelible black ink pen to write on the form.
- Print all information on the form.
- Ensure that all information is spelled correctly.
- Review the metric notation guidelines presented in the box *Metric Notation Guidelines.* (Most prescriptions are written in metric units.)
- Always ask the physician if you have questions about the prescription.
- Complete all of the required information on the form; it includes the following:

  1. **Patient's name, address, and age**
     - Clearly print all of this information on the form. Never leave the address and age categories blank.
  2. **Date**
     - Indicate today's date on the prescription form.
  3. **Name of the medication**
     - The physician may prescribe the medication using either the generic or brand name.
     - Make sure to spell the name of the drug correctly. If you are unsure, use a drug reference to find the correct spelling of a drug.
  4. **Medication dosage**
     - Never leave a decimal point "naked." If the dosage is a fraction of a unit, a zero must be placed before the decimal point as a means of focusing on the fractional dose. This reduces the possibility of misreading the dose as a whole number. *Example:* 0.5 ml (*not* .5 ml).
     - Never place a decimal point and a zero after a whole number because the decimal point may be overlooked, resulting in a 10-fold overdose error. *Example:* 5 mg (*not* 5.0 mg).
  5. **Quantity to dispense**
     - Use numbers and letters to indicate the quantity to be dispensed. *Example:* Disp: #30 (thirty).
     - Ensure that the quantity is correct. The number of prescribed pills should match the duration of treatment. *Example:* If the patient has been prescribed 3 tablets a day for 7 days, the quantity should be written as follows: Disp: #21 (twenty-one).
  6. **Directions for taking the medication**
     - Clearly indicate the directions for taking the medication. Many authorities recommend writing the directions without abbreviations. *Example:* Sig: Take 1 capsule 3 times a day for 10 days.
     - If abbreviations are used, use only commonly accepted abbreviations, and print the information clearly. *Example:* Sig: ī cap po tid × 10 days.
  7. **Refills**
     - Never leave this category blank.
     - If there are no refills, indicate this clearly on the form. The method for doing this is based on the setup of the preprinted form.
       Example: Refill: ⓝⓡ 1 2 3 4 5
       (on this form the information is circled)
       Example: Refill: Ø
       (on this form the information is written in)
  8. **Dispense as written**
     - If the physician does not allow a substitution (e.g., generic equivalent) for this medication, check this category.
  9. **DEA number**
     - If the prescription is for a controlled drug, clearly indicate the physician's DEA number on the form.
  10. **Group practice**
     - If there is more than one physician in the practice, circle (or check) the name of the physician prescribing the medication. This avoids confusion if the pharmacist cannot read the physician's signature.

  Example:
  James Ortman, MD, (Mark Rothstein, MD), Richard Bontrager, MD
  - Give the prescription to the physician to review and sign.
  - Document the prescription order in the patient's medication record if directed by the physician. Some offices use multiple-copy prescription pads. In this case, file the copy of the prescription in the patient's medical record.
  - Give the prescription to the patient. Provide the patient with guidelines for taking the medication (see Patient Teaching box on prescription medications).
  - Ask the patient whether he or she has any questions about the medication.

MEDICATION RECORD

The medical office may use a preprinted form to record the medications (Rx and OTC) that a patient is taking; vitamin supplements and herbal products the patient is taking should also be recorded on the form. A medication record form (Figure 26-3) includes detailed information about each medication so that the physician can tell at a glance what medications and how much the patient is taking. The medication record is part of the patient's medical record. The medical assistant may be responsible for documenting medication information on this form. Care must be taken to ensure the information is correct and clearly written.

A medication record form typically includes the following information:

- Patient's name and date of birth
- Any drug allergies
- Date the medication was prescribed (Rx) or date the patient started taking the medication (OTC)
- Name and dose of the medication
- Frequency of administration of the medication
- Route of administration
- Prescription or OTC medication category

What Would You Do? What Would You *Not* Do?

Case Study 2

Linda Cardwell calls the medical office. Her daughter Rachel, 9 years old, was seen in the office 10 days ago. Rachel was diagnosed with strep throat, and the physician ordered Amoxil 250 mg tid × 7 days. Mrs. Cardwell says that after 3 days of taking the medication, Rachel was much better, so she stopped giving her the Amoxil because it was causing her to have diarrhea. Mrs. Cardwell says that her 12-year-old son started feeling achy all over and she gave him the Amoxil for 2 days, and it seemed to help. She also says that her husband started complaining of sinus problems, so she also gave him the Amoxil for 2 days. Mrs. Cardwell says that now Rachel's throat is hurting again, and she has a fever. She wants to know whether Rachel has developed another case of strep throat. Mrs. Cardwell says she does not know what to do because she does not have any Amoxil left to give Rachel. ■

MEDICATION RECORD

Patient: John Walsh
Birthdate: 6/10/49

ALLERGY: Ø

DATE	MEDICATION AND DOSAGE	FREQUENCY	RX	OTC	REFILLS			STOP
2/18/09	Cipro 250 mg	⊤̄ q 12 h po × 10 days	X					2/28/09
6/10/09	Prevacid 15 mg	⊤̄ qd po	X					7/10/09
6/10/09	Lipitor 10 mg	⊤̄ qd po	X		1/6/07			
6/10/09	Prozac 20 mg	⊤̄ qd po	X		1/6/07			
12/3/09	Tobrex Ophthalmic Solution	⊤̄ gtt q 3 h OD	X					12/10/09
2/5/10	Echinacea	⊤̄ qd po		X				
3/15/10	Nitrostat 0.4 mg	⊤̄ prn pain SL Rep q 5 min prn pain, not to exceed 3 tabs	X					
3/15/10	Inderal 40 mg	⊤̄ bid po	X					
3/15/10	St Joseph ASA Enteric Coated 81 mg	⊤̄ qd po		X				

Figure 26-3. Example of a medication record. (From Bonewit-West K: *Clinical procedures for medical assistants,* ed 7, St. Louis, 2008, Saunders.)

- Refills (Rx medication only)
- Date the patient stopped taking the medication

FACTORS AFFECTING DRUG ACTION
Therapeutic Effect

Each drug has an intended therapeutic effect—the reason the patient takes the medication. Certain factors affect the therapeutic action of drugs in the body, causing patients to respond differently to the same drug. Because of this, the drug therapy may need to be adjusted to meet these variations, which include the following.

Age

Children and the elderly tend to respond more strongly to drugs than do young and middle-aged adults. The physician may calculate smaller doses for very young and old patients.

Route of Administration

Medications administered by different routes are absorbed at different rates. Drugs administered orally are absorbed slowly because they must be digested first. Parenterally administered drugs are absorbed more quickly than orally administered drugs because they are injected directly into the body.

Size

A patient's body size has an effect on drug action. A thin individual may require a smaller quantity of a drug, and an obese individual may require more.

Time of Administration

A drug administered through the oral route is absorbed more rapidly when the stomach is empty than when it contains food. A drug may not produce the desired effect or may be absorbed too slowly if it is taken when food is present. Some drugs irritate the stomach's lining, however, and must be taken with food. The drug package insert or a drug reference should always be consulted to determine when a drug should be taken.

Tolerance

A patient taking a certain drug over a period of time may develop a tolerance to it. This means that the same dose of a drug no longer produces the desired effect after prolonged administration. The physician should be notified to determine whether a change of drug or dosage is necessary.

Undesirable Effects of Drugs

A drug may cause undesirable effects, which may occur immediately or be delayed hours or even days after administration of the medication.

Adverse Reactions

Most drugs produce unintended and undesirable effects known as **adverse reactions.** Adverse reactions are secondary effects that occur along with the therapeutic effect of the drug. Some adverse reactions, referred to as *side effects,* are harmless and often tolerated by the patient to obtain the therapeutic effect of the drug. Most patients are willing to tolerate the dry mouth and drowsiness that may accompany an antihistamine to obtain its therapeutic effect. Other adverse reactions, such as a decrease in blood pressure or an allergic reaction, can be harmful to the patient and warrant discontinuing the medication.

Drug Interactions

When certain medications are used at the same time, drug interactions may produce undesirable effects. The medical assistant should inquire about other medications the patient is taking and record this information in the patient's chart for review by the physician.

Allergic Drug Reaction

The patient may exhibit an allergic reaction to a drug. The reaction is usually mild and takes the form of a rash, rhinitis, or pruritus. Occasionally, a patient has a severe allergic reaction that occurs suddenly and immediately. This is known as an **anaphylactic reaction.**

An anaphylactic reaction is the least common but the most serious type of allergic reaction. Symptoms begin with sneezing, urticaria (hives), itching, *angioedema, erythema,* and disorientation. Erythema is the reddening of the skin caused by dilation of superficial blood vessels in the skin. Angioedema is a localized urticaria of the deeper tissues of the body. If not treated, the symptoms of anaphylaxis quickly increase in severity and progress to dyspnea, cyanosis, and shock. Blood pressure decreases, and the pulse becomes weak and thready. Convulsions, loss of consciousness, and death may occur if treatment is not initiated promptly.

To prevent an anaphylactic reaction to a drug or to reduce its danger, the medical assistant should stay with the patient after administration of the medication. The medical assistant should be especially alert for signs of an anaphylactic reaction after administering allergy skin tests or a penicillin or allergy injection. If a reaction occurs, the physician should be notified immediately so that he or she can begin treatment immediately. Treatment generally consists of one or more injections of epinephrine, depending on the severity of the reaction. Epinephrine goes to work immediately to reverse the life-threatening symptoms of anaphylaxis. When the patient is stabilized, he or she is usually given an injection of an antihistamine. The antihistamine takes longer to begin working but helps alleviate urticaria, itching, angioedema, and erythema. The medical assistant must ensure that an ample supply of epinephrine is on hand at all times. Many offices maintain emergency crash carts for this purpose.

Idiosyncratic Reaction

An idiosyncratic reaction is an abnormal or peculiar response to a drug that is unexplained and unpredictable. Elderly patients are most prone to idiosyncratic reactions to drugs and should be monitored closely when they are taking a new medication.

Memories *from* Externship

Theresa Cline: I can clearly remember the first time I gave an injection at my externship site. I was worried that I would forget how to give an injection and look bad in front of my externship supervisor and the patient. What made things worse was that the patient was a woman with very thin arms. I was giving her a flu shot, and I was so scared that the needle would hit her bone even though I was only using a 1-inch needle. When I walked into the room, my supervisor told the woman that I was a student and asked her if it was all right if I gave her the flu injection. The woman laughed and said, "Well, I guess so." That made me feel even more nervous. The patient then asked if it was my first shot. I told her "yes" and she said, "Just don't hurt me." When it came time to give the injection, everything that I had ever learned about injections came back to me. I gave the injection, and the woman told me I did a good job and that she didn't even feel it. That made me feel so good! My supervisor said, "If you can give a shot to her, you can give a shot to anyone." Every injection after that was a "piece of cake." I've learned just to take a deep breath before each difficult situation encountered in the office, and everything will work out. ■

Prepare for Success

GUIDELINES FOR PREPARATION AND ADMINISTRATION OF MEDICATION

To prevent medication errors, the medical assistant should follow these guidelines when preparing and administering any drug:

1. Work in a quiet, well-lit atmosphere that is free of distractions.
2. Always ask if you have a question about the medication order.
3. Know the drug to be given.
4. Select the proper drug. Check the label of the medication three times—as it is taken from its storage location, before preparing the medication, and after preparing the medication. Do not use a drug if the label is missing or is difficult to read.
5. Do not use a drug if the color has changed, if a precipitate has formed, or if it has an unusual odor.
6. Check the expiration date before preparing the drug for administration.
7. Prepare the proper dose of the drug. The term **dose** refers to the quantity of a drug to be administered at one time. Each medication has a dose range, or range of quantities of the drug that can produce therapeutic effects. It is important to administer the exact dose of the drug. A dose that is too small would not produce a therapeutic effect, and a dose that is too large could be harmful or even fatal to the patient.
8. Correctly identify the patient so that the drug is administered to the intended patient. When administering medication, the patient should be identified by his or her full name and date of birth.

9. Before administering the medication, check the patient's records or question the patient to ensure that he or she is not allergic to the medication.
10. If you are giving an injection, determine the appropriate route and site at which to administer the injection; the route and site are dictated by the type of injection being given. An allergy injection is given through the SC route, and an antibiotic injection is given through the IM route. The site must be free from abrasions, lesions, bruises, and edema.
11. Use the proper technique to administer the medication.
12. Stay with the patient after administering the medication.
13. Document information properly in the patient's chart immediately after administering the drug. Make sure the recording is clear and legible to avoid confusion by others who read it. Include the date and time, name of the medication, lot number (if required), dose given, route of administration, site of administration, and any unusual observations or patient reactions. Sign the recording with your name and credentials. If you administer a medication that contains a fraction of a unit, place a 0 before the decimal point (e.g., 0.5 mg, not .5 mg) so that the dosage is not misread as 5 mg. A decimal point and a zero should never be placed after a whole number. The decimal point may be overlooked and misread, resulting in a 10-fold overdose error (e.g., 20 mg, not 20.0 mg).
14. Always follow the seven "rights" of preparing and administering medication in the medical office:
    Right drug
    Right dose
    Right time
    Right patient
    Right route
    Right technique
    Right documentation

ORAL ADMINISTRATION

The oral route is the most convenient and the most used method of administering medication. **Oral administration** means that the drug is given by mouth in either a solid form (e.g., a tablet or capsule) or a liquid form (e.g., a suspension or a syrup). Absorption of most oral medication occurs in the small intestine, although some may be absorbed in the mouth and stomach.

Many patients find it easier to swallow a tablet or capsule with a glass of water. Water should not be offered after the patient has received a cough syrup, however, because the water would dilute the medication's beneficial effects. Unless the patient has a malabsorption problem or is unable to swallow, the oral route is considered the safest and most desirable route for administering medication. Procedure 26-1 outlines the procedure for the administration of oral medications.

PROCEDURE 26-1   Administering Oral Medication

Outcome Administer oral solid and liquid medications.

Equipment/Supplies

- Medication ordered by the physician
- Medicine cup
- Medication tray

1. **Procedural Step.** Sanitize your hands.
2. **Procedural Step.** Assemble the equipment.
3. **Procedural Step.** Work in a quiet, well-lit atmosphere.
   Principle. Good lighting aids the medical assistant in reading the medication label.
4. **Procedural Step.** Select the correct medication from the shelf. Compare the medication with the physician's instructions. Check the drug label three times—while removing the medication from storage, while preparing the medication, and after preparing the medication. Check the expiration date.
   Principle. If the medication is outdated, consult the physician because it may produce undesirable effects for which the medical assistant could be held responsible. To prevent a drug error, the medication should be carefully compared with the physician's instructions.

Compare the medication with the physician's instructions. (From Bonewit-West K: *Clinical procedures for medical assistants, ed 7,* St. Louis, 2008, Saunders.)

5. **Procedural Step.** Calculate the correct dose to be given, if necessary.
6. **Procedural Step.** Remove the bottle cap, touching the outside of the lid only.
   Principle. Touching the inside of the lid contaminates it.

7. **Procedural Step.** Check the drug label again, and pour the medication.
   Solid Medications. Pour the correct number of capsules or tablets into the bottle cap. Transfer the medication to a medicine cup, being careful not to touch the inside of the cup.
   Principle. Pouring the medication into the lid prevents contamination of the medication and lid.
   Liquid Medications. Place the lid of the bottle on a flat surface with the open end facing up. Palm the surface of the label. With the opposite hand, place the

Pour the correct number of capsules or tablets into the bottle cap. (From Bonewit-West K: *Clinical procedures for medical assistants,* ed 7, St. Louis, 2008, Saunders.)

Place the lid of the bottle on a flat surface with the open end facing up. (From Bonewit-West K: *Clinical procedures for medical assistants,* ed 7, St. Louis, 2008, Saunders.)

Continued

PROCEDURE 26-1   Administering Oral Medication—cont'd

7 (3)

Hold the cup at eye level, and pour the medication. (From Bonewit-West K: *Clinical procedures for medical assistants,* ed 7, St. Louis, 2008, Saunders.)

thumbnail at the proper calibration on the medicine cup, and hold the cup at eye level. Pour the medication, and read the dose at the lowest level of the meniscus. (The meniscus is the curved surface of the liquid in a container. When a liquid is poured into a medicine cup, capillary action causes the liquid in contact with the cup to be drawn upward, resulting in a curved surface in the middle.)

Principle. Placing the bottle cap with the open end up prevents contamination of the inside of the cap. Palming the medication label prevents the medication from dripping on the label and obscuring it.

8. **Procedural Step.** Replace the bottle cap, and check the drug label a third time to ensure it is the correct medication. Return the medication to its storage location.

9. **Procedural Step.** Greet the patient and introduce yourself. Identify the patient by full name and date of birth and explain the procedure. Explain the purpose of administering the medication.
   Principle. It is crucial that no error be made in patient identity.

10. **Procedural Step.** Hand the medicine cup containing the medication to the patient, along with a glass of water. (If the medication is a cough syrup, do not offer water.)
    Principle. Water helps the patient swallow the medication.

11. **Procedural Step.** Remain with the patient until the medication is swallowed. If the patient experiences any unusual reaction, notify the physician.

12. **Procedural Step.** Sanitize your hands.

13. **Procedural Step.** Chart the procedure. Include the date and time, the name of the medication, the dosage given, the route of administration, and any significant observations or patient reactions. The Latin abbreviation *po,* which means "by mouth," can be used to indicate the route of administration.

CHARTING EXAMPLE

Date	
2/12/10	9:30 a.m. Acetaminophen, 650 mg, po.
	———————————— T. Cline, CMA (AAMA)

PARENTERAL ADMINISTRATION

The parenteral route of drug administration has several advantages. Medications given subcutaneously, intramuscularly, and intravenously are absorbed more rapidly and completely than medications given orally. In some cases, the parenteral route is the only way a drug can be given. If the patient is unconscious or has a gastric disturbance, such as nausea or vomiting, the parenteral route would be used. If state laws permit, the medical assistant is usually responsible for administering SC, IM, and intradermal injections. IV medications are sometimes administered in the medical office and are discussed in more detail later in the section on IV therapy.

The parenteral route also has disadvantages, such as pain and the possibility of infection as a result of breaking the skin. The medical assistant can minimize pain by inserting and withdrawing the needle quickly and smoothly and by withdrawing the needle at the same angle as for insertion. If injections are given repeatedly (e.g., allergy injections),

the sites should be rotated to prevent the overuse of one site, which may cause irritation and tissue damage. Rotating sites also allows better absorption of the drug.

When recording the administration of a medication in the patient's chart, the medical assistant must include the site of injection (e.g., right upper arm, left dorsogluteal). This assists in proper site rotation for patients who receive repeated injections. In addition, the information provides a reference point should a problem arise with the injection site.

Medical asepsis must be used when parenteral medications are administered. In addition, the needle and inside of the syringe must remain sterile. These practices reduce the danger of microorganisms entering the patient's body during the administration of medication. The medical assistant must follow the Occupational Safety and Health Administration (OSHA) standard when administering medication as a means of protecting himself or herself from bloodborne pathogens (see Chapter 17). Procedure 26-2 describes how to prepare an injection.

Figure 26-4. Diagram of a needle and a 3-cc syringe, with parts identified. (From Bonewit-West K: *Clinical procedures for medical assistants,* ed 7, St. Louis, 2008, Saunders.)

Figure 26-5. Examples of syringe and needle packages labeled according to contents. (From Bonewit-West K: *Clinical procedures for medical assistants,* ed 7, St. Louis, 2008, Saunders.)

Parts of a Needle and Syringe

Needle

The needle consists of several parts (Figure 26-4). The *hub* of the needle fits onto the top of the syringe. The *shaft* is inserted into the body tissue. The opening in the shaft of the needle, known as the *lumen,* is continuous with the needle hub. Medication flows from the syringe and through the lumen of the needle. The *point* of the needle is located at the end of the needle shaft. The point is sharp so that it can penetrate body tissues easily. The top of the needle is slanted and is called the *bevel.* The bevel is designed to make a narrow, slitlike opening in the skin. This narrow opening closes quickly when the needle is removed to prevent leakage of medication, and it heals quickly.

Each needle has a certain **gauge;** needle gauges for administering medication range between 18 G and 27 G. The gauge of a needle is determined by the diameter of the lumen: As the size of the gauge increases, the diameter of the lumen decreases. A needle with a gauge of 23 has a smaller lumen diameter than a needle with a gauge of 21. Thick or oily preparations must be given with a large lumen because they are too thick to pass through a smaller one. A needle with a larger lumen makes a larger needle track in the tissues. To reduce pain and tissue damage, a needle with the smallest gauge appropriate for the solution and route of administration is always chosen.

The length of the needle ranges between 3/8 and 3 inches; the length used is based on the type of injection being given and the size of the patient. To administer an IM injection to an obese adult requires a longer needle to reach the muscle tissue than would be required for a normal-size adult. To administer an IM injection to a thin patient requires a shorter needle to avoid inserting a needle too deeply and possibly penetrating the bone. The needle used to give an IM injection must be longer than one used for an SC injection so that it penetrates deeply enough to reach the muscle tissue.

Syringe

The syringe is used for inserting fluids into the body. It is made of plastic and must be disposed of after one use. The syringe with an attached needle is packaged in a cellophane wrapper or a rigid plastic container. Information regarding the syringe's capacity and the needle's length and gauge is printed on the wrapper of the syringe and needle (Figure 26-5). Syringes and needles are also available in separate packages. In this case, the medical assistant must attach a needle to the syringe before drawing medication into the syringe.

The parts of a syringe are the barrel, flange, and plunger (see Figure 26-4). The *barrel* of the syringe holds the medication and contains calibrated markings to measure the proper amount of medication. Most syringes are calibrated in cubic centimeters (cc), the unit of measurement used most often to administer parenteral medication. The medical assistant should become familiar with reading the graduated scales on syringes. At the end of the barrel is a rim known as the *flange,* which helps in injecting the medication. The flange also prevents the syringe from rolling when it is placed on a flat surface. The *plunger* is a movable cylinder that slides back and forth in the barrel. It is used to draw medication into the syringe when preparing an injection and to push medication out of the syringe when administering an injection.

Various types of syringes are available to administer injections. The choice is based on the type of injection being given (e.g., tuberculin skin test, allergy injection, antibiotic injection) and the amount of medication being administered. The types of syringes used most often in the

Figure 26-6. Various syringes used to administer injections. **A,** Hypodermic. **B,** Insulin (U-100). **C,** Tuberculin. (From Bonewit-West K: *Clinical procedures for medical assistants,* ed 7, St. Louis, 2008, Saunders.)

medical office include hypodermic, insulin, and tuberculin (Figure 26-6).

Hypodermic syringes are available in 2-, 2.5-, 3-, and 5-cc sizes and are calibrated in cubic centimeters. They are commonly used to administer IM injections.

The *insulin syringe* is designed especially for the administration of an insulin injection, and the barrel is calibrated in units. The most common type is the U-100 syringe, which is calibrated into 100 units in increments of 2.

Tuberculin syringes are employed to administer a small dose of medication, such as when administering a tuberculin test. The tuberculin syringe has a capacity of 1 cc, and the calibrations are divided into tenths (0.10) and hundredths (0.01) of a cubic centimeter.

Syringes are also available with capacities of 10, 20, 30, 50, and 60 cc; however, they are not used for administering medication, but rather for medical treatments, such as irrigating wounds and draining fluid from cysts.

Safety-Engineered Syringes

OSHA stipulates requirements to reduce needlestick and other sharps injuries among health care workers. As discussed in Chapter 17, employers are required to evaluate and implement commercially available safer medical devices that reduce occupational exposure to the lowest extent feasible.

Safer medical devices include safety-engineered syringes. *Safety-engineered syringes* incorporate a built-in safety feature to reduce the risk of a needlestick injury. Figure 26-7 illustrates types of safety-engineered syringes and the methods for using them.

Preparation of Parenteral Medication

Medication used for injections is available in various types of dispensing units—vials, ampules, and prefilled syringes and cartridges.

Vials

A **vial** is a closed glass container with a rubber stopper; a soft metal or plastic cap protects the rubber stopper and must be removed the first time the medication is used. An injectable medication may be available in a single-dose vial, a multiple-dose vial, or both (Figure 26-8).

Before the medication can be withdrawn, some vials require mixing (e.g., reconstituting a powdered drug, mixing a vial that separates on standing). Vials that require mixing should be rolled between the hands rather than shaken because shaking would cause the medication to foam, creating air bubbles that may enter the syringe when the medication is withdrawn.

To remove medication from a vial, an amount of air exactly equal to the amount of liquid to be removed is injected into the vial. The air should be inserted above the fluid level to avoid creating bubbles in the medication. If air is not injected first, a partial vacuum is created, and it is difficult to remove the medication. During the withdrawal of medication, the needle opening should be inserted below the fluid level to prevent the entrance of air bubbles. Air bubbles can be removed by tapping the barrel of the syringe with the fingertips. If the bubbles are allowed to remain, they take up space that the medication should occupy, which would prevent the patient from receiving the full dose of medication.

Ampules

An **ampule** is a small, sealed glass container that holds a single dose of medication (see Figure 26-8). An ampule has a constriction in the stem, known as the *neck,* which helps in opening it. Before opening, the medical assistant must ensure that there is no medication in the stem by tapping it lightly. A colored ring around the neck indicates where the ampule is prescored for easy opening. The ampule is opened by holding it firmly with gauze and breaking off the stem with a strong steady pressure.

A hazard with medication in ampules is the possibility of small glass particles getting into the ampule as the stem is broken off. When the medication is withdrawn into the syringe, the glass particles might also be withdrawn. To prevent this problem, a needle with a filter that filters out small glass particles should be used (Figure 26-9).

The needle opening is inserted into the base of the ampule below the fluid level to withdraw medication. To prevent contamination, the needle should not be permitted to touch the outside of the ampule. Air should never be injected into the ampule because it could force out some of the medication.

Prefilled Syringes

Some drugs come in *prefilled disposable syringes.* Using this type of dispensing unit does not require drawing up the medication. The name of the drug, dose, and expiration date are printed on the syringe (Figure 26-10).

Storage

The medical assistant should always read the drug package insert to determine the proper method for storing each

A, Safety-Engineered Syringes Hinged Shield Syringe (Becton-Dickinson Safety Glide Syringe).
1. After administering the injection, push the lever of the hinged-shield forward.
2. Continue pushing until the needle tip is fully covered by the shield, then discard the syringe in a biohazard sharps container.

B, Sliding Shield Syringe (Monoject Safety Syringe).
1. After administering the injection, extend the sliding shield forward fully until a click is heard.
2. Lock the shield by twisting it in either direction until a click is heard. Discard the syringe in a biohazard sharps container.

Figure 26-7. Safety-engineered syringes. (From Bonewit-West K: *Clinical procedures for medical assistants,* ed 7, St. Louis, 2008, Saunders.)

Continued

parenteral medication because improper storage may alter the effectiveness of the medication.

Reconstitution of Powdered Drugs

Some parenteral medications are stable for only a short time in liquid form; these medications are prepared and stored in powdered form and require the addition of a liquid before administration. The process of adding a liquid to a powdered drug is known as *reconstitution.* The liquid used to reconstitute a powdered drug is known as the *diluent* and usually consists of sterile water or normal saline. The pow-

dered drug is contained in a single-dose or multiple-dose vial and is accompanied by specific instructions for reconstitution. An example of a parenteral medication that requires reconstitution is the measles, mumps, and rubella (MMR) immunization (Figure 26-11). The procedure for reconstituting powdered drugs is outlined in Procedure 26-3.

Subcutaneous Injections

A **subcutaneous (SC) injection** is made into the subcutaneous tissue, which consists of adipose (fat) tissue and is

C, Retractable Needle (Vanish Point Syringe).

1. Administer the injection following the proper technique.
2. After administering the medication, continue depressing the plunger with the thumb. Use firm pressure past the point of initial resistance. This action delivers the full dose of medication to the patient and activates the needle retraction device, causing the needle to retract automatically from the patient's skin and into the barrel of the syringe.
3. Discard the syringe in a biohazard sharps container.

Figure 26-7, cont'd.

Figure 26-8. The multiple-dose vial *(left)* and the single-dose vial *(middle)* consist of a closed glass container with a rubber stopper. The ampule *(right)* consists of a small, sealed glass container that holds a single dose of medication. (From Bonewit-West K: *Clinical procedures for medical assistants,* ed 7, St. Louis, 2008, Saunders.)

Figure 26-9. Filter needle used to withdraw medication from an ampule. (From Bonewit-West K: *Clinical procedures for medical assistants,* ed 7, St. Louis, 2008, Saunders.)

Figure 26-10. A prefilled disposable syringe. (From Bonewit-West K: *Clinical procedures for medical assistants,* ed 7, St. Louis, 2008, Saunders.)

Figure 26-11. The measles, mumps, and rubella (MMR) vaccine is a parenteral medication that requires reconstitution before administration. The vial on the left contains the medication in powdered form, and the vial on the right contains the sterile diluent. (From Bonewit-West K: *Clinical procedures for medical assistants,* ed 7, St. Louis, 2008, Saunders.)

Figure 26-12. Angle of insertion for intradermal, subcutaneous, and intramuscular injections. (From Bonewit-West K: *Clinical procedures for medical assistants,* ed 7, St. Louis, 2008, Saunders.)

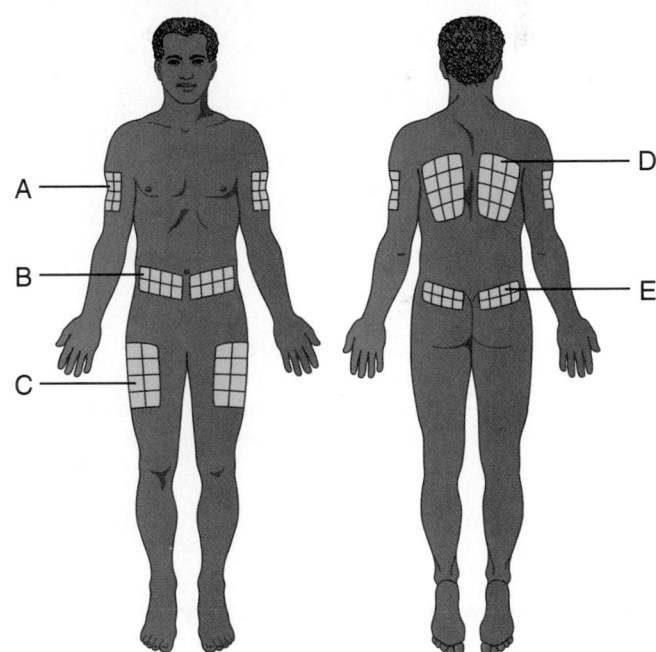

Figure 26-13. Common sites for subcutaneous injections. **A,** Upper outer arm. **B,** Lower abdomen. **C,** Upper outer thigh. **D,** Upper back. **E,** Flank region. (From Bonewit-West K: *Clinical procedures for medical assistants,* ed 7, St. Louis, 2008, Saunders.)

located just under the skin (Figure 26-12). Subcutaneous tissue is located all over the body; however, certain sites are more commonly used because they are located where bones and blood vessels are not near the surface of the skin. These sites include the upper lateral part of the arms, the anterior thigh, the upper back, and the abdomen (Figure 26-13). Absorption of medication from an SC injection occurs mainly through capillaries, resulting in a slower absorption rate than with IM injections. To ensure proper absorption, tissue that is grossly adipose, hardened, inflamed, or edematous should not be used as an injection site.

The needle length varies from ½ to ⁵⁄₈ inch, and the gauge ranges from 23 G to 25 G. Elderly and dehydrated patients tend to have less subcutaneous tissue, and obese patients have more. The length of the needle should be adjusted accordingly to ensure the medication is administered into the subcutaneous tissue and not into muscle tissue.

Subcutaneous tissue is sensitive to irritating solutions and large volumes of medications; therefore drugs given subcutaneously must be isotonic, nonirritating, nonviscous, and water soluble. The amount of medication injected through the SC route should not exceed 1 cc. More than this amount results in pressure on sensory nerve endings, causing discomfort and pain.

Medications commonly administered through the SC route include epinephrine, insulin, and allergy injections. Patients who receive allergy injections must wait in the medical office for 15 to 20 minutes after the injection to be observed for an allergic reaction. Procedure 26-4 outlines the administration of an SC injection.

Intramuscular Injections

Intramuscular (IM) injections are made into the muscular layer of the body, which lies below the skin and subcutaneous layers (Figure 26-14). The amount of medication that

Figure 26-14. Sites of intramuscular injections. **A,** Dorsogluteal muscle. **B,** Deltoid muscle. **C,** Vastus lateralis. **D,** Ventrogluteal muscle. (From Leahy JM, Kizilay PE: *Foundations of nursing practice: a nursing process approach,* Philadelphia, 1988, Saunders.)

can be injected into muscle tissue is more than the amount that can be injected into subcutaneous tissue. An amount up to 3 cc can be injected into the gluteal or vastus lateralis muscles, although older and very thin adults can tolerate only 2 cc or less in these sites.

Absorption is more rapid by this route than by the SC route because there are more blood vessels in muscle tissue. Medication that is irritating to subcutaneous tissue is often given intramuscularly because there are fewer nerve endings in deep muscle tissue. Most parenteral medications administered in the medical office are given through the IM route; examples include immunizations, antibiotics, injectable contraceptives, vitamin B_{12}, and corticosteroids.

The length of the needle for an adult must be long enough to reach muscle tissue and varies from 1 to 3 inches. A 1½-inch needle is typically used for an average-sized adult, whereas a 1-inch needle is often used for a thin adult or child and a needle of 2 to 3 inches may be necessary for an obese adult. The gauge of the needle used ranges from 18 G to 23 G, depending on the viscosity of the medication. Procedure 26-5 outlines the technique for the administration of an IM injection.

Intramuscular Injection Sites

The sites chosen for IM injections are away from large nerves and blood vessels. The medical assistant should practice locating these sites to become familiar with them. The area should always be fully exposed to permit clear visualization of the injection site.

Dorsogluteal Site

The dorsogluteal site is often used to administer IM injections in the medical office. In adults and children older than 3 years of age, the gluteal muscles are well developed and can absorb a large amount of medication. The patient should lie on the abdomen with the toes pointed inward, which aids in relaxation of the gluteal muscles. The medication is injected into the upper outer quadrant of the gluteal area, in the area located above and outside a diagonal line drawn from the greater trochanter to the posterior superior iliac spine. These landmarks should be identified through palpation. The medical assistant must be *extremely* careful to maintain the proper boundary lines to avoid injection into the sciatic nerve or superior gluteal artery (see Figure 26-14).

Deltoid Site

The deltoid area is easily accessible and can be used when the patient is sitting or lying down. This site is small because major nerves and blood vessels surround it, and large amounts of medication (no more than 1 cc) and repeated injections should not be given in this area. The medication is injected into the deltoid muscle.

The medical assistant should ensure that the entire arm is exposed by having the patient's sleeve completely pulled up or by removing the sleeve from the arm if it cannot be pulled up. A tight sleeve constricts the arm and causes unnecessary bleeding from the puncture site.

The deltoid site is located by palpating the lower edge of the acromion process, which forms the base of a triangle in line with the midpoint of the lateral side of the arm, opposite the axilla (see Figure 26-14). This site may also be located by placing four fingers horizontally across the deltoid muscle with the top finger along the acromion process. The injection site is located three finger widths below the acromion process.

Vastus Lateralis Site

The vastus lateralis is used because it is not near major nerves and blood vessels and is a relatively thick muscle (see Figure 26-14). This site is particularly desirable for infants and children younger than 3 years old whose gluteal muscles are not yet well developed. The area is bounded by the midanterior thigh on the front of the leg and the midlateral thigh on the side. The proximal boundary is a hand's breadth below the greater trochanter, and the distal boundary is a hand's breadth above the knee. It is easier to give an injection in the vastus lateralis if the patient is lying down, but a sitting position can also be used.

Ventrogluteal Site

The ventrogluteal site is growing in acceptability as an IM injection site because the subcutaneous layer is relatively small and the muscle layer is thick. The site is located away from major nerves and blood vessels. Through palpation, the greater trochanter of the femur, anterior superior iliac spine, and iliac crest can be located. If the injection is being made into the patient's left side, the palm of the right hand is placed on the greater trochanter and the index finger is placed on the anterior superior iliac spine. The middle finger is spread posteriorly as far as possible away from the index finger, to touch the iliac crest. The hand position is reversed if the injection is being made into the patient's right side. The triangle formed by the fingers is the area into which the injection is given. An injection into the ventrogluteal site can be administered when the patient is lying prone or on one side (see Figure 26-14).

Z-Track Method

Medications that are irritating to subcutaneous and skin tissue or that discolor the skin must be given intramuscularly using the Z-track method; one medication that is administered by this method is iron dextran (Imferon). The dorsogluteal, ventrogluteal, and vastus lateralis sites all can be used as areas to administer a Z-track injection.

The Z-track method is similar to the IM injection procedure except that the skin and subcutaneous tissue at the injection site are pulled to the side before the needle is inserted. This causes a zigzag path through the tissues when the needle is removed and the skin is released. The zigzag path prevents the medication from reaching the subcutaneous layer or skin surface by sealing off the needle track (Figure 26-15). The procedure for administering medication using the Z-track method is outlined in Procedure 26-6.

Text continued on p. 617

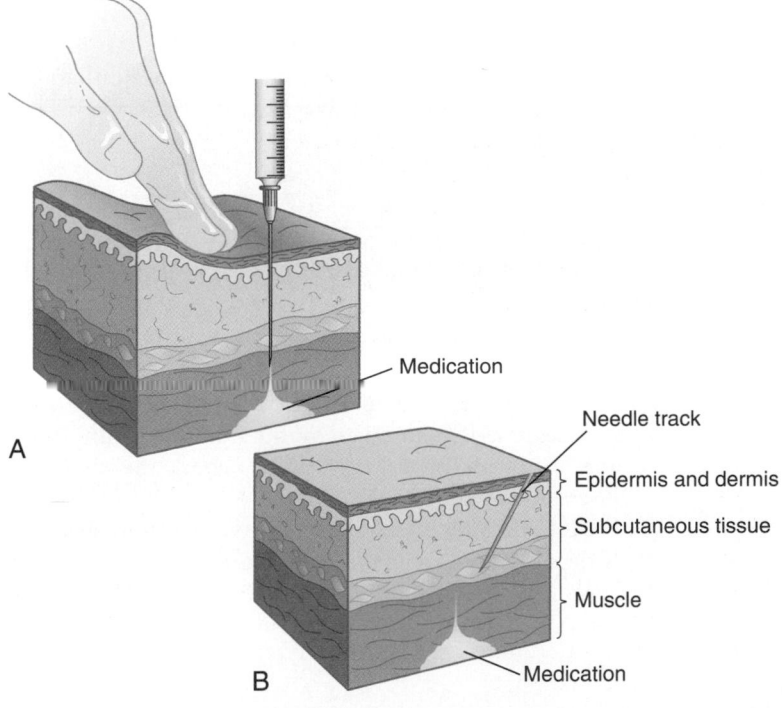

Figure 26-15. Z-track intramuscular injection method. **A,** The skin and subcutaneous tissue are pulled to the side before the needle is inserted. **B,** This causes a zigzag path through the tissue when the skin is released, which seals off the needle track. (From Bonewit-West K. *Clinical procedures for medical assistants,* ed 7, St. Louis, 2008, Saunders.)

PROCEDURE 26-2   Preparing an Injection

Outcome Prepare an injection from an ampule and a vial.

Equipment/Supplies

- Medication ordered by the physician
- Appropriate needle and syringe

- Antiseptic wipe
- Medication tray

1. **Procedural Step.** Sanitize your hands.
2. **Procedural Step.** Assemble the equipment.
3. **Procedural Step.** Work in a quiet and well-lit atmosphere.
   Principle. Good lighting aids the medical assistant in reading the medication label.
4. **Procedural Step.** Select the proper medication. Compare the medication with the physician's instructions. Check the drug label three times—while removing the medication from storage, before withdrawing the medication into the syringe, and after preparing the medication. Check the expiration date.
   Principle. The medication should be carefully identified to prevent the administration of the wrong medication. Outdated medication should not be used because it could produce undesirable effects.

Check the drug label three times. (From Bonewit-West K: *Clinical procedures for medical assistants,* ed 7, St. Louis, 2008, Saunders.)

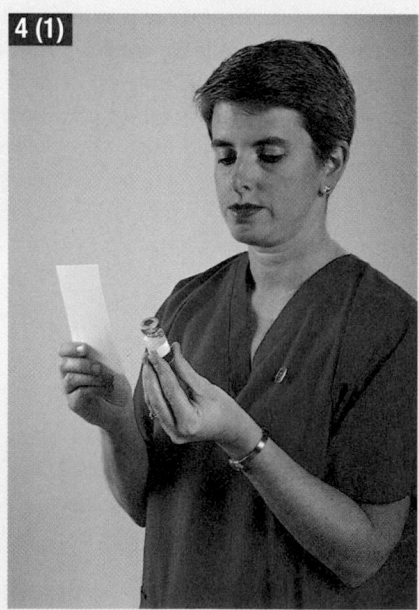

Compare the medication with the physician's instructions. (From Bonewit-West K: *Clinical procedures for medical assistants,* ed 7, St. Louis, 2008, Saunders.)

Check the expiration date. (From Bonewit-West K: *Clinical procedures for medical assistants,* ed 7, St. Louis, 2008, Saunders.)

5. **Procedural Step.** Calculate the correct dose to be given, if necessary. If you have any questions regarding the administration of the medication, check the package insert accompanying the drug.
6. **Procedural Step.** Open the syringe and needle package. If necessary, assemble the needle and syringe.

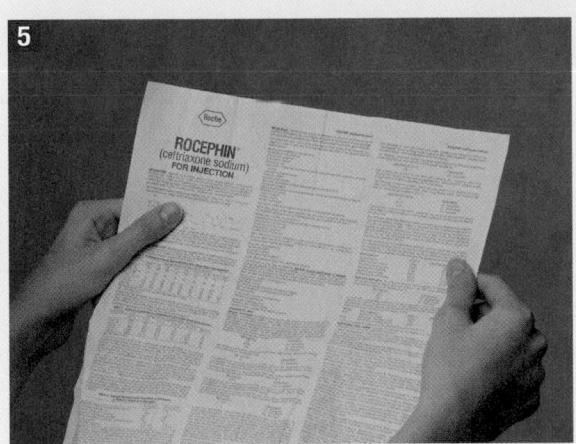

Check the package insert. (From Bonewit-West K: *Clinical procedures for medical assistants,* ed 7, St. Louis, 2008, Saunders.)

Principle. Disposable needles and syringes may come already assembled together in a package or in separate packages that require assembly of the needle and syringe.

7. Procedural Step. Check to ensure that the needle is attached firmly to the syringe by loosening the guard on the needle, grasping the needle at the hub, and tightening it. Break the seal on the syringe by moving the plunger back and forth several times.

8. Procedural Step. Check the drug label again to ensure it is the correct medication. If required, mix the medication by rolling the vial between your hands to obtain a uniform suspension of the medication.

9. Procedural Step. Withdraw the medication following these steps.

Withdrawing Medication from a Vial

a. Procedural Step. Remove the soft metal or plastic cap protecting the rubber stopper of the vial. Open the antiseptic; wipe and cleanse the rubber stopper.
Principle. Cleansing the top of the vial removes dust and bacteria.

Cleanse the rubber stopper. (From Bonewit-West K: *Clinical procedures for medical assistants,* ed 7, St. Louis, 2008, Saunders.)

b. Procedural Step. Place the vial in an upright position on a flat surface. Remove the needle guard. Pull

back on the plunger to draw an amount of air into the syringe equal to the amount of medication to be withdrawn from the vial.
Principle. Air must be injected into the vial first to prevent the formation of a partial vacuum in the vial, which would make it difficult to remove medication.

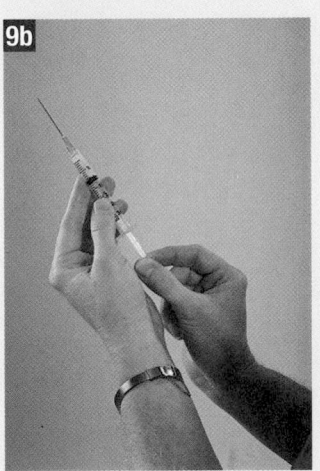

Draw air into the syringe. (From Bonewit-West K: *Clinical procedures for medical assistants,* ed 7, St. Louis, 2008, Saunders.)

c. Procedural Step. Using moderate pressure, insert the needle through the center of the rubber stopper at a 90-degree angle, until it reaches the empty space between the stopper and fluid level. Be careful not to bend the needle. Push down on the plunger to inject the air into the vial, keeping the needle opening above the fluid level. (*Note:* If you are using a retractable safety syringe, do not push too hard on the plunger to avoid activating the retracting mechanism prematurely.)
Principle. The air must be inserted above the fluid level to avoid creating air bubbles in the medication.

Inject air into the vial. (From Bonewit-West K: *Clinical procedures for medical assistants,* ed 7, St. Louis, 2008, Saunders.)

Continued

PROCEDURE 26-2 **Preparing an Injection—cont'd**

d. Procedural Step. Invert the vial while holding onto the syringe and plunger. Hold the syringe at eye level, and withdraw the proper amount of medication. Keep the needle opening below the fluid level.
Principle. The needle opening must be below the fluid level to prevent the entrance of air bubbles into the syringe.

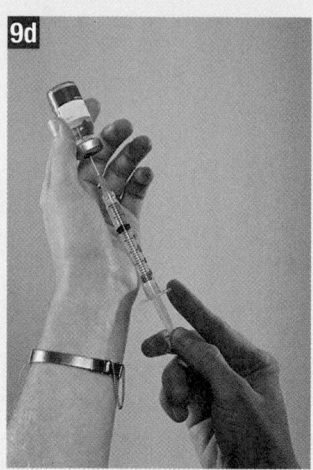

Withdraw the proper amount of medication. (From Bonewit-West K: *Clinical procedures for medical assistants,* ed 7, St. Louis, 2008, Saunders.)

e. Procedural Step. Remove any air bubbles in the syringe by holding the syringe in a vertical position and tapping the barrel with the fingertips until they disappear.
Principle. Air bubbles take up space the medication should occupy, preventing the patient from getting the proper dose of medication.

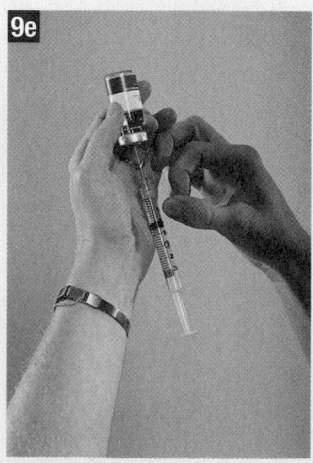

Tap the barrel with the fingertips to remove air bubbles. (From Bonewit-West K: *Clinical procedures for medical assistants,* ed 7, St. Louis, 2008, Saunders.)

f. Procedural Step. Remove any air remaining at the top of the syringe by slowly pushing the plunger forward and allowing the air to flow back into the vial. Carefully remove the needle from the rubber stopper, and replace the needle guard.
Principle. The needle must remain sterile. The needle guard prevents the needle from becoming contaminated.

g. Procedural Step. Check the drug label for the third time, and return the medication to its proper storage location.

Withdrawing Medication from an Ampule

a. Procedural Step. Remove the needle (and needle guard) from the syringe, and attach a filter needle (and needle guard).

b. Procedural Step. Open the antiseptic wipe, and cleanse the neck of the ampule.
Principle. Cleansing the neck of the ampule removes dust and bacteria.

c. Procedural Step. Tap the stem of the ampule lightly to remove any medication in the neck of the ampule.

d. Procedural Step. Check the medication label a second time and place a piece of gauze around the neck of the ampule. Hold the base of the ampule between the first two fingers and the thumb of one hand. Hold the neck of the vial between the first two fingers and the thumb of the other hand. Apply a strong, steady pressure with the thumbs, and break off the stem by snapping it quickly and firmly away from the body. Discard the stem and gauze in a biohazard sharps container.

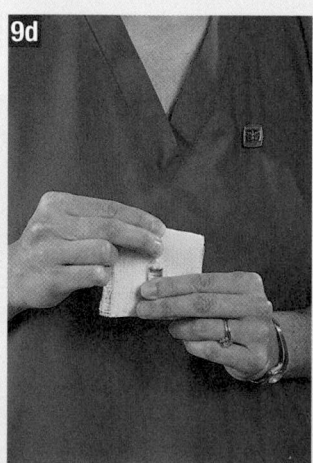

Snap off the stem away from the body. (From Bonewit-West K: *Clinical procedures for medical assistants,* ed 7, St. Louis, 2008, Saunders.)

e. Procedural Step. Place the ampule on a flat surface. Remove the needle guard. Insert the filter needle opening below the fluid level.

Principle. The filter needle prevents glass particles from being withdrawn into the syringe.

f. Procedural Step. Withdraw the proper amount of medication by pulling back on the plunger. Keep the needle opening below the fluid level to prevent the entrance of air bubbles into the syringe. Tilt the ampule as needed to keep the needle opening immersed in the fluid.

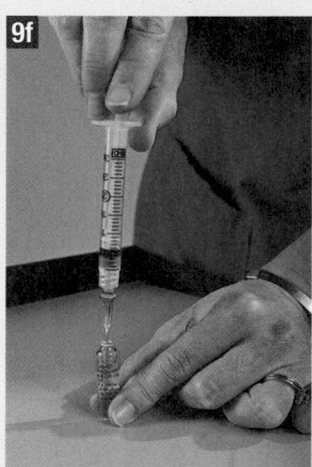

Withdraw the medication. (From Bonewit-West K: *Clinical procedures for medical assistants,* ed 7, St. Louis, 2008, Saunders.)

Principle. Air bubbles take up space the medication should occupy, resulting in an inaccurate measurement of medication.

Note: Another method can be used to remove medication from an ampule. Choose the method that is easiest for you. To perform this method, invert the ampule, making sure to keep the needle opening below the fluid level. Withdraw the proper amount of medication by pulling back on the plunger. Move the needle downward as needed to keep the needle opening immersed in the fluid.

g. Procedural Step. Remove the needle from the ampule, and replace the needle guard. Check the drug label for the third time, and dispose of the glass ampule in a biohazard sharps container.

h. Procedural Step. Remove the filter needle (and guard) from the syringe, and discard it in a biohazard sharps container. Reapply the needle (and guard) for administering the medication.

i. Procedural Step. If air bubbles are in the syringe, remove the needle guard, hold the syringe in a vertical position, and tap the barrel with the fingertips until the bubbles disappear. Remove the air at the top of the syringe by slowly pushing the plunger forward. If the syringe contains excess fluid, hold the syringe vertically over a sink with the needle tip up and slanted toward the sink. Slowly eject the excess fluid into the sink. Replace the needle guard.

PROCEDURE 26-3

PROCEDURE 26-3 Reconstituting Powdered Drugs

Outcome Reconstitute a powdered drug for parenteral administration.

Equipment/Supplies

- Medication ordered by the physician
- Appropriate needle and syringe
- Antiseptic wipe
- Medication tray

1. Procedural Step. Follow steps 1 through 8 of Procedure 26-2.

2. Procedural Step. From the vial of the powdered drug, withdraw an amount of air equal to the amount of liquid to be injected into the vial.

Principle. Removing air from the powdered drug vial allows room for injection of the diluent.

3. Procedural Step. Inject the air removed from the powdered drug vial into the vial of diluent.

Principle. Air must be injected into the vial to prevent formation of a partial vacuum in the vial, which would make it difficult to remove the diluent.

4. Procedural Step. Invert the diluent vial, and withdraw the proper amount of liquid into the syringe. Remove air bubbles from the syringe, and carefully remove the needle from the vial.

5. Procedural Step. Insert the needle into the powdered drug vial, and inject the diluent into the vial. Remove the needle from the vial, and replace the needle guard.

6. Procedural Step. Roll the vial between the hands to mix the powdered drug and liquid (unless indicated otherwise by the drug package insert).

Principle. Shaking the vial may cause air bubbles to form.

7. Procedural Step. Label multiple-dose vials with the date of preparation and your initials.

8. Procedural Step. Follow step 9 (a through g) of Procedure 26-2.

9. Procedural Step. Store multiple-dose vials as indicated by the manufacturer's instructions. Because reconstituted drugs are stable for a short time, carefully check the date of preparation on the multiple-dose vial before administering it again.

Continued

PROCEDURE 26-3 **Reconstituting Powdered Drugs—cont'd**

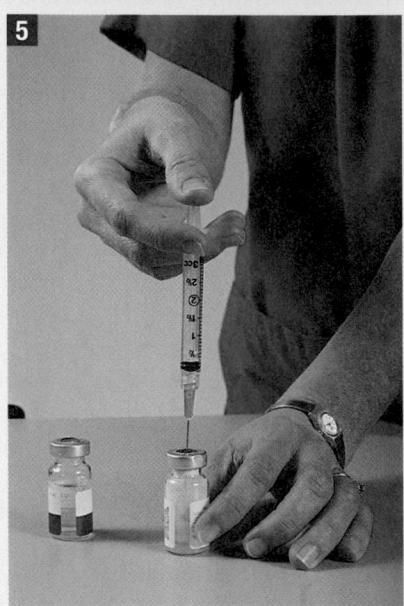

Inject the diluent into the vial. (From Bonewit-West K: *Clinical procedures for medical assistants,* ed 7, St. Louis, 2008, Saunders.)

Roll the vial between the hands. (From Bonewit-West K: *Clinical procedures for medical assistants,* ed 7, St. Louis, 2008, Saunders.)

PROCEDURE 26-4 **Administering a Subcutaneous Injection**

Outcome Administer an SC injection.

Equipment/Supplies

- Medication ordered by the physician
- Appropriate needle and syringe
- Antiseptic wipe
- Sterile 2 × 2 gauze pad
- Disposable gloves
- Biohazard sharps container

1. **Procedural Step.** Sanitize your hands, and prepare the injection.
2. **Procedural Step.** Greet the patient and introduce yourself. Identify the patient by full name and date of birth. Explain the procedure and purpose of the injection.
   Principle. It is crucial that no error be made in patient identity. An apprehensive patient may need reassurance.
3. **Procedural Step.** Select an appropriate injection site. The upper arm, thigh, back, and abdomen are recommended sites for an SC injection. See Figure 26-14.
   Principle. The entire area should be exposed to ensure a safe and comfortable injection.
4. **Procedural Step.** Prepare the injection site. Cleanse the area with an antiseptic wipe. Using a circular motion, start with the injection site and move outward. Do not touch the site after cleansing it.
   Principle. Using a circular motion carries contaminants away from the injection site. Touching the site after cleansing contaminates it, and the cleansing process needs to be repeated.

Cleanse the area with an antiseptic wipe. (From Bonewit-West K: *Clinical procedures for medical assistants,* ed 7, St. Louis, 2008, Saunders.)

5. **Procedural Step.** Allow the area to dry completely.
   Principle. If the area is not permitted to dry, the antiseptic may enter the tissues when the skin is

pierced, resulting in irritation and patient discomfort.

6. Procedural Step. Apply gloves, and remove the needle guard. Position your nondominant hand on the area surrounding the injection site. The skin may be held taut, or the area surrounding the injection site may be grasped and held in a cushion fashion.

Principle. Gloves provide a barrier against bloodborne pathogens. In normal adults, the needle enters the subcutaneous tissue when the skin is held taut. Grasping the area around the injection site is recommended for a thin or dehydrated patient. This ensures that the subcutaneous tissue, and not muscle tissue, is entered.

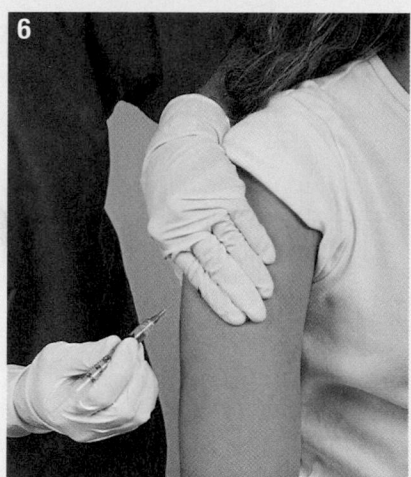

Grasp the area surrounding the injection site. (From Bonewit-West K: *Clinical procedures for medical assistants,* ed 7, St. Louis, 2008, Saunders.)

7. Procedural Step. Hold the barrel of the syringe between your thumb and index finger. Insert the needle quickly and smoothly at a 45-degree or 90-degree angle, depending on the length of the needle. With a ½-inch needle, a 90-degree angle should be used; with a ⅝-inch needle, a 45-degree angle should be used. Insert the needle to the hub.

Insert the needle at a 45-degree angle. (From Bonewit-West K: *Clinical procedures for medical assistants,* ed 7, St. Louis, 2008, Saunders.)

Principle. Inserting the needle quickly and smoothly minimizes tissue trauma and pain. Needle length determines the angle of insertion to ensure placement of the medication in subcutaneous tissue.

8. Procedural Step. Remove your hand from the skin.

Principle. Medication injected into compressed tissue causes pressure against nerve fibers and is uncomfortable for the patient.

9. Procedural Step. Hold the syringe steady and pull back gently on the plunger to determine whether the needle is in a blood vessel, in which case blood would appear in the syringe. If blood appears, withdraw the needle, prepare a new injection, and begin again.

Principle. Moving the syringe after the needle has entered the tissue causes patient discomfort. Drugs intended for SC administration but injected into a blood vessel are absorbed too quickly, and undesirable results may occur.

Pull back gently to determine whether the needle is in a blood vessel. (From Bonewit-West K: *Clinical procedures for medical assistants,* ed 7, St. Louis, 2008, Saunders.)

10. Procedural Step. Inject the medication slowly and steadily by depressing the plunger. If you are using a retractable safety syringe, activate it at this time following the steps outlined in Figure 26-7, and continue to step 12.

Principle. Rapid injection creates pressure and destroys tissue, which are uncomfortable for the patient.

11. Procedural Step. Place the antiseptic wipe or a gauze pad gently over the injection site, and quickly remove the needle, keeping it at the same angle as for insertion.

Principle. Withdrawing the needle quickly and at the same angle as for insertion reduces patient discomfort. The antiseptic wipe or gauze pad placed over the injection site helps prevent tissue movement as the needle is withdrawn, reducing patient discomfort. Using a gauze pad prevents a stinging sensation from the alcohol.

Continued

PROCEDURE 26-4

PROCEDURE 26-4 **Administering a Subcutaneous Injection—cont'd**

12. Procedural Step. Apply gentle pressure to the injection site with the antiseptic wipe or gauze pad. If you are using a safety syringe with a shield, activate the safety feature at this time following the steps outlined in Figure 26-7.
Principle. Gentle pressure helps distribute the medication so that it is completely absorbed. Avoid vigorous massaging because it could damage underlying tissue.

13. Procedural Step. Properly dispose of the needle and syringe in a biohazard sharps container.
Principle. Proper disposal is required by the ⊙SHA standard to prevent accidental needlestick injuries.

14. Procedural Step. Remove gloves, and sanitize your hands.

15. Procedural Step. Chart the procedure. Include the date and time, the name of the medication, the lot number (if required), the dosage given, the route of administration, the injection site used, and any significant observations or patient reactions.
Principle. The lot number indicates the batch in which the medication was made. Should a problem arise with that batch, the drug can be recalled, and individuals who received it can be identified.

16. Procedural Step. Stay with the patient to ensure that he or she is not experiencing any unusual reactions. (*Note:* If an allergy injection has been given, the patient should remain at the medical office for at least 15 minutes to ensure that an allergic reaction does not occur.) Check the patient's arm after the waiting period and observe for induration and redness. If the patient experiences such a reaction, notify the physician immediately.

CHARTING EXAMPLE	
Date	
2/17/10	3:30 p.m. Ragweed allergy inj, 0.20 cc, SC Ⓡ upper arm. Arm checked 15 min. after admin. No reaction noted. ——— T. Cline, CMA (AAMA)

PROCEDURE 26-5 **Administering an Intramuscular Injection**

Outcome Administer an IM injection.

Equipment/Supplies

- Medication ordered by the physician
- Appropriate needle and syringe
- Antiseptic wipe
- Sterile 2 × 2 gauze pad
- Disposable gloves
- Biohazard sharps container

1. Procedural Step. Sanitize your hands, and prepare the injection.

2. Procedural Step. Greet the patient and introduce yourself. Identify the patient by full name and date of birth and explain the procedure.
Principle. Make sure that you administer the medication to the right patient. Explain the purpose of the injection. Assistance may be necessary for restraining infants and children.

3. Procedural Step. Select an appropriate IM injection site. See Figure 26-15 for the recommended IM injection sites. Remove the patient's clothing as needed to ensure the entire area is exposed.
Principle. Major nerves and blood vessels may lie in close proximity to the IM injection sites. The medical assistant should develop skill and accuracy in locating the proper sites.

4. Procedural Step. Prepare the injection site. Cleanse the area with an antiseptic wipe. Using a circular motion, start with the injection site and move outward. Do not touch the site after cleansing it.
Principle. Using a circular motion carries contaminants away from the injection site. Touching the site after cleansing contaminates it, and the cleansing process needs to be repeated.

5. Procedural Step. Allow the area to dry completely.
Principle. If the area is not permitted to dry, the antiseptic may enter the tissues when the skin is pierced, resulting in irritation and patient discomfort.

6. Procedural Step. Apply gloves, and remove the needle guard. Using the thumb and first two fingers of the nondominant hand, stretch the skin taut over the injection site.

Cleanse the site with an antiseptic wipe. (From Bonewit-West K: *Clinical procedures for medical assistants,* ed 7, St. Louis, 2008, Saunders.)

Principle. Gloves provide a barrier against blood-borne pathogens. Stretching the skin taut permits easier insertion of the needle and helps ensure that the needle enters muscle tissue.

7. **Procedural Step.** Hold the barrel of the syringe like a dart, and insert the needle quickly and smoothly at a 90-degree angle to the patient's skin with a firm motion. Insert the needle to the hub.

Insert the needle at a 90-degree angle. (From Bonewit-West K: *Clinical procedures for medical assistants,* ed 7, St. Louis, 2008, Saunders.)

Principle. The needle is inserted at a 90-degree angle to ensure that it reaches muscle tissue. Inserting the needle quickly and smoothly minimizes tissue trauma and pain.

8. **Procedural Step.** Hold the syringe steady, and pull back gently on the plunger to determine whether the needle is in a blood vessel. If blood appears, withdraw the needle, prepare a new injection, and begin again.

Principle. Moving the syringe after the needle has penetrated the tissue causes patient discomfort. If drugs intended for IM administration are injected into a blood vessel, the result is faster absorption of the medication. This may produce undesirable results.

Aspirate to determine whether the needle is in a blood vessel. (From Bonewit-West K: *Clinical procedures for medical assistants,* ed 7, St. Louis, 2008, Saunders.)

9. **Procedural Step.** Inject the medication slowly and steadily by depressing the plunger. If you are using a retractable safety syringe, activate it at this time following the steps outlined in Figure 26-7, and continue to step 11.

Principle. Rapid injection creates pressure and destroys tissue, causing discomfort for the patient.

10. **Procedural Step.** Place the antiseptic wipe or gauze pad gently over the injection site, and remove the needle quickly, keeping it at the same angle as for insertion.

Principle. Withdrawing the needle quickly and at the same angle as for insertion reduces patient discomfort. Placing the antiseptic wipe or gauze pad over the injection site helps prevent tissue movement as the needle is withdrawn, also reducing patient discomfort. Using a gauze pad prevents a stinging sensation from the alcohol.

PROCEDURE 26-5

Continued

Inject the medication slowly and steadily. (From Bonewit-West K: *Clinical procedures for medical assistants,* ed 7, St. Louis, 2008, Saunders.)

11. Procedural Step. Apply gentle pressure to the injection site with an antiseptic wipe or gauze pad. If you are using a safety syringe with a shield, activate the safety feature at this time following the steps outlined in Figure 26-7.

Principle. Gentle pressure helps distribute the medication so that it is absorbed by the muscle tissue. Avoid vigorous massaging because it could damage underlying tissues.

12. Procedural Step. Properly dispose of the needle and syringe in a biohazard sharps container.

Principle. Proper disposal is required by the OSHA standard to prevent accidental needlestick injuries.

Apply gentle pressure to the injection site. (From Bonewit-West K: *Clinical procedures for medical assistants,* ed 7, St. Louis, 2008, Saunders.)

13. Procedural Step. Remove the gloves, and sanitize your hands.

14. Procedural Step. Chart the procedure. Include the date and time, the name of the medication, the lot number (if required), the dosage given, the route of administration, the injection site used, and any significant observations or patient reactions.

Principle. The lot number indicates the batch in which the medication was made. Should a problem arise with that batch, the drug can be recalled, and individuals who received it can be identified.

15. Procedural Step. Stay with the patient to ensure he or she is not experiencing any unusual reactions. If the patient experiences an unusual reaction, notify the physician immediately.

CHARTING EXAMPLE

Date	
2/20/10	9:30 a.m. Rocephin (Lot #: U6261). Admin 1 gram, IM, Ⓛ dorsogluteal. Tolerated injection well.
	———————————— T. Cline, CMA (AAMA)

PROCEDURE 26-6   Z-Track Intramuscular Injection Technique

Outcome Administer an IM injection using the Z-track method.

Equipment/Supplies

- Medication ordered by the physician
- Appropriate needle and syringe
- Antiseptic wipe
- Disposable gloves
- Biohazard sharps container

1. **Procedural Step.** Follow steps 1 through 5 of Procedure 26-5.
2. **Procedural Step.** Apply gloves, and remove the needle guard. With the nondominant hand, pull the skin away laterally from the injection site approximately 1 to 1½ inches.
3. **Procedural Step.** Insert the needle quickly and smoothly at a 90-degree angle.
4. **Procedural Step.** Aspirate to determine whether the needle is in a blood vessel.
5. **Procedural Step.** Inject the medication slowly and steadily.
6. **Procedural Step.** After injecting the medication, wait 10 seconds before withdrawing the needle to allow initial absorption of the medication.
7. **Procedural Step.** Withdraw the needle quickly, keeping it at the same angle as for insertion.

8. **Procedural Step.** Release the traction on the skin to seal off the needle track; doing so prevents the medication from reaching the subcutaneous tissue and skin surface.
9. **Procedural Step.** Do not apply pressure to the site because it could cause the medication to seep out.
10. **Procedural Step.** Complete the procedure by following steps 12 through 15 of Procedure 26-2.

CHARTING EXAMPLE

Date	
2/20/10	10:30 a.m. Iron dextran (Lot #: 1445). Admin 100 mg, IM, Z-track into Ⓡ dorsogluteal. No complaints of discomfort.
	——————— T. Cline, CMA (AAMA)

PROCEDURE 26-6

What Would You Do? What Would You *Not* Do?

Case Study 3

Danielle Roush, 16 years old, has come to the office with her mother. Danielle is complaining of a painful sore throat, fever, and aching in both of her ears. The physician diagnoses her with strep throat and otitis media and orders 2 cc of an antibiotic to be given deep IM. Danielle says that she's a basketball player and on the varsity team at her high school. She says that she is always too embarrassed to change or take a shower in front of the other girls because she's so skinny. Danielle would like to have the injection in her arm because it would be too embarrassing to have it in the buttocks. ■

Intradermal Injections

An **intradermal injection** is given into the dermal layer of the skin, at an angle almost parallel to the skin (see Figure 26-12). Absorption is slow; only a small amount of medication may be injected (0.01 to 0.2 cc). The sites most often used for an intradermal injection are areas where the skin is thin, such as the anterior forearm and the middle of the back. The upper arm is also used to administer an intradermal injection.

The needle used is short, usually ³/₈ to ⁵/₈ inch long, and the lumen has a small diameter, usually 25 G to 27 G. A

tuberculin syringe is often used for administering the injection. The capacity of the syringe is small (1 cc), and the calibrations are divided into tenths and hundredths of a cubic centimeter. The fine calibrations allow a very small amount of medication to be administered, which is required with an intradermal injection. Procedure 26-7 outlines the technique for the administration of an intradermal injection.

The most frequent use of intradermal injections is to administer a skin test, such as an allergy test or a tuberculin test. The medication for the appropriate test is placed into the skin layers, and a small, raised area known as a **wheal** is produced at the injection site, owing to distention of the skin (Figure 26-16). At a time dictated by the type of test being administered, the results are read and interpreted. Most allergy tests can be read and interpreted at the medical office a short time (usually 15 to 20 minutes) after administration of the test, whereas tuberculin testing requires 48 hours before the results can be read.

The skin testing medication interacts with the body tissues; if no reaction occurs, the wheal disappears within a short time, and the only visible sign left is the puncture site. If a reaction to the skin test occurs, induration results, indicating a positive reaction. Erythema may also be present at the test site; however, for most skin tests, the extent of induration is the only criterion used to assess a positive reaction.

Figure 26-16. Intradermal injections are used to administer skin tests. Enough medication must be deposited in the skin layers to form a wheal. (From Bonewit-West K: *Clinical procedures for medical assistants,* ed 7, St. Louis, 2008, Saunders.)

TUBERCULIN TESTING

Tuberculosis

Tuberculosis (TB) is an infectious disease that usually attacks the lungs, although it can occur in almost any other part of the body, particularly the brain and kidneys. The causative agent of TB is the tubercle bacillus, *Mycobacterium tuberculosis,* which is a rod-shaped bacterium. Symptoms of active pulmonary TB include fatigue, weakness, unexplained weight loss, low-grade fever, night sweats, a cough that produces mucopurulent sputum, and occasional hemoptysis (coughing up blood) and chest pain.

TB is not a highly contagious disease, and many people who are infected with the tubercle bacillus do not develop the disease because their body defenses protect them. This protective mechanism involves building a fibrous wall around the TB organisms to encapsulate them. Some of the TB bacteria may remain alive inside the capsule in a dormant or inactive state. During this time, the patient experiences no symptoms and cannot spread the disease to others. The individual is said to have a *latent tuberculosis infection* and usually has a positive reaction to a tuberculin test.

Latent TB may develop into active TB shortly after infection or many years after infection. The TB bacteria break out of the capsule and cause the symptoms of active TB. This occurs in approximately 10% of individuals with latent TB infection. It is most apt to occur when the body defenses are weakened, such as during a serious illness, or in patients who have an immune disorder, such as acquired immunodeficiency syndrome (AIDS).

Purpose of Tuberculin Testing

The purpose of tuberculin testing is to detect the presence of a tuberculin infection. The tuberculin test is recommended for individuals who have close day-to-day contact with someone who has active TB, individuals who have symptoms of TB, and individuals with lowered immunity, such as patients infected with the human immunodefi-

ciency virus (HIV). The test is also recommended as a screening measure to assist in the early detection of unsuspected cases of TB before the patient becomes symptomatic. In this way, appropriate therapeutic measures can be instituted, leading to early treatment, which also helps prevent the spread of the disease. Tuberculin testing is usually part of a regular health screen, or it may be required as a prerequisite for employment, college entrance, or entrance into the military service.

The medical assistant is responsible for administering the tuberculin test and interpreting the test results. Although tuberculin testing is relatively easy to perform, the procedure must be followed exactly to ensure accurate results. A patient with a TB infection may fail to react to the test if it is not performed correctly.

Tuberculin Test Reactions

The substance used in the test is *tuberculin,* which consists of a purified protein derivative (PPD) extracted from a culture of tubercle bacilli (the causative agent of TB), to test for sensitivity to the microorganism. When introduced into the skin of an individual with an active or latent case of TB, tuberculin causes a localized thickening of the skin, resulting in induration. **Induration** is an abnormally hard spot caused by an accumulation of small, sensitized lymphocytes that occurs in the area in which the tuberculin was injected into the skin. Tuberculin test reactions are based on the amount of induration present and are interpreted according to the manufacturer's instructions that accompany the test.

A positive reaction to a tuberculin test indicates the presence of a tuberculous infection; however, it does not differentiate between the active and latent forms of the infection. A positive reaction warrants further diagnostic procedures before the physician can make a final diagnosis. Additional procedures used to detect an active tuberculous infection include a chest x-ray and microbiologic examination of the patient's sputum for tubercle bacilli.

Tuberculin Testing Methods

Two methods can be used for tuberculin testing: the *Mantoux* test and the *tine* test. The Mantoux test is the more common method used for tuberculin testing. The Mantoux test is administered using an intradermal needle and syringe. The Mantoux test is considered a more specific and accurate test because it uses a known amount of tuberculin to perform the test.

The tine test uses a sterile plastic unit containing four stainless-steel tines for puncturing the skin. The tines are approximately 2 mm long and are impregnated with tuberculin. The patient is inoculated intradermally to a depth of 1 to 2 mm by pressing the disc onto the skin, causing the tuberculin on the tines to be deposited into the skin layers. The amount of tuberculin injected into the patient's skin cannot be precisely controlled with the tine test, and it is rarely used at present. Because of this, the focus here is on the Mantoux test.

Highlight on Tuberculosis

Tuberculosis (TB) has made an unwelcome comeback in the United States among certain high-risk groups. Until more recently, public health officials considered TB a disease that had been conquered. Worldwide, 8 million people are infected with TB every year, and an estimated 3 million die from this disease annually. In addition, outbreaks of drug-resistant strains of TB have appeared in patients in hospitals, prisons, and community health clinics across the United States.

What Part of the Body Becomes Infected?

Although any part of the body can be infected, the TB organism prefers body tissues with high oxygen concentrations, such as the lungs. That is why approximately 85% of individuals with TB have *pulmonary tuberculosis.*

Is TB Contagious?

TB is not highly contagious, and prolonged contact with an infected individual is usually required before the disease develops. The natural defense mechanisms in the upper respiratory tract prevent most inhaled TB organisms from reaching the lungs.

Who Is at Risk for TB?

Individuals at greatest risk for contracting TB from infected patients are young children, whose immune systems are not fully developed; elderly individuals, whose immune systems are diminished; and individuals with immune deficiency diseases, such as AIDS. There also has been an increased incidence in long-term care environments, such as nursing homes and prisons, which are conducive to the transmission of TB.

Why Is the Mantoux Test the Preferred Method of Testing?

The tuberculin test is used to identify individuals infected with the TB organism. A positive reaction occurs 2 to 10 weeks after infection with TB. Most authorities believe that the Mantoux tuberculin test method is more specific and accurate than the tine test. The Mantoux test uses a known amount of tuberculin (0.10 ml of purified protein derivative) compared with the tine test, in which the tuberculin cannot be as precisely controlled. Because of this, authorities recommend that the tine test be used only for screening individuals at low risk for TB infection.

How Is TB Treated?

Active TB can be treated if it is diagnosed early. Antibiotics have been available since the 1940s to cure TB and help prevent its spread. Unless antibiotic drug resistance occurs, most patients are able to leave the hospital shortly after beginning drug therapy. Discharge does not mean that the patient is cured, however. Compared with most other infectious diseases, treatment for TB is lengthy, typically lasting 6 months to 1 year. After 2 to 4 weeks of drug therapy, the disease is no longer contagious, and the patient can resume a normal lifestyle. If the patient does not comply with the drug therapy regimen, however, some of the TB organisms will survive and the patient will be at risk for a recurrence of the disease. Many physicians recommend treating individuals with latent TB infection to prevent it from developing into active TB.

Is TB a Reportable Disease?

TB is a reportable disease; physicians must notify the local health department of cases of TB. The physician is also required to keep public health officials informed of the patient's compliance with the drug therapy regimen. To help prevent the spread of TB, public health officials conduct investigations to locate people who may have been infected by individuals known to have TB. ■

Mantoux Test

The Mantoux test is administered through an intradermal injection using a tuberculin syringe with a capacity of 1 ml and a short ($3/8$ to $1/2$ inch) needle with a gauge of 26 G to 27 G. The standard injected dose is 0.10 ml of PPD solution containing 5 TU (tuberculin units). Brand names for Mantoux tests include Tubersol and Aplisol.

It is important that the medical assistant draw up the proper amount of tuberculin solution. Injecting too much of the solution might elicit a reaction not caused by a tuberculous infection, and injecting too little of the solution results in insufficient solution being injected into the skin to elicit a reaction. This invalidates the test because if no reaction occurs, it cannot be accepted as a negative reaction.

The medical assistant must inject the solution into the superficial skin layers to form a wheal. If the injection is made into the subcutaneous layer, a wheal does not form, whereas a too-shallow injection may cause leakage of the tuberculin solution onto the skin. In either case, to prevent the possibility of a false-negative test result, the medical assistant must repeat the test at a site at least 2 inches away.

The medical assistant should not apply pressure to the site after injecting the solution because the solution is not intended to be absorbed into the tissues. In addition, applying pressure may cause leakage of the tuberculin solution through the needle puncture site. The wheal disappears on its own within a few minutes and should not be covered with an adhesive bandage.

Guidelines for Administering a Mantoux Test

1. Use the anterior forearm, approximately 4 inches below the bend in the elbow, as the site of administration of

the test. Avoid the following areas because they make the test harder to perform and interfere with good visualization and palpation of test reactions:

- Hairy areas of the skin
- Areas with visible veins
- Scar tissue
- Red or swollen areas
- Bruised areas
- Areas with dermatitis or other skin irritations

2. Cleanse the skin thoroughly with an antiseptic wipe, and allow it to dry completely before administering the test.

3. Inject the tuberculin into the superficial layers of the skin. If blood appears at the puncture site when the test has been administered, it is not significant and will not interfere with the test.

4. When the test has been administered, the results must be read within 48 to 72 hours.

Guidelines for Reading Mantoux Test Results

1. The test results must be read in good lighting within 48 to 72 hours.
2. Use inspection and palpation to read the test results.
3. If induration is present, rub your finger lightly from the area of normal skin (without induration) to the indurated area to assess its size. Measure the area of induration in millimeters.
4. The extent of induration present is the only criterion used to determine a positive reaction. If erythema is present without induration, the results are interpreted as negative.
5. The diameter of induration should be measured horizontally to the long axis of the forearm, and the results should be recorded in millimeters. Record all reactions in millimeters. If no induration is present, record 0 mm. Results should never be recorded as positive or negative.
6. The interpretation of the test results depends on the following:
   - Measurement (in millimeters) of the induration
   - The individual's risk of being infected with TB
   - The individual's risk of progression to disease if infected

Mantoux tuberculin test results are interpreted as follows:

1. **Positive reaction.** The following reactions might indicate tuberculous infection:
   - *Vesiculation* is the formation of vesicles, which are fluid-containing lesions of the skin. If vesiculation is present, the test is interpreted as strongly positive and warrants further diagnostic procedures to determine whether active TB is present.
   - *Induration of 10 mm or more* constitutes a positive reaction and warrants further diagnostic procedures to determine whether active TB is present.
   - *Induration of 5 mm* should be interpreted as a positive reaction for an individual who lives in close contact

with a person with infectious TB; an HIV-infected individual; and an individual at risk for HIV infection but whose HIV status is unknown.

2. **Doubtful reaction.** Induration measuring 5 to 9 mm means that retesting is recommended using a different site of injection.
3. **Negative reaction.** Induration of less than 5 mm constitutes a negative reaction.

The procedure for administering and reading a Mantoux test is presented in Procedure 26-7.

ALLERGY TESTING
Allergy

An **allergy** is an abnormal hypersensitivity of the body to substances that are ordinarily harmless; these substances are known as **allergens.** Allergens enter the body by being inhaled, being swallowed, being injected, or contact with the skin. Almost any substance in the environment can be an allergen. Some common allergens are plant pollens, molds, house dust, animal danders, feather pillows, dyes, soaps, detergents, cosmetics, certain foods and medications, and insect stings.

The exact cause of allergies is not fully understood. In many cases, the tendency to develop allergies seems to be inherited because children of allergic parents tend to exhibit more allergic symptoms than children of nonallergic parents. Although allergies can develop at any age, children are more apt to develop allergies than are older individuals.

Allergic Reaction

The first time an allergen enters the body of an allergic individual, it stimulates the body to produce antibodies to that allergen. These antibodies are usually of a type known as *IgE antibodies.* After the initial sensitization, allergic antibodies combine with the allergen in the body, resulting in an allergen-antibody reaction. When such a reaction occurs, histamine is released in significant amounts, causing allergic symptoms. Allergen-antibody reactions may involve any system of the body; however, they most frequently affect the respiratory and integumentary systems. Allergic symptoms can range from mild to very severe, as is the case with the potentially fatal anaphylactic reaction.

Depending on the allergen and the body system affected, allergies appear in different forms in an individual. Table 26-6 lists the common clinical forms and symptoms of allergies.

Diagnosis and Treatment

The best way to prevent allergic symptoms is to identify and avoid the offending allergen or allergens. The first and most important step in this process is the completion of a careful and detailed medical history by the physician. Of particular importance to the diagnosis of an allergy are the patient's home and work environments, diet, and living habits. The physician also performs a thorough physical examination to detect conditions resulting from aller-

Highlight on Allergens

House Dust

There are many components in house dust to which an individual may be allergic; the most significant of these is the house dust mite. Dust mites thrive in warm, humid conditions and feed on scales shed from human skin; they are often found in mattresses, carpets, stuffed animals, and upholstered furniture. An individual who is allergic to house dust reacts to the waste products of these dust mites.

There is no shortage of food for the dust mite because one person sheds up to 1 g of scales per day, which is enough to feed thousands of mites for months. *Dermatophagoides pteronyssinus* and *Dermatophagoides farinae* are the most common house dust mites and are present in varying numbers in virtually every home. Mites occur in greatest numbers in bedding, particularly in mattresses; there may be 5000 mites in each gram of dust from a mattress. Sufferers often notice that symptoms become much worse when the bedding is disturbed and allergenic material becomes airborne. Practices that eliminate dust also reduce the number of dust mites in a household.

Insect Stings

It is estimated that 1 of every 125 Americans is allergic to insect stings. Approximately 40 people in the United States die each year from a severe allergic reaction to insect stings. The incidence of deaths is low because most people know they need to obtain medical attention immediately if an allergic reaction begins.

Almost all insects whose venom can cause allergic reactions belong to the group Hymenoptera, which includes honeybees and bumblebees, wasps, yellow jackets, and hornets. When a honeybee stings, its stinger remains embedded in the victim's skin, causing the bee to die as it tries to tear itself away. Wasps, yellow jackets, and hornets are more aggressive than bees and can sting repeatedly. Hornets are the most aggressive of the group and may sting even when not provoked. Yellow jackets are close behind in aggressiveness, but wasps usually sting only if someone interferes with them near their nest.

If an insect sting does not cause an allergic reaction within 30 minutes, chances are excellent that no problem will occur. A normal reaction to an insect sting includes localized pain, redness, swelling, and itching lasting 1 to 2 days. Any generalized reaction not arising directly from the area of the sting is almost certain to be an anaphylactic reaction, which begins with such symptoms as sneezing, urticaria, itching, angioedema, erythema, and disorientation and progresses to difficulty in breathing, dizziness, faintness, and loss of consciousness. Medical care should be sought immediately because most fatalities occur within 2 hours following the sting. Because time is a factor, individuals who are known to have a severe allergy to insect stings are provided with an anaphylactic emergency treatment kit that contains epinephrine in a prefilled syringe and oral antihistamines. They can carry the kit with them so that treatment for a severe allergic reaction can be started as soon as possible.

Penicillin

Penicillin is a common cause of allergic drug reactions. Approximately 2% to 5% of individuals are allergic to penicillin. The reaction may be mild and completely overlooked or confused with the symptoms of the disease being treated with penicillin, or it can be more serious and take the form of severe dermatitis or an anaphylactic reaction. Death as a result of a severe anaphylactic reaction is rare, occurring only in 0.01% of patients being treated with penicillin.

Penicillin was discovered in 1929 by Sir Alexander Fleming, but it was not used as a therapeutic drug until 1940. By 1944, it was evident that some of the side effects of penicillin were allergic reactions; the first recorded death as a result of an anaphylactic reaction to penicillin occurred in 1945.

Oral administration of penicillin is safer than a penicillin injection because it has a lower frequency of severe allergic reactions. There have been only six reported deaths from oral administration of penicillin.

Approximately 95% of serious reactions occur within 1 hour after a penicillin injection. The best preventive measure is to keep the patient under direct observation for at least 30 minutes after administration of the injection. ■

---

gies, such as nasal polyps, wheezing, skin rashes, and urticaria.

When the medical history and physical examination have been completed, the physician may order diagnostic tests. Allergy testing is performed to confirm information obtained through the medical history and physical examination. The allergy tests ordered most often are direct skin testing and the radioallergosorbent assay (RAST) test, which are described in more detail in the following section. The general treatment of allergies includes avoiding of the allergen (if possible); alleviating of the symptoms through drug therapy, such as antihistamines, decongestants, bronchodilators, and inhaled steroids; and decreasing the sensitivity of the body to the allergen by the administration of allergy injections, or desensitization injections.

Types of Allergy Tests

The purpose of allergy testing is to determine the specific substances or allergens that are causing the patient's allergic symptoms. The two main categories of allergy tests are direct skin tests and the RAST test. The medical assistant is often responsible for performing direct skin testing in the medical office. The RAST test is performed by an outside laboratory on a blood specimen. The medical assistant may be responsible for performing a venipuncture to obtain the blood specimen.

Table 26-6 Clinical Forms of Allergies

Allergic rhinitis	Inflammation of mucous membrane of nose caused by allergies. Symptoms include nasal congestion, sneezing, and runny nose. An individual may have seasonal allergic rhinitis, meaning that nasal mucosa is inflamed only during certain seasons of the year, as typically occurs with hay fever. An individual may have perennial rhinitis, in which nasal mucosa is inflamed year-round. This type of allergic rhinitis is commonly caused by allergens that are always present in the environment, such as house dust and animal danders
Hay fever	Caused by allergy to molds or pollen of trees, grasses, or weeds. The term *hay fever* is misleading because hay fever is not caused by hay, and it does not result in fever. English physicians first used term *hay fever* in early 1800s when treating patients with allergies to grass pollens. Symptoms of hay fever and common cold are almost identical: episodes of sneezing, itching and watery eyes, runny and stuffy nose, and burning sensation of palate and throat. Hay fever is seasonal, occurring when there is pollen in the air. Depending on geographic location, hay fever may occur in spring, summer, or fall and last until first frost
Asthma	Condition characterized by wheezing, coughing, and dyspnea. During asthmatic attack, bronchioles constrict and become clogged with mucus, which accounts for many symptoms of asthma. Asthma can occur at any age but is more common in children and young adults and, if not treated, can lead to serious complications such as permanent lung damage. It is frequently, but not always, associated with family history of allergy. Any common allergen, such as house dust, pollens, molds, or animal danders, may trigger asthmatic attack. Asthmatic attacks also can be caused by nonspecific factors, such as air pollutants, tobacco smoke, chemical fumes, vigorous exercise, respiratory infections, exposure to cold, and emotional stress
Urticaria	Urticaria, or hives, is outbreak on skin of welts of varying sizes that are redder or paler than surrounding skin and are accompanied by intense itching. When swellings are large and invade deeper tissues, condition is known as *angioedema*. Hives may develop on face or lips or even internally. Allergies to food or drugs (especially penicillin and aspirin) and insect bites often cause hives, but they may also result from underlying disease or occur after exercise. In many cases, exact cause of urticaria cannot be determined
Contact dermatitis	Rash caused by direct contact with skin of allergen, such as cosmetics, perfumes, deodorants, rubber, plastics, and clothing treated with certain preservatives or dyes. Symptoms include swelling, blistering, oozing, and scaling. Rash usually occurs only on area of body that has been in contact with allergen. The most common causes of contact dermatitis are poison ivy, poison oak, and sumac
Eczema	Noncontagious rash accompanied by redness, itching, vesicles, oozing, crusting, and scaling. Eczema is common allergic reaction in children, but it may also occur in adults, usually in more severe form. Rash commonly appears on face, neck, and folds of elbows and knees. Eczema is frequently associated with allergies, and substances to which a person is allergic may aggravate it. Foods may be important factors, particularly milk, fish, or eggs. Allergens that are inhaled, such as dust and pollen, rarely cause eczema

From Bonewit-West K: *Clinical procedures for medical assistants*, ed 7, St. Louis, 2008, Saunders.

Direct Skin Testing

Direct skin testing involves applying extracts of common allergens to the skin and observing the body's reaction to them. The extract is applied either topically to the skin (patch testing) or into the superficial skin layers (skin-prick and intradermal testing). The advantage of direct skin testing is that test results are obtained immediately. This in vivo administration of allergens has the potential, however, to cause adverse reactions, the least common but most serious being an anaphylactic reaction. The medical assistant should have a thorough knowledge of the symptoms of an anaphylactic reaction and alert the physician immediately if the patient begins to exhibit them.

Regardless of the specific type of direct skin test (patch, skin-prick, or intradermal), some general guidelines should be followed:

1. Instruct the patient to discontinue the use of antihistamines for 3 days before the skin testing; otherwise, false-negative results may occur.
2. Verify that the area of application is free from hair, scar tissue, and dermatitis to permit good visualization and palpation of test reactions. Recommended sites include the anterior forearm, the upper arm, and the middle of the back. The back is usually used for patch and skin-prick testing, and the upper arm and forearm are typically used for intradermal skin testing.
3. Cleanse the area of application thoroughly with an antiseptic wipe, and allow it to dry completely.
4. Wear gloves when the allergy testing involves puncture of the skin, which includes skin-prick testing and intradermal skin testing. Gloves protect the medical assistant from exposure to bloodborne pathogens, as required by the OSHA standard.
5. Space the allergen extracts at least 1 inch apart to provide enough surface area for a sizable reaction. If not enough surface area is available, large adjacent reactions may run together, making it difficult to read test results.
6. Label the test sites so that the application site of each allergen extract can be identified later when reading results.
7. Make the patient aware that the skin testing may cause a mild allergic reaction, such as a runny nose, sneezing,

and mild wheezing 8 to 24 hours after skin-prick and intradermal skin testing. Instruct the patient to contact the physician if a more severe reaction than this occurs.

Types of Direct Skin Tests

Patch Testing

Patch testing is primarily used to identify allergens that cause contact dermatitis. Patch testing involves the topical application of each allergen to the skin, using a "patch." A patch consists of a small piece of gauze or filter paper impregnated with the allergen, which is applied to the skin and taped in place with hypoallergenic tape (Figure 26-17). Allergens commonly applied include plants, topical drugs, resins, metals, cosmetics, dyes, and chemicals. The patient should be instructed to leave the patches in place, keep them dry, and return to the medical office in 48 hours to have the results read. When the patient returns to the office, the patches are carefully removed and the results are read 20 minutes later. The delayed reading time allows lessening of redness that may occur from the tape removal.

Test results are recorded as positive or negative. Positive reactions are characterized by itching, erythema, and induration, often accompanied by vesiculation. In strongly positive responses, the reaction may extend beyond the margin of the patch. Positive results are graded further on a quantitative 1+ to 3+ scoring system according to the type of reaction (Table 26-7).

Skin-Prick Testing

Skin-prick testing is usually performed to diagnose allergies to common allergens, particularly those that are inhaled, such as house dust, pollens, and molds. Skin-prick testing involves the application of numerous allergen extracts to the skin, followed by the pricking of each with a sterile needle or other sharp instrument (Figure 26-18). The number of allergen extracts applied during one office visit usually ranges between 20 and 30. Pricking the skin deposits the allergens in the outer layers of the skin to allow each to react with the body tissues.

The following guidelines should be followed for skin-prick testing: The extracts should be placed on the skin in rows in a specific pattern. This, along with labeling the test sites with a felt-tipped pen, tracks the location of each extract. Only a single drop of extract should be placed on the skin; more than this amount may cause the extracts to diffuse and run together. A sterile needle should be passed

Table 26-7 Guidelines for Recording Direct Skin Test Results	
Patch Test	
−	No reaction
+1	Presence of erythema and edema, possibly papules
+2	Presence of erythema, edema, and vesicles, possibly papules
+3	Erythema, vesicles, and severe edema
Skin-Prick Testing and Intradermal Testing	
−	No reaction
±1	Induration 1 mm or less
+1	Induration greater than 1 mm and up to 5 mm in diameter
+2	Induration greater than 5 mm and up to 10 mm in diameter
+3	Induration greater than 10 mm and up to 15 mm in diameter
+4	Induration greater than 15 mm in diameter

From Bonewit-West K: *Clinical procedures for medical assistants*, ed 7, St. Louis, 2008, Saunders.

Figure 26-17. Patch testing. A patch consists of a small piece of gauze or filter paper impregnated with the allergen, which is applied to the skin and taped in place. (From Bonewit-West K: *Clinical procedures for medical assistants,* ed 7, St. Louis, 2008, Saunders.)

Figure 26-18. Skin-prick testing. Skin-prick testing involves the application of numerous allergen extracts to the skin, followed by the pricking of each with a sterile needle. (From Bonewit-West K: *Clinical procedures for medical assistants,* ed 7, St. Louis, 2008, Saunders.)

through the drop, and the point should lightly lift the top layer of skin without causing bleeding. It is important to wipe the needle dry with a sterile swab between each prick to prevent one extract from mixing with the next, leading to inaccurate test results.

The maximum reaction is usually seen in 15 to 20 minutes. During this time, the test sites should be left uncovered, and the patient should be instructed not to touch them. The area should not be wiped because this removes the allergen extract, resulting in false-negative results. The results are read (after 15 to 20 minutes) using a millimeter ruler.

An area of induration surrounded by redness and itching characterizes a positive reaction. Positive results are recorded by measuring the size of the induration in millimeters and converting it to a numeric scale based on the extent of the induration (see Table 26-7). Any redness should be ignored. See Figure 26-20 for an illustration of skin test results. If only a mild reaction occurs, the physician may perform more specific intradermal skin testing.

Intradermal Skin Testing

Intradermal skin testing is similar to skin-prick testing, but it is more specific. The number of skin tests performed during one office visit ranges from 5 to 30. Because there is a greater chance of adverse allergic reactions to intradermal skin testing, the physician often starts with skin-prick testing in individuals who are suspected of being highly allergic as determined by the medical history and the results of the physical examination.

Intradermal skin testing involves the injection of a small amount (0.02 to 0.05 ml) of allergen extract into the superficial skin layers through the intradermal route of administration (Figure 26-19). A tuberculin syringe is used to administer the test, and the allergen extract is injected until a wheal forms (see Procedure 26-7). After 15 to 20 minutes, the test sites are observed for reactions. Positive reactions are characterized by an area of induration surrounded by redness and itching. As with skin-prick testing, positive results are recorded by measuring the size of the induration in millimeters and converting it to a numeric scale based

on the amount of induration present (Figure 26-20; see Table 26-7).

RAST Testing

The RAST measures the amount of IgE antibodies in the blood to common allergens. A sample of the patient's blood is sent to an outside laboratory, where it is exposed to radioactively tagged allergens. A radiation detection device is used to measure the amount of IgE antibodies to the allergens. The advantages of the RAST test over direct skin testing are as follows: The results are not affected by medications (e.g., antihistamines); there is no danger of adverse allergic reactions because the test is performed in vitro, meaning outside the body; and RAST testing can be performed on patients who have skin eruptions and are unable to undergo direct skin testing because of a lack of an intact skin surface area. RAST testing is expensive, however, and does not provide immediate test results, which are available with direct skin testing.

Figure 26-19. Intradermal skin testing. Intradermal testing involves the injection of a small amount of allergen extract into the superficial skin layers through the intradermal route of administration. (From Bonewit-West K: *Clinical procedures for medical assistants*, ed 7, St. Louis, 2008, Saunders.)

NEG   ±1   +1   +2   +3   +4

Figure 26-20. Skin-prick and intradermal skin test results. (Copyright and courtesy Hollister-Stier, Spokane, Wash.)

PROCEDURE 26-7 Administering an Intradermal Injection

Outcome Administer an intradermal injection, and read the test results.

Equipment/Supplies

- Medication ordered by the physician
- Appropriate needle and syringe
- Antiseptic wipe
- Sterile 2 × 2 gauze pad
- Disposable gloves
- Biohazard sharps container

1. **Procedural Step.** Sanitize your hands, and prepare the injection.

2. **Procedural Step.** Greet the patient and introduce yourself. Identify the patient by full name and date of birth and explain the procedure.
   Principle. It is crucial that no error be made in patient identity. Explain the purpose of the injection to reassure an apprehensive patient.

3. **Procedural Step.** Select an appropriate injection site. The anterior forearm and the middle of the back are recommended sites for an intradermal injection.
   Principle. The entire area should be exposed to ensure a safe and comfortable injection.

4. **Procedural Step.** Prepare the injection site. Cleanse the area with an antiseptic wipe. Using a circular motion, start with the injection site, and move outward. Do not touch the site after cleansing it.
   Principle. Using a circular motion carries material away from the injection site. Touching the site after cleansing contaminates it, and the cleansing process needs to be repeated.

5. **Procedural Step.** Allow the area to dry completely.
   Principle. If the area is not permitted to dry, the antiseptic may enter the tissue when the skin is pierced, resulting in irritation and patient discomfort. In addition, the antiseptic may cause a reaction that could be mistaken for a positive test response.

6. **Procedural Step.** Apply gloves, and remove the needle guard. With the nondominant hand, stretch the skin taut at the proposed site of administration. Insert the needle at a 10- to 15-degree angle (almost parallel to

the skin), with the bevel upward. The needle should be inserted about ⅛ inch until the bevel of the needle just penetrates the skin. Slight resistance may be felt as the needle is inserted. No aspiration is necessary.
   Principle. Gloves provide a barrier against bloodborne pathogens. Stretching the patient's skin taut permits easier insertion of the needle. The needle should be inserted at an angle almost parallel to the skin, to ensure penetration within the dermal layer of the skin. The needle must be inserted with the bevel facing up to allow proper wheal formation. If the needle is inserted with the bevel facing down, the medication is absorbed into the underlying tissues and a wheal does not form.

7. **Procedural Step.** Hold the syringe steady, and inject the medication slowly and steadily by depressing the plunger until a firm, tense, white wheal forms (approximately 6 to 10 mm in diameter). Expect to feel a certain amount of resistance as you inject the medication; this helps in indicating that the needle is properly located in the superficial skin layers rather than in the deeper subcutaneous tissue. If a wheal does not form, repeat the test at a site at least 2 inches away from the first test site.
   Principle. Moving the syringe after the needle has entered the skin causes patient discomfort. Test results are considered reliable only if a wheal forms.

Inject the medication to form a wheal. (From Bonewit-West K: *Clinical procedures for medical assistants*, ed 7, St. Louis, 2008, Saunders.)

8. **Procedural Step.** Place the antiseptic wipe or gauze pad gently over the injection site, and remove the

Insert the needle at a 10- to 15-degree angle with the bevel upward. (From Bonewit-West K: *Clinical procedures for medical assistants*, ed 7, St. Louis, 2008, Saunders.)

Continued

PROCEDURE 26-7 **Administering an Intradermal Injection—cont'd**

needle quickly and at the same angle as for insertion.

Principle. Withdrawing the needle quickly and at the angle of insertion reduces patient discomfort. The antiseptic wipe or gauze pad placed over the injection site helps prevent tissue movement as the needle is withdrawn, also reducing patient discomfort.

9. **Procedural Step.** Do not apply pressure to the injection site. If you are using a safety syringe with a shield, activate the safety feature at this time following the steps outlined in Figure 26-7.

Principle. Applying pressure may cause leakage of the testing solution through the needle puncture site, resulting in inaccurate test results.

10. **Procedural Step.** Properly dispose of the needle and syringe in a biohazard sharps container.

Principle. Proper disposal of the needle and syringe is required by the OSHA standard to prevent accidental needlestick injuries.

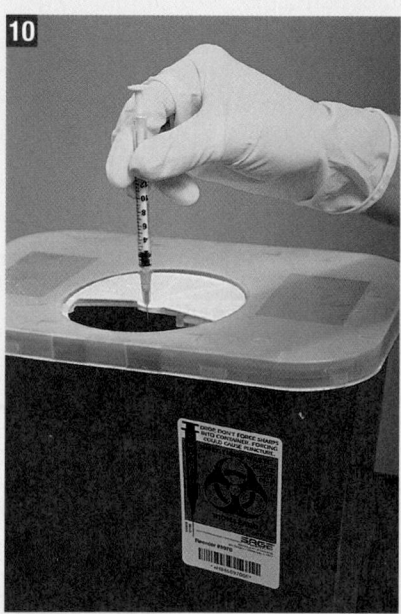

Properly dispose of the needle and syringe. (From Bonewit-West K: *Clinical procedures for medical assistants,* ed 7, St. Louis, 2008, Saunders.)

11. **Procedural Step.** Remove gloves, and sanitize your hands.
12. **Procedural Step.** Stay with the patient to ensure that he or she is not experiencing any unusual reactions. The medical assistant should be especially careful and alert for any sign of a patient reaction when administering allergy skin tests. If the patient experiences an unusual reaction, notify the physician immediately.
13. **Procedural Step.** Perform one of the following, based on the type of skin test being administered:

Allergy Skin Tests

a. Read the test results within 20 to 30 minutes, using inspection and palpation at the site of the injection to assess the presence of and to determine the amount of induration. Interpret the skin test results according to the information outlined in Table 26-7.

b. Chart the procedure. Include the date and time, the injection site used, the names of the skin tests, the skin test results, and any significant observations or patient reactions.

CHARTING EXAMPLE	
Date	
2/15/10	Allergy skin tests, ID, Ⓡ ant forearm.
	Results: House dust +2
	Cat dander +4
	Dog dander –
	Ragweed +4
	Mixed fungi +3
	———————— T. Cline, CMA (AAMA)

Mantoux Tuberculin Test

a. Instruct the patient in the care of the test site as follows:

- Continue your normal daily personal hygiene activities, such as showering or bathing.
- Do not cover the test site with a Band-Aid.
- Avoid the use of ointments, lotions, and sunscreens.
- Do not touch, scratch, press on, or rub the test site. This could alter the test results. If the test site itches, apply a cold compress to the area.
- Pat the arm dry after washing it. Do not rub it dry.
- If blisters occur, do not break them.

b. Inform the patient of the date and time to return to the medical office to have the results read. Results must be read within 48 to 72 hours after the test has been administered. Stress the importance of returning to the office to have the results read, even if the test site does not exhibit a reaction. Failure to return warrants having to repeat the test.

c. Chart the procedure. Include the date and time, the name of the medication, the dosage given, the manufacturer and lot number, the route of administration, the injection site used, and any significant observations or patient reactions.

Principle. The lot number indicates the batch in which the medication was made. Should a problem arise with that batch, the drug can be recalled, and individuals who received it can be identified.

CHARTING EXAMPLE

Date	
2/15/10	10:00 a.m. Tubersol Mantoux test 5 TU,
	0.10 ml, ID. Connaught Laboratories,
	Lot #: C0832AA. Admin Ⓡ ant forearm.
	Pt to return on 2/17/10 to have results
	read. —————— T. Cline, CMA (AAMA)

Reading Mantoux Test Results

Equipment/Supplies

- Millimeter ruler
- Disposable gloves
- Tuberculin test record card

1. **Procedural Step.** Greet the patient and introduce yourself. Identify the patient by full name and date of birth and explain the procedure.
2. **Procedural Step.** Work in a quiet, well-lit atmosphere. Check the patient's chart to determine which arm was used to administer the test.
3. **Procedural Step.** Sanitize your hands, and apply gloves.
4. **Procedural Step.** Ask the patient to flex the arm at the elbow.
5. **Procedural Step.** Locate the application site. The result should be read horizontally to the long axis of the forearm, meaning "across" the forearm.
6. **Procedural Step.** Gently rub your finger over the test site, and lightly palpate for the presence of induration. If induration is present, the area should be lightly rubbed from the area of normal skin (without induration) to the indurated area to assess the size of the area of induration.

   Principle. Induration is the only criterion used in determining a positive reaction. If erythema is present without induration, the results are interpreted as negative.

Lightly palpate for induration. (From Bonewit-West K: *Clinical procedures for medical assistants,* ed 7, St. Louis, 2008, Saunders.)

7. **Procedural Step.** Measure the diameter of the induration with a flexible millimeter ruler (supplied by the

manufacturer). The results of the Mantoux test are interpreted as follows:

Positive Reaction: Vesiculation or induration 10 mm or more.
Doubtful Reaction: Induration 5 to 9 mm.
Negative Reaction: Induration less than 5 mm.

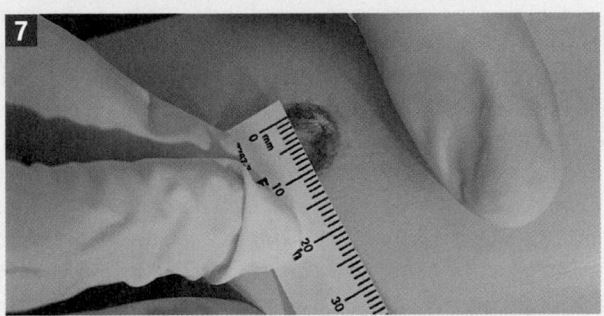

Measure the induration. (From Bonewit-West K: *Clinical procedures for medical assistants,* ed 7, St. Louis, 2008, Saunders.)

8. **Procedural Step.** Remove gloves, and sanitize your hands.
9. **Procedural Step.** Chart the results. Include the date and time, the name of the test (Mantoux), and the test results (recorded in millimeters). If no induration is present, 0 mm should be recorded.
10. **Procedural Step.** Complete a tuberculin test record card, and give it to the patient.

    Principle. The record card provides the patient with a permanent record of the test results.

TUBERCULOSIS TEST RECORD

Name		Date Admin:	2/15/10
Carrie Fee		Date Read:	2/17/10

MANTOUX TEST	RESULT		
	Negative	Doubtful	Positive
Tubersol, 5 TU	___ mm	_9_ mm	___ mm

Logan Family Practice
401 St. George St.
St. Augustine, FL 32084
(904) 555-3933

Performed by *T. Cline, CMA (AAMA)*

(From Bonewit-West K: *Clinical procedures for medical assistants,* ed 7, St. Louis, 2008, Saunders.)

CHARTING EXAMPLE

Date	
2/17/10	3:00 p.m. Tubersol Mantoux test: 9mm.
	Pt provided c̄ TB record card. Scheduled
	for TB retesting on 2/28/10. ————
	—————— T. Cline, CMA (AAMA)

[Handwritten margin notes:] Drug Dose Time Patient Route Technic

INTRAVENOUS THERAPY

Intravenous (IV) therapy is the administration of a liquid agent directly into a patient's vein, where it is distributed throughout the body by way of the circulatory system (Figure 26-21). The veins most commonly used for IV therapy are the peripheral veins of the arm and hand. The liquid agent may consist of basic fluids, medication, nutrients, blood, or blood products. When fluids, medications, or nutrients are administered through the IV route, the technique is called an **infusion.** When whole blood or blood products are administered through the IV route, the procedure is called a **transfusion.**

Most IV therapy occurs in a hospital setting on an inpatient and outpatient basis. IV therapy is also administered in outpatient ambulatory settings, such as medical offices and clinics, urgent care centers, ambulatory infusion clinics, and the patient's home (Figure 26-22).

Advantages of Outpatient Intravenous Therapy

Administration of IV therapy in an outpatient setting is growing in acceptance by patients and the medical community. Outpatient IV therapy is more convenient for the patient and reduces medical costs through earlier discharge from the hospital or by avoiding hospitalization altogether.

Earlier Hospital Discharge

When a hospitalized patient is receiving IV therapy and requires continued therapy, it is not always necessary or cost effective to keep the patient in the hospital. If the patient is medically stable, he or she may no longer need the careful observation and daily nursing care provided by a hospital. By receiving IV therapy in an outpatient setting, the patient can be discharged earlier. Most patients, particularly children, are more comfortable in their home environment, which often contributes to faster healing. An example of this is a hospitalized patient with an infection who still needs IV antibiotic therapy, but no longer needs

to be hospitalized, and receives the therapy at an infusion clinic.

Avoidance of Hospitalization

Outpatient IV therapy provides an alternative to patients with an acute or chronic illness that requires IV therapy. Patients who do not require hospitalization for their condition can obtain their IV therapy in an outpatient setting. This allows patients the option of being able to continue their daily routine without major interruptions and provides them with more independence and control over their condition. An example of this is a patient with rheumatoid arthritis who needs IV infliximab (Remicade) therapy and receives that therapy at the rheumatology medical office.

Medical Office–Based Intravenous Therapy

Some medical offices provide outpatient IV therapy. Outpatient IV therapy may be provided in an oncology office for the administration of IV chemotherapy. With the advent of newer rheumatology medications that must be given intravenously, some rheumatology offices have started to provide this service. Medical office–based IV therapy has distinct advantages. It allows the physician to provide closer monitoring of a patient's response to the IV therapy and any adverse reactions exhibited by the patient. These benefits have prompted more physicians to consider office-based IV therapy.

Based on the potential future growth of IV therapy in the medical office and the current growth of other IV outpatient settings, such as infusion clinics and the patient's home, there is a need for medical assistants to acquire some basic knowledge in IV therapy. The medical assistant is often responsible for scheduling IV therapy and providing the patient with IV therapy instructions, such as the length of time required for the therapy. In addition, patients may have questions that the medical assistant may need to answer (or refer to the proper individual for answering) regarding their outpatient IV therapy. The entry-level medical

Figure 26-21. Intravenous therapy. (From Potter PA, Perry AG: *Basic nursing: essentials for practice,* ed 5, St. Louis, 2002, Mosby.)

Figure 26-22. Patient receiving intravenous therapy in an outpatient setting. (Photo by Margaret Hartshorn: Courtesy Arizona Arthritis Center [www.arthritis.arizona.edu].)

assistant should be familiar with the basic theory of outpatient IV therapy, which is presented here.

Advanced IV theory and initiating, maintaining, and discontinuing IV therapy are not entry-level medical assisting competencies and are not addressed in this text. Certain requirements must be met before the medical assistant can perform IV therapy in the medical office. The medical assistant should first check the laws of his or her state to determine whether it is legally permissible for the medical assistant to perform this procedure. The medical assistant must acquire the proper training (theory and skills) by completing a recognized IV therapy training program including supervised clinical practice. Although the IV procedure can appear simple when performed by an expert, it is a difficult skill that requires considerable practice to perfect.

Indications for Outpatient Intravenous Therapy

Outpatient IV therapy has been shown to be a safe and effective alternative to inpatient IV therapy for the treatment of certain conditions. Before prescribing outpatient IV therapy, the physician assesses the need for the therapy by determining whether the following criteria are met: The patient's condition warrants the use of IV therapy, no alternative routes are feasible or appropriate to deliver the therapy, and the patient does not need to be hospitalized to receive the IV therapy. After determining the need for outpatient IV therapy, the physician prescribes the appropriate medication or fluid and treatment plan, orders laboratory tests to monitor the patient's progress, and assesses the patient after the IV therapy.

Scheduling the IV Therapy

If the patient receives the IV therapy at an outpatient site other than the medical office (e.g., an infusion clinic), the medical assistant may be responsible for scheduling the necessary services and providing the patient with IV therapy instructions, such as the length of time required for the therapy, any dietary restrictions, whether to wear loose-fitting comfortable clothing, and whether someone needs to transport the patient to and from the appointment.

Medical Office Guidelines

Medical offices that provide IV therapy on-site usually set up a special room to deliver the therapy, which often includes a lounge chair to provide for patient comfort during the therapy. With office-based IV therapy, the entry-level medical assistant is responsible for scheduling the IV therapy and providing the patient with the IV therapy instructions listed previously. The medical office employs an IV practitioner, such as a nurse or specially trained medical assistant, to initiate, maintain, and discontinue the IV therapy. This practitioner must be completely familiar with all aspects of the IV therapy, including indications and uses, actions, dose and rate of infusion, incompatibilities, contraindications and precautions, antidote, and adverse effects. During the IV therapy, the practitioner must monitor carefully the patient's response to the therapy and be alert for adverse or allergic reactions. After the therapy is completed, the IV practitioner provides the patient with follow-up instructions, such as normal side effects that may occur when the patient returns home and any adverse reactions that need to be reported to the medical office.

Administration of IV Therapy

IV therapy may be administered in an outpatient setting for a variety of reasons. These include the following, which are discussed in more detail in the next section:
- Administration of IV medication
- Replacement of fluids and electrolytes
- Administration of nutritional supplements
- Administration of blood products
- Emergency administration of IV medication and fluids

Administration of Intravenous Medication

IV medication administration is the process of delivering medication directly into a patient's vein. The IV route provides a rapid and effective method for administering medication to a patient. It also provides more accurate dosing than other routes because the medication enters the body directly from the circulatory system. This allows the medication to bypass barriers to drug absorption, such as the digestive tract (from oral administration) or muscle tissue (from IM administration), which makes it easier to control the actual amount of drug delivered to the body.

Medication may have to be administered through the IV route, as opposed to other, less invasive routes, such as oral administration, for many reasons, including the following:
- A rapid systemic response to the medication is desired.
- Therapeutic blood levels of the medication need to be maintained.
- The medication is destroyed by stomach acids, digestive enzymes, or both.
- The medication cannot be absorbed into the body through the gastrointestinal tract.
- The medication is toxic and could damage the lining of the gastrointestinal tract.
- The medication is painful or irritating when given by other parenteral routes (IM or SC injection).

Intravenous Administration Methods

IV medication can be administered by three methods: direct IV injection, intermittent IV administration, and continuous IV administration.

Direct Intravenous Injection

The direct IV injection method (known as an *IV push*) involves the administration of the medication as a single dose into the vein over a short time, usually less than 10 minutes. It is usually administered through a vascular access device that is already in place. Medication administered through this method produces immediate and predictable results and is a good way to administer lifesaving medications in an emergency.

Intermittent Intravenous Administration

Intermittent IV administration is employed frequently in outpatient settings. It involves the administration of a medication over a specific amount of time (termed the *rate of infusion*) and at specified intervals. Before administering, the medication first must be diluted in a moderate amount of an IV fluid (25 to 250 ml). The amount and type of IV fluid are indicated in the drug insert accompanying the medication. The intermittent IV administration of ceftriaxone (Rocephin) (an antibiotic) requires that it first be reconstituted and then diluted in 50 to 100 ml of an IV fluid, such as sterile water or 0.9% sodium chloride.

The rate of infusion for administering an IV medication intermittently depends on the medication being administered and typically ranges from 15 minutes to several hours. This information is also specified in the drug insert accompanying the medication. The recommended rate for the intermittent infusion of ceftriaxone is 15 to 30 minutes. The recommended rate of infusion for IV infliximab is at least 2 hours.

The interval of time between doses is determined by the physician and depends on the medication being administered and the patient's condition. The physician may prescribe the following outpatient treatment plan for a patient with Lyme disease: IV ceftriaxone intermittently once a day for 14 days. In this instance, the interval of time between doses is 24 hours, or 1 day.

Continuous Intravenous Administration

Continuous IV administration, also known as an *IV drip,* is most often used in a hospital or home setting. It involves the infusion of medication over a continuous period of time (4 to 24 hours). Continuous IV administration is used to maintain a constant therapeutic blood level of the medication. The medication is diluted in a large quantity (250 to 1000 ml) of an IV fluid (Figure 26-23), such as 0.9%

Figure 26-23. Intravenous fluid bags. (From Bonewit-West K: *Clinical procedures for medical assistants,* ed 7, St. Louis, 2008, Saunders.)

sodium chloride (normal saline) or 5% dextrose in water (D5W). Because of the time required for continuous administration, this method of administration is not generally used to administer IV medications in the medical office.

Intravenous Medications Administered in an Outpatient Setting

Medications that are most commonly administered intravenously in an outpatient setting are listed next, along with the conditions each is used to treat.

Antibiotics

The physician may prescribe IV antibiotic therapy to treat a serious infection to prevent the infection from spreading and to avoid the development of serious complications. The IV route allows the antibiotic to achieve high blood concentrations quickly, permitting it to go to work on the infection immediately.

Examples of infections for which the physician may prescribe IV antibiotic therapy in an outpatient setting include osteomyelitis, cellulitis endocarditis, bacterial meningitis, Lyme disease, bacterial pneumonia, bacterial septicemia, pyelonephritis, pelvic inflammatory disease, AIDS-related infections, severe urinary tract infections, and nonhealing wound infections.

Chemotherapy

Chemotherapy is broadly defined as the use of chemicals to treat disease. More specifically, chemotherapy refers to the use of antineoplastic medications to treat different types of cancer. In most cases, chemotherapy works by interfering with the ability of the cancer cells to grow or reproduce. The IV route is commonly used to administer chemotherapy because most antineoplastic medications are toxic and irritating and must be delivered to the body through a vein. These types of medications cause pain and trauma to the tissues if administered by other parenteral routes (i.e., IM, SC).

IV chemotherapy may take only a few minutes to administer or several hours and may be given on a daily, weekly, or monthly basis. The frequency and length of the chemotherapy treatment depend on the type of cancer being treated, the medications that are being administered, and the patient's overall health and ability to tolerate the medications. IV chemotherapy is often administered in an outpatient setting, such as a medical oncology office or an infusion clinic.

Monoclonal Antibodies

One use of monoclonal antibodies is to treat inflammatory diseases; infliximab (Remicade) is a monoclonal antibody. Individuals with certain inflammatory disease have too much of a normally occurring protein (tumor necrosis factor [TNF]) in their bodies. TNF causes inflammation in the body, but in too large amounts, it attacks healthy tissues. Infliximab works by binding with TNF and blocking its action, reducing the inflammatory response of the body. In doing so, however, infliximab also lowers the ability of the body to fight infection.

IV infliximab therapy is often administered in an outpatient setting for treatment of the following conditions: Crohn's disease, rheumatoid arthritis, ulcerative colitis, ankylosing spondylitis, and psoriatic arthritis. Infliximab works to reduce the symptoms of the patient's condition and to initiate and maintain remission of the disorder. Infliximab has some undesirable side effects and is very expensive, so it is administered only when patients with these conditions have had an inadequate response to conventional therapy.

Analgesics

When a patient cannot manage pain using oral pain medication, the physician may prescribe a narcotic pain medication administered through the IV route. Conditions for which the physician may prescribe IV analgesic therapy in an outpatient setting include migraine headaches, cancer-related pain, and the pain associated with AIDS conditions.

Some patients receive IV narcotic analgesics at home through the use of an ambulatory IV pump (Figure 26-24) that is controlled by the patient. This type of IV analgesic therapy is known as *patient-controlled analgesia* (PCA). When the patient experiences pain, he or she presses a button attached to the PCA pump. The PCA pump is programmed to deliver a predetermined dose of the

Figure 26-24. Patient-controlled analgesia pump. (From Elkin MK, Perry AG, Potter PA: *Nursing interventions and clinical skills,* ed 3, St. Louis, 2004, Mosby.)

narcotic analgesic intravenously to the patient to relieve the pain. The pump is preset to prevent overmedication, and it includes a locking device for security of the medication.

Replacement of Fluids and Electrolytes

To remain healthy, the body must maintain an adequate fluid and electrolyte balance. This balance can be altered by a variety of conditions. Conditions that may cause a depletion of fluids and electrolytes include vomiting and diarrhea, excessive perspiration (from fever or hot weather), and starvation. If an individual experiences an excessive loss of fluids or electrolytes, he or she must recover the loss as soon as possible to prevent dehydration. Infants and children are especially vulnerable to dehydration.

The best way to replace fluids and electrolytes is through oral consumption; however, this may not always be possible, such as when the patient is experiencing excessive vomiting. In these instances, IV fluid therapy may be prescribed. The physician determines the specific IV fluid and amount of fluid to treat the patient's condition using the following information:

- Patient's diagnosis (e.g., prolonged diarrhea)
- Other coexisting medical conditions
- Length of the current illness
- Patient's body size and weight
- Physician's findings from the physical examination
- Laboratory test results

Examples of IV fluids commonly used to replace fluids and electrolytes include 0.9% sodium chloride (see Figure 26-23) and Ringer's solution. IV fluids are administered by continuous administration in the following outpatient settings: urgent care centers, infusion clinics, and the patient's home. Because of the length of time required for continuous administration, the medical office does not typically administer IV fluids and electrolytes except in an emergency situation (see later).

Administration of Nutritional Supplements

IV therapy can be used to administer nutritional supplements to patients in an outpatient setting who are unable to eat or have conditions causing poor absorption of nutrients from the gastrointestinal tract. IV nutritional therapy provides the nutrients necessary for basic health maintenance and to promote healing. The IV route is used only when the patient has a condition that prevents other routes of administration, such as the oral or enteral routes. **Enteral nutrition** is the delivery of nutrients through a tube inserted into the gastrointestinal tract.

Examples of specific conditions that may require the IV administration of nutritional supplements include ulcerative colitis, Crohn's disease, short bowel syndrome, celiac disease, pancreatitis, esophageal cancer, AIDS-related malnutrition, and malnutrition related to an eating disorder. Parenteral IV nutrition is often administered in the following outpatient settings: infusion clinics and the patient's home.

Administration of Blood Products

Blood products can be administered to a patient in an out-patient setting. The most frequently administered blood products are discussed next.

Immune Globulin

Immune globulin consists of antibodies that must be given through the IV route of administration. Immune globulin is obtained from pooled human plasma that has been tested and found to be safe and free of bloodborne pathogens, such as HIV and the hepatitis viruses.

Intravenous immune globulin (IVIG) therapy is used to treat patients with immune deficiencies who are unable to produce their own antibodies, such as chronic inflammatory demyelinating polyneuropathy. It is also used in the treatment of a variety of autoimmune diseases, such as multiple sclerosis, myasthenia gravis, and lupus erythematosus. An **autoimmune disease** is a condition in which, for some unknown reason, the body's immune system attacks the body's own cells.

The IVIG dose is based on the patient's weight, and the medication is infused slowly over many hours. The number and frequency of treatments depend on the patient's condition. Patients who cannot produce their own antibodies usually receive an IVIG treatment once a month, whereas patients with autoimmune diseases may require a treatment only when there is a flare-up of their condition to boost their immune system.

Hemophilia Factors

Hemophilia is an inherited bleeding disorder characterized by a deficiency of a clotting factor needed for proper coagulation of the blood. Without this factor, a hemophiliac may bleed spontaneously or after trauma to any tissues or organs of the body. The most common sites of bleeds are joints and muscles. The missing blood clotting factor must be periodically administered intravenously to an individual with hemophilia. If treatment is delayed, it can lead to irreversible damage to the affected tissues and even death. Many patients with hemophilia receive their intravenous clotting factors at home, making it more convenient and easier for them to manage their condition.

Emergency Administration of Intravenous Medication and Fluids

Having the capability to initiate an IV line is important in an emergency situation. It provides an access route for the IV administration of lifesaving medications and fluids. Emergency situations sometimes arise in the medical office. While waiting for the emergency medical services to transport the patient to the hospital, an IV line may be established to administer medication and fluids to the patient as soon as possible. Situations occurring in the medical office that may benefit from establishing IV access include myocardial infarction, stroke, anaphylactic reaction, diabetic emergencies, and heat-related injuries such as heatstroke.

MEDICAL PRACTICE *and the* LAW

Medications have the potential to do great good and great harm. Many lawsuits are medication related, so the medical assistant has a tremendous responsibility to follow all procedures to avoid doing harm.

Many patients are prescribed multiple medications from various physicians. When performing a medication evaluation, ask the patient to bring in all medications he or she is currently taking. Include over-the-counter medications such as aspirin, vitamins, and herbal products.

When administering medications, first check a current medication reference to determine potential adverse effects. See the *Physician's Desk Reference* or package insert for this information. This information may also be available on a computer program. Next, check for patient allergies. Check the chart, and then ask the patient about allergies before administering the medication. Be sure the patient knows why the drug is being given, its name, and common side effects. Watch the patient take the drug if given orally. If given parenterally, use proper technique to prevent injury. Follow the seven "rights" of medication administration, and check the medication label three times before administering any medication. This all may seem cumbersome, but if any steps are omitted and the patient has a serious adverse reaction, you could be held liable.

Controlled drugs have specific laws that regulate their ordering, storing, and dispensing. Failure to adhere to these regulations could cause the physician to lose his or her license. Be aware of drug-seeking behavior of patients and physical symptoms of addiction. You also have a duty to be aware of coworkers' behavior and to report to the physician any individual who appears chemically impaired or whom you suspect of diverting medications for personal use. ■

What Would You Do? What Would You *Not* Do?   RESPONSES

Case Study 1
Page 578

What Did Theresa Do?

❑ Asked Mrs. Okasinski what pharmacy she uses. Called the pharmacy and asked them to fax a copy of her medications to the medical office. Used the information from the pharmacy and the Product Identification section of the PDR to identify Mrs. Okasinski's medications.

❑ Wrote the names of her medications in her chart for the physician to review.

❑ Explained to Mrs. Okasinki that when she has her prescriptions filled, she should request nonchildproof containers so that she can use the original containers, which have the name and prescription information on them. This would make it easier to tell her medications apart.

❑ After the physician was finished with Mrs. Okasinski, made a list of all the medications she would be taking based on the physician's order. Went over each medication with Mrs. Okasinski and gave her a copy of the medication list to keep as a reference.

What Did Theresa Not *Do?*

❑ Did not criticize Mrs. Okasinski for taking her medications out of their original containers.

What Would You Do?/What Would You *Not* Do? Review Theresa's response and place a checkmark next to the information you included in your response. List additional information you included in your response.

_____

_____

_____

_____

Case Study 2
Page 596

What Did Theresa Do?

❑ Explained to Mrs. Cardwell that for the infection to be completely eliminated from Rachel's body, she needed to be given all of the medication.

❑ Stressed to Mrs. Cardwell that medication prescribed to one person should never be given to someone else because it might cause him or her to have a bad reaction.

❑ Explained to Mrs. Cardwell that if side effects of medication ever occur, it is important to call the medical office for information on what to do.

❑ Told Mrs. Cardwell that Rachel needs to be seen by the doctor again and scheduled an appointment for her. Asked if any other family members needed an appointment with the doctor.

What Did Theresa Not *Do?*

❑ Did not tell Mrs. Cardwell that she should have known better than to give Rachel's antibiotic to the other family members.

What Would You Do?/What Would You *Not* Do? Review Theresa's response and place a checkmark next to the information you included in your response. List additional information you included in your response.

_____

_____

_____

_____

Case Study 3
Page 617

What Did Theresa Do?

❑ Explained to Danielle that if the injection were given in her arm, it would not be absorbed very well and she might not get better.

❑ Explained to Danielle that injections are given to patients every day at the office and that Danielle does not need to be embarrassed.

❑ Told Danielle that she would be draped extra well and that it would only take a minute to give the injection.

What Did Theresa Not *Do?*

❑ Did not disregard Danielle's concerns.

❑ Did not give the injection in the deltoid.

What Would You Do?/What Would You *Not* Do? Review Theresa's response and place a checkmark next to the information you included in your response. List additional information you included in your response.

_____

_____

_____

_____

TERMINOLOGY REVIEW

Adverse reaction An unintended and undesirable effect produced by a drug.

Allergen A substance that is capable of causing an allergic reaction.

Allergy An abnormal hypersensitivity of the body to substances that are ordinarily harmless.

Ampule A small sealed glass container that holds a single dose of medication.

Anaphylactic reaction A serious allergic reaction that requires immediate treatment.

Autoimmune disease A condition in which the body's immune system produces antibodies that attack the body's own cells. The cause is unknown.

Chemotherapy The use of chemicals to treat disease. Chemotherapy is most often used to refer to the treatment of cancer using antineoplastic medications.

Controlled drug A drug that has restrictions placed on it by the federal government because of its potential for abuse.

Conversion Changing from one system of measurement to another.

Cubic centimeter (cc) The amount of space occupied by 1 milliliter (1 ml = 1 cc).

DEA number A registration number assigned to physicians by the Drug Enforcement Administration for prescribing or dispensing controlled drugs.

Dose The quantity of a drug to be administered at one time.

Drug A chemical used for the treatment, prevention, or diagnosis of disease.

Enteral nutrition The delivery of nutrients through a tube inserted into the gastrointestinal tract.

Gauge The diameter of the lumen of a needle used to administer medication.

Hemophilia An inherited bleeding disorder caused by a deficiency of a clotting factor needed for proper coagulation of the blood.

Immune globulin A blood product consisting of pooled human plasma containing antibodies.

Induration An area of hardened tissue.

Infusion The administration of fluids, medications, or nutrients into a vein. *or IV route*

Inhalation administration The administration of medication by way of air or other vapor being drawn into the lungs.

Inscription The part of a prescription that indicates the name of the drug and the drug dosage.

Intradermal injection Introduction of medication into the dermal layer of the skin.

Intramuscular (IM) injection Introduction of medication into the muscular layer of the body.

Intravenous (IV) therapy The administration of a liquid agent directly into a patient's vein, where it is distributed throughout the body via the circulatory system.

Oral administration Administration of medication by mouth.

Parenteral Administration of medication by injection.

Pharmacology The study of drugs.

Prescription A physician's order authorizing the dispensing of a drug by a pharmacist.

Signatura The part of a prescription that indicates the information to print on the medication label.

Subcutaneous (SC) injection Introduction of medication beneath the skin, into the subcutaneous or fatty layer of the body.

Sublingual administration Administration of medication by placing it under the tongue, where it dissolves and is absorbed through the mucous membrane.

Subscription The part of the prescription that gives directions to the pharmacist and usually designates the number of doses to be dispensed.

Superscription The part of a prescription consisting of the symbol Rx (from the Latin word *recipe,* meaning "take").

Topical administration Application of a drug to a particular spot, usually for a local action.

Transfusion The administration of whole blood or blood products through the intravenous route.

Vial A closed glass container with a rubber stopper that holds medication.

Wheal A small raised area of the skin.

ON THE WEB

For Information on Pharmacology:

Food and Drug Administration: www.fda.gov

Drug Enforcement Administration: www.usdoj.gov/dea

RxList: The Internet Drug Index: www.rxlist.com

Drug Topics: www.drugtopics.com

Medline Plus: www.medlineplus.gov

Health Square: www.healthsquare.com

For Information on Alcohol and Drug Abuse:

Alcoholics Anonymous (AA): www.aa.org

National Institute on Alcohol Abuse and Alcoholism (NIAAA): www.niaaa.nih.gov

National Council on Alcoholism and Drug Dependence (NCADD): www.ncadd.org

National Clearinghouse for Alcohol and Drug Information: www.health.org

Partnership for a Drug Free America: www.drugfree.org

Institute for a Drug-Free Workplace: www.drugfreeworkplace.org

Al-Anon/Alateen: www.al-anon.alateen.org

Mothers Against Drunk Driving (MADD): www.madd.org

For Information on Tuberculosis:

American Lung Association: www.lungusa.org

American Thoracic Society: www.thoracic.org

National Center for TB Prevention: www.cdc.gov/tb

For Information on Allergies:

American Academy of Allergy, Asthma, and Immunology: www.aaaai.org

National Institute of Allergy and Infectious Diseases (NIAID): www.niaid.nih.gov

Asthma and Allergy Foundation of America: www.aafa.org

 PREPARE FOR CERTIFICATION Visit the Evolve site at http://evolve.elsevier.com/Bonewit/today/ to actively Prepare for your Certification.

 *Check out the **Companion CD** bound with the book to access additional interactive activities.*

27

Cardiopulmonary Procedures

LEARNING OBJECTIVES

Electrocardiography

1. State the purpose of electrocardiography.
2. Identify each of the following components of the ECG cycle:
   - P wave
   - QRS complex
   - T wave
   - P-R segment
   - S-T segment
   - P-R interval
   - Q-T interval
   - Baseline following the T wave
3. State the purpose of the standardization mark.
4. State the function of the electrodes, amplifier, and galvanometer.
5. List the 12 leads that are included in an ECG.
6. Describe the function served by each of the following:
   - Three-channel recording
   - Teletransmission
   - Interpretive electrocardiography
7. Identify each of the following types of artifacts, and state their causes:
   - Muscle
   - Wandering baseline
   - Alternating current
   - Interrupted baseline

Holter Monitor Electrocardiography

1. List the reasons for applying a Holter monitor.

Cardiac Dysrhythmias

1. List the three categories of cardiac dysrhythmias.
2. State examples of cardiac dysrhythmias.

Pulmonary Function Testing

1. List the different pulmonary function tests.
2. List indications for performing spirometry testing.
3. Describe the following: FVC, FEV_1, and FEV_1/FVC ratio.
4. Explain the difference between predicted values and measured values.
5. Describe the patient preparation for spirometry.
6. Explain how to calibrate a spirometer.
7. Explain the purpose of postbronchodilator spirometry.

PROCEDURES

Record a 12-lead, three-channel electrocardiogram (ECG).

Identify cardiac dysrhythmias on a 12-lead ECG.

Perform spirometry testing.

CAAHEP COMPETENCIES

Clinical Competencies
Diagnostic Testing
- Perform electrocardiography.
- Perform respiratory testing.

ABHES COMPETENCIES

Clinical Duties
- Perform electrocardiograms.
- Perform respiratory testing.

KEY TERMS

amplitude (AM-pli-tood)
artifact (AR-tih-fakt)
atherosclerosis (ath-roe-skler-OH-sus)
baseline
cardiac cycle
dysrhythmia (dis-RITH-mee-ah)
ECG cycle
electrocardiogram (ee-LEK-troe-KAR-dee-oh-gram) (ECG)
electrocardiograph (ee-LEK-troe-KAR-dee-oh-graf)

electrode (ee-LEK-trode)
electrolyte (ee-LEK-troe-lite)
interval (IN-ter-val)
ischemia (is-KEEM-ee-ah)
normal sinus rhythm
segment
spirometer (spih-ROM-ih-ter)
spirometry (spih-ROM-ih-tree)

Introduction to Electrocardiography

The **electrocardiograph** is an instrument used to record the electrical activity of the heart. The **electrocardiogram (ECG)** is the graphic representation of this activity. The ECG exhibits the amount of electrical activity produced by the heart and the time required for the impulse to travel through the heart.

Electrocardiography is used for the following purposes:
- To detect an abnormal cardiac rhythm (**dysrhythmia**)
- To help diagnose damage to the heart caused by a myocardial infarction
- To assess the effect on the heart of digitalis or other cardiac drugs
- To determine the presence of electrolyte disturbances
- To assess the progress of rheumatic fever
- To determine the presence of hypertrophy of the heart chambers
- Performed before surgery to assess cardiac risk during surgery

[handwritten: calcium, potassium, Potassium,]

Figure 27-1. A three-channel electrocardiograph. (From Bonewit-West K: *Clinical procedures for medical assistants*, ed 7, St. Louis, 2008, Saunders.)

Putting It All into Practice

My name is Janet Canterbury, and I work in the medical laboratory of an internal medicine office. I also run ECGs, hook up and read Holter monitors, and perform pulmonary function tests and assist with cardiac stress testing.

One of my most rewarding experiences was when a young woman came into the office with severe chest pains. I immediately helped her back to an examining room. I ran an ECG as ordered by the physician. After the physician read the ECG, he indicated the results did not look good and that the patient would have to be transported to the hospital. I went into the patient's room to comfort her. She asked me if she was going to have to go to the hospital. I replied, "Possibly." She immediately said, "No!" Then I began to explain to her how important it was to have more tests to make sure she would be all right. She finally agreed to go. After being taken to the hospital by an ambulance, she was later transferred to another hospital for a heart catheterization. A few weeks passed, and she came into the office. She hugged me and thanked me for possibly saving her life. It felt so good that I could help make a difference in a patient's life. ■

Prepare for Success

An ECG cannot detect all cardiovascular disorders. In addition, it cannot always detect impending heart disease. The ECG is generally used in combination with other diagnostic and laboratory tests to assess cardiac functioning.

The medical assistant is frequently responsible for recording ECGs in the medical office. Because of this, knowledge and skill must be acquired in the following aspects of electrocardiography: preparation of the patient, operation of the electrocardiograph, identification and elimination of artifacts, labeling the completed ECG, and care and maintenance of the electrocardiograph.

Electrocardiographs are available in single-channel and three-channel recording formats. Because most medical offices use a three-channel ECG, the information in this chapter focuses on the three-channel electrocardiograph (Figure 27-1).

CARDIAC CYCLE

The **cardiac cycle** represents one complete heartbeat. It consists of contraction of the atria, contraction of the ventricles, and relaxation of the entire heart (as described in Chapter 12). The electrocardiograph records the electrical activity that causes these events in the cardiac cycle. The **ECG cycle** is the graphic representation of the cardiac cycle (Figure 27-2).

Waves

The normal ECG cycle consists of a P wave; the Q, R, and S waves (known as the *QRS complex*); and a T wave. The ECG cycle is recorded from left to right, beginning with the P wave.

P wave The P wave represents the electrical activity associated with contraction of the atria, or atrial depolarization.

QRS complex The QRS complex represents the electrical activity associated with the contraction of the ventricles, or ventricular depolarization, and consists of the Q wave, the R wave, and the S wave.

T wave The T wave represents the electrical recovery of the ventricles, or ventricular repolarization. The muscle cells are recovering in preparation for another impulse.

U wave Occasionally, a U wave follows a T wave. It is a small wave that is associated in some as yet undefined way with repolarization.

Baseline, Segments, and Intervals

The flat, horizontal line that separates the various waves is known as the **baseline.** The waves deflect either upward (positive deflection) or downward (negative deflection) from the baseline. The baseline is divided into segments and intervals for the purpose of interpretation and analysis of the ECG by the physician. A **segment** is the portion of the ECG between two waves, and an **interval** is the length of a wave or the length of a wave with a segment.

Segments

P-R segment The P-R segment represents the time interval from the end of the atrial depolarization to the beginning of the ventricular depolarization. It is the time needed for the impulse to be delayed at the AV node and then travel through the bundle of His and Purkinje fibers to the ventricles.

S-T segment The S-T segment represents the time interval from the end of the ventricular depolarization to the beginning of repolarization of the ventricles.

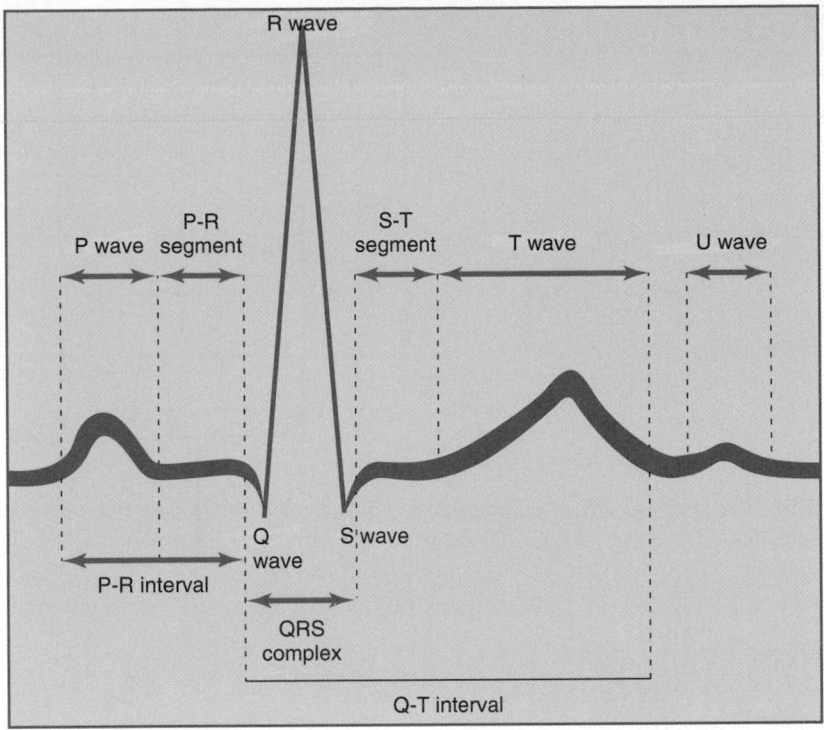

Figure 27-2. Electrocardiogram cycle. (From Bonewit-West K: *Clinical procedures for medical assistants,* ed 7, St. Louis, 2008, Saunders.)

Intervals

P-R interval   The P-R interval represents the time interval from the beginning of the atrial depolarization to the beginning of the ventricular depolarization.

Q-T interval   The Q-T interval is the time interval from the beginning of the ventricular depolarization to the end of repolarization of the ventricles.

Baseline   The baseline after the T wave (or U wave, if present) represents the period when the entire heart returns to its resting, or polarized, state.

ELECTROCARDIOGRAPH PAPER

Electrocardiograph paper is divided into two sets of squares for accurate and convenient measurement of the waves, intervals, and segments (Figure 27-3). Each small square is 1 mm high and 1 mm wide. Each large square (made up of 25 small squares) is 5 mm high and 5 mm wide. By measuring the various waves, intervals, and segments of the graph cycle, the physician can determine whether the electrical activity of the heart falls within normal limits.

Electrocardiograph paper consists of a black or blue base with a white plastic coating. A black or red graph is printed on top of the plastic coating. A heated stylus moves over the heat-sensitive paper and melts away the plastic coating, resulting in the recording of the ECG cycles. In addition to being heat sensitive, the paper is pressure sensitive and should be handled carefully to avoid making impressions that would interfere with the proper reading of the ECG.

STANDARDIZATION OF THE ELECTROCARDIOGRAPH

The electrocardiograph machine must be standardized when recording an ECG. This is a quality control measure that ensures an accurate and reliable recording. It means that an ECG run on one electrocardiograph compares inaccuracy with a recording run on another machine.

By international agreement, 1 millivolt (mV) of electricity should cause the stylus to move 10 mm high in **amplitude** (10 small squares). A three-channel electrocardiograph automatically records standardization marks on the tracing. During the recording, the machine allows 1 mV to enter the electrocardiograph machine, which should result in an upward deflection of 10 mm. The marking on the ECG paper is known as the *standardization mark* (Figure 27-4). The width of the mark made by the machine is approximately 2 mm (two small squares). If the standardization mark is more or less than 10 mm in amplitude, it can be adjusted. The manufacturer's operating manual must be consulted for proper adjustment information. An electrocardiograph must never be adjusted without use of the operating manual.

ELECTROCARDIOGRAPH LEADS

The standard ECG consists of 12 leads. Each lead provides an electrical "photograph" of the heart's activity from a different angle. Together, the 12 leads, or "photographs," facilitate a thorough interpretation of the heart's activity.

Figure 27-3. Diagram of electrocardiogram paper with a section enlarged to indicate the size of the large and small squares. (From Bonewit-West K: *Clinical procedures for medical assistants,* ed 7, St. Louis, 2008, Saunders.)

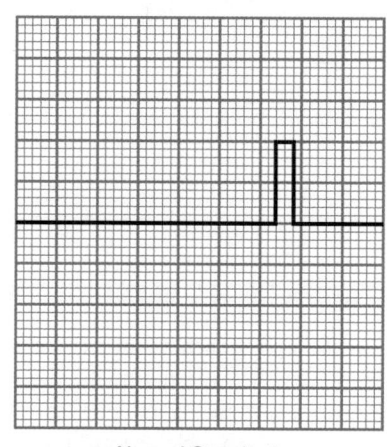

Normal Standard
Standardization mark is
10 mm high

Figure 27-4. Standardization mark. (From Bonewit-West K: *Clinical procedures for medical assistants,* ed 7, St. Louis, 2008, Saunders.)

The electrical impulses given off by the heart are picked up by **electrodes** and conducted into the machine through lead wires. Electrodes are composed of a substance that is a good conductor of electricity. The impulses given off by the heart are very small. To produce a readable ECG, they must be made larger, or amplified, by a device known as an *amplifier,* located within the electrocardiograph. The amplified voltages are changed into mechanical motion by the *galvanometer* and recorded on the electrocardiograph paper by a heated stylus (Figure 27-5).

There are four limb electrodes: the right arm electrode (RA), the left arm electrode (LA), the right leg electrode (RL), and the left leg electrode (LL). The right leg electrode is known as the *ground.* It is not used for the actual recording, but serves as an electrical reference point. The chest leads are abbreviated V or C and use six chest electrodes.

Disposable electrodes are typically used with a three-channel electrocardiograph. A disposable electrode consists of a self-adhesive tab that contains an electrolyte. An **electrolyte** is a substance that facilitates the transmission of the heart's electrical impulse. The electrode is applied to the skin and held in place with its adhesive backing; it is thrown away after use.

Bipolar Leads

The first three leads of the 12-lead ECG are the bipolar leads; they are leads I, II, and III. The bipolar leads use two of the limb electrodes to record the heart's electrical activity. Lead I records the heart's voltage difference between the right arm and the left arm, lead II records the difference between the right arm and the left leg, and lead III records the difference between the left arm and left leg (Figure 27-6).

Lead II shows the heart's rhythm more clearly than the other leads. Because of this, the physician often requests a *rhythm strip,* which is a longer recording (approximately 12 inches) of lead II.

Augmented Leads

The next three leads are the augmented leads: aVR (augmented voltage—right arm), aVL (augmented voltage—left arm), and aVF (augmented voltage—left leg or foot). Lead aVR records the heart's voltage difference between the right arm electrode and a central point between the left arm and left leg. Lead aVL records the heart's voltage difference between the left arm electrode and a central point between the right arm and left leg. Lead aVF records the heart's voltage difference between the left leg electrode and a central point between the right and left arms. Leads I, II, III, aVR, aVL, and aVF record the voltage from side to side and from the top to the bottom of the heart (see Figure 27-6).

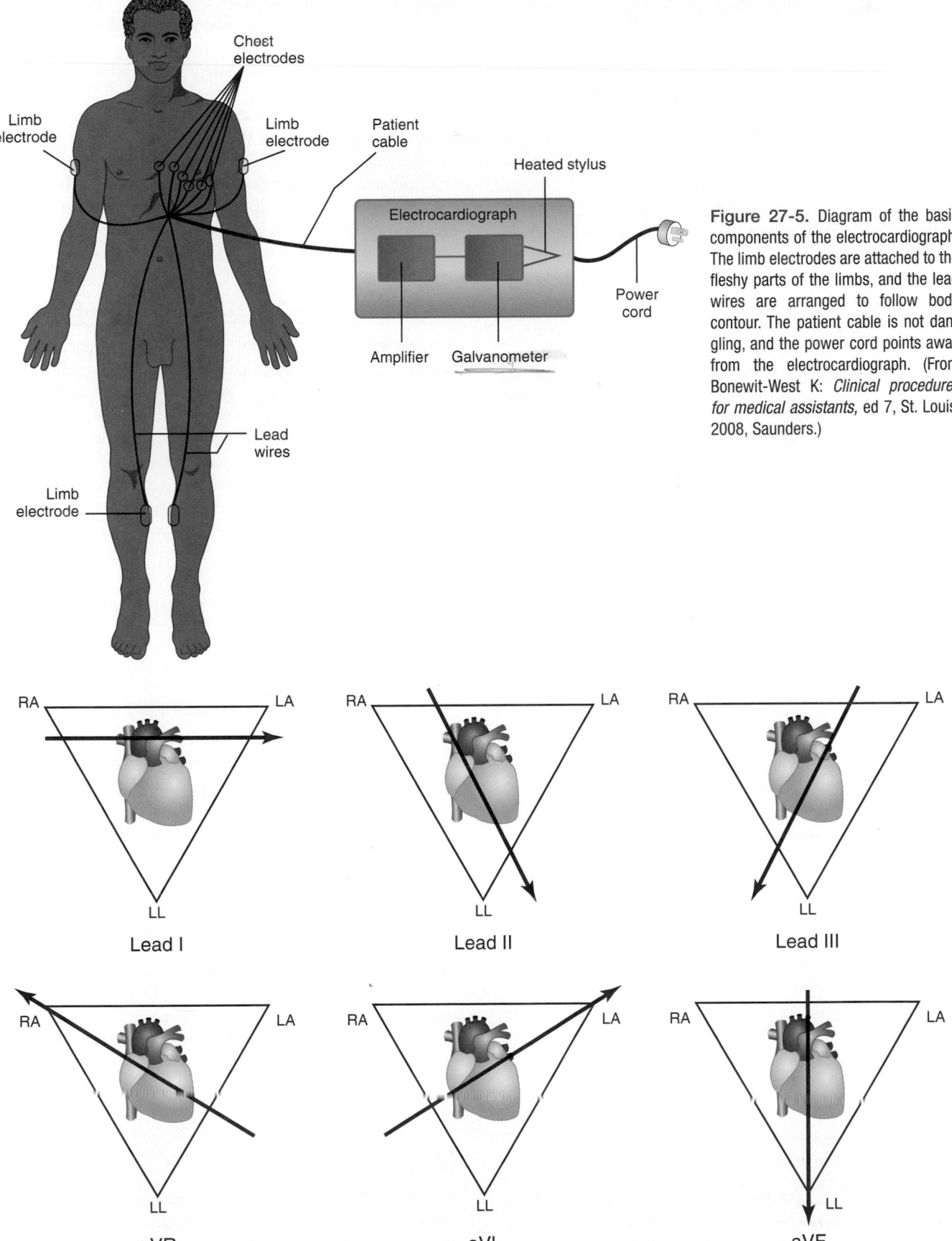

Figure 27-5. Diagram of the basic components of the electrocardiograph. The limb electrodes are attached to the fleshy parts of the limbs, and the lead wires are arranged to follow body contour. The patient cable is not dangling, and the power cord points away from the electrocardiograph. (From Bonewit-West K: *Clinical procedures for medical assistants,* ed 7, St. Louis, 2008, Saunders.)

Lead I

Lead II

Lead III

aVR

aVL

aVF

Figure 27-6. Diagram of the heart's voltage for leads I, II, III, augmented voltage—right arm *(aVR),* augmented voltage—left arm *(aVL),* and augmented voltage—left leg or foot *(aVF). LA,* Left arm electode; *LL,* left leg electrode; *RA,* right arm electrode. (From Bonewit-West K: *Clinical procedures for medical assistants,* ed 7, St. Louis, 2008, Saunders.)

est Leads

The last six leads are the chest, or precordial, leads: V_1, V_2, V_3, V_4, V_5, and V_6. These leads record the heart's voltage from front to back. The voltage is recorded from a central point "inside" the heart to a point on the chest wall where the electrode is placed. These points correspond to the chest leads. Figure 27-7 shows the proper location of the six chest

---

What Would You Do? What Would You *Not* Do?

Case Study 1

Camilla Rossi is 22 years old and works at a waffle house during the day and goes to business school at night. She comes to the office because she has been experiencing some heart problems. Over the past month, she has had three episodes of tachycardia, palpitations, trouble breathing, and profuse sweating. She is really scared that she has heart disease. Her beloved grandfather just died from a heart attack, and she is afraid she will die next. The physician orders an ECG, but Camilla is reluctant to have the procedure. She is embarrassed about having to take her top off, and she is worried that she will get shocked by all the wires coming out of the machine. She says that she does not have health insurance, and she does not know how she would pay for such a fancy test. She wants to know whether there is a cheaper way to find out what is wrong with her. ∎

Figure 27-7. Recommended positions for electrocardiogram chest leads:

1. V_1, fourth intercostal space at right margin of sternum
2. V_2, fourth intercostal space at left margin of sternum
3. V_3, midway between positions 2 and 4
4. V_4, fifth intercostal space at junction of left midclavicular line
5. V_5, at horizontal level of position 4 at left anterior axillary line
6. V_6, at horizontal level of position 4 at left midaxillary line

(From Bonewit-West K: *Clinical procedures for medical assistants*, ed 7, St. Louis, 2008, Saunders.)

---

leads. To ensure an accurate and reliable recording, the medical assistant must be able to locate them accurately. When first learning to locate the chest leads, it helps to mark their location on the patient's chest with a felt-tipped pen.

Normally, the ECG is recorded with the paper moving at a speed of 25 mm/sec. Occasionally, the ECG cycles are close together, making the recording difficult to read. The medical assistant can change the paper speed to 50 mm/sec to spread out the cycles. To alert the physician to the change, the medical assistant must make a notation of it on the recording.

MAINTENANCE OF THE ELECTROCARDIOGRAPH

Electrocardiographs require very little maintenance. The casing of the electrocardiograph should be cleaned frequently with a soft cloth, slightly dampened with a mild detergent, to remove dust and dirt. Commercial solvents and abrasives should not be used because they can damage the finish of the casing. The patient cables, lead wires, and power cord should be cleaned periodically with a cloth moistened with a disinfectant cleaner. The cables should never be immersed in the cleaning solution because this could damage them.

ELECTROCARDIOGRAPHIC CAPABILITIES

Electrocardiographs have a variety of capabilities that permit specific recording options.

Three-Channel Recording Capability

An electrocardiograph with a three-channel recording capability can record electrical activity through three leads simultaneously. This is in contrast to a single-channel electrocardiograph, which records only one lead at a time. The advantage of a three-channel electrocardiograph is that an ECG can be produced in less time than would be required if each lead were recorded separately.

The leads that are recorded simultaneously are leads I, II, and III; followed by aVR, aVL, and aVF; followed by V_1, V_2, and V_3; followed by V_4, V_5, and V_6. Recording three leads at one time requires three-channel recording paper, which is designed in a standard $8\frac{1}{2} \times 11$-inch format. This size of the printout fits easily into the patient's chart. Most three-channel electrocardiographs have a *copy capability* that quickly produces an accurate tracing of the last ECG recorded. Figure 27-8 is an example of a three-channel ECG recording that also includes a rhythm strip. Procedure 27-1 describes how to run a 12-lead three-channel ECG.

Teletransmission

An electrocardiograph with teletransmission capabilities can transmit a recording performed at the medical office over the telephone line to an ECG data interpretation site. The recording is interpreted by a cardiologist (often along with a computer analysis) at the ECG site, and a printout of the

Highlight on Stress Testing

Description

Exercise tolerance testing, also called *stress testing,* is a diagnostic procedure used to evaluate the cardiovascular system. It is usually performed in a hospital under the direction of a cardiologist and an exercise tolerance technician so that emergency equipment and trained personnel are available to deal with unusual situations that might arise.

Purpose

The purpose of exercise tolerance testing is as follows:

1. To diagnose ischemic heart disease that cannot be detected by a standard resting electrocardiogram (ECG). Ischemic heart disease is heart disease that occurs as a result of inadequate blood supply to the myocardium, as in a myocardial infarction and angina pectoris.
2. To assist in evaluating the cause of cardiac symptoms, such as chest discomfort and dysrhythmias.
3. To assess the effectiveness of cardiac drug therapy.
4. To follow the course of rehabilitation after a myocardial infarction or a cardiac surgical procedure, such as a coronary bypass operation or a coronary stent placement.
5. To determine an individual's fitness for a strenuous exercise program, such as jogging.

How the Test Works

Exercise tolerance testing involves the continuous electrocardiographic monitoring of an individual during physical exercise. The patient's blood pressure, heart rate, and physical symptoms are also monitored during the test. The tolerance testing is accomplished by having the patient use a treadmill. The intensity of the physical exertion is increased gradually until the patient's target heart rate is reached, unless the signs and symptoms of cardiac **ischemia** appear, in which case the test is stopped. These symptoms include claudication (severe leg pain), severe dyspnea, chest discomfort or pain, pallor, and dizziness.

Interpretation of Results

The patient's response to the exercise tolerance testing is used to determine normal or abnormal results. A normal response is a gradual increase in the patient's blood pressure as the physical exertion increases, whereas an abnormal response is a sudden increase or decrease of the patient's blood pressure. The ECG of a normal individual exhibits a shortened P-R interval and a compressed QRS complex. An abnormal tracing indicative of myocardial ischemia results in a depressed S-T segment and an inverted T wave. An abnormal exercise tolerance test usually warrants further testing, such as a coronary angiogram. ∎

Name : Jane Doe
ID   : 34
Date : 04/06/73   Time : 11:37
Age   : 20   Sex : Female
Hgt   : 64 IN   Wgt : 130 LBS
Med1 :
Med2 :
Ccl1 :
Ccl2 :
Cmnt :

Vent rate : 81

- - Durations - -
P   : 84
QRS : 92
- - Intervals - -
PR   : 138
QT   : 356
QTc : 393
- - Axes - -
P   : 45
QRS : 10
T   : 16

SINUS RHYTHM
WITHIN NORMAL LIMITS

SUMMARY: NORMAL

Speed: 25 mm/s   Freq: 60~ .05-30Hz   E350i Rev.1.26 GRI 10.1
Gain : Limb 10   Chest 10 mm/mv

Figure 27-8. A three-channel electrocardiogram with a rhythm strip.

recording along with the interpretation is electronically transmitted to the sending office the same day. Patient information (e.g., age, sex, height, weight, medications) must be relayed to the ECG site to assist in the interpretation. This information is entered into the electrocardiograph by the medical assistant (using a keyboard) and transmitted automatically with the ECG recording.

Interpretive Electrocardiograph

An electrocardiograph with interpretive capabilities has a built-in computer program that analyzes the recording as it is being run. Interpretive electrocardiographs provide immediate information on the heart's activity, leading to earlier diagnosis and treatment. Patient data are used in the interpretation of the ECG and must be entered into the electrocardiograph using a keyboard before running the recording. The data generally required are the patient's age, sex, height, weight, and medications. The computer analysis of the ECG is printed at the top of the recording, along with the reason for each interpretation (Figure 27-9).

The results are reviewed and interpreted further by the physician before a diagnosis is made and treatment is initiated.

ARTIFACTS

The medical assistant is responsible for producing a clear and concise ECG recording that can be read and interpreted easily by the physician. Structures sometimes appear in the recording that are not natural and interfere with the normal appearance of the ECG cycles. They are known as **artifacts** and represent additional electrical activity that is picked up by the electrocardiograph. The medical assistant should be able to identify artifacts and correct them. There are several types of artifacts; the most common are muscle, wandering baseline, and alternating current (AC) (Figure 27-10).

In some circumstances, as when individuals have trouble holding still or in buildings with older electrical systems, normal methods to eliminate muscle and AC artifacts may

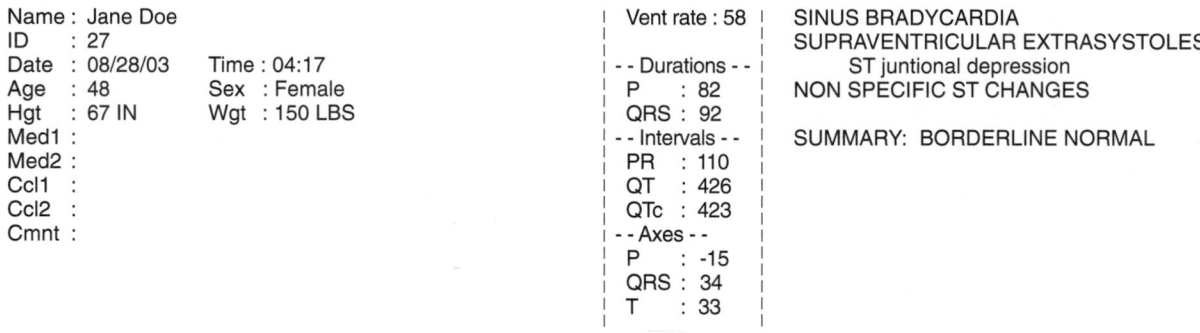

```
Name : Jane Doe                              | Vent rate : 58 |    SINUS BRADYCARDIA
ID   : 27                                    |                |    SUPRAVENTRICULAR EXTRASYSTOLES
Date : 08/28/03    Time : 04:17              | - - Durations - - |      ST juntional depression
Age  : 48          Sex  : Female             | P    : 82       |    NON SPECIFIC ST CHANGES
Hgt  : 67 IN       Wgt  : 150 LBS            | QRS  : 92       |
Med1 :                                       | - - Intervals - - |   SUMMARY:  BORDERLINE NORMAL
Med2 :                                       | PR   : 110      |
Ccl1 :                                       | QT   : 426      |
Ccl2 :                                       | QTc  : 423      |
Cmnt :                                       | - - Axes - -    |
                                             | P    : -15      |
                                             | QRS  : 34       |
                                             | T    : 33       |
```

Figure 27-9. An electrocardiogram that has been analyzed by an interpretive electrocardiograph. The computer analysis is printed at the top of the recording, along with the reason for each interpretation.

60~ .05-30Hz
10 mm/mv

E350i R

A   Muscle artifact

E350i Rev. 1.26 GR1 10.1

B   Wandering baseline

aVR   V1

C   Alternating current artifacts

Figure 27-10. A-C, Examples of electrocardiogram artifacts.

[handwritten: Which one error EKG Do not run cable under the bed]

be unsuccessful. Electrocardiographs have an artifact filter that can reduce artifacts when all else fails. Because the *artifact filter* also affects the diagnostic accuracy of the ECG, it should be used as little as possible.

If the medical assistant is unable to correct an artifact, the physician should be consulted. It is possible that the machine is broken. If an electrocardiograph service technician has to be contacted, the medical assistant should have the following information available to aid the service technician in locating the problem:

1. What already has been done to locate and correct the problem
2. Leads in which the artifact occurs
3. A sample of the artifact recorded by the machine

Muscle Artifact

A muscle artifact (see Figure 27-10A) can be identified by its fuzzy, irregular baseline. There are two types of

muscle artifacts: those caused by involuntary muscle movement (somatic tremor) and those caused by voluntary muscle movement. Muscle artifacts may be caused by the following:

1. **An apprehensive patient.** To reduce the patient's apprehension and relax muscles, explain the procedure and reassure the patient that having an ECG recorded is a painless procedure.
2. **Patient discomfort.** Ensure that the table is wide enough to support the patient's arms and legs adequately. The patient can be made more comfortable by placing a pillow under his or her head. Check that the room temperature is comfortable for the patient. A temperature that is warm enough for the medical assistant may be too cold for the patient who has removed clothing. This could result in shivering, which also would produce a muscle artifact on the ECG.
3. **Patient movement.** The patient must be instructed to lie still and not talk during the recording.

4. **A physical condition.** Several nervous system disorders, such as Parkinson's disease, prevent relaxation, and the patient trembles continually. The medical assistant must be understanding and try to record while the tremor is at a minimum.

Wandering Baseline Artifact

A wandering baseline artifact (see Figure 27-10B) can be caused by the following:

1. **Loose electrodes.** The medical assistant should ensure that the disposable adhesive electrodes are attached firmly to the patient's skin. If an electrode pulls loose, it can be reattached with hypoallergenic tape or replaced with a new electrode. The alligator clips should be attached firmly to the electrodes. To prevent pulling or twisting of the patient cable, it should be well supported on the table or the patient's abdomen and not be allowed to dangle.
2. **Body creams, oils, or lotions** on the skin in the area where the electrode is applied. The medical assistant should remove these by rubbing with alcohol, using friction.

Alternating Current Artifact *Which one cause*

AC artifacts (see Figure 27-10C) are caused by electrical interference. Alternating electric current can "leak" or spread out from the power used by electrical appliances in the room in which the ECG is being run. This current may be picked up by the patient and carried into the electrocardiograph, where it would show up on the ECG recording as an AC artifact. An AC artifact appears as small, straight, spiked lines that are consistent. AC artifacts can be caused by the following:

1. **Lead wires not following body contour.** Dangling lead wires can pick up AC. Arrange the wires to follow body contour and to lie flat.
2. **Other electrical equipment in the room.** Lamps, autoclaves, electrically powered examining tables, or other electrical equipment that is plugged in may be leaking AC. Unplug all nearby electrical equipment.
3. **Wiring in the walls, ceilings, or floors.** Try moving the patient table away from the walls.
4. **Improper grounding of the electrocardiograph.** The machine is automatically grounded when it is plugged in. Ensure that the plug is securely in the wall outlet. The right leg electrode is not used for recording the leads, but it picks up AC that has "leaked" onto the patient and carries it into the electrocardiograph. The AC is carried away by the machine's grounding system.

Interrupted Baseline Artifact

Occasionally, an interrupted baseline occurs. It may be caused by the metal tip of a lead wire becoming detached or by a broken patient cable. If the latter is the case, a new patient cable should be ordered from the manufacturer.

 PROCEDURE 27-1

PROCEDURE **27-1**   **Running a 12-Lead, Three-Channel Electrocardiogram**

Outcome Record a 12-lead ECG.

Equipment/Supplies

- Three-channel electrocardiograph
- Disposable electrodes
- ECG paper

1. **Procedural Step.** Work in a quiet, relaxing atmosphere away from sources of electrical interference.
2. **Procedural Step.** Sanitize your hands, and assemble the equipment. Greet the patient and introduce yourself. Identify the patient by full name and date of birth.
3. **Procedural Step.** Help the patient relax by explaining the procedure. Tell the patient that having an ECG recording is painless. Explain that he or she must lie still and not talk while the ECG is being recorded so that an accurate ECG can be obtained.
   Principle. Explaining the procedure helps reassure apprehensive patients. The patient should be mentally and physically relaxed for an accurate ECG recording; an apprehensive or moving patient produces muscle artifacts.
4. **Procedural Step.** Prepare the patient. Ask him or her to remove clothing from the waist up. The lower legs must also be uncovered. Assist the patient into a supine position on the table. The table should support the arms and legs adequately so that they do not dangle. Properly drape the patient to prevent exposure and provide warmth. A pillow can be used to support the patient's head.
   Principle. The chest, upper arms, and lower legs must be uncovered to allow proper placement of the electrodes. The patient should be kept warm, and the arms and legs should not be allowed to dangle; otherwise, muscle artifacts could result.
5. **Procedural Step.** Position the electrocardiograph so that the power cord points away from the patient and does not pass under the table. It is usually easier for

the medical assistant to work on the left side of the patient.

Principle. Proper positioning of the electrocardiograph reduces AC artifacts.

6. Procedural Step. Prepare the patient's skin for application of the disposable electrodes. If the patient has oily skin or has used lotion, wipe the area to which the electrode will be applied with alcohol, and allow it to dry. If the patient's chest is hairy, dry shave it at each electrode site before applying the electrode.

Principle. The patient's skin must be dry and free of oil and body hair so that the adhesive backing of the electrodes sticks to the patient's skin and stays on during the procedure.

7. Procedural Step. Apply limb electrodes. Firmly apply the adhesive backing of the electrodes to the fleshy part of each of the four limbs (upper arms and lower legs). The tabs of the arm electrodes should point downward, and the tabs of the leg electrodes should point upward. The adhesive backing of the electrode allows it to adhere firmly to the patient's skin.

Principle. The tab of the electrodes should be positioned toward the cable to provide a more stable connection when the lead wire is attached to the electrode and to prevent the lead wires from pulling and causing artifacts.

A, Apply the leg electrodes. **B,** Apply the arm electrodes. (From Bonewit-West K: *Clinical procedures for medical assistants,* ed 7, St. Louis, 2008, Saunders.)

8. Procedural Step. Apply the chest electrodes. Properly locate each chest position, and apply the electrode with the tab pointing downward. Continue until all six of the chest electrodes have been applied.

Principle. Positioning the tabs of the electrodes downward prevents the lead wires from pulling and causing artifacts.

Apply the chest electrodes. (From Bonewit-West K: *Clinical procedures for medical assistants,* ed 7, St. Louis, 2008, Saunders.)

9. Procedural Step. Connect the lead wires to the electrodes. This is accomplished by inserting an alligator clip onto the metal tip of each electrode. The alligator clip is attached to the tab of each electrode. The ends of the lead wires are usually color coded and identified with abbreviations to help the medical assistant connect the proper lead to each electrode. Arrange the lead wires to follow body contour.

Principle. Arranging the lead wires to follow body contour reduces the possibility of AC artifacts.

Connect the lead wires to the electrodes. (From Bonewit-West K: *Clinical procedures for medical assistants,* ed 7, St. Louis, 2008, Saunders.)

10. Procedural Step. Plug the patient cable into the machine. The cable should be supported on the table or on the patient's abdomen to prevent pulling or twisting.

Continued

PROCEDURE 27-1

PROCEDURE 27-1   Running a 12-Lead, Three-Channel Electrocardiogram—cont'd

PROCEDURE 27-1

11. Procedural Step. Turn on the electrocardiograph. Enter patient data using the soft-touch keypad. Always use your fingertips to enter the data. Pencils or other sharp objects can damage the keyboard. As the data are entered, they are displayed on the LCD screen. The patient data to be entered generally include the patient's name, a patient identification number, age, sex, height, weight, and medications.

Principle. The patient data and the date and time of the recording are printed at the top of the recording. If the electrocardiograph is equipped with interpretive capabilities, this information is also used in the computer-assisted interpretation of the ECG.

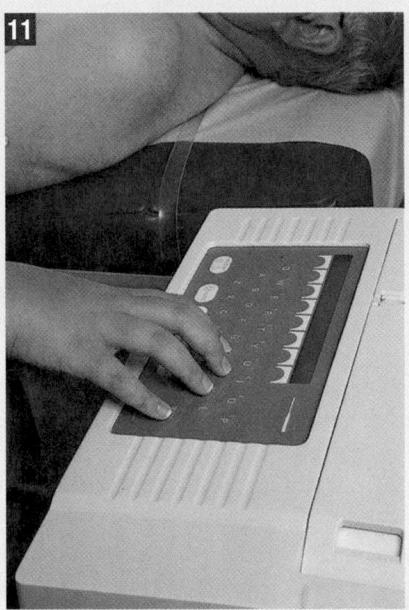

Enter patient data. (From Bonewit-West K: *Clinical procedures for medical assistants,* ed 7, St. Louis, 2008, Saunders.)

12. Procedural Step. Remind the patient to lie still and not talk. Press the AUTO (automatic) button, and run the recording. The machine automatically inserts a standardization mark at the beginning of the recording, followed by the recording of the 12-lead ECG in a three-channel format.

13. Procedural Step. After the ECG has been recorded, do the following:

a. Check the printout to ensure the standardization mark is 10 mm high. If it is more or less than 10 mm, adjust the standardization mark according to the manufacturer's instructions and run another ECG.

b. Check the direction of the R wave in Lead 1. If your patient's limb leads are attached correctly, the

R wave on Lead 1 should have a positive deflection. If it has a negative deflection, the limb leads are not attached correctly. Reattach the limb leads properly and run another recording.

c. Observe the recording for artifacts. If an artifact is present, determine the cause of the artifact, correct the problem, and run another ECG.

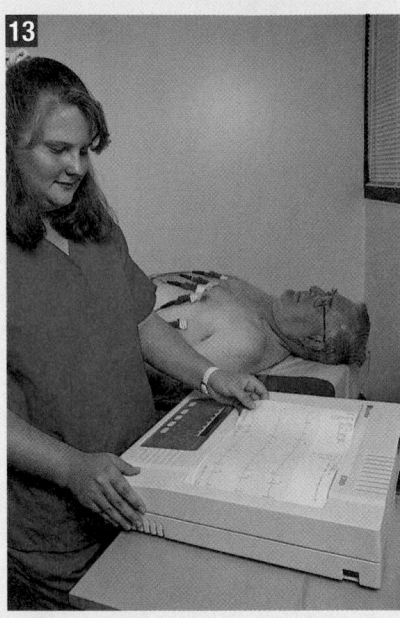

Check the standardization mark. (From Bonewit-West K: *Clinical procedures for medical assistants,* ed 7, St. Louis, 2008, Saunders.)

14. Procedural Step. Inform the patient that you are finished and he or she can now talk or move. Turn the machine off. Disconnect the lead wires. Remove and discard the electrodes.

15. Procedural Step. Assist the patient in stepping down from the table.

16. Procedural Step. Sanitize your hands. Chart the procedure. Include the date and time and the name of the procedure (12-lead ECG). Place the recording in the patient's medical record, and put the record in the appropriate place to be reviewed by the physician.

17. Procedural Step. Return all equipment to its proper storage place.

CHARTING EXAMPLE

Date	
6/12/10	10:30 a.m. Completed a 12-lead ECG.
	Recording to physician for review. ———
	——————— J. Canterbury, CMA (AAMA)

HOLTER MONITOR ELECTROCARDIOGRAPHY

A Holter monitor is a portable ambulatory monitoring system for recording the cardiac activity of a patient for 24 hours. The system is designed so that the patient can maintain his or her usual daily activities with minimal inconvenience while being monitored. Holter monitor electrocardiography is an important noninvasive procedure used to diagnose cardiac rhythm and conduction abnormalities. Specifically, it is most frequently used to evaluate patients with unexplained syncope, to discover intermittent cardiac dysrhythmias not picked up on a routine 12-lead ECG, to assess the effectiveness of antidysrhythmic medications (e.g., digitalis and antianginal medications), and to assess the effectiveness of an artificial pacemaker.

The Holter monitor consists of electrodes placed on the patient's chest and a special portable recorder that continually monitors the heart's activity. The portable recording device is available in two formats: a magnetic tape recorder that uses a cassette tape to record the heart's activity (Figure 27-11) and a newer computerized digital recorder that uses a compact flash memory card to document the heart's activity.

The lightweight, battery-powered recorder is held in a protective case, which is worn on a belt around the patient's waist or hung over the patient's shoulder by a strap. Throughout the 24-hour period, the system continuously records the patient's heartbeat on a magnetic cassette tape or the compact flash memory card.

CARDIAC DYSRHYTHMIAS

The normal ECG graph cycle consists of a P wave, a QRS complex, and a T wave, which repeats in a regular pattern (see Figure 27-2). The term **normal sinus rhythm** refers to an ECG that is within normal limits. This means that the waves, intervals, segments, and cardiac rate fall within normal range. The normal heart rate ranges from 60 to 100 beats per minute. A rate slower than 60 beats per minute is *sinus bradycardia,* and a rate faster than 100 beats per minute is *sinus tachycardia.*

Each ECG graph cycle is separated from the next one by a flat length of baseline termed the *T-P segment.* Any change in the baseline distance between graph cycles indicates a cardiac abnormality known as a *dysrhythmia* that falls into one of the following categories: (1) extra beats, (2) an abnormal rhythm, or (3) an abnormal heart rate. Cardiac dysrhythmias include atrial premature contraction, paroxysmal atrial tachycardia, atrial flutter, atrial fibrillation, premature ventricular contraction, ventricular tachycardia, and ventricular fibrillation.

PULMONARY FUNCTION TESTS

The purpose of a pulmonary function test (PFT) is to assess lung functioning, assisting in the detection and evaluation of pulmonary disease. Pulmonary function tests include spirometry, lung volumes, diffusion capacity, arterial blood gas studies, pulse oximetry, and cardiopulmonary exercise tests. The most frequently performed pulmonary function test is spirometry, which is described in detail in the next section. Procedure 27-2 outlines how to use a spirometer.

Spirometry

Spirometry is a simple, noninvasive screening test that is often performed in the medical office. A computerized electronic instrument known as a **spirometer** is used to conduct the test. A spirometer measures how much air is pushed out of the lungs and how fast it is pushed out. The spirometry report is printed out as a table and graph. Spirometry is considered a screening test, and abnormal test results require that the patient undergo additional pulmonary function tests and possibly a computed tomography scan before a diagnosis can be made. Indications for performing spirometry include the following:

1. Patients who exhibit symptoms of lung dysfunction such as dyspnea

Figure 27-11. Holter monitor and supplies required for its application. (From Bonewit-West K: *Clinical procedures for medical assistants,* ed 7, St. Louis, 2008, Saunders.)

Memories *from* Externship

Janet Canterbury: During my externship, I was at an office where ECGs were one of the many procedures that were performed. For my first ECG, the patient was a man who had a lot of hair on his chest, and I would need to shave the electrode placement sites on his chest. I was very nervous, but the procedure went well. When the ECG was run, he told me that I did a wonderful job and that it did not hurt at all to have his chest shaved. I realized then that it was not so bad after all. That patient made me feel so good about what I do and helped me feel confident in the procedures I had ahead of me. ■

Prepare for Success

PATIENT TEACHING Angina Pectoris

Answer questions the patient has about angina pectoris.

What is angina pectoris?

Angina pectoris is a symptom rather than a disease. Its name is a Latin term that means "pain in the chest." Angina pectoris occurs when the muscle tissue of the heart does not receive enough oxygenated blood, resulting in discomfort or pain under the sternum.

What causes angina pectoris?

For most patients, the cause of angina is **atherosclerosis**, a condition in which fibrous plaques of fatty deposits and cholesterol build up on the inner walls of the coronary arteries, causing a narrowing and obstruction of the lumen of these arteries. This results in a reduction of oxygenated blood flow to the heart. Despite the narrowing, enough oxygen may still reach the heart for normal needs. More oxygen is necessary, however, when situations occur that increase the workload of the heart, such as physical activity, emotional stress, a heavy meal, and exposure to cold weather. If the coronary arteries cannot deliver enough oxygen during these times of increased need, angina pectoris results.

What happens during an angina episode?

Individuals experience angina in different ways, including the following: severe indigestion or burning, heaviness, ache, or squeezing or crushing pressure in the chest. The chest discomfort varies greatly. It can feel only mildly uncomfortable, or it may be intense and accompanied by a feeling of suffocation and doom. The pain is usually felt beneath the sternum and may radiate to the neck, throat, jaw, left shoulder, arm, or back. In most cases, the pain lasts no longer than a few minutes and is relieved by resting.

Severe and prolonged anginal pain generally suggests a myocardial infarction (heart attack) and requires immediate medical attention.

What type of treatment might be prescribed by the physician?

The goal of treating angina is to reduce the workload of the heart and to increase the oxygen supply to the heart. This is accomplished by resting when an angina attack occurs. In addition, the physician often prescribes medications, the most common one being nitroglycerin. Nitroglycerin is usually taken sublingually. It works by reducing the workload of the heart and increasing the oxygen supply to the heart by dilating the coronary arteries. Nitroglycerin can also be administered through patches worn on the skin or an ointment rubbed into the skin.

What tests might be ordered by the physician?

For patients who exhibit angina pectoris, the physician may order one or more of the following: a 12-lead electrocardiogram, chest x-ray, blood tests, and an exercise tolerance test. These tests assist in detecting coronary artery narrowing and blockage. To determine the exact location and extent of blockage, a more specific test, known as *coronary angiography*, may be performed. To help prevent more serious heart disease from developing, the physician generally recommends lifestyle changes, such as a diet low in cholesterol and saturated fat, weight reduction, smoking cessation, and stress reduction. For patients with severe blockage of the coronary arteries, coronary artery bypass surgery, coronary stent placement, or balloon angioplasty may be recommended.

Provide the patient with educational materials on angina pectoris and coronary artery disease. ∎

---

2. Individuals at high risk for lung disease because of smoking or exposure to environmental pollutants, such as coal dust, asbestos, and exhaust fumes
3. Patients with lung disease, such as asthma, chronic bronchitis, and emphysema
4. Patients who are to undergo surgery (to assess probable lung performance during an operation)
5. Patients who need to be evaluated for lung disability or impairment for a compensation program (e.g., coal miners)

Spirometry Test Results

The results obtained from spirometry testing provide numerous measurements that help the physician assess lung functioning. The most important parameters are described next.

Forced Vital Capacity

Forced vital capacity (FVC) is the maximum volume of air (measured in liters) that can be expired when the patient exhales as forcefully and rapidly as possible and for as long as possible. FVC is obtained by having the patient perform a breathing maneuver. The patient is instructed to take a deep breath until the lungs are completely full. Following this, the patient is told to blow all the air out of the lungs and into the mouthpiece as hard and as fast as possible until no more air can be expelled. To be considered an adequate test, the patient must forcibly blow out all the air from the lungs and continue smooth, continuous exhaling for at least 6 seconds. To be considered a valid test, a minimum of three acceptable efforts must be obtained.

Some patients have difficulty performing the FVC breathing maneuver because they have a physical impairment or poor motivation, or they do not understand the instructions. The medical assistant should be patient and work with these individuals to help them perform the maneuver. If patients are unable to perform the maneuver after eight attempts, however, testing should be discontinued. At this point, fatigue may affect the accuracy of the results and additional efforts are not recommended.

Forced Expiratory Volume after 1 Second

Forced expiratory volume after 1 second (FEV₁) is the volume of air (in liters) that is forcefully exhaled during the first second of the FVC breathing maneuver. The spirometer automatically determines this parameter from the FVC maneuver.

FEV₁/FVC Ratio

In patients with healthy lungs, 70% to 75% of the air exhaled (FVC) is exhaled in the first second (FEV₁) of the breathing maneuver. This comparison is known as the *FEV₁/FVC ratio*, and it is expressed as a percentage. A patient with healthy lungs may have an FEV₁/FVC ratio of 85%. This means that 85% of the exhaled air was exhaled during the first second of the breathing maneuver.

What Would You Do? What Would You *Not* Do?

Case Study 2

Joel Matthews, 48 years old, is at the office for a biannual checkup. Joel had a mild heart attack 2 years ago. Since then, he has completely changed his life. He's become a vegetarian and practices yoga every morning before going to work. After he gets home, he jogs 10 miles. He also lifts weights every other day and takes herbal vitamin supplements. Since his heart attack, he has lost 40 lb and says that he has never felt better. The only thing he cannot seem to do is give up smoking. He started smoking when he was 17 years old and has cut back from 2 packs to 1 pack a day. He keeps trying to stop but says that he has been smoking so long that it might not be possible. Besides, with all the other healthy stuff he is doing, he thinks it probably cancels out the bad effect of the cigarettes. Joel is very concerned that if he does stop smoking, he will gain back all of the weight that it took him so long to lose. ■

In patients with chronic obstructive pulmonary disease, the FEV₁/FVC ratio is less than 70% to 75%. These patients are unable to move most of their exhaled air out of the lungs during the first second because of an obstruction to the airflow, such as inflammation or damaged lung tissue. Based on the FEV₁/FVC ratio, the obstruction is characterized as mild (61% to 69%), moderate (45% to 60%), or severe (less than 45%). Figure 27-12 shows a graph of spirometry parameters in a patient with healthy lungs and in a patient with obstructive pulmonary disease.

Evaluation of Results

To evaluate the spirometry test results fully, certain demographic factors must be taken into consideration, including the patient's age, sex, weight, and height. These demographic factors are used to calculate the *predicted values,* which is what the results should be for a patient with healthy lungs. When the test is run, the physician compares the patient's *measured values* with the predicted values. For example, the FVC predicted value is 6 liters, and the FVC measured value is 4 liters. This means that the patient should have been able to exhale 6 liters of air (based on age, sex, weight, and height), but he or she was able to exhale only 4 liters of air.

The computerized spirometer automatically calculates predicted values using demographic information entered into the machine by the medical assistant. The predicted values and the measured values are printed on the spirometry report. Figure 27-13 shows an example of these results. Comparing the measured values with the predicted values assists the physician in detecting the presence of pulmonary disease.

Patient Preparation

Patient preparation is essential to obtain accurate test results. To prepare for the test, the patient should be instructed to do the following:

Figure 27-12. Spirometry parameters. *FEV₁,* Forced expiratory volume after 1 second; *FVC,* forced vital capacity. (From Bonewit-West K: *Clinical procedures for medical assistants,* ed 7, St. Louis, 2008, Saunders.)

Parameter	Predicted Values	Measured Values
FVC	6.00 liters	4.00 liters
FEV$_1$	5.00 liters	2.00 liters
FEV$_1$/FVC	83%	50%

Figure 27-13. Predicted values compared with measured values. This individual exhibits a moderate airflow obstruction. *FEV$_1$*, Forced expiratory volume after 1 second; *FVC*, forced vital capacity. (From Bonewit-West K: *Clinical procedures for medical assistants,* ed 7, St. Louis, 2008, Saunders.)

1. Do not eat a heavy meal for 8 hours before the test. (The patient must exert the diaphragm muscles, and a full stomach may interfere with this action.)
2. Stop smoking at least 8 hours before the test.
3. Do not take bronchodilators for 4 hours before the test.
4. Do not engage in strenuous activity for 4 hours before the test.
5. Wear loose, nonrestrictive clothing to keep the chest area as free as possible, which makes it easier to perform the breathing maneuver.

Highlight on Smoking and Chronic Obstructive Pulmonary Disease

COPD Defined

Chronic obstructive pulmonary disease (COPD) comprises a group of diseases that includes emphysema, chronic bronchitis, and chronic asthma. It is a chronic, debilitating, and sometimes fatal disease. The primary characteristics associated with COPD are airflow obstruction and shortness of breath.

Currently, 16 million people in the United States have been diagnosed with some form of COPD. Smoking tobacco is the primary cause of COPD, specifically emphysema and chronic bronchitis. In the United States, approximately 80% to 90% of the cases of COPD are caused by smoking. According to the American Lung Association, COPD is the fourth leading cause of death in the United States, behind heart disease, cancer, and strokes. Although COPD is much more common in men than in women, the greatest increase in death rates is occurring in women. This is a direct reflection of an increase in the number of women who smoke cigarettes.

Emphysema

Emphysema is most often seen in older individuals with a long history of smoking. Emphysema is caused by irreversible damage to the alveoli in the lungs from toxins present in cigarette smoke. As alveoli continue to be damaged, the lungs transfer less and less oxygen to the bloodstream. In addition, air becomes trapped in the damaged alveoli, making it difficult to remove during exhalation. Because of this, the primary symptom of emphysema is shortness of breath. Other symptoms include a chronic cough and tiredness. An estimated 2 million people in the United States have emphysema; of these 55% are men, and 45% are women. The reason is not yet understood, but fortunately only 10% to 15% of long-term smokers develop emphysema.

Chronic Bronchitis

Chronic bronchitis is an inflammation of the lining the bronchiole tubes that causes swelling and excess production of mucus. The swelling and excess mucus narrow the bronchiole tubes and restrict airflow into and out of the lungs. Symptoms include a chronic cough, shortness of breath, and coughing up of mucus. To be classified as chronic bronchitis, the symptoms must last 3 months or more out of the year for at least 2 years. As the disease progresses, the lips and skin may exhibit cyanosis resulting from a lack of oxygen in the blood. Chronic bronchitis affects individuals of all ages and often precedes or accompanies emphysema. It is estimated that 12 million Americans have chronic bronchitis.

Symptoms of COPD

Damage to the lungs caused by smoking occurs gradually over many years. Because there are no early symptoms, many people do not know they have COPD. By the time an individual experiences symptoms, it is usually a sign that irreversible lung damage has already occurred. The first symptoms of COPD include mild shortness of breath on exertion and occasional coughing. The disease slowly becomes more pronounced with severe episodes of dyspnea and coughing even after modest activity. As the disease progresses, the heart can also be affected, and the shortness of breath is present all the time, even while sitting quietly. At this point, the individual's quality of life is greatly diminished. When the lungs and heart are no longer able to deliver oxygen to the body's tissues, death occurs.

Treatment for COPD

The best treatment for COPD caused by smoking is for the patient to stop smoking. Continued smoking makes the COPD worse; quitting smoking slows the disease process. Programs, support groups, and stop-smoking aids (e.g., nicotine patch) are available to help individuals quit smoking. Other forms of treatment depend on the patient's condition and degree of lung impairment and may include the following:

1. Bronchodilators to relax and widen the bronchial tubes to increase airflow. They may be inhaled as aerosol sprays or taken orally.
2. Expectorants to thin the mucus so that is easier to expel.
3. Antibiotics to treat infections that could interfere further with breathing and lung function.
4. Breathing exercises to strengthen the muscles used to breathe.
5. Postural bronchial drainage to remove mucus from the bronchial tubes. The patient lies in positions that allow gravity to drain different parts of the bronchiole tubes.
6. Maintaining overall good health habits, which include proper nutrition, adequate sleep, and regular exercise.
7. Oxygen therapy for patients with low blood oxygen to help with shortness of breath, allowing them to be more active.
8. Special measures include avoiding extremes (heat and cold) of temperature, getting an annual influenza immunization, avoiding individuals with respiratory infections, and reducing exposure to air pollution.
9. Lung transplantation surgery is being performed on some patients who are in the later stages of COPD. ∎

What Would You Do? What Would You *Not* Do?

Case Study 3

Walter Conrad, 62 years old, comes to the office because he has been getting short of breath when he goes up and down stairs. He has worked in coal mines his whole life and has just retired. The physician orders a pulmonary function test. Walter tries to breathe like he is supposed to during the test, but he cannot do it and is getting dizzy from trying so hard. He is also having problems with the nose clips. He says they pinch his nose, and he feels like he is being smothered. After four attempts, he puts down the spirometer in frustration and wants to know if he can come back some other time. He says that he is thinking his symptoms are not that bad after all, and maybe he will just wait and see what happens and come back if it they get worse. ■

Calibration of the Spirometer

To ensure accurate and valid test results, the spirometer should be calibrated each day that the machine is used. Calibration is performed by injecting a known quantity of

better result

air into the spirometer. A large 3-liter spirometry syringe is used to inject 3 liters of air into the machine. The output should read 3 L, and the reading should not vary by more than 3%. If the machine is not properly calibrated, the medical assistant should consult the operating manual and adjust the machine as required.

Postbronchodilator Spirometry

If the results of the spirometry test indicate a possible obstruction, the physician usually orders a postbronchodilator spirometry test. This test is performed by having the patient inhale a bronchodilator and running a spirometry test approximately 10 to 15 minutes later. The purpose of this test is to inform the physician as to how treatment would work in patients whose airways are obstructed. If the FVC or FEV_1 parameter increases by at least 15%, the result is reported as positive for bronchodilator responsiveness. This means that the obstruction may be reversible or partially reversible through the use of medication.

---

see DVD

PROCEDURE 27-2   Spirometry Testing

Outcome Perform a spirometry test.

Equipment/Supplies

- Spirometer
- Disposable tubing
- Disposable mouthpiece
- Disposable nose clips
- Waste container

---

1. **Procedural Step.** Sanitize your hands. Assemble and prepare the equipment. Calibrate the spirometer according to the manufacturer's instructions. Apply a disposable mouthpiece to the mouthpiece holder, which is attached to the spirometer by a cable.
   Principle. Calibration of the spirometer ensures accurate and valid test results.

2. **Procedural Step.** Greet the patient and introduce yourself. Identify the patient and explain the procedure. Tell the patient that he or she will be wearing nose clips and performing a breathing maneuver several times to see how well his or her lungs are functioning. Ask the patient whether he or she prepared properly for the procedure.

3. **Procedural Step.** Prepare the patient. Have the patient remove any heavy or constricting clothing, such as a jacket or a sweater. Also, ask the patient to loosen tight clothing, such as a necktie or a tight collar.
   Principle. Heavy outer clothing and tight clothing may make it difficult for the patient to perform the breathing maneuvers.

4. **Procedural Step.** Measure the patient's weight and height precisely.

   Principle. Precise weight and height measurements are required for the accurate calculation of predicted values.

5. **Procedural Step.** Have the patient sit near the machine. The patient should be seated to prevent dizziness or possible fainting during the procedure. Enter the following data into the computer database of the spirometer: patient's age, sex, weight, height, and any other information required, such as the patient's identification number and whether the patient smokes.
   Principle. Demographic data need to be entered for the computer to calculate the predicted values.

6. **Procedural Step.** Instruct the patient in the breathing maneuver. The following procedure should be described and demonstrated to the patient:
   a. Relax and take the deepest breath possible until your lungs are completely filled with air.
   b. Place the mouthpiece in your mouth, and seal your lips tightly around it.
   c. Blow out as hard as you can and for as long as possible until your lungs are completely empty. Do not block the opening of the mouthpiece with your tongue.

Continued

PROCEDURE 27-2   Spirometry Testing—cont'd

d. Remove the mouthpiece from your mouth.
Principle. The lips must be tightly sealed around the mouthpiece so that all of the air leaving the mouth enters the mouthpiece.

7. **Procedural Step.** Tell the patient you will repeat the instructions during the test. Encourage the patient to remain calm during the procedure. Gently apply nose clips to the patient's nose. Hand the mouthpiece to the patient, and tell him or her to hold it close to the mouth.
Principle. Fear or anxiety can make the results less reliable. Nose clips prevent air from escaping from the nostrils and ensure that all breathing is done through the mouth.

8. **Procedural Step.** Begin the test. When the patient is ready, press the start button on the spirometer. Actively coach the patient as follows:
a. "Now relax and take in a big breath—in—in—in—more—keep inhaling."
b. "Put the mouthpiece in your mouth and blow hard. Keep going—keep going—keep going—more—more—more—you're almost there—a little more. That's good. You can stop now."

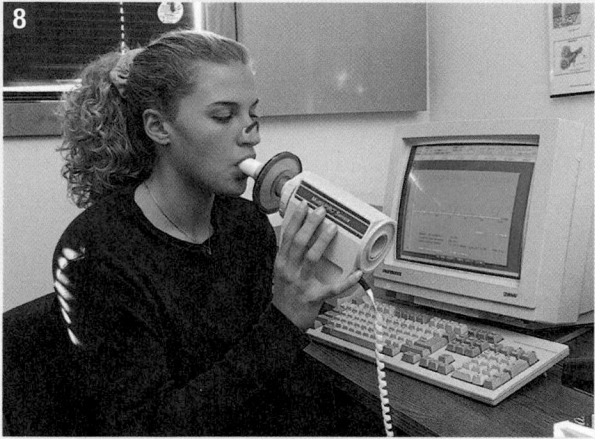

Instruct the patient to blow into the mouthpiece. (From Bonewit-West K: *Clinical procedures for medical assistants,* ed 7, St. Louis, 2008, Saunders.)

c. "Take out the mouthpiece and rest for awhile. You did a great job."
Principle. Coaching the patient helps to obtain accurate test results.

9. **Procedural Step.** If the patient does not perform the breathing maneuver correctly, inform him or her of what modifications are necessary for the next effort. Continue until three acceptable efforts have been obtained.
Principle. Three acceptable efforts must be obtained to ensure valid test results.

10. **Procedural Step.** Gently remove the nose clips from the patient's nose. Remove the mouthpiece from the mouthpiece holder. Dispose of the mouthpiece and nose clips in a regular waste container.

11. **Procedural Step.** Allow the patient to remain seated for a few minutes.
Principle. The patient may feel lightheaded after the procedure.

12. **Procedural Step.** Sanitize your hands. Print the report, and label it with the patient's name, the date, and your initials. Chart the procedure. Include the date, the time, the name of the procedure, and the patient's reaction. Place the spirometry report in the patient's medical record, and put the record in the appropriate place for review by the physician.

13. **Procedural Step.** Clean the spirometer according to the manufacturer's instructions.

CHARTING EXAMPLE

Date	
6/20/10	9:00 a.m. Spirometry test run. Obtained 3 acceptable efforts. Pt stated she was tired following the test. Report to physician for review. ———————— J. Canterbury, CMA (AAMA)

MEDICAL PRACTICE *and the* LAW

Cardiopulmonary procedures are frightening for many patients because of the potential for unfavorable results. These results must never be given to the patient by the medical assistant. Only a physician can interpret results of electrocardiographic and pulmonary function tests. If results indicate a life-threatening condition, your duty is to calmly to notify the physician at once, without alarming the patient. All offices have emergency supplies; be sure you know where they are and how to use them. While you are attending to the machinery and technology, remember the human dignity of the patient and attend to all of his or her needs for privacy, comfort, respect, and caring. ■

What Would You Do? What Would You *Not* Do? RESPONSES

Case Study 1
Page 642

What Did Janet Do?
❑ Tried to reduce Camilla's fears by talking with her calmly and quietly.
❑ Explained to Camilla that an ECG is the best screening test available to check for heart problems.
❑ Reassured Camilla that she would be draped during the procedure and that she would be exposed as little as possible.
❑ Told Camilla that the wires may look a little scary, but there is no chance of being shocked by them. Explained that she won't feel anything when the test is being run.
❑ Told Camilla that she could talk with the billing clerk about setting up a payment plan for the test. Provided her with information about community resources that might help her pay for the test.

What Did Janet Not *Do?*
❑ Did not tell Camilla that she was too young to have heart problems.
❑ Did not tell Camilla that she needed to act more mature about being tested.

What Would You Do?/What Would You *Not* Do? Review Janet's response and place a checkmark next to the information you included in your response. List additional information you included in your response.

_____
_____
_____
_____

Case Study 2
Page 651

What Did Janet Do?
❑ Commended Joel on his weight loss and positive lifestyle changes.
❑ Shared a positive story with Joel about a patient who stopped smoking and did not gain weight.
❑ Asked Joel whether he would like any of the latest information on smoking cessation.

What Did Janet Not *Do?*
❑ Did not agree that Joel's positive lifestyle changes would counteract the bad effects of smoking.

❑ Did not lecture Joel on the dangers of smoking because if he has been smoking since age 17 and has been trying to quit, he already knows what they are.

What Would You Do?/What Would You *Not* Do? Review Janet's response and place a checkmark next to the information you included in your response. List additional information you included in your response.

_____
_____
_____
_____

Case Study 3
Page 653

What Did Janet Do?
❑ Removed the nose clips and empathized with Mr. Conrad that the test is hard to do and that the nose clips do fit very snugly.
❑ Explained to Mr. Conrad that it is normal to feel dizzy and that it is only temporary.
❑ Allowed Mr. Conrad to rest for awhile. Tried to relax and calm him by talking with him about his family and interests.
❑ Talked to Mr. Conrad about the importance of performing the test. Told him that detecting a problem early would help him get the treatment he needs as soon as possible so that his condition will not get worse.
❑ Asked Mr. Conrad whether he would try the test one more time.

What Did Janet Not *Do?*
❑ Did not criticize Mr. Conrad for not being able to perform the test.
❑ Did not force Mr. Conrad to stay if he did not want to, but scheduled another pulmonary function test for him before he left the office.

What Would You Do?/What Would You *Not* Do? Review Janet's response and place a checkmark next to the information you included in your response. List additional information you included in your response.

_____
_____
_____
_____

TERMINOLOGY REVIEW

Amplitude Refers to amount, extent, size, abundance, or fullness.

Artifact Additional electrical activity picked up by the electrocardiograph that interferes with the normal appearance of the electrocardiogram cycles.

Atherosclerosis Buildup of fibrous plaques of fatty deposits and cholesterol on the inner walls of the coronary arteries.

Baseline The flat horizontal line that separates the various waves of the electrocardiogram cycle.

Cardiac cycle One complete heartbeat.

Dysrhythmia An irregular heart rhythm; also termed *arrhythmia.*

ECG cycle The graphic representation of a heartbeat.

Electrocardiogram (ECG) The graphic representation of the electrical activity of the heart.

Electrocardiograph The instrument used to record the electrical activity of the heart.

Electrode A conductor of electricity, which is used to promote contact between the body and the electrocardiograph.

Electrolyte A chemical substance that promotes conduction of an electrical current.

Interval The length of a wave or the length of a wave with a segment.

Ischemia Deficiency of blood in a body part.

Normal sinus rhythm Refers to an electrocardiogram that is within normal limits.

Segment The portion of the electrocardiogram between two waves.

Spirometer An instrument for measuring air taken into and expelled from the lungs.

Spirometry Measurement of an individual's breathing capacity by means of a spirometer.

ON THE WEB

For Information on Heart Disease:

American Heart Association: www.americanheart.org

National Heart, Lung, and Blood Institute: www.nhlbi.nih.gov

American Association of Cardiovascular and Pulmonary Rehabilitation: www.aacvpr.org

Health Centers Online: www.healthcentersonline.com

Heart Information Network: www.heartinfo.org

Cardiology Channel: www.cardiologychannel.com

American College of Cardiology: www.acc.org

The National Coalition for Women with Heart Disease: www.womenheart.org

For Information on Lung Disease:

American Lung Association: www.lungusa.org

Pulmonary Channel: www.pulmonarychannel.com

Lung Cancer Online: www.lungcanceronline.org

American Association for Respiratory Care: www.aarc.org

For Information on Smoking Cessation:

The Foundation for a Smokefree America: www.antismoking.org

Quit Net: www.quitnet.com

Habitrol Support Program: www.habitrol.com

National Center for Tobacco-Free Kids: www.tobaccofreekids.org

Why Quit.com: www.whyquit.com

Quit Smoking Now: www.smokefree.gov

The Quit Smoking Company: www.quitsmoking.com

PREPARE FOR CERTIFICATION   Visit the Evolve site at http://evolve.elsevier.com/Bonewit/today/ to actively Prepare for your Certification.

 *Check out the **Companion CD** bound with the book to access additional interactive activities.*

28

Specialty Examinations and Procedures:
Colon Procedures
Male Reproductive Health
Radiology and Diagnostic Imaging

LEARNING OBJECTIVES

Fecal Occult Blood Testing
1. Explain the purpose of a fecal occult blood test.
2. Describe the patient preparation for fecal occult blood testing.
3. Explain the purpose of each type of preparation for fecal occult blood testing.

Flexible Sigmoidoscopy
1. Explain the purpose of a digital rectal examination (DRE) before a sigmoidoscopic examination.
2. Explain the purpose of a flexible sigmoidoscopy.
3. Describe the patient preparation for a flexible sigmoidoscopy.
4. State the responsibilities of the medical assistant during a sigmoidoscopy.

Male Reproductive Health
1. List the symptoms of prostate cancer.
2. Explain how the DRE is used for the early detection of prostate cancer.
3. Describe how the PSA test is used to screen for the presence of prostate cancer.

Radiology
1. State the function of radiographs in medicine.
2. Explain the importance of proper patient preparation for a radiographic examination.
3. Explain how to prevent the radiograph from becoming obscured or blurred.
4. Explain the function of a contrast medium.
5. Describe the purpose of a fluoroscope.
6. Explain the purpose of each of the following types of radiographic examinations:
   Mammography
   Upper GI
   Lower GI
   Intravenous pyelography

PROCEDURES

Instruct a patient in the procedure for a fecal occult blood test.
Develop a fecal occult blood test.

Instruct a patient in the preparation for a flexible sigmoidoscopy.
Assist the physician with flexible sigmoidoscopy.

Assist the physician with a DRE.
Instruct a patient in the preparation for a prostate-specific antigen (PSA) test.
Teach a patient how to perform a testicular self-examination.

Instruct a patient in the proper preparation necessary for each of the following types of radiographic examinations:
   Mammography
   Upper gastrointestinal (GI)
   Lower GI
   Intravenous pyelography

LEARNING OBJECTIVES

Diagnostic Imaging

1. Explain the purpose of each of the following diagnostic imaging procedures:
   - Ultrasonography
   - Computed tomography (CT)
   - Magnetic resonance imaging (MRI)
   - Nuclear medicine
2. Explain how nuclear medicine is used to produce an image of a body part or organ.
3. State the guidelines that may be required for nuclear medicine.

Digital Radiology

1. Explain the advantages of digital radiology.

PROCEDURES

Instruct a patient in the purpose and advance preparation for each of the following diagnostic imaging procedures:
- Ultrasonography
- CT
- MRI
- Nuclear medicine

CHAPTER OUTLINE

COLON PROCEDURES
Introduction to Colon Procedures
Fecal Occult Blood Testing
   Guaiac Slide Test
Flexible Sigmoidoscopy
   Patient Preparation for Sigmoidoscopy
   Digital Rectal Examination
   Flexible Sigmoidoscope
MALE REPRODUCTIVE HEALTH
Introduction to Male Reproductive Health
Prostate Cancer Screening
   Digital Rectal Examination
   Prostate-Specific Antigen Test
Testicular Self-Examination
RADIOLOGY AND DIAGNOSTIC IMAGING
Introduction to Radiology
Contrast Media

Fluoroscopy
Positioning the Patient
Specific Radiographic Examinations
   Mammography
   Gastrointestinal Series
   Intravenous Pyelography
   Other Types of Radiographs
Introduction to Diagnostic Imaging
Ultrasonography
   Patient Preparation
Computed Tomography
   Patient Preparation
Magnetic Resonance Imaging
   Patient Preparation
Nuclear Medicine
   Guidelines
Digital Radiology

CAAHEP COMPETENCIES

Clinical Competencies
Specimen Collection
- Instruct patients in the collection of fecal specimens.

Patient Care
- Prepare and maintain examination and treatment areas.
- Prepare patients for and assist with routine and specialty examinations.

General Competencies
Patient Instruction
- Instruct individuals according to their needs.
- Provide instruction for health maintenance and disease prevention.

Operational Functions
- Use methods of quality control.

ABHES COMPETENCIES

Clinical Duties
- Prepare patients for procedures.
- Prepare and maintain examination and treatment areas.
- Prepare patient for and assist physician with routine and specialty examinations and treatments and minor office surgeries.
- Use quality control.
- Instruct patient in the collection of fecal specimen.

Instruction
- Instruct patients with special needs.
- Teach patients methods of health promotion and disease prevention.

KEY TERMS

biopsy (BIE-op-see)
colonoscopy (KOL-un-OS-koe-pee)
contrast medium
echocardiogram (EK-oh-KAR-dee-oh-gram)
endoscope (EN-doe-skope)
enema (EN-em-ah)
fluoroscope (FLOOR-oh-skope)
fluoroscopy (floor-OS-koe-pee)
insufflate (IN-suf-flate)
melena (ma-lee-na)
occult (ah-KULT) blood

peroxidase (per-OKS-ih-dase)
radiograph (RAY-dee-oh-graf)
radiography (ray-dee-OG-rah-fee)
radiologist (ray-dee-AH-lah-jist)
radiology (ray-dee-AH-lah-jee)
radiolucent (ray-dee-oh-LOO-sent)
radiopaque (ray-dee-oh-PAYK)
sigmoidoscope (sig-MOYD-oh-skope)
sigmoidoscopy (sig-moyd-OS-koe-pee)
sonogram (SON-oh-gram)
ultrasonography (ul-trah-son-AH-grah-fee)

Colon Procedures

Introduction to Colon Procedures

Colon procedures are performed in the medical office and include the fecal occult blood test and the flexible sigmoidoscopic examination, which are presented in this chapter. Some patients initially may be reluctant to perform a fecal occult blood test at home. The medical assistant can help by explaining the purpose of the test to the patient. If the patient understands the beneficial results to be derived from the test, he or she is more likely to participate as required. The medical assistant aids the physician during a sigmoidoscopy, and he or she should have a thorough knowledge of the responsibilities accompanying this procedure.

FECAL OCCULT BLOOD TESTING

Blood in the stool can indicate a number of conditions, including hemorrhoids, diverticulosis, polyps, colitis, upper gastrointestinal (GI) ulcers, and colorectal cancer. Some of these conditions produce visible red blood on the outside of the stool, making it easy to detect. Blood entering the stool from the upper GI tract in an amount of 50 ml or greater causes the stool to exhibit **melena,** meaning it is black and tarlike. The dark color is a result of the oxidation of the iron in the blood (heme) by intestinal and bacterial enzymes. If a minute quantity of blood is present, however, it is not possible to detect it with the unaided eye. This hidden, or nonvisible, blood is termed **occult blood,** and its presence can be determined only through chemical or microscopic analysis.

Colorectal cancer is one of the most common forms of cancer in individuals older than the age of 40 years. During the early asymptomatic stages, almost all neoplasms of the colon and rectum bleed a small amount on an intermittent basis, and this takes the form of occult blood. Discovering occult blood is of particular importance for the early diagnosis and treatment of colorectal cancer, which increases the patient's survival rate. In most cases, when more pronounced symptoms of colorectal cancer start appearing (e.g., visible bleeding, a change in bowel habits, abdominal pain), the condition has reached an advanced stage.

Guaiac Slide Test

Routine screening of stool specimens for occult blood is frequently performed in the medical office. The guaiac slide test is most often used and is commercially available with brand names of Hemoccult and ColoScreen (Figure 28-1). Fecal blood loss greater than 5 ml per day results in a positive reaction. Patients may normally lose up to 3 ml per day of blood in the feces, owing to minor insignificant abrasions of the nasopharynx and GI tract. To allow for normal blood loss, the test does not show a positive reaction until it reaches a level of 5 ml (or more) per day.

The guaiac slide test is a simple and inexpensive method to screen for the presence of occult blood; however, care must be taken to reduce the occurrence of false-positive or false-negative results. This test is designed to assess the presence of blood in stool specimens collected from three bowel movements on 3 different days. The purpose of using three specimens is to provide for the detection of blood from GI lesions that exhibit intermittent bleeding, meaning they do not bleed every day. Because three stool specimens are required, the patient must collect the specimens at home and return the prepared slides to the medical office for developing. The medical assistant is responsible for providing the patient with instructions on patient preparation and collection and proper care and storage of the slides until they are returned to the medical office.

Figure 28-1. Examples of fecal occult blood testing kits. Hemoccult *(top)* and ColoScreen *(bottom).* (From Bonewit-West K: *Clinical procedures for medical assistants*, ed 7, St. Louis, 2008, Saunders.)

Although the primary use of the guaiac slide test is to screen for colorectal cancer, other important uses include screening for occult blood for the detection of an upper GI ulcer or for disorders causing gastric and intestinal irritation. A positive test result on the guaiac slide test indicates blood in the stool, although the cause of the bleeding still must be determined. Further diagnostic procedures must be performed before the physician can make a final diagnosis; these tests may include flexible sigmoidoscopy, **colonoscopy,** and a double-contrast barium enema radiographic study.

Patient Preparation

Patient preparation plays an important role in ensuring accurate test results. The patient must follow a special diet, beginning 3 days before the guaiac slide test and continuing until all three slides have been prepared. The patient is placed on a high-fiber, meat-free diet. Meat contains animal blood that could lead to a false-positive test result. A high-fiber diet is used because it encourages bleeding from lesions that may bleed only occasionally. In addition, the fiber adds bulk, which promotes bowel elimination and ensures adequate specimen collection.

Certain medications irritate the GI tract, which may result in a small amount of bleeding and thus result in a false-positive test result on the guaiac slide test. Medications that irritate the GI tract include aspirin, indomethacin, phenylbutazone, and corticosteroids. In addition, an iron supplement could cause a false-positive result, and a vitamin C supplement (greater than 250 mg per day) can cause a false-negative result. All of these substances should be discontinued before testing. The Patient Teaching box *Patient Preparation for Fecal Occult Blood Testing* lists the specific patient preparation requirements and their purposes.

Putting It All into Practice

My name is Megan Baer, and I work in a large medical office that includes the specialties of family practice, proctology, allergies, and internal medicine. I am the medical office clinical supervisor and oversee all of the clinical medical assistants and our "in-house" laboratory. I work closely with all physicians to meet the growing needs of the medical office.

Working with a proctologist has been interesting and educational. When preparing a patient for a flexible sigmoidoscopy, you must help the patient feel relaxed. This is an embarrassing situation for the patient, so you need to make him or her feel as comfortable as possible and maintain the patient's privacy and modesty. During the procedure, I talk to the patients about the weather, their pets, and other interests to make them feel more relaxed and comfortable with me. This can help take their mind off the procedure.

One day I was assisting with a sigmoidoscopic examination, and a few minutes into the procedure the look on the physician's face told me something was wrong. When the examination was finished, the physician and I left the room and went back to his office. He informed me that what he saw on his examination was colorectal cancer, and at this stage, not much could be done for the patient. The worst thing a physician has to do is give unpleasant news to a patient and see the look on the patient's face. This is something you don't forget, going into the room of a patient who has just received life-threatening information. All you can do is be sympathetic and understanding and be a good listener. You have to be strong and not show your emotions even though your heart is breaking for the patient and the family. Always let patients know you are there for them.

Being with a patient who receives bad news about his or her health can make you think about your own life, and how it not only affects you, but also your family and friends. I often think of how I would feel about receiving such news. I try to put myself in the patient's place and be sincere and understanding and willing to lend an ear. ∎

Prepare for Success

Quality Control

Quality control methods must be employed with the guaiac slide test to ensure reliable and valid results. The quality control procedure should be performed after the patient's slide test has been developed, read, and interpreted. The Hemoccult slide test contains an on-slide performance monitor that consists of positive and negative monitor areas. This monitor is located on the developing side of the filter paper under the back flap of the cardboard slide. The positive monitor area contains a control chemical that has been impregnated into the filter paper during the manufacturing process.

The medical assistant should apply 1 drop of the developing solution between the positive and negative

| PATIENT TEACHING | Patient Preparation for the Fecal Occult Guaiac Slide Test |

Testing

Beginning 3 days before obtaining the first stool specimen, the patient should follow certain diet and medication modifications. These modifications should be followed until all three slides have been prepared.

Meats. Eat no red or rare meat (beef and lamb) or processed meats and liver. Small amounts of well-cooked pork, poultry, and fish are permitted. Red meat contains animal blood that could cause a false-positive test result.

Vegetables. Eat moderate amounts of raw and cooked vegetables. Especially advised are lettuce, spinach, corn, and celery. Do not consume horseradish, turnips, broccoli, cauliflower, and radishes. These foods contain **peroxidase,** which could cause a false-positive test result.

Fruits. Eat moderate amounts of apples, bananas, oranges, peaches, pears, and plums. Avoid vitamin C in excess of 250 mg a day from citrus fruits and juices. Do not consume melons because they contain peroxidase.

Miscellaneous high-fiber foods. Eat moderate amounts of whole-wheat bread, bran cereal, and popcorn. Foods high in fiber provide roughage to promote bowel elimination and encourage bleeding from lesions that bleed only occasionally.

Medications. Do not take medications that contain iron or vitamin C in excess of 250 mg for 3 days before and during the collection period. In addition, based on the patient's medication therapy, the physician may stipulate additional medication restrictions. Certain medications cause irritation of the gastrointestinal (GI) tract, which may result in a small amount of bleeding. Aspirin and other nonsteroidal antiinflammatory drugs should be avoided for at least 7 days before and continuing through the test period. Acetaminophen (Tylenol) can be taken as needed.

Special guidelines

Inform the physician, and do not consume any of the food items listed previously if you know, from past experience, that they cause you severe GI discomfort or serious diarrhea. Ensure that the diet modifications have been followed for 3 days before collecting the first stool specimen.

Do not initiate the test during a menstrual period or in the first 3 days after a menstrual period. The test should not be conducted when there is visible blood in the stool or urine, such as from bleeding from hemorrhoids or a urinary tract infection. These conditions would result in false-positive test results.

If you are using a toilet bowel cleaning device, remove the device and flush the toilet twice before proceeding with the first bowel movement.

Store the slides at room temperature, and protect them from heat, sunlight, and fluorescent light to prevent deterioration of the active reagents on the slides. ■

Highlight on Colorectal Cancer

Incidence

Colorectal cancer is the second leading cause of cancer-related deaths in the United States, with the most common being lung cancer. According to the American Cancer Society, every year approximately 150,000 people are diagnosed with colorectal cancer, and approximately 56,000 die every year from this disease. As the U.S. population ages, these numbers will increase.

Risk Factors

The risk of colorectal cancer begins to increase after age 40 years and reaches a peak from age 60 to 75 years. Other factors that increase the risk of colorectal cancer include a family history of colorectal cancer, personal history of colorectal polyps, and history of inflammatory bowel disease of a long duration (e.g., ulcerative colitis, Crohn's disease). Most colorectal cancer arises from polyps that gradually become malignant over many years. A polyp is a grapelike growth that protrudes from the inner lining of the colon or rectum. Polyps are fairly common in individuals older than 50 years of age. Approximately 1 in 20 polyps can become cancerous if not removed.

Symptoms

There are no symptoms during the early stages of colorectal cancer. If colorectal cancer is detected and treated while the patient is still asymptomatic, the patient has an 80% chance of 5-year survival. By comparison, the 5-year survival rate for patients in whom colorectal cancer is diagnosed after symptoms appear is only 40%.

Symptoms that may occur when colorectal cancer has developed include the following:

- Bleeding from the rectum
- Blood in the stool
- A change in the shape of the stool (e.g., stools that are narrower than usual)
- A change in bowel habits (e.g., diarrhea, constipation)
- General abdominal discomfort (e.g., aches, pains, cramps)
- Unexplained weight loss
- Constant fatigue

Recommendations for Early Detection

For the early detection of colorectal cancer, the American Cancer Society recommends that all adults 50 years old and older who are at average risk for colorectal cancer be screened according to the following schedule:

Beginning at age 50, have a fecal occult blood test and a flexible sigmoidoscopy; repeat the fecal occult blood test annually and the sigmoidoscopy every 5 years,

Continued

PROCEDURE 28-1

Highlight on Colorectal Cancer—cont'd

or have a colonoscopy at 10-year intervals,

or have a double-contrast barium enema every 5 to 10 years.

Individuals who have a family history of colorectal cancer should begin screening at 40 years of age.

Cause

The cause of colorectal cancer is unknown, but studies have shown that there is a higher incidence of this disease in countries, such as the United States, whose populations have a diet that is high in meat and animal fat and low in fiber. This finding is supported by the fact that in countries such as Japan, in which the diet is high in fiber and low in fat, the incidence of colorectal cancer is much lower. ◼

What Would You Do? What Would You *Not* Do?

Case Study 1

Beatrice Bernard is 52 years old and has come to the office for a physical examination. The physician wants Mrs. Bernard to perform a Hemoccult test. After being told the purpose of the test and how to prepare for it, Mrs. Bernard expresses some concerns. She does not like the idea of what she has to do to perform the test because it does not seem sanitary to her. She also thinks it will be a lot of work to prepare for the test. She has red meat for dinner at least four times a week, and she does not understand why she has to eliminate it from her meals. She says she takes a baby aspirin every day for "heart health" and would prefer not to stop taking it. Mrs. Bernard says that she has always taken very good care of herself, and she has never had problems with her colon. She also says that there is no history of colon cancer in her family. Mrs. Bernard is too embarrassed to talk about this topic with the physician. She says she may just throw the test away when she gets home. ◼

performance monitor areas. The results must be read within 10 seconds after application of the developer. If the slide and developer are functioning properly, the positive area turns blue, whereas the negative area shows no color change. Failure of the expected control results to occur indicates an error, and the test results are not considered valid; possible causes include the use of outdated cards or developing solution; an error in technique; and subjection of the slides to heat, sunlight, or strong fluorescent light. Procedure 28-1 outlines the medical assistant's responsibilities related to fecal occult blood testing. Procedure 28-2 describes the development of a Hemoccult slide test.

PROCEDURE 28-1 Fecal Occult Blood Testing: Guaiac Slide Test

Outcome Instruct a patient in specimen collection for a Hemoccult guaiac slide test.

Equipment/Supplies

- Hemoccult slide testing kit

1. Procedural Step. Obtain a Hemoccult slide testing kit. Check the expiration date on the slides.
Principle. Outdated slides can lead to inaccurate test results.

2. Procedural Step. Greet the patient and introduce yourself. Identify the patient and explain the purpose of the test. Tell the patient that the test should not be conducted during a menstrual period or when hemorrhoids are bleeding or a urinary tract infection is present.
Principle. Bleeding from other (identifiable) sources causes a false-positive test result.

3. Procedural Step. Instruct the patient in the proper preparation for the test. See the box *Highlight on Colorectal Cancer* for the specific guidelines the patient should follow. Tell the patient to begin the diet

Check the expiration date. (From Bonewit-West K: *Clinical procedures for medical assistants,* ed 7, St. Louis, 2008, Saunders.)

modifications 3 days before collecting the first stool specimen. Encourage the patient to adhere to the diet modifications.

Principle. The diet modifications may discourage patient compliance. The medical assistant should reinforce the importance of adhering to the diet requirements. Improper patient preparation can lead to inaccurate test results.

4. **Procedural Step.** Provide the patient with the Hemoccult slide test kit. The kit consists of three identical cardboard slides attached to one another; each slide contains two squares, labeled "A" and "B." Three wooden applicator sticks and written instructions are also included in the testing kit.

Principle. Three slides are provided so that three stool specimens can be collected. The two squares in each slide (A and B) contain filter paper impregnated with guaiac, a chemical necessary for detection of blood in the stool.

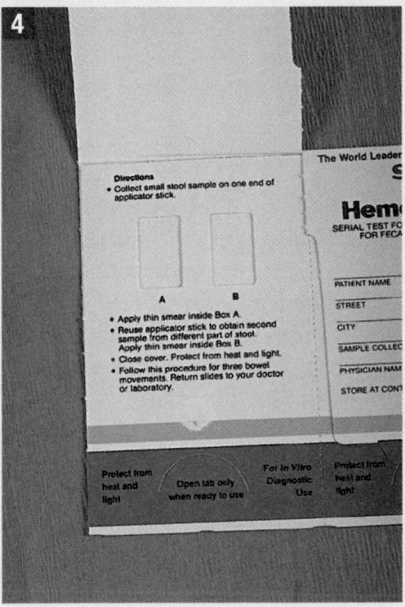

Each slide contains two squares labeled "A" and "B." (From Bonewit-West K: *Clinical procedures for medical assistants,* ed 7, St. Louis, 2008, Saunders.)

5. **Procedural Step.** Instruct the patient in the completion of the information required on the front flap of each card. This includes the patient's name, address, phone number, and age and the date of the specimen collection. A ballpoint pen should be used to write this information.

6. **Procedural Step.** Provide instructions on the proper care and storage of the slides. Make it clear that the slides must be stored at room temperature and protected from heat, sunlight, and strong fluorescent light.

Principle. Adverse storage conditions can result in deterioration of the active reagents impregnated on the filter paper, leading to inaccurate test results.

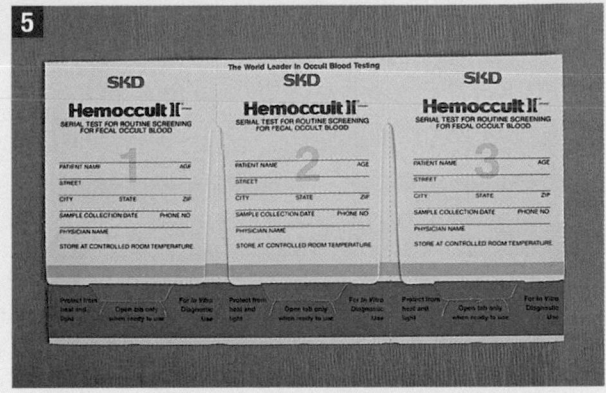

Instruct the patient on how to complete the information section on the slides. (From Bonewit-West K: *Clinical procedures for medical assistants,* ed 7, St. Louis, 2008, Saunders.)

7. **Procedural Step.** Instruct the patient in the initiation of the test by telling him or her to begin the diet modifications and then to collect a stool specimen from the first bowel movement after the 3-day preparatory period.

8. **Procedural Step.** Instruct the patient in the proper collection of the stool specimen:
   a. Fill in the sample collection date on the front flap of the first cardboard slide.
   b. Use a clean, dry container to collect the stool sample. The sample must be collected before it comes in contact with toilet bowl water. Allow the stool to fall into the collection container.
   c. Use one of the wooden applicators to obtain a specimen from one part of the stool sample.
   d. Open the front flap of the first cardboard slide (located on the left in the series of three).
   e. Spread a very thin smear of the specimen over the filter paper in the square labeled "A."
   f. Using the other end of the same wooden applicator, obtain another specimen from a different area of the stool.
   g. Spread a thin smear of the specimen over the filter paper in the square labeled "B."

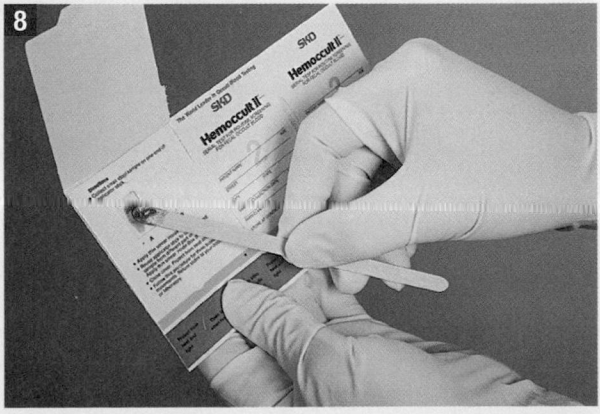

Spread a thin smear of the specimen over the filter paper. (From Bonewit-West K: *Clinical procedures for medical assistants,* ed 7, St. Louis, 2008, Saunders.)

Continued

PROCEDURE 28-1

PROCEDURE 28-1   Fecal Occult Blood Testing: Guaiac Slide Test—cont'd

h. Close the front flap of the cardboard slide.

i. Discard the wooden applicator in a waste container. Do not flush it down the toilet.

j. Place the slides in a regular paper envelope to air-dry overnight.

Principle. Two squares are included in each slide to allow specimen collection from different parts of the stool because occult blood is not always uniformly distributed throughout the stool (e.g., when bleeding occurs from the lower GI tract). Thick specimens prevent adequate light penetration through the filter paper, making it difficult to interpret the test results.

9. **Procedural Step.** Instruct the patient to continue the testing period on 3 different days until all three specimens have been obtained as follows.

a. Repeat Procedural Step 8 after the second bowel movement the next day. If you do not have a bowel movement on the next day, then collect the specimen on the following day. The specimens should be collected on 3 different days. Use the cardboard slide located in the middle of the series of three.

b. Repeat Procedural Step 8 after the third bowel movement, using the cardboard slide located to the right in the series of three.

c. Allow the completed slides to air-dry overnight in the paper envelope.

10. **Procedural Step.** Instruct the patient to place the cardboard slides in the envelope lined with foil, seal carefully, and return them as soon as possible to the medical office. Emphasize to the patient that only the foil-lined envelope can be used to mail the slides; a standard envelope cannot be used.

Principle. Standard paper envelopes are not approved by U.S. postal regulations for mailing fecal occult blood testing slides.

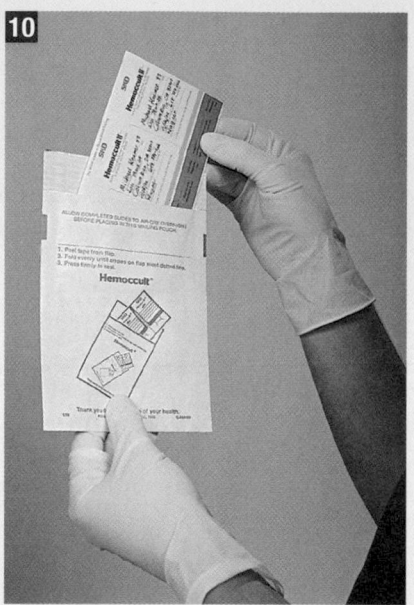

Place the cardboard slides in the envelope. (From Bonewit-West K: *Clinical procedures for medical assistants,* ed 7, St. Louis, 2008, Saunders.)

11. **Procedural Step.** Give the patient an opportunity to ask questions; ensure that the patient understands the instructions for patient preparation and collection of the stool specimen and for storage of the slides.

Principle. Improper patient preparation and poor collection technique can lead to inaccurate test results.

12. **Procedural Step.** Record in the patient's chart. Include the date and documentation that the Hemoccult test and instructions were given to the patient.

Note: The ColoScreen guaiac slide test uses a procedure similar to that of Hemoccult.

PROCEDURE 28-2   Developing the Hemoccult Slide Test

Outcome Develop a Hemoccult slide test.

Equipment/Supplies

- Disposable gloves
- Prepared cardboard slides
- Hemoccult developing solution
- Waste container

1. **Procedural Step.** Assemble the equipment. The reference card provides an illustration of positive and negative test results, which can be used as a guide in interpreting results. *Note:* The slides may be developed immediately or stored (at room temperature) for up to 14 days before developing.

2. **Procedural Step.** Check the expiration date on the developing solution bottle. The developing solution contains hydrogen peroxide. It should be stored away from heat and light and tightly capped when not in use.

Principle. Outdated solution should not be used because it can lead to inaccurate test results. The solution should be stored properly because it is flammable and evaporates easily.

3. **Procedural Step.** Sanitize your hands, and apply gloves. Open the back flap of the cardboard slides. Apply 2

drops of the developing solution to the guaiac test paper underlying the back of each smear.

Principle. The developing solution is absorbed through the filter paper and into the stool specimen. This solution could irritate the skin and eyes; if contact occurs, immediately rinse the area with water.

Apply 2 drops of developing solution. (From Bonewit-West K: *Clinical procedures for medical assistants,* ed 7, St. Louis, 2008, Saunders.)

4. Procedural Step. Read the results within 60 seconds. Fecal blood loss greater than 5 ml per day results in a positive reaction, which is indicated by any trace of blue on or at the edge of the fecal smear. If no detectable color change occurs, the result is considered negative.

Principle. In the presence of hydrogen peroxide, the heme compound in hemoglobin oxidizes guaiac,

causing it to turn blue within 60 seconds after adding the developer. The reading time is important because the color reaction may fade after 2 to 4 minutes.

5. Procedural Step. Perform the quality control procedure.

Principle. Quality control procedures ensure the accuracy and reliability of the test results.

6. Procedural Step. Properly dispose of the Hemoccult slides in a regular waste container.

Principle. Fecal material is not considered regulated medical waste and can be discarded in a regular waste container.

7. Procedural Step. Remove gloves, and sanitize your hands. Chart the results. Include the date and time, the brand name of the test (Hemoccult), and the test results for each slide (recorded as positive or negative).

PROCEDURE 28-2

CHARTING EXAMPLE

Date	*Patient verblize understad*
9/08/10	9:00 a.m. Pt provided with a Hemoccult test and instructions for the procedure.
	——————————— M. Baer, CMA (AAMA)
9/14/10	10:30 a.m. Hemoccult test:
	Slide 1: Negative
	Slide 2: Negative
	Slide 3: Positive
	——————————— M. Baer, CMA (AAMA)

4 **INTERPRETING THE HEMOCCULT® TEST**

Negative Smears

Sample report: negative
No detectable blue on or at the edge of the smears indicates the test is negative for occult blood. (See **LIMITATIONS OF PROCEDURE**.)

Negative and Positive Smears

Positive Smears

Sample report: positive
Any trace of blue on or at the edge of one or more of the smears indicates the test is positive for occult blood.

SKD **SmithKline Diagnostics, Inc.**
A SMITHKLINE BECKMAN COMPANY
San Jose, CA 95134-1622

(From Bonewit-West K: *Clinical procedures for medical assistants,* ed 7, St. Louis, 2008, Saunders.)

FLEXIBLE SIGMOIDOSCOPY

Flexible **sigmoidoscopy** is the visual examination of the mucosa of the rectum and lower third of the colon using a flexible fiberoptic **sigmoidoscope**. The Sims position is recommended for flexible sigmoidoscopy. Sigmoidoscopy may be performed to detect lesions, polyps, hemorrhoids, fissures, infection, and inflammation or to determine the cause of rectal bleeding. It is especially valuable as a diagnostic procedure for the early detection of symptomatic and asymptomatic colorectal cancer. If an abnormal area is detected, a **biopsy** is performed for histologic examination. Early detection of colorectal cancer leads to early diagnosis and treatment, which increases the chance of survival for patients with this disease.

Patient Preparation for Sigmoidoscopy

The physician may want the patient to prepare the colon before the sigmoidoscopy. The preparation generally involves eating a light, low-residue meal the evening before the examination. Foods high in residue that should be avoided include raw fruits and vegetables and whole-grain breads and cereals. The patient may also be instructed to take a laxative and perform an enema (e.g., Fleet's enema) the evening before the examination. On the morning of the examination, the patient should consume a light breakfast and perform another enema until the returns are clear. The fecal material must be removed for the physician to visualize the mucosa of the colon.

Some physicians prefer that the patient not take a laxative or perform an enema because it may change the appearance of the intestinal mucosa of the colon, making diagnosis difficult. In this case, the patient is examined after normal defecation. The medical assistant should consult the physician to determine his or her preference.

Digital Rectal Examination

With the patient in Sims position, a digital examination of the anal canal and rectum is performed before sigmoidoscopy. Using a well-lubricated, gloved index finger, the physician palpates the rectum for the presence of tenderness, hemorrhoids, polyps, and tumors. Any palpable abnormality is viewed directly when the endoscope is inserted. An **endoscope** is an instrument (e.g., sigmoidoscope) that consists of a tube and an optical system that is used for direct visual inspection of organs or cavities. The digital examination also helps relax the sphincter muscles of the anus and prepares the patient for the insertion of the endoscope.

Flexible Sigmoidoscope

The flexible fiberoptic sigmoidoscope is composed of extremely thin fibers of bendable glass that transmit light and images back to the physician. The image, magnified 10 times by the fiberoptic system, is viewed by the physician through the eye lens located in the handle of the sigmoidoscope. Videoscopes available for flexible sigmoidoscopy permit viewing of the images on a display screen.

Flexible sigmoidoscopes consist of a control head and a long flexible insertion tube attached to a light source (Figure 28-2). The insertion tube is ½ inch in diameter and 65 cm long, which allows the physician to view approximately one third of the colon. To perform the procedure, the distal end of the sigmoidoscope is lubricated and inserted into the anus and rectum and then slowly advanced into the colon.

Figure 28-2. Flexible fiberoptic sigmoidoscope. (From Bonewit-West K: *Clinical procedures for medical assistants,* ed 7, St. Louis, 2008, Saunders.)

A small amount of air is usually blown, or **insufflated,** into the colon through tubing attached to the air control valve located on the head of the sigmoidoscope. The function of the air is to distend the lumen of the colon for better visualization.

In addition, suction equipment can be used to remove secretions, such as mucus, blood, and liquid feces, which interfere with proper visualization of the intestinal mucosa. The physician performs the visual examination of the intestinal mucosa as the sigmoidoscope is being inserted and as it is being withdrawn.

The medical assistant must prepare the patient for the procedure and assist the physician during the sigmoidoscopy. These responsibilities include the following:

- Determine whether the patient has prepared properly for the sigmoidoscopy.
- Ask the patient whether he or she needs to void before the procedure.
- Position and drape the patient in Sims position.
- Reassure the patient and help him or her to relax.
- Lubricate the physician's gloved index finger for the digital examination.
- Lubricate the distal end of the sigmoidoscope before the physician inserts it.
- Assist with suction equipment.
- Assist with the collection of a biopsy by holding the specimen container to accept the specimen.
- Assist the patient after the examination.
- Prepare the biopsy specimen for transport to the laboratory.
- Clean the examining room.
- Sanitize and disinfect the sigmoidoscope.

Male Reproductive Health

Introduction to Male Reproductive Health

Two important areas related to male reproductive health are prostate screening and testicular self-examination. Preventive examinations and tests can detect prostate and testicular cancer early, leading to early treatment, which often results in a cure. Both of these areas are described in the following section.

PROSTATE CANCER SCREENING

According to the American Cancer Society, prostate cancer is the second most common cause of cancer deaths in men, lung cancer being the most common. Every year, more than 230,000 men are diagnosed with prostate cancer, and approximately 27,000 die from this disease. The incidence of prostate cancer increases after age 50. Prostate cancer is found more often in African-American men and men with a family history of prostate cancer.

The prostate gland surrounds the urethra and is located just below the bladder and in front of the rectum (see Figure

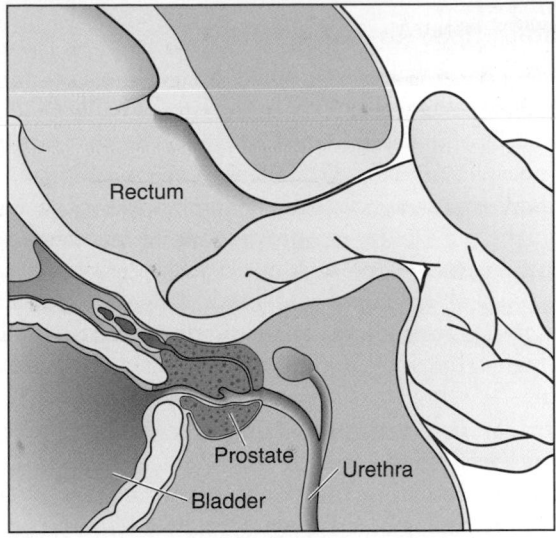

Figure 28-3. Digital rectal examination. (From Bonewit-West K: *Clinical procedures for medical assistants,* ed 7, St. Louis, 2008, Saunders.)

28-3). It is approximately the size and shape of a walnut, and its function is to secrete fluid that transports sperm.

In the early stages, prostate cancer often causes no symptoms. Symptoms that occur when the cancer is more developed include the following:

- Difficulty in urinating
- Weak or interrupted urinary flow
- Pain or burning during urination
- Frequent urination, especially at night
- Blood in the urine
- Pain in the lower back, pelvis, or upper thighs

When prostate cancer is diagnosed early, the chances for a cure are very good. Because of this, the American Cancer Society recommends that men older than age 50 undergo annual prostate screening. The primary screening tests for prostate cancer are the DRE and the prostate-specific antigen (PSA) test. The American Cancer Society recommends that both of these tests be offered annually to men older than 50 so that if cancer does develop, it is found at an early stage.

Digital Rectal Examination

The DRE is a quick and simple procedure that causes only momentary discomfort. During the examination, the physician inserts a lubricated gloved finger into the patient's rectum. Because the prostate gland is located in front of the rectum, the physician is able to palpate the surface of the prostate gland through the rectal wall (Figure 28-3). The physician palpates the gland to determine whether it is enlarged or has an abnormal consistency. Normally, the prostate gland should feel soft, whereas malignant tissue is firm and hard. The sensitivity of the DRE is limited, however, because the physician can palpate only the posterior and lateral aspects of the prostate gland.

Prostate-Specific Antigen Test

The PSA test is a screening test that measures the amount of PSA in the blood. PSA is a protein normally produced by the cells of the membrane that covers the prostate gland. The normal range for PSA is 0 to 4 ng/ml of blood. The PSA level becomes elevated in men who have a benign or malignant growth in the prostate. A PSA level of 4 to 10 ng/ml is considered slightly elevated; levels between 10 and 20 ng/ml are considered moderately elevated; and a value greater than 20 ng/ml is considered highly elevated. The higher the PSA level, the more likely that cancer is present.

The PSA level may normally increase after vigorous exercise, such as jogging or biking. The medical assistant should instruct the patient to engage only in normal activity for 2 days before having blood drawn for a PSA test. The patient also should be instructed not to have sexual intercourse for 2 days before the test because it can change the PSA level.

If the physician determines the likelihood of cancer through prostate screening, further testing is performed to determine whether prostate cancer is present and, if so, the type of cancer and its location and stage of development. To make this assessment, one or more of the following tests may be performed: transrectal ultrasound (TRUS), biopsy of the prostate gland, bone scan, and computed tomography (CT) scan.

TESTICULAR SELF-EXAMINATION

The purpose of testicular self-examination (TSE) is early detection of testicular cancer. In the past 40 years, testicular cancer among young Caucasian men has more than doubled. Although testicular cancer can develop at any age, it is most common in males 15 to 34 years old. If detected early, it has a very high cure rate. Most cases of testicular cancer are detected by men themselves, either by accident or when performing a TSE. Certain factors increase a man's chance of getting testicular cancer, including the following:

- A history of cryptorchidism (undescended testicles)
- Family history of testicular cancer
- Cancer of the other testicle
- Caucasian race (testicular cancer is five times more common in Caucasian men than in African-American men)

The TSE should be performed monthly starting at 15 years of age. A good idea is for the patient to choose an easy-to-remember date each month, such as the first day of the month. The best time to perform the examination is after taking a warm bath or shower. Heat allows the scrotal skin to relax and become soft, making it easier to palpate the underlying testicular tissues.

The most common sign of testicular cancer is a small, hard, painless lump (about the size of a pea) located on the front or side of the testicle. Any abnormalities should be reported to the physician immediately. It does not mean that the patient has cancer, however; the physician must make that determination. Figure 28-4 outlines the procedure for a TSE.

Radiology and Diagnostic Imaging

Introduction to Radiology

Wilhelm Konrad Roentgen, a German physicist, discovered x-rays on November 8, 1895, while working with a cathode ray tube. He noticed that these rays could pass through solid materials, such as paper, wood, and human skin. Because he did not know what they were, he named them *x-rays*. The rays have since been renamed *roentgen rays* after their discoverer; however, they are better known as "x-rays."

X-rays are high-energy electromagnetic waves that are invisible and have a short wavelength that enables them to penetrate solid materials. A special radiographic film is placed behind the part being examined, and a shadow or image of the internal body structure photographed is produced on the film. **Radiograph** is the term for the permanent record of the picture produced on the radiographic film.

X-rays are used to visualize internal organs and structures and serve as a diagnostic aid in determining the presence of disease. They are also used therapeutically in the treatment of disease conditions, such as malignant neoplasms.

Radiology is the branch of medicine that deals with the use of radiant energy in the diagnosis and treatment of disease. A **radiologist** is a physician who specializes in the diagnosis and treatment of disease with any of various forms of radiant energy, such as x-rays, radium, and radioactive material.

A medical office may have its own radiograph machine, but more often radiographs are taken in a hospital by radiology personnel. Some radiographs, such as a chest x-ray, require no advance preparation, whereas others, such as a lower GI study, require a great deal of special preparation. Medical assistants are usually responsible for patient instruc-

---

What Would You Do? What Would You *Not* Do?

Case Study 2

Peter Bota, a 62-year-old retired Caucasian man, came to the medical office 1 week ago for a physical examination. The physician performed a DRE but did not palpate anything abnormal. At that visit, Mr. Bota's blood was drawn for a PSA test, and the results came back as slightly elevated (8 ng/ml). Mr. Bota has returned to the office and is waiting to talk with the physician about his test results and possible follow-up testing. Mr. Bota is extremely worried that he has cancer and wants to know the symptoms of prostate cancer. He also wants to know whether there's anything he did to cause prostate cancer. He says he does not smoke and drinks very little and that he walks his dog twice a day for exercise. ∎

TESTICULAR SELF-EXAMINATION

1
Take a warm bath or shower.

2
Stand in front of a mirror. Look for any swelling of the skin of the scrotum.

3
Place the index and middle fingers of both hands on the underside of one testicle and the thumbs on top of the testicle.

4
Apply a small amount of pressure and gently roll the testicle between the thumb and fingers of both hands, feeling for lumps, swelling, or any change in the size, shape, or consistency of the testicle. A normal testicle should feel smooth, egg-shaped and rather firm. It is also normal for one testicle to be larger or hang lower than the other testicle.

5
Find the epididymis so that you do not confuse it with a lump. The epididymis is a soft tubular cord, located behind the testicle, that functions in storing and carrying sperm.
(Note: Tenderness in the area of the epididymis is considered normal.)

6
Repeat the examination outlined above on the other testicle.

7
Report any of the following abnormalities to the physician: any unusual lump, a feeling of heaviness in the scrotum, a dull ache in the lower abdomen or groin, enlargement of one of the testicles, tenderness or pain in a testicle, or any change in the way the testicle feels.

Figure 28-4. Testicular self-examination. (From Bonewit-West K: *Clinical procedures for medical assistants,* ed 7, St. Louis, 2008, Saunders.)

---

tion in the type of preparation necessary for a particular radiographic examination and for ensuring that the patient understands the importance of the preparation. If the patient does not prepare properly, the radiograph may be of poor quality, and the procedure may need to be rescheduled. This section provides an introduction to the study of radiographs, with a focus on the patient preparation necessary for common radiographs.

CONTRAST MEDIA

Radiography relies on differences in density between various body structures to produce shadows of varying intensities on the radiographic film. A difference in density exists between bone and flesh (bone is denser than flesh). The bone absorbs more x-rays and does not allow them to reach the radiographic film. This leaves that part of the film unexposed and causes white areas to appear on the processed film. If the x-rays penetrate an organ or structure, a black area appears on the film. Because the lungs contain air, x-rays can penetrate them easily. As a result, the lungs appear black on the processed film. The ribs absorb the x-rays and appear as white shadows on the film (Figure 28-5). A structure, such as lung tissue, that permits the passage of x-rays is **radiolucent.** A structure, such as bone, that obstructs the passage of x-rays and causes an image to be cast on the film is **radiopaque.**

In many cases, the natural densities of two adjacent organs or structures are similar. In this instance, a **contrast medium** must be used to make a particular structure visible on the radiograph. Contrast media are usually radiopaque chemical compounds that cause the body tissue or organ to absorb more radiation. This absorption provides a contrast in density between the tissue or organ and the surrounding area. The tissue or organ becomes visible and appears white on the processed radiograph. Substances used as contrast media must be able to be ingested or injected into the body tissues or organs without causing harm to the patient.

Barium sulfate and inorganic iodine compounds are commonly used radiopaque contrast media. Barium sulfate is a chalky compound that is water insoluble and does not allow penetration by x-rays. It is frequently used for examination of the GI tract because barium is not absorbed into the body through the GI tract and does not alter its normal function. Iodine salts are radiopaque and are combined with other compounds for radiographic examination of structures such as the gallbladder and kidneys. Iodine may produce an allergic reaction, so before administration, patients should be asked whether they have an allergy to iodine or foods containing iodine. Patients with known allergies may be given an iodine-sensitivity test as a precautionary measure.

Another type of contrast medium causes the structure to become less dense than the surrounding area. The x-rays

Figure 28-5. Posteroanterior view of the chest. Position of patient and radiograph. (From Meschan I: *Synopsis of radiologic anatomy with computed tomography,* Philadelphia, 1980, Saunders.)

can easily penetrate the structure, which appears as a darker area on the radiograph. This type of contrast medium includes substances such as air and carbon dioxide.

FLUOROSCOPY

A **fluoroscope** is an instrument used to view internal organs and structures of the body directly on a display screen. Examination of a patient with a fluoroscope is known as **fluoroscopy.** A radiopaque medium is often used with fluoroscopy to outline various parts of the body. The patient is positioned between the radiographic tube and a fluorescent screen composed of zinc cadmium sulfide crystals. When the x-rays pass through the body and strike the crystals, visible light is emitted so that the radiologist can view (on a screen) the action of body organs or structures, such as the stomach and intestines. During fluoroscopy, the radiologist can take radiographs that permit the study of the structure in detail and serve as a permanent record.

POSITIONING THE PATIENT

The position of the patient is determined by the purpose of the examination and the area examined. The patient is generally positioned so that several different views can be taken to provide a complete three-dimensional picture of the part examined. Articles such as jewelry and hairpins must be removed so that the image on the radiograph is not obscured. To prevent blurring of the image on the film, patients must maintain the position in which they are placed and not move during the radiographic examination. Blurring prevents good visualization of the part and may warrant retaking of the film.

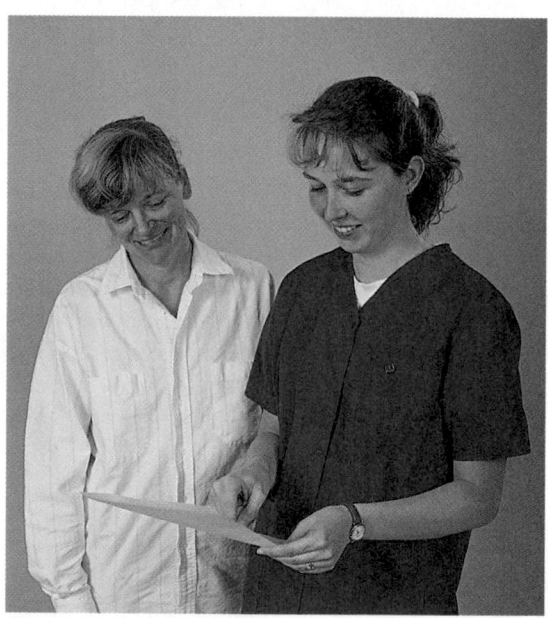

Figure 28-6. Instructing a patient in proper preparation for a radiographic examination. (From Bonewit-West K: *Clinical procedures for medical assistants,* ed 7, St. Louis, 2008, Saunders.)

SPECIFIC RADIOGRAPHIC EXAMINATIONS

The medical assistant should understand the purpose of commonly performed radiographic examinations and should be able to instruct a patient in the proper preparation for each (Figure 28-6). Frequently performed radiographic examinations and the special advance preparation necessary for each are described. The preparation may vary, depending on the medical office.

Mammography

Mammography is a radiographic examination of the breasts used to detect many forms of breast disease, such as benign breast masses, breast calcifications, fibrocystic breast disease, and particularly breast cancer. It is also used to monitor the effects of surgery and radiation therapy on breast tumors.

Mammography uses low doses of x-rays that pass through the breast and create an image on a film. On the radiograph, an abnormal area appears noticeably different from normal breast tissue. Mammography can be used to detect a breast tumor when the growth is less than 1 cm in diameter (about the size of a pea) and before it is clinically palpable. A malignant lump can be removed at an early stage, which usually results in conservative treatment with less disfigurement and a high survival rate. With early diagnosis and treatment, breast cancer survival rates for women can reach as high as 94%.

No specific preparation is necessary for mammography. The patient should not wear any lotions, powders, or deodorants because they may contain small amounts of metal that can be seen on the radiograph and may interfere with interpretation. For the mammogram, the patient must remove clothing from the waist up; the patient should be told to wear a two-piece outfit so that the procedure is easier and more comfortable.

A radiology technician generally performs the mammogram. The patient's breast is positioned on the mammography machine, and pressure is applied with a plastic compression paddle that flattens the breast (Figure 28-7). Compression of the breasts is necessary to obtain a clear radiograph and to lower the radiation dosage as much as possible. During the procedure, the patient must hold her breath and remain still momentarily because any type of motion, even breathing, can blur the image and make a repeat radiograph necessary.

Two radiographs are taken of each breast—one from above and one from the side. A radiologist then checks the mammogram (Figure 28-8) and occasionally orders additional images to obtain a more complete view of the breast tissue. After the procedure, the radiologist studies the mammogram for any signs of breast cancer or other breast problems and sends a written report of the findings to the patient's physician.

Gastrointestinal Series

Upper Gastrointestinal

An upper GI is an examination of the upper digestive tract using fluoroscopy and radiography. The examination is helpful in the diagnosis of disorders of the esophagus, stomach, duodenum, and small intestine, such as peptic ulcers or benign and malignant tumors.

Proper patient preparation is important for this procedure. The patient's stomach must be empty at the beginning of the study so that food does not obscure the radiographic image. To prepare for the examination, the patient must eat a light evening meal and then not eat or drink anything, including water and medications, after midnight the day before the examination. Food and fluid in the GI tract have a degree of density and could cause confusing shadows on the radiograph.

The stomach varies little in density from the structures around it, and to make it show up on a radiograph, a contrast medium must be used. The patient drinks a suspension of barium mixed with water and flavoring. The mixture, which has a chalky taste, is known as the *barium swallow*.

Figure 28-7. Patient positioning for mammography. (From Ballinger PW, Frank ED, eds: *Merrill's atlas of radiographic positions and radiologic procedures,* vol 2, ed 10, St. Louis, 2003, Mosby.)

Figure 28-8. Mammogram. Arrows indicate suspicious area of increased density that needs further evaluation. (From Prue L: *Atlas of mammographic positioning,* Philadelphia, 1994, Saunders.)

PATIENT TEACHING Mammography

Answer questions patients may have about mammography.

What is the purpose of mammography?

Mammography is a safe, low-dose radiographic examination used to screen for abnormal changes in the breasts. Mammography allows the physician to detect small lumps in the breast long before they can be felt. Although most breast lumps are not cancerous, breast cancer can be removed at an early stage when detected early, which usually results in treatment that is less deforming and has a much higher survival rate.

Who should have a mammogram?

The American Cancer Society recommends women 40 years old and older have an annual mammogram because the risk of breast cancer increases after this age. Women with a family history of, or other risk factors for, breast cancer should follow the advice of the physician regarding mammography; the age guidelines do not apply because these women undergo examination on a more frequent basis.

What occurs during the mammography procedure?

During mammography, the breast is positioned on a special machine and flattened with a compression paddle. Breast compression may be uncomfortable for some women. The discomfort can be reduced with avoidance of caffeine several days before the procedure and by scheduling the mammography the week after a menstrual period, when the breasts are less tender. Each breast is radiographed from above and from the side. A radiologist studies the resulting mammogram to detect any abnormalities. The results are reported to the physician.

Does mammography take the place of breast self-examination?

Mammography is not a substitute for breast self-examination. Women should continue to examine their breasts once a month and undergo a periodic breast examination by a physician. Most breast lumps are detected by women themselves.

- Encourage the patient to have a mammogram according to the schedule recommended by the American Cancer Society.
- Instruct the patient in the procedure for a breast self-examination.
- Provide the patient with educational materials on breast self-examination and mammography. ■

As the patient swallows the barium, the radiologist observes its passage down the esophagus and into the stomach and duodenum with fluoroscopy. Radiographs are taken periodically during the examination to allow a detailed study of the upper GI tract and to provide a permanent record. The patient's position is changed at various times so that the upper digestive tract can be visualized from different profiles. If the radiologist wants to observe the passage of the barium through the small and large intestines, the patient must wait at the facility and return to the radiology examination room several times for additional radiographs.

The medical assistant should explain to the patient that the barium suspension will appear in the stool the following day and will cause it to have a lighter color. The barium mixture may cause constipation and the need for a laxative. To help prevent constipation, the patient should be instructed to drink water after the procedure.

Lower Gastrointestinal

A lower GI involves filling the colon with a barium sulfate mixture with a tube inserted into the colon. The examination uses fluoroscopy and radiography to observe and obtain permanent pictures of the colon (Figure 28-9). A lower GI assists in diagnosis of disorders of the lower intestines, such as polyps, tumors, lesions, and diverticulosis. The colon must be thoroughly cleansed in advance to remove gas and fecal material. Gas has a certain degree of density and shows up as confusing shadows on the radiograph. If fecal material appears on the film, the image of the colon is obscured.

The instructions for cleansing the colon may vary from one medical office to another, but in general the patient is instructed to consume only clear liquids the day before the examination, such as water, coffee, tea, clear broth, and strained fruit juice. A laxative should be taken on the day before the scheduled examination; an enema also may be necessary. An **enema** is an injection of fluid into the rectum to aid in the elimination of feces from the colon. The patient should not drink anything (except water) after midnight on the day before the examination. On the morning of the examination, the patient may be required to perform a warm water-cleansing enema until the returns are clear.

The patient should report at the scheduled time and is instructed to relax on one side while the rectal tube is inserted. As the barium enters the colon, the radiologist watches it on the fluoroscopic screen and periodically takes radiographs. The patient has a sensation of fullness and the urge to defecate as the barium enters the colon. The patient is moved into various positions to allow the barium to fill the colon completely and to obtain better visualization of the colon. The patient is allowed to evacuate the barium, and another radiograph is taken to finish the radiographic examination.

Figure 28-9. Lower gastrointestinal series. Colon is distended with barium. Positioning of patient and radiograph. (From Meschan I: *Synopsis of radiologic anatomy with computed tomography*, Philadelphia, 1980, Saunders.)

Intravenous Pyelography

An intravenous pyelogram (IVP) is a radiograph of the kidneys and urinary tract (Figure 28-10). An IVP is used to assist in the diagnosis of kidney stones, blockage or narrowing of the urinary tract, and growths within or near the urinary system.

The patient should eat a light evening meal and not eat or drink anything after 9:00 PM. The patient must remove gas and fecal material from the intestines with a laxative and cleansing enemas. Removal of gas and fecal material permits proper visualization of the urinary tract. Unless the patient is allergic to iodine, a contrast medium consisting of iodine is used and is administered intravenously to the patient. As the iodine enters the bloodstream, the patient may feel warm and flushed and have a metallic or salty taste in the mouth. This reaction is normal and lasts only for a few minutes. If the patient is allergic to iodine or foods containing iodine, such as shellfish, a different type of contrast medium must be used.

Other Types of Radiographs

Other types of radiographs that the medical assistant may encounter include the following:

Angiocardiogram A radiograph of the heart in which valves and vessels are examined with radiography and fluoroscopy after the introduction of a radiopaque contrast medium.

Bronchogram A radiograph of the lungs after introduction of a radiopaque contrast medium.

Cerebral angiogram A radiograph of the major arteries of the brain after injection of a radiopaque contrast medium.

Figure 28-10. Intravenous pyelogram obtained 15 minutes after intravenous injection of a suitable contrast agent. (From Meschan I: *Synopsis of radiologic anatomy with computed tomography*, Philadelphia, 1980, Saunders.)

Cholangiogram A radiograph of the bile ducts after administration of a radiopaque contrast medium.

Coronary angiogram A radiograph of the coronary arteries after the injection of a radiopaque contrast medium.

Cystogram   A radiograph of the urinary bladder after injection of a radiopaque contrast medium.

Hysterosalpingogram   A radiograph of the uterus and fallopian tubes after injection of an oily radiopaque contrast medium.

Retrograde pyelogram   A radiograph of the kidneys and urinary tract after injection of radiopaque contrast medium directly into the ureter through a ureteral catheter. The dye flows to the kidneys through the ureters.

Introduction to Diagnostic Imaging

Diagnostic imaging procedures are performed frequently because they allow for the visualization of internal body structures in great detail. The most common diagnostic imaging procedures are ultrasonography, CT, magnetic resonance imaging (MRI), and nuclear medicine. Diagnostic imaging procedures are almost always performed in a hospital; however, information may need to be relayed to a patient scheduled for such a procedure, including what to expect during the procedure and any patient preparation that may be required. A medical assistant should have a basic knowledge of diagnostic imaging procedures and the preparation necessary for each.

ULTRASONOGRAPHY

Ultrasonography, also called "ultrasound," is the oldest of the diagnostic imaging procedures. Ultrasound uses high-frequency sound waves for the study of soft tissue structures. It is frequently used in the diagnosis of conditions of the abdominal and pelvic organs, particularly the liver, gallbladder, spleen, pancreas, kidneys, uterus, and ovaries. An ultrasound examination of the heart is called an **echocardiogram** and is used to determine the size, shape, and position of the heart and the movement of the heart valves and chambers.

Ultrasonography offers many advantages as a diagnostic imaging procedure. It shows movement, allows for continuous viewing of a structure, and uses sound waves rather than radiation. Ultrasound does have some minor limitations. Because sound waves are unable to penetrate bone and gas-filled cavities, such as the lungs, ultrasound cannot be used in the evaluation of these structures. In addition, ultrasound may be difficult with obese patients because adipose tissue can interfere with sound wave transmission.

During the ultrasound examination, the examiner places a probe containing a transducer firmly on the patient's skin and moves it over the body areas to be examined. The transducer generates sound waves that are directed into the patient's tissues. The sound waves are reflected back to the transducer, similar to an echo. Deep structures of the body, such as the kidneys, are visualized by recording the reflections, or echoes, of the sound waves directed into the tissues (Figure 28-11). The image is displayed on an oscilloscope, which is a special type of viewing screen. The image can also be permanently recorded on film and videotape. The recording is called a **sonogram,** and the patient is often permitted to view the sonogram on the oscilloscope as the procedure is performed.

Although ultrasound is commonly used for a wide variety of noninvasive imaging procedures, individuals are most familiar with its use in obstetrics. Obstetric ultrasound is most frequently used to determine gestational age of a fetus and to confirm the due date; to detect congenital abnormalities, ectopic pregnancy, and multiple pregnancy; and to determine the fetus' position and size late in pregnancy. Because the ultrasound machine is a compact unit, some obstetricians perform this procedure in their medical offices.

Patient Preparation

The medical assistant should tell the patient what to expect during an ultrasound examination and instruct the patient in the preparation required for the procedure, as follows:

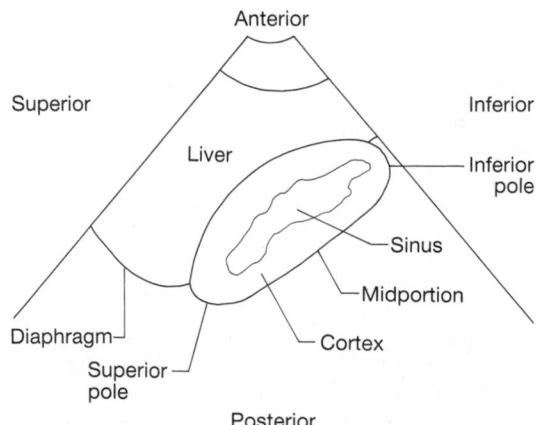

Figure 28-11. Sonogram of right kidney. (From Tempkin BB: *Ultrasound scanning: principles and protocols,* ed 2, Philadelphia, 1999, Saunders.)

1. Ultrasound is a safe and painless procedure that takes approximately 15 to 45 minutes to complete, depending on the body part examined.
2. The patient may need to prepare for the procedure, depending on the part of the body examined. An ultrasound of the gallbladder and liver necessitates that the patient fast for 8 to 12 hours. In obstetric ultrasound, the patient needs to have a full bladder. This patient should be instructed to consume approximately 32 oz of fluid about 1 hour before the procedure.
3. The patient must remain still when requested during the procedure because movement can interfere with accurate results. In addition, the patient may be asked to change positions so that the organs can be seen at different angles.

COMPUTED TOMOGRAPHY

Computed tomography (also known as a *CT* or *CAT* scan) is an advanced radiographic examination that uses only a minimal amount of radiation. It produces a series of cross-sectional images of a body part, permitting the imaging of structures that cannot be visualized with conventional radiographic procedures. A CT scan allows the radiologist to view the bones and organs of the head and body in fine detail and has been used most successfully in diagnostic studies of the brain. CT scans are used primarily to detect and evaluate tumors and other abnormalities and to monitor the effects of surgery, radiation therapy, or chemotherapy on tumors.

The scan is conducted by a skilled diagnostic imaging technician. The patient is positioned on a special motorized table (Figure 28-12). From an adjoining room, the technician mechanically moves the table into a doughnut-shaped device known as the *CT scanner* until the part of the body to be examined is inside the tubular opening of the scanner.

During the scan, two examinations are often performed. The first examination is a plain scan, and the second is a repeat scan after a contrast dye has been injected through a vein in the arm. The dye makes a sharper image of internal structures of the body possible. The CT scanner takes multiple radiographic images in a rapid sequence at different angles. The series of radiographs is processed with a computer to produce cross-sectional images, which are permanently recorded on film or stored digitally on electronic media for evaluation by a radiologist (Figure 28-13).

Patient Preparation

The medical assistant should tell the patient what to expect during the CT scan and instruct the patient in the preparation required for the procedure, as follows:
1. If a contrast agent is to be used, the patient should fast for 4 hours before the procedure. It is important to ask the patient whether he or she is allergic to radiographic contrast media, iodine, or shellfish to avoid an adverse reaction to the contrast medium.

Figure 28-12. Positioning patient for computed tomography scan. (From Kowalczyk N, Donnett K: *Integrated patient care for the imaging professional,* St. Louis, 1996, Mosby.)

2. Before the procedure, the patient must remove all radiopaque objects, such as metal and jewelry, because they would interfere with a clear image of the body part examined.
3. The patient should lay motionless and breathe normally during the procedure. When a radiograph is being taken, the patient is asked to hold his or her breath so that the radiograph is not blurred. The patient hears mechanical clacking sounds from the scanner as pictures are taken.

MAGNETIC RESONANCE IMAGING

MRI is the newest of the advanced diagnostic imaging procedures. It is used for imaging tissues of high fat and water content that cannot be seen with other radiologic techniques. MRI assists in the diagnosis of intracranial and spinal lesions and cardiovascular and soft tissue abnormalities, such as herniated discs and joint diseases. MRI allows the examiner to see through bone and view fluid-filled soft tissue in great detail.

MRI is a safe and painless procedure in which a strong magnetic field and ordinary radiowaves produce computer-processed images of internal body structures. The patient lies on a table inside the bore of the cylindric MRI machine while a diagnostic imaging technician in an adjoining room monitors the procedure (Figure 28-14). Because of the closed space, some patients may have difficulty with claustrophobia. The physician may order a sedative for these patients.

The high-resolution, three-dimensional images that are obtained with MRI are permanently recorded on film or

Figure 28-13. The computed tomography scanner takes multiple cross-sectional radiographic images. The images shown here are cross-sectional pictures of the head used to evaluate the orbits and sinuses. (From Snopek A: *Fundamentals of special radiographic procedures,* ed 4, Philadelphia, 1999, Saunders.)

Figure 28-14. Magnetic resonance imaging (MRI). The patient lies on a table inside the bore of the cylindric MRI machine while MRI technicians in an adjoining room monitor the procedure. (From Ballinger PW, Frank ED, eds: *Merrill's atlas of radiographic positions and radiologic procedures,* vol 3, ed 10, St. Louis, 2003, Mosby.)

stored digitally on electronic media for evaluation by a radiologist. Because MRI does not involve radiation, the U.S. Food and Drug Administration has classified the MRI machine as a low-risk device.

Patient Preparation

The medical assistant should tell the patient what to expect during MRI and instruct the patient in the preparation required for the procedure, as follows:

1. MRI is a safe and painless procedure with a usual completion time of approximately 1 hour.
2. No special preparation is necessary for the MRI examination. The patient may eat or drink before the examination and take any prescribed medication. The patient should wear loose, comfortable clothing, such as a jogging suit, for the procedure.

What Would You Do? What Would You *Not* Do?

Case Study 3

Michael Wendl is an 18-year-old high school varsity football player. For the past 3 months, he has had pain and swelling in his left shoulder. The physician schedules an MRI to assist in determining the cause of the problem. Michael has had several radiographs over the past 2 years and is worried about the radiation exposure to his body. He wants to know how much radiation will be involved with the procedure. Michael has problems with claustrophobia and wants to know whether he can play his Game Boy during the procedure to distract him. He also wants to know whether he is allowed to eat anything before the procedure. ■

Memories *from* Externship

Megan Baer: My first externship was terrifying, but at the same time I was overwhelmed with excitement. I remember worrying how I was going to remember all my clinical and administrative skills. I was worried that I would hurt someone or forget to do something important.

One day a patient came into our office upset and crying. The examination rooms were full, so I took her into our staff lounge. I sat her down, fixed her a cup of coffee, and asked her if I could help. She told me that her son had drowned 2 years ago on that day, her mother had cancer, and her husband had passed away 8 months previously. I listened to everything she had to say, and I comforted her until the physician was ready to see her. She walked over to me, hugged me, and said my smile and people skills were the best treatment for her depression that she had ever had. Her telling me that made me feel good about my career choice, and it made me realize how fulfilling it was. It did not take me long to realize that all the skills that I was taught were not forgotten, and I learned that a smile and listening to people were just as important as my skills. ■

Prepare for Success

3. Because the procedure involves a strong magnet, the patient should remove any metal or magnetic-sensitive objects, such as watches, rings, or other metallic jewelry and credit cards.
4. The patient must remain completely still for 15- to 20-minute intervals during the procedure. The patient hears a metallic clacking sound like a muffled drumbeat during the procedure. Earplugs or headphones are available for use if the patient desires.

NUCLEAR MEDICINE

Nuclear medicine is an advanced diagnostic imaging procedure in which a tiny bit of radioactive material is introduced into the patient. The radiation is introduced into the body by a diagnostic imaging technician using one of the following methods: injection, ingestions, or inhalation. The technologist places the patient on a specialized piece of equipment known as a *gamma camera*. A gamma camera can detect the radiation being given off by the body part that has been targeted by the radiation. This is accomplished through the use of scintillation crystals. These crystals convert the radiation being given off by the body into light. This light is converted into electrical impulses, which are interpreted by a computer program contained within the gamma camera. The resulting information is displayed as still images or functional animations of body parts and organs. The ability of nuclear medicine to show the actual function of organs provides more detailed information for certain conditions than other diagnostic imaging examinations (e.g., CT, MRI).

During the nuclear medicine examination, a radioactive material is used to target certain body parts. This material is known as a *radiopharmaceutical* (or radionuclide); examples of radiopharmaceuticals include technetium-99m, iodine-123, and thallium-201. Most radiopharmaceuticals are chemically bound to a complex known as a *tracer*. A tracer is designed to be attracted to specific areas of the body or, in some cases, to types of diseased tissue.

The most common nuclear medicine procedures include bone scans and cardiac studies. *Bone scans* are performed to detect small fractures (e.g., stress fractures) or lesions that may not be visible on other diagnostic imaging examinations. To perform a bone scan, the patient is injected with a radiopharmaceutical. The patient is instructed to wait at the facility for a predetermined period of time based on the area being examined. The purpose of the waiting period is to allow the radiopharmaceutical to be absorbed sufficiently so that an accurate diagnosis can be made.

Cardiac studies in nuclear medicine typically involve two phases—a resting phase and a stress phase, which is a functional study. The resting phase is performed with the heart at a normal rate, whereas the stress phase is performed immediately after exercising at a level determined by the patient's condition and personal history.

Guidelines

Specific guidelines that may be required for nuclear medicine examinations are as follows:

1. Depending on the type of nuclear medicine examination being performed, the patient may be required to be in a fasting state or to abstain from consuming certain foods for a period of time. The medical assistant should check with the institution performing the examination so that proper dietary instructions can be relayed to the patient.
2. Nuclear medicine examinations are time consuming because most examinations require multiple scans. The interval between each scan is determined by the part being examined and the type of equipment and radiopharmaceutical being used. There may be a delay between the administration of the radiopharmaceutical and when

the patient is actually placed on the gamma camera. There may also be the need for follow-up images that may be done later the same day or, in some cases, the following morning. Because of this, the medical assistant must inform the patient of the amount of time required for the examination so that arrangements can be made with work and home schedules if needed.

3. Because most nuclear medicine examinations require that the patient lie still on a table for a prolonged time, the patient should be advised to wear comfortable clothing to the examination. If a nuclear medicine examination requires exercise as a component of the test, the patient should be instructed to wear appropriate exercise clothing, including athletic shoes.

DIGITAL RADIOLOGY

Modern advances in digital imaging technology have made inroads into the field of radiology. The result is the transformation of film-based radiology into a system of computer-displayed and stored digital images. This change allows for increased efficiency and cost savings and better patient care. Higher-quality images and the ability to transfer these digital images electronically over the phone lines are two important benefits that affect the patient directly. As a result of this digital revolution, the medical assistant may be required to use the medical office computer to access, display, and permanently save images taken by the facilities providing diagnostic imaging services.

MEDICAL PRACTICE *and the* LAW

Colon procedures can be embarrassing for the patient. Most colon procedures can be diagnostic for cancer. This combination makes these procedures very stressful for the patient. Professionalism, compassion, and a caring attitude can alleviate many fears. Many invasive procedures require a written informed consent.

While assisting with a flexible sigmoidoscopy, assist the patient and maintain proper positioning as comfortably as possible. Be aware of the patient's condition, and inform the physician if the patient is not tolerating the procedure well.

Radiology and diagnostic imaging involve high-technology equipment and procedures that can be frightening and uncomfortable to the patient. Be aware of the patient's reactions, and provide

assistance and comfort whenever possible. Be specific in providing the patient with instructions to ensure the best imaging results.

Procedures that involve injectable contrast media or that are invasive usually require written informed consent. Check office policy for procedures that require signed consent forms.

With procedures that use radiation, federal laws regulate usage and exposure testing and record keeping. The acronym ALARA (As Low As Reasonably Able) reminds workers to minimize exposure to themselves and patients. Ask female patients whether they may be pregnant before starting any radiologic procedure. ■

What Would You Do? What Would You *Not* Do? RESPONSES

Case Study 1
Page 662

What Did Megan Do?
❑ Relayed to Mrs. Bernard that this is not the most fun test to perform, but that if colon cancer is detected early, the cure rate is very high.
❑ Explained to Mrs. Bernard that colon cancer increases after age 40, and that an individual can develop colon cancer without a family history of it.
❑ Told Mrs. Bernard that during the early stages of colon cancer, there are no symptoms, so it is possible to feel fine but still have a problem.
❑ Explained to Mrs. Bernard in more detail the reason for not eating red meat or taking aspirin during the testing period.
❑ Told Mrs. Bernard that disposable gloves could be given to her to take home to wear when she collected the specimens.
❑ Explained to Mrs. Bernard that the physician talks with patients every day about these types of things, and it is important to talk with him about all aspects of her health so that she receives the best care possible.
❑ Told Mrs. Bernard that the office would call her in 3 days to see whether she has any questions or is having any problems with the test.

What Did Megan Not Do?
❑ Did not tell Mrs. Bernard that she is getting older and needs to be more concerned about performing health screening tests.

What Would You Do?/What Would You *Not* Do? Review Megan's response and place a checkmark next to the information you included in your response. List additional information you included in your response.

_____
_____
_____
_____

Case Study 2
Page 668

What Did Megan Do?
❑ Listened patiently and tried to reassure and calm Mr. Bota. Told him that physicians do not yet know what causes prostate cancer.
❑ Explained that the PSA test is a screening test and that he should not jump to conclusions about the results.
❑ Told Mr. Bota that the physician would talk with him about his test results in a short while.

What Would You Do? What Would You *Not* Do?   RESPONSES—cont'd

❑ Commended Mr. Bota on his healthy lifestyle habits and encouraged him to continue with them.

❑ Gave Mr. Bota some brochures on male reproductive health to read while he waited to be seen by the physician.

What Did Megan Not *Do*?

❑ Did not tell Mr. Bota that there was nothing to worry about.

What Would You Do?/What Would You *Not* Do? Review Megan's response and place a checkmark next to the information you included in your response. List additional information you included in your response.

_____

_____

_____

_____

Case Study 3
Page 677

What Did Megan Do?

❑ Explained to Michael that an MRI does not use radiation, so he would not be exposed to any radiation during the procedure.

❑ Told Michael that he would not be able to play his Game Boy during the procedure. Explained that the MRI works with a strong magnet that might damage the Game Boy and also interfere with a good image of the shoulder. Told Michael that he would also need to lie still during the procedure.

❑ Told Michael the physician would be informed of his problem with claustrophobia. Explained that the physician may want to give him something to help him relax during the procedure.

❑ Told Michael that it was fine to eat before the procedure.

What Did Megan Not *Do*?

❑ Did not overlook or minimize Michael's concern about claustrophobia.

What Would You Do?/What Would You *Not* Do? Review Megan's response and place a checkmark next to the information you included in your response. List additional information you included in your response.

_____

_____

_____

_____

⟳ TERMINOLOGY REVIEW

Biopsy The surgical removal and examination of tissue from the living body. Biopsies are generally performed to determine whether a tumor is benign or malignant.

Colonoscopy The visualization of the entire colon using a colonoscope.

Contrast medium A substance used to make a particular structure visible on a radiograph.

Echocardiogram An ultrasound examination of the heart.

Endoscope An instrument that consists of a tube and an optical system that is used for direct visual inspection of organs or cavities.

Enema An injection of fluid into the rectum to aid in the elimination of feces from the colon.

Fluoroscope An instrument used to view internal organs and structures directly.

Fluoroscopy Examination of a patient with a fluoroscope.

Insufflate To blow a powder, vapor, or gas (e.g., air) into a body cavity.

Melena The darkening of the stool caused by the presence of blood in an amount of 50 ml or greater.

Occult blood Blood in such a small amount that it is not detectable by the unaided eye.

Peroxidase (as it pertains to the guaiac slide test) A substance that is able to transfer oxygen from hydrogen peroxide to oxidize guaiac, causing the guaiac to turn blue.

Radiograph A permanent record of a picture of an internal body organ or structure produced on radiographic film.

Radiography The taking of permanent records (radiographs) of internal body organs and structures by passing x-rays through the body to act on a specially sensitized film.

Radiologist A physician who specializes in the diagnosis and treatment of disease using radiant energy, such as x-rays, radium, and radioactive material.

Radiology The branch of medicine that deals with the use of radiant energy in the diagnosis and treatment of disease.

Radiolucent Describing a structure that permits the passage of x-rays.

Radiopaque Describing a structure that obstructs the passage of x-rays.

Sigmoidoscope An endoscope that is specially designed for passage through the anus to permit visualization of the rectum and sigmoid colon.

Sigmoidoscopy The visual examination of the rectum and sigmoid colon using a sigmoidoscope.

Sonogram The record obtained with ultrasonography.

Ultrasonography The use of high-frequency sound waves to produce an image of an organ or tissue.

ON THE WEB

For Information on Colorectal Cancer:

American Cancer Society: www.cancer.org

National Cancer Institute: www.cancer.gov

Colon Cancer Alliance: www.ccalliance.org

Oncology Channel: www.oncologychannel.com

For Information on Prostate Cancer:

Prostate Health: www.prostatehealth.com

Prostate Information: www.prostateinfo.com

Prostate.com: www.prostate.com

Prostate.org: www.prostatitis.org

Male Health: www.malehealthcenter.com

For Information on Radiography and Diagnostic Imaging:

BrighamRAD: www.brighamrad.harvard.edu

Society for Computer Applications in Radiology: www.scarnet.org

Whole Brain Atlas: www.med.harvard.edu/AANLIB/home.html

Radiology Information: www.radiologyinfo.org

For Information on Breast Cancer:

American Cancer Society: www.cancer.org

PREPARE FOR CERTIFICATION Visit the Evolve site at http://evolve.elsevier.com/Bonewit/today/ to actively Prepare for your Certification.

*Check out the **Companion CD** bound with the book to access additional interactive activities.*

29

Introduction to the Clinical Laboratory

LEARNING OBJECTIVES

Clinical Laboratory

1. Explain the general purpose of a laboratory test.
2. List and explain specific uses of laboratory test results.
3. Describe the relationship between the medical office and an outside laboratory.
4. List the information included in a laboratory directory.
5. Identify the purpose of a laboratory request form. List and explain the function of each type of information included on the form.
6. Identify the use of each of the following profiles, and list the tests included in each:

   Comprehensive metabolic profile
   Electrolyte profile
   Hepatic profile
   Renal profile
   Lipid profile
   Thyroid profile
   Rheumatoid profile
   Prenatal profile
   Hepatitis profile

7. Identify the purpose of the laboratory report form, and list the information included on it.

Collecting, Transporting, and Handling Specimens

1. Explain the purpose of advance patient preparation for the collection of a laboratory specimen.
2. List examples of specimens.
3. Identify and explain the guidelines that should be followed during specimen collection.
4. Explain why specimens must be handled and stored properly.
5. Identify the proper handling and storage techniques for the following specimens: blood, urine, microbiologic specimen, and stool specimen.

Physician's Office Laboratory

1. List the six basic steps involved in testing a specimen.
2. Describe the methods that are used to test a specimen.
3. Explain the purpose of quality control in the laboratory, and list quality control methods that should be used for each of the following: advance patient preparation; specimen collection, handling, and transportation; and laboratory testing.
4. List the laboratory safety guidelines that should be followed in the medical office to prevent accidents.

PROCEDURES

Use a laboratory directory.
Complete a laboratory request form.
Read a laboratory report.
Instruct a patient in the preparation necessary for a laboratory test that requires fasting.

Collect a specimen.
Handle and store a specimen.

Use quality control methods.
Practice laboratory safety.

CAAHEP COMPETENCIES

Clinical Competencies
Patient Care
- Screen and follow up test results.

General Competencies
Patient Instruction
- Instruct individuals according to their needs.
- Provide instruction for health maintenance and disease prevention.
- Identify community resources.

Operational Functions
- Use methods of quality control.

ABHES COMPETENCIES

Clinical Duties
- Use quality control.
- Collect and process specimens.
- Screen and follow up patient test results.

Office Management
- Operate and maintain facilities and perform routine maintenance of administrative and clinical equipment safely.

Instruction
- Teach patients methods of health promotion and disease prevention.

KEY TERMS

automated method
fasting
homeostasis (hoe-mee-oh-STAY-sis)
in vivo (in-VEE-voe)
laboratory test
manual method
normal range

plasma (PLAZ-ma)
profile
quality control
routine test
serum (SERE-um)
specimen (SPES-i-men)

Introduction to the Clinical Laboratory

Clinical laboratory test results are often used along with a thorough health history and physical examination to provide essential data needed by the physician for accurate diagnosis and management of a patient's condition. Clinical **laboratory tests** provide objective and quantitative information regarding the status of body conditions and functions. When the body is healthy, its systems function normally, and a state of equilibrium of the internal environment is said to exist; this is termed **homeostasis.** When the body is in a state of homeostasis, the physical and chemical characteristics of the body substances (e.g., fluids, secretions, excretions) are within an acceptable range known as the **normal range** or reference range.

When a pathologic condition exists, biologic changes occur within the body, altering the normal physiology or functioning of the body and resulting in an imbalance. These changes cause the patient to experience the symptoms of that particular pathologic condition. Iron deficiency anemia usually causes the patient to experience weakness, fatigue, pallor, irritability, and, in some cases, shortness of breath on exertion. In addition, these changes in the body's biologic processes may cause an alteration in the characteristics of body substances, such as an alteration of the chemical content of the blood or urine, an alteration in the antibody level, or an alteration in cell counts or cellular morphology.

The physical and chemical alterations of body substances become evident through abnormal values or results in laboratory tests—in other words, values outside the accepted normal range or limit for that particular test. Just as certain pathologic conditions cause specific symptoms to occur, certain pathologic conditions cause abnormal values to occur for specific laboratory tests. Iron deficiency anemia causes an alteration in normal red blood cell morphology and a decreased hemoglobin level.

An important realization is that an abnormal value for a particular test may be seen with more than one pathologic condition. A decrease in the hemoglobin level is found with hyperthyroidism and cirrhosis of the liver. In this regard, the physician cannot rely solely on laboratory test results to make a final diagnosis, but rather must rely also on the combination of the data obtained from the health history, the physical examination, and diagnostic and laboratory test results.

LABORATORY TESTS

The number of laboratory tests ordered for a patient varies depending on the physician's clinical findings. A clinical diagnosis of a urinary tract infection usually necessitates only a urine culture for confirmation. Many diseases cause more than one alteration in the physical and chemical characteristics of body substances, however, and a series of laboratory tests is often necessary to establish the pattern of abnormalities characteristic of a particular disease.

The medical assistant should realize that not all pathologic conditions necessitate the use of laboratory test results for arrival at a final diagnosis; the information obtained from the patient's clinical signs and symptoms can be sufficient for a final diagnosis of some conditions. In these instances, the physician is so certain of the clinical diagnosis that therapy can be instituted without laboratory confirmation. Most physicians diagnose acute purulent otitis media with the information obtained from patient symptoms (earache, fever, feeling of fullness in the ear) and from an otoscopic examination of the tympanic membrane (the tympanic membrane is red and bulging). The information

obtained through the clinical signs and symptoms is sufficiently specific to otitis media to allow the physician to make a final diagnosis and to prescribe treatment.

The medical assistant must acquire knowledge and skill in basic clinical laboratory methods and techniques. It is important that the medical assistant have knowledge of the laboratory tests that are performed most often, including the purpose of these tests; the normal value or range for each test; any advance patient preparation or special instructions; and any substances that might interfere with accurate test results, such as food or medication.

The medical assistant frequently works with this information when collecting, handling, and storing **specimens;** performing laboratory tests; typing health histories; and receiving and filing laboratory reports. It is essential that the medical assistant understand the value of laboratory tests and alert the physician to any abnormal results as soon as the test is performed or the laboratory report is received.

This chapter serves as an introduction to the clinical laboratory by providing an overview of methods and general guidelines to follow and by focusing on the relationship between the medical office and an outside laboratory. Specific information for collection, handling, storing, and testing of biologic specimens is presented in subsequent chapters.

PURPOSE OF LABORATORY TESTING

The most frequent use of laboratory test results is to assist in the diagnosis of a patient's condition. Laboratory test results also have many other significant medical uses. A summary of the purpose and function of laboratory testing follows:

1. Laboratory tests are most frequently ordered by the physician *to assist in the diagnosis of pathologic conditions.* Along with the health history and physical examination, laboratory test results provide the physician with essential data needed to arrive at the final diagnosis and prescribe treatment. After obtaining the health history and performing the physical examination, the physician may order laboratory tests for these reasons:
   - *To confirm a clinical diagnosis.* The patient's signs and symptoms may provide a strong clinical diagnosis of a particular condition, and the physician may order laboratory tests simply to confirm that diagnosis. For example, the patient may have the typical signs and symptoms of diabetes mellitus, which would provide the physician with a fairly certain clinical diagnosis. In this instance, a glucose tolerance test (GTT) would be ordered to confirm the diagnosis and institute therapy.
   - *To assist in the differential diagnosis of a patient's condition.* Two or more diseases may have similar signs and symptoms; the physician orders laboratory tests to assist in the differential diagnosis of the patient's condition. A final diagnosis of streptococcal sore throat

must be made with a laboratory test to differentiate it from other pathologic conditions with similar signs and symptoms, such as pharyngitis.

- *To obtain information regarding a patient's condition* when not enough concrete evidence exists to support a clinical diagnosis. The patient sometimes may have vague signs and symptoms, and laboratory tests are ordered to provide information on what may be causing the patient's problem. For example, the patient may have nonspecific abdominal pain, and the physical examination may not yield enough information to support a clinical diagnosis. In this case, the physician may order a series of laboratory and diagnostic tests to assist in pinpointing the cause of the patient's problems.

2. When the final diagnosis has been made, laboratory testing may be performed *to evaluate the patient's progress and to regulate treatment.* On the basis of the laboratory results, the therapy may need to be adjusted or further treatment prescribed. A patient undergoing iron therapy for iron deficiency anemia should have a complete blood count (CBC) performed every month to assess response to the treatment and ensure the condition is improving. Another example is a patient with thrombophlebitis who is taking warfarin (Coumadin), an anticoagulant used to inhibit blood clotting. The patient must have a prothrombin time test at regular intervals to assess the clotting ability of the blood. On the basis of the test results, the medication may need to be adjusted to ensure the dosage is at a safe level. A patient with diabetes who measures the blood glucose level each day to regulate insulin dosage provides another example of laboratory tests used to regulate treatment.

3. On the basis of such factors as age, gender, race, and geographic location, individuals have different normal levels within the established normal range for a particular test. In this respect, laboratory tests also can serve *to establish each patient's baseline or normal level* with which future results can be compared. A patient who is going to receive warfarin (Coumadin) therapy should have a blood specimen drawn for a prothrombin time test before administration of this anticoagulant. The results serve as a baseline recording for that particular patient with which future prothrombin time test results can be compared.

4. Laboratory tests also can help *to prevent or reduce the severity of disease* by early detection of abnormal findings. Certain conditions, such as high cholesterol, anemia, and diabetes, are relatively common disorders and sometimes may exist undetected in a patient, especially early in the development of the disease. Laboratory tests known as **routine tests** are performed on a routine basis on apparently healthy patients (usually as part of a general physical examination) to assist in the early detection of disease. These tests are relatively easy to perform and present a minimal hazard to the patient. The most commonly used routine tests are urinalysis, CBC, and routine blood chemistries.

5. Another reason for a laboratory test is its *requirement by state law.* The statutes of most states require a gonorrhea and syphilis test to be performed on pregnant women. The purpose of these tests is to protect the mother and fetus from harm by screening for the presence of these venereal diseases.

TYPES OF CLINICAL LABORATORIES

The medical office may use an outside laboratory for testing, or the office may contain its own laboratory, known as a *physician's office laboratory* (POL), in which the medical assistant performs various tests. Most medical offices use a combination of the two to fulfill the physician's needs for test results.

Physician's Office Laboratory

Generally, laboratory tests that are convenient to perform and commonly required, such as a glucose determination and urinalysis, are performed in the POL. Most physicians consider it too time-consuming and expensive in terms of equipment, supplies, medical laboratory personnel, and **quality control** to perform highly sophisticated and complex tests, such as serologic studies and microbiologic studies, in the medical office. These tests are usually performed at an outside laboratory. These laboratories use automated equipment to perform the tests, providing the medical offices with fast and reliable test results.

Outside Laboratories

Because the medical assistant usually works closely with an outside laboratory, a basic knowledge of the relationship between the medical office and the laboratory, as described in the following paragraphs, is important. Outside laboratories include hospital and privately owned commercial laboratories, which employ individuals specifically trained in clinical laboratory techniques and methods. If the specimen is collected at the medical office, the laboratory provides the medical office with the supplies and forms necessary to collect the specimen and prepare it for transport to the laboratory. The medical assistant is responsible for checking these supplies periodically and for reordering them from the laboratory as needed.

Laboratory Directory

The outside laboratory provides the medical office with a laboratory directory that serves as a valuable reference source for the proper collection and handling of specimens in the medical office for transport to the outside laboratory. Directories vary in organization, depending on the laboratory. The following information is generally included, however: names of the tests performed by the laboratory, the normal range for each test, instructions on completion of forms, patient preparation necessary for each test, supplies necessary for the collection of each specimen, amount and type of specimen required for each test, techniques to use for the collection of the specimen, proper handling and storage of the specimen, and instructions for transporting specimens.

Table 29-1 is a sample of representative tests taken from a laboratory directory. If the medical assistant has a question regarding any aspect of the collection and handling of the specimen, the laboratory should be called before proceeding.

Collection and Testing Categories

Collection and testing of a specimen can be categorized as follows: (1) the specimen is collected and tested at the medical office, (2) the specimen is collected at the medical office and transferred to an outside medical laboratory for testing, or (3) the patient is given a laboratory request to have the specimen collected and tested at an outside laboratory. The medical assistant's responsibilities depend on which of these methods is used in the medical office. For example, a specimen collected at the medical office and transferred to an outside laboratory for testing involves a series of individual steps different from the steps followed when it is collected and tested at the medical office. The

Table 29-1 Representative Tests from a Laboratory Directory

Test	Specimen Requirements	Normal Values
Albumin, serum	2 ml serum in SST or transfer tube	3.5-5.5 g/dL
ALT	2 ml serum in SST or transfer tube	45 U/L or less
AST	2 ml serum in SST or transfer tube	40 U/L or less
Bilirubin, total	2 ml serum in SST or transfer tube. Protect from light	1.2-1.3 mg/dL or less
Blood group (ABO)	5 ml lavender stoppered tube	—
BUN, serum	2 ml serum in transfer tube	7-25 mg/dL
Calcium, serum	2 ml serum in transfer tube	8.5-108 mg/dL
CBC with differential	5 ml lavender stoppered tube. Tube should be inverted 8-10 times immediately after drawing. Two blood smears	Values given with report
Chloride, serum	2 ml serum in SST or transfer tube	96-109 mmol/L
CPK	3 ml serum in SST or transfer tube	Male: 17-148 U/L Female: 10-70 U/L
Creatinine, serum	2 ml serum in SST or transfer tube	0.6-6 mg/dL
CRP	1 ml serum in SST or transfer tube. Avoid hemolysis	0.8 mg/dL or less
Glucose, **plasma**	5 ml gray stoppered tube. Tube should be inverted 6-8 times immediately after drawing	70-110 mg/dL
LDH	3 ml serum in SST or transfer tube. Hemolysis invalidates results	Less than 240 U/L
Potassium, serum	2 ml serum in SST or transfer tube. Hemolysis invalidates results	3.5-5.3 mmol/L
Prothrombin time	1- to 5-ml blue stoppered tube. Tube should be inverted 8-10 times immediately after drawing	9-12 sec
RPR	2 ml serum in SST or white-topped transfer tube	Nonreactive
Sedimentation rate	5 ml lavender stoppered tube. Tube should be inverted 6-8 times immediately after drawing	Male: 0-15 mm/hr Female: 0-20 mm/hr
Sodium, serum	2 ml serum in SST or transfer tube	135-147 mmol/L
Triiodothyronine (T_3)	2 ml serum in SST or transfer tube	85-205 mg/ml
Thyroxine (T_4)	1 ml serum in SST or transfer tube	4.5-12 µg/dL
Total protein, serum	2 ml serum in SST or transfer tube	6-8.5 g/dL
Triglycerides	2 ml serum in SST or transfer tube. Patient should be fasting 12-14 hr	Less than 150 mg/dL
Uric acid, serum	2 ml serum in SST or transfer tube	Male: 3.9-9 mg/dL Female: 2.2-7.7 mg/dL
Urinalysis, routine	Random sample. First morning specimen preferred (10 ml)	—

From Bonewit-West K: *Clinical procedures for medical assistants*, ed 7, St. Louis, 2008, Saunders.
ALT, Alanine aminotransferase; *AST,* aspartate aminotransferase; *BUN,* blood urea nitrogen; *CBC,* complete blood count; *CPK,* creatine phosphokinase; *CRP,* C-reactive protein; *LDH,* lactate dehydrogenase; *RPR,* rapid plasma reagin; *SST,* serum separator tube.

following clinical laboratory methods are presented in the remainder of this chapter to provide the student with the information needed to function competently in all three modes just described as follows:

1. Completing laboratory request forms and reviewing laboratory reports
2. Informing the patient of any necessary advance preparation or special instructions
3. Collecting, handling, and transporting specimens
4. Testing the specimens in the medical office
5. Practicing quality control and laboratory safety

LABORATORY REQUESTS

Purpose

A laboratory request is a printed form that contains a list of the most frequently ordered laboratory tests (Figure 29-1). A laboratory request is required when the specimen is collected at the medical office and transferred to an outside laboratory for testing, or when the specimen is to be collected and tested at an outside laboratory, in which case the request is given to the patient at the medical office to take to the laboratory. The request provides the outside laboratory with essential information necessary for accurate testing, reporting of results, and billing. The organizational formats for the request forms vary, depending on the laboratory. In general, most outside laboratories find it more convenient and economical to provide the medical office with one form for designating all tests, with the possible exception of the Pap test, in which case a separate form, known as a *cytology request,* is provided.

Parts of Laboratory Request Form

The request form can be completed manually by the medical assistant by writing in all information required, or it may be completed on a computer screen by entering the information using a keyboard. Specific information that is required on the laboratory request form follows.

1. *Physician's name and address.* The physician's name and address should be clearly indicated on the laboratory request form to facilitate the reporting of test results to the physician. Most laboratories provide request forms with the physician's name and address preprinted on the form. In addition, the forms are usually prenumbered with the physician's account number, which assists in identification, reporting, and billing of laboratory tests.
2. *Patient's name and address.* The patient's name and address should be printed (or entered) as requested by the laboratory; for example, the laboratory may want the patient's name designated with the last name first, middle initial, and then first name. The patient's address is needed for billing purposes and must include the city, state, and zip code.
3. *Patient's age and gender.* The normal ranges for some tests vary depending on the patient's age and gender. The normal range for hemoglobin concentration varies according to gender (12 to 16 g/dL for a woman; 14 to 18 g/dL for a man).
4. *Date and time of collection of the specimen.* The date of the specimen collection indicates to the laboratory the number of days that have passed since the collection, providing the laboratory with information regarding the freshness of the specimen. A time lapse that is too long between collection and testing of a specimen may affect the accuracy of some test results. The time of collection is significant with respect to selected laboratory tests. The normal range for serum cortisol varies depending on whether the specimen is collected in the morning or afternoon.
5. *Laboratory tests desired.* The tests desired by the physician are usually indicated by marking a box adjacent to those tests (see Figure 29-1). The boxes should be clearly marked to avoid any confusion. A space designated as "additional tests" or "other tests" is provided on the laboratory request form for specifying a test that is desired but not listed on the request form. As previously indicated, most laboratory request forms include only the tests most frequently ordered. The laboratory directory contains a complete listing of all the tests performed.

   Laboratory tests termed **profiles** contain many tests; the profiles performed by the laboratory and the tests included in each are listed in the directory. A profile may be specific in nature—that is, all the tests included relate to a specific organ of the body or a particular disease state. A specific profile is usually ordered when the physician does not have a definite clinical diagnosis but has a good idea of what organ or organs are involved in the patient's condition. The physician orders a profile of the organ in question. An example of this type of profile is the hepatic profile, which is used to assess liver function and to assist in the diagnosis of a pathologic condition that affects the liver.

   A profile may also be general in nature. A general metabolic profile contains numerous routine laboratory tests and is primarily used in a routine health screen of a patient. General metabolic profiles are used to detect any changes in the body's biologic processes that may be present, although the patient may not have had any symptoms to indicate that these changes have occurred. General metabolic profiles are also used when the patient's symptoms are so vague that the physician does not have enough concrete evidence to support a clinical diagnosis of a specific organ or disease state. An example of a general profile is the comprehensive metabolic profile; refer to Table 29-2 for a list of the tests included in this profile.

   The medical assistant should have knowledge of the names of common profiles and the tests generally contained in each, which are listed in Table 29-2. The tests contained in each profile may vary slightly from one laboratory to another.

6. *Source of the specimen.* Certain tests require that the source of the specimen (e.g., throat, wound, ear, eye,

Cronological

LABORATORY REQUISITION
Biomedical Laboratories, Inc.
100 Main Street
Athens, Georgia 45760

☐ Fax Send additional copy of report to:
☐ Call Client Number/Physician's Name   ( ) Phone/Fax number
☐ Mail Physician's Address   City, State, Zip

| Patient's Name (Last) | (First) | (MI) | Sex | Date of Birth MO│DAY│YEAR | Collection Time : AM PM | Fasting YES NO | Collection Date MO│DAY│YEAR |

| NPI/UPIN | Physician's ID # | Patient's SS # | Patient's ID # | Urine hrs/vol hrs___ vol___ |

Physician's Name (Last, First) | Physician's Signature | Patient's Address | Phone

Medicare # (Include prefix/suffix) ☐ Primary ☐ Secondary | City | State | ZIP

Medicaid # | State | Physician's Provider # | Name of Responsible Party (if different from patient)

Diagnosis/Signs/Symptoms in ICD-9 Format (Highest Specificity) **REQUIRED** | Address of Responsible Party (if different from patient) APT # | City | State | ZIP

Patient's Relationship to Responsible Party ☐ 1–Self ☐ 2–Spouse ☐ 3–Child ☐ 4–Other

Performance Lab ☐ | Carrier | Group # | Employee # | Mem

Insurance Company Name | Plan | Carrier Code
Subscriber/Member # | Location | Group #
Insurance Address | Physician's Provider #
City | State | ZIP
Employer's Name or Number | Insured SS # (If not patient) | Worker's Comp ☐ Yes ☐ No

I hereby authorize the release of medical information related to the service subscribed herein and authorize payment directed to LabCorp.
X ___ Patient's Signature ___ Date

MEDICARE ADVANCE BENEFICIARY NOTICE
I have read the ABN on the reverse. If Medicare denies payment, I agree to pay for the identified test(s).
X ___ Patient's Signature ___ Date

NOTE: WHEN ORDERING TESTS FOR WHICH MEDICARE OR MEDICAID REIMBURSEMENT WILL BE SOUGHT, PHYSICIANS SHOULD ONLY ORDER TESTS THAT ARE MEDICALLY NECESSARY FOR THE DIAGNOSIS OR TREATMENT OF THE PATIENT. COMPONENTS OF THE ORGAN OR DISEASE PANELS/COMBINATIONS PRINTED BELOW ARE SHOWN ON THE REVERSE SIDE AND MAY ALSO BE ORDERED INDIVIDUALLY BELOW. COMPONENTS MAY BE BILLED SEPARATELY PER CARRIER POLICY.

PROFILES (See reverse for components)
80049	Basic Metabolic Profile	SST
80054	Comp Metabolic Profile	SST
80051	Electrolyte Profile	SST
80058	Hepatic Profile	SST
80059	Hepatitis Profile	SST
80061	Lipid Profile	SST
80091	Thyroid Profile	SST
80055	Prenatal Profile	RED LAV
80072	Rheumatoid Profile	SST

HEMATOLOGY
85025	CBC w Diff	LAV
85027	CBC w/o Diff	LAV
85014	Hematocrit	LAV
85018	Hemoglobin	LAV
85595	Platelet Count	LAV
85041	RBC Count	LAV
85048	WBC Count	LAV
85007	WBC Differential	LAV
89190	Nasal Smear, Eosin	Nasal Smear
85060	Pathologist Consult–Peripheral Smear	LAV

ALPHABETICAL/COMBINATION TESTS
86900/86901	ABO and Rh	LAV
82040	Albumin	SST
84075	Alkaline Phosphatase	SST
84460	ALT (SGPT)	SST
82150	Amylase, Serum	SST
86038	Antinuclear Antibodies	SST
84450	AST (SGOT)	SST
82607/82746	B12 and Folate	SST
82250	Bilirubin, Total	SST

ALPHABETICAL TESTS CON'T
84520	BUN	SST
82310	Calcium	SST
80156	Carbamazepine (Tegretol®)	SER
82378	CEA	SST
82465	Cholesterol, Total	SST
82565	Creatinine	SST
80162	Digoxin	SER
82670	Estradiol	SST
82728	Ferritin, Serum	SST
82985	Fructosamine	SST
83001	FSH	SST
83001/83002	FSH and LH	SST
82977	GGT	SST
82947	Glucose, Plasma	GRY
82947	Glucose, Serum	SST
82950	Glucose, 2-hr. PP	SST
83036	Glycohemoglobin, Total	LAV
84703	hCG, Beta Subunit, Qual	SST
84702	hCG, Beta Subunit, Quant	SST
83718	HDL Cholesterol	SST
86677	Helicobacter pylori, IgG	SST
86706	Hep B Surface Antibody	SST
87340	Hep B Surface Antigen	SST
86803	Hep C Antibody	SST
83036	Hemoglobin A1C	LAV
86701	HIV Antibodies	SST
83540	Iron, Total	SST
83540/83550	Iron and IBC	SST
83615	LDH	SST

ALPHABETICAL TESTS CON'T
83002	LH	SST
83690	Lipase	SER
80178	Lithium (Eskalith®)	SER
83735	Magnesium, Serum	SST
80184	Phenobarbital (Luminal®)	SER
80185	Phenytoin (Dilantin®)	SER
84132	Potassium	SST
84146	Prolactin, Serum	SST
84153	Prostate-Specific Antigen	SST
84066	Prostatic Acid Phos	SST
84155	Protein, Total	SST
85610	Prothrombin Time (PT)	BLU
85610/85730	PT and PTT Activated	BLU
85730	PTT Activated	BLU
86431	Rheumatoid Arthritis Factor	SST
86592	RPR	SST
86762	Rubella Antibodies, IgG	SST
85651	Sed Rate	LAV
84295	Sodium	SST
84403	Testosterone	SST
80198	Theophylline	SER
84436	Thyroxine (T4)	SST
84478	Triglycerides	SST
84480	Triiodothyronine (T3)	SST
84443	TSH, High Sensitivity	SST
84550	Uric Acid	SST
81003	Urinalysis Microscopic on Positives	URN
81001	Urinalysis with Microscopic	URN
80164	Valproic Acid (Depakene®)	SER

MICROBIOLOGY See Reverse Side
☐ ENDOCERVICAL ☐ THROAT ☐ URINE
☐ STOOL ☐ URETHRAL   INDICATE SOURCE
87070	Aerobic Bacterial Culture	Bact Trnspt
87490/87590	Chlamydia/GC DNA Probe w/ Confirmation on Positives	Probe Trnspt
87490/87590	Chlamydia/GC DNA Probe Without Confirmation	Probe Trnspt
87490	Chlamydia DNA Probe	Probe Trnspt
87081	Genital, Beta-Hemolytic Strep Cult, Group B	Bact Trnspt
87070	Genital Culture, Routine	Bact Trnspt
87070	Lower Respiratory Culture	Steril Trnspt
87590	N. gonorrhoeae DNA Probe	Probe Trnspt
87015/87211	Ova and Parasites	O & P Kit
87081 X2/87045	Stool Culture	Fecal Trnspt
87081	Throat, Beta-Hemolytic Strep Cult, Group A	Bact Trnspt
87060	Upper Respiratory Culture, Routine	Bact Trnspt
87086	Urine Culture, Routine	Urn Cul Trnspt

Clinical Information/Comments

OTHER TESTS/INDIVIDUAL COMPONENTS
TEST #   TEST NAMES

LAB USE ONLY | STAT ☐998074 | VENIPUNCTURE ☐998085 | TRAVEL ☐998096 | NON LABCORP ☐998239 | VERBAL ORDER ☐998250 | CHART ORDER ☐998261 | HANDWRITTEN ☐998272 | 24 HR TLV ☐998283 | PST/PSC #

CONTAINERS RECEIVED → SST SPUN | USST UNSPUN | SER SERUM TRNSPT | FRZ FRZ TRNS | RED RED | LAV LAVENDER | SLD SLIDE | BLU LT. BLUE | GRY GREY | GRN GREEN | RYB RYL BLU | YEL ACD | PLS PLASMA | URN URINE | 24U 24 HR URINE | TA-U TART. ACID | FL FLUID | OT OTHER | BACT TRNSP | O & P KIT | PROBE TRNSP | URN CULT TRNSP | STERIL TRNSP | FECAL TRNSP | VIRAL TRNSP

300-0384

Figure 29-1. Laboratory request form. (From Bonewit-West K: *Clinical procedures for medical assistants,* ed 7, St. Louis, 2008, Saunders.)

Table 29-2 Laboratory Profiles

Profile	Tests Included	Use
Comprehensive metabolic profile	Albumin ALP ALT AST Bilirubin BUN Calcium Carbon dioxide Chloride Creatinine Glucose Potassium Sodium Total protein	General health screen that provides information on kidneys, liver, acid-base balance, blood glucose level, and blood proteins. Used to evaluate organ function and check for conditions such as diabetes, liver disease, and kidney disease Routinely ordered as part of blood workup for physical examination or medical examination (particularly when patient's symptoms are vague) Abnormal test results are usually followed up with more specific tests before final diagnosis is made
Electrolyte profile	Carbon dioxide Chloride Potassium Sodium	Screen for electrolyte or acid-base imbalance and monitor effect of treatment on disease or condition that causes electrolyte imbalance This profile is also used to evaluate patient taking medication that can cause electrolyte imbalance
Hepatic profile	Albumin ALP ALT AST Direct bilirubin Total bilirubin Total protein	Detection of pathologic conditions affecting liver This test is often ordered when symptoms indicating liver condition occur, such as jaundice, dark urine, light-colored bowel movements, or pain or swelling in abdomen This profile may be ordered when individual has been exposed to hepatitis, has family history of liver disease, has excessive alcohol consumption, or is taking medication that can result in liver damage
Hepatitis profile	HBsAg Anti-HBc IgM Anti-HAV IgM	Detection of viral hepatitis
Kidney function profile	Albumin BUN Calcium Carbon dioxide Chloride Creatinine Phosphatase Potassium Sodium	Detection of kidney problems This profile shows how well kidneys are functioning to remove excess fluid and waste When problem is detected, diagnostic imaging tests may be used for further evaluation and diagnosis
Lipid profile	Total cholesterol LDL cholesterol HDL cholesterol Triglycerides VLDL cholesterol (calculation) Total cholesterol/HDL ratio (calculation)	Determine risk of coronary artery disease
Prenatal profile	ABO grouping and Rh typing Antibody screen CBC HBsAg Rubella antibodies Syphilis serology	Establish baseline recordings and screenings of prenatal patients for disease or potential problems
Rheumatoid profile	Rheumatoid factor ESR CRP Uric acid ANA	Assist in diagnosis of rheumatoid arthritis and to help distinguish it from other forms of arthritis and conditions with similar symptoms This profile also is used to evaluate severity of rheumatoid arthritis, to monitor the condition and its complications, and to assess response to treatment
Thyroid function profile	FTI Thyroxine (T_4) Triiodothyronine (T_3) uptake	Detection of conditions affecting thyroid gland

From Bonewit-West K: *Clinical procedures for medical assistants*, ed 7, St. Louis, 2008, Saunders.

ALP, Alkaline phosphatase; *ALT,* alanine aminotransferase; *ANA,* antinuclear antibody; *AST,* aspartate aminotransferase; *BUN,* blood urea nitrogen; *CBC,* complete blood count; *CRP,* C-reactive protein; *ESR,* erythrocyte sedimentation rate; *FTI,* free thyroxine index; *HAV,* hepatits A virus; *HBc,* hepatitis B core; *HBsAg,* hepatitis B surface antigen; *HDL,* high-density lipoprotein; *IgM,* immunoglobulin M; *LDL,* low-density lipoprotein; *VLDL,* very-low-density lipoprotein.

urine, vagina) be recorded on the laboratory request form. This is for identification of the origin of the specimen for the laboratory because this information is not available from looking at the specimen. In many instances, the source dictates the test method used by the laboratory to evaluate the specimen for the presence of a possible pathogen. The test method used to detect the presence of *Streptococcus* in a specimen obtained from the throat would be different from that used to detect *Candida albicans* in a vaginal specimen.

7. *Physician's clinical diagnosis.* The clinical diagnosis assists the laboratory in correlating the clinical laboratory data with the needs of the physician. In some instances, further testing is performed by the laboratory if one test method proves inconclusive with respect to providing the physician with the information necessary to confirm or reject the clinical diagnosis. Another function of the clinical diagnosis is to assure laboratory personnel that the test results are within the framework of the diagnosis. When the results of a test disagree with the physician's clinical diagnosis, the laboratory repeats the test on the same or another specimen. The clinical diagnosis also alerts laboratory personnel to the possibility of the presence of a potentially dangerous pathogen, such as the hepatitis virus. In addition, this information is necessary for third-party billing by the laboratory. If the laboratory bills an insurance company for the tests, the clinical diagnosis needs to be on the insurance form. The processing of insurance forms is facilitated by having the information at hand and not having to contact the medical office to obtain it.

8. *Medications.* Certain medications may interfere with the accuracy and validity of the test results. The laboratory should be notified on the request form of any medications taken by the patient.

9. *STAT.* Sometimes the physician wants the laboratory test results reported as soon as possible. In this case, "STAT" should be clearly written in bold letters (or the appropriate STAT box checked) on the laboratory request form. Requests that are marked STAT are performed as soon as possible after receipt by the laboratory, and the results are telephoned or faxed to the physician as soon as they are available.

After the specimen has been collected, the completed request form must be placed with the specimen for transport to the outside laboratory. The medical assistant should realize the significance of this simple but important step. Numerous possible tests can be performed on one particular specimen, and without the request form, the laboratory does not have the information it needs to carry out the physician's orders, causing delays in completing the tests and reporting results.

LABORATORY REPORTS

Laboratory report forms are used to relay the results of the laboratory tests to the physician (Figure 29-2). The report

Putting It All into Practice

My name is Korey McGrew, and I am employed by a group of physicians in a family practice medical office. Some of my duties include showing patients to examining rooms, taking the patient's vital signs, administering medications, transcription, filing, and many other duties that medical assistants perform. I have found that being a medical assistant has been challenging and rewarding, and I wish you the best of luck in reaching your goals.

As a practicing medical assistant, I had a challenging venipuncture experience. The patient was a kind and personable 64-year-old man with hardening of the arteries. I tried two times to obtain the blood specimen from his arms but was not successful. The patient was calm and not bothered at all with the two sticks. He said that it was hard to draw blood on him and to go ahead and try again. I decided to try taking blood from a vein on the back of his hand with a butterfly setup. To my relief, I obtained the blood specimen. I think that I was more nervous about this experience than the patient was. It is important to remain calm on the outside around patients even if you are nervous on the inside. ■

Prepare for Success

is usually in the form of a computer printout. It may consist of a preprinted form with the test results printed in the appropriate spaces on the form by a computer (as illustrated in Figure 29-2), or the entire report may be generated by the computer. The report includes the following information:

1. Name, address, and telephone number of the laboratory
2. Physician's name and address
3. Patient's name, age, and gender
4. Patient accession number
5. Date the specimen was received by the laboratory
6. Date the results were reported by the laboratory
7. Names of the tests performed
8. Results of the tests
9. Normal range for each test performed

A patient accession number or laboratory number is assigned to each specimen received by the laboratory. Its purpose is to provide positive identification of each specimen within the laboratory and to allow easy access to the patient's laboratory records should a test result need to be located again. If the physician desires to have the laboratory test repeated, the accession number listed on the original report form must be included on the laboratory request form.

A normal range, rather than a single value, is necessary for laboratory test results because of individual differences among a general population due to factors such as age,

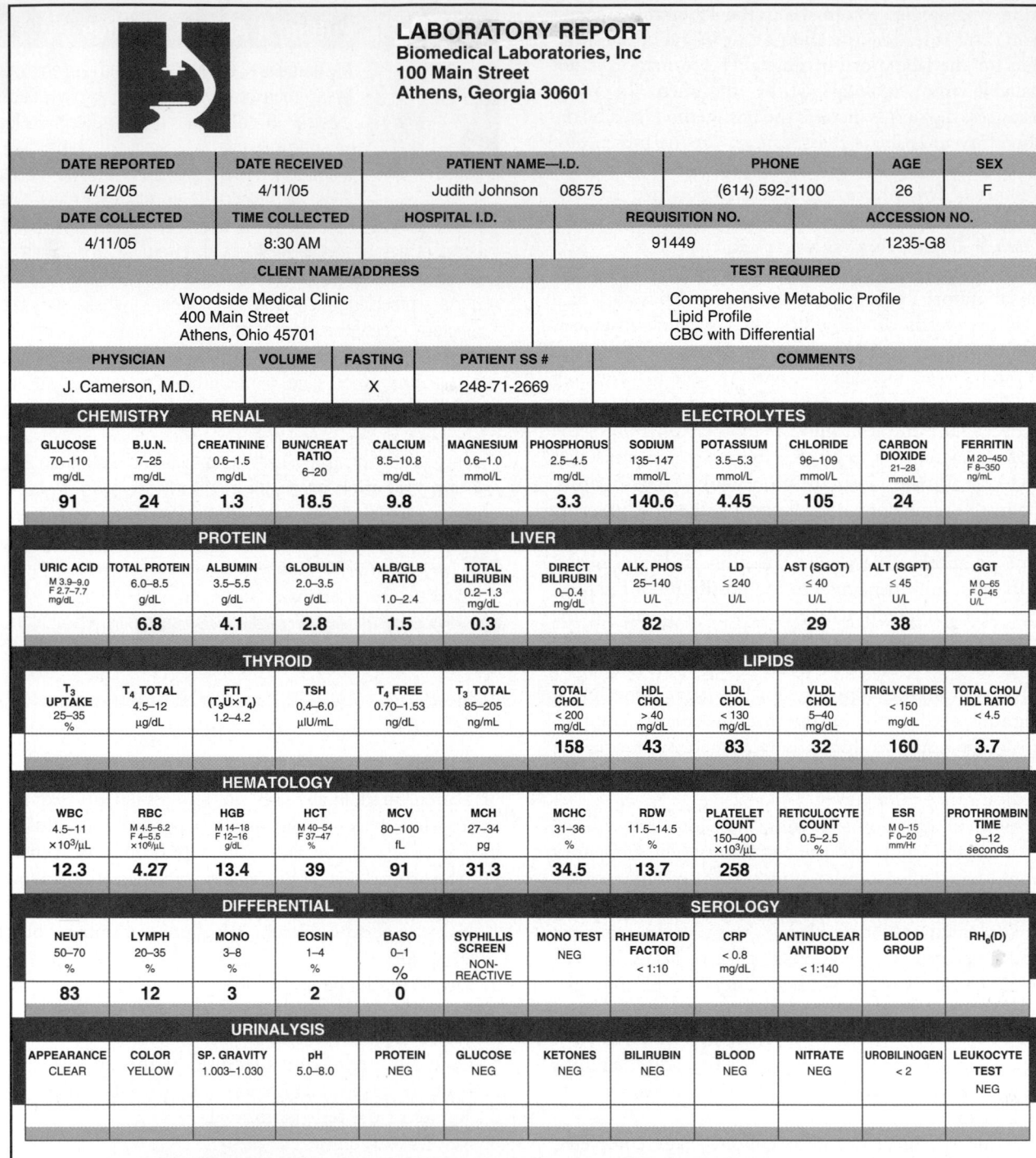

LABORATORY REPORT
Biomedical Laboratories, Inc
100 Main Street
Athens, Georgia 30601

DATE REPORTED	DATE RECEIVED	PATIENT NAME—I.D.		PHONE	AGE	SEX
4/12/05	4/11/05	Judith Johnson	08575	(614) 592-1100	26	F

DATE COLLECTED	TIME COLLECTED	HOSPITAL I.D.	REQUISITION NO.	ACCESSION NO.
4/11/05	8:30 AM		91449	1235-G8

CLIENT NAME/ADDRESS	TEST REQUIRED
Woodside Medical Clinic 400 Main Street Athens, Ohio 45701	Comprehensive Metabolic Profile Lipid Profile CBC with Differential

PHYSICIAN	VOLUME	FASTING	PATIENT SS #	COMMENTS
J. Camerson, M.D.		X	248-71-2669	

CHEMISTRY   RENAL / **ELECTROLYTES**

GLUCOSE 70–110 mg/dL	B.U.N. 7–25 mg/dL	CREATININE 0.6–1.5 mg/dL	BUN/CREAT RATIO 6–20	CALCIUM 8.5–10.8 mg/dL	MAGNESIUM 0.6–1.0 mmol/L	PHOSPHORUS 2.5–4.5 mg/dL	SODIUM 135–147 mmol/L	POTASSIUM 3.5–5.3 mmol/L	CHLORIDE 96–109 mmol/L	CARBON DIOXIDE 21–28 mmol/L	FERRITIN M 20–450 F 8–350 ng/mL
91	24	1.3	18.5	9.8		3.3	140.6	4.45	105	24	

PROTEIN / **LIVER**

URIC ACID M 3.9–9.0 F 2.7–7.7 mg/dL	TOTAL PROTEIN 6.0–8.5 g/dL	ALBUMIN 3.5–5.5 g/dL	GLOBULIN 2.0–3.5 g/dL	ALB/GLB RATIO 1.0–2.4	TOTAL BILIRUBIN 0.2–1.3 mg/dL	DIRECT BILIRUBIN 0–0.4 mg/dL	ALK. PHOS 25–140 U/L	LD ≤ 240 U/L	AST (SGOT) ≤ 40 U/L	ALT (SGPT) ≤ 45 U/L	GGT M 0–65 F 0–45 U/L
	6.8	4.1	2.8	1.5	0.3		82		29	38	

THYROID / **LIPIDS**

T_3 UPTAKE 25–35 %	T_4 TOTAL 4.5–12 µg/dL	FTI ($T_3U \times T_4$) 1.2–4.2	TSH 0.4–6.0 µIU/mL	T_4 FREE 0.70–1.53 ng/dL	T_3 TOTAL 85–205 ng/mL	TOTAL CHOL < 200 mg/dL	HDL CHOL > 40 mg/dL	LDL CHOL < 130 mg/dL	VLDL CHOL 5–40 mg/dL	TRIGLYCERIDES < 150 mg/dL	TOTAL CHOL/ HDL RATIO < 4.5
						158	43	83	32	160	3.7

HEMATOLOGY

WBC 4.5–11 ×10³/µL	RBC M 4.5–6.2 F 4–5.5 ×10⁶/µL	HGB M 14–18 F 12–16 g/dL	HCT M 40–54 F 37–47 %	MCV 80–100 fL	MCH 27–34 pg	MCHC 31–36 %	RDW 11.5–14.5 %	PLATELET COUNT 150–400 ×10³/µL	RETICULOCYTE COUNT 0.5–2.5 %	ESR M 0–15 F 0–20 mm/Hr	PROTHROMBIN TIME 9–12 seconds
12.3	4.27	13.4	39	91	31.3	34.5	13.7	258			

DIFFERENTIAL / **SEROLOGY**

NEUT 50–70 %	LYMPH 20–35 %	MONO 3–8 %	EOSIN 1–4 %	BASO 0–1 %	SYPHILLIS SCREEN NON-REACTIVE	MONO TEST NEG	RHEUMATOID FACTOR < 1:10	CRP < 0.8 mg/dL	ANTINUCLEAR ANTIBODY < 1:140	BLOOD GROUP	RH₀(D)
83	12	3	2	0							

URINALYSIS

APPEARANCE CLEAR	COLOR YELLOW	SP. GRAVITY 1.003–1.030	pH 5.0–8.0	PROTEIN NEG	GLUCOSE NEG	KETONES NEG	BILIRUBIN NEG	BLOOD NEG	NITRATE NEG	UROBILINOGEN < 2	LEUKOCYTE TEST NEG

Figure 29-2. Laboratory report form. (From Bonewit-West K: *Clinical procedures for medical assistants,* ed 7, St. Louis, 2008, Saunders.)

gender, race, and geographic location. In addition, no test can be so accurate that a single value is possible. The normal range for each test varies slightly from one laboratory to another, depending on the test method, equipment, and reagents used to perform the test. In this regard, it is essential that the medical assistant compare the test results with the normal ranges supplied by the laboratory performing the test, rather than with a reference source such as a medical laboratory textbook.

Laboratory reports are faxed, mailed, hand delivered, or sent electronically to the medical office by the laboratory. Abnormal results that pose a threat to the patient's health and laboratory reports marked STAT are telephoned or faxed to the medical office as soon as the tests are completed, and a complete written report follows immediately thereafter. The laboratory usually supplies the medical office with telephone reporting pads to transcribe the results from the telephone report to reduce errors.

What Would You Do? What Would You *Not* Do?

Case Study 1

Three days ago, Hildy McNicle was given a laboratory requisition at the medical office to have blood drawn and tested at an outside medical laboratory. Hildy calls the medical office and says she is a little confused. She called the laboratory for her test results, and they would not give them to her. They told her to call the medical office. She does not understand this because her blood was collected and tested at the laboratory, and it would seem logical to her that they would give her the test results, especially because she is paying the laboratory to perform the tests. The test results have come back with abnormal values, and the physician is at a medical convention and will not return until tomorrow. ■

The medical assistant may be responsible for reviewing the laboratory reports as they are received. The medical assistant should compare the patient's test results with the normal ranges supplied by the laboratory and notify the physician of any abnormal test results. Most computer systems automatically flag abnormal results on the laboratory report; if not, the physician may want the medical assistant to identify them by circling them with a red pen. The physician reviews the reports, and the data obtained are correlated with the information obtained from the health history and physical examination. The physician indicates that he or she is finished with the report usually by placing his or her initials on it. The medical assistant is then responsible for filing the laboratory report in the patient's chart, according to the medical office policy.

PATIENT PREPARATION AND INSTRUCTIONS

Factors such as food consumption, medication, activity, and time of day affect the laboratory results of certain tests. For some laboratory tests, advance patient preparation is necessary to obtain a quality specimen suitable for testing, which leads to accurate results and assists the physician in accurate diagnosis and treatment. The quality of the laboratory test results can be only as good as the quality of the specimen obtained from the patient. A specimen obtained from a patient who has not prepared properly may invalidate the test results and necessitate calling the patient back to collect the specimen again.

The medical assistant is usually responsible for instructing the patient in any advance preparation that might be necessary. A complete and thorough explanation of the instructions should be relayed clearly to the patient. The medical assistant should explain the reason for the advance preparation so that the patient will be more likely to comply with the preparation necessary. It should be emphasized to the patient that the preparation is essential to obtain accurate test results and to avoid having to collect the specimen again.

After the instructions have been explained, the medical assistant needs to verify that the patient completely understands them and offer to answer any questions. It is also advisable to provide the patient with a written instruction sheet to serve as a reference, should the patient forget some of the information after leaving the medical office. Some specimen collections may require that the patient remain at the collection site for a specified time; an example of this is the GTT, which requires several hours for the collection of multiple, timed specimens. The patient should be told in advance of the time requirement so that any necessary arrangements can be made with an employer or babysitter.

Sometimes the patient collects the specimen at home. The medical assistant is responsible for explaining detailed instructions to the patient on the proper techniques for collection of the specimen. For example, if a first-voided morning urine specimen is necessary for the laboratory test, the medical assistant needs to provide the patient with the appropriate specimen container and to instruct the patient in the proper collection, handling, and storage of the specimen until it reaches the medical office.

The specific type of preparation necessary for a particular test depends on the test ordered and the method used to run it. If the medical office uses an outside laboratory, the patient preparation necessary for each test can be found in the laboratory directory. If the test is performed in the medical office, the medical assistant should consult the manufacturer's instructions that accompany the testing product to obtain specific information regarding patient preparation. Advance patient preparation is usually in the form of fasting, a diet modification (e.g., low-fat diet), or medication restrictions.

Fasting

Some venous blood specimens require the patient to fast before collection. The composition of blood is altered by the consumption of food because the digested food is absorbed into the circulatory system, changing the results of certain laboratory tests. Food intake causes blood glucose and triglyceride laboratory tests to yield falsely high results. Any individual test (e.g., fasting blood sugar, GTT) or profile including these tests (e.g., comprehensive metabolic profile, lipid profile) requires the patient to fast before the specimen is collected.

Fasting involves abstaining from food and fluids (except water) for a specified amount of time before the collection of the specimen (usually 12 to 14 hours). Fasting specimens are usually collected in the morning to allow the food from the previous evening meal to be completely digested and absorbed. In addition, collection of the specimen in the morning causes the least amount of inconvenience to the patient in terms of abstaining from food and fluid.

The medical assistant must give detailed instructions to the patient, ensuring that the patient understands that fasting includes abstaining from food and fluid. The patient should be told, however, that it is permissible—in fact

What Would You Do? **What Would You *Not* Do?**

Case Study 2

Hans Volkman is leaving the medical office after being seen by the physician. The physician gave him a laboratory requisition for a CBC and a lipid profile. Hans notices that the clinical diagnosis on the form indicates iron deficiency anemia and wants to know why the physician did not prescribe any medication for him if he thought he had anemia. Hans says that he told the physician his father had a heart attack at age 53 years and asked whether he would order a cholesterol test. He says the physician must have forgotten because the test was not marked on the laboratory form. Hans has been instructed to fast for the laboratory tests. He says that he stops every morning at the Coffee Cup restaurant and has coffee with cream and sugar, orange juice, and two doughnuts. He would like to know whether he could just have the coffee before the tests. Hans says he has a hard time functioning in the morning without coffee. ■

What Would You Do? **What Would You *Not* Do?**

Case Study 3

Kathleen O'Leary is scheduled for a follow-up appointment today at the office. She was seen last week with fatigue, shortness of breath, weight loss, increased urination, and blurred vision. Kathleen was given a laboratory requisition to have blood drawn at an outside medical laboratory. The physician ordered a CBC with differential and a comprehensive metabolic profile. When the charts are prepared for the day, Kathleen's laboratory results are not in her chart. Kathleen is contacted by phone; she says she knows she should have gone to the laboratory to have her blood drawn, but she is afraid of needles and panics at the sight of blood. She says that the last time she had her blood drawn she started feeling hot and lightheaded and had to lie down on a table and was embarrassed. Kathleen says she also is worried the laboratory results might show something is wrong with her. She is thinking of not coming for her appointment today and hopes that she starts feeling better on her own. ■

advisable—to drink water because dehydration caused by water abstinence can also alter certain test results.

The medical assistant should indicate a specific time to the patient for initiation of the fast. If the specimen is to be collected in the morning, the patient should be instructed to begin fasting at 6:00 PM on the previous evening. The patient must also be told the time to report for collection of the specimen.

Medication Restrictions

Many medications affect the physical and chemical characteristics of body substances; medications taken by the patient may lead to inaccurate test results. Antibiotic therapy administered before collection of a throat specimen for strep testing may cause a falsely negative test result. The physician generally asks the patient to avoid taking medication for a period of time before the collection of the specimen if discontinuing the medication would not cause any health threat or serious discomfort to the patient. Because medication is more likely to interfere with test results on urine than on blood, the patient is recommended to discontinue medication 48 to 72 hours before the collection of a urine specimen and 4 to 24 hours before the collection of a blood specimen.

If the patient cannot be taken off medication, this information should be recorded on the laboratory request form for specimens transported to an outside laboratory for testing. This alerts the laboratory personnel to the presence of the medication. If the medication taken by the patient interferes with the method normally used to perform the test, the laboratory may be able to use an alternative method to obtain valid results. If the test is being performed in the medical office, the medical assistant should consult the manufacturer's instructions that accompany the testing device or kit for the names of the medications that interfere with test results.

The physician determines the need for a patient to discontinue medication before specimen collection. The medical assistant is responsible for ensuring that the patient understands any instructions regarding restrictions on medication and for recording medications the patient is taking on the laboratory request form.

COLLECTING, HANDLING, AND TRANSPORTING SPECIMENS

Clinical laboratory tests are performed on specimens obtained from the body. A **specimen** is a small sample or part taken from the body to represent the nature of the whole. Most laboratory tests are performed on specimens that are easily obtained from the body, such as blood, urine, feces, sputum, a cervical and vaginal scraping of cells, or a sample of a secretion or discharge from various parts of the body (e.g., nose, throat, wound, ear, eye, vagina, urethra) for microbiologic analysis. Other examples of specimens analyzed in the laboratory but more difficult to obtain from the body include gastric juices, cerebrospinal fluid, pleural fluid, peritoneal fluid, synovial fluid, and tissue specimens for biopsy. The source of the specimen may not be indicative of the pathologic condition in question; for example, triiodothyronine and thyroxine tests are performed on blood **serum** but are used to detect a condition that affects the thyroid gland.

The medical assistant is responsible for the collection of most specimens obtained from patients in the medical office; of these, blood and urine constitute the largest percentage of specimens collected. Certain specimens, such as a sample of vaginal or urethral discharge, cerebrospinal fluid, or a tissue specimen, must be collected by the physician; in these cases, the medical assistant aids with the collection. Procedure 29-1 describes the collection of a specimen for transport to an outside laboratory.

The most important aspect of specimen collection and handling is to provide the laboratory with a sample that is as biologically representative as possible of the body substance collected. If the specimen is collected or handled improperly, the **in vivo** characteristics of the specimen may be adversely affected, which may cause inaccurate and unreliable test results; this may interfere with the accurate diagnosis and treatment of the patient's condition. General guidelines for handling and storing biologic specimens most frequently collected in the medical office are presented in Table 29-3.

Table 29-3 Handling and Storage of Biologic Specimens*

Specimen	Handling	Storage
Blood	**All Blood Specimens** Prevent hemolysis Collect specimen in tube at room temperature	**For Most Blood Specimens** Refrigerate at 39°F (4°C) to retard alterations in physical and chemical composition of specimen Plasma and serum may be frozen; however, whole blood should not be frozen because it would cause hemolysis
	Serum Separate serum from blood within 30-45 min after collection	
	Plasma Mix anticoagulant gently but thoroughly with blood specimen immediately after collection	
Urine	Avoid contamination of inside of specimen container Do not leave specimen standing out for more than 1 hr after collection	If urine specimen cannot be tested within 1 hr after collection, refrigerate it or add appropriate preservative
Microbiologic specimens	Avoid contamination of swab used to collect specimen Avoid contamination of inside of microbiologic specimen container Protect yourself from contamination from microbiologic specimen Protect anaerobic specimens from exposure to air	Transport specimen as soon as possible. If not possible, place specimen in transport medium or inoculate it on appropriate culture medium and (for most specimens) place it in refrigerator at 39°F (4°C) to prevent drying and death of specimen or overgrowth of specimen with extraneous microorganisms
Stool	Collect specimen in clean container For detection of ova and parasites, keep stool warm	For most accurate test results, deliver specimen to laboratory immediately. If transportation of specimen is delayed, mix stool with appropriate preservative or place it in transport medium

From Bonewit-West K: *Clinical procedures for medical assistants*, ed 7, St. Louis, 2008, Saunders.
*For all specimens: Do not expose to extreme temperature changes.

PROCEDURE **29-1**   Collecting a Specimen for Transport to an Outside Laboratory

Outcome Collect a specimen for transport to an outside laboratory. A summary of the series of individual steps required for collecting a specimen in the medical office and transporting it to an outside laboratory is presented in this procedure.

1. Procedural Step. Inform the patient of any advance preparation or special instructions, which may include:
 a. Diet modification
 b. Fasting
 c. Medication restriction
 d. Collection of a specimen at home
Explain the instructions thoroughly, and provide the patient with written instructions to take home as a reference. Notify the patient of the time to report to the medical office for the specimen collection.

Principle. The patient must prepare properly to provide a quality specimen that would lead to accurate test results and would avoid a return to have another specimen collected.

2. Procedural Step. Review the requirements in the laboratory directory for the collection and handling of the specimens ordered by the physician, which include:
 a. Collection materials required
 b. Type of specimen to be collected
 c. Amount of the specimen necessary for laboratory analysis

Continued

PROCEDURE 29-1

PROCEDURE 29-1 Collecting a Specimen for Transport to an Outside Laboratory—cont'd

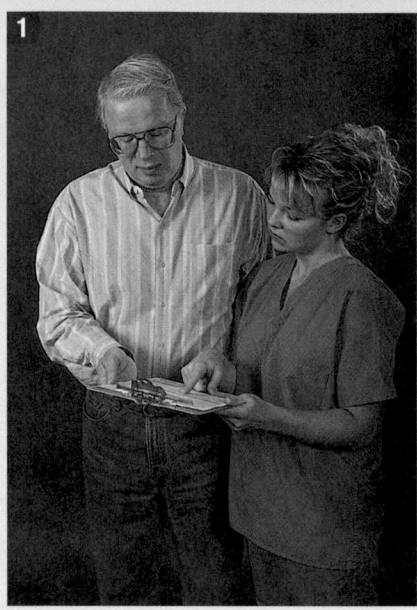

Instruct the patient in advance preparation. (From Bonewit-West K: *Clinical procedures for medical assistants,* ed 7, St. Louis, 2008, Saunders.)

    d. Procedure to follow to collect the specimen

    e. Proper handling and storage of the specimen

    Telephone the laboratory with any questions you have regarding any aspect of the collection or handling of the specimen.

    Principle. A review of the requirements beforehand prevents errors in collection and handling of the specimen.

3. Procedural Step. Complete the laboratory request form, which must include the following information printed in legible handwriting:

    a. Physician's name and address

    b. Patient's name (and address if required)

    c. Patient's age and gender

    d. Date and time of the collection

    e. Laboratory tests ordered by the physician

    f. Type of specimen

    g. Source of specimen

    h. Physician's clinical diagnosis

    i. Any medications the patient is taking

    j. Third-party billing information

    If the physician needs the test results as soon as possible, mark "STAT" on the request in bold letters.

    Principle. The completed form provides the laboratory with the information necessary to perform the tests accurately.

4. Procedural Step. Sanitize your hands.

5. Procedural Step. Assemble the equipment and supplies. Use the appropriate specimen container required by the outside laboratory. Ensure the container is sterile, and check that it is not broken, chipped, or cracked.

Principle. The appropriate specimen container must be used to ensure the collection of the proper type of specimen required by the laboratory. Damaged specimen containers are unsuitable for collection and should be discarded.

6. Procedural Step. Clearly label the tubes and containers with the patient's name, the date, your initials, and any other information required by the laboratory, such as the source of the specimen.

Principle. Properly labeled tubes and containers prevent mix-ups of specimens.

Label the tubes. (From Bonewit-West K: *Clinical procedures for medical assistants,* ed 7, St. Louis, 2008, Saunders.)

7. Procedural Step. Greet the patient and introduce yourself. Identify the patient by full name and date of birth and explain the procedure. Verify that you have the correct patient. If patient preparation was required for the test, determine whether the patient prepared properly.

Principle. Identification of the patient prevents collection of a specimen from the wrong person by mistake. Specimen collection is often an anxiety-producing experience for the patient, and reassurance should be offered to help reduce apprehension.

8. Procedural Step. Collect the specimen according to the following guidelines:

    a. Follow the OSHA standard.

    b. Collect the specimen with the proper technique.

    c. Collect the proper type and amount of the specimen required for the test.

    d. Process the specimen further if required by the outside laboratory (e.g., separating serum from whole blood).

    e. Place the lid tightly on the specimen container.

Principle. Proper collection of a specimen maintains its in vivo qualities and provides the laboratory with

PROCEDURE 29-1

a biologically representative sample of the body substance collected.

8

Collect the specimen. (From Bonewit-West K: *Clinical procedures for medical assistants,* ed 7, St. Louis, 2008, Saunders.)

9. **Procedural Step.** Prepare the specimen for transport to an outside laboratory for testing by performing the following:

a. Place the specimen in a biohazard specimen bag.
b. Place the laboratory request in the outside pocket of the specimen bag.
c. Properly handle and store the specimen while awaiting pick-up by a laboratory courier.
d. Record information in the patient's chart, including the date and time of the collection, the type and source of the specimen, the laboratory tests ordered by the physician, and information indicating its transport to the outside laboratory, including the date the specimen was sent.

Principle. The biohazard bag protects the laboratory courier from the possibility of an exposure incident. The outside laboratory must have the completed request form to know which laboratory tests have been ordered by the physician. The specimen must be handled and stored properly to maintain the in vivo characteristics of the specimen.

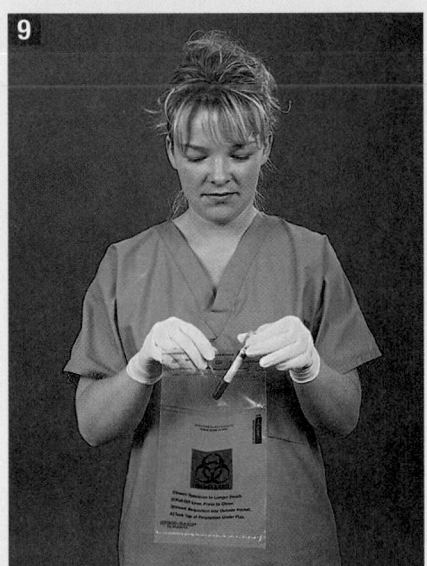

9

Prepare the specimen for transport. (From Bonewit-West K: *Clinical procedures for medical assistants,* ed 7, St. Louis, 2008, Saunders.)

10. **Procedural Step.** Review the laboratory report when it is returned to the medical office. Compare each test result with the normal range provided by the laboratory, and notify the physician of any abnormal results. File the laboratory report in the patient's chart after the physician has reviewed it.

CHARTING EXAMPLE	
Date	
3/10/10	8:00 a.m. Venous blood specimen collected from ⓡ arm. Tests ordered: total cholesterol, HDL, and triglycerides. Pt was in a fasting state. Courier pick-up by Medical Center Laboratory on 3/10/10. ————————
	——————— K. McGrew, CMA (AAMA)

PROCEDURE 29-1

CLINICAL LABORATORY IMPROVEMENT AMENDMENTS

Purpose of CLIA 1988

In 1988, Congress passed the Clinical Laboratory Improvement Amendments (CLIA 1988) to improve the quality of laboratory testing in the United States. CLIA 1988 consists of federal regulations governing all facilities that perform laboratory tests for health assessment or for the diagnosis, prevention, or treatment of disease. CLIA 1988 includes facilities not previously covered under federal legislation, such as POLs and nursing homes. The regulations for

implementing CLIA, developed by the Department of Health and Human Services (DHHS), consist of four separate sets of rules: laboratory standards, application and user fees, enforcement procedures, and approval of accreditation programs. The Centers for Medicare and Medicaid Services (CMS) is a division of DHHS. The CMS is responsible for monitoring compliance with the CLIA regulations.

Categories of Laboratory Testing

The CLIA regulations establish three categories of laboratory testing on the basis of the complexity of the testing methods.

1. *Waived tests.* Waived tests are simple procedures that are easy to perform and include procedures that patients can perform at home (e.g., blood glucose testing). POLs that perform only waived tests must apply for a certificate of waiver from the CMS, which exempts them from many of the CLIA oversight requirements. POLs with certificates of waiver are still expected to adhere to good laboratory practices, which include following the manufacturer's recommended instructions for each product or testing kit. To assist individuals in keeping up with new waived test additions and new methodologies for waived tests, the CMS maintains the following website: www.cms.hhs.gov/clia. The following tests are examples of waived tests:

   - Dipstick or tablet reagent urinalysis
   - Fecal occult blood testing
   - Ovulation testing with visual color comparisons
   - Urine pregnancy tests with visual color comparisons
   - Erythrocyte sedimentation rate, nonautomated
   - Hemoglobin using a CLIA-waived analyzer
   - Spun microhematocrit
   - Blood glucose determination using a Food and Drug Administration–approved blood glucose
   - Rapid streptococcus testing

2. *Moderate-complexity tests.* Moderate-complexity tests account for 75% of the estimated 10,000 laboratory tests performed in the United States every day. Examples of moderate-complexity tests performed in the medical office include hematology and blood chemistry tests performed on automated blood analyzers that are not CLIA-waived and microscopic analysis of urine sediment.

3. *High-complexity tests.* High-complexity tests include all procedures related to cytogenetics, histopathology, histocompatibility, and cytology (includes Pap testing). These tests are not usually performed in medical offices; most of these tests are done in laboratories already subject to federal regulation.

Requirements for Moderate-Complexity and High-Complexity Testing

Laboratories that perform moderate-complexity or high-complexity tests or both must meet the CLIA regulations and are subject to unannounced inspections every 2 years by the CMS. The major components of the CLIA 1988 regulations relating to laboratory standards are as follows:

1. *Patient test management.* A system must be established to maintain the optimal integrity and identification of patient specimens throughout the testing process. This system must also ensure accurate reporting of results.

2. *Quality control.* To ensure accurate and reliable test results, each laboratory must establish and follow written quality control procedures that monitor and evaluate the quality of each testing process. These include the following:

   - Developing a laboratory procedures manual, following the manufacturer's instructions for each product

   - Performing calibration procedures at least every 6 months and documenting results
   - Performing two levels of controls daily and documenting results
   - Performing and documenting actions taken when problems or errors are identified
   - Documenting all quality control activities

3. *Quality assurance.* Each laboratory must establish and follow written policies and procedures to monitor and evaluate the overall quality of the total testing process to ensure the accuracy and reliability of patient test results.

4. *Proficiency testing.* Proficiency testing (PT) is a form of external quality control in which laboratory specimens are prepared by an approved PT agency. Three times a year, the POL must test a shipment of these unknown specimens with the same procedure as for testing a patient's specimen. The results are forwarded to the PT agency for evaluation.

5. *Personnel requirements.* The CLIA regulations specify qualifications and responsibilities for personnel for laboratory directors, technical consultants, clinical consultants, and testing personnel. The regulations list specific education and training qualifications for the various positions and define the responsibilities for the persons who fill these positions. Personnel requirements are most stringent for high-complexity testing.

PHYSICIAN'S OFFICE LABORATORY

As previously discussed, a POL consists of an in-house medical office laboratory. The testing of a specimen in a POL involves following a series of steps to measure or identify the presence of a specific substance in the specimen, such as the measurement of a chemical or the identification of a microorganism. The medical assistant may be responsible for performing the laboratory tests and recording the

Memories *from* **Externship**

Korey McGrew: One of my most difficult situations as a medical assisting student was taking the temperature of a patient who went into seizures. I was scared because I was only a student, and I had never been in a situation like that before. I knew I had to act immediately, and luckily one of the certified medical assistants was nearby. We immediately put the patient on the floor and moved things away from him to prevent him from hurting himself. We then notified the physician, who was with a patient in another examining room. The seizures lasted only about 4 minutes, and the patient was fine. The certified medical assistant told me that the patient had a history of seizures and that I was not to be alarmed. That surely was a difficult but valuable learning experience for me. ∎

Prepare for Success

results, or the physician may employ a medical laboratory technologist or a medical technician to perform the tests. The decision is based on the number of tests performed in the medical office, the complexity of these tests, and the CLIA regulations. The medical assistant is qualified to perform waived laboratory tests; more sophisticated tests require the knowledge and skill of the medical laboratory technologist or technician.

Specimens can be analyzed with the **manual method** or the **automated method.** The manual method of laboratory testing involves performing the series of steps included in the test method by hand or manually. With the automated method, the series of steps are performed automatically by a self-operating system known as an *automated analyzer.* The method the physician uses to test biologic specimens in the medical office is based on the number and type of laboratory tests performed in the office. Regardless of the method used, a series of basic steps must be followed in testing each specimen, as follows:

1. The specific amount of the specimen necessary for the test method is measured from the specimen sample.
2. The necessary chemical reagents necessary for the test are combined with the specimen.
3. The specimen/reagents may require further processing, such as centrifugation, incubation, air drying, or heat fixing.
4. The substance undergoing assessment is manually or automatically measured or identified.
5. The results of the laboratory testing are obtained from a direct readout or with a mathematic calculation.
6. The results are recorded on a laboratory report form or in the patient's chart. The entry includes the patient's name, date, time, name of each laboratory test, results of the tests, and name of the individual performing the tests.

These steps are stated in general terms, but a basis is provided for understanding the process of laboratory testing. Textbooks such as this one and the manufacturer's instructions included with testing equipment should be consulted as reference sources to obtain the procedure for performing specific tests. The medical assistant must follow the procedure exactly to ensure accurate and reliable test results.

QUALITY CONTROL

The ultimate goal in the clinical laboratory is to ensure the laboratory test accurately measures what it is supposed to measure; this involves practicing and maintaining a quality control program. **Quality control** may be defined as the application of methods and means to ensure that test results are reliable and valid and errors that may interfere with obtaining accurate test results are detected and eliminated. Quality control is an ongoing process that encompasses every aspect of patient preparation and specimen collection, handling, transport, and testing. The quality control methods that should be used to obtain precision and accuracy in these areas have already been presented in this

chapter under their respective headings, with the exception of testing, which is discussed here.

Quality control methods used in testing the specimen include the following:
1. Using standards to check the precision and accuracy of laboratory equipment
2. Using controls to identify reagents that are outdated or have been improperly stored or to detect any errors in technique of the individual performing the test
3. Discarding outdated reagents
4. Following the procedure exactly to test the specimen
5. Performing tests in duplicate
6. Periodically checking the accuracy of the test results with a reference laboratory (PT)
7. Maintaining equipment by having it checked periodically for proper working order

Practicing quality control methods ensures that the test results represent the true status of the patient's condition and body functions and provides the physician with reliable information with which to make a diagnosis and prescribe treatment.

LABORATORY SAFETY

Laboratory safety is an important aspect of clinical laboratory testing in the medical office. Many of the laboratory tests performed in the medical office involve the use of strong chemical reagents, the handling of specimens that may contain pathogens, and the use of laboratory equipment. Practicing good techniques in testing laboratory specimens and recognizing potential hazards help reduce accidents in the laboratory. Some areas specifically related to laboratory safety in the medical office are described here.

The careful handling and storing of glassware to prevent breakage should be performed as follows:
1. Carefully arrange glassware in storage cabinets to prevent breakage.
2. Carefully remove glassware from storage cabinets.
3. If glassware does break, dispose of it in a puncture-resistant container to protect trash handlers from the shards.

The medical assistant should handle all chemical reagents carefully by adhering to the following instructions:
1. Ensure that all reagent containers are clearly and properly labeled.
2. If a label is loose, reattach it immediately.
3. Recap reagent containers immediately after use to prevent spills.

Laboratory specimens should be handled carefully as follows:
1. Follow the OSHA Bloodborne Pathogens Standard in collecting and handling of laboratory specimens.
2. Wash hands immediately if some of the material contained in the specimen is accidentally touched.
3. Avoid hand-to-mouth contact while working with specimens.

4. Immediately clean up any specimen spilled on the work-table, and cleanse the table with a disinfectant.
5. Properly dispose of all contaminated needles, syringes, specimen containers, and infectious waste.
6. Cover any break in the skin, such as a cut or scratch, with a bandage.

7. Ensure that all specimen containers are tightly capped to prevent leakage.
8. Handle all laboratory equipment and supplies properly and with care as indicated by the manufacturer. For example, wait until the centrifuge comes to a complete stop before opening it.

MEDICAL PRACTICE *and the* LAW

Laboratory procedures must be performed with precision to obtain accurate test results. Pay particular attention to each step in the procedure. Inaccurate laboratory results may cause the physician to incorrectly diagnose a patient's condition, which could lead to the wrong treatment. This situation could lead to a lawsuit.

Certain federal regulations govern laboratory testing, including those from CLIA and OSHA. These regulations help ensure stan-

dardization of laboratory tests and safe handling of reagents, blood, and body fluids to prevent contamination of specimens and infection of health care workers. Know and follow all regulations. Failure to do so could result in a legal liability. ■

What Would You Do? What Would You *Not* Do?   RESPONSES

Case Study 1
Page 691

What Did Korey Do?
❏ Told Hildy that the laboratory cannot release test results. Explained that they are experts in performing tests but do not have the medical knowledge to know their meanings.
❏ Told Hildy that the physician needed to give her the test results. Explained that the physician was out of town today but that an appointment could be made for her for tomorrow with the physician to discuss the results.

What Did Korey Not *Do?*
❏ Did not give Hildy the test results.
❏ Did not alarm Hildy that something might be wrong.

What Would You Do?/What Would You *Not* **Do?** Review Korey's response and place a checkmark next to the information you included in your response. List additional information you included in your response.

_____
_____
_____
_____

Case Study 2
Page 692

What Did Korey Do?
❏ Told Hans that the term "clinical diagnosis" means what the physician "thinks" is wrong before the laboratory tests are performed. Explained that when the test results are returned, the physician would be able to make a final diagnosis and then he would determine what treatment is necessary.
❏ Told Hans that a lipid profile includes several tests, one of which is a cholesterol test. Explained that the tests in a lipid profile

all help to determine whether someone is at risk for heart disease.
❏ Told Hans that he could not have any coffee until after his blood was drawn because it would affect the test results. Told him that his test could be scheduled first thing in the morning if that would help.

What Did Korey Not *Do?*
❏ Did not tell Hans he could have a cup of coffee before the laboratory tests.
❏ Did not tell Hans that he should not be eating doughnuts if he was concerned about his heart.

What Would You Do?/What Would You *Not* **Do?** Review Korey's response and place a checkmark next to the information you included in your response. List additional information you included in your response.

_____
_____
_____

Case Study 3
Page 692

What Did Korey Do?
❏ Stressed to Kathleen that if the laboratory test results are abnormal, it is better to know so that the physician can help make her better.
❏ Told Kathleen that many patients feel the same way about having blood drawn, so she is not alone. Relayed to her that her fear is normal, and she has no reason to be embarrassed.
❏ Told Kathleen that she should tell the laboratory about her last experience so that they could make it easier for her. Explained that they would probably put her in a reclining position to draw her blood so that she would not get light-headed.

What Would You Do? What Would You *Not* Do? RESPONSES—cont'd

❑ Gave Kathleen some suggestions on how to relax during the venipuncture. Told her to turn her head when the blood was drawn.

❑ Asked Kathleen whether she had any additional symptoms.

❑ Checked with the physician to see whether he wanted to keep her appointment for today or have her appointment rescheduled after the laboratory work is completed.

What Did Korey *Not* Do?

❑ Did not ignore or minimize Kathleen's concerns and fears.

❑ Did not tell Kathleen that her test results would probably be fine.

What Would You Do?/What Would You *Not* Do? Review Korey's response and place a checkmark next to the information you included in your response. List additional information you included in your response.

_____

_____

_____

_____

TERMINOLOGY REVIEW

Automated method *(for testing laboratory specimens)* A method of laboratory testing in which the series of steps in the test method is performed with an automated analyzer.

Fasting Abstaining from food or fluids (except water) for a specified amount of time before the collection of a specimen.

Homeostasis The state in which body systems are functioning normally, and the internal environment of the body is in equilibrium; the body is in a healthy state.

In vivo Occurring in the living body or organism.

Laboratory test The clinical analysis and study of materials, fluids, or tissues obtained from patients to assist in diagnosis and treatment of disease.

Manual method A method of laboratory testing in which the series of steps in the test method is performed by hand.

Normal range *(for laboratory tests)* A certain established and acceptable parameter or reference range within which the laboratory test results of a healthy individual are expected to fall.

Plasma The liquid part of the blood, consisting of a clear, yellowish fluid that comprises approximately 55% of the total blood volume.

Profile Numerous laboratory tests providing related or complementary information used to determine the health status of a patient.

Quality control The application of methods to ensure that test results are reliable and valid and that errors are detected and eliminated.

Routine test A laboratory test performed routinely on apparently healthy patients to assist in the early detection of disease.

Serum The clear, straw-colored part of the blood (plasma) that remains after the solid elements and the clotting factor fibrinogen have been separated out of it.

Specimen A small sample of something taken to show the nature of the whole.

ON THE WEB

For Information on Aging:

National Institute on Aging: www.nia.nih.gov

Administration on Aging: www.aoa.dhhs.gov

American Association of Retired Persons: www.aarp.org

Social Security Administration: www.ssa.gov

Centers for Medicare and Medicaid Services: www.cms.hhs.gov

Growth House: www.growthhouse.org

The AGS Foundation for Health in Aging: www.healthinaging.org

The Institute for Geriatric Social Work: www.bu.edu/igsw

Geriatrics at Your Fingertips: www.geriatricsatyourfingertips.org

Family Caregiver Alliance: www.caregiver.org

Senior Citizens Resources: www.firstgov.gov

Medicare: www.medicare.gov

Aging Statistics: www.agingstats.gov

Alzheimer's Foundation of America: www.alzfdn.org

 PREPARE FOR CERTIFICATION Visit the Evolve site at http://evolve.elsevier.com/Bonewit/today/ to actively Prepare for your Certification.

 *Check out the **Companion CD** bound with the book to access additional interactive activities.*

30

Urinalysis

LEARNING OBJECTIVES

Composition of Urine
1. List conditions that may cause polyuria and oliguria.
2. Define the terms used to describe symptoms of the urinary system.

Collection of Urine
1. Explain why a first-voided morning specimen is often preferred for urinalysis.
2. Explain the purpose of collecting a clean-catch midstream specimen.
3. Explain the purpose of a 24-hour urine collection.
4. List changes that may occur if urine is allowed to remain standing for more than 1 hour.

Analysis of Urine
1. List factors that may cause urine to have an unusual color or become cloudy.
2. Identify the various tests that are included in the physical and chemical examination of urine.
3. List the structures that may be found in a microscopic examination of urine.

Urine Pregnancy Testing
1. Explain the basis for urine pregnancy tests.
2. List the guidelines that must be followed in a urine pregnancy test to ensure accurate test results.

PROCEDURES

Instruct a patient in the procedure for collecting a clean-catch midstream urine specimen.

Assess the color and appearance of a urine specimen.

Perform a chemical assessment of a urine specimen.

Prepare a urine specimen for microscopic analysis by the physician.

Perform a urine pregnancy test.

CHAPTER OUTLINE

Composition of Urine
Terms Relating to the Urinary System
Collection of Urine
Guidelines for Urine Collection
Urine Specimen Collection Methods
Twenty-Four-Hour Urine Specimen
Analysis of Urine
Physical Examination of Urine
Chemical Examination of Urine

Reagent Strips
Microscopic Examination of Urine
Urine Pregnancy Testing
Human Chorionic Gonadotropin
Immunoassay Tests
Guidelines for Urine Pregnancy Testing
Serum Pregnancy Test

CAAHEP COMPETENCIES

Clinical Competencies
Specimen Collection
- Instruct patients in the collection of a clean-catch midstream urine specimen.

Diagnostic Testing
- CLIA-waived tests (perform urinalysis).

Patient Care
- Screen and follow up test results.

700

General Competencies

Patient Instruction

- Instruct individuals according to their needs.
- Provide instruction for health maintenance and disease prevention.

Operational Functions

- Use methods of quality control.

ABHES COMPETENCIES

Clinical Duties

- Use quality control.
- Perform selected CLIA-waived tests that assist with diagnosis and treatment.
- Screen and follow up patient test results.
- Instruct patients in the collection of a clean-catch midstream urine specimen.
- Perform urinalysis.

Office Management

- Operate and maintain facilities and perform routine maintenance of administrative and clinical equipment safely.

Instruction

- Teach patients methods of health promotion and disease prevention.

KEY TERMS

bilirubinuria (bill-ih-roo-bin-YUR-ee-ah)
bladder catheterization
glycosuria (glie-koe-SOO-ree-ah)
ketonuria (kee-toe-NOO-ree-ah)
ketosis (kee-TOE-sis)
micturition (mik-tur-ISH-un)
nephrons (NEF-rons)
oliguria (oh-lig-YUR-ee-ah)
pH (PEE-AYCH)
polyuria (pol-ee-YUR-ee-ah)

proteinuria (PRO-teen-YUR-ee-ah)
refractive index
refractometer (reh-frak-TOM-ih-tur)
renal threshold (REE-nul-THRESH-hold)
specific gravity
supernatant (soo-per-NAY-tent)
suprapubic aspiration
urinalysis (yur-in-AL-ih-sis)
void (VOYD)

COMPOSITION OF URINE

A physiologic change in the body caused by disease can create a disturbance in one or more of the functions of the kidney. Detection of such a disturbance can be made with the examination of urine and other body fluids such as blood.

Urine is composed of 95% water and 5% organic and inorganic waste products. Organic waste products consist of urea, uric acid, ammonia, and creatinine. Urea is present in the greatest amounts and is derived from the breakdown of proteins. Inorganic waste products include chloride, sodium, potassium, calcium, magnesium, phosphate, and sulfate.

A normal adult excretes approximately 750 to 2000 ml of urine per day. This amount varies according to the amount of fluid consumed and the amount of fluid lost through other means, such as perspiration, feces, and water vapor from the lungs. An excessive increase in urine output is known as **polyuria,** with the urine volume exceeding 2000 ml in 24 hours. Polyuria may be caused by the excessive intake of fluids or the intake of fluids that contain caffeine (e.g., coffee, tea, cola), which is a mild diuretic. Certain drugs, such as diuretics, and the pathologic conditions of diabetes mellitus, diabetes insipidus, and renal disease may also result in polyuria. A decreased or scanty urine output is known as **oliguria.** In the case of oliguria, the urine volume is less than 400 ml in 24 hours. Oliguria may occur with decreased fluid intake, dehydration, profuse perspiration, vomiting, diarrhea, or kidney disease. The normal act of voiding urine is known as **micturition.**

Terms Relating to the Urinary System

The medical assistant should have a thorough knowledge of the following terms used to describe symptoms associated with the urinary system:

Anuria   Failure of the kidneys to produce urine.

Diuresis   Secretion and passage of large amounts of urine.

Dysuria   Difficult or painful urination.

Frequency   The condition of having to urinate often.

Hematuria   Blood present in the urine.

Nocturia   Excessive (voluntary) urination during the night.

Nocturnal enuresis   Inability of an individual to control urination at night during sleep (bedwetting).

Oliguria   Decreased output of urine.

Polyuria   Increased output of urine.

Pyuria   Pus present in the urine.

Retention   The inability to empty the bladder. The urine is being produced normally but is not being voided.

Urgency   The immediate need to urinate.

Urinary incontinence   The inability to retain urine.

COLLECTION OF URINE

The advantage of urine testing is that urine is readily available and does not require an invasive procedure or the use of special equipment to obtain. For accurate test results, however, the medical assistant must adhere to proper urine collection procedures to obtain the proper specimen as ordered by the physician.

Guidelines for Urine Collection

The guidelines listed should be followed in collection of a urine specimen:

1. The medical assistant must obtain an adequate volume of urine as needed for the type of test (usually 30 to 50 ml of urine).

2. Each specimen must be labeled properly with the patient's name, the date and time of collection, and the type of specimen (i.e., urine) to avoid any mixups in specimens.

3. Any medication the patient is taking should be recorded on the laboratory requisition and in the patient's chart because some medications may interfere with the accuracy of the test results.

4. If possible, the collection of a urine specimen should be avoided in women during menstruation and for several days thereafter because the specimen may become contaminated with blood. This results in a false-positive test result for blood in the urine.

5. The medical assistant should take into consideration that voiding may be difficult for patients under stress and anxiety. In these instances, understanding and patience should be conveyed to the patient.

6. A urine specimen may be difficult to obtain from a child, even with the assistance of a parent. In this case, the physician should be informed because another collection method may be used, such as a urine collection bag, suprapubic aspiration, or catheterization of the patient.

Urine Specimen Collection Methods

The type of test to be performed often dictates the method used to collect the urine specimen. A first-voided morning specimen is recommended for pregnancy testing, and a clean-catch midstream specimen is necessary for identification of the presence of a urinary tract infection (UTI).

Most offices use disposable plastic urine specimen containers. These containers are available in different sizes and come with lids to prevent spillage and reduce bacterial and other types of contamination.

What Would You Do? What Would You *Not* Do?

Case Study 1

Yusuke Urameshi is at the office with fever and chills, dysuria, frequency, and difficulty urinating. The physician suspects that Mr. Urameshi has prostatitis and orders a clean-catch urine specimen for a complete urinalysis, including a microscopic examination of the sediment. Mr. Urameshi tries to collect the specimen but is able to collect only 5 ml of urine. He says that he is worried about what is wrong with him and that he thinks his nervousness is making it hard to get a specimen. Mr. Urameshi says that it is probably just as well because he did not understand how to cleanse himself, and he is not sure that he did it right. ■

Random Specimen

Urine testing in the medical office is often performed on freshly voided, random specimens. The medical assistant instructs the patient to **void** into a clean, dry, wide-mouthed container, and the urine is tested immediately at the medical office.

First-Voided Morning Specimen

In many cases, a first-voided morning specimen may be desired for testing because it contains the greatest concentration of dissolved substances, and a small amount of an abnormal substance that is present would be more easily detected. The patient should be instructed to collect the first specimen of the morning after rising and to preserve the specimen by refrigerating it until it is brought to the medical office. It is important to provide the patient with a specimen container to prevent the patient's use of a container from home that might harbor contaminants and affect the test results.

Clean-Catch Midstream Specimen

The urinary bladder and most of the urethra are normally free of microorganisms, whereas the distal urethra and urinary meatus normally harbor microorganisms. If the urine is being cultured and examined for bacteria, a clean-catch midstream specimen is necessary to prevent contamination of the specimen with these normally present microorganisms. Only microorganisms that may be causing the patient's condition are desired in the urine specimen. A clean-catch midstream collection may be ordered for the detection of a UTI and the evaluation of the effectiveness of drug therapy in a patient undergoing treatment for such an infection.

The purpose of the clean-catch midstream collection is the removal of microorganisms from the urinary meatus and the distal urethra. This is accomplished by instructing the patient to thoroughly cleanse the area surrounding the meatus and to void a small amount of urine into the toilet, which flushes out microorganisms in the distal urethra. The urine specimen is collected in a sterile container with medically aseptic conditions. A properly collected specimen reduces the possibility of having to do a bladder catheterization or a suprapubic aspiration of the bladder. **Bladder catheterization** involves the passing of a sterile tube (the catheter) through the urethra and into the bladder to remove urine. **Suprapubic aspiration** involves the passing of a sterile needle through the abdominal wall into the bladder to remove urine. Both of these procedures must be performed using sterile technique.

Guidelines

Guidelines that should be followed when collecting a clean-catch midstream specimen are listed:

1. A clean-catch midstream specimen is collected by the patient at the medical office. The medical assistant must provide complete instructions for the collection of this specimen. Failure to instruct the patient adequately may necessitate a return to the medical office for the collection of another specimen because of bacterial contamination. Patient instructions for obtaining a clean-catch midstream specimen are presented in Procedure 30-1.

2. The medical assistant must label the container with the patient's name, date, time of the collection, and type of specimen (clean-catch midstream specimen).

3. For reliable test results, the specimen should be tested immediately and not be allowed to stand. If this is not possible, the specimen should be refrigerated or a preservative should be added.

4. If the specimen is to be tested at an outside laboratory, completion of a laboratory requisition to accompany it is necessary. A urinalysis laboratory request form is shown in Figure 30-1.

5. The procedure is completed by sanitizing the hands and recording the procedure in the patient's chart. The information to be charted for specimens tested at the medical office includes the date and time, type of specimen collected, and laboratory test results. If the specimen is being transported to an outside laboratory for testing, record the date and time, type of specimen collected, and date the specimen was transported to the laboratory.

Twenty-Four-Hour Urine Specimen

A 24-hour urine specimen is used for quantitative measurement of specific urinary components. With collection of urine over a 24-hour period, a greater accuracy of measurement exists than with a random specimen. This is because body metabolism, exercise, and hydration can affect the excretion rate of substances in the urine. In addition, at certain times during a 24-hour period, an increased excretion of substances (e.g., electrolytes, hormones, proteins, urobilinogen) is seen, and at other times a decreased excretion is seen. Examples of substances measured in a 24-hour specimen include calcium, creatinine, lead, potassium, protein, and urea nitrogen. A 24-hour specimen is often used in the diagnosis of the cause of kidney stone formation

NAME:	ADDRESS:	UR- **183900**
		ICDA
	DATE:	REQUESTING PHYSICIAN
		PHYSICIAN HAS SEEN-INITIAL

	ROUTINE URINALYSIS - 001			MICROSCOPIC - 022			QUANTITATIVE	
	APPEARANCE COLOR			WBC'S	/HPF	024	SULKOWITCH	
023	SPECIFIC GRAVITY			RBC'S	/HPF	026	BILE	
004	PH			CASTS (Hyaline)	/LPF		PHENYLPYRUVIC ACID	
	PROTEIN			CASTS (Granular)	/LPF	027	PHENESTIX	
	GLUCOSE			CASTS (Cellular)	/LPF	028	UROBILINOGEN	
007	KETONES (ACETONE)			CASTS (Waxy)	/LPF	029	PORPHOBILINOGEN	
3	OCCULT BLOOD			EPITHELIAL CELLS	/LPF	030	PORPHYRIN	
	RII F			BACTERIA		031	BENCE-JONES	
	UROBILINOGEN			MUCUS		025	TOTAL PROTEIN 24HR. SPECIMEN	
	LEUKOCYTE			CRYSTALS			TOTAL VOLUME REQUIRED:	
COMMENTS				AMORPHOUS				
URINALYSIS				OTHER:			SIGNATURE:	
DMH-0067 (Rev. 3/83)		33		**F P N**			DATE:	

DMH-MedR-1065-A

Figure 30-1. Urinalysis laboratory request form. (From Bonewit-West K: *Clinical procedures for medical assistants,* ed 7, St. Louis, 2008, Saunders.)

and in the control and prevention of new stone formation.

A large container (3000 ml) is used to collect the specimen. To prevent changes in the quality of the urine specimen, the specimen must be kept refrigerated or placed in an ice chest. Some containers also contain a preservative to assist in maintaining the quality of the specimen.

The medical assistant should provide the patient with verbal and written instructions for the collection of the urine specimen. The patient should be advised to limit fluid intake moderately during the collection period and to avoid alcohol intake for 24 hours before and during the collection period. Certain medications, such as thiazides, phosphorus-binding antacids, allopurinol, and vitamin C, could alter the specimen's test results. The physician may want the patient to discontinue these medications for 1 week before the test.

PROCEDURE 30-1   Clean-Catch Midstream Specimen Collection Instructions

Outcome Instruct a patient in the procedure for collecting a clean-catch midstream urine specimen.

Equipment/Supplies

- Sterile specimen container and label
- Personal antiseptic towelettes
- Tissues

1. Procedural Step. Sanitize your hands. Greet the patient and introduce yourself. Identify the patient and explain the procedure.

2. Procedural Step. Assemble equipment. Label the specimen container with the patient's name, date, type of specimen (clean-catch midstream), and your initials.

Assemble the equipment. (From Bonewit-West K: *Clinical procedures for medical assistants,* ed 7, St. Louis, 2008, Saunders.)

3. Procedural Step. Instruct a female patient in the collection of the specimen as follows:
a. Wash the hands, open the package of towelettes, and place them on their wrapper.
b. Remove the lid from the specimen container and place it on a paper towel with the opening of the lid facing upward. Do not touch the inside of the lid or the inside of the specimen container.
c. Pull undergarments down and sit on the toilet. Expose the urinary meatus by spreading apart the labia with one hand.
d. Cleanse each side of the urinary meatus with an antiseptic towelette using a front-to-back motion (from pubis to anus). Use a separate antiseptic towelette for each side of the meatus. After use, discard each towelette in the toilet.
Principle. Cleansing removes microorganisms from the urinary meatus. A front-to-back motion must be used for cleansing to avoid drawing microorganisms from the anal region into the area that is being cleansed.
e. Cleanse directly across the meatus (front to back) with a third antiseptic towelette.
f. Continue to hold the labia apart, and void a small amount of urine into the toilet.
Principle. Voiding a small amount flushes microorganisms out of the distal urethra.
g. Collect the next amount of urine by voiding into the sterile container. Do not touch the inside of the container. Fill the specimen container about half full with urine.
Principle. Touching the inside of the container contaminates it with microorganisms that normally reside on the skin.
h. Void the last amount of urine into the toilet. This means that the first and last portion of the urine flow is not included in the specimen. Replace the lid of the specimen container.
i. Wipe the area dry with a tissue, and discard it in the toilet. Flush the toilet and wash the hands.

4. Procedural Step. *Instruct a male patient as follows:*
a. Wash the hands, open the towelettes, remove the lid from the specimen container, and remove undergarments.
b. Stand in front of the toilet. Retract the foreskin of the penis (if uncircumcised).
c. Cleanse the area around the meatus (glans penis) and the urethral opening (meatal orifice) by wiping each side of the meatus with a separate antiseptic towelette.

d. Cleanse directly across the meatus with a third antiseptic towelette. After use, discard each towelette in the toilet.

e. Void a small amount of urine into the toilet.

f. Collect the next amount of urine by voiding into the sterile container without touching the inside of the container with the hands or penis. Fill the container about half full with urine.

g. Void the last amount of urine into the toilet and replace the lid on the container.

h. Wipe the area dry with a tissue, and discard it in the toilet. Flush the toilet and wash the hands.

5. **Procedural Step.** Provide the patient with instructions about what to do with the specimen after it has been collected (e.g., placing it in a designated area or directly handing it to the medical assistant).

6. **Procedural Step.** Record the procedure in the patient's chart. Include the date and time and the type of specimen collected (clean-catch midstream collection).

7. **Procedural Step.** Test the specimen at the office or prepare the specimen for transport to an outside laboratory for testing. If the specimen is to be transported to an outside laboratory, perform the following:

a. Place the specimen container in a biohazard specimen bag.

b. Place the laboratory request in the outside pocket of the specimen bag.

c. Properly preserve the specimen while awaiting pickup by a laboratory courier by placing it in a refrigerator.

d. Chart the date the specimen was transported to the laboratory and the tests requested.

CHARTING EXAMPLE	
Date	
3/24/10	10:15 a.m. Clean-catch midstream collected by pt. Sent to Medical Center Laboratory for C & S on 3/24/10. —L. Proffitt, CMA (AAMA)

ANALYSIS OF URINE

Urinalysis is the analysis of urine and is the laboratory test most commonly performed in the medical office because a urine specimen is readily obtainable and can be tested easily. Urinalysis consists of a *physical, chemical,* and *microscopic examination.* A deviation from normal in any of the three areas assists the physician in the diagnosis and treatment of pathologic conditions, not only of the urinary system, but also of other body systems. Urinalysis may be performed as a screening measure as part of a general physical examination or to assist in the diagnosis of a pathologic condition. It may also assist in the evaluation of effectiveness of therapy after treatment has been initiated for a pathologic condition.

The urinalysis should be performed on a fresh or preserved specimen. If a specimen cannot be examined within 1 hour of voiding, it should be preserved at once in the refrigerator in a closed container and later returned to room temperature and mixed before testing. Chemical additives are also used to preserve urine specimens but are generally used only with specimens that require prolonged storage, such as specimens that must be shipped a long distance, because the chemical preservative sometimes interferes with the chemicals used to perform the urine test.

If the urine is allowed to stand at room temperature for more than 1 hour, some of the following changes may occur:

1. Bacteria in the environment that get into the urine specimen work on the urea present in the urine, converting it to ammonia. Because ammonia is alkaline, an acidic urine becomes alkaline, increasing the pH. In addition, an alkaline pH may result in a false-positive result on the protein test.

2. Bacteria multiply rapidly in the urine, resulting in a cloudy specimen and an increase in the nitrite.

3. If glucose is present in the specimen, it decreases in amount because microorganisms use the glucose as a source of food.

4. If any red or white blood cells are present, they may break down.

5. Casts decompose after several hours.

Physical Examination of Urine

The physical examination of urine includes determination of the color, appearance, and specific gravity. The color and appearance of the urine specimen may be evaluated during preparation for another testing procedure, such as the chemical testing of the urine or before centrifugation of the specimen in preparation for microscopic analysis. For an accurate evaluation of the color and appearance, the urine specimen must be in a clear plastic container.

Color

The normal color of urine ranges from almost colorless to dark yellow. Dilute urine tends to be a lighter yellow in color, whereas concentrated urine is a darker yellow. The first-voided morning specimen is usually the most concentrated because consumption of fluids is decreased during the night. The urine becomes more dilute as the day progresses and more fluids are consumed.

The color of the urine is the result of the presence of a yellow pigment known as *urochrome,* produced by the breakdown of hemoglobin. It is common for the color of urine to vary among different shades of yellow within the course of a day. Classifications that can be used to describe the color of urine include light yellow, yellow, dark yellow, light amber, amber, and dark amber (Figure 30-2).

The color of the urine specimen assists in determining additional tests that may be necessary. Abnormal colors may be caused by the presence of hemoglobin or blood (resulting in a red or reddish color), bile pigments (resulting in a yellow-brown or greenish color), and fat droplets or pus (resulting in a milky color). Some foods and medications may also cause the urine to change to an abnormal color. Phenazopyridine (Pyridium), a urinary tract analgesic, causes the urine to change to an orange to red color.

Appearance

The evaluation of the appearance of urine is usually performed at the same time as the color evaluation. Fresh urine is usually clear, or transparent, but becomes cloudy on standing out too long. Cloudiness in a freshly voided specimen may be the result of the presence of bacteria, pus, blood, fat, yeast, sperm, mucous threads, or fecal contaminants. A microscopic examination of the urine sediment should be performed on all cloudy specimens to determine the cause of the cloudiness. Cloudiness resulting from bacteria may be caused by a UTI.

Classifications used to describe the appearance of urine include clear, slightly cloudy, cloudy, and very cloudy (Figure 30-3). The medical assistant should develop skill in recognizing the varying degrees of urine clarity.

Odor

Freshly voided urine normally should have a slightly aromatic odor. Urine that has been standing for a long time develops an ammonia odor from the breakdown of urea by bacteria in the specimen. The urine of a patient with diabetes mellitus may have a fruity odor from the presence of ketones. The urine of a patient with a UTI is usually foul smelling, and the odor becomes worse on standing. Certain

foods, such as asparagus, can cause the urine to have a musty smell. Although urine may have many characteristic odors, as a rule the odor of urine is not generally used in the diagnosis of a patient's condition.

Specific Gravity

The **specific gravity** of urine measures the weight of the urine compared with the weight of an equal volume of distilled water. Specific gravity indicates the amount of dissolved substances present in the urine, providing information on the ability of the kidneys to dilute or concentrate the urine. Specific gravity is decreased in conditions in which the kidneys cannot concentrate the urine, such as chronic renal insufficiency, diabetes insipidus, and malignant hypertension. The specific gravity is increased in patients with adrenal insufficiency, congestive heart failure, hepatic disease, diabetes mellitus with glycosuria, and conditions that cause dehydration, such as fever, vomiting, and diarrhea.

The normal specific gravity of urine ranges from 1.003 to 1.030 but is usually between 1.010 and 1.025 (the specific gravity of distilled water is 1.000). Specific gravity varies greatly with fluid intake and the state of hydration of an individual. Dilute urine contains fewer dissolved substances and has a lower specific gravity. Concentrated urine has a higher specific gravity because of the increased amount of dissolved substances. A urine specimen is generally more concentrated in the morning and becomes more dilute after fluid consumption.

Measurement of Specific Gravity

In the medical office, specific gravity is measured with one of the following methods:

- *Reagent strip method.* This is the most common method used to measure specific gravity. It involves a color comparison determination with a reagent strip that contains a reagent area for specific gravity. The reagent strip is dipped into the urine specimen, and the results are compared with a color chart (see Procedure 30-2 later).

Figure 30-2. Color of urine. (From Bonewit-West K: *Clinical procedures for medical assistants,* ed 7, St. Louis, 2008, Saunders.)

Figure 30-3. Appearance of urine. (From Bonewit-West K: *Clinical procedures for medical assistants,* ed 7, St. Louis, 2008, Saunders.)

• *Refractometer method.* The amount of dissolved substances in urine can also be measured with a clinical **refractometer,** which is a hand-held optical instrument that consists of a lens and prism system. The refractometer measures the **refractive index** of urine, which is directly correlated with the specific gravity of urine; the results are read directly from a calibrated scale (Figure 30-4A and B). The advantage of a refractometer is that only 1 to 2 drops of urine are necessary to perform the test.

Chemical Examination of Urine

Substances present in excess (abnormal) amounts in the blood are usually removed by the urine. For example, glucose is normally present in the blood, but if it exceeds a certain level or threshold, the excess amount is excreted in the urine. The chemical testing of urine is an indirect means of detecting abnormal amounts of chemicals in the body, indicating a pathologic condition. The chemical examination of urine can also be used to detect the presence of

Figure 30-4. **A,** Measuring specific gravity using a refractometer. **B,** Calibration scale of a refractomer. The results are read at the boundary line that shows the distinct division of the light and dark areas. The specific gravity reading on this scale is 1.020. (From Bonewit-West K: *Clinical procedures for medical assistants,* ed 7, St. Louis, 2008, Saunders.)

substances that, in the absence of disease, do not normally appear in the urine, such as blood and nitrite.

Chemical tests that are routinely performed during a urinalysis include testing for pH, glucose, protein, and ketones. Other chemical tests that may be performed include testing for blood, bilirubin, urobilinogen, nitrite, and leukocytes.

• *Qualitative tests.* The chemical analysis of urine involves the use of qualitative and quantitative tests. Qualitative tests indicate whether a substance is present in the urine and also provide an approximate indication of the amount of the substance present. The interpretation of qualitative tests usually involves the use of a color chart, with results recorded in terms of trace, 1+, 2+, or 3+; trace, small, moderate, or large; or negative or positive. Qualitative tests are useful for screening purposes in the medical office because they are easy to perform and can be used to screen large numbers of individuals, a procedure that otherwise might be too expensive and time consuming.

• *Quantitative tests.* Quantitative tests indicate the exact amount of a chemical substance that is present in the body; the results are reported in measurable units (e.g., milligrams per deciliter). Quantitative urine tests usually involve the use of more complex equipment and testing procedures than are found in the medical office; they are also more time consuming to run.

Urine Testing Kits

Commercially prepared urine testing kits are most frequently used in the medical office for the chemical testing of urine. These kits are usually preferred because they contain premeasured reagents, the procedure is easy to follow, and they provide an immediate answer. Most of these tests are qualitative, and a positive result may indicate the need for further testing. Most of the tests are manufactured in the form of reagent strips, and they rely on a color change for interpretation of results. A color chart is provided with the kit for making a visual comparison. Brand names of urine testing kits include Multistix 10 SG, Chem-

---

What Would You Do? What Would You *Not* Do?

Case Study 2

Nora Sheridan is at the clinic with frequency, urgency, dysuria, and blood in the urine. During the past 6 months, Nora has been having problems with UTIs. She wants to know why these infections continue to occur and whether she can do anything to prevent them. Nora says that she has a lot of deadlines at work and that it is difficult to find time to come to the medical office. She says that her drugstore sells urine testing strips. Nora wants to know whether she could get a bottle of the strips and test her urine at home when she is having problems. That way she could just contact the office when she has positive test results, and the physician could call in a prescription for an antibiotic for her. ■

Putting It All into Practice

My name is Linda Proffitt, and I work for a urologist and his wife, who is a pediatrician. I work primarily in the urology practice and only occasionally in pediatrics. I am responsible for having the charts ready when the patients are seen and for doing their urinalysis. Another one of my responsibilities is to assist with special procedures, such as catheter insertions, male and female dilations, ultrasound (US) examinations of the bladder, and prostate examinations.

When I first started working in the urology office, I had to learn to assist with transrectal ultrasounds of the prostate in case the US technician was sick. When she retired, I inherited the position whether I wanted it or not. At first I dreaded doing the procedures and would be so nervous that I would get the shakes and forget the order in which things were supposed to be done. My physician was understanding and would help by talking me through it. I think the main reason I was so nervous was that sometimes the patients have trouble and we have to administer oxygen and run IVs. One time, a patient had a reaction to the pain medication we gave before the procedure.

Time, practice, and confidence in myself have improved my nerves, even with the occasional emergency situation. ∎

Prepare for Success

strip 10 SG, and Uristix. When results are recorded, the brand name of the test that was used should be specified.

For accurate and reliable test results, the medical assistant should carefully read and follow the instructions that accompany each kit. Test strips that contain more than one reagent may require different time intervals for reading results. Certain medications that the patient is taking may interfere with the test results. These medications are listed in the manufacturer's instructions accompanying the test.

Before a test is used, its expiration date must be checked. If the test is outdated, it must not be used to prevent inaccurate test results. Test material must not be used if a color change has occurred or if the *tested* strip gives off a color that does not match the shades on the color chart. Light, heat, and moisture can alter the effectiveness of the strips; care must be taken to store the test materials in a cool, dry area. Most test materials are packaged in light-resistant containers to protect them from light. The test materials must never be transferred from their original container to another because the other container may harbor traces of moisture, dirt, or chemicals that could affect the test results.

pH

The **pH** is the unit that indicates the acidity or alkalinity of a solution. The pH scale ranges from 0.0 to 14.0. The lower the number, the greater the acidity; the higher the number, the greater the alkalinity. A pH reading of 7.0 is neutral; a reading below 7.0 indicates acidity; and a reading above 7.0 indicates alkalinity.

The kidneys help regulate the acid-base balance of the body. For an accurate pH reading of the urine, the measurement should be performed on freshly voided urine. If the urine is allowed to remain standing, it becomes more alkaline as urea is converted to ammonia by bacterial action.

Although the pH of urine can normally range from 4.6 to 8.0, the pH of a freshly voided specimen of a patient on a normal diet is usually acidic and has a pH reading of about 6.0. An abnormally high pH reading on a fresh specimen (i.e., an alkaline urine) may indicate a bacterial infection of the urinary tract.

Glucose

Normally, no glucose should be detectable in the urine. Glucose in the blood is filtered through the **nephrons** and is reabsorbed into the body. If the glucose concentration in the blood becomes too high, the kidney is unable to reabsorb all of it back into the blood, the renal threshold is exceeded, and glucose is spilled into the urine—a condition known as **glycosuria.** (The **renal threshold** is the concentration at which a substance in the blood that is not normally excreted by the kidney begins to appear in the urine.) The renal threshold for glucose is generally 160 to 180 mg/dL (100 ml of blood), but this number may vary among individuals. Diabetes mellitus is the most common cause of glycosuria. Some individuals have a low renal threshold, and glucose may appear in their urine after the consumption of a large quantity of foods containing sugar. This condition is known as *alimentary glycosuria.*

Protein

The presence of protein in the urine is known as **proteinuria.** Protein in the urine usually indicates a pathologic condition if found in several samples over time. A temporary increase in urine protein may be caused by stress or strenuous exercise. Some of the conditions that may cause proteinuria include glomerular filtration problems, renal diseases, and bacterial infections of the urinary tract. If proteinuria occurs, the physician usually requests an examination of the sediment to determine, through visual observation, what is causing protein to be in the urine.

Ketones

Three types of ketone bodies exist: β-hydroxybutyric acid, acetoacetic acid, and acetone. *Ketones* are the normal products of fat metabolism and can be used by muscle tissue as a source of energy. When larger than normal amounts of fat are metabolized by the body, the muscles cannot handle all of the ketones that result. Large amounts of ketones accumulate in the tissues and body fluids; this condition is known as **ketosis.** The body rids itself of these excess ketones by excreting them in the urine. **Ketonuria** is the term that refers to the presence of ketone bodies in the urine. Conditions that may lead to ketonuria include uncontrolled dia-

Highlight on Drug Testing in the Workplace

Statistics

Statistics suggest that the problem of drug abuse is growing in the workplace. On any one day, 8.9 to 16 million employees are estimated to be working under the influence of drugs. The effects of on-the-job drug use extend into every segment of the population and touch every business and industry. The Occupational Safety and Health Administration estimates that 65% of all work-related accidents can be traced to substance abuse. The Metropolitan Insurance Company states that drug abuse costs industry $85 billion annually because of absenteeism, lowered productivity, and higher health care costs.

Testing Programs

Because of these economic and safety factors, businesses across the United States are adopting a less permissive attitude toward drug use and are beginning compulsory drug testing in the workplace. Approximately one third of U.S. employers have implemented drug testing programs in the workplace. Employers include utility companies, transportation operations, sports associations, and governmental agencies. Currently, many companies test blue-collar and white-collar employees for drug use. Companies with drug testing programs report a significant reduction in employee accidents, fewer sick days, and healthier employees.

A comprehensive drug testing program includes the detection of drug use in the workplace, policies to discourage further abuse, and the referral of employees for treatment and rehabilitation. Drug testing may be performed for one or more of the following purposes: (1) preemployment drug screening, (2) testing for probable cause after unexplained behavior or incident (e.g., an accident on the job), and (3) random sample testing of the workforce to detect use of controlled substances by employees on the job.

Testing Methods

Blood testing is the best means for determining precise information concerning the amount of the drug used and when the drug was taken. Blood tests are costly, however, and are time consuming to perform. Urine drug testing offers the next best alternative; it is noninvasive and technically easier and cheaper to perform. The current urine screening tests target the most common drugs of abuse: amphetamines, barbiturates, benzodiazepines, cocaine, marijuana, opiates, PCP, methaqualone, and methadone.

Chain of Custody

The usual procedure for urine drug testing involves screening the specimen and confirming positive results with more specific urine tests. The specimen may be collected at the workplace, at the medical office, or at an outside laboratory. To help ensure reliable and valid drug testing results, a security system or "chain of custody" must be followed in the collection and handling of the specimen. This typically includes ensuring the identification of the individual undergoing drug testing, taking precautions to avoid falsifying or tampering with specimens, properly labeling the urine specimen, sealing the sample in the specimen container after collection, and immediately sending it to the laboratory for analysis or refrigerating it at once for any delay in transporting. Urine drug testing kits are available for testing the specimen in the medical office. These kits provide immediate results and only take a few minutes to perform.

Disadvantages

The main disadvantage of urine drug testing is that a positive test result indicates only the presence of a drug in the urine; it does not provide any information regarding when the drug was taken. Drugs that are detected in the urine may or *may not* still be present in the blood, where they can affect an individual's behavior and impair performance. A positive urine test result does not reveal whether an individual is impaired by drugs. In addition, the initial urine screening tests are sometimes unreliable; unless positive results are confirmed with a more specific test, an individual may be unjustly accused of drug use. These factors and the violation of an individual's right to privacy are the main areas of dispute for individuals who oppose drug testing in the workplace.

Intervention

Companies with drug testing programs have various options when results are positive, such as recommendations for drug treatment programs or disciplinary action. Many companies have established in-house employee assistance programs that include counseling and drug withdrawal therapy for employees who desire help. Most companies prefer to help current employees with rehabilitation instead of discharging them and hiring and training new employees. Studies show a 35% to 60% recovery rate for employees enrolled in drug treatment programs. ■

---

betes mellitus, starvation, and a diet composed almost entirely of fat.

Bilirubin

The average life span of a red blood cell is 120 days. When a red blood cell breaks down, one of the substances released from the breakdown of hemoglobin is a vivid yellow pigment known as *bilirubin*. Normally, bilirubin is transported to the liver and excreted into the bile, and it eventually leaves the body through the intestines in the feces. Certain liver conditions, such as gallstones, hepatitis, and cirrhosis, may result in the presence of bilirubin in the urine, or **bilirubinuria.** The urine becomes yellow-brown or greenish, and a yellow foam appears when the urine is shaken.

Urobilinogen

Normally, bilirubin is excreted by the liver into the intestinal tract. Bacteria present in the intestines convert it to urobilinogen. Approximately 50% of the urobilinogen is reabsorbed into the body for reexcretion by the liver. Small amounts may appear in the urine, but most of the urobilinogen is excreted in the feces. An increase in the production of bilirubin increases the amount of urobilinogen excreted in the urine. Conditions such as excessive hemolysis of red blood cells, infectious hepatitis, cirrhosis, congestive heart failure, and infectious mononucleosis may increase the level of urobilinogen in the urine.

Blood

Blood is considered an abnormal constituent of urine, unless it is present as a contaminant during menstruation. The condition in which blood is found in the urine is termed *hematuria*. Hematuria may be the result of injury or disorders such as cystitis, tumors of the bladder, urethritis, kidney stones, and certain kidney disorders.

Nitrite

Nitrite in the urine indicates the presence of a pathogen in the (normally sterile) urinary tract, which results in a UTI. The pathogen possesses the ability to convert nitrate, which normally occurs in the urine, to nitrite, which is normally absent. The nitrite test must be performed with urine that has been in the bladder for at least 4 to 6 hours to ensure that bacteria have converted nitrate to nitrite. Therefore, use of a first-voided morning specimen is recommended. The test should *not* be performed on specimens that have been left standing out because a false-positive result may occur from bacterial contamination from the environment. The nitrite test is a screening test and is usually followed by a quantitative culture and identification of the invading pathogen.

Leukocytes

The presence of leukocytes in the urine is known as *leukocyturia* and accompanies inflammation of the kidneys and the lower urinary tract. Examples of specific conditions include acute and chronic pyelonephritis, cystitis, and urethritis. Reagent strips are available that contain a reagent area that permits the chemical detection of intact and lysed leukocytes in the urine. The advantage of detecting lysed leukocytes is that these cells cannot be observed during a microscopic examination of urine sediment and would otherwise remain undetected. The recommended urine specimen, particularly for women, is a clean-catch midstream collection to prevent contamination of the specimen with leukocytes from vaginal secretions leading to false-positive test results.

Reagent Strips

In the medical office, reagent strips are the most commonly used diagnostic urine testing kit. Reagent strips consist of disposable plastic strips on which separate reagent areas are affixed for testing specific chemical constituents that may be present in the urine during pathologic conditions. The results provide the physician with information to assist in the diagnosis of the following:

- Conditions affecting kidney function (e.g., kidney stones)
- UTIs

- Conditions affecting carbohydrate metabolism (e.g., diabetes mellitus)
- Conditions affecting liver function (e.g., hepatitis)

The test results also provide the physician with information related to the status of the patient's acid-base balance and urine concentration. Reagent strips are considered qualitative tests, and a positive result necessitates further testing. Table 30-1 presents an outline of reagent strip parameters and the diagnoses in which they assist.

The number and type of reagent areas included on the reagent strip depend on the particular brand of reagent strips. Multistix 10 SG (Bayer Corporation, Tarrytown, NY) contains 10 reagent areas for testing pH, protein, glucose, ketones, bilirubin, blood, urobilinogen, nitrite, specific gravity, and leukocytes.

The reagent strip procedure in this chapter (Procedure 30-2) is specifically for Multistix 10 SG; however, the procedure can be followed for the chemical testing of urine with most reagent strips. In all instances, the medical assistant should read the manufacturer's instructions before performing the test.

Guidelines for Reagent Strip Urine Testing

Testing urine with reagent strips is a relatively easy procedure to perform. Specific guidelines must be used, however, to obtain accurate test results.

1. *Type of specimen.* The best results are obtained with a freshly voided and thoroughly mixed urine specimen. If the medical assistant is unable to test the specimen within 1 hour of voiding, the specimen should be refrigerated immediately and then allowed to return to room temperature before testing.

2. *Type of collection.* Most reagent strips are designed to be used with a random specimen collection; however, clean-catch midstream and first-voided morning specimens are suggested for specific tests. The nitrite test results are optimized with a first-voided morning specimen, whereas a clean-catch midstream collection is recommended for the leukocyte test.

3. *Specimen container.* The specimen container used must be thoroughly clean and free from any detergent or disinfectant residue because cleansing agents contain oxidants that react with the chemicals on the reagent strip, leading to inaccurate test results. The container should be large enough to allow for complete immersion of all reagent strip areas.

4. *Interpretation of results.* Of particular importance is the comparison of the reagent strip with the color chart. The reagent strip must be compared with the color chart in good lighting to obtain a good visual match of the color reactions with the color chart provided with the test kit.

5. *Storage of reagent strips.* The reagents on the strips are sensitive to light, heat, and moisture, and the bottle containing the strips must be stored in a cool, dry area with the cap tightly closed to maintain reactivity of the reagent. The bottle may contain a desiccant that should

not be removed because its purpose is to promote dryness by absorbing moisture. The bottle of reagent strips must be stored at a temperature less than 86°F (less than 30°C) but should not be stored in the refrigerator or freezer. A tan-to-brown discoloration or darkening on the reagent areas indicates deterioration of the chemical reagent strips, in which case the strips should not be used because the test results would be inaccurate.

Quality Control

Quality control should be used in a chemical examination of urine with a reagent strip. Quality control ensures the reliability of test results by (1) determining whether the reagent strips are reacting properly and (2) confirming that the test is being properly performed and accurately interpreted.

To check the reliability of Multistix reagent strips, the Chek-Stix control (Bayer Corporation) should be used. Each Chek-Stix control consists of a firm plastic strip to which are affixed seven synthetic ingredients (Figure 30-5). The control strip is reconstituted by immersing it in distilled water for 30 minutes, which allows the ingredients on the strip to dissolve in the water. After reconstitution, the resulting solution is tested in the same manner as a urine specimen. The values to be expected are outlined on a reference sheet that accompanies the control strips. If the expected values are not obtained, the cause of the problem must be determined and corrected. Factors that can cause a problem include outdated reagent strips, improper storage of the strips, or an error in testing technique. The quality control test should be performed when each bottle of strips is opened for the first time or when there is a question of reliability regarding the testing strips.

Urine Analyzer

Urine analyzers are used to perform an automatic chemical examination of urine with reagent strips. They offer the advantage of the ability to perform the chemical analysis quickly and to interpret results automatically. These analyzers are used most often in medical offices that perform moderate-volume to large-volume urine testing.

The Clinitek Analyzer (Bayer Corporation) is an example of a urine analyzer that automatically reads Multistix SG and other (Bayer) urinalysis reagent strips (Figure 30-6A). The results are printed out, and abnormal results are flagged to call attention to them (Figure 30-6B). Different models are available; some can be used to perform a color and appearance analysis and a microscopic examination of the urine.

Text continued on p. 716

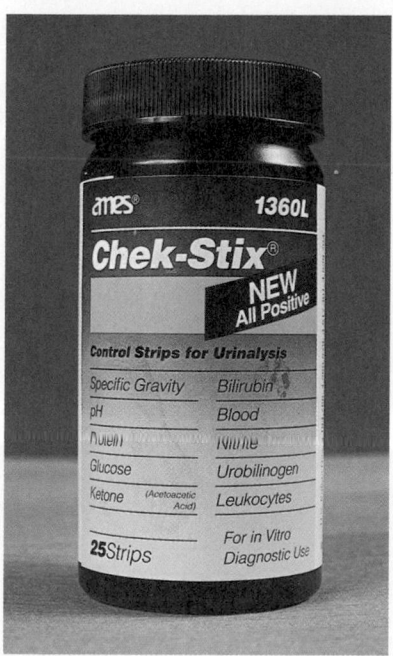

Figure 30-5. Chek-Stix control strips. (From Bonewit-West K: *Clinical procedures for medical assistants,* ed 7, St. Louis, 2008, Saunders.)

Figure 30-6. A, Clinitek Urine Analyzer. **B,** Clinitek printout. (From Bonewit-West K: *Clinical procedures for medical assistants,* ed 7, St. Louis, 2008, Saunders.)

Table 30-1 Urine Test Strip Parameters and the Diagnoses They Assist*

System/Source	Leukocytes	Nitrite	Urine pH		Protein
Genitourinary	Renal infection or inflammation • Acute/chronic pyelonephritis • Glomerulonephritis • Urolithiasis • Tumors • Lower urinary tract infection (cystitis, urethritis, prostatitis)	Bacteriuria • Urinary tract infection (cystitis, urethritis, prostatitis, pyelonephritis)	Up (greater than 6) in: • Renal failure • Bacterial infection (e.g., *Proteus* bacteriuria) • Renal tubular acidosis	—	Renal, glomerular, or tubular disease • Glomerulonephritis • Glomerulosclerosis (e.g., in diabetes) • Nephrotic syndrome • Pyelonephritis • Renal tuberculosis
Hepatobiliary	—	—	—	—	—
Gastrointestinal	—	—	Up in: • Pyloric obstruction	Down in: • Diarrhea • Malabsorption	—
Cardiovascular	—	—	—	—	Congestive heart failure
Hormonal, metabolic, and other systems	—	—	Up in: • Alkalosis (metabolic, respiratory)	Down in: • Acidosis (metabolic, respiratory, diabetic) • Pulmonary emphysema • Dehydration	Gout Hypokalemia Preeclampsia Severe febrile infection
Environmental (diet, drugs, stress)	Phenacetin-induced nephritis	—	Up in: • Diet high in vegetables, citrus fruits • Alkalizing drug use (sodium bicarbonate, acetazolamide)	Down in: • Diet high in meats or other protein, cranberries • Acidifying drug use (e.g., ammonium chloride, methenamine mandelate therapy)	Nephrotoxic drugs

Courtesy Roche Diagnostics, Indianapolis.
Modified from Conn HF, Conn RB (eds): *Current diagnosis 5,* Philadelphia, 1977, Saunders; Davidson I, Henry JB (eds): *Todd-Stanford clinical diagnosis by laboratory methods,* ed 15, Philadelphia, 1974, Saunders; Raphael SS, et al: *Lynch's medical laboratory technology,* ed 3, Philadelphia, 1976, Saunders; Wallach J: *Interpretation of diagnostic tests,* ed 2, Boston, 1974, Little, Brown; Widmann FK: *Goodale's clinical interpretation of laboratory tests,* ed 7, Philadelphia, 1973, Davis.
*Reagent strip detection of abnormal urine constituent or concentration characteristic of disease (e.g., glycosuria in diabetes mellitus) may provide useful screen or monitor, but requires confirmation with other laboratory and clinical evidence.

Glucose	Ketones	Urobilinogen	Bilirubin	Blood, Erythrocytes (Hematuria)	Hemoglobin
Renal glycosuria (e.g., during pregnancy Renal tubular disease (e.g., in Fanconi's syndrome) Decreased renal glucose threshold (e.g., in old age)	—	—	—	Renal infection, inflammation, or injury • Renal tuberculosis • Renal infarction • Calculi (urethral, renal) • Polycystic kidneys • Tumors (bladder, renal pelvis, prostate) • Salpingitis • Cystitis	Renal intravascular Hemolysis Acute glomerulonephritis
—	—	Liver cell damage Chronic liver stasis Cirrhosis Dubin-Johnson syndrome Note: May be 0 or down in biliary obstruction	Biliary dysfunction • Gallstones Obstructive jaundice Hepatitis (viral toxic) Dubin-Johnson syndrome	Cirrhosis	—
—	Vomiting Diarrhea	Note: May be negative with inhibition of intestinal flora by antimicrobial agents	—	Colon tumor Diverticulitis	—
Myocardial infarction	—	—	—	Bacterial endocarditis	—
Diabetes mellitus Hemochromatosis Hyperthyroidism Cushing's syndrome Pheochromocytomas	Diabetic ketosis Glycogen storage disease Preeclampsia Acute fever	Sickle cell anemia Hemolytic disease • Pernicious anemia Leptospirosis	Hemolytic disease Leptospirosis	Blood dyscrasias • Hemophilia • Thrombocytopenia • Sickle cell anemia Disseminated lupus erythematosus Malignant hypertension	Hemolytic disease Plasmodium (malaria) Clostridium (tetanus)
Sudden shock or pain Steroid therapy	Weight-reducing diet Ketogenic diet (e.g., in anticonvulsant therapy) Starvation	—	—	Hemorrhagenic drugs (e.g., anticoagulant, salicylate) Nephrotoxic agents Internal injury or foreign body Vitamin C or K deficiency	Overexertion Exposure to cold Incompatible blood transfusion Drug-induced hemolysis

PROCEDURE 30-2   Chemical Testing of Urine with the Multistix 10 SG Reagent Strip

Outcome Perform a chemical assessment of a urine specimen.

Equipment/Supplies

- Disposable gloves
- Multistix 10 SG reagent strips
- Urine container
- Timer
- Laboratory report form

1. **Procedural Step.** Obtain a freshly voided urine specimen from the patient with a clean container. The specimen should be uncentrifuged and at room temperature.
   Principle. The best results are obtained with a freshly voided specimen. The container should be clean because contaminants could affect the results. Uncentrifuged specimens ensure a homogeneous sample.

2. **Procedural Step.** Sanitize your hands.

3. **Procedural Step.** Assemble the equipment. Check the expiration date of the reagent strips.
   Principle. Outdated reagent strips may lead to inaccurate test results.

4. **Procedural Step.** Apply gloves. Remove a reagent strip from its plastic container, and recap the container immediately. Do not touch the test areas with your fingers or lay the strip on the table. It is permissible, however, to lay the reagent strip on a clean, dry paper towel.
   Principle. Recapping the container is necessary to prevent exposing the strips to environmental moisture, light, and heat, which cause altered reagent reactivity. Contamination of the test areas by the hands or table surface may affect the accuracy of the test results.

5. **Procedural Step.** Thoroughly mix the urine specimen and remove the lid from the container. Using the dominant hand, completely immerse the reagent strip in the urine specimen and remove it immediately. While removing, run the edge of the strip against the rim of the urine container to remove excess urine.
   Principle. The strip should be completely immersed to ensure that all test areas are moistened for accurate test results. Prolonged immersion of the reagent strip and failure to remove excess urine may cause the reagents to dissolve and leach onto adjacent test areas, affecting the accuracy of the test results.

6. **Procedural Step.** With the nondominant hand, start the timer, pick up the reagent strip container, and rotate it to the color chart. Hold the reagent strip in a horizontal position and place it as close as possible to the corresponding color blocks on the color chart. Do not lay the strip directly on the color chart because this would result in the urine soiling the chart. Read the results carefully and at the exact reading times specified on the color chart and as indicated here:

Completely immerse the reagent strip in the urine. (From Bonewit-West K: *Clinical procedures for medical assistants,* ed 7, St. Louis, 2008, Saunders.)

Run the edge of the strip against the urine container. (From Bonewit-West K: *Clinical procedures for medical assistants,* ed 7, St. Louis, 2008, Saunders.)

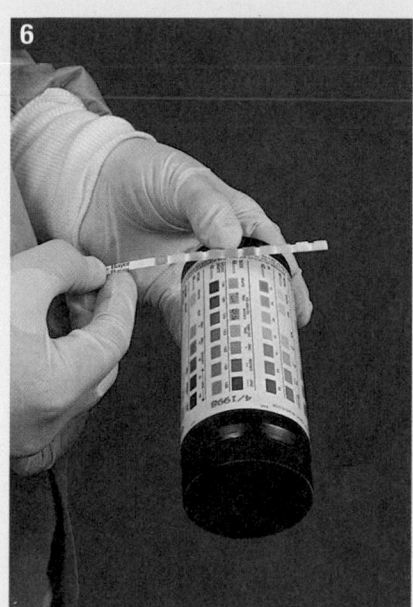

Hold the strip horizontally and read the results. (From Bonewit-West K: *Clinical procedures for medical assistants,* ed 7, St. St. Louis, 2008, Saunders.)

Glucose: 30 seconds　　pH: 60 seconds
Bilirubin: 30 seconds　　Protein: 60 seconds
Ketones: 40 seconds　　Urobilinogen: 60 seconds
Specific gravity: 45　　Nitrite: 60 seconds
　seconds　　Leukocytes: 2 minutes
Blood: 60 seconds

Principle. Holding the strip in a horizontal position avoids soiling your gloves with urine and prevents reagents from running over into the adjacent testing areas, causing inaccurate test results. The strip must be read at the proper time to avoid dissolving out reagents, leading to inaccurate test results.

7. **Procedural Step.** Dispose of the strip in a regular waste container.
8. **Procedural Step.** Remove gloves, and sanitize your hands.
9. **Procedural Step.** Chart the results. The results should be charted following the interpretation guide provided above each color block on the color chart. Most offices use a preprinted reporting form to make it easier to record results. The recording should include the date and time, the brand name of the test used (Multistix 10 SG), and the results.

PROCEDURE 30-2

CHARTING EXAMPLE

Multistix® 10 SG *Reageant Strips for Urinalysis*

PATIENT　Annette Ross

DATE　3/22/10　　　　　　　　　　　TIME　9:45 a.m.

LEUKOCYTES	NEGATIVE ☑		TRACE ☐	SMALL + ☐	MODERATE ++ ☐	LARGE +++ ☐
NITRITE	NEGATIVE ☑		POSITIVE ☐	POSITIVE ☐	(Any degree of uniform pink color is found)	
UROBILINOGEN	NORMAL 0.2 ☑	NORMAL 1 ☐	mg/dL 2 ☐	4 ☐	8 ☐ (1mg = approx. 1 BU)	
PROTEIN	NEGATIVE ☐	TRACE ☑	mg/dL 30 ☐	100 ++ ☐	300 +++ ☐ 2000 OR MORE ☐	
pH	5.0 ☑	6.0 ☐	6.5 ☐	7.0 ☐	7.5 ☐ 8.0 ☐	8.5 ☐
BLOOD	NEGATIVE ☑	NON-HEMOLYZED ☐ TRACE	NON-HEMOLYZED ☐ MODERATE	HEMOLYZED ☐ TRACE	SMALL + ☐ MODERATE ++ ☐	LARGE +++ ☐
SPECIFIC GRAVITY	1.000 ☐	1.006 ☐	1.010 ☐	1.015 ☑	1.020 ☐ 1.025 ☐	1.030 ☐
KETONE	NEGATIVE ☑	mg/dL	TRACE 5 ☐	SMALL 15 ☐	MODERATE 40 ☐ LARGE 80 ☐	LARGE 160 ☐
BILIRUBIN	NEGATIVE ☑		SMALL ☐	MODERATE ++ ☐	LARGE +++ ☐	
GLUCOSE	NEGATIVE ☑	g/L (%) mg/dL	1/10 tr.) 100 ☐	1/6 250 ☐	1/2 500 ☐ 1 1000 ☐	2 or more 2000 or more ☐

(Modified and printed by permission of Siemens Healthcare Diagnostics, Deerfield, Ill, 60015.)

Continued

(From Bonewit-West K: *Clinical procedures for medical assistants,* ed 7, St. Louis, 2008, Saunders.)

Microscopic Examination of Urine

Urine sediment is the solid material contained in the urine. A microscopic examination of the urine sediment performed by the physician helps clarify results of the physical and chemical examinations. A first-voided morning specimen is generally preferred because it is more concentrated and contains more dissolved substances; small amounts of abnormal substances are more likely to be detected. Use of a fresh specimen is important because changes occur in a specimen left standing out, as previously discussed. These changes affect the reliability of the test results. The medical assistant is responsible for preparing the urine specimen for microscopic examination by the physician, as presented in Procedure 30-3. Structures that may be found in a microscopic examination of urine are described next.

Red Blood Cells

Red blood cells appear as round, colorless, biconcave discs that are highly refractile (Table 30-2). The presence of 0 to 5 per high-power field (HPF) is considered normal. More than this amount may indicate bleeding somewhere along the urinary tract. Table 30-2 lists the possible causes of an abnormal number of red blood cells in the urine. Concentrated urine causes the red blood cells to become shrunken or *crenated,* whereas dilute urine causes them to swell and become rounded, which may cause them to hemolyze. If the red blood cells have hemolyzed, they cannot be seen under the microscope. The presence of blood in the urine can still be identified, however, with a reagent strip, such as Multistix, designed to detect free hemoglobin.

White Blood Cells

White blood cells are round and granular and have a nucleus (see Table 30-2). They are approximately 1.5 times as large as a red blood cell. The presence of 0 to 8 per HPF is considered normal. More than this amount may indicate inflammation of the genitourinary tract. Table 30-2 lists the possible causes of an abnormal number of white blood cells in the urine.

Epithelial Cells

Most structures that make up the urinary system are composed of several layers of epithelial cells. The outer

Table 30-2 Structures in Urine Sediment

Structure	Possible Causes	Microscopic Appearance
Red blood cells	Inflammatory diseases Acute glomerulonephritis Pyelonephritis Hypertension Renal infarction Trauma Stones Tumor Bleeding diseases Use of anticoagulants	 Red blood cells

White blood cells	Pyelonephritis
	Cystitis
	Urethritis
	Prostatitis
	Transplant rejection (manifested by lymphocytes in urine)
	Tissue injury accompanied by severe inflammation
	   (manifested by monocytes in urine)
	Inflammation, immune mechanisms, and other host defense
	   mechanisms (manifested by histiocytes in urine)
		
		White blood cells

Squamous epithelial cells	Vaginal contamination	 Squamous epithelial cells
Renal tubular epithelial cells	Acute tubular necrosis Glomerulonephritis Acute infection Renal toxicity Viral infection	 Renal tubular epithelial cells
Amorphous urate	Nonpathologic	 Amorphous urate crystals

Continued

Table 30-2 Structures in Urine Sediment—cont'd

Structure	Possible Causes	Microscopic Appearance
Uric acid	Usually nonpathologic; in large numbers, may indicate gout	 Uric acid crystals
Calcium oxalate	Usually nonpathologic; may be associated with stone formation	 Calcium oxalate crystals
Bacteria	More than 100,000 bacteria/ml indicates urinary tract infection 10,000-100,000 bacteria/ml indicates that tests should be repeated Less than 10,000 bacteria/ml may signify urine in which any bacteria are due to urethral organisms or contamination Bacteria accompanied by white blood cells or white blood cell or mixed casts may indicate acute pyelonephritis	 Bacteria (small rod structures)
Yeast	May indicate contamination by yeasts from skin or hair May indicate diabetes mellitus or urinary tract infection *Candida albicans* may occur in patients with diabetes mellitus or in the contaminated urine of female patients with candidal vaginitis	 *Candida albicans* (yeast)
Parasites and parasitic ova	Usually indicate fecal or vaginal contamination and should be reported *Trichomonas* may be found in patients with urethritis and in contaminated urine of women with *Trichomonas* vaginitis Pinworm is a common contaminant and should be reported	 *Trichomonas* (parasite)
Spermatozoa	Nonpathologic	 Spermatozoa

Table 30-2 Structures in Urine Sediment—cont'd

Structure	Possible Causes	Microscopic Appearance
Urinary artifacts	Nonpathologic	Hair (a)†
Hair (a) Pollen grains Bubbles Oil droplets Fibers (b) Powder (c) Dust Mucous threads (d) Glass particles	May result from improper urine collection, improper slide preparation, or outside contamination	Fiber (b)* Powder (c)* Mucous threads (d)‡

Text courtesy Roche Diagnostics, Indianapolis.
*Photomicrographs courtesy Bayer Corporation, Tarrytown, NY.
†Photomicrographs from Stepp CA, Woods M: *Laboratory procedures for medical office personnel,* Philadelphia, 1998, Saunders.
‡Photomicrographs from Henry JB: *Clinical diagnosis and management by laboratory methods,* ed 20, Philadelphia, 2001, Saunders.

layer is constantly sloughed off and replaced by the cells underneath it. *Squamous epithelial cells* are large, clear, flat cells with an irregular shape. They contain a small nucleus and come from the urethra, bladder, and vagina. Squamous epithelial cells are normally present in small amounts in the urine. *Renal epithelial cells* are round and contain a large nucleus. They come from the deeper layers of the urinary tract, and their presence in the urine is considered abnormal. Table 30-2 lists the types of epithelial cells and possible causes of the presence of abnormal amounts in the urine.

Casts

Casts are cylindric structures formed in the lumen of the tubules that make up the nephron. Materials in the tubules harden, are flushed out, and appear in the urine in the form of casts. Various types of casts may be present in the urine. Their presence generally indicates a diseased condition.

Casts are named according to what they contain. *Hyaline casts* are pale, colorless cylinders with rounded edges that vary in size (see Table 30-2). *Granular casts* are hyaline casts that contain granules and are described as "coarsely granular" or "finely granular," depending on the size of the granules. *Fatty casts* are hyaline casts that contain fat droplets. *Waxy casts* are light yellow and have serrated edges; their name is derived from the fact that they appear to be made of wax. *Cellular casts* contain organized structures and are named according to what they contain. Examples include red blood cell casts, which are hyaline casts containing red blood cells; white blood cell casts, which are hyaline casts containing white blood cells; epithelial casts, which are hyaline casts containing epithelial cells; and bacterial casts, which are hyaline casts containing bacteria.

Crystals

A variety of crystals may be found in the urine. The type and number vary with the pH of the urine. Abnormal crystals include leucine, tyrosine, cystine, and cholesterol. Crystals that commonly appear in acid urine include amorphous urates, uric acid, and calcium oxalate (see Table 30-2). Crystals that commonly appear in alkaline urine include amorphous phosphate, triple phosphate, calcium phosphate, and ammonium urate crystals.

Miscellaneous Structures

Mucous threads are normally present in small amounts in the urine. They appear as long, wavy, threadlike structures with pointed ends.

Bacteria should not normally exist in the urinary tract. The presence of more than a few bacteria may indicate either contamination of the specimen during collection or a UTI. Bacteria are small structures and may be rod shaped or round.

Yeast cells are smooth, refractile bodies with an oval shape. A distinguishing feature of yeast cells is small buds that project from the cells involved with reproduction. Yeast cells in the urine of female patients are usually a vaginal contaminant caused by the yeast *Candida albicans* and produce the vaginal infection known as *candidiasis*. They may also be present in the urine of patients with diabetes mellitus.

Parasites may be present in the urine sediment as a contaminant from fecal or vaginal material. *Trichomonas vaginalis* is a parasite that causes trichomoniasis vaginitis.

Spermatozoa may be present in the urine of a man or woman after intercourse. The spermatozoa have round heads and long, slender, hairlike tails.

Table 30-2 lists the miscellaneous structures that may be present in the urine and the significance when found.

Memories *from* Externship

Linda Proffitt: My main problem as a student on externship was that I was a little shy. I learned that when your patient is relaxed, he or she is more likely to give you additional and important information about what is wrong. If your patient tenses up during a procedure, it can cause pain for the patient and make the procedure more difficult. When I started to make myself talk more to the patients and staff, things went more smoothly. ■

Prepare for Success

PATIENT TEACHING | Urinary Tract Infections

Answer questions patients may have about urinary tract infections (UTIs).

What is a UTI?

UTI is a general term for the presence of bacteria in any portion of the urinary tract. UTIs, particularly those involving the bladder (cystitis) and urethra (urethritis), are common and treatable. A UTI is usually treated with an antibiotic. Use of the entire antibiotic for the full number of days prescribed by the physician is important, even if the symptoms disappear. If the medication is stopped too soon, the infection may recur and be more difficult to treat than the original infection.

What are the symptoms of a UTI?

The symptoms of a simple UTI (cystitis) commonly include the frequent need to urinate, urgency (meaning the immediate need to urinate), a burning sensation during urination, and sometimes blood in the urine. The symptoms of a more complicated UTI involving the kidneys (pyelonephritis) include the above symptoms, as well as lower abdominal discomfort, low back pain, fever, cloudy or foul-smelling urine, and blood in the urine.

Why do women have UTIs more frequently than do men?

Women are more prone to the type of UTI called *cystitis* than are men because the urethra of a woman is much shorter than that of a man, which makes travel up the urethra and into the bladder easier for bacteria. The most common source of infection is bacteria *(Escherichia coli)*. This organism is normally found in the large intestine but can travel from the anal area to the urinary bladder, often as the result of poor hygienic practices. Cystitis occurs if *E. coli* organisms are able to overcome the body's natural defenses when the bacteria reach the urinary bladder and set up an infection.

What can women do to prevent a UTI?

Women prone to development of UTIs should practice the following prevention measures:

- Practice good hygienic measures by always cleaning the genital area from front to back after a bowel movement.
- Avoid possible irritants, such as bubble baths, perfumed soaps, feminine hygiene sprays, or the use of strong powders and bleaches for washing underclothes.

PATIENT TEACHING Urinary Tract Infections—cont'd

- Avoid clothing that traps moisture and encourages the growth of microorganisms, such as tight, constricting clothing; nylon panties; and pantyhose.
- Avoid activities that can contribute to irritation of the urinary meatus, such as prolonged bicycling, motorcycling, horseback riding, and traveling that involves prolonged sitting.
- Urinate as soon as possible when you feel the urge. Holding urine in the bladder gives the bacteria more time to grow, which can cause more infection. The more often you urinate, the quicker the bacteria are removed from the bladder.
- Seek prompt treatment if you experience any of the symptoms of a UTI.

The medical assistant should do the following:
- Encourage the patient with a UTI to drink plenty of water to help flush the bacteria out of the urinary tract.
- Emphasize to the patient the importance of taking the entire antibiotic for the duration of time prescribed by the physician.
- Emphasize the importance of practicing preventive measures to prevent the occurrence of UTIs.
- Provide the patient with educational materials on UTIs. ∎

PROCEDURE 30-3 Prepare a Urine Specimen for Microscopic Examination: Kova Method

Outcome Prepare a urine specimen for microscopic analysis.

Equipment/Supplies

- Disposable gloves
- Urine specimen (first-voided morning specimen)
- Kova urine centrifuge tube
- Kova cap
- Kova pipet

- Kova slide
- Kova stain
- Test tube rack
- Urine centrifuge
- Mechanical stage microscope

Preparing the Specimen

1. Procedural Step. Sanitize the hands, and assemble the equipment.

Assemble the equipment. (From Bonewit-West K: *Clinical procedures for medical assistants,* ed 7, St. Louis, 2008, Saunders.)

2. Procedural Step. Apply gloves. Mix the urine specimen with the Kova pipet.
Principle. The specimen must be well mixed to ensure accurate test results.

3. Procedural Step. Pour the urine specimen into the urine centrifuge tube. Fill it to the 12-ml graduation mark, and cap the tube.

Pour the specimen into the urine tube. (From Bonewit-West K: *Clinical procedures for medical assistants,* ed 7, St. Louis, 2008, Saunders.)

4. Procedural Step. Centrifuge the tube for 5 minutes at approximately 1500 revolutions per minute (rpm).
Principle. Centrifuging the specimen causes the solid elements in the urine to settle to the bottom of the tube.

5. Procedural Step. Remove the urine tube from the centrifuge; do not disturb or dislodge the sediment.

6. Procedural Step. Remove the cap. Insert the Kova pipet into the urine tube, and push it to the bottom

Continued

PROCEDURE **30-3**   **Prepare a Urine Specimen for Microscopic Examination:
Kova Method—cont'd**

of the tube until it seats firmly. Ensure that the clip on the bulb is hooked over the outside edge of the tube.

Centrifuge the specimen. (From Bonewit-West K: *Clinical procedures for medical assistants,* ed 7, St. Louis, 2008, Saunders.)

Insert the pipet until it seats firmly. (From Bonewit-West K: *Clinical procedures for medical assistants,* ed 7, St. Louis, 2008, Saunders.)

7. **Procedural Step.** Decant the specimen by inverting the tube and pouring off the **supernatant** fluid. Approximately 1 ml of sediment is retained in the bottom of the tube.

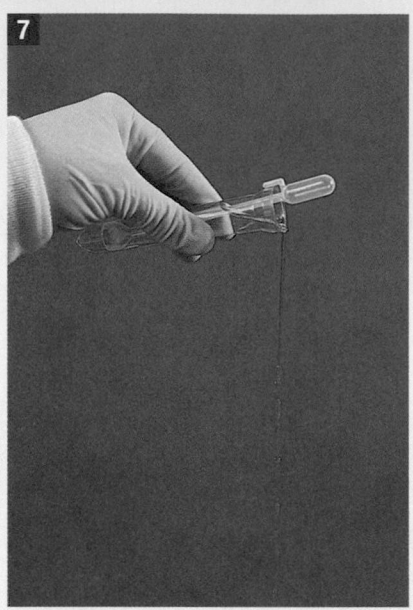

Pour off the supernatant fluid. (From Bonewit-West K: *Clinical procedures for medical assistants,* ed 7, St. Louis, 2008, Saunders.)

8. **Procedural Step.** Remove the pipet from the tube. Add 1 drop of Kova stain to the tube. Place the pipet back in the tube, and mix the sediment and stain together vigorously with the pipet. Ensure that the sediment and stain are well mixed. Place the urine tube in a test tube rack.

Principle. Kova stain improves the detail of the sediment for better visualization of structures under the microscope.

Mix the sediment and stain. (From Bonewit-West K: *Clinical procedures for medical assistants,* ed 7, St. Louis, 2008, Saunders.)

9. **Procedural Step.** Transfer a sample of the sediment to the Kova slide as follows:

a. Place the Kova slide on a flat surface with the open "envelope" areas facing upward.

b. Squeeze the bulb of the pipet to draw a sample of the sediment into the tip of the pipet.

c. Place the tip of the pipet so that it just touches the notched corner edge of the slide.

d. Gently squeeze the bulb to allow the specimen to fill the well. Do not overfill or underfill the well.

e. Place the pipet in the urine tube.

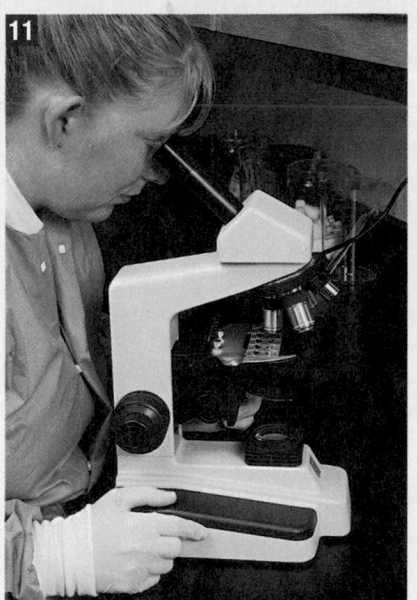

Focus the specimen under the microscope. (From Bonewit-West K: *Clinical procedures for medical assistants,* ed 7, St. Louis, 2008, Saunders.)

Fill the well with the specimen. (From Bonewit-West K: *Clinical procedures for medical assistants,* ed 7, St. Louis, 2008, Saunders.)

10. Procedural Step. Allow the specimen to sit for 1 minute to permit the sediment to settle in the well. *Principle.* Allowing the sediment to settle prevents structures from moving when viewing the slide under the microscope.

11. Procedural Step. Place the slide on the stage of the microscope. Focus the specimen for the physician under the microscope following the procedures presented in Procedure 34-1, Using the Microscope.

12. Procedural Step. When the physician is finished examining the urine sediment, remove the slide from the stage.

13. Procedural Step. Dispose of the plastic slide and pipet in a regular waste container. Rinse the remaining urine down the sink. Cap the empty plastic urine tube, and dispose of it in a regular waste container.

14. Procedural Step. Remove gloves, and sanitize your hands.

LAB REPORT

Date	Time	Name	
3/18/10	10:00 a.m.	Tanya Howe	
		MICROSCOPIC	
	WBCs		20 /HPF
	RBCs		3 /HPF
	CASTS (Hyaline)		0 /LPF
	CASTS (Granular)		0 /LPF
	CASTS (Cellular)		0 /LPF
	CASTS (Waxy)		0 /LPF
	EPITHELIAL CELLS		0 /LPF
	BACTERIA		Freq
	MUCUS		Occ
	CRYSTALS		0 WBCs
			— T. Bach, MD

PROCEDURE 30-3

URINE PREGNANCY TESTING

The diagnosis of pregnancy can be accomplished several ways. By the eighth week after fertilization, pregnancy can be confirmed with the medical history and physical examination. The physician may desire an earlier diagnosis, however, with a pregnancy test to initiate early prenatal care. A pregnancy test may also be necessary before certain medications are ordered or procedures are performed that may cause injury to a fetus.

In the medical office, immunologic tests are often used for pregnancy testing. These tests are performed on a concentrated urine specimen and rely on the presence of a hormone known as *human chorionic gonadotropin* (HCG) for a positive reaction.

Human Chorionic Gonadotropin

HCG is produced by the developing fertilized egg, and small amounts of it are secreted into the urine and blood. Immediately after conception and implantation of the fertilized egg, the plasma level of HCG increases rapidly and can be used to detect pregnancy with a serum pregnancy test as early as 6 days before the first missed menstrual period. The highest plasma levels of HCG occur at about 8 weeks after conception. After this time, the production of HCG declines and remains at a lower level for the duration of the pregnancy. Within 72 hours of delivery, HCG disappears entirely from the plasma. As a result, pregnancy tests are more sensitive during the first trimester and may show a negative reaction when the level of HCG begins to decline during the second and third trimesters.

Immunoassay Tests

Immunoassay tests provide for the rapid, qualitative detection of HCG in a urine specimen; brand names include QuickVue, Clearview, OSOM, and ICON. Early prediction pregnancy tests may be able to detect pregnancy 1 week after implantation, or 4 to 5 days before a first missed menstrual period. Urine pregnancy tests performed this early, however, may show a false-negative result and should be repeated later to confirm the results. Accurate results are much more probable if the urine is tested 1 week after a missed period.

Immunoassay tests take approximately 5 minutes to perform and are easier to read than agglutination tests because the results are easily observed as a color change. Specific instructions for the test are included with each commercially available testing kit. The procedure for performing an immunoassay test with QuickVue (Quidel) is outlined in Procedure 30-4.

Guidelines for Urine Pregnancy Testing

Specific guidelines must be followed in a urine pregnancy test to ensure accurate test results:
1. Use clean, preferably disposable, urine containers to collect the specimen. Traces of urine detergent in the specimen container may cause inaccurate test results.

2. The preferred specimen for a urine pregnancy test is a first-voided morning specimen because it contains the highest concentration of HCG. If the urine specimen cannot be tested immediately after voiding, it should be preserved in the refrigerator. A patient who collects the specimen at home should be given instructions on preserving the specimen.
3. The specific gravity of the urine specimen should be determined before the test is performed. A specific gravity of less than 1.010 is considered too dilute for pregnancy testing because it may lead to a false-negative test result.
4. The urine specimen should be at room temperature before the procedure is performed.
5. The urine pregnancy testing kit should be stored according to the manufacturer's instructions. Most testing kits are stored at room temperature.
6. Testing kits past their expiration dates should not be used.

SERUM PREGNANCY TEST

The radioimmunoassay for HCG is used to detect HCG in the serum of the blood. This test can detect pregnancy earlier and with more accuracy than a urine pregnancy test. A serum pregnancy test can usually detect pregnancy at approximately the eighth day after fertilization, which is 6 days before the first missed menstrual period. This test uses a radioisotope technique and is capable of detecting minute amounts of HCG in the blood. This test is generally used to diagnose abnormalities, such as ectopic pregnancy; to follow the course of early pregnancy when abnormalities of embryonic development are suspected; and to provide an early diagnosis of pregnancy in individuals at high risk, such as patients with diabetes.

What Would You Do? What Would You *Not* Do?

Case Study 3

Rita Lavelle is 8½ months pregnant and is at the clinic for a prenatal appointment. Lately, she has been having difficulty obtaining a urine specimen at the medical office because of her enlarged abdomen. At her last appointment, the office provided her with a urine specimen container so that she could obtain her specimen more easily at home. Rita brings in a first-voided urine specimen in a glass jar. She says her dog chewed up the specimen container from the office, so she used an empty peanut butter jar. The urine testing results from her specimen show that her glucose level is normal, but her protein level is +4. Until this time, her urine test results all have been normal. Rita is concerned about her baby. She says that she was cleaning her bathroom cabinet yesterday and came across a pregnancy test; just for the fun of it, she decided to run the test. The results were negative, and now she is worried that something is wrong. Rita says that she has not been sleeping as well at night, and that she has noticed more Braxton Hicks contractions, but that the baby has been kicking and moving as usual. ∎

PROCEDURE 30-4 Performing a Urine Pregnancy Test

Outcome Perform a urine pregnancy test.

Equipment/Supplies

- Disposable gloves
- Urine pregnancy testing kit (QuickVue by Quidel)
- Urine specimen (first-voided morning specimen)

1. Procedural Step. Sanitize the hands, and assemble the equipment. Check the expiration date on the urine pregnancy test. It should not be used if the expiration date has passed. When a new testing kit is opened, an external positive and negative control should be performed according to the manufacturer's instructions. If the control does not produce the expected results, the testing kit should not be used.

Principle. An expired pregnancy test may produce inaccurate test results. Running positive and negative test results ensures that the test results are valid and reliable.

Assemble the equipment. (From Bonewit-West K: *Clinical procedures for medical assistants,* ed 7, St. Louis, 2008, Saunders.)

2. Procedural Step. Apply gloves. Rotate the urine specimen cup to mix the urine. Remove the test cassette from its foil pouch, and place it on a clean, dry, level surface.

3. Procedural Step. Add 3 drops of urine to the round sample well on the test cassette with a disposable pipet supplied with the kit. The test cassette should not be handled again until the test is ready for interpretation. Dispose of the pipet in a regular waste container.

4. Procedural Step. Wait 3 minutes, and read the results by observing the result window.

5. Procedural Step. Interpret the test results as follows:

Negative: The appearance of the blue procedural control line next to the letter "C" only and no pink-to-purple test line next to the letter "T."

Add 3 drops of urine to the test well. (From Bonewit-West K: *Clinical procedures for medical assistants,* ed 7, St. Louis, 2008, Saunders.)

Negative   Positive

Interpret the results. (From Bonewit-West K: *Clinical procedures for medical assistants,* ed 7, St. Louis, 2008, Saunders.)

Positive: The appearance of any pink-to-purple line next to the letter "T" along with a blue procedural control line next to the letter "C."

No result: If no blue procedural control line appears, the test result is invalid, and the specimen must be retested. The blue procedural control line is an internal quality-control indicator designating that the test is working properly and the result is valid and reliable.

Continued

PROCEDURE 30-4

PROCEDURE 30-4 Performing a Urine Pregnancy Test—cont'd

6. **Procedural Step.** Dispose of the test cassette in a regular waste container. Remove gloves, and sanitize your hands.
7. **Procedural Step.** Chart the results. Include the date and time of the patient's last menstrual period (LMP), the name of the test, and the results recorded as either positive or negative.

CHARTING EXAMPLE

Date	
3/25/10	10:30 a.m. LMP: 2/20/10.
	QuickVue preg test: Positive. _____
	_____ L. Proffitt, CMA (AAMA)

MEDICAL PRACTICE *and the* **LAW**

In collection and analysis of patient urine, meticulous attention should be paid to patient instructions, such as cleansing and collecting first morning, midstream, or 24-hour specimens. Patients are often embarrassed to have someone else see their urine, so handle urine specimens in a professional, matter-of-fact manner, with universal precautions to protect yourself. As with all diagnostic procedures, care must be taken to perform the test correctly and treat results confidentially.

Civil versus Criminal Law

Civil law involves a conflict with another person, and if found guilty by a preponderance of evidence (greater than 50%), the loser may lose money or property. Malpractice is a type of civil law. Civil law is divided into *torts,* or wrongs, and *contracts,* or promises. Malpractice is a tort, and nonpayment for services is a contract.

Criminal law involves a conflict with society as a whole (local, state, or federal law). If found guilty beyond a reasonable doubt, the loser may lose money, property, freedom (jail), or life (execution). Violation by the physician of licensure laws and failure to report child abuse are criminal suits. ■

What Would You Do? What Would You *Not* Do? RESPONSES

Case Study 1
Page 702

What Did Linda Do?
- ❑ Took some time to try to calm and relax Mr. Urameshi. Reassured him that the physician would do everything he could to make him better.
- ❑ Offered Mr. Urameshi something to drink and told him it might help him obtain a specimen.
- ❑ Went over the directions again with Mr. Urameshi.
- ❑ Asked Mr. Urameshi if he would try again to obtain a specimen.

What Did Linda Not *Do?*
- ❑ Did not tell Mr. Urameshi that he was not trying hard enough.

What Would You Do?/What Would You *Not* Do? Review Linda's response and place a checkmark next to the information you included in your response. List additional information you included in your response.

_____
_____
_____
_____

Case Study 2
Page 707

What Did Linda Do?
- ❑ Asked Nora whether she takes all of the antibiotic she is prescribed when she has a UTI.
- ❑ Explained to Nora in terms she can understand why women seem to be more prone to development of UTIs.
- ❑ Explained to Nora what she could do to help prevent UTIs. Gave her a patient education brochure on UTIs to take home.
- ❑ Told Nora that the physician is not legally or ethically permitted to call in a prescription for her without seeing her. Also explained that it is in the best interests of her health care to be seen by the physician.

PROCEDURE 30-4

What Would You Do? What Would You *Not* Do?   RESPONSES—cont'd

What Did Linda Not Do?

❑ Did not tell Nora that she could not test her urine at home.

What Would You Do?/What Would You *Not* Do? Review Linda's response and place a checkmark next to the information you included in your response. List additional information you included in your response.

_____

_____

_____

_____

Case Study 3
Page 724

What Did Linda Do?

❑ Told Rita that some peanut butter residue might have been left in the jar she used and might have affected the test results. Asked her to try to collect another specimen at the office so that the urine could be tested again.

❑ Told Rita that if something happens to the specimen container again, she should come to the office and get another one.

❑ Told Rita that several things could have caused her pregnancy test result to be negative. Explained to her that the test could have been outdated or not stored properly. Also explained that as a pregnancy gets farther along, less of the hormone that causes the test to be positive is secreted, so negative test results at the end of a pregnancy are not unusual.

❑ Reassured Rita that many women have trouble sleeping during the last month of pregnancy and that it is normal to have more Braxton-Hicks contractions as she gets closer to delivery.

❑ Told Rita that Linda would inform the physician of her symptoms so that he could discuss them in more detail with her.

What Did Linda Not Do?

❑ Did not criticize Rita for collecting her specimen in a peanut butter jar.

❑ Did not ignore or minimize Rita's concerns.

What Would You Do?/What Would You *Not* Do? Review Linda's response and place a checkmark next to the information you included in your response. List additional information you included in your response.

_____

_____

_____

_____

✪ TERMINOLOGY REVIEW

Bilirubinuria The presence of bilirubin in the urine.

Bladder catheterization The passing of a sterile catheter through the urethra and into the bladder to remove urine.

Glycosuria The presence of glucose in the urine.

Ketonuria The presence of ketone bodies in the urine.

Ketosis An accumulation of large amounts of ketone bodies in the tissues and body fluids.

Micturition The act of voiding urine.

Nephron The functional unit of the kidney.

Oliguria Decreased or scanty output of urine.

pH The unit that describes the acidity or alkalinity of a solution.

Polyuria Increased output of urine.

Proteinuria The presence of protein in the urine.

Refractive index The ratio of the velocity of light in air to the velocity of light in a solution.

Refractometer *(clinical)* An instrument used to measure the refractive index of urine, which is an indirect measurement of the specific gravity of urine.

Renal threshold The concentration at which a substance in the blood that is not normally excreted by the kidneys begins to appear in the urine.

Specific gravity The weight of a substance compared with the weight of an equal volume of a substance known as the standard. In urinalysis, the *specific gravity* refers to the measurement of the amount of dissolved substances present in the urine compared with the same amount of distilled water.

Supernatant The clear liquid that remains at the top after a precipitate settles.

Suprapubic aspiration The passing of a sterile needle through the abdominal wall into the bladder to remove urine.

Urinalysis The physical, chemical, and microscopic analysis of urine.

Void To empty the bladder.

ON THE WEB

For Information on Kidney Disease:

National Kidney Foundation: www.kidney.org

National Institute of Diabetes and Digestive and Kidney
  Diseases: www.niddk.nih.gov

Renal Net: www.renalnet.org

For Information on Drug Abuse:

National Institute on Drug Abuse: www.nida.nih.gov

American Council for Drug Education: www.acde.org

Research Institute on Addictions: www.ria.buffalo.edu

Alcohol and Drug Free Workplace: www.dol.gov/
  workingpartners

Alcohol and Drug Abuse: www.alcoholanddrugabuse.
  com

DARE: www.dare.com

Dependency Free: www.dependencyfree.com

 PREPARE FOR CERTIFICATION   Visit the Evolve site at http://evolve.elsevier.com/Bonewit/today/ to actively Prepare for your Certification.

CD *Check out the* **Companion CD** *bound with the book to access additional interactive activities.*

31

Phlebotomy

Butterfly Method of Venipuncture
    Guidelines for the Butterfly Method
Problems Encountered with Venipuncture
    Failure to Obtain Blood
    Inappropriate Puncture Sites
    Scarred and Sclerosed Veins
    Rolling Veins
    Collapsing Veins
    Premature Needle Withdrawal
    Hematoma
    Hemolysis
    Fainting
Obtaining a Serum Specimen
    Serum

    Tube Selection
    Preparation of the Specimen
    Removal of Serum
    Serum Separator Tubes
Skin Puncture
Puncture Sites
Skin Puncture Devices
    Disposable Semiautomatic Lancet
    Reusable Semiautomatic Lancet
Microcollection Devices
    Capillary Tubes
    Microcollection Tubes
Guidelines for Performing a Finger Puncture

CAAHEP COMPETENCIES

Clinical Competencies
Specimen Collection
- Perform venipuncture.
- Perform capillary puncture.

ABHES COMPETENCIES

Clinical Duties
- Collect and process specimens.
- Perform venipuncture.
- Perform capillary puncture.

KEY TERMS

antecubital space (an-tih-KYOO-bih-tul SPAYS)
anticoagulant (an-tih-koe-AG-yoo-lent)
buffy coat
evacuated tube
hematoma (hee-mah-TOE-mah)
hemoconcentration (hee-moe-kon-sen-TRAY-shun)
hemolysis (hee-MOL-ih-sis)
osteochondritis (OS-tee-oh-kon-DRY-tis)

osteomyelitis (OS-tee-oh-mie-LIE-tis)
phlebotomist (fleh-BOT-oe-mist)
phlebotomy (fleh-BOT-oe-mee)
plasma
serum
venipuncture (VEN-ih-punk-chur)
venous reflux (VEEN-us-REE-fluks)
venous stasis (VEEN-us-STAE-sis)

Introduction to Phlebotomy

The purpose of phlebotomy is to collect a blood specimen for laboratory analysis. The word *phlebotomy* is derived from the Greek words for "vein" *(phlebos)* and "incision" *(tome)* and literally means "making an incision into a vein." As used in the clinical laboratory sciences, **phlebotomy** is defined generally as the collection of blood. An individual who collects a blood sample is a **phlebotomist.**

Some blood specimens are tested in the medical office, and others are picked up and taken to an outside laboratory for testing. The latter specimens need to be placed in a biohazard specimen bag along with a laboratory request so that the laboratory personnel know what type of test the physician desires. The medical assistant may be responsible for completing the laboratory request form either on the computer or manually. The request form includes the physician's name and address; the patient's name, address, age, and gender; the date and time of collection of the specimen; the physician's clinical diagnosis; and a mark next to the type of test or tests to be performed.

Phlebotomy encompasses three major areas of blood collection:

- Arterial puncture
- Venipuncture
- Skin puncture

An arterial puncture is typically performed in a hospital to assess the oxygen level, carbon dioxide level, and acid-base balance of arterial blood; medical assistants do not perform arterial punctures. In the medical office, medical assistants perform venipunctures and skin punctures. This chapter focuses on these two ways to obtain blood.

VENIPUNCTURE

Venipuncture means the puncturing of a vein for the removal of a venous blood sample. In the medical office, a venipuncture is performed when a large blood specimen is necessary for testing. Venipuncture can be performed by the following methods:

- Vacuum tube method
- Butterfly method

The vacuum tube method is the fastest and most convenient of the three methods and is used most often. This method relies on the use of an **evacuated tube,** which is a closed glass or plastic tube that contains a vacuum. The butterfly method is used for difficult draws, such as when a vein is small or sclerosed (hardened). This chapter presents the theory and procedure for each method.

GENERAL GUIDELINES FOR VENIPUNCTURE

General guidelines that are common to all three methods of venipuncture include any advance preparation, identification of the patient, reassuring the patient, positioning the patient, applying the tourniquet, selecting a site for the venipuncture, obtaining the type of blood specimen required, and following the Occupational Safety and Health Administration (OSHA) Bloodborne Pathogens Standard.

Patient Preparation for Venipuncture

The patient should be given instructions an appropriate number of days before the specimen collection on any advance preparation that is required. Although most tests require no preparation, some tests require fasting or the avoidance of certain medications. *Fasting* involves abstaining from food or fluids (except water) for a specified amount of time before the collection of a specimen. If the medical assistant is unsure whether a laboratory test requires advance patient preparation, an appropriate reference source should be consulted. If the specimen is being tested at an outside laboratory, references consist of a laboratory directory and the laboratory's technical support staff. If the specimen is being tested at the medical office, references include instructions included with blood analyzers and testing kits.

When a laboratory test requires advance preparation, before performing the venipuncture, verify that the patient has prepared properly. If the patient has not properly prepared, do not collect the specimen unless directed otherwise by the physician. If the venipuncture is to be rescheduled, carefully review the preparation requirements with the patient.

Identification of the Patient

It cannot be emphasized enough how important it is to identify the patient before performing a venipuncture. Proper patient identification is essential to avoid collecting a specimen on the wrong patient by mistake. After greeting the patient, the medical assistant should ask the patient to state his or her full name and date of birth. This information should be compared with the demographic data indicated in the patient's chart. The patient should *not* be asked whether he or she is a certain patient. For example, the patient should not be asked: "Are you Brad Thompson?" The patient may not hear the medical assistant correctly or not be paying attention and answer in the affirmative even if he is not that patient. A specimen that is not identified correctly could lead to an inaccurate patient diagnosis and the wrong treatment.

Reassuring the Patient

Venipuncture is often a frightening experience for the patient. For many patients, the anticipation of the procedure is worse than the actual drawing of the blood. The medical assistant should take time to explain the procedure to the patient in an unhurried and confident manner. This helps to alleviate the patient's fears, which relaxes the patient's veins. Relaxed veins make venipuncture easier to perform and result in less pain for the patient.

Instruct the patient to remain still during the procedure. Explain to the patient that a small amount of pain is associated with a venipuncture, but it is brief. Never tell the patient that the venipuncture will not hurt. Just before inserting the needle, tell the patient that he or she will "feel a small stick." This prevents startling the patient, which could cause the patient to move. Movement causes pain for the patient, and it may damage the venipuncture site.

Patient Position for Venipuncture

The patient position for venipuncture is especially important to the successful collection of a blood specimen. Proper positioning allows easy access to the vein and is more comfortable for the patient. The patient position depends on the vein to be used. The most common site for venipuncture is the **antecubital space,** and the information presented next refers to this site.

The patient should be seated comfortably in a chair. The arm should be extended downward to form a straight line from the shoulder to the wrist with the palm facing up; the arm should not bend at the elbow. The arm should be well supported on the armrest by a rolled towel or by having the patient place the fist of the other hand under the elbow (Figure 31-1).

A venipuncture should never be performed with the patient sitting on a stool or standing. The patient may faint and injure himself or herself. If the patient appears nervous or has fainted in the past from a venipuncture, it is best to

Figure 31-1. Patient position for obtaining a blood specimen from the antecubital veins. (From Bonewit-West K: *Clinical procedures for medical assistants,* ed 7, St. Louis, 2008, Saunders.)

place the patient in a semireclining position (semi-Fowler's position) on the examining table. A pillow or a cushion should be placed under the patient's arm to support the arm in a straight line from the shoulder to the wrist.

Although unusual, it is possible for blood to flow from the evacuated tube back into the patient's vein during the procedure. This condition is known as **venous reflux.** Venous reflux could cause the patient to have an adverse reaction to a tube additive, particularly if the additive in the tube is ethylenediaminetetraacetic acid. Venous reflux can occur only if the contents of the evacuated tube are in contact with the tube stopper while the specimen is being drawn. Venous reflux is prevented by keeping the patient's arm in a downward position so that the evacuated tube remains below the venipuncture site and fills from the bottom up.

Application of the Tourniquet

An important step in the venipuncture procedure is the application of the tourniquet. The tourniquet makes the patient's veins stand out so that they are easier to palpate. The tourniquet acts as a "dam," which causes the venous blood to slow down and pool in the veins in front of the tourniquet. This pooling of blood makes the veins more prominent so that they are more visible and can be palpated.

When applying a tourniquet, it is important to obtain the correct tourniquet tension. The tourniquet should be applied with enough tension to slow the venous flow without affecting the arterial flow. A tourniquet that is too tight obstructs both the venous blood flow and the arterial flow, which may result in a specimen that produces inaccurate test results. A tourniquet that is too loose fails to cause the veins to stand out enough to be palpated. A correctly applied tourniquet should fit snugly and not pinch the patient's skin.

Putting It All into Practice

My name is Dori Glover, and I work in a very busy, fast-paced family practice office for two physicians. I love my job. The physicians are great, with very different styles; the pace is fast; and the time flies by. I am constantly challenged, learning new things, meeting and helping people, and being a part of a team that works well together.

While performing a venipuncture for a routine blood chemistry profile (a procedure I have performed many times), I accidentally stuck myself. I could see the blood inside my glove, and I could see the patient's blood clinging to the point of the needle—my heart sank. I placed the needle and holder in the sharps container and tried to keep my cool and not alarm the patient. I mentally assessed the patient. He was an older man from a rural community, but I know you cannot always judge a book by its cover.

I excused myself and immediately proceeded to wash my hands thoroughly with soap and water and rinse, rinse, rinse! I then notified the physician. The physician questioned the patient regarding operations he had had in the previous year. He had undergone bypass surgery and had received 2 units of blood. Although blood is effectively screened, I thought about that one-in-a-zillion chance that it could have been contaminated. Thankfully, I had received the hepatitis B immunization series, but there was still concern regarding hepatitis C and, of course, HIV.

The patient was gracious and complied with our request to be tested for hepatitis and HIV. The physician and I discussed the situation, and we determined the risk to be low, but he nonetheless offered me the option of getting the HIV postexposure prophylactic treatment. The window of time for this to be effective is only 1 to 2 hours after the stick. It is very toxic and not something you want to receive needlessly. I declined and proceeded to wait 5 agonizing days for the patient's test results. The word *relief* hardly describes how I felt when the laboratory results came back negative!

This incident confirmed the importance of getting the hepatitis B immunization and paying attention to good technique when performing procedures involving blood. ■

Prepare for Success

Guidelines for Applying the Tourniquet

The following guidelines help to ensure the successful application of the tourniquet:
1. Do not apply the tourniquet over sores or burned skin.
2. Place the tourniquet 3 to 4 inches above the bend in the elbow. This allows adequate room for cleansing the site and performing the venipuncture without the tourniquet getting in the way.
3. Apply the tourniquet so that it is snug, but not so tight that it pinches the patient's skin or is otherwise painful to the patient.
4. When applying the tourniquet, ask the patient to clench his or her fist. This pushes blood from the lower arm

into the veins and makes them easier to palpate. You can ask the patient to clench and unclench the fist a few times; however, vigorous pumping should be avoided because it could lead to hemoconcentration, which could produce inaccurate test results.

5. Never leave the tourniquet on for more than 1 minute because it would be uncomfortable for the patient. In addition, prolonged application of the tourniquet causes the venous blood to stagnate, or pool in one place too long, a condition known as **venous stasis.** When venous stasis occurs, the plasma portion of the blood filters into the tissues, causing hemoconcentration. **Hemoconcentration** is an increase in the concentration of nonfilterable blood components in the blood vessels, such as red blood cells, enzymes, iron, and calcium, as a result of a decrease in the fluid content of the blood. This can result in inaccurate results for a variety of laboratory tests.

6. Ideally, you should remove the tourniquet as soon as a good blood flow is established; however, this may not be practical when first learning the venipuncture procedure. Removing the tourniquet may cause the needle to move such that no more blood can be obtained, and the blood has to be redrawn. When learning the venipuncture procedure, it is better to wait until just before the needle is removed before removing the tourniquet.

7. *Always* remove the tourniquet before removing the needle from the patient's arm. If the needle is removed first, the pressure of the tourniquet causes blood to be forced out of the puncture site and into the surrounding tissue, resulting in a **hematoma.**

8. After use, wipe a tourniquet thoroughly with a disinfectant such as alcohol. Disposable tourniquets that are thrown away after one use are available.

Types of Tourniquets

The most common tourniquets are the *rubber* tourniquet and the *Velcro-closure* tourniquet. The type of tourniquet used is a matter of individual preference.

Rubber Tourniquet

The rubber tourniquet consists of a flat, soft band of rubber approximately 1 inch (2.5 cm) wide and 15 to 18 inches (38 to 45 cm) long. Rubber tourniquets are commercially available in latex or nonlatex rubber. They offer the advantage of being easily removable with one hand. The technique for applying a rubber tourniquet is described next and illustrated in Figure 31-2.

Procedure: Rubber Tourniquet

1. Hold each end of the tourniquet with one hand. Position the tourniquet 3 to 4 inches (7.5 to 10 cm) above the bend in the elbow, making sure that the tourniquet lies flat against the patient's skin. Pull the ends away from each other to create tension (see Figure 31-2A).

2. Bring the ends of the tourniquet toward each other and cross one over the other at the point of your grasp, with enough tension so that the tourniquet is snug but not pinching the patient's skin (see Figure 31-2B).

3. Tuck a portion of the top length into the bottom length, forming a loop between the tourniquet and the patient's arm. This allows for a one-handed release of the tourni-

Figure 31-2. Application of a rubber tourniquet. **A,** Create tension by pulling the ends of the tourniquet away from each other. **B,** With tension, cross one flap over the other at the point of your grasp. **C,** Form a loop by tucking a portion of the top length into the bottom length. (From Bonewit-West K: *Clinical procedures for medical assistants,* ed 7, St. Louis, 2008, Saunders.)

quet when pulled on one end. Make sure the flaps are directed upward so that they do not dangle into the working area (see Figure 31-2C).

Velcro-Closure Tourniquet

The Velcro-closure tourniquet consists of a band of rubber or elastic material with Velcro attached at the ends. This type of tourniquet is easier to apply and is more comfortable for the patient than the rubber tourniquet. The disadvantage to the Velcro-closure tourniquet is that it is more difficult to remove with one hand than the rubber tourniquet. In addition, this type of tourniquet may not fit around the arms of extremely obese patients. The technique for applying a Velcro-closure tourniquet is described next and illustrated in Figure 31-3.

Procedure: Velcro-Closure Tourniquet

1. Hold each end of the tourniquet with one hand. Position the tourniquet 3 to 4 inches (7.5 to 10 cm) above the bend in the elbow.
2. Wrap the tourniquet around the arm, and secure it with the Velcro fastener. The tourniquet should be applied with enough tension so that it is snug but not pinching the patient's skin.

Site Selection for Venipuncture

For most patients, the best site to use is the veins in the antecubital space (Figure 31-4). If the patient has large, visible antecubital veins, drawing blood is easy. If the patient has small veins or veins that cannot be palpated, obtaining a blood specimen can be quite a challenge, even for the most experienced medical assistant.

The antecubital space is the surface of the arm in front of the elbow. The antecubital veins generally have a wide lumen and are close to the surface of the skin, which makes them easily accessible. In addition, these veins typically have thick walls, making them less likely to collapse. Using the antecubital space spares the patient unnecessary pain because the skin is less sensitive there than at other sites, such as the back of the hand. The medical assistant should not be misled by the presence in some patients of many small, very blue, "spidery" veins that lie close to the surface of the skin. These veins are not suitable for performing a venipuncture. The antecubital veins lie beneath these veins.

The best vein to use in the antecubital space is the *median cubital*. The median cubital is a prominent vein in the middle of the antecubital space and does not roll (see Figure 31-4). At times, however, the median cubital vein cannot be used (e.g., when it lies deep in the tissues and cannot be palpated or is scarred from repeated venipunctures).

The *cephalic* and *basilic* veins are located on opposite sides of the antecubital space and provide an alternative site when the median cubital vein is unavailable. The cephalic vein is located on the thumb side of the antecubital space, and the basilic vein is located on the little finger side of the antecubital space. The disadvantage of these "side" veins is that they tend to roll or move away from the needle, escaping puncture. To prevent rolling, firm pressure should be applied below the vein to stabilize it as the needle is inserted.

Figure 31-3. Application of a Velcro-closure tourniquet. (From Bonewit-West K: *Clinical procedures for medical assistants,* ed 7, St. Louis, 2008, Saunders.)

Figure 31-4. Antecubital veins. (From Bonewit-West K: *Clinical procedures for medical assistants,* ed 7, St. Louis, 2008, Saunders.)

The brachial artery is also located in the antecubital space, but it lies deeper in the tissues. This is the artery that is used to measure blood pressure. Before performing a venipuncture, palpate for the presence of this artery. In contrast to a vein, an artery pulsates, is more elastic, and has a thicker wall than a vein. If the brachial artery is inadvertently punctured, the patient feels more than the usual amount of pain and the blood is bright red and comes out in pulsing movements. If this situation occurs, the tourniquet should be removed and then the needle. Pressure with a gauze pad should be applied for 4 to 5 minutes.

Guidelines for Site Selection

Specific guidelines should be followed to facilitate the selection of a good vein:

1. Ensure that the lighting is adequate. Good lighting facilitates inspection of the veins.
2. Ensure that the veins "stand out" as much as possible. Before locating a venipuncture site, always apply the tourniquet and have the patient make a fist. This combination makes the veins more prominent.
3. Examine the antecubital veins of both arms. The best site to perform a venipuncture varies with each individual. The patient may have larger veins in one arm than in the other. It is advisable to ask the patient whether he or she has had a venipuncture before. Most adults have had previous venipunctures and know which of their veins are best to use and which should be avoided. Listen to and evaluate information offered by the patient.
4. Use inspection and particularly palpation to select a vein. A vein does not have to be seen to be a good selection. If you cannot see a vein, palpation alone can be used to locate it. A vein feels like an elastic tube that "gives" under the pressure of the fingertips.
5. Always palpate for the median cubital vein (middle vein) first. It is usually bigger, is anchored better, bruises less, and poses the smallest risk of injuring underlying structures (e.g., nerves, arteries) than the other veins. Because of this, if the patient's median cubital vein cannot be seen but still can be palpated, it should be used as the first choice when selecting a vein. If the median cubital vein is good in both arms, select the one that appears the fullest. The cephalic vein located on the thumb side is the next best vein choice because it does not roll and bruise as easily as the basilic vein. The basilic vein, located on the little finger side of the antecubital space, is the least desirable venipuncture site in the antecubital space. Branches of the median nerve may lie close to this vein in some individuals. In addition, the basilic vein lies in close proximity to the brachial artery. Both of these conditions pose a risk of injuring underlying structures when drawing blood from the basilic vein.
6. Thoroughly assess the patient's veins. To assess a vein as a possible site for the venipuncture, place one or two fingertips (index and middle finger) over it and press lightly, then release pressure. Do not use your thumb to palpate the vein because it is not as sensitive as the index finger. To be suitable for a venipuncture, the vein should feel round, firm, elastic, and engorged. When you depress and release an engorged vein, it should spring back in a rounded, filled state.
7. Determine the size, depth, and direction of the vein. When a suitable vein has been located, it should be palpated thoroughly and carefully to determine the direction of the vein and to estimate the size and depth of the vein. Palpate and trace the path of the vein several times by rolling your index finger back and forth over the vein to determine its size. Inspect and palpate the vein for problems. Some veins that appear suitable at first sight feel small, hard, bumpy, or flat when palpated.
8. Map the location of the site. After locating an acceptable vein, mentally "map" the location of the puncture site on the patient's arm with "skin marks." This technique is particularly helpful if the vein cannot be seen, but only palpated. The puncture site may be located on or next to a skin mark, such as a freckle, a small wrinkle, or a pigmented area.
9. Do not leave the tourniquet on for more than 1 minute. When first learning the venipuncture procedure, you may need to perform numerous assessments of the patient's arms to locate the best vein. After each assessment, remove the tourniquet for approximately 2 minutes to allow normal circulation of the blood to occur. This prevents patient discomfort and hemoconcentration, which can lead to inaccurate results for a variety of laboratory tests.
10. If a good vein cannot be found, the following techniques can be employed to make the veins more prominent:
    - Remove the tourniquet, and have the patient dangle the arm over the side of the chair for 1 to 2 minutes.
    - Tap the vein site sharply a few times with your index finger and second finger.
    - Gently massage the arm from the wrist to the elbow.
    - Apply a warm, moist washcloth to the area for 5 minutes.

Alternative Venipuncture Sites

If it is impossible to locate a suitable vein in the antecubital space, alternative sites are available, including the inner forearm, the wrist area above the thumb, and the back of the hand (Figure 31-5). These alternative veins are smaller and have thinner walls than the antecubital veins and should be used for venipuncture only when all possibilities for obtaining the blood specimen at the antecubital site have been considered. If the medical assistant is able to palpate a small vein in the antecubital space, it may be possible to obtain blood there using the butterfly method of venipuncture.

The hand veins, in particular, should be used only as a last resort. The veins of the hand tend to roll because they are not supported by much tissue and are close to the surface of the skin. This makes them more difficult to stick. In addition, there is an abundant supply of nerves in the hands, which makes this procedure more uncomfortable for the patient. Hand veins tend to have thin walls, which makes them more susceptible to collapsing, bruising, and phlebitis. In some patients, however, especially the obese and the elderly, the hand veins may be the only accessible site.

What Would You Do? What Would You *Not* Do?

Case Study 1

Angela Castillo is 21 years old and comes to the office at 9:00 AM to have her blood drawn for a CBC and a thyroid profile. She has brought a friend along with her. Angela seems nervous, and her voice is shaking. She says this is the first venipuncture she has ever had. Angela asks whether her friend could stay with her to give her moral support while her blood is being drawn. Angela says that the blood has to be taken out of her left arm. She says she is right-handed and has a softball game this evening. When the veins of Angela's left arm are examined, a suitable vein cannot be located; however, she has a good median cubital vein in her right arm. Angela then wants to know whether the blood could be drawn from her left hand like they do on hospital television shows. ∎

Types of Blood Specimens

The type of blood specimen required depends on the type of test to be performed. Serum is required for most blood chemistry studies, whereas whole blood is required for a complete blood count (CBC). The various types of blood specimen that the medical assistant would be required to obtain through the venipuncture procedure are as follows:

1. **Clotted blood.** Clotted blood is obtained from a tube that does not contain an **anticoagulant.** A tube without an anticoagulant causes the blood cells to clot.
2. **Serum.** Serum is obtained from clotted blood by allowing the specimen to stand and then centrifuging it. Centrifuging a blood specimen that does not contain an anticoagulant causes the blood to separate into the following layers (Figure 31-6A):
   - Top layer—serum
   - Bottom layer—clotted blood cells
3. **Whole blood.** Whole blood is obtained by using a tube that contains an anticoagulant. The anticoagulant prevents clotting of the blood cells. It is important to mix the anticoagulant with the blood by gently inverting the tube back and forth 8 to 10 times after collection.
4. **Plasma.** Plasma is obtained from whole blood that has been centrifuged. Centrifuging a blood specimen that contains an anticoagulant causes the blood to separate into the following layers (Figure 31-6B):
   - Top layer—plasma
   - Middle layer—**buffy coat** (contains white blood cells and platelets)
   - Bottom layer—red blood cells

Figure 31-5. Alternative venipuncture sites: the inner forearm, the wrist area above the thumb, and the back of the hand. (From Bonewit-West K: *Clinical procedures for medical assistants,* ed 7, St. Louis, 2008, Saunders.)

Serum

Plasma

Buffy coat

Cells
(clot)

Cells

A

B

No anticoagulant   Anticoagulant

Figure 31-6. Layers into which the blood separates when there is no anticoagulant **(A)** and when an anticoagulant is present **(B).** (From Bonewit-West K: *Clinical procedures for medical assistants,* ed 7, St. Louis, 2008, Saunders.)

Plastic
holder

Evacuated   Rubber   Flange   Posterior   Anterior
tube   stopper   needle   needle

Figure 31-7. Vacuum tube system. (From Bonewit-West K: *Clinical procedures for medical assistants,* ed 7, St. Louis, 2008, Saunders.)

OSHA Safety Precautions

The OSHA Bloodborne Pathogens Standard presented in Chapter 17 must be carefully followed during the venipuncture procedure to avoid exposure to bloodborne pathogens. The following OSHA requirements apply specifically to the venipuncture procedure and to separation of serum or plasma from whole blood (see later):

1. Wear gloves when it is reasonably anticipated that you will have hand contact with blood.
2. Wear a face shield or mask in combination with an eye protection device whenever splashes, spray, splatter, or droplets of blood may be generated.
3. Perform all procedures involving blood in a manner so as to minimize splashing, spraying, splattering, and generating droplets of blood.
4. Bandage cuts and other lesions on the hands before gloving.
5. Sanitize hands as soon as possible after removing gloves.
6. If your hands or other skin surfaces come in contact with blood, wash the area as soon as possible with soap and water.
7. If your mucous membranes (e.g., eyes, nose, mouth) come in contact with blood, flush them with water as soon as possible.
8. Do not bend, break, or shear contaminated venipuncture needles.
9. Do not recap a contaminated venipuncture needle.

10. Locate the sharps container as close as possible to the area of use. Immediately after use, place the contaminated venipuncture needle (and plastic holder) in the biohazard sharps container.
11. Place blood specimens in containers that prevent leakage during collection, handling, processing, storage, transport, and shipping.
12. If you are exposed to blood, report the incident immediately to your physician-employer.

VACUUM TUBE METHOD OF VENIPUNCTURE

The vacuum tube method is frequently used to collect venous blood specimens. This method is considered ideal for collecting blood from normal healthy antecubital veins that are adequate in size to withstand the pressure of the vacuum in the evacuated tube. Procedure 31-1 outlines the venipuncture vacuum tube method. The vacuum tube system consists of a collection needle, a plastic holder, and an evacuated tube (Figure 31-7). One commercially available vacuum tube system is the Vacutainer (Becton Dickinson, Tarrytown, NY).

Needle

The needle used with the vacuum tube method consists of a double-pointed, stainless steel needle with a threaded hub near its center (Figure 31-8). The needle is coated with silicon, enabling it to penetrate the skin smoothly. The threaded hub of the needle screws into the plastic holder. Vacuum tube needles are packaged in sealed twist-apart plastic containers. The needle gauge and length are printed on the paper seal on the container (see Figure 31-8). A needle should not be used if the seal has been broken.

The double-pointed needle consists of an anterior needle and a posterior needle. The *anterior needle* is longer and has

[Handwritten notes in left margin: "5 mL", "2.5 mL", "12.5", "need blood", "2 mL x 2.5 = 5 mL", "if not in quality not sufficient"]

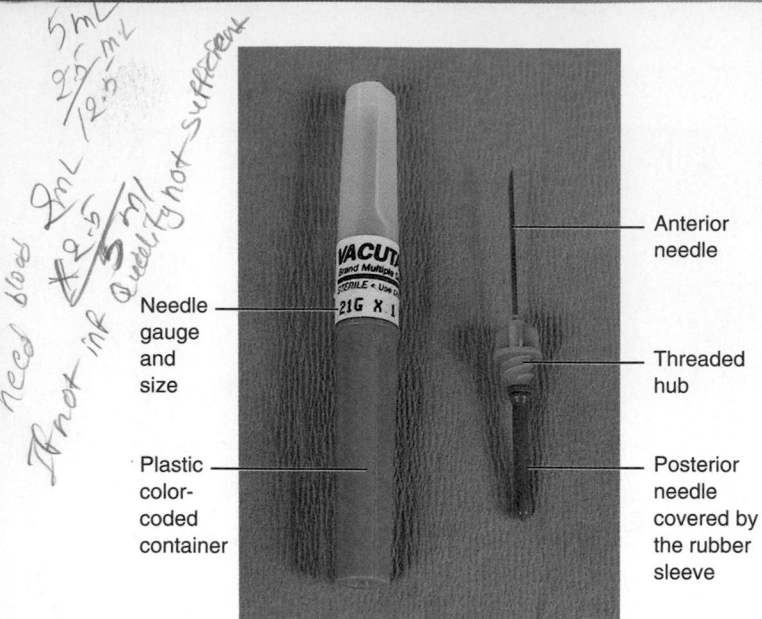

Needle gauge and size

Plastic color-coded container

Anterior needle

Threaded hub

Posterior needle covered by the rubber sleeve

Figure 31-8. Vacuum tube needle in its container showing the gauge and size of the needle. The gauge of this needle is 21 G, and the size is 1 inch. (From Bonewit-West K: *Clinical procedures for medical assistants,* ed 7, St. Louis, 2008, Saunders.)

a beveled point designed to facilitate entry into the skin and the vein. The *posterior needle* is shorter, and its purpose is to pierce the rubber stopper of the evacuated tube. The posterior needle has a rubber sleeve that functions as a valve. Pushing the tube stopper of an evacuated tube onto the posterior needle compresses this rubber sleeve and exposes the opening of the needle, allowing blood to enter the tube. When a tube is removed, the sleeve slides back over the needle opening and stops the flow of blood.

Vacuum tube needles are available in sizes 20 G to 22 G, with 21 G needles used most often for a routine venipuncture. Vacuum tube needles come in two lengths, 1 inch and 1½ inch. The length used is based on individual preference; most medical assistants prefer the 1-inch needle for routine venipunctures. A 1-inch needle is less intimidating to the patient and tends to offer more control because it allows the medical assistant to rest the fourth and fifth fingers on the patient's arm for stability. A 1½-inch needle allows more room for stabilizing the vein.

Safety-Engineered Venipuncture Devices

OSHA stipulates requirements to reduce needlestick and other sharps injuries among health care workers. As discussed in Chapter 17, employers are required to evaluate and implement commercially available safer medical devices that reduce occupational exposure to the lowest extent feasible.

Safer medical devices include safety-engineered venipuncture devices. These devices incorporate a built-in safety feature to reduce risk of a needlestick injury. Figure 31-9 illustrates a safety-engineered venipuncture device and method for using it.

Plastic Holder

The plastic holder consists of a plastic cylinder with two openings. The small opening is used to secure the double-pointed needle, and the large opening is used to hold the evacuated tube. The large opening has a plastic extension known as the *flange.* The flange assists in the insertion and removal of evacuated tubes and prevents the plastic holder from rolling when it is placed on a flat surface.

The plastic holder has an indentation about ½ inch from the hub of the needle. This marks the point at which the posterior needle starts to enter the rubber stopper of the tube. If a tube stopper is inserted past this point before the vein is entered, the tube fills with air, which prevents blood from entering the tube.

Evacuated Tubes

Evacuated tubes consist of a glass tube with a rubber stopper. The tube contains a premeasured vacuum that creates suction to pull the blood specimen into the tube. Evacuated tubes use a color-coded stopper system for ease in identifying the additive (or no additive) content of the tube. The additive content of evacuated tubes is described in the box *Additive Content of Evacuated Tubes* and illustrated in Figure 31-10. A tube additive must not alter the blood components or affect the laboratory test to be performed.

The color of the tube stopper used depends on the type of test to be performed. The medical assistant must determine the correct stopper color to use for each collection. The color-coded stoppered tubes must not be substituted for one another because inaccurate test results could occur. If a CBC has been ordered by the physician, a lavender stoppered tube must be used and a different color stoppered tube cannot be substituted for it.

Evacuated tubes are available in varying capacities, the most common being the 2-, 3-, 5-, 7-, 10-, and 15-ml sizes (see Figure 31-10). The capacity of the tube used depends on the amount of the specimen required for the test. If the medical assistant is working with an outside laboratory, information on the amount of specimen required for a laboratory test and the stopper color of the tube required is indicated in the laboratory directory. If the test is being performed in the medical office, this information is indicated in the instructions accompanying the blood analyzer or testing kit.

Information regarding additive content, expiration date, and tube capacity is on the label of each box of evacuated tubes. In addition, evacuated tubes have a label affixed to them indicating the additive content, expiration date, tube capacity, and a fill indicator to indicate when the vacuum has been exhausted and the tube is full.

Hemogard closure tubes, manufactured by Becton Dickinson, are a newer type of evacuated tube (Figure 31-11). A Hemogard tube consists of a special rubber stopper and a plastic closure that overhangs the outside of the tube. Together, these components act as a single unit to reduce the likelihood of coming in contact with the contents of the

Figure 31-9. Safety-engineered venipuncture device. **A,** Perform the venipuncture with the shield in a downward position. **B,** After performing the venipuncture, push the shield forward. **C,** Continue pushing until the needle tip is fully covered by the shield. Discard the needle and holder in a biohazard sharps container. (From Bonewit-West K: *Clinical procedures for medical assistants,* ed 7, St. Louis, 2008, Saunders.)

Red:
No anticoagulant

Lavender:
EDTA

Light Blue:
Sodium citrate

Green:
Heparin

Gray:
Sodium fluoride/
potassium
oxalate

Dark Blue:
Specially
refined glass

Figure 31-10. Vacutainer evacuated tubes. The stoppers of the evacuated tubes are color coded for ease in identifying the additive content. The lavender, light-blue, green, gray, and dark-blue stoppered tubes contain an anticoagulant and are used to obtain whole blood or plasma. The red stoppered tube contains no additive and is used to obtain clotted blood or serum. *EDTA,* Ethylenediaminetetraacetic acid. (From Bonewit-West K: *Clinical procedures for medical assistants,* ed 7, St. Louis, 2008, Saunders.)

tube. After collecting a blood specimen, the medical assistant may need to gain access to the blood in the tube for testing it or for further processing, such as in separating serum from whole blood. A regular evacuated tube "pops" as the top is removed, which may result in splattering of blood. The design of the Hemogard tube works to prevent

Gray: Sodium fluoride/potassium oxalate

Red: No anticoagulant

Lavender: EDTA

Gold: Serum separator tube

Figure 31-11. Hemogard tubes. *EDTA,* Ethylenediaminetetraacetic acid. (From Bonewit-West K: *Clinical procedures for medical assistants,* ed 7, St. Louis, 2008, Saunders.)

splattering of blood when the top is removed. In addition, closure tubes are made of plastic, which reduces the possibility of tube breakage under normal conditions. The color coding of Hemogard stoppers is similar to that of rubber stoppered tubes (refer to Figure 31-10).

Order of Draw for Multiple Tubes

When using the vacuum tube system, and when multiple tubes of blood are to be drawn, the following order of draw is recommended by the Clinical Laboratory Standards Institute:

1. **Blood culture tube** (and other tests that require sterile specimens)
   - *Rationale:* To prevent contamination of the specimen by other tubes, which may lead to inaccurate test results
2. **Coagulation tube:** Light-blue stoppered tube for coagulation tests
   - *Rationale:* To prevent additives from other tubes from getting into the tube
   - *Note:* When the needle penetrates the patient's skin, thromboplastin, a clotting factor, is released because of tissue trauma. It was previously thought that thromboplastin entering the blood specimen could alter coagulation test results. To avoid this problem, it was recommended that a red stoppered tube be drawn first to collect the thromboplastin, followed by the collection of the blue stoppered tube. Current studies show that tissue thromboplastin entering the blood specimen does not affect coagulation test results. Further studies show, however, that a modification in technique is required when a butterfly setup

Additive Content of Evacuated Tubes

The vacuum tube method uses a color-coded system for ease in identifying the additive content of each type of tube. The most frequently used vacuum tubes are classified here according to the color of the stopper and additive content.

1. **Red.** Red stoppered tubes do not contain an anticoagulant and are used to obtain clotted blood or serum. Serum is required for serologic tests and most blood chemistries.
2. **Red/gray** (gold if using Hemoguard tubes). These tubes do not contain an anticoagulant and are used to obtain serum. Red/gray and gold stoppered tubes contain a gel that separates the cells from the serum when the tube is centrifuged.
3. **Lavender.** Lavender stoppered tubes contain the anticoagulant ethylenediaminetetraacetic acid and are used to obtain whole blood or plasma. The most common use is to collect a blood specimen for a complete blood count.
4. **Light blue.** Light-blue stoppered tubes contain the anticoagulant sodium citrate and are used to obtain whole blood or

plasma; the most common use is for coagulation tests, such as the prothrombin time.
5. **Green.** Green stoppered tubes contain the anticoagulant heparin and are commonly used to collect blood specimens to perform blood gas determinations and pH assays.
6. **Gray.** Gray stoppered tubes contain the anticoagulant sodium fluoride/potassium oxalate and are used to obtain whole blood or plasma; the most common use is to collect blood specimens to perform a glucose tolerance test.
7. **Dark blue.** Dark blue stoppered tubes contain either heparin or no additive at all. These tubes are made of a specially refined glass and rubber stopper and are used for the detection of trace elements, such as lead, zinc, arsenic, and copper, which are contracted through occupational or environmental exposure.

is used to obtain the specimen for a coagulation test. The tubing of the butterfly setup contains 0.3 to 1 cc of air. If a blue stoppered tube is the first or only tube to be drawn, a 5-ml red stoppered tube must be drawn first and discarded. This is because some of the tube's vacuum is exhausted by the air in the tubing (rather than blood), resulting in underfilling of the tube. If the blue stoppered tube is filled first, the underfilled tube results in an incorrect anticoagulant-to-blood ratio. An incorrect ratio when performing a coagulation test leads to inaccurate coagulation test results.

3. **Serum tubes:** Tubes with or without a clot activator and serum separator tubes (e.g., red stoppered tube and red/slate-gray stoppered tube)
   - *Rationale:* To prevent contamination of nonadditive tubes by tubes with an anticoagulant
4. **Anticoagulant tubes** in this order of stopper color: green, lavender, gray
   - *Rationale:* To prevent cross-contamination between different types of anticoagulants, which may lead to inaccurate test results

Evacuated Tube Guidelines

Certain guidelines should be followed when using evacuated tubes, as follows:
1. Select the proper evacuated tubes according to the tests to be performed and amount of specimen required.
2. Check to ensure the tube is not cracked. A cracked tube no longer has a vacuum.
3. Check the expiration date of each tube. Outdated tubes may no longer contain a vacuum, and, as a result, they would not be able to draw blood into the tube.
4. Label each tube with the patient's name, the date, and your initials. Proper labeling avoids mixing up specimens. Advances in specimen identification include the use of computer bar codes to identify specimens (Figure 31-12). The laboratory instruments that do the testing are able to read the bar codes and automatically record results onto the laboratory report form.
5. Before using tubes that contain powdered additives (e.g., gray stoppered tube), gently tap the tube just below the stopper so that all of the additive is dislodged from the stopper. If an additive remains trapped in the stopper, erroneous test results may occur.
6. Take precautions to avoid premature loss of the tube's vacuum. Premature loss of vacuum can occur from the following:
   - Dropping the tube
   - Pushing the posterior needle through the tube stopper before puncturing the vein
   - Partially pulling the needle out of the vein after penetrating the patient's vein
7. Use a continuous, steady motion to make the puncture. Performing the puncture with a slow, timid motion or

Figure 31-12. Identifying a blood specimen using a computer bar code. (From Bonewit-West K: *Clinical procedures for medical assistants,* ed 7, St. Louis, 2008, Saunders.)

a rapid, jabbing motion is painful for the patient. In addition, a rapid motion could cause the needle to go completely through the vein, resulting in a failure to obtain blood and possibly a hematoma.
8. When multiple tubes are to be drawn, follow the proper *order of draw.* This prevents contamination of nonadditive tubes by additive tubes and cross-contamination between different types of additive tubes, which could lead to inaccurate test results.
9. Fill evacuated tubes until the vacuum is exhausted, as evidenced by the cessation of the blood flow into the tube. The tube is almost, but not quite, full when the vacuum is exhausted. If the evacuated tube is removed before the vacuum is exhausted, a rush of air enters the tube, damaging the red blood cells. A tube that contains an anticoagulant must be filled completely to ensure the proper ratio of anticoagulant to the blood specimen.
10. Remove the last tube from the plastic holder before removing the needle from the patient's vein. This prevents blood from dripping out of the tip of the needle after it is withdrawn from the patient's skin.
11. Mix tubes that contain an anticoagulant immediately after drawing by gently inverting the tube back and forth 8 to 10 times. This provides adequate mixing without causing **hemolysis,** or breakdown of blood cells. Inadequate mixing or not mixing the tubes immediately after drawing them may result in clotting of the blood, leading to inaccurate test results.
12. After the venipuncture, the top of the stopper may contain residual blood. Take precautions following the OSHA standard when handling these tubes.

Text continued on p. 746

PROCEDURE 31-1 Venipuncture—Vacuum Tube Method

Outcome Perform a venipuncture using the vacuum tube method.

Equipment/Supplies

- Disposable gloves
- Tourniquet
- Antiseptic wipe
- Double-pointed needle
- Plastic holder
- Evacuated tubes with labels

- Sterile 2 × 2 gauze pad
- Adhesive bandage
- Biohazard sharps container
- Biohazard specimen bag
- Laboratory request form

1. Procedural Step. Sanitize your hands.

2. Procedural Step. Greet the patient and introduce yourself. Identify the patient by asking the patient to state his or her full name and date of birth. Compare this information with the demographic data in the patient's chart. If the patient was required to prepare for the test (e.g., fasting, medication restriction), determine whether he or she has prepared properly. If the patient has not followed the patient preparation requirements, notify the physician for instructions on handling this situation.

Principle. It is important to confirm that you have the correct patient to avoid collecting a specimen on the wrong patient. The patient must prepare properly to obtain a quality specimen that would lead to accurate test results.

3. Procedural Step. Assemble the equipment. Select the proper evacuated tubes for the tests to be performed. Check the expiration date of the tubes. Label each tube using one of the following methods: (a) attaching a computer bar code label to each tube to be drawn and labeling it with your initials, or (b) manually labeling each tube with the patient's name, the date, and your initials. If the specimen is to be tested at an outside laboratory, complete a laboratory request form.

Principle. Outdated tubes may no longer contain a vacuum and, as a result, they may not be able to draw blood into the tube. Proper labeling of blood specimens avoids a mixup of specimens.

Assemble the equipment. (From Bonewit-West K: *Clinical procedures for medical assistants,* ed 7, St. Louis, 2008, Saunders.)

4. Procedural Step. Prepare the vacuum tube system. Remove the cap from the posterior needle using a twisting and pulling motion. Insert the posterior needle into the small opening on the plastic holder. Screw the plastic holder onto the Luer adapter, and tighten it securely.

Principle. An unsecured needle can fall out of its plastic holder.

Screw the needle into the holder. (From Bonewit-West K: *Clinical procedures for medical assistants,* ed 7, St. Louis, 2008, Saunders.)

5. Procedural Step. Open the sterile gauze packet, and lay it flat to allow the gauze pad to rest on the inside of its wrapper. Position the evacuated tubes in the correct

Tap tubes with powdered additives. (From Bonewit-West K: *Clinical procedures for medical assistants,* ed 7, St. Louis, 2008, Saunders.)

order of draw. If the evacuated tube contains a pow-dered additive, tap the tube just below the stopper to release any additive adhering to the stopper.

Principle. If an additive remains trapped in the stopper, erroneous test results may occur.

6. **Procedural Step.** Place the first tube loosely in the plastic holder.

7. **Procedural Step.** Explain the procedure to the patient, and reassure the patient. Perform a preliminary assess-ment of both arms to determine the best vein to use. It is also helpful to ask the patient which arm has been used in the past to obtain blood.

Principle. Venipuncture is often a frightening experi-ence for the patient, and reassurance should be offered to reduce apprehension.

8. **Procedural Step.** Apply the tourniquet. Position the tourniquet 3 to 4 inches above the bend in the elbow. The tourniquet should be snug but not tight. Ask the patient to clench the fist of the arm to which the tourniquet has been applied.

Principle. The combined effect of the pressure of the tourniquet and the clenched fist should cause the antecubital veins to stand out so that accurate selec-tion of a puncture site can be made.

Apply the tourniquet. (From Bonewit-West K: *Clinical procedures for medical assistants,* ed 7, St. Louis, 2008, Saunders.)

9. **Procedural Step.** With a tourniquet in place, thor-oughly assess the veins of first one arm and then the other to determine the best vein to use.

10. **Procedural Step.** Position the patient's arm. The arm with the vein selected for the venipuncture should be extended and placed in a straight line from the shoul-der to the wrist with the antecubital veins facing ante-riorly. The arm should be supported on the armrest by a rolled towel or by having the patient place the fist of the other hand under the elbow.

Principle. This position allows easy access to the ante-cubital veins.

11. **Procedural Step.** Thoroughly palpate the selected vein. Gently palpate the vein with the fingertips to determine the direction of the vein and to estimate its size and depth. Never leave the tourniquet on an arm for more than 1 minute at a time. (*Note:* If you need to perform several assessments to locate the best vein, the tourniquet must be removed and reapplied after a 2-minute waiting period.)

Principle. Leaving the tourniquet on for more than 1 minute is uncomfortable for the patient and may alter the test results.

Palpate the vein. (From Bonewit-West K: *Clinical procedures for medical assistants,* ed 7, St. Louis, 2008, Saunders.)

12. **Procedural Step.** Remove the tourniquet and cleanse the site with an antiseptic wipe. Cleansing should be done in a circular motion, starting from the inside and moving away from the puncture site. Allow the site to air dry; after cleansing, do not touch the area, wipe the area with gauze, or fan the area with your hand. Place the remaining supplies within comfortable reach of your nondominant hand.

Principle. Using a circular motion helps carry foreign particles away from the puncture site. The site must be allowed to air dry to allow the alcohol enough time to destroy microorganisms on the patient's skin. Residual alcohol entering the blood specimen can cause hemolysis, leading to inaccurate test results. In addition, residual alcohol causes the patient to experi-ence a stinging sensation when the puncture is made. Touching or fanning the area causes contamination of the puncture site, and the cleansing process must be repeated. Items used during the procedure should be positioned so that you do not have to reach over the

Continued

patient and possibly move the needle, resulting in pain, injury, or both.

13. **Procedural Step.** Reapply the tourniquet. Apply gloves. If you are using a needle with a safety shield, rotate the shield backwards toward the holder (refer to Figure 31-9A). Remove the cap from the needle using a twisting and pulling motion. Hold the vacuum tube system by placing the thumb of the dominant hand on top of the plastic holder and the pads of the first three fingers underneath the holder and evacuated tube. The needle should be positioned with the bevel facing up. Position the evacuated tube so that the label is facing down.

Principle. Gloves provide a barrier against blood-borne pathogens. Positioning the needle with the bevel up allows easier entry into the skin and the vein, resulting in less pain for the patient. With the label facing down, you would be able to observe the blood as it fills the tube, which allows you to know when the tube is full.

14. **Procedural Step.** Anchor the vein. Grasp the patient's arm with the nondominant hand. Your thumb should be placed 1 to 2 inches below and to the side of the puncture site. Using your thumb, draw the skin taut over the vein in the direction of the patient's hand.

Principle. The thumb helps hold the skin taut for easier entry and helps stabilize the vein to be punctured. Placing the thumb to the side keeps it out of the way of the vacuum tube setup so that you can maintain a 15-degree angle when entering the vein.

15. **Procedural Step.** Position the needle at a 15-degree angle to the arm. Rest the backs of the fingers on the patient's forearm. Ensure that the needle points in the same direction as the vein to be entered. The needle should be positioned so that it enters the vein approximately $\frac{1}{8}$ inch below the place where the vein is to be entered.

Principle. An angle of less than 15 degrees may cause the needle to enter above the vein, preventing puncture. An angle of more than 15 degrees may cause the needle to go through the vein by puncturing the posterior wall. This could result in a hematoma.

16. **Procedural Step.** Tell the patient that he or she will "feel a small stick," and with one continuous steady motion, enter the skin and then the vein. You will feel a sensation of resistance followed by a "release" as the vein is entered. When the "release" is felt, you have entered the vein and should not advance the needle any further.

Principle. Using one continuous steady motion helps to prevent tissue damage.

17. **Procedural Step.** Stabilize the vacuum tube setup by firmly grasping the holder between the thumb and the underlying fingers to prevent the needle from moving. Do *not* change hands during the procedure.

Position the needle. (From Bonewit-West K: *Clinical procedures for medical assistants,* ed 7, St. Louis, 2008, Saunders.)

Make the puncture. (From Bonewit-West K: *Clinical procedures for medical assistants,* ed 7, St. Louis, 2008, Saunders.)

Principle. Stabilizing the holder helps prevent the needle from moving when a tube is inserted or removed. Changing hands may cause the needle to move, which is painful for the patient.

18. **Procedural Step.** With the nondominant hand, place the first two fingers on the underside of the flange on the plastic holder, and with the thumb, slowly push the tube forward to the end of the holder. This allows the posterior needle to puncture the rubber stopper.

Blood begins flowing into the tube if the (anterior) needle is in a vein.

Principle. Not using the flange may cause the needle to advance forward and go completely through the vein, resulting in failure to obtain blood; internal bleeding may also occur, resulting in a hematoma.

19. Procedural Step. Allow the evacuated tube to fill to the exhaustion of the vacuum, as indicated by the cessation of the blood flow into the tube. The suction of the evacuated tube automatically draws the blood into the tube.

Principle. If the evacuated tube is removed before the vacuum is exhausted, a rush of air enters the tube, damaging the red blood cells. Also, a tube containing an additive, such as an anticoagulant, must be filled completely to ensure accurate test results.

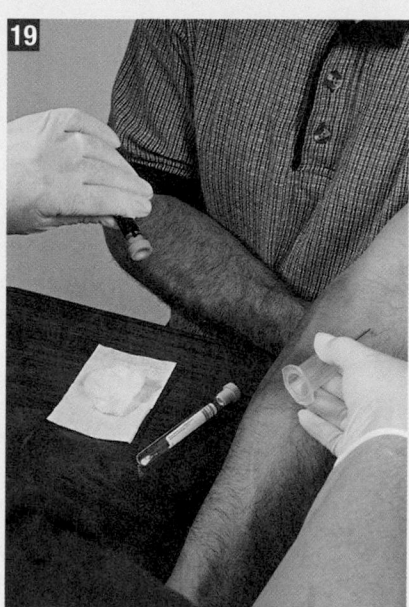

Invert tubes with additives back and forth 8 to 10 times. (From Bonewit-West K: *Clinical procedures for medical assistants,* ed 7, St. Louis, 2008, Saunders.)

20. Procedural Step. Remove the tube from the holder by grasping the tube with the fingers, placing the thumb or index finger against the flange, and pulling the tube off the posterior needle. Do not change the position of the needle in the vein. If the tube contains an anticoagulant, gently invert the tube back and forth 8 to 10 times before laying it down.

Principle. The rubber sheath covers the point of the needle, stopping the flow of blood until the next tube is inserted. Not using the flange to remove the tube can cause the needle to come out of the vein prematurely, resulting in blood being forced out of the puncture site. A tube containing an anticoagulant must be inverted immediately to prevent the blood from clotting. Careful mixing of the blood with the anticoagulant prevents hemolysis.

21. Procedural Step. Using the flange, carefully insert the next tube into the holder. Continue in this manner until the last tube has been filled.

22. Procedural Step. Remove the tension from the tourniquet by pulling upward on one of the flaps of the tourniquet. Ask the patient to unclench the fist.

Principle. The tourniquet tension must be removed before the needle. Otherwise, the pressure on the vein from the tourniquet could cause internal and external bleeding around the puncture site.

23. Procedural Step. Remove the last tube from the holder. Immediately invert the tube back and forth 8 to 10 times if it contains an anticoagulant.

Principle. Removing the last tube prevents blood from dripping out of the tip of the needle after it is removed from the patient's arm.

Remove the tourniquet, and withdraw the needle. (From Bonewit-West K: *Clinical procedures for medical assistants,* ed 7, St. Louis, 2008, Saunders.)

24. Procedural Step. Place a sterile gauze pad slightly above the puncture site, and carefully withdraw the needle at the same angle as that for penetration. Immediately move the gauze over the puncture site, and apply firm pressure. (Do not apply any pressure to the puncture site until the needle is completely removed.) If you are using a needle with a safety shield, push the shield forward with your thumb until you hear an audible click, which indicates the shield has locked into place. Do not push the shield forward by pressing it against a hard surface. (Refer to Figure 31-9B,C.)

Principle. Placing the gauze pad above the puncture helps prevent tissue movement as the needle is withdrawn and reduces patient discomfort. Careful withdrawal prevents further tissue damage.

Continued

PROCEDURE 31-1

PROCEDURE **31-1** Venipuncture—Vacuum Tube Method—cont'd

25. Procedural Step. Immediately discard the plastic holder and attached needle in a biohazard sharps container. Do not remove the needle from the holder; the holder must be discarded and not reused.

Principle. Immediate disposal of the needle and holder unit is required by the OSHA standard to prevent a needlestick injury; even if a safety shield has been activated to encase the anterior needle, a needlestick injury can still occur from the posterior needle, which is only covered with a rubber sleeve. Plastic holders are often contaminated with blood and must not be reused.

26. Procedural Step. Continue to apply pressure with the gauze pad. Cooperative patients can be asked to assist by applying pressure with the gauze pad for 1 to 2 minutes. The arm can be elevated to facilitate clot formation. Do not allow the patient to bend the arm at the elbow because this increases blood loss from the puncture site.

Principle. Applying pressure reduces the leakage of blood from the puncture site externally or internally. Internal leakage of blood into the tissues could result in a hematoma.

27. Procedural Step. Stay with the patient until the bleeding has stopped. Remove the gauze, and inspect the puncture site to ensure that the opening is sealed with a clot. Apply an adhesive bandage to the puncture site. As an alternative, the gauze pad can be folded into quarters and taped on the puncture site to be used as a pressure bandage. Instruct the patient not to pick up anything heavy for about an hour. (*Note:* If swelling or discoloration occurs, apply an ice pack to the site after bandaging it.)

Principle. Lifting a heavy object causes pressure on the puncture site, which could result in bleeding.

28. Procedural Step. Remove the gloves, and sanitize your hands.

29. Procedural Step. Chart the procedure. Include the date and time, which arm and vein were used, unusual patient reaction, and your initials.

30. Procedural Step. Test the specimen or prepare the specimen for transport to an outside laboratory for testing according to the medical office policy. If the specimen is to be transported to an outside laboratory, perform the following:
a. Place the specimen tube in a biohazard specimen bag.
b. Place the laboratory request in the outside pocket of the specimen bag.
c. Properly handle and store the specimen while awaiting pick-up by a laboratory courier.
d. Chart the date the specimen was transported to the laboratory in the patient's record.

Principle. The biohazard bag protects the laboratory courier from the possibility of an exposure incident. The outside laboratory must have the completed request form to know which laboratory tests have been ordered by the physician. The specimen must be handled and stored properly to maintain the in vivo characteristics of the specimen.

CHARTING EXAMPLE

Date	
4/5/10	9:00 a.m. Venous blood specimen collected from Ⓛ arm. Picked up by Medical Center Laboratory on 4/5/10. ——————————— D. Glover, CMA (AAMA)

BUTTERFLY METHOD OF VENIPUNCTURE

The butterfly method of venipuncture also is called the *winged infusion method.* This is because a winged infusion set is used to perform the procedure. The term *butterfly* is derived from the plastic "wings" located between the needle and the tubing of the winged infusion set (Figure 31-13).

The butterfly method is used to collect blood from patients who are difficult to stick by conventional methods because it provides better control when making the puncture and also less pressure is exerted on the vein wall from the evacuated tube. The butterfly method is recommended for adults with small antecubital veins and children, who typically have small antecubital veins. The butterfly method is also used when the antecubital veins are unavailable, and the veins in the forearm, wrist area, or back of the hand are used, as may occur with elderly and obese patients. These

Figure 31-13. Winged infusion set. **A,** Luer adapter with evacuated tube. **B,** Hub adapter with syringe. (From Bonewit-West K: *Clinical procedures for medical assistants,* ed 7, St. Louis, 2008, Saunders.)

alternative veins are usually smaller and sometimes have a thin wall (e.g., hand veins), making them more likely to collapse when using the vacuum tube method of venipuncture. With the vacuum tube method, the "sucking action" exerted on the vein when the pressure in the vacuum is released causes the vein to collapse, blocking the flow of blood into the tube. The butterfly method results in less pressure on the vein wall because the pressure exerted by the evacuated tube must travel through a length of tubing before reaching the vein. Because the pressure against the vein wall is minimized, the vein is less likely to collapse with the butterfly method. Procedure 31-2 describes the venipuncture procedure using the butterfly method.

The gauge of the winged infusion needle ranges from 21 G to 23 G, and the length of the needle ranges from ½ to ¾ inch. The needle is short and sharp, making it easier to stick difficult veins. For extremely small veins, a 23 G needle should be used to prevent rupture of the vein by a larger needle. In this case, it is preferable to use smaller-volume tubes (e.g., 2-ml evacuated tubes) because large evacuated tubes may put too much vacuum pressure on the vein, causing it to collapse.

The winged infusion needle is attached to a 6- or 12-inch length of tubing and a *Luer adapter,* attached to a (posterior) needle with a rubber sleeve. A plastic holder is screwed onto the Luer adapter, which allows it to be used with evacuated tubes (see Figure 31-13A). Winged infusion sets are also available with a hub adapter that allows them to be used with a syringe (see Figure 31-13B). Safety needles are available with a shield that covers the contaminated needle after it is withdrawn from the patient's vein (Figure 31-14).

Guidelines for the Butterfly Method

Certain guidelines should be followed when performing the butterfly method of venipuncture, as follows:

1. Position the patient according to the site selected for the venipuncture as follows:
   - **Antecubital, wrist, and forearm veins.** Position the arm in a straight line from the shoulder to the wrist as described in the vacuum tube method of venipuncture.
   - **Hand veins.** Position the patient's hand on the armrest, and ask the patient to make a loose fist or to grasp a rolled towel. This combination causes the hand veins to stand out so that accurate selection of a puncture site can be made. Locate a suitable vein between the knuckles and the wrist bones. Hand veins are usually visible and easy to locate.
2. Position the tourniquet according to the venipuncture site as follows: If the veins of the forearm or wrist are used, apply the tourniquet to the forearm, approximately 3 inches above the puncture site. For hand veins, position the tourniquet on the arm just above the wrist bone (Figure 31-15).

Figure 31-14. Butterfly safety needle. The safety needle has a shield that covers the contaminated needle after it is withdrawn from the patient's vein. **A,** The medical assistant has covered half of the needle with the shield. **B,** The needle is completely covered with the shield. (From Bonewit-West K: *Clinical procedures for medical assistants,* ed 7, St. Louis, 2008, Saunders.)

What Would You Do? What Would You *Not* Do?

Case Study 2

Buzz Braydon had a heart attack 4 weeks ago and is taking the anticoagulant warfarin (Coumadin). He is at the office for a checkup and to have his prothrombin time tested. Blood is collected from a small vein in Buzz's left arm using the butterfly method. After the specimen is collected, Buzz wants to know why a red-stoppered tube was used to draw blood from him and then thrown away. Buzz says that they used something called a Vacutainer to draw his blood in the hospital and wants to know if a Vacutainer is ever used in the medical office. Buzz says that he is going on vacation in North Carolina for 2 weeks. He says that they explained to him at the hospital why he should have his blood tested every week, but he's not sure where to go to get his blood tested while he's on vacation. Buzz wants to know if as long as he takes his medication exactly as he should, it would be all right to skip his weekly prothrombin test during that time. ■

PROCEDURE 31-2

3. Grasp the needle by compressing the plastic wings together. Insert the needle with the bevel facing up at a 15-degree angle to the skin. When the vein has been entered, decrease the angle to 5 degrees.

4. After decreasing the needle angle to 5 degrees, slowly thread the needle inside the vein an additional ¼ inch. This anchors or seats the needle in the center of the vein and allows the medical assistant to use both hands to change tubes.

5. To prevent venous reflux, keep the evacuated tube and holder in a downward position as in the vacuum tube venipuncture procedure. This technique ensures that the blood fills from the bottom up and not near the rubber stopper.

6. When multiple tubes are to be drawn, follow the proper order of draw. The order of draw for the butterfly method is identical to that for the vacuum tube method (previously presented). Following this order of draw prevents contamination of nonadditive tubes and cross-contamination of additive tubes.

Text continued on p. 753

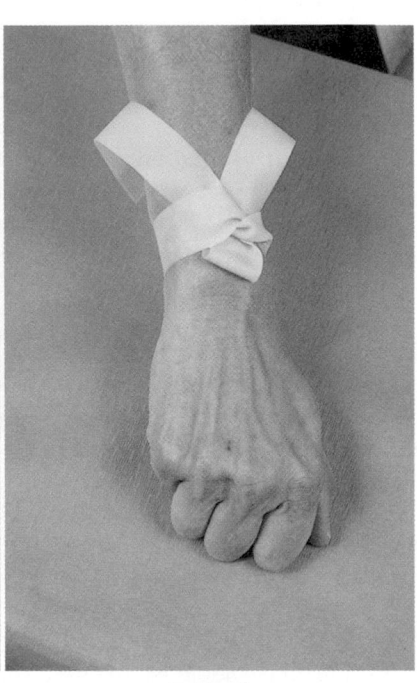

A. Forearm site	B. Wrist site	C. Hand

Figure 31-15. Application of the tourniquet for alternative venipuncture sites. (From Bonewit-West K: *Clinical procedures for medical assistants,* ed 7, St. Louis, 2008, Saunders.)

 PROCEDURE 31-2   Venipuncture—Butterfly Method

Outcome Perform a venipuncture using the butterfly method.

Equipment/Supplies

- Disposable gloves
- Tourniquet
- Antiseptic wipe
- Winged infusion set with a Luer adapter
- Plastic holder
- Evacuated tubes with labels

- Sterile 2 × 2 gauze pad
- Adhesive bandage
- Biohazard sharps container
- Biohazard specimen bag
- Laboratory request form

1. Procedural Step. Sanitize your hands.

2. Procedural Step. Greet the patient and introduce yourself. Identify the patient by asking the patient to state his or her full name and date of birth. Compare this information with the demographic data in the patient's chart. If the patient was required to prepare for the test (e.g., fasting, medication restriction), determine whether he or she has prepared properly. If the patient has not followed the patient preparation requirements, notify the physician for instructions on handling this situation.

Principle. It is important to confirm that you have the correct patient to avoid collecting a specimen on the wrong patient. The patient must prepare properly to obtain a quality specimen that would lead to accurate test results.

3. Procedural Step. Assemble the equipment. Select the proper evacuated tubes for the tests to be performed. Check the expiration date of the tubes. Label each tube using one of the following methods: (a) attaching a computer bar code label to each tube and labeling it with your initials, or (b) manually labeling each tube with the patient's name, the date, and your initials. If the specimen is to be tested at an outside laboratory, complete a laboratory request form.

Principle. Outdated tubes may no longer contain a vacuum, and, as a result, they may not be able to draw blood into the tube. Proper labeling of blood specimens avoids a mixup of specimens.

Assemble the equipment. (From Bonewit-West K: *Clinical procedures for medical assistants,* ed 7, St. Louis, 2008, Saunders.)

4. Procedural Step. Prepare the winged infusion set. Remove the winged infusion set from its package. Extend the tubing to its full length, and stretch it slightly to prevent it from recoiling. Insert the posterior needle into the small opening on the plastic holder. Screw the plastic holder onto the Luer adapter, and tighten it securely.

Principle. Extending the tubing straightens it to permit a free flow of blood in the tubing. An unsecured needle can fall out of its plastic holder.

5. Procedural Step. Open the sterile gauze packet, and lie it flat to allow the gauze pad to rest on the inside of its wrapper. Position the evacuated tubes in the correct order of draw. If the evacuated tube contains a powdered additive, tap the tube just below the stopper to release any additive adhering to the stopper.

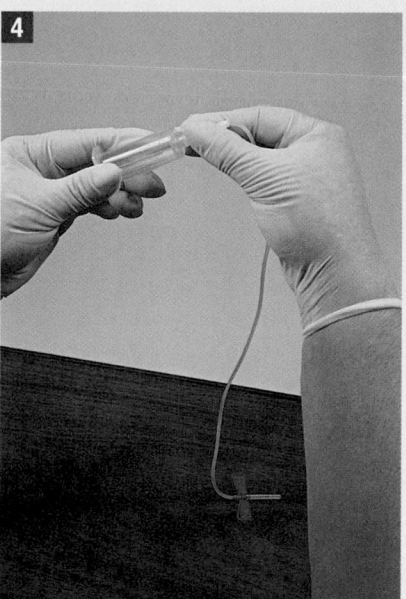

Screw the Luer adapter into the holder. (From Bonewit-West K: *Clinical procedures for medical assistants,* ed 7, St. Louis, 2008, Saunders.)

Principle. If an additive remains trapped in the stopper, erroneous test results may occur.

6. Procedural Step. Place the first tube loosely in the plastic holder with the label facing down.

Principle. With the label facing down, you can observe the blood as it fills the tube, which allows you to know when the tube is full.

7. Procedural Step. Explain the procedure to the patient, and reassure the patient. Perform a preliminary assessment of both arms to determine the best vein to use. It is also helpful to ask the patient which arm has been used in the past to obtain blood.

Principle. Venipuncture is often a frightening experience for the patient, and reassurance should be offered to reduce apprehension.

8. Procedural Step. Apply the tourniquet. Position the tourniquet 3 to 4 inches above the bend in the elbow. The tourniquet should be snug but not tight. Ask the patient to clench the fist of the arm to which the tourniquet has been applied.

Principle. The combined effect of the pressure of the tourniquet and the clenched fist should cause the antecubital veins to stand out so that accurate selection of a puncture site can be made.

9. Procedural Step. With a tourniquet in place, thoroughly assess the veins of first one arm and then the other to determine the best vein to use.

10. Procedural Step. Position the patient's arm. The arm with the vein selected for the venipuncture should be extended and placed in a straight line from the shoulder to the wrist with the antecubital veins facing anteriorly. The arm should be supported on the armrest

Continued

PROCEDURE 31-2   Venipuncture—Butterfly Method—cont'd

by a rolled towel or by having the patient place the fist of the other hand under the elbow.

Principle. This position allows easy access to the antecubital veins.

11. **Procedural Step.** Thoroughly palpate the selected vein. Gently palpate the vein with the fingertips to determine the direction of the vein and to estimate its size and depth. Never leave the tourniquet on an arm for more than 1 minute at a time. (*Note:* If you need to perform several assessments to locate the best vein, the tourniquet must be removed and reapplied after a 2-minute waiting period.)

    Principle. Leaving the tourniquet on for more than 1 minute is uncomfortable for the patient and may alter the test results.

12. **Procedural Step.** Remove the tourniquet and cleanse the site with an antiseptic. Cleansing should be done in a circular motion, starting from the inside and moving away from the puncture site. Allow the site to air dry, and after cleansing, do not touch the area, wipe the area with gauze, or fan the area with your hand. Place your remaining supplies within comfortable reach.

    Principle. Using a circular motion helps carry foreign particles away from the puncture site. The site must be allowed to air dry to allow the alcohol enough time to destroy microorganisms on the patient's skin. Residual alcohol entering the blood specimen can cause hemolysis, leading to inaccurate test results. In addition, residual alcohol causes the patient to experience a stinging sensation when the puncture is made. Touching or fanning the area causes contamination of the puncture site, and the cleansing process must be repeated. Items used during the procedure should be positioned so that you do not have to reach over the patient and possibly move the needle, resulting in patient pain, injury, or both.

13. **Procedural Step.** Reapply the tourniquet. Apply gloves. With the dominant hand, grasp the winged infusion set by pressing the butterfly tips together. Remove the protective sheath from the needle of the infusion set. The needle should be positioned with the bevel facing up.

    Principle. Gloves provide a barrier against bloodborne pathogens. Positioning the needle with the bevel up allows easier entry into the skin and the vein, resulting in less pain for the patient.

14. **Procedural Step.** Anchor the vein. Grasp the patient's arm with the nondominant hand. The thumb should be placed 1 to 2 inches below and to the side of the puncture site. Using the thumb, draw the skin taut over the vein in the direction of the patient's hand.

Remove the protective shield from the needle. (From Bonewit-West K: *Clinical procedures for medical assistants,* ed 7, St. Louis, 2008, Saunders.)

Principle. The thumb helps hold the skin taut for easier entry and helps stabilize the vein to be punctured. Placing the thumb to the side keeps it out of the way of the winged infusion setup so that you can maintain a 15-degree angle when entering the vein.

15. **Procedural Step.** Position the needle at a 15-degree angle to the arm. Rest the backs of the fingertips on the patient's skin. Make sure the needle points in the same direction as the vein to be entered. The needle should be positioned so that it enters the vein approximately ⅛ inch below the place where the vein is to be entered.

    Principle. An angle of less than 15 degrees may cause the needle to enter above the vein, preventing puncture. An angle of more than 15 degrees may cause the needle to go through the vein by puncturing the posterior wall. This could result in a hematoma.

16. **Procedural Step.** Tell the patient that he or she will "feel a small stick," and with one continuous steady motion, enter the skin and then the vein. You will feel a sensation of resistance followed by a "release" as the vein is entered. After penetrating the vein, decrease the angle of the needle to 5 degrees. If the needle is in the vein, a flash of blood appears at the top of the tubing.

    Principle. Using one continuous motion reduces tissue damage.

Make the puncture. (From Bonewit-West K: *Clinical procedures for medical assistants,* ed 7, St. Louis, 2008, Saunders.)

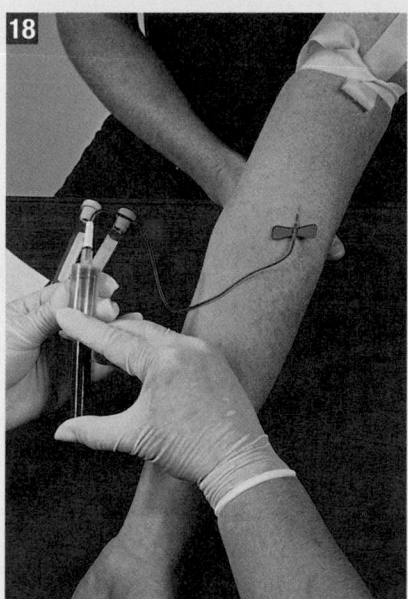

Fill the tubes in a downward position. (From Bonewit-West K: *Clinical procedures for medical assistants,* ed 7, St. Louis, 2008, Saunders.)

17. Procedural Step. Seat the needle by threading it forward an additional ¼ inch inside the center of the vein so that it does not twist out of the vein, even if you let go of it. Open the butterfly wings and securely rest the wings flat against the skin. Ensure that the needle does not move.

Principle. Seating the needle anchors the needle in the center of the vein and allows the use of both hands for changing tubes. Moving the needle is painful for the patient.

18. Procedural Step. Keep the tube and holder in a downward position so that the tube fills from the bottom up and not near the rubber stopper. Slowly push the tube forward to the end of the holder. This allows the needle to puncture the rubber stopper. Blood begins flowing into the tube. Allow the evacuated tube to fill to the exhaustion of the vacuum, as indicated by the cessation of the blood flow into the tube. The suction of the evacuated tube automatically draws the blood into the tube.

Principle. The tube must fill from the bottom up to prevent venous reflux. If the evacuated tube is removed before the vacuum is exhausted, a rush of air enters the tube, damaging the red blood cells. Also, a tube containing an anticoagulant must be filled completely to ensure accurate test results.

19. Procedural Step. Remove the tube from the plastic holder. If the tube contains an additive, gently invert the tube back and forth 8 to 10 times before laying it down.

Principle. The rubber sheath covers the point of the needle, stopping the flow of blood until the next tube is inserted. A tube containing an anticoagulant must be inverted before laying it down to prevent the blood

Remove the tube from the holder. (From Bonewit-West K: *Clinical procedures for medical assistants,* ed 7, St. Louis, 2008, Saunders.)

from clotting. Careful mixing of the blood with the anticoagulant prevents hemolysis.

20. Procedural Step. Using the flange, carefully insert the next tube into the holder. Continue in this manner until the last tube has been filled.

21. Procedural Step. Remove the tension from the tourniquet by pulling upward on one of the flaps of the tourniquet. Ask the patient to unclench the fist.

Principle. The tourniquet tension must be removed before the needle. Otherwise, the pressure on the vein

Continued

PROCEDURE 31-2   Venipuncture—Butterfly Method—cont'd

from the tourniquet could cause internal and external bleeding around the puncture.

22. Procedural Step. Remove the last tube from the holder. Immediately invert the tube back and forth 8 to 10 times if it contains an additive.

Principle. This prevents blood from dripping out of the tip of the needle after it is removed from the patient's arm.

23. Procedural Step. Place a sterile gauze pad slightly above the puncture site. Grasp the setup just below the wings, and slowly withdraw the needle at the same angle as that for penetration. Immediately move the gauze over the puncture site, and apply firm pressure. (*Note:* Do not apply pressure to the puncture site until the needle is completely removed.) Cooperative patients can be asked to assist by applying pressure with the gauze pad. If you are using a butterfly needle with a safety shield, grasp the base of the shield with the thumb and index finger of one hand and, with the other hand, grasp either wing. Slide the wing back into the rear slot of the safety shield until you hear an audible click, which indicates the shield has locked into place (refer to Figure 31-14A,B).

Principle. Placing the gauze pad above the puncture site helps prevent tissue movement as the needle is withdrawn and reduces patient discomfort. Careful withdrawal prevents further tissue damage.

24. Procedural Step. Immediately discard the winged infusion set and attached plastic holder. Holding onto the plastic holder, first drop the needle into a biohazard sharps container, followed by the tubing and holder. Do not remove the plastic holder from the setup; the plastic holder must be discarded and not reused.

Principle. Proper disposal is required by the OSHA Standard to prevent a needlestick injury; even if a safety shield has been activated to encase the butterfly needle, a needlestick injury can still result from the posterior needle, which is covered with only a rubber sleeve. Plastic holders are often contaminated with blood and must not be reused.

25. Procedural Step. Continue to apply pressure with the gauze pad. The arm can be elevated to facilitate clot formation. Do not allow the patient to bend the arm at the elbow because this increases blood loss from the puncture site.

Principle. Applying pressure reduces the leakage of blood from the puncture site externally or internally. Internal leakage into the tissues could result in a hematoma.

26. Procedural Step. Stay with the patient until the bleeding has stopped. Remove pressure, and inspect the puncture site to ensure that the opening is sealed with a clot. Apply an adhesive bandage to the puncture site. As an alternative, the gauze pad can be folded into quarters and taped on the puncture site to be used as a pressure bandage. Instruct the patient not to pick up anything heavy for about an hour. (*Note:* If swelling or discoloration occurs, apply an ice pack to the site after bandaging it.)

Principle. Lifting a heavy object causes pressure on the puncture site, which could result in bleeding.

27. Procedural Step. Remove the gloves, and sanitize your hands.

28. Procedural Step. Chart the procedure. Include the date and time, which arm and vein were used, unusual patient reactions, and your initials.

29. Procedural Step. Test the specimen or prepare the specimen for transport to an outside laboratory for testing according to the medical office policy. If the specimen is to be transported to an outside laboratory, perform the following:

a. Place the specimen tube in a biohazard specimen bag.

b. Place the laboratory request in the outside pocket of the specimen bag.

c. Properly handle and store the specimen while awaiting pickup by a laboratory courier.

d. Chart the date the specimen was transported to the laboratory in the patient's record.

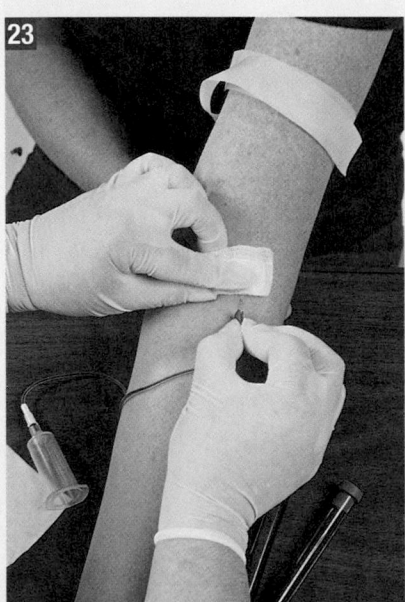

Release the tourniquet, and remove the needle. (From Bonewit-West K: *Clinical procedures for medical assistants,* ed 7, St. Louis, 2008, Saunders.)

Principle. The biohazard bag protects the laboratory courier from the possibility of an exposure incident. The outside laboratory must have the completed request form to know which laboratory tests have been ordered by the physician. The specimen must be handled and stored properly to maintain the in vivo characteristics of the specimen.

CHARTING EXAMPLE

Date	
4/10/10	10:30 a.m. Venous blood specimen collected from Ⓛ arm. Picked up by Medical Center Laboratory on 4/10/10. ———————————————— ———————————⌒———— D. Glover, CMA (AAMA)

Memories *from* Externship

Dori Glover: One of the most terrifying things for me as a student was learning venipuncture. Even though I would practice during classroom laboratory hours and felt comfortable with it, it still scared me to know I would have to draw on a real person one day. When the day arrived to draw on my laboratory partner, I became sick to my stomach. In the end, we both got through it just fine and walked away without hurting each other. I spent days trying to prepare myself for that first experience, but after it was over, I felt more confident and relaxed that I could do this. At my externship site, I was able to perform several venipunctures a day, which raised my confidence level. Today venipuncture is my favorite responsibility of all. I would draw blood all day if I could. I know I could even draw with my eyes closed, but never would, of course! ∎

Prepare for Success

What Would You Do? What Would You *Not* Do?

Case Study 3
Maud Gabriel is at the office complaining of persistent headaches and abdominal pain over the past 3 months. The physician gives Mrs. Gabriel a laboratory requisition to have her blood drawn and tested at an outside laboratory. Mrs. Gabriel says that her daughter, who lives with her, works as a phlebotomist at the local hospital. Mrs. Gabriel wants to know whether her daughter can draw her blood at home and then drop it off at the laboratory. She says that the last time she had her blood drawn they had to stick her two times and then she got a big bruise on her arm afterward. She says the laboratory technician kept digging around in her arm to find the vein and that it was quite painful. ∎

PROBLEMS ENCOUNTERED WITH VENIPUNCTURE

Sometimes the medical assistant encounters problems when attempting to draw blood from a patient. The appropriate response depends on the type of problem.

Failure to Obtain Blood

Periodically, even individuals highly skilled at performing venipuncture have difficulty obtaining blood. Although large and prominent veins make it easier to collect the blood specimen, conditions often exist that make the procedure more difficult.

It is often difficult to draw blood from obese patients who have small, superficial veins and whose veins suitable for venipuncture are buried in adipose tissue. Elderly patients with arteriosclerosis may have veins that are thick and hard, making them difficult to puncture. Other patients have veins that are small or have a thin wall, making the veins likely to collapse. After two unsuccessful attempts at venipuncture, the medical assistant should seek assistance in obtaining the blood specimen.

Factors that result in a failure to obtain blood after the needle has been inserted include not inserting the needle far enough, preventing it from entering the vein (Figure 31-16); insertion of the needle too far, causing it to go through the vein; and the bevel opening becoming lodged against the wall of the vein. In these instances, most authorities recommend removal of the needle, rather than trying to probe the vein. Probing is often uncomfortable for the patient and can affect the integrity of the blood specimen, leading to inaccurate test results. Occasionally, an evacuated tube loses its vacuum because of a manufacturing defect or through improper handling of the tube. If suspected, this problem can be corrected by removing the defective tube and inserting another vacuum tube.

Inappropriate Puncture Sites

If a patient complains of pain or soreness in a potential venipuncture site, this area should be avoided. In addition, any skin areas that are scarred, bruised, burned, or adjacent to areas of infection should not be used. A venipuncture should not be performed on an arm with edema or an arm on the same side as a mastectomy. Swelling makes it more difficult to locate a vein and results in a longer time for healing of the puncture site to occur. Other sites to avoid include an arm that has a cast applied to it or an arm on the same side as a radical mastectomy.

Scarred and Sclerosed Veins

An individual who has had many venipunctures over a period of years often develops scar tissue in the wall of the vein. Elderly patients may have veins that have become

A. Correct insertion of the needle into the vein.

B. Improper angle of insertion (<15 degrees), causing the needle to enter above the vein.

C. Improper angle of insertion (>15 degrees), causing the needle to go through the vein.

D. Collapsed vein (most likely to occur in persons with small veins).

E. The beveled opening is partially within and partially outside of the vein, causing a hematoma.

Figure 31-16. Problems encountered with venipuncture. (From Bonewit-West K: *Clinical procedures for medical assistants,* ed 7, St. Louis, 2008, Saunders.)

thickened from arteriosclerosis. In both cases, the veins feel stiff and hard when palpated. A scarred or sclerosed vein is difficult to stick, and the blood return may be poor owing to a narrowed lumen; it is recommended that another vein be used for the venipuncture. If this is impossible, the needle should be inserted with careful pressure to avoid going completely through the vein.

Rolling Veins

The median cubital vein, located in the center of the ante-cubital space, is considered the best vein for a venipuncture. Sometimes it is impossible to use this vein, however, such as when it lies deep in the tissues and cannot be palpated or is scarred from repeated venipunctures. The veins on either side of the median cubital (cephalic or basilic) can be used, but they tend to "roll," or move away from the needle, escaping puncture. To prevent rolling, firm pressure should be applied below the vein to stabilize it as the needle is inserted.

Collapsing Veins

Veins are most likely to collapse in individuals who have small veins or veins with thin walls. This is particularly true when the vacuum tube method is being used. The "sucking action" exerted on the vein when the pressure in the vacuum is released causes the vein to collapse, blocking the flow of blood into the tube (see Figure 31-16). The typical result observed is that a small amount of blood enters the tube and then stops. Because better control and less pressure on the vein is possible, the butterfly method of venipuncture is recommended to obtain the specimen in patients with small veins.

Premature Needle Withdrawal

Patient movement or improper venipuncture technique can cause the needle to come out of the vein prematurely. Because of the pressure exerted by the tourniquet, blood may be forced out of the puncture site, and immediate action is required to prevent a hematoma. The tourniquet should be removed at once, a gauze pad placed on the puncture site, and pressure applied until the bleeding has stopped.

Hematoma

A hematoma is caused by blood leaking from the puncture site of the vein and into the surrounding tissues, resulting in a bruise. A hematoma is caused by a needle that is inserted too far and that goes through the vein, a bevel opening that is partially in the vein and partially out of the vein (see Figure 31-16), and insufficient pressure applied to the puncture site after removing the needle. The first sign of a hematoma is a sudden swelling around the puncture site. If this occurs when the needle is in the patient's vein, the tourniquet and needle should be removed immediately, and pressure should be applied to the puncture site until the bleeding stops.

Hemolysis

The blood specimen should be handled carefully at all times. Blood cells are fragile, and rough handling may cause hemolysis, or breakdown of the blood cells. Hemolyzed blood specimens produce inaccurate test results. To prevent hemolysis, these guidelines should be followed:

1. Store the vacuum tubes at room temperature because chilled tubes can result in hemolysis.
2. Allow the alcohol to air dry completely before performing the venipuncture. Alcohol entering a blood specimen can cause hemolysis.
3. Use an appropriate-gauge needle to collect the specimen; a needle with a gauge between 20 G and 22 G should be used. Using a small-gauge needle (e.g., 25 G) can cause the blood cells to rupture as they pass through the lumen of the needle.
4. Practice good technique in collecting the specimen; excessive trauma to the blood vessel can result in hemolysis.
5. Always handle the blood tube carefully; do not shake it or handle it roughly.

Fainting

Occasionally, a patient experiences dizziness or fainting during or after a venipuncture. Should this occur, the most immediate concern is to protect the patient from injury (e.g., by preventing the patient from falling). The patient should be placed in a position that promotes blood flow to the brain, and the physician should be notified for further treatment; see the box *Highlight on Vasovagal Syncope (Fainting)*.

OBTAINING A SERUM SPECIMEN
Serum

Serum is plasma from which the clotting factor fibrinogen has been removed.

Highlight on Vasovagal Syncope (Fainting)

Most people experience no change in their sense of well-being when they have blood taken. A very small percentage of individuals experience a type of fainting, however, known as *vasovagal syncope*.

Cause and Symptoms
Vasovagal syncope is caused by unpleasant physical or emotional stimuli, such as pain, fright, and the sight of blood. A sudden pooling of blood occurs, which results in a sudden decrease in the blood pressure. This momentarily deprives the brain of blood, causing a temporary loss of consciousness, usually lasting only 1 to 2 minutes. Vasovagal syncope usually occurs when an individual is in an upright position, as in standing or sitting. Before fainting, the patient usually experiences some warning signals, such as sudden lightheadedness, nausea, weakness, yawning, paleness, blurred vision, a feeling of warmth, and sweating followed by drooping eyelids, weak, rapid pulse, and finally unconsciousness.

Treatment
A person who is about to faint should be placed in a position that facilitates blood flow to the brain and told to breathe deeply. The preferred position is lying down (supine) with the legs elevated and the collar and clothing loosened. This position may not always be possible, such as when a patient is seated and the venipuncture needle has already been inserted. In this case, the tourniquet and then the needle should be removed, and the patient's head should be lowered between the legs. An individual who has fainted should be protected from injury by falling and be placed in a position that facilitates blood flow to the brain, as just described.

Prevention
Fainting during or after venipuncture is more likely in the following individuals: patients having a venipuncture for the first time, young patients, thin patients, patients with a low diastolic or high systolic blood pressure, patients with a history of fainting, nervous and apprehensive patients, and patients who are very quiet or very talkative. Fainting can often be prevented by identifying and closely observing individuals who are more likely to faint (as described). Talking to the patient often helps relax him or her and diverts attention from the venipuncture procedure. If a patient has a history of fainting, he or she should be in a semi-Fowler's position for the venipuncture procedure because people rarely faint in this position. Other factors that contribute to fainting and that should be avoided include fatigue, lack of sleep, hunger, and environmental factors, such as a noisy, crowded, or overheated room. ∎

Serum contains many dissolved substances, such as glucose, cholesterol, sodium, potassium, chloride, antibodies, hormones, and enzymes. As a result, many laboratory tests require a serum specimen to determine whether these substances are within normal limits and to detect substances that should not normally be in the serum, and that, if present, indicate a pathologic condition. To perform laboratory tests on serum, it must be separated from the blood specimen, which is usually the responsibility of the medical assistant.

Tube Selection

A tube without an anticoagulants (red stoppered) must be used to collect the blood specimen, to allow the specimen to separate into serum and clotted blood cells. Because the amount of serum recovered is only a portion of the specimen, a blood specimen must be drawn that is 2.5 times the amount required for the test. If 2 ml of serum is required, a 5-ml red stoppered tube of blood must be collected; if 4 ml of serum is required, a 10-ml red stoppered tube is collected, and if 6 ml of serum is required, a 15-ml red stoppered tube is necessary.

Preparation of the Specimen

After the blood specimen has been collected, the tube must be allowed to stand upright at room temperature for 30 to 45 minutes before being centrifuged. This allows clot formation, which yields more serum from the specimen. If the specimen is centrifuged immediately after collection, the clotting factors do not have an opportunity to settle down into the cell layer to form a whole blood clot. The result of this is the formation of a *fibrin clot* in the serum layer. A fibrin clot is a spongy substance that occupies space, interfering with adequate serum collection. The blood specimen should not be allowed to stand for longer than 1 hour, however, because leaching of substances from the cell layer into the serum may occur. This leaching of substances changes the integrity of the serum, leading to inaccurate test results.

Removal of Serum

After the blood cells have clotted by allowing the specimen to stand, the specimen is centrifuged. The serum is removed from the clot using a pipet and placed in a separate transfer tube. It is important that proper technique be employed in removing the serum, to avoid disturbing the cell layer of the clot and drawing red blood cells into the serum layer. If cells do enter the serum, the entire specimen must be recentrifuged.

When the serum has been removed from the blood specimen, the medical assistant should hold the specimen in the transfer tube up to good light. The serum specimen should be inspected for the presence of intact red blood cells or hemolyzed blood; in both cases, the specimen has a reddish appearance. A specimen having a reddish appearance must be recentrifuged. If the specimen contains intact red blood cells, they settle to the bottom of the tube, and the serum

can be removed. If the blood is hemolyzed, recentrifugation would not make the red color disappear because the red blood cells have ruptured and released hemoglobin into the serum. Hemolyzed serum is unsuitable for laboratory tests because the results would be inaccurate; another blood specimen must be collected.

Serum Separator Tubes

A serum separator tube (SST) is an evacuated tube specially designed to facilitate the collection of a serum specimen. The SST glass tube is identified by a red/gray stopper (or gold stopper if using Hemoguard tubes) and is used for collection and separation of blood. The SST contains a thixotropic gel, which is in a solid state in the bottom of the unused tube (Figure 31-17A).

The blood specimen is collected and processed following the appropriate venipuncture method. The specimen must be allowed to stand in an upright position for 30 to 45 minutes for proper clot formation and centrifuged as previously described. During centrifugation, the gel temporarily becomes fluid and moves to the dividing point between the serum and clotted cells, where it reforms into a solid gel, serving as a physical and chemical barrier between the serum and clot (Figure 31-17B).

The serum can be transported or stored in the separator tube; the medical assistant must inspect the tube carefully to ensure that the gel barrier is firmly attached to the glass

Figure 31-17. Serum separator tubes. **A,** An unused tube that contains the thixotropic gel in the bottom of the tube. **B,** A tube that has been used to collect a blood specimen. During centrifugation, the gel temporarily becomes fluid and moves to the dividing point between the serum and blood cells in a fibrin clot. (From Bonewit-West K: *Clinical procedures for medical assistants,* ed 7, St. Louis, 2008, Saunders.)

wall. If a complete barrier has not formed, the serum specimen must be removed and placed in a transfer tube to prevent leaching of substances from the cell layer into the serum, affecting the accuracy of the test results.

SKIN PUNCTURE

A skin puncture is used to obtain a capillary blood specimen and is also called a *capillary puncture*. Laboratory testing of a capillary blood specimen is usually performed at the medical office. Examples of such tests are hemoglobin, hematocrit, blood glucose, mononucleosis, and prothrombin time.

A skin puncture is performed when a test requires only a small blood specimen. Skin puncture is the method preferred for obtaining blood from infants and young children. Collecting blood in this age group by venipuncture is often difficult and may damage veins and surrounding tissues. In addition, infants and young children have such a small blood volume that removing large quantities of blood may cause anemia. A skin puncture might be performed as a last resort on an adult when a blood specimen is necessary and there are no acceptable veins. Before collecting a capillary blood specimen, the medical assistant must (1) select a puncture site, (2) select the skin puncture device, and (3) obtain the proper microcollection device to collect the specimen.

PUNCTURE SITES

The puncture site varies depending on the age of the patient. The fingertip of the third or fourth finger is the preferred site for a skin puncture on an adult. In the past, the earlobe was recommended as a skin puncture site for an adult. This is no longer true. Blood obtained by puncturing the earlobe has been found to contain a higher concentration of hemoglobin than fingertip blood. In addition, the earlobe produces a slower flow of blood, making it more difficult to obtain a blood specimen.

In an infant (birth to 1 year old), the skin puncture should be performed on the plantar surface of the heel. A finger puncture should *never* be performed on infants. The amount of tissue between skin surface and bone is so small that an injury to the bone is likely. After a child is walking, the skin puncture can be performed on the fingertip.

SKIN PUNCTURE DEVICES

According to OSHA, a skin puncture should be performed in the medical office using either a disposable or reusable semiautomatic retractable lancet device. The device used to perform the skin puncture is a matter of personal preference, and the technique for performing the puncture depends on the device that is used. A description of skin puncture devices is presented next, and the procedures for using them are presented at the end of this section.

Regardless of the skin puncture device, the puncture must not penetrate deeper than 3.1 mm on adults and 2.4 mm on infants and children. If the puncture is deeper than this, the bone may be penetrated, which could result in the painful and serious conditions of osteochondritis or osteomyelitis. **Osteochondritis** is inflammation of bone and cartilage, and **osteomyelitis** is an inflammation of the bone caused by bacterial infection. To avoid these complications, skin puncture devices are used with a spring-loaded blade available in different lengths to control the depth of puncture. The blade length used to perform a skin puncture is based on the size of the patient's fingers and the amount of blood specimen required. Adults with thin fingers and children require a shorter blade to avoid penetrating the bone. A longer blade must be used to obtain enough blood to fill a microcollection device, whereas a shorter blade can be used if only a drop of blood is necessary.

OSHA does not recommend the use of lancets that are not retractable. A lancet that is not retractable increases the possibility that the medical assistant will stick himself or herself accidentally, resulting in an exposure incident. A disadvantage of a lancet that is spring loaded and does not retract automatically is that some patients may become apprehensive and flinch when they see the point of the lancet coming. Children might pull their hands out of the medical assistant's grasp.

Disposable Semiautomatic Lancet

A disposable semiautomatic retractable lancet consists of a spring-loaded plastic holder with a metal blade inside the holder. Disposable lancets are available in different lengths of blades to control the depth of the puncture. The plastic holder is color coded by the manufacturer for ease in identifying the blade length of the lancet device. The plastic holder conceals the blade so that the patient cannot see it during the puncture. One such lancet device is the Microtainer Brand Safety Flow Lancet (Becton Dickinson) (Figure 31-18A). Another example is the Tenderlette (International Technidyne Corporation, Edison, NJ), which is used for heel punctures on infants.

To perform the skin puncture, the lancet device is placed on the patient's skin and the device is activated. Depending on the brand, this is accomplished by one of the following methods:

- Depressing an activation button located on the top or side of the lancet until an audible click is heard (Microtainer BD Genie Lancet)
- Pushing the lancet firmly onto the puncture site until an audible click is heard (e.g., Surgilance Safety Lancet)

When the device is activated, the spring forces the blade into the skin and retracts the blade into the holder. The concealed blade and automatic puncture tend to result in less patient apprehension. After the puncture, the entire lancet device is discarded in a biohazard sharps container. Procedure 31-3 describes the skin puncture procedure using a disposable semiautomatic lancet.

A. Microtainer Brand
Safety Flow Lancet

B. Glucolet II

Figure 31-18. Lancet devices. (From Bonewit-West K: *Clinical procedures for medical assistants*, ed 7, St. Louis, 2008, Saunders.)

Reusable Semiautomatic Lancet

A wide variety of reusable semiautomatic lancets are commercially available; however, not all are appropriate for use in the medical office. Some of these devices are suitable for use only by an individual patient to perform home blood glucose monitoring. When used by more than one patient in the medical office, they have been associated with the transmission of hepatitis B. The safest reusable device is one in which the part that becomes contaminated is retractable and can be disposed of easily. This type of device reduces the risk of a sharps injury and infection from a contaminated sharp. An example of a reusable lancet that is safe to use in the medical office is the Glucolet II (Bayer Corporation).

The Glucolet II consists of a plastic spring-loaded lancet holder and a retractable lancet/endcap (Figure 31-18B). The lancet holder is reusable, whereas the lancet/endcap is retractable and disposable and meant for only one use. To perform the puncture, the lancet/endcap is placed on the patient's skin and a release button is depressed. The spring forces the blade into the skin and retracts the blade into the endcap. After the procedure, the lancet/endcap is discarded in a biohazard sharps container (Procedure 31-4).

MICROCOLLECTION DEVICES

After the skin has been punctured, a capillary blood specimen must be collected. The blood specimen can be collected directly onto a reagent strip, such as occurs with blood glucose monitors. It can also be collected in a small container known as a *microcollection device*. The device depends on the laboratory equipment running the test. Common microcollection devices are capillary tubes and microcollection tubes.

A. Microcollection tubes   B. Capillary tubes

Figure 31-19. Microcollection devices. (From Bonewit-West K: *Clinical procedures for medical assistants*, ed 7, St. Louis, 2008, Saunders.)

Capillary Tubes

A capillary tube consists of a disposable glass or plastic tube (see Figure 31-19). Depending on the size of the tube, it can hold 5 to 75 µl of blood. In the medical office, a capillary tube is used to collect a blood specimen for a hematocrit determination. This procedure is presented in Chapter 32.

Microcollection Tubes

A microcollection tube consists of a small plastic tube with a removable blood collector tip. The tip is designed to collect capillary blood from a skin puncture and results in a relatively large blood specimen. After the specimen has been collected, the collector tip is removed, discarded, and replaced by a plastic plug. Microcollection tubes are available with or without additives. The plugs are color coded and correspond to the color-coded evacuated tube system used in venipuncture. One such device is the Microtainer (Becton-Dickinson) (Figure 31-19).

GUIDELINES FOR PERFORMING A FINGER PUNCTURE

1. If a laboratory test requires advance preparation, before you perform the finger puncture, verify that the patient has prepared properly. If not, do not collect the specimen unless directed otherwise by the physician. If the finger puncture is to be rescheduled, carefully review the preparation requirements with the patient.

2. The patient should be seated comfortably in a chair. The arm should be firmly supported and extended with the palmar surface of the hand facing up. Never perform a skin puncture with the patient sitting on a stool or standing. The patient may faint and injure himself or herself.

3. Instruct the patient to remain still during the procedure. Explain to the patient that the procedure should be relatively quick and only slightly uncomfortable. Just before making the puncture, tell the patient that he or she will "feel a small stick." This prevents startling the patient, which could cause the patient to move.

4. Use the lateral part of the tip of the third or fourth finger (middle or ring finger) of the nondominant hand for the puncture site. The capillary bed in these fingers is large, and the skin is easy to penetrate. The puncture site should be free of lesions, scars, bruises, and edema. The index finger is not recommended as a puncture site. The index finger is more calloused, which makes it harder to penetrate than the other fingers. Also, the patient uses that finger more and would notice the pain longer. The little finger should also not be used as a puncture site. The amount of tissue between the skin surface and the bone is so small that using this finger as a puncture site could result in an injury to the bone.

5. After selecting the puncture site, warm the site to increase the blood flow to the capillary bed. Warming the site can be accomplished by gently massaging the finger five or six times from base to tip or by placing the hand in warm water for a few minutes (105°F [40°C]). Warming the site promotes bleeding after an effective puncture.

6. Cleanse the site with an antiseptic wipe, and allow it to dry thoroughly. The site must be dry to allow a round drop of blood to form on the finger. Otherwise, the drop would leach out onto the skin of the patient's finger and be difficult to collect. In addition, alcohol entering the capillary specimen contaminates it, leading to inaccurate test results. Alcohol also causes the patient to experience a stinging sensation when the puncture is made.

7. Firmly grasp the finger in front of the most distal knuckle joint. Apply enough pressure to cause the fingertip to become hard and red so that adequate penetration and depth of puncture will occur.

8. Make the puncture in the fleshy portion of the fingertip, slightly to the side of center. To prevent injury to the bone, do not puncture the side or very tip of the finger. The blade of the lancet should be positioned so that the puncture is perpendicular to the lines of the fingerprint rather than parallel to the fingerprint (Figure 31-20). This facilitates the formation of a well-formed drop of blood that is easy to collect. A puncture that is not perpendicular causes the blood flow to follow the lines of the fingerprint and run down the finger, making it difficult to collect.

9. Firmly press the lancet device against the puncture site, and activate the spring-loaded puncturing device. If a good puncture has been made, the blood flows freely. When learning this procedure, many individuals do not apply enough pressure to obtain a puncture that is deep enough. If this occurs, a poor blood flow results and the patient has to be punctured again. A deep puncture hurts no more than a superficial one and provides a much better blood flow.

10. Wipe away the first drop of blood with a gauze pad. The first drop of blood is diluted with alcohol and tissue fluid and is not a suitable specimen for testing. Using the first drop of blood may lead to inaccurate test results.

11. Allow a large drop of blood to form by applying continual gentle pressure near the puncture site. Collect the blood specimen using a reagent strip or the appropriate microcollection device. If the required amount of blood is not obtained, you can gently massage the tissue surrounding the puncture site to promote blood flow. Do not squeeze or massage excessively because doing so causes dilution of the blood specimen with tissue fluids, which can affect the accuracy of the test results.

12. Check the puncture site to make sure the bleeding has stopped. Apply an adhesive bandage, if needed. A bandage is not recommended for children younger than 2 years old. The bandage may irritate the skin of a young child, and the child might put the bandage in his or her mouth, aspirate it, and choke.

Figure 31-20. Recommended sites for a finger puncture. (From Bonewit-West K: *Clinical procedures for medical assistants*, ed 7, St. Louis, 2008, Saunders.)

PROCEDURE 31-3   Skin Puncture—Disposable Semiautomatic Lancet Device

Outcome Obtain a capillary blood specimen.

Equipment/Supplies

- Disposable gloves
- Antiseptic wipe
- Microtainer brand safety flow lancet device

- Sterile 2 × 2 gauze pad
- Adhesive bandage
- Biohazard sharps container

1. **Procedural Step.** Sanitize your hands.
2. **Procedural Step.** Greet the patient and introduce yourself. Identify the patient by asking the patient to state his or her full name and date of birth. Compare this information with the demographic data in the patient's chart. If the patient was required to prepare for the test (e.g., fasting, medication restriction), determine whether he or she has prepared properly. If the patient has not followed the patient preparation requirements, notify the physician for instructions on handling this situation.
3. **Procedural Step.** Assemble the equipment. Open the sterile gauze packet and lay it flat to allow the gauze pad to rest on the inside of its wrapper.

Assemble the equipment. (From Bonewit-West K: *Clinical procedures for medical assistants,* ed 7, St. Louis, 2008, Saunders.)

4. **Procedural Step.** Explain the procedure to the patient, and reassure the patient.
   Principle. Reassurance should be offered to reduce apprehension.
5. **Procedural Step.** Seat the patient comfortably in a chair. The patient's arm should be firmly supported and extended with the palmar surface of the hand facing up.
6. **Procedural Step.** Select an appropriate puncture site. Use the lateral part of the tip of the third or fourth finger of the nondominant hand to make the puncture. If the patient's finger is cold, you can warm it by gently massaging the finger five or six times from base to tip or by placing the hand in warm water for a few minutes.
   Principle. Warming the site increases the blood flow to the area and promotes bleeding from the puncture site.

7. **Procedural Step.** Cleanse the site with an antiseptic wipe. Allow the site to air dry, and after cleansing it, do not touch the area, wipe the area with gauze, or fan the area with your hand.
   Principle. The site must be allowed to air dry to allow enough time for the alcohol to destroy microorganisms on the patient's skin. If the site is dry, a round drop of blood forms on the finger, making it easy to collect the specimen. If the site is not dry, the blood leaches out and runs down the finger, making it difficult to collect. Residual alcohol entering the blood specimen can cause hemolysis, leading to inaccurate test results. In addition, residual alcohol causes the patient to experience a stinging sensation when the puncture is made. Touching or fanning the area causes contamination, and the cleansing process has to be repeated.
8. **Procedural Step.** Apply gloves.
   Principle. Gloves provide a barrier precaution against bloodborne pathogens.
9. **Procedural Step.** Without touching the puncture site, firmly grasp the patient's finger in front of the most distal knuckle joint. Apply enough pressure to cause the fingertip to become hard and red. Position the

Make the puncture. (From Bonewit-West K: *Clinical procedures for medical assistants,* ed 7, St. Louis, 2008, Saunders.)

blade of the lancet perpendicular to the lines of the fingerprint on the fleshy portion of the fingertip, slightly to the side of center.

Principle. The site must be grasped with enough pressure so that adequate penetration and depth of puncture can occur. Punctures that are not perpendicular cause the blood to run down the finger, making it difficult to collect. Puncturing the side or tip of the finger may cause the lancet to penetrate the bone.

10. **Procedural Step.** Firmly depress the activation button, without moving the lancet or finger, until an audible click is heard. Pressing the activation button causes the lancet to puncture the skin and then retract into its plastic casing. A well-made puncture results in a free-flowing wound that needs only slight pressure to make it bleed.

    Principle. Moving the lancet or finger before the process is complete can result in an inadequate puncture and poor blood flow.

11. **Procedural Step.** Immediately dispose of the lancet device in a biohazard sharps container.

    Principle. Proper disposal of contaminated sharps is required by the OSHA standard to prevent exposure to bloodborne pathogens.

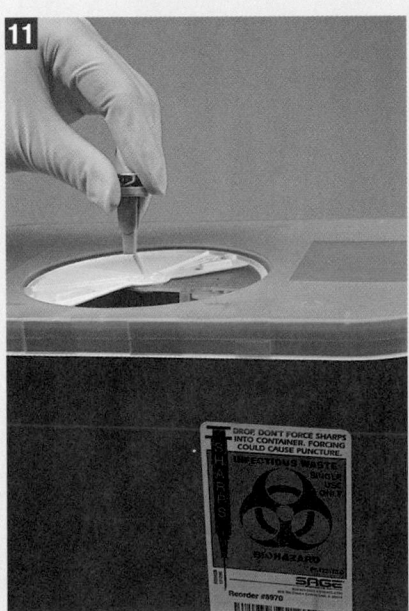

Discard the lancet. (From Bonewit-West K: *Clinical procedures for medical assistants,* ed 7, St. Louis, 2008, Saunders.)

12. **Procedural Step.** Wait a few seconds to allow blood flow to begin. Wipe away the first drop of blood with a gauze pad.

    Principle. The first drop of blood is diluted with alcohol and tissue fluid and is not a suitable specimen.

13. **Procedural Step.** Use the second drop of blood for the test. Allow a large, well-rounded drop of blood to

form by holding the hand in a downward position and applying gentle, continuous pressure without squeezing the finger. You can massage the tissue surrounding the puncture firmly but gently to encourage blood flow.

Principle. Squeezing or massaging the site excessively causes dilution of the blood sample with tissue fluid, leading to inaccurate test results.

Wipe away the first drop of blood. (From Bonewit-West K: *Clinical procedures for medical assistants,* ed 7, St. Louis, 2008, Saunders.)

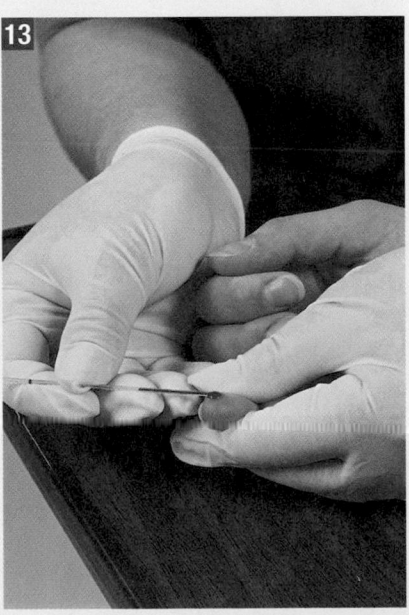

Collect the specimen. (From Bonewit-West K: *Clinical procedures for medical assistants,* ed 7, St. Louis, 2008, Saunders.)

Continued

PROCEDURE 31-3

PROCEDURE **31-3** Skin Puncture—Disposable Semiautomatic Lancet Device—cont'd

14. Procedural Step. Collect the blood specimen on a test strip or in the appropriate microcollection device.

15. Procedural Step. Have the patient hold a gauze pad over the puncture and apply pressure until the bleeding stops. As a safety precaution, remain with the patient until the bleeding stops. If needed, apply an adhesive bandage.

16. Procedural Step. Test the blood specimen following the manufacturer's instructions that accompany the blood analyzer or testing kit.

17. Procedural Step. Remove the gloves, and sanitize your hands.

PROCEDURE **31-4** Skin Puncture—Reusable Semiautomatic Lancet Device

Outcome Obtain a capillary blood specimen.

Equipment/Supplies

- Disposable gloves
- Antiseptic wipe
- Glucolet II lancet device
- Disposable retractable lancet/endcap
- Sterile 2 × 2 gauze pad
- Biohazard sharps container

1. Procedural Step. Sanitize your hands.

2. Procedural Step. Greet the patient and introduce yourself. Identify the patient by asking the patient to state his or her full name and date of birth. Compare this information with the demographic data in the patient's chart. If the patient was required to prepare for the test (e.g., fasting, medication restriction), determine whether he or she has prepared properly. If the patient has not followed the patient preparation requirements, notify the physician for instructions on handling this situation.

3. Procedural Step. Assemble the equipment. Push the transparent barrel of the lancet device toward the release button until it clicks into place.

4. Procedural Step. Insert the retractable lancet/endcap onto the lancet device. Open the sterile gauze packet and lay it flat to allow the gauze pad to rest on the inside of its wrapper.

5. Procedural Step. Explain the procedure to the patient, and reassure the patient.
Principle. Reassurance should be offered to reduce apprehension.

6. Procedural Step. Seat the patient comfortably in a chair. The patient's arm should be firmly supported and extended with the palmar surface of the hand facing up.

Assemble the equipment. (From Bonewit-West K: *Clinical procedures for medical assistants,* ed 7, St. Louis, 2008, Saunders.)

7. Procedural Step. Select an appropriate puncture site. Use the lateral part of the tip of the third or fourth finger of the nondominant hand to make the puncture. If the patient's finger is cold, you can warm it by gently massaging the finger five or six times from base to tip or by placing the hand in warm water for a few minutes.

Push the barrel until it clicks into place. (From Bonewit-West K: *Clinical procedures for medical assistants,* ed 7, St. Louis, 2008, Saunders.)

Insert the retractable lancet onto the device. (From Bonewit-West K: *Clinical procedures for medical assistants,* ed 7, St. Louis, 2008, Saunders.)

Principle. Warming the site increases the blood flow to the area and promotes bleeding from the puncture site.

8. **Procedural Step.** Cleanse the site with an antiseptic wipe. Allow the site to air dry, and after cleansing it, do not touch the area or fan the area with your hand.

   Principle. The site must be allowed to air dry to allow enough time for the alcohol to destroy microorganisms on the patient's skin. If the site is dry, a round drop of blood forms on the finger, making it easy to collect the specimen. If the site is not dry, the blood leaches out and runs down the finger, making it difficult to collect. Residual alcohol entering the blood specimen can cause hemolysis, leading to inaccurate test results. In addition, residual alcohol causes the

patient to experience a stinging sensation when the puncture is made. Touching or fanning the area causes contamination, and the cleansing process has to be repeated.

9. **Procedural Step.** Apply gloves. Using a twisting motion, remove the plastic post from the lancet/endcap.

   Principle. Gloves provide a barrier against bloodborne pathogens.

Remove the plastic port. (From Bonewit-West K: *Clinical procedures for medical assistants,* ed 7, St. Louis, 2008, Saunders.)

10. **Procedural Step.** Without touching the puncture site, firmly grasp the patient's finger in front of the most distal knuckle joint. Apply enough pressure to cause the fingertip to become hard and red. Position the blade of the lancet perpendicular to the lines of the fingerprint on the fleshy portion of the fingertip slightly to the side of center.

    Principle. The site must be grasped with enough pressure so that adequate penetration and depth of puncture can occur. Punctures that are not perpendicular cause the blood to run down the finger, making it difficult to collect. Puncturing the side or tip of the finger may cause the lancet to penetrate the bone.

11. **Procedural Step.** Firmly depress the activation button without moving the Glucolet or finger. Pressing the activation button causes the lancet to puncture the skin and then retract into the endcap. A well-made puncture results in a free-flowing wound that needs only slight pressure to make it bleed.

    Principle. Moving the lancet or finger before the process is complete can result in an inadequate puncture and poor blood flow.

12. **Procedural Step.** Wait a few seconds to allow blood flow to begin. Wipe away the first drop of blood with a gauze pad.

    Principle. The first drop of blood is diluted with alcohol and tissue fluid and is not a suitable specimen.

Continued

PROCEDURE 31-4

Make the puncture. (From Bonewit-West K: *Clinical procedures for medical assistants,* ed 7, St. Louis, 2008, Saunders.)

Collect the specimen. (From Bonewit-West K: *Clinical procedures for medical assistants,* ed 7, St. Louis, 2008, Saunders.)

13. **Procedural Step.** Use the second drop of blood for the test. Allow a large well-rounded drop of blood to form by holding the hand in a downward position and applying gentle, continuous pressure without squeezing the finger. The tissue surrounding the puncture site can be massaged firmly but gently to encourage blood flow.
    Principle. Squeezing or massaging the site excessively causes dilution of the blood sample with tissue fluid, leading to inaccurate test results.

14. **Procedural Step.** Collect the blood specimen on a test strip or in the appropriate microcollection device as required by the test being performed.

15. **Procedural Step.** Have the patient hold a gauze pad over the puncture site, and apply pressure until the bleeding stops. As a safety precaution, remain with the patient until the bleeding stops. If needed, apply an adhesive bandage.

16. **Procedural Step.** Remove the endcap from the lancet device, and discard it in a biohazard sharps container.

17. **Procedural Step.** Test the blood specimen following the manufacturer's instructions that accompany the blood analyzer or testing kit.

18. **Procedural Step.** Remove the gloves, and sanitize your hands.

19. **Procedural Step.** Sanitize and disinfect the Glucolet II according to the manufacturer's instructions. Store the Glucolet II in its resting position.

MEDICAL PRACTICE and the LAW

Phlebotomy is an invasive procedure that can harm the patient if performed incorrectly. Sharps and medical waste contaminated with blood must be disposed of according to federal regulations. Laboratory tests involving blood must be performed correctly for accurate results. Incorrect results can lead to an inaccurate diagnosis and treatment. Currently, performing HIV testing requires the patient's written consent. If the patient has questions regarding HIV, refer him or her to the physician for discussion. Never give out laboratory results without checking with the physician. Medical assistants are usually given permission by the physician to relay negative laboratory test results; however, abnormal laboratory results should be relayed by the physician. The medical assistant does not have the medical knowledge to answer the questions the patient may have when the results are abnormal. HIV results (negative or positive) should be given only by the physician. Never speculate to the patient or coworkers about the results of any test. All test results must remain confidential.

Use appropriate personal protective equipment to prevent the transmission of bloodborne pathogens to protect yourself, your coworkers, and your patients. ■

What Would You Do? What Would You *Not* Do? RESPONSES

Case Study 1
Page 736

What Did Dori Do?
❑ Told Angela that it was fine to have her friend there while she gets her blood drawn.
❑ Told Angela that she could not have the blood drawn out of her left arm because a good vein could not be located in that arm.
❑ Told Angela that using the hand veins are always the last choice when drawing blood. Explained that there are many nerve endings in the hand, which makes it hurt more.
❑ Told Angela that most of the time what she sees on TV is someone getting an IV started in the hand, not their blood being drawn.
❑ Explained to Angela that there will just be a small stick and that it would heal quickly, and there should be no reason it would affect her softball game this evening.
❑ Tried to relax and reassure Angela before the venipuncture. Carefully explained the procedure to her because it was her first one.
❑ Because Angela was nervous, took precautions to prevent her from fainting by placing her in a semi-Fowler's position on the examining table.
❑ Had Angela's friend stand near the head of the table to help calm her down.

What Did Dori Not *Do?*
❑ Did not try to draw Angela's blood from her left arm or hand.
❑ Did not ignore the fact that Angela was nervous about the venipuncture.

What Would You Do?/What Would You *Not* Do? Review Dori's response and place a checkmark next to the information you included in your response. List additional information you included in your response.

_____

_____

_____

_____

Case Study 2
Page 747

What Did Dori Do?
❑ Told Buzz that when a butterfly setup is used, the air in the tubing alters the test results. Explained that the red tube is used get rid of the air, and because it is not needed for testing, it is thrown away.
❑ Told Buzz that Vacutainer setups are also used in the medical office, and that the choice of what to use depends on the size of a patient's veins and the policy of the health care facility.
❑ Stressed to Buzz how important it is to have his blood tested every week to ensure there is not too much or too little of the Coumadin in his body. Explained to him again what might occur if his Coumadin were at the wrong level.
❑ Told Buzz that the office would help him locate a medical laboratory where he will be vacationing so that he could have his test done.
❑ Made sure that Buzz had a laboratory requisition so that he could have his test done while he was on vacation.

What Did Dori Not *Do?*
❑ Did not tell Buzz that it would be all right to skip his prothrombin test during his vacation.

What Would You Do?/What Would You *Not* Do? Review Dori's response and place a checkmark next to the information you included in your response. List additional information you included in your response.

_____

_____

_____

Case Study 3
Page 753

What Did Dori Do?
❑ Told Mrs. Gabriel that only the laboratory can accept specimens drawn at the laboratory or the medical office.

Continued

What Would You Do? What Would You *Not* Do?   RESPONSES—cont'd

❑ Told Mrs. Gabriel that if it would make her feel more comfortable, the laboratory could drop off the blood-drawing supplies at the office, and her blood could be drawn tomorrow at the office.

❑ Informed the physician about Mrs. Gabriel's experience at the laboratory.

What Did Dori Not *Do?*

❑ Did not tell Mrs. Gabriel that probing a vein could cause the test results to be inaccurate.

What Would You Do?/What Would You *Not* Do? Review Dori's response and place a checkmark next to the information you included in your response. List additional information you included in your response.

_____

_____

_____

_____

TERMINOLOGY REVIEW

Antecubital space The surface of the arm in front of the elbow.

Anticoagulant A substance that inhibits blood clotting.

Buffy coat A thin, light-colored layer of white blood cells and platelets that lies between a top layer of plasma and a bottom layer of red blood cells when an anticoagulant has been added to a blood specimen.

Evacuated tube A closed glass or plastic tube that contains a premeasured vacuum.

Hematoma A swelling or mass of coagulated blood caused by a break in a blood vessel.

Hemoconcentration An increase in the concentration of the nonfilterable blood components in the blood vessels, such as red blood cells, enzymes, iron, and calcium, as a result of a decrease in the fluid content of the blood.

Hemolysis The breakdown of blood cells.

Osteochondritis Inflammation of bone and cartilage.

Osteomyelitis Inflammation of the bone as a result of bacterial infection.

Phlebotomist A health care professional trained in the collection of blood specimens.

Phlebotomy Incision of a vein for the removal of blood; the collection of blood.

Plasma The liquid part of the blood consisting of a clear, straw-colored fluid that comprises approximately 55% of the blood volume.

Serum Plasma from which the clotting factor fibrinogen has been removed.

Venipuncture Puncturing of a vein.

Venous reflux The backflow of blood (from an evacuated tube) into the patient's vein.

Venous stasis The temporary cessation or slowing of the venous blood flow.

ON THE WEB

For Information on Phlebotomy:

Clinical Laboratory Standards Institute: www.clsi.org

National Accrediting Agency for Clinical Laboratory Sciences: www.naacls.org

Lab Explorer: www.labexplorer.com

American Society for Clinical Laboratory Science (ASCLS): www.ascls.org

American Society for Clinical Pathology (ASCP): www.ascp.org

American Society of Phlebotomy Technicians (ASPT): www.aspt.org

Becton, Dickinson and Company: www.bd.com

National Phlebotomy Association (NPA): www.national-phlebotomy.org

The Safety Lady: www.safetylady.com

My Blood Draw: www.myblooddraw.com

Phlebotomy Pages: www.phlebotomypages.com

PREPARE FOR CERTIFICATION   Visit the Evolve site at http://evolve.elsevier.com/Bonewit/today/ to actively Prepare for your Certification.

 *Check out the **Companion CD** bound with the book to access additional interactive activities.*

32

Hematology

KEY TERMS

anemia (ah-NEE-mee-ah)
hematology (hee-mah-TOL-oe-jee)
hemoglobin (HEE-moe-gloe-bin)

leukocytosis (loo-koe-sie-TOE-sis)
leukopenia (loo-koe-PEE-nee-ah)
polycythemia (pol-ee-sie-THEE-mee-ah)

Introduction to Hematology

Hematology is the study of blood, including the morphologic appearance and function of blood cells and diseases of the blood and blood-forming tissues. Before beginning a study of this chapter, it is suggested that you review the components and function of blood presented in Chapter 12.

Laboratory analysis in hematology is concerned with the examination of blood for the purpose of detecting pathologic conditions. It includes performing blood cell counts, evaluating the clotting ability of the blood, and identifying cell types. These tests are valuable tools that allow the physician to determine whether each blood component falls within its normal value or range.

Examples of hematologic tests include the hemoglobin, hematocrit, white blood cell count, red blood cell count, differential white blood cell count, prothrombin time, erythrocyte sedimentation rate, and platelet count. Table 32-1 summarizes common hematologic tests, including specimen requirements, normal values, and conditions that cause abnormal test results.

Hematologic laboratory tests may be performed in the medical office. Advances in automated blood analyzers designed for use in the medical office have made this possible. Automated blood analyzers perform laboratory tests with accurate test results in a short time. Each automated analyzer is accompanied by a detailed operating manual that explains its operation, test parameters, care, and maintenance.

The most frequently performed hematologic laboratory test is the *complete blood count* (CBC). A CBC is routinely performed on new patients and on patients with a pathologic condition. The test results provide valuable information to assist the physician in making a diagnosis, evaluating the patient's progress, and regulating treatment. The tests included in a CBC are as follows:

- White blood cell (WBC) count
- Red blood cell (RBC) count
- Platelet count
- Hemoglobin (Hgb)
- Hematocrit (Hct)
- Differential WBC count (diff)
- RBC indices

HEMOGLOBIN DETERMINATION

Hemoglobin (Hgb) is a major component of RBCs. Hemoglobin transports oxygen to the tissue cells of the body and is responsible for the color of the RBC.

The hemoglobin determination is used to measure indirectly the oxygen-carrying capacity of the blood. The normal range for an adult female is 12 to 16 g/dL, and the normal range for an adult male is 14 to 18 g/dL. A hemoglobin determination is performed as an individual test or as part of the CBC. A hemoglobin determination is often performed as a routine test on individuals, such as children younger than 2 years of age and pregnant women, who are at risk for developing anemia.

A decreased hemoglobin level occurs with **anemia** (especially iron deficiency anemia), hyperthyroidism, cirrhosis of the liver, severe hemorrhaging, hemolytic reactions, and certain systemic diseases such as leukemia and Hodgkin's disease. Increased levels of hemoglobin are present with **polycythemia,** chronic obstructive pulmonary disease, and congestive heart failure.

The hemoglobin determination can be performed on capillary or venous blood. The most accurate and reliable method for measuring hemoglobin concentration involves the use of a blood analyzer. An office blood analyzer permits the processing of the specimen in a short time, allowing the physician to evaluate the condition while the patient is still at the medical office.

HEMATOCRIT

The hematocrit (Hct) is a simple, reliable, and informative test that is frequently performed in the medical office. The word *hematocrit* means "to separate blood." The solid or cellular elements are separated from the plasma by centrifuging an anticoagulated blood specimen. The heavier RBCs become packed and settle to the bottom of a tube. The top layer contains the clear, straw-colored plasma. Between the plasma and the packed RBCs is a small, thin, yellowish-gray layer known as the *buffy coat,* which contains the platelets and WBCs (Figure 32-1).

The purpose of the hematocrit is to measure the percentage volume of packed RBCs in whole blood. The normal hematocrit range for a woman is 37% to 47%; for a man, 40% to 54%. A low hematocrit reading may indicate

Table 32-1 Common Hematologic Tests

Name of Test (Abbreviation)	Purpose	Normal Range	Increased with	Decreased with
White blood cell count (WBC)	Assist in diagnosis and prognosis of disease	4,500-11,000/mm³ (or 10⁹ cells/L)	Leukocytosis Acute infections (appendicitis, chickenpox, diphtheria, infectious mononucleosis, meningitis, pneumonia, rheumatic fever, smallpox, tonsillitis) Hemorrhaging Trauma Malignant disease Leukemia Polycythemia vera	Leukopenia Viral infections Hypersplenism Bone marrow depression Infectious hepatitis Cirrhosis Chemotherapy Radiation therapy
Red blood cell count (RBC)	Assist in diagnosis of anemia and polycythemia	*Male:* 4.5-6.2 million/mm³ (or 10¹² cells/L) *Female:* 4-5.5 million/mm³ (10¹² cells/L) MCV 80-100 fL MCH 27-34 pg MCHC 1%-36% RDW 11.5%-14.5%	Polycythemia vera Secondary polycythemia Severe diarrhea Dehydration Acute poisoning Pulmonary fibrosis Severe burns	Iron deficiency anemia Hodgkin's disease Multiple myeloma Leukemia Hemolytic anemia Pernicious anemia Lupus erythematosus Addison's disease
Hemoglobin (Hgb or Hb)	To screen for anemia, determine its severity, monitor response to treatment	*Male:* 14-18 g/dL (SI units: 2.17-2.79 mmol/L) *Female:* 12-16 g/dL (SI units: 1.86-2.48 mmol/L)	Severe burns Chronic obstructive pulmonary disease Congestive heart failure	Anemia Hyperthyroidism Cirrhosis Severe hemorrhage Hemolytic reactions Hodgkin's disease Leukemia
Hematocrit (Hct)	Assist in diagnosis and evaluation of anemia	*Male:* 40%-54% *Female:* 37%-47%	Polycythemia vera Severe dehydration Shock Severe burns	Anemia Leukemia Hyperthyroidism Cirrhosis Acute blood loss Hemolytic reactions
Differential WBC count (diff)	Assist in diagnosis and prognosis of disease	Neutrophils 50%-70% Eosinophils 1%-4% Basophils 0%-1% Lymphocytes 20%-35% Monocytes 3%-8%	**Neutrophilia** Acute bacterial infections Parasitic infections Liver disease **Eosinophilia** Allergic conditions Parasitic infections Addison's disease Lung and bone cancer **Basophilia** Leukemia Chronic inflammation Polycythemia vera Hemolytic anemia Hodgkin's disease **Lymphocytosis** Acute and chronic infections Hematopoietic disorders Addison's disease Carcinoma Hyperthyroidism	**Neutropenia** Acute viral infections Blood diseases Hormone diseases Chemotherapy **Eosinopenia** Infectious mononucleosis Hypersplenism Congestive heart failure Aplastic and pernicious anemia **Basopenia** Acute allergic reactions Hyperthyroidism Steroid therapy **Lymphopenia** HIV infection Cardiac failure Cushing's disease Hodgkin's disease Leukemia

Continued

Table 32-1 Common Hematologic Tests—cont'd

Name of Test (Abbreviation)	Purpose	Normal Range	Increased with	Decreased with
			Monocytosis Viral infections Bacterial and parasitic infections Collagen diseases Cirrhosis Polycythemia vera Polycythemia	**Monocytopenia** Prednisone treatment Hairy cell leukemia
Prothrombin time (PT)	Screen for coagulation disorders and regulate treatment of patients taking oral anticoagulant therapy with warfarin sodium (Coumadin)	11-16 sec	**Thrombocytosis** Prothrombin deficiency Vitamin K deficiency Hemorrhagic disease of the newborn Liver disease Anticoagulant therapy Biliary obstruction Acute leukemia Polycythemia vera	**Thrombocytopenia** Acute thrombophlebitis Diuretics Multiple myeloma Pulmonary embolism Vitamin K therapy
Erythrocyte sedimentation rate (ESR)	Nonspecific test for connective tissue diseases, malignancy, and infectious diseases; also used to evaluate progress of inflammatory diseases (elevated test results warrant further testing)	Westergren's method *Male:* younger than age 50, 0-20 mm/hr; age 50 or older, 0-20 mm/hr *Female:* younger than age 50, 0-20 mm/hr; age 50 or older, 0-30 mm/hr	Collagen diseases Infections Inflammatory diseases Carcinoma Cell or tissue destruction Rheumatoid arthritis	Polycythemia vera Sickle cell anemia Congestive heart failure
Platelet count (Plt)	Assist in evaluation of bleeding disorders that occur with liver disease, thrombocytopenia, uremia, and anticoagulant therapy	150,000-400,000/mm^3 (SI units: 150-400 × 10^9/L)	**Thrombocytosis** Cancer Leukemia Polycythemia vera Splenectomy Acute blood loss Rheumatoid arthritis Trauma (fractures)	**Thrombocytopenia** Pernicious anemia Aplastic anemia Hemolytic anemia Pneumonia Allergic conditions Infection Bone marrow— depressant drugs

From Bonewit-West K: *Clinical procedures for medical assistants,* ed 7, St. Louis, 2008, Saunders.
SI units, International System of Units.

Putting It All into Practice

My name is Latisha Sharpe, and I work in a multiphysician office as a laboratory technician. I have worked in the office for 2 years. My job duties include venipuncture, preparing blood for transport to an outside laboratory, operating laboratory equipment, and performing laboratory tests.

When I first started working in a physician's office, the patients were apprehensive about someone new drawing their blood. It made me a little nervous because it seemed they were questioning my ability to perform the procedure. I explained to the patients that I had the proper training. I showed that I was confident, and that I could perform the procedure with success. By doing this, I gained their trust. Before long, they were requesting that I draw their blood. ■

Prepare for Success

PATIENT TEACHING   Iron Deficiency Anemia

Answer questions patients have about iron deficiency anemia.

What is anemia?

Anemia is a shortage of red blood cells (RBCs) or hemoglobin. Hemoglobin, the part of the blood that gives RBCs their color, carries oxygen to all the cells in the body. There are many types of anemia, of which iron deficiency anemia is the most common. Other types of anemia are pernicious anemia, sickle cell anemia, hemolytic anemia, and aplastic anemia.

What causes iron deficiency anemia?

In general, iron deficiency anemia is caused by conditions that deplete the iron stored in the body; it can result from an increased need for iron by the body or an increased loss of iron from the body. Iron deficiency anemia may occur in children younger than 2 years old if there is not enough iron in their diet to meet their demands of rapid growth. This is especially true in children whose main source of nutrition during these years is breast milk or bottle milk because milk contains very little iron. Adolescent girls are prone to iron deficiency anemia because of their growth spurts during puberty and the loss through menstruation. In adults, the most common cause of anemia is chronic blood loss, such as from a bleeding ulcer, bleeding hemorrhoids, and heavy menstrual bleeding. Pregnant women are also at increased risk because of the demands of the growing fetus.

What can be done for individuals at risk for iron deficiency anemia?

Individuals prone to developing iron deficiency anemia are encouraged to increase foods in their diet that contain iron, such as beef, liver, spinach, eggs, and iron-fortified breads and cereals. As a preventive measure, the physician usually prescribes vitamin supplements for individuals at an increased risk for developing iron deficiency anemia, such as pregnant women, infants, and young children. Also, infant formulas and cereals that have been supplemented with iron are available.

What are the symptoms of anemia?

All types of anemia have the same general symptoms. Often these symptoms do not develop right away; when they do develop, feeling tired and run down may be the only sign of anemia. Other symptoms that may occur, particularly as the anemia becomes worse, are paleness of the skin, fingernail beds, and mucous membranes; shortness of breath, especially during physical activity; dizziness; headache; irritability; and inability to concentrate. These symptoms result from the diminished ability of the blood to carry oxygen to the cells of the body. Blood tests are necessary to diagnose anemia and to determine the specific type of anemia present.

How is iron deficiency anemia treated?

The most important part of treating anemia is to determine its cause, such as not enough iron consumed in the diet or chronic blood loss, and to correct that condition. The physician usually prescribes an iron supplement to replace the iron that has been depleted from the body. It is generally prescribed in oral form, but it is given through an injection in special situations. An oral iron supplement causes the stool to turn a black, tarlike color. This is normal and should not be a cause for concern. Also, an effort should be made to consume foods high in iron content.

- For patients who have had a vitamin supplement prescribed to *prevent* iron deficiency anemia, such as children younger than 2 years old and pregnant women: Emphasize the importance to the patient of taking the vitamin supplement every day to prevent the development of iron deficiency anemia.
- For patients who have had an iron supplement prescribed to treat iron deficiency anemia: Emphasize to the patient the importance of taking the iron supplement for the period of time prescribed by the physician because replacement of iron takes time.
- Instruct patients to keep iron supplements out of the reach of children to prevent iron poisoning.
- Provide patients with written educational materials about anemia. ∎

What Would You Do? What Would You *Not* Do?

Case Study 1

Theodore Pascal is at the office for a general physical examination. The physician orders a routine urinalysis and a hemoglobin determination be done on Theodore at the office. Theodore wants to know whether the physician thinks there is something wrong with him. He also wants to know the purpose of the blood test and how it is done. When Theodore realizes that a hemoglobin determination involves a fingerstick, he says that he does not like having his finger stuck and wants to know whether the blood can be taken out of his earlobe instead. ∎

PROCEDURE 32-1

Capillary tube

Plasma

The results are read at the top of the packed cell column — Buffy coat

Packed red blood cells

Sealing compound

Figure 32-1. Hematocrit test results. The blood cells are separated from the plasma by centrifuging an anticoagulated blood specimen, and the results are read at the top of the packed cell column. (From Bonewit-West K: *Clinical procedures for medical assistants,* ed 7, St. Louis, 2008, Saunders.)

anemia, and a high reading may indicate polycythemia. The hematocrit, in conjunction with other hematologic tests, is an aid to the physician in the diagnosis of a patient's condition. The hematocrit is also used as a screening measure for the early detection of anemia and is often included in a general physical examination.

The *microhematocrit method* is used most often in the medical office to perform a hematocrit determination. Through capillary action, blood is drawn directly from a free-flowing skin puncture into a disposable capillary tube lined with an anticoagulant. An anticoagulated blood specimen collected by venipuncture can be used as well; through capillary action, the blood specimen is drawn into the capillary tube from the evacuated collection tube. After collecting the specimen, one end of the capillary tube is sealed with a commercially prepared sealing compound (e.g., Cha-Seal, Seal-Ease). The capillary tube is then placed in a microhematocrit centrifuge. The centrifuge spins the blood at an extremely high speed and requires only 3 to 5 minutes to pack the RBCs. The results are read at the top of the packed cell column. Procedure 32-1 describes how to perform a hematocrit determination.

PROCEDURE 32-1 Hematocrit

Outcome Perform a hematocrit determination.

Equipment/Supplies

- Microhematocrit centrifuge
- Disposable gloves
- Lancet
- Antiseptic wipe
- Gauze pads

- Capillary tubes
- Sealing compound
- Adhesive bandage
- Biohazard sharps container

---

1. **Procedural Step.** Sanitize your hands. Greet the patient and introduce yourself. Identify the patient by full name and date of birth, and explain the procedure.
2. **Procedural Step.** Assemble equipment. Cleanse the puncture site with an antiseptic wipe, and allow it to air dry. Apply gloves and perform a finger puncture, then dispose of the lancet in a biohazard sharps container.
   Principle. Personal protective equipment and proper disposal of the lancet are required by the OSHA standard to prevent exposure to bloodborne pathogens.
3. **Procedural Step.** Wipe away the first drop of blood with a gauze pad. Fill the capillary tube by holding one end of it horizontally, but slightly downward, next to the free-flowing puncture. Keep the tip of the capillary tube in the blood, but do not allow it to press

Fill the capillary tube. (From Bonewit-West K: *Clinical procedures for medical assistants,* ed 7, St. Louis, 2008, Saunders.)

against the patient's skin. Calibrated tubes are filled to the calibration line; uncalibrated tubes are filled approximately three quarters (within 10 to 20 mm of the end of the tube). The blood is drawn into the tube through capillary action. Fill a second tube using the method just described.

Principle. Not keeping the tip of the capillary tube in the blood can cause air bubbles in the stem of the tube, which leads to inaccurate test results. Allowing the capillary tube to press against the skin closes the opening of the capillary tubes and does not allow blood to enter it. The type of tube (calibrated or uncalibrated) is based on the method used to read the test results. The hematocrit should be performed in duplicate to ensure accurate and reliable test results.

4. **Procedural Step.** Seal one end of each tube with a small amount of sealing compound. The sealing compound can be used to hold the capillary tubes until they are ready to be placed in the microhematocrit centrifuge. To do this, the sealing compound should be placed on a flat surface with the tubes in a vertical position. Before removing a capillary tube from the sealing compound, rotate the tube between the thumb and index finger to prevent the sealing compound from pulling out when the tube is lifted out of the sealing compound.

Principle. The capillary tubes must be sealed properly to prevent leakage of the blood specimen during centrifugation.

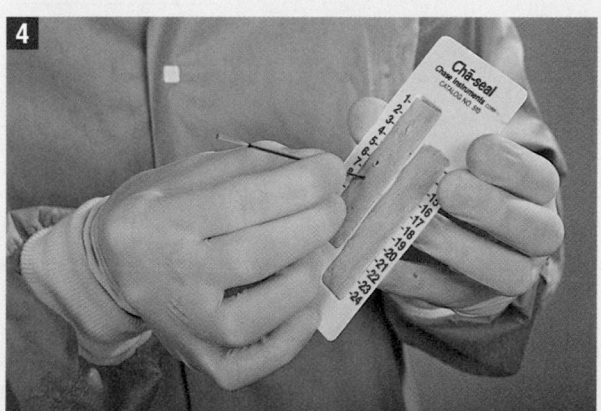

Seal one end of the tube. (From Bonewit-West K: *Clinical procedures for medical assistants,* ed 7, St. Louis, 2008, Saunders.)

5. **Procedural Step.** Place the capillary tubes in the microhematocrit centrifuge with the sealed end facing out. Balance one tube with the other capillary tube placed on the opposite side of the centrifuge.

Principle. Placing the sealed end toward the outside prevents the blood specimen from spinning out of the capillary tube when the centrifuge is in operation.

Place the tube in the centrifuge. (From Bonewit-West K: *Clinical procedures for medical assistants,* ed 7, St. Louis, 2008, Saunders.)

6. **Procedural Step.** Place the cover on the centrifuge, and lock it securely. Centrifuge the blood specimen for 3 to 5 minutes at a speed of 10,000 rpm.

Principle. Centrifuging the blood specimen causes the RBCs to become packed and to settle on the bottom of the tube.

7. **Procedural Step.** Allow the centrifuge to come to a complete stop. Read the results, as follows:

Calibrated tube. If a capillary tube with a calibration line was used, read the results using the special graphic reading device that is part of the centrifuge. Adjust the capillary tube so that the bottom of the RBC column (just above the sealing compound) is placed on the 0 line. With a magnifying glass, read the results at the top of the packed RBC column, and you will see a percentage on the reading device.

Uncalibrated tube. If an uncalibrated tube was used, you must use a microhematocrit reader card to determine the results; place the top of the plasma column on the 100% mark and the bottom of the cell column on the 0 line. Read the results on the scale, which corresponds to the top of the packed cell column.

In both cases, the buffy coat should not be included in the reading. The answer represents the percentage of blood volume occupied by the RBCs. (The hematocrit determination on this reading device is 38.)

Principle. Stopping the centrifuge with your hands can injure you and damage the machine.

8. **Procedural Step.** Read the second tube in the manner just described; the results of the tubes should agree within 4 percentage points. If not, the hematocrit procedure must be repeated. If they are within 4 percentage points, the two values are averaged to derive the test results.

9. **Procedural Step.** Properly dispose of the capillary tubes in a biohazard sharps container. Remove gloves and sanitize your hands. Chart the results. Include the date and time and the hematocrit results.

Continued

PROCEDURE 32-1

PROCEDURE 32-1 Hematocrit—cont'd

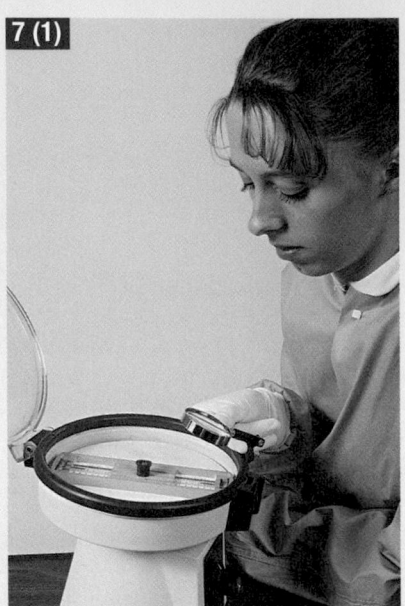

7 (1)

Align the bottom of the red cell column with the 0 line. (From Bonewit-West K: *Clinical procedures for medical assistants,* ed 7, St. Louis, 2008, Saunders.)

7 (2)

Read the results. (From Bonewit-West K: *Clinical procedures for medical assistants,* ed 7, St. Louis, 2008, Saunders.)

10. **Procedural Step.** Return the equipment to its proper storage place. Store the sealing compound at room temperature. Exposing it to a temperature above 80°F adversely affects its consistency.

   Normal Range for Hematocrit:
   Female: 37% to 47%
   Male: 40% to 54%

CHARTING EXAMPLE

Date	
5/5/10	11:15 a.m. Hct: 38%. ————————
	———————— L. Sharpe, CMA (AAMA)

What Would You Do? What Would You *Not* Do?

Case Study 2
Baylee Frasure brings in her 6-month-old son, Travis, for a well-child visit. Mrs. Frasure has been breastfeeding Travis since he was born, and he is not yet on solid food. She says that Travis has been doing just fine, but he did not like his liquid vitamins, so she stopped giving them to him. Mrs. Frasure says that she is eating a well-balanced diet and takes a multivitamin every day, so she did not think it would be a problem. Travis's hemoglobin is checked during the visit, and it is 8 g/dL. The physician prescribes ferrous sulfate drops for Travis. After the physician leaves the room, Mrs. Frasure becomes quite upset. She says she does not understand why Travis' hemoglobin is so low. She says that she thought that breast milk provided the best nutrition possible for infants. ■

WHITE BLOOD CELL COUNT

The WBC count is used by the physician to assist in the diagnosis and prognosis of disease. The WBC count is an approximate measurement of the number of WBCs in the circulating blood. The normal range for a WBC count is 4500 to 11,000 WBCs per cubic millimeter of blood, which is expressed as 4.5 to 11 ($\times 10^3$/mm^3) on laboratory reports. An increase in the WBC count, or **leukocytosis,** is most commonly seen in acute infections, such as appendicitis, chickenpox, diphtheria, infectious mononucleosis, meningitis, and rheumatic fever. A normal elevation of the WBC count can occur with pregnancy, strenuous exercise, stress, and treatment with corticosteroids. Conditions that result in leukopenia, or a decrease in the WBC count, include viral infections, chemotherapy, and radiation therapy.

If the WBC count is performed in the medical office, an automated blood cell counter is used. Blood cell counters are also able to perform an RBC count, platelet count, hemoglobin, hematocrit, differential WBC count, and calculation of RBC indices. Examples of blood cell counters include the QBC Autoread (Beckton-Dickinson), the Cell-

Dyn (Abbott), and the Coulter (Coulter Company) (Figure 32-2).

RED BLOOD CELL COUNT

The RBC count is a measurement of the number of RBCs in whole blood. The range for the RBC count in a healthy woman is 4 to 5.5 million RBCs per cubic millimeter of blood, expressed as 4 to 5.5 ($\times 10^6/mm^3$) on laboratory reports. The range for a healthy man is 4.5 to 6.2 million RBCs per cubic millimeter of blood, expressed as 4.5 to 6.2 ($\times 10^6/mm^3$) on a laboratory report. In the medical office, the RBC count is performed using an automated blood cell counter.

Conditions that cause a decrease in the RBC count include anemia, Hodgkin's disease, and leukemia; conditions that cause an increase of RBCs include polycythemia, dehydration, and pulmonary fibrosis.

WHITE BLOOD CELL DIFFERENTIAL COUNT

WBCs, or leukocytes, are of five types, each having a certain size, shape, appearance, and function: neutrophils, eosinophils, basophils, lymphocytes, and monocytes (Figure 32-3). The purpose of the differential cell count is to identify and count the five types of WBCs in a representative blood sample. An increase or decrease in one or more types may occur in pathologic conditions, which assists the physician in making a diagnosis.

The differential cell count can be performed automatically or manually. The automatic method is faster and more convenient and, because of this, is growing in popularity.

Automatic Method

The automatic method involves the use of a blood cell counter, such as the Coulter cell counter (see Figure 32-2). The specimen requirement is an ethylenediaminetetraacetic acid (EDTA)–anticoagulated blood specimen, which is obtained through venipuncture using a lavender stoppered

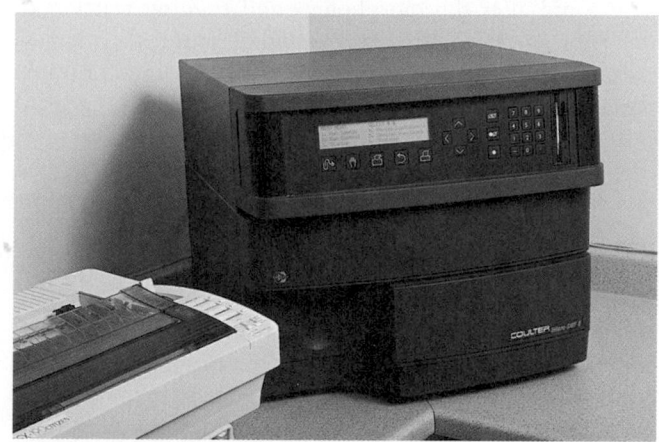

Figure 32-2. Coulter blood cell counter. (From Bonewit-West K: *Clinical procedures for medical assistants,* ed 7, St. Louis, 2008, Saunders.)

Figure 32-3. Types of human blood cells. *1* to *7,* White blood cells (leukocytes) stained as they are in the laboratory to show the many types. They play the active role in immune response or in defense against disease. *1,* Neutrophil; *2,* neutrophilic band; *3,* eosinophil; *4,* basophil; *5,* lymphocyte; *6,* (large) lymphocyte; *7,* monocyte; *8,* platelets (thrombocytes), which are responsible for clotting; *9,* red blood cells (erythrocytes), which carry oxygen. (From Custer RP: *An atlas of the blood and bone marrow,* ed 2, Philadelphia, 1974, Saunders.)

PROCEDURE 32-2

tube. The blood cell counter automatically performs the differential cell count, and the results are printed on a laboratory report.

Manual Method

The manual method requires that the medical assistant make two blood smears. The preparation of a blood smear is outlined in Procedure 32-2. Fresh whole blood is preferred for blood smears; however, a satisfactory smear can be made from an EDTA-anticoagulated blood specimen, provided that the smear is made within 2 hours after collection. Other anticoagulants should not be used because they could alter the morphology and staining reaction of the WBCs. After preparing the blood smear, the medical assistant places the slides in a protective container for transportation to an outside laboratory. The blood smear is evaluated at the laboratory by medical laboratory personnel. Because WBCs are clear and colorless, they must be stained first with an appropriate dye (usually Wright's stain) before a differential count is performed. The nucleus, cytoplasm, and any granules in the cytoplasm take on the characteristic color of their cell type, which aids in proper identification. A minimum of 100 WBCs is identified on the blood smear, and each is assigned to its appropriate category (neutrophil, eosinophil, basophil, lymphocyte, or monocyte). The number of each type of leukocyte is recorded as a percentage and reflects the overall distribution of WBCs in the patient's bloodstream.

Normal Range

The healthy adult range for each type of WBC making up the total number of leukocytes is listed here:

> Neutrophils: 50% to 70%
> Eosinophils: 1% to 4%
> Basophils: 0% to 1%
> Lymphocytes: 20% to 35%
> Monocytes: 3% to 8%

Memories *from* **Externship**

Latisha Sharpe: During my externship experience, I had a female patient who drank too much the night before and had been vomiting for 3 hours before coming to the physician's office. Although this incident was self-inflicted, I still found myself feeling deeply sorry for the patient. She was so weak she could not hold her head up, so I stayed with her and held her head up while she was vomiting. I stayed with her throughout this time, and my sympathy for her really made a difference. No matter what the situation is, I always let the patient know that I care. ■

Prepare for Success

What Would You Do? What Would You *Not* Do?

Case Study 3

Marjorie Merrick comes to the office for a follow-up visit to discuss her laboratory results with the physician. Marjorie is in perimenopause and has been having problems with heavy menstrual periods, hot flashes, insomnia, fatigue, and shortness of breath. Marjorie's laboratory tests indicate that she has iron deficiency anemia. The physician orders an injection of iron dextran, Z-track technique, and instructs Marjorie to take an iron supplement every day and to return in 3 months for a recheck. Marjorie says she has heard that an iron injection can stain the skin and wants to know whether that is true. She says she has a friend who has anemia, and he has to go in every week for a vitamin B_{12} shot. Marjorie wants to know whether she will have to do that, too. Marjorie signed up to donate blood this week at her church's Red Cross blood drive. She wants to know whether it is all right for her to donate. ■

 PROCEDURE 32-2   Preparation of a Blood Smear for a Differential Cell Count

Outcome   Prepare a blood smear for a differential WBC count.

Equipment/Supplies

- Disposable gloves
- Supplies to perform a finger puncture or venipuncture
- Slides with a frosted edge
- Slide container
- Biohazard specimen bag
- Laboratory request form
- Biohazard sharps container

---

1. **Procedural Step.** Sanitize your hands. Greet the patient and introduce yourself. Identify the patient by full name and date of birth, and explain the procedure.

2. **Procedural Step.** Assemble the equipment. Using a pencil, label two slides on the frosted edge with the patient's name and the date.

Principle. Laboratories request the preparation of two blood smears as a means of quality control.

3. **Procedural Step.** Cleanse the puncture site with an antiseptic wipe. Apply gloves, obtain a blood sample from the patient, and place a drop of fresh whole blood on each slide as follows:

From a venipuncture. You can obtain the blood specimen from the fresh whole blood left in the needle immediately after performing a venipuncture as follows: After withdrawing the needle from the patient's arm, deposit the drops of blood remaining in the needle onto the middle of each slide, approximately ¼ inch from the slide's frosted edge.

From a skin puncture. Perform a finger puncture, and wipe away the first drop of blood. Place a drop of blood from the patient's finger in the middle of each slide, approximately ¼ inch from the slide's frosted edge, by touching the slide to the drop of blood. Do not allow the patient's finger to touch the slide.

Principle. If the patient's finger touches the slide, it will spread out the blood specimen, producing an uneven smear. In addition, moisture or oil from the patient's finger could interfere with the smear.

4. **Procedural Step.** Make the blood smear as follows:

a. Hold a second "spreader" slide in front of the drop of blood and at a 30-degree angle to the first slide.

b. Move the spreader slide until it touches the drop of blood. The blood distributes itself along the edge of the spreader by capillary action.

c. Using a smooth, continuous motion, spread the blood thinly and evenly across the surface of the first slide, ending the motion by lifting the spreader slide off the specimen in a smooth, low arc. The smear should be approximately 1½ inches long. The blood smear is thickest at the beginning and gradually thins to a very fine "feathered" edge.

If the blood smear has been prepared correctly, it exhibits the following characteristics: (a) It is smooth and even with no ridges, holes, lines, streaks, or clumps; (b) it is not too thick or too thin; (c) there is a feathered edge at the thin end of the smear; and (d) there is a margin on all sides of the smear. Repeat this step with the other slide.

Principle. An angle of more than 30 degrees causes the smear to be too thick; the cells overlap, do not stain well, and are smaller than normal, making them difficult to count. If the angle is smaller than 30 degrees, the smear would be too thin, and the cells would be spread out, increasing the time needed to count them.

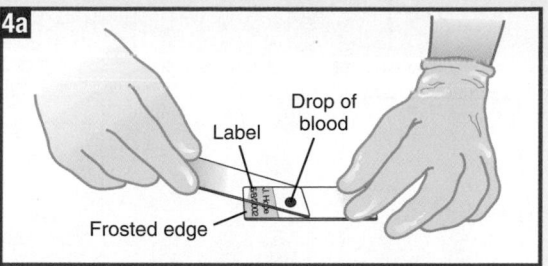

Hold the spreader slide in front of the drop of blood.

Move the spreader into the drop of blood.

Spread the blood across the slide. (From Bonewit-West K: *Clinical procedures for medical assistants,* ed 7, St. Louis, 2008, Saunders.)

5. **Procedural Step.** Dispose of the spreader slide in a biohazard sharps container.

6. **Procedural Step.** Lay the blood smears on a flat surface, and allow them to dry. Never blow on the slides to dry them.

Principle. The blood smears must be dried immediately to prevent shrinkage of the blood cells, which makes them difficult to identify. Blowing on the slide might cause exhaled water droplets to make holes in the smears.

7. **Procedural Step.** Prepare the blood tube and slides for transportation to the laboratory.

8. **Procedural Step.** Remove the gloves, and sanitize your hands.

Continued

PROCEDURE 32-2

PROCEDURE **32-2** Preparation of a Blood Smear for a Differential Cell Count—cont'd

Properly prepared blood smear.

Slide contains ridges

Slide contains holes

Slide contains streaks

Slide is too thin

The length of the smear is too short

Improperly prepared blood smears. (From Rodak BF: *Hematology: clinical principles and applications,* Philadelphia, 1995, Saunders.)

CHARTING EXAMPLE

Date	
5/05/10	11:15 a.m. Venous blood specimen collected
	from Ⓡ arm. Specimen to Medical Center
	Laboratory for CBC c̄ diff on 5/05/10. ———
	————————— L. Sharpe, CMA (AAMA)

MEDICAL PRACTICE *and the* LAW

When dealing with blood, any specimen can contain bloodborne pathogens, such as hepatitis B and HIV. If spraying or splashing of blood is a possibility, use personal protective equipment, including gloves, mask, and goggles.

Laboratory test results are confidential. Giving out results without the patient's permission can result in an invasion of privacy lawsuit. Usually only the physician gives these results so that he or she can explain their meaning to the patient. ■

What Would You Do? What Would You *Not* Do? RESPONSES

Case Study 1
Page 771

What Did Latisha Do?

❑ Told Theodore that the physician was running some routine screening tests on him to make sure he is in good health. Explained that all patients have these tests run as part of a physical examination.

❑ Told Theodore that it was not possible to get the specimen from the earlobe. Explained that the earlobe is not recommended as a good site to obtain blood.

❑ Reassured Theodore that the fingerstick would be made on the least sensitive part of his finger. Told him that it would hurt for just a second, and then it would be all over and it would heal quickly.

❑ Told Theodore that the purpose of the blood test is for the early detection of anemia. Explained that if anemia is present, it can be caught early and treated before symptoms develop.

What Did Latisha Not *Do?*

❑ Did not collect the specimen from Theodore's earlobe.

❑ Did not tell Theodore that he is healthy and does not have anything wrong with him.

What Would You Do?/What Would You *Not* Do? Review Latisha's response and place a checkmark next to the information you included in your response. List additional information you included in your response.

_____

_____

_____

_____

Case Study 2
Page 774

What Did Latisha Do?

❑ Commended Mrs. Frasure on eating nutritiously.

❑ Told Mrs. Frasure that breast milk does not contain very much iron. Explained that because of that, it is important to give Travis his liquid vitamins because they have iron in them.

❑ Reassured Mrs. Frasure that breastfeeding does provide very good nutrition for Travis.

❑ Explained to Mrs. Frasure that the iron supplement may cause Travis's stool to be a dark, tarlike color, and she should not be alarmed because this is normal.

What Did Latisha Not *Do?*

❑ Did not criticize Mrs. Frasure for not giving Travis his vitamins or make her feel it was her fault that his hemoglobin was low.

What Would You Do?/What Would You *Not* Do? Review Latisha's response and place a checkmark next to the information you included in your response. List additional information you included in your response.

_____

_____

_____

_____

Case Study 3
Page 776

What Did Latisha Do?

❑ Told Marjorie that the iron injection can stain the skin but that it would be given in a special way to prevent that from happening.

❑ Told Marjorie vitamin B$_{12}$ injections are given for pernicious anemia and that her type of anemia is iron deficiency anemia.

❑ Gave Marjorie a patient education brochure on iron deficiency anemia to take home with her.

❑ Told Marjorie that the Red Cross requires a blood donor's hemoglobin level to be within normal range. Explained that she could not donate this time, but when her hemoglobin was back to normal she would be able to donate.

❑ Explained to Marjorie that the iron supplement may cause her stool to be a dark, tarlike color, and she should not be alarmed because this is normal.

What Did Latisha Not *Do?*

❑ Did not tell Marjorie that her friend has pernicious anemia because there is no way of knowing this.

What Would You Do?/What Would You *Not* Do? Review Latisha's response and place a checkmark next to the information you included in your response. List additional information you included in your response.

_____

_____

_____

_____

↻ TERMINOLOGY REVIEW

Anemia A condition in which there is a decrease in the erythrocytes or amount of hemoglobin in the blood.

Hematology The study of blood and blood-forming tissues.

Hemoglobin The iron-containing pigment of erythrocytes that transports oxygen in the body.

Leukocytosis An abnormal increase in the number of white blood cells (greater than 11,000 per cubic millimeter of blood).

Leukopenia An abnormal decrease in the number of white blood cells (less than 4500 per cubic millimeter of blood).

Polycythemia A disorder in which there is an increase in the red blood cell mass.

🖾 ON THE WEB

For Information on Stress and Stress Management:

American Institute of Stress: www.stress.org

The Medical Basis of Stress, Depression, Anxiety, Sleep Problems, and Drug Use: www.teachhealth.com

The Anxiety Panic Internet Resource: www.algy.com/anxiety

Stress Tips: www.stresstips.com

𝄜 PREPARE FOR CERTIFICATION
Visit the Evolve site at http://evolve.elsevier.com/Bonewit/today/ to actively Prepare for your Certification.

*Check out the **Companion CD** bound with the book to access additional interactive activities.*

33

Blood Chemistry and Serology

LEARNING OBJECTIVES

Blood Chemistry

1. Explain the purpose of a blood chemistry test.
2. Describe the function of LDL cholesterol and HDL cholesterol in the body.
3. State the desirable ranges for each of the following tests: total cholesterol, LDL cholesterol, and HDL cholesterol.
4. State the patient preparation for a triglyceride test.
5. Explain the functions of glucose and insulin in the body.
6. State the patient preparation for an FBS.
7. Identify the normal range for an FBS.
8. State the purpose of each of the following tests: FBS, 2-hour postprandial glucose test, and glucose tolerance test (GTT).
9. Describe the procedure for a 2-hour postprandial blood sugar test.
10. Identify the patient preparation required for a GTT.
11. State the restrictions that must be followed by the patient during a GTT.
12. List three advantages of self-monitoring of blood glucose by diabetic patients.
13. Explain the purpose of the hemoglobin A_{1c} test.
14. State the A_{1c} level for an individual without diabetes.
15. State the recommended blood glucose level and hemoglobin A_{1c} percentage for an individual with diabetes.
16. Explain the storage requirements for blood glucose reagent strips.

Serology

1. Explain the purpose of each of the following serologic tests: hepatitis tests, syphilis test, mononucleosis test, rheumatoid factor, antistreptolysin test, C-reactive protein, cold agglutinins, ABO and Rh blood typing, and Rh antibody titer.
2. List the symptoms of infectious mononucleosis.

PROCEDURES

Perform blood chemistry testing, using an automated blood chemistry analyzer and operating manual.
Perform a fasting blood sugar (FBS) using a glucose monitor.
Instruct a patient in how to measure blood glucose using a glucose monitor.

Demonstrate the proper care and maintenance of a glucose monitor.

Perform a rapid mononucleosis test.

CHAPTER OUTLINE

CAAHEP COMPETENCIES

Clinical Competencies
Diagnostic Testing
- CLIA-waived tests (perform chemistry testing).
- CLIA-waived tests (perform immunology testing).

Patient Care
- Screen and follow up test results.

General Competencies
Patient Instruction
- Instruct individuals according to their needs.
- Provide instruction for health maintenance and disease prevention.

Operational Functions
- Use methods of quality control.

ABHES COMPETENCIES

Clinical Duties
- Use quality control.
- Perform selected CLIA-waived tests that assist with diagnosis and treatment.
- Screen and follow up patient test results.
- Perform chemistry testing.
- Perform immunology testing.

Instruction
- Teach patients methods of health promotion and disease prevention.

KEY TERMS

agglutination (ah-gloo-ti-NAY-shun)
antibody (AN-ti-bod-ee)
antigen (AN-ti-jen)
glycogen (GLIE-koe-jen)
glycosylation
HDL cholesterol

hemoglobin A$_{1c}$
hyperglycemia (hie-per-glie-SEE-me-ah)
hypoglycemia (hie-poe-glie-SEE-me-ah)
LDL cholesterol
lipoprotein (lie-poe-PROE-teen)

Introduction to Blood Chemistry and Serology

Blood chemistry and serologic laboratory tests are often performed in the medical office. Advances in automated blood analyzers designed for use in the medical office have made this possible. Automated blood analyzers perform laboratory tests in a short time with accurate test results.

Each automated analyzer is accompanied by a detailed operating manual explaining its operation, test parameters, care, and maintenance.

This chapter is divided into two units. The first presents blood chemistry laboratory tests, and the second presents serologic tests. The material in this chapter about blood testing is intended to serve only as a basic guide for the medical assistant and should be supplemented by much well-supervised practice in a classroom laboratory, the medical office, or both.

BLOOD CHEMISTRY

Blood chemistry testing involves the quantitative measurement of chemical substances in the blood. These chemicals are dissolved in the liquid portion of the blood; most blood chemistry tests require a serum specimen for analysis. Numerous types of blood chemistry tests are available; the type of test (or tests) the physician orders depends on the clinical diagnosis. Table 33-1 lists common blood chemistry tests with specimen requirements, normal values, and conditions that cause abnormal test results. The most frequently performed blood chemistry tests are described in more detail in this chapter.

AUTOMATED BLOOD CHEMISTRY ANALYZERS

In the medical office, automated blood chemistry analyzers may be used to perform blood chemistry testing. A blood chemistry analyzer consists of a reflectance photometer that quantitatively measures the amount of chemical substances, or *analytes,* in the blood. Specifically, a reflectance photometer measures light intensity to determine the exact amount of an analyte in a specimen. Examples of blood chemistry analyzers used to perform moderately complex blood chemistry tests in the medical office include the ATAC Lab System (Rankin Biomedical Corporation, Holly, Mich.) (Figure 33-1) and the Reflotron Analyzer (Roche Diagnostics, Indianapolis). Examples of blood chemistry analyzers used to run CLIA-waived blood chemistry tests in the medical office include the Accu-Check Advantage blood glucose meter (Roche Diagnostics) and the Cholestech LDX Cholesterol System (Cholestech Corporation, Hayward, Calif.).

The manufacturer of each automated analyzer provides a detailed operating manual with the instrument that includes the information necessary to collect, handle, and

Table 33-1 Common Blood Chemistry Tests

Name of Test (Abbreviation)	Purpose	Normal Range	Increased with	Decreased with
Alanine aminotransferase (ALT)	To detect liver disease	45 U/L or less	Hepatocellular disease Active cirrhosis Metastatic liver tumor Obstructive jaundice Pancreatitis	—
Alkaline phosphatase (ALP)	Assists in diagnosis of liver and bone diseases	25-140 U/L	Liver disease Bone disease Hyperparathyroidism Infectious mononucleosis	Hypophosphatasia Malnutrition Hypothyroidism Chronic nephritis
Aspartate aminotransferase (AST)	To detect tissue damage	40 U/L or less	Myocardial infarction Liver disease Acute pancreatitis Acute hemolytic anemia	Beriberi Uncontrolled diabetes mellitus with acidosis
Blood urea nitrogen (BUN)	Screens for renal disease, especially glomerular functioning	7-25 mg/dL (SI units: 2.5-6.4 mmol/L)	Kidney disease Urinary obstruction Dehydration Gastrointestinal bleeding	Liver failure Malnutrition Impaired absorption
Calcium (Ca)	To assess parathyroid functioning and calcium metabolism and evaluate malignancies	8.5-10.8 mg/dL (SI units: 2.13-2.76 mmol/L)	**Hypercalcemia** Hyperparathyroidism Bone metastases Multiple myeloma Hodgkin's disease Addison's disease Hyperthyroidism	**Hypocalcemia** Hypoparathyroidism Acute pancreatitis Renal failure
Chloride (Cl)	Assists in diagnosing disorders of acid-base and water balance	96-109 mmol/L	Dehydration Cushing's syndrome Hyperventilation Preeclampsia Anemia	Severe vomiting Severe diarrhea Ulcerative colitis Pyloric obstruction Severe burns Heat exhaustion

Table 33-1 Common Blood Chemistry Tests—cont'd

Name of Test (Abbreviation)	Purpose	Normal Range	Increased with	Decreased with
Cholesterol (Chol)	To screen for atherosclerosis related to coronary heart disease; secondary aid in study of thyroid and liver functioning	**Total Cholesterol** Less than 200 mg/dL (SI units: less than 5.18 mmol/L)—*desirable* 200-239 mg/dL (SI units: 5.18-6.19 mmol/L)—*borderline high* 240 mg/dL or greater (6.22 mmol/L or greater)—*high* **LDL Cholesterol** Less than 100 mg/dL (SI units: less than 2.6 mmol/L)—*optimal* 100-129 mg/dL (SI units: 2.6-3.34 mmol/L)—*near optimal* 130-159 mg/dL (SI units: 3.4-4.14 mmol/L)—*borderline high* 160-189 mg/dL (SI units: 4.14-4.9 mmol/L)—*high* 190 mg/dL or greater (SI units: 4.92 mmol/L or greater)—*very high* **HDL Cholesterol** 60 mg/dL or greater (SI units: 1.55 mmol/L or greater)—*optimal* 45-59 mg/dL (SI units: 1.16-1.53 mmol/L)—*desirable* 40-45 mg/dL (SI units: 1.04-1.17 mmol/L)—*borderline low* Less than 40 mg/dL (SI units: less than 1.04 mmol/L)—*increased risk for coronary heart disease*	Atherosclerosis Cardiovascular disease Obstructive jaundice Hypothyroidism Nephrosis	Malabsorption Liver disease Hyperthyroidism Anemia
Creatinine (Creat)	Screening test of renal functioning	0.6-1.5 mg/dL (SI units: 46-115 μmol/L)	Impaired renal function Chronic nephritis Obstruction of urinary tract Muscle disease	Muscular dystrophy
Globulin (Glob)	To identify abnormalities in rate of protein synthesis and removal	2-3.5 g/dL (SI units: 20-35 g/L)	Brucellosis Chronic infections Rheumatoid arthritis Dehydration Hepatic carcinoma Hodgkin's disease	Agammaglobulinemia Severe burns

Continued

Table 33-1 Common Blood Chemistry Tests—cont'd

Name of Test (Abbreviation)	Purpose	Normal Range	Increased with	Decreased with
Glucose	To detect disorders of glucose metabolism	—	**Hyperglycemia**	**Hypoglycemia**
Fasting blood sugar (FBS)	—	**FBS:** 70-110 mg/dL (SI units: 3.9-6.1 mmol/L)	Diabetes mellitus	Excess insulin
2-hour postprandial blood sugar (2-hr PPBS)	—	**2-hr PPBS:** less than 140 mg/dL (SI units: less than 7.8 mmol/L)	Hepatic disease	Addison's disease
Glucose tolerance test (GTT)	—	**GTT** **FBS:** 70-110 mg/dL (SI units: 3.9-6.1 mmol/L)—*normal* **FBS:** greater than 120 mg/dL (SI units: greater than 6.7 mmol/L)—*diabetic* **30 min:** 150-160 mg/dL (SI units: 8.4-8.9 mmol/L)—*normal* **30 min:** greater than 200 mg/dL (SI units: greater than 11.1 mmol/L)—*diabetic* **1 hr:** 160-170 mg/dL (SI units: 8.9-9.5 mmol/L)—*normal* **1 hr:** greater than 200 mg/dL (SI units: greater than 11.1 mmol/L)—*diabetic* **2 hr:** 120 mg/dL (SI units: 6.7 mmol/L)—*normal* **2 hr:** greater than 140 mg/dL (SI units: greater than 7.8 mmol/L)—*diabetic* **3 hr:** 70-110 mg/dL (SI units: 3.9-6.1 mmol/L)—*normal* **3 hr:** greater than 140 mg/dL (SI units: greater than 7.8 mmol/L)—*diabetic*	Brain damage Cushing's syndrome	Bacterial sepsis Pancreatic carcinoma Hepatic necrosis Hypothyroidism
Lactate dehydrogenase, 30°C (LD)	Assists in confirming myocardial or pulmonary infarction; also used in differential diagnosis of muscular dystrophy and pernicious anemia	240 U/L or less	Acute myocardial infarction Acute leukemia Muscular dystrophy Pernicious anemia Hemolytic anemia Hepatic disease Extensive cancer	—

Table 33-1 Common Blood Chemistry Tests—cont'd

Name of Test (Abbreviation)	Purpose	Normal Range	Increased with	Decreased with
Phosphorus (P)	Assists in proper evaluation and interpretation of calcium levels; used to detect disorders of endocrine system, bone diseases, and kidney dysfunction	2.5-4.5 mg/dL (SI units: 0.81-1.45 mmol/L)	**Hyperphosphatemia** Renal insufficiency Severe nephritis Hypoparathyroidism Hypocalcemia Addison's disease	**Hypophosphatemia** Hyperparathyroidism Rickets and osteomalacia Diabetic coma Hyperinsulinism
Potassium (K)	To diagnose disorders of acid-base and water balance in the body	3.5-5.3 mmol/L	**Hyperkalemia** Renal failure Cell damage Acidosis Addison's disease Internal bleeding	**Hypokalemia** Diarrhea Pyloric obstruction Starvation Malabsorption Severe vomiting Severe burns Diuretic administration Chronic stress Liver disease with ascites
Sodium (Na)	To detect changes in water and salt balance in the body	135-147 mmol/L	**Hypernatremia** Dehydration Conn's syndrome Primary aldosteronism Coma Cushing's disease Diabetes insipidus	**Hyponatremia** Severe burns Severe diarrhea Addison's disease Severe nephritis Pyloric obstruction
Total bilirubin (TB)	To evaluate liver functioning and hemolytic anemia	0.2-1.3 mg/dL (SI units: 3.4-22.4 μmol/L)	Liver disease Obstruction of common bile or hepatic duct Hemolytic anemia	—
Total protein (TP)	Screens for diseases that alter protein balance and assesses state of body hydration	6-8.5 g/dL (SI units: 60-85 g/L)	Dehydration (vomiting, diarrhea) Chronic infections Acute liver disease Multiple myeloma Lupus erythematosus	Severe hemorrhaging Hodgkin's disease Severe liver disease Malabsorption
Total thyroxine (Total T$_4$)	To assess thyroid functioning and evaluate thyroid replacement therapy	4.5-12 μg/dL (SI units: 58-155 nmol/L)	**Hyperthyroidism** Graves' disease Thyrotoxicosis Thyroiditis	**Hypothyroidism** Cretinism Goiter Myxedema Hypoproteinemia
Triglycerides (Trig)	To evaluate patients with suspected atherosclerosis	Less than 150 mg/dL— *desirable* 150-199 mg/dL— *borderline high* 200-499 mg/dL—*high* 500 mg/dL or greater— *very high*	Liver disease Nephrotic syndrome Hypothyroidism Poorly controlled diabetes Pancreatitis	Malnutrition Congenital lipoproteinemia
Uric acid (UA)	To evaluate renal failure, gout, and leukemia	Male: 3.9-9 mg/dL (SI units: 232-596 μmol/L) Female: 2.2-7.7 mg/dL (SI units: 131-458 μmol/L)	Renal failure Gout Leukemia Severe eclampsia Lymphomas	Patients undergoing treatment with uricosuric drugs

From Bonewit-West K: *Clinical procedures for medical assistants,* ed 7, St. Louis, 2008, Saunders.

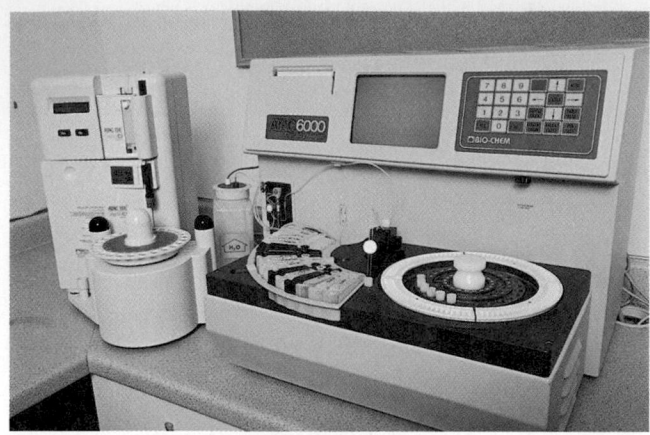

Figure 33-1. Blood chemistry analyzer (ATAC Lab System by Rankin Biomedical Corporation, Holly, Mich.).

test the specimen and to perform quality control procedures. In addition, the manufacturer has personnel available for on-site training and service.

QUALITY CONTROL

Quality control consists of methods and means to ensure that test results are reliable and valid. Two important quality control measures must be performed routinely when using a blood chemistry analyzer: calibration of the instrument and running controls.

Calibration involves the use of a standard to check the precision of the blood chemistry analyzer. If an analyzer is not properly calibrated, it cannot produce accurate test results. If this occurs, the operating manual should be consulted to determine the action that should be taken to correct the problem. Calibration of a blood chemistry analyzer can be compared with placing a scale at zero before weighing a patient. In other words, if the scale is not at zero, the results will not be accurate.

A *control* consists of a sample of a known value. The control is processed in the same manner as a patient specimen, and the results should fall within a specified range as indicated on a reference sheet that accompanies each control. Normal and abnormal controls are commercially available. Normal controls fall within the normal range, whereas abnormal controls fall outside the normal range. Low abnormal controls fall below the normal range, and high abnormal controls fall above the normal range. If the control does not fall within its specified range, problems or errors exist, either with the analyzer itself or with the technique or chemical reagents used to perform the testing procedure. The operating manual should be consulted to determine the action to take to correct the situation. A control can be compared with placing an object with a known weight of 5 lb on a scale. The scale should weigh the object at 5 lb; otherwise, the results are not valid.

The Clinical Laboratory Improvement Amendments of 1988 (CLIA 1988) require the following for moderately complex laboratory tests: The calibration procedure must be performed and documented at least every 6 months, and two levels of controls must be performed daily (e.g., running a normal control and a high control). In addition, when problems or errors are identified, the action taken to correct them must be documented. Medical offices running CLIA-waived tests are required to follow the manufacturer's instructions for each testing procedure. The instructions include the quality control procedures (calibration and controls) that must be performed when running the test.

CHOLESTEROL

Cholesterol is a white, waxy, fatlike substance (lipid) that is essential for normal functioning of the body. It is an important component of cell membranes and is used in the production of hormones and bile. Most of the cholesterol circulating in the blood is manufactured by the liver; however, a portion of it comes from an individual's diet and is known as *dietary cholesterol.* Dietary cholesterol is found only in animal products, such as organ meats, egg yolks, and dairy products.

High blood cholesterol means there is an excessive amount of cholesterol in the blood. An individual's cholesterol level is determined by his or her genetic makeup and by the amount of dietary cholesterol and saturated fat consumed. High blood cholesterol may cause fatty deposits, or plaque, to build up on the walls of the arteries, a condition known as *atherosclerosis.* As the atherosclerosis progresses, the arteries become more occluded, which eventually could lead to a heart attack or stroke. Because of this, high blood cholesterol is considered a risk factor for coronary heart disease (see *Highlight on Coronary Heart Disease*), and efforts should be made to reduce the cholesterol level (see *Highlight on Lowering Cholesterol*).

HDL and LDL Cholesterol

Cholesterol is transported in the blood as a complex molecule known as a **lipoprotein.** Two types of lipoproteins contain cholesterol: low-density lipoprotein (LDL) and high-density lipoprotein (HDL).

LDL picks up cholesterol from ingested fats and from the liver and delivers it to blood vessels and muscles, where it is deposited in the cells. **LDL cholesterol** is often referred to as "bad" cholesterol because an excess amount of it in the blood can cause plaque to build up on the arterial walls, resulting in atherosclerosis. See Table 33-1 for an interpretation of LDL cholesterol values.

HDL removes excess cholesterol from the cells and carries it to the liver to be excreted. Because HDL removes excess cholesterol from the walls of the blood vessels, it is protective and beneficial to the body and is often called "good" cholesterol. A high **HDL cholesterol** level has been shown to reduce the risk of heart disease, whereas a low level

Highlight on Coronary Heart Disease

Coronary heart disease (CHD) affects 6.6 million Americans. The chief forms of CHD are atherosclerosis, high blood pressure, heart attacks, strokes, congestive heart failure, congenital heart disease, and rheumatic heart disease. These various forms of heart disease are interrelated and have elements in common; for example, atherosclerosis can lead to a stroke or heart attack.

Heart disease is the number one killer of adults in the United States today. Because of the national focus on heart disease and cholesterol reduction, since 1985 there has been a decline in heart attacks by 25% and strokes by nearly 40%; however, heart disease is likely to remain the number one cause of death until more Americans adopt a more heart-healthy lifestyle.

Risk Factors

Not everyone is equal when it comes to CHD. Some individuals have a much higher risk of developing it than others. The following are risk factors for CHD:

- High total blood cholesterol (greater than 200 mg/dL confirmed by repeated measurement)
- High blood pressure
- Cigarette smoking (more than 10 cigarettes per day)
- Family history of premature CHD (definite heart attack or sudden death in a parent or sibling before age 55 years)
- Diabetes mellitus
- History of blood vessel disease
- Obesity (30% or more overweight)
- Low HDL cholesterol (less than 40 mg/dL confirmed by repeated measurement)
- Being a man older than 45 years
- Being a woman older than 55 years or postmenopausal

Some of these risk factors can be modified; others, such as age, gender, and a family history of CHD, cannot be modified or controlled. The three major risk factors for CHD are high total blood cholesterol, high blood pressure, and cigarette smoking, which all are modifiable.

Each person's overall risk of CHD must be assessed individually by the physician, based on the type and number of risk factors present. A 47-year-old man with a cholesterol level of 220 mg/dL who smokes a pack of cigarettes a day and is overweight is at greater risk than a 28-year-old man who is within normal weight, does not smoke, and exercises regularly but has a cholesterol level of 250 mg/dL. ∎

Highlight on Lowering Cholesterol

Research has shown, beyond doubt, that high total blood cholesterol is a major risk factor for coronary heart disease, and the higher the cholesterol, the greater the risk. The National Institutes of Health (NIH) has established guidelines on safe levels of blood cholesterol. The NIH recommends that adults not exceed 200 mg/dL of blood cholesterol.

The National Cholesterol Educational Program (NCEP) was established in 1985 by the federal government to reduce the prevalence of elevated blood cholesterol levels in the United States by educating the public about the health risks associated with high blood cholesterol and to make recommendations for helping individuals reduce their cholesterol levels. It has been shown that for every 1% that an individual lowers his or her total blood cholesterol, the risk of coronary heart disease is reduced by 2%. Taking the following measures can help individuals reduce their level of "bad" LDL cholesterol and increase their level of "good" HDL cholesterol.

Diet

Dietary therapy is the first line of treatment of high blood cholesterol. The NCEP recommends that all individuals (older than 2 years of age) reduce dietary cholesterol and saturated fats. Many foods high in fat tend to be high in cholesterol. Reading nutrition labels on packaged products helps provide information on the cholesterol and fat content of a food.

Dietary Cholesterol

The body manufactures all the cholesterol it needs for normal functioning, and dietary intake of cholesterol (in foods) serves only to increase the blood cholesterol. According to the NCEP, dietary cholesterol should be limited to 300 mg daily, which is slightly more than the amount of cholesterol in one egg (270 mg). Cholesterol is found only in animal foods and shellfish. Egg yolks, dairy products, and organ meats, such as liver and kidneys, are especially high in cholesterol.

Saturated Fat

The intake of saturated fat is the most important dietary factor leading to high blood cholesterol, even more so than consuming dietary cholesterol. In general, the more saturated a fat is, the harder and more solid it is at room temperature. The main source of saturated fat is animal products, including meat fat, poultry skin, and the fat in dairy products (butter, cream, ice cream, cheese, whole milk). Unsaturated fats have little or no effect on the blood cholesterol level; they include olive oil, canola oil, peanut oil, and sunflower, safflower, and corn oil. The NCEP recommends that no more than 30% of the calories consumed each day come from fat, with no more than 10% of calories coming from saturated fat and the remaining 20% from unsaturated fat.

Continued

Highlight on Lowering Cholesterol—cont'd

Soluble Fiber

Soluble fiber has been shown to lower the cholesterol level by keeping the cholesterol consumed from being absorbed by the body. Examples of foods high in soluble fiber are bran, oats, and beans.

Weight Reduction

An estimated one in four Americans is overweight. It is recommended that these individuals follow a sensible eating plan along with an exercise program to reach and maintain desirable weight. Losing weight reduces total cholesterol and triglyceride levels. Overweight and obese people are at very high risk for coronary heart disease because their hearts have to work harder to pump blood through the body.

Exercise

An aerobic exercise program is especially beneficial for weight control because it improves cardiovascular fitness and lowers blood cholesterol level. People who exercise regularly generally have higher HDL cholesterol levels in their blood. Health experts recommend exercising at least three times a week for 20 to 30 minutes at your target heart rate.

Smoking Cessation

Smoking is one of the three main risk factors for coronary heart disease. By quitting smoking, an individual may be able to strengthen the heart and lower the cholesterol level. Also, nonsmokers tend to have higher HDL levels in their blood. A variety of smoking cessation programs are usually available in the community. Some people have succeeded by using nicotine patches, which help them adjust gradually to lower levels of nicotine.

Generally, the cholesterol level begins to decrease 2 to 3 weeks after beginning a cholesterol-lowering diet and other cholesterol-lowering measures. Over time, it is possible to reduce the total cholesterol level by 30 to 55 mg/dL or even more through these lifestyle changes. If the blood cholesterol level cannot be lowered to an acceptable level, the physician may prescribe cholesterol-lowering medications along with the continuation of the aforementioned measures. ■

---

of HDL cholesterol (less than 40 mg/dL) is a risk factor for coronary heart disease.

Cholesterol Testing

All adults older than 20 years old should have a cholesterol test at least once every 5 years. Initial testing includes a *total cholesterol* determination, which is a combined measurement of LDL cholesterol and HDL cholesterol in the blood. To obtain a fuller picture of a patient's cholesterol status, physicians typically also order an HDL cholesterol determination, which measures only the HDL cholesterol in the blood. Cholesterol tests are considered screening tests, and elevated results usually require confirmation through repeat testing before a diagnosis of high blood cholesterol is made.

Interpretation of Results

Cholesterol test results are interpreted as follows: Total cholesterol levels less than 200 mg/dL are desirable. Levels between 200 and 239 mg/dL are borderline high, and levels of 240 mg/dL and greater are high. Based on confirmed testing, individuals in the high category are clearly at increased risk for coronary heart disease, and individuals in the borderline high category are at increased risk if they have other risk factors, such as being overweight or smoking. An HDL cholesterol level greater than 60 mg/dL is considered optimal, and a level less than 40 mg/dL is a risk factor for coronary heart disease (45 to 59 mg/dL is considered desirable and 40 to 45 mg/dL is considered borderline low).

Patient Preparation

Because the total cholesterol and the HDL cholesterol determinations are not affected significantly by food consumption, the patient is usually not required to fast before the collection of the blood specimen. Some physicians prefer the patient to be in a fasting state, however.

If the total cholesterol level is 200 mg/dL or greater, the physician usually orders a *lipid profile,* which includes total cholesterol, HDL cholesterol, LDL cholesterol, and triglycerides. (The LDL cholesterol level is usually determined as a calculation from the results of the triglyceride and HDL cholesterol levels.) Because triglyceride levels are affected by the consumption of food, the patient must be instructed to fast for at least 12 hours before collection of this blood specimen. An elevated triglyceride level (greater than 150 mg/dL) places an individual at an increased risk for coronary heart disease, particularly when the LDL cholesterol is high and the HDL cholesterol is low.

Although the primary use of cholesterol testing is to screen for the presence of high blood cholesterol related to coronary heart disease, this test is also used as a secondary aid in the study of thyroid and liver function. See Table 33-1 for a list of specific conditions that cause abnormal cholesterol test results.

BLOOD UREA NITROGEN

The blood urea nitrogen (BUN) is a kidney function test. Urea is the end product of protein metabolism and is nor-

What Would You Do? What Would You *Not* Do?

Case Study 1

Karen Scrimshaw is at the office. She is 20 years old and mildly obese. Karen had her cholesterol tested at a health fair and it was 325. The physician orders a complete blood count, lipid profile, and thyroid profile on Karen and instructs her to return in 1 week for a follow-up visit to discuss the test results. Karen is very concerned about her cholesterol. She says that she had a candy bar and some potato chips before going to the health fair and wants to know whether that could have caused her cholesterol to be so high. She also wants to know the accuracy of machines that are used at health fairs. Karen says that if she has to go on cholesterol medication, it would be hard to decide between Lipitor and Zocor. She says she has seen them advertised on television, and they both seem pretty good to her. ■

Putting It All into Practice

My name is **Michelle Villers**, and I work for a physician in an internal medicine medical office. My primary job responsibility includes running the laboratory at the office. I mainly draw blood and perform blood chemistry tests. I also work up patients, run electrocardiograms, apply Holter monitors, and perform pulmonary function tests.

When performing a venipuncture, you need to make sure all the necessary equipment is on hand and ready. Sometimes you may have a tube that has no vacuum in it. In cases like these, it is always better to have a couple of spare tubes on hand. I recently had an experience in which one of my tubes had no vacuum. Luckily, I had a few extra tubes within arm's reach, so I did not have to interrupt the procedure to get a new one. I have learned that you can never be too prepared. ■

Prepare for Success

mally present in the blood. Certain kidney diseases may interfere with the ability of the body to excrete the urea properly, causing an increased level of urea in the blood. See Table 33-1 for a list of specific conditions that cause abnormal BUN test results.

BLOOD GLUCOSE

Glucose is the end product of carbohydrate metabolism; it is the chief source of energy for the body. Energy is necessary to perform normal functions and maintain body temperature. The body maintains a constant blood glucose level to ensure a continuous source of energy for the body. Ingested glucose that is not necessary for energy can be stored in the form of **glycogen** in muscle and liver tissue for later use. When no more tissue storage is possible, excess glucose is converted to fat and stored as adipose tissue.

Insulin is a hormone secreted by the beta cells of the pancreas and is required for normal use of glucose in the body. Insulin enables glucose to enter the body's cells and be converted to energy. Insulin is also necessary for the proper storage of glycogen in liver and muscle cells.

Blood Glucose Testing

Measuring the amount of glucose in a blood specimen is one of the most common blood chemistry tests. It is used to detect abnormalities in carbohydrate metabolism such as occur in diabetes mellitus, **hypoglycemia,** and liver and adrenocortical dysfunction. Blood glucose is measured by several different testing methods, which include the fasting blood sugar, the 2-hour postprandial blood sugar test, and the glucose tolerance test. Each of these methods serves a specific role in diagnosing and evaluating abnormalities in carbohydrate metabolism and is described in more detail here.

Fasting Blood Sugar

Blood glucose is usually measured when the patient is in a fasting state. This type of test is termed a *fasting blood sugar*

(FBS), which involves collecting a fasting blood sample and measuring the amount of glucose in it. The patient should not have anything to eat or drink except water for 12 hours preceding the test. Certain medications, such as oral contraceptives, salicylates, diuretics, and steroids, may affect the test results; the physician may also place the patient on medication restrictions for a specific period before the test—usually 3 days. The patient should be scheduled for the test in the morning to minimize the inconvenience of abstaining from food and fluid.

The normal range for an FBS test varies among laboratories and with the specific type of test, but it usually falls between 70 and 110 mg of glucose per 100 ml of blood (or mg/dL). An FBS is often performed on patients diagnosed with diabetes to evaluate their progress and regulate treatment and on patients as a routine screening test to detect diabetes mellitus. FBS greater than 120 mg/dL, considered the dividing point between normal and hyperglycemic values, indicates diabetes mellitus. An elevated test result warrants further testing with the glucose tolerance test.

Two-Hour Postprandial Blood Sugar

The 2-hour postprandial blood sugar (2-hour PPBS) test is used to screen for diabetes mellitus and to monitor the effects of insulin dosage in patients with diabetes. The patient is required to fast, beginning at midnight preceding the test and continuing until breakfast. For breakfast, the patient must consume a prescribed meal that contains 100 g of carbohydrate, which consists of orange juice, cereal with sugar, toast, and milk. An alternative to this is the consumption of a 100-g test-load glucose solution. A blood specimen is collected from the patient exactly 2 hours after consumption of the meal or glucose solution.

In a nondiabetic patient, the glucose level returns to the fasting level within 1½ to 2 hours of glucose consumption, whereas the glucose level in a diabetic patient does not return to the fasting level. A postprandial glucose level of 140 g/dL or higher suggests diabetes mellitus and warrants further testing, such as the glucose tolerance test.

Glucose Tolerance Test

The glucose tolerance test (GTT) provides more detailed information about the ability of the body to metabolize glucose by assessing the insulin response to a glucose load. The GTT is used to assist in the diagnosis of diabetes mellitus, hypoglycemia, and liver and adrenocortical dysfunction. It provides a more thorough analysis of glucose use than either the FBS or the 2-hour PPBS test.

Testing Requirements

The patient is usually required to consume a high-carbohydrate diet, consisting of 150 g of carbohydrate per day, for 3 days before the GTT. The patient must be in a fasting state when the test begins. On the morning of the test, a blood specimen is drawn from the patient for an FBS, and a urine specimen is taken to measure the amount of glucose in each of these samples. If the FBS indicates **hyperglycemia,** the physician should be notified because this situation is a contraindication for the administration of a large test load of glucose.

After the FBS has been performed, the patient is instructed to drink a measured amount of a glucose solution (1.75 g of glucose per kilogram of body weight, or the standard adult dose of 100 g). Thereafter at regular intervals (generally 30, 60, 120, and 180 minutes), blood and urine specimens are taken to determine the patient's ability to handle the increased amount of glucose. Each blood and urine specimen must be labeled carefully with the exact time of collection. The patient is permitted to eat and drink normally after the completion of the test.

It is important that the patient adhere to certain restrictions during the test to ensure accurate results. Because food and fluid affect blood glucose levels, the patient must not eat or drink anything except water during the test. Consumption of water should be encouraged to make it easier for the patient to produce a urine specimen. Smoking is not permitted during the test because tobacco is a stimulant that increases the blood glucose level. The patient should remain at the testing site so that he or she is present when needed for the collection of the blood and urine specimens and to minimize activity. Activity affects the test results by using up glucose; the patient should remain relatively inactive during the test. Sitting and reading is an activity that would be recommended.

Side Effects

Particularly during the second and third hours of the test, the patient may experience some normal side effects, including weakness, a feeling of faintness, and perspiration. These are considered normal reactions of the body to a

What Would You Do? What Would You *Not* Do?

Case Study 2

Crystal Louellen is at the medical office for a GTT. She says that she tried not to eat anything, but she started shaking, so she stopped at McDonald's on the way over and got a sausage biscuit and orange juice. Crystal gets quite upset when she learns that she has to come back again to have her test run. She said that she hired a babysitter to watch her four preschool-age children. She demands to know why this test takes so long and why she can't have anything to eat before the test. Crystal wants to know if she can bring her children next time so she doesn't have to hire a babysitter. Crystal says that she's a "nicotine" addict and when she's not needed for testing she could take the kids outside to play. She says that way the kids won't bother anyone and she can have a cigarette at the same time. ■

decrease in the glucose level as insulin is secreted in response to the glucose load. The patient should be reassured that this is a temporary condition. Serious symptoms of severe hypoglycemia should be reported immediately to the physician, including headache; pale, cold, and clammy skin; irrational speech or behavior; profuse perspiration; and fainting.

Interpretation of Results

The test results are interpreted by evaluating the data obtained for each collection period. If the glucose level is abnormally high compared with established norms for the various blood collection times, a disorder of glucose metabolism, such as diabetes mellitus, may be present. Individuals with diabetes are unable to remove glucose from the bloodstream at the same rate as a nondiabetic individual.

As glucose is absorbed into the bloodstream, the blood glucose level of a nondiabetic individual increases to a peak level of 160 to 180 mg/dL approximately 30 to 60 minutes after the glucose solution is consumed. The pancreas secretes insulin to compensate for this rise, and the blood glucose returns to the fasting level within 2 to 3 hours of ingestion of the glucose solution. In addition, the urine specimens exhibit negative test results for glucose.

The individual with diabetes does not exhibit the normal use of glucose just described. The blood glucose peaks at a much higher level, and glucose is present in the urine. In addition, blood glucose levels are above normal throughout the test because of the lack of insulin. See Table 33-1 for normal and diabetic glucose values. The GTT is generally not used for diagnostic purposes in patients with an FBS greater than 140 mg/dL or a 2-hour postprandial test result greater than 180 mg/dL because results greater than these values would qualify for the diagnosis of diabetes mellitus, and the GTT would not be required.

Hypoglycemia

Hypoglycemia is a condition in which the glucose in the blood is abnormally low. During the GTT, patients with this condition exhibit an abnormally low blood glucose level beginning at the 2-hour interval and continuing for 4 or 5 hours. Hypoglycemia results from glucose removal from the blood at an excessive rate or from a decreased secretion of glucose into the blood, which can be caused by an overdose of insulin, Addison's disease, bacterial sepsis, carcinoma of the pancreas, hepatic necrosis, or hypothyroidism.

TESTS FOR MANAGEMENT OF DIABETES

It is important for individuals with diabetes to manage their condition effectively. This is best accomplished by keeping their blood glucose levels as close to normal as possible. Diabetic patients who maintain good blood glucose control generally experience fewer symptoms and delay or prevent long-term complications of the disease; these results can lead to a longer life.

Two testing methods are used for the management of diabetes—self-monitoring of blood glucose and the hemoglobin A_{1c} test. Self-monitoring of blood glucose is performed by diabetic patients at home and measures day-to-day fluctuations in blood glucose levels. The hemoglobin A_{1c} test must be ordered by the physician and provides an average or overall picture of the patient's blood glucose levels over time. These testing methods assist the patient and physician in determining whether the diabetes management plan is working or whether it needs to be adjusted.

Self-Monitoring of Blood Glucose

Individuals with diabetes cannot usually tell by the way they feel whether or not their blood glucose levels are within normal range. The only way for them to know for certain is by self-monitoring of blood glucose (SMBG). SMBG not only provides diabetic patients with feedback for maintaining normal blood glucose levels, but it also assists them in anticipating and treating day-to-day, or even hour-to-hour,

4 times a day
some doctor do 2 times a day

PATIENT TEACHING | **Diabetes Mellitus**

Answer questions patients have about diabetes mellitus.

What is diabetes?

Diabetes mellitus is a lifelong condition that occurs when the body is not able to use glucose for energy because of a problem with insulin. Diabetes develops when the body produces little or no insulin or when the body cannot use the insulin it does produce (known as *insulin resistance*). According to the American Diabetes Association, almost 21 million Americans have diabetes; of these, nearly 6 million are not yet diagnosed and are unaware that they have diabetes. The cause of diabetes is not completely understood, but it seems that the predisposition to develop diabetes is inherited. Diabetes increases the risk of developing serious complications, including heart disease, blindness (retinopathy), nerve damage (neuropathy), kidney damage (nephropathy), and poor circulation, which can result in amputation of a limb.

What is the function of insulin?

Insulin is a hormone produced and secreted by the beta cells of the pancreas. The pancreas is a gland located just behind the stomach and is about the size of a hand. Insulin is required for the normal use of glucose in the body. Through the process of digestion, carbohydrates are broken down into glucose. Shortly after eating a meal containing carbohydrates, glucose levels in the blood begin to increase. This sends a message to the pancreas to secrete insulin. Insulin "unlocks" the cells of the body and allows glucose to enter the cells. Inside the cells, glucose is converted into energy. Glucose is the main source of energy for the body and is necessary to carry out normal body functions and assist in maintaining body temperature.

What are the symptoms of diabetes?

Individuals with diabetes produce little or no insulin or cannot use the insulin they do produce. Without insulin, glucose cannot get into the cells of the body and builds up in the bloodstream, resulting in a high blood glucose level, known as *hyperglycemia.* Although the blood glucose levels are increased, the body is unable to use the glucose for energy. This results in increased hunger, weight loss, and fatigue. The body attempts to get rid of the excess glucose by expelling it in the urine. To be excreted, the glucose must be diluted in large amounts of water. This results in increased urination and increased thirst to replace the water being lost. A summary of the symptoms of diabetes follows:

    Increased urination
    Excessive thirst
    Weight loss
    Constant hunger
    Nausea and vomiting
    Abdominal pain
    Fatigue
    Blurred vision

What is the difference between type 1 diabetes and type 2 diabetes?

There are two main categories of diabetes: type 1 diabetes and type 2 diabetes. Type 2 diabetes is the most common form of diabetes. Approximately 90% of individuals with this condition have type 2 diabetes.

Type I Diabetes

Type 1 diabetes can occur at any age but is most apt to begin in childhood, adolescence, or early adulthood (before age 30). Type

Continued

PATIENT TEACHING Diabetes Mellitus—cont'd

1 diabetes is an autoimmune disease in which the body produces antibodies that attack and gradually destroy the insulin-producing beta cells of the pancreas. This results in the body not being able to produce any insulin at all or very little insulin. The symptoms are usually severe and occur rapidly—typically over weeks or months. Individuals with type 1 diabetes almost always require insulin therapy. The insulin is administered subcutaneously using an insulin syringe/needle or an insulin pen. An insulin pen is an insulin injection device that contains a needle and holds a vial of insulin. Insulin can also be administered through an insulin pump, which is a small, battery-operated device about the size of a cell phone that is clipped to a belt or carried in a pocket. The pump continuously delivers insulin into the subcutaneous tissue of the abdomen. An insulin pump can also be programmed to deliver varying doses of insulin as a patient's need for insulin changes during the day (e.g., before exercise or meals).

Type II Diabetes

Type 2 diabetes can affect people at any age, but the chance of developing it increases with age and it is more likely to occur in individuals who are 40 years of age or older. The biggest risk factor for developing type 2 diabetes is excess body weight. As a result of the more recent increase in childhood obesity combined with a sedentary lifestyle, type 2 diabetes is starting to appear in younger age groups. Individuals with type 2 diabetes do not produce enough insulin or are not able to use the insulin they do produce (insulin resistance), resulting in high blood glucose levels. Type 2 diabetes almost always has a slow onset with mild symptoms that appear gradually over a long time (often years). Some individuals have no symptoms at all (except for high blood glucose levels). Because of this, they may be unaware that they have diabetes until a complication from prolonged hyperglycemia occurs, such as a vision problem or foot pain. Type 2 diabetes is first treated by dietary adjustments, weight reduction, and exercise. These changes can sometimes restore insulin sensitivity, even if the weight loss is modest. Approximately 20% of cases of type 2 diabetes can be managed by lifestyle changes alone. The next step, if necessary, is treatment with oral hypoglycemics, which are medications taken by mouth that stimulate the release of insulin from the pancreas, help the body use its own insulin better, or both. If this treatment is ineffective, insulin therapy becomes necessary to maintain normal or near-normal glucose levels.

What factors increase the risk of developing type 2 diabetes?

The cause of type 2 diabetes is unknown, although certain factors, known as *risk factors,* make a person more prone to developing type 2 diabetes. The more risk factors present, the more likely an individual will develop type 2 diabetes. Some of these factors can be controlled, and others cannot.

Risk Factors That Can Be Controlled

1. **Weight.** The risk factor that contributes most to the development of type 2 diabetes is excess body weight. Approximately 80% of individuals with type 2 diabetes are overweight. Being overweight (body mass index of 25 or greater) makes it harder for the body to use insulin. A research study by the Diabetes Prevention Program showed that people who followed a low-fat, low-calorie diet; lost a moderate amount of weight; and engaged in regular physical activity (five times a week for 30 minutes) sharply reduced their chances of developing type 2 diabetes.
2. **Smoking.** Smoking makes it harder for the body to control the blood glucose level.
3. **Lack of physical activity.** Regular exercise helps the body to use insulin normally, whereas a sedentary lifestyle contributes to insulin resistance.
4. **High blood pressure, abnormal lipid profile, or both.** The following factors contribute to insulin resistance: a blood pressure greater than 130/80 mm Hg; HDL cholesterol of 35 mg/dL or less, and triglyceride level of 250 mg/dL or greater. Decreasing blood pressure can also reduce the risk of cardiovascular complications.

Risk Factors That Cannot Be Controlled

1. **Family history.** The risk of developing type 2 diabetes is increased if a close relative (parent, brother, sister) has diabetes.
2. **Gestational diabetes or giving birth to a large infant.** Women who have diabetes during pregnancy or gave birth to an infant weighing more than 9 lb are at greater risk for developing type 2 diabetes.
3. **Age.** Type 2 diabetes is more common in people 40 years and older, but it is increasing among young people who are overweight and inactive.
4. **Ethnic group.** The following ethnic groups are more likely to develop type 2 diabetes: African Americans, Latinos, Hispanics, Native Americans, Asian Americans, and Pacific Islanders.

Can diabetes be cured?

There is no cure for diabetes, but the outlook for individuals with this condition is improving. This is primarily due to better patient education, advances in blood glucose monitoring, and newer methods for insulin delivery that help simplify management of the disease. Today, most individuals with diabetes under good control have life expectancies comparable to individuals without diabetes. ■

fluctuations in glucose levels brought on by food, exercise, stress, and infection.

Diabetic patients who take insulin (insulin-dependent) must monitor their blood glucose levels each day. Based on the results of SMBG, decisions can be made regarding insulin and dietary adjustments that may be necessary to maintain normal glucose levels and to avoid the extremes of hypoglycemia and hyperglycemia (see Chapter 35). Satisfactory control of the blood glucose level on a day-to-day basis through SMBG reduces symptoms of the disease and helps delay or prevent long-term complications that can occur with diabetes.

Memories *from* Externship

Michelle Villers: During my externship experience, I was assigned to a four-physician pediatric practice. The office was constantly busy with screaming children. As if I were not nervous enough, I was asked to assist in the removal of sutures. When I walked into the room with the physician, beads of sweat began to form on my forehead. A child was lying on the examining table—a little boy no more than 7 years old. He was there to have sutures removed from a recent surgery. The sutures had been tied very well, and it was difficult for the physician to cut them. The little boy lay there with tears streaming down his cheeks. I reassured him and talked to him, and his tears began to subside. "A few more minutes and it will be all over," I told him. And within those next few minutes, the physician cut the last suture. The little boy eagerly hopped down off the examining table and gave me a big hug. I learned that day how a little reassurance can make everyone involved feel better. ■

Prepare for Success

What Would You Do? What Would You *Not* Do?

Case Study 3

Dave Felden has recently been diagnosed with type 1 diabetes and is taking insulin. He has come to the office for an FBS. A finger-stick will be performed to collect the specimen, and a glucose meter will be used to test the specimen. Dave has been performing this test on himself at home now for 2 weeks and wants to know whether he can stick his own finger. Dave says that he's been having a few problems giving himself his insulin injections. He says that he has been getting some very large air bubbles in his syringe when he draws up the insulin. He says he's been having trouble getting them out and wants to know how important that is. Dave says he is on a limited income and wants to know whether he could use his needle and syringe for more than one injection. He also wants to know whether he should throw his used needle and syringes in the regular trash. ■

Frequency of Testing

The frequency of blood glucose testing depends on numerous factors, including the severity of the diabetes, diet, activity level, and special conditions such as pregnancy. Ideally, the blood glucose level for an insulin-dependent diabetic patient should be measured four times a day: in the morning (after an 8-hour fast), before lunch, before dinner, and at bedtime. The FBS test result (obtained in the morning) is the best overall indicator of control, and the other determinations provide guidance for adjusting insulin dosage, diet, and exercise.

Test Results

Blood glucose levels are measured using a glucose meter, and the results are displayed in mg/dL. Table 33-2 lists recommended blood glucose levels for patients with diabetes based on when the testing is performed. Diabetic patients should be instructed to maintain a cumulative record of their daily SMBG test results for periodic review by the physician. This record assists the physician in making decisions regarding the patient's diabetes management plan.

Advantages

Research shows that SMBG is the most effective way for a diabetic patient to maintain a normal blood glucose level and delay or prevent long-term complications associated with diabetes. High blood glucose levels (greater than 180 mg/dL) for a long time can cause progressive damage to the body organs, resulting in blindness, kidney disease, nerve damage, and circulation problems. Because of the necessity of performing a skin puncture and the fact that the patient must assume responsibility in self-management decisions, the medical assistant may need to reinforce the advantages of SMBG, as follows:

1. **Convenience of testing.** The patient is able to test his or her blood at any time of the day without a laboratory order from the physician. This provides a distinct advantage because patients are able to check their blood glucose level when a side effect common to diabetes occurs, such as hypoglycemia. In these situations, treatment can be instituted immediately to prevent the problem from getting worse.
2. **More involvement in self-management decisions.** The patient is able to become more involved in self-

Table 33-2 Recommended Blood Glucose Levels for Patients with Diabetes

Time of Day	Recommended Blood Glucose Level (mg/dL)
Before meals	80-120
1-2 hr after meals	100-180
At bedtime	100-140

From Bonewit-West K: *Clinical procedures for medical assistants,* ed 7, St. Louis, 2008, Saunders.

management decisions regarding insulin dosage, meal planning, and physical activity. Initially some patients lack confidence in making insulin and dietary adjustments based on the blood glucose test results. The medical assistant should provide encouragement and stress the benefits to be derived in terms of improved regulation of the blood glucose level.

3. **Reliable decisions regarding insulin dosage.** More reliable decisions regarding insulin needs can be made during situations that affect the blood glucose level, such as illness, emotional stress, increased physical activity, or suspected hypoglycemia.

4. **Delay or prevent long-term complications.** The medical assistant should emphasize to patients how important it is to perform daily SMBG testing to increase their chances of staying healthy. As previously discussed, diabetic patients who maintain good blood glucose control generally experience fewer symptoms and a delay or prevention of long-term complications of the disease.

Hemoglobin A₁c Test

The hemoglobin A_{1c} test (Hb A_{1c} test or A_{1c} test) provides valuable information for determining whether a diabetic patient's blood glucose level is under control. The A_{1c} test supplies the physician with an assessment of the average amount of glucose in the blood over a 3-month period.

When an individual consumes food containing glucose, the glucose is absorbed from the digestive tract and into the circulatory system. Glucose (sugar) has a "sticky" quality to it and thus has a tendency to stick to protein in the body. One of the proteins it attaches to is the protein comprising hemoglobin. Hemoglobin is found in red blood cells and functions in transporting oxygen in the body. The process of glucose attaching to hemoglobin is known as **glycosylation.**

When glucose attaches or glycosylates to the protein in hemoglobin, it forms a compound known as **hemoglobin A_{1c}.** Glycosylation occurs in all individuals; hemoglobin A_{1c} is formed in diabetic patients and healthy individuals. The amount of glucose that attaches to hemoglobin is proportional to the amount of glucose in the blood; the more glucose in the blood, the more hemoglobin that becomes glycated and the higher the A_{1c} level. Individuals with undiagnosed or poorly controlled diabetes have a higher than normal blood glucose level, and more hemoglobin A_{1c} forms in these individuals. The percentage of hemoglobin A_{1c} in the blood can be measured by the A_{1c} laboratory test. The attachment of the glucose to the hemoglobin is permanent for the life of the red blood cell (90 to 120 days); the A_{1c} test result is able to provide an overall picture of the patient's blood glucose level for the past 3 months.

Interpretation of Results

The normal A_{1c} level for an individual without diabetes is 4% to 6%. Patients with diabetes usually have a higher A_{1c} level than this. The American Diabetes Association strongly recommends that patients with diabetes maintain an A_{1c}

Table 33-3 Comparison of Hemoglobin A₁c Percentages with Average Blood Glucose Levels	
Hemoglobin A₁c (%)	Average Daily Blood Glucose Level (mg/dL)
4	65
5	100
6	135
7	170
8	205
9	240
10	275
11	310
12	345

From Bonewit-West K: *Clinical procedures for medical assistants,* ed 7, St. Louis, 2008, Saunders.

level of less than 7%. Table 33-3 shows the correlation between hemoglobin A_{1c} percentages and average blood glucose levels. A change in a patient's diabetes management plan is almost always required if the A_{1c} test result is greater than 8%.

Patients who keep their hemoglobin A_{1c} levels close to 7% have a much better chance of delaying or preventing diabetic complications than patients with A_{1c} levels that are 8% or greater. Studies show that for every 1 percentage point drop in the A_{1c} value, there is a 35% reduction in risk for diabetes-related complications.

The physician orders an A_{1c} test when a patient is first diagnosed with diabetes to determine how elevated the blood glucose level has been before being diagnosed. The test is usually ordered several times after a diabetes management plan has been prescribed to verify that blood glucose control is being achieved. The A_{1c} test is ordered periodically for patients already diagnosed with diabetes to evaluate the effectiveness of their diabetes management plan. For stable diabetic patients under good control, the test is typically ordered at least two times a year (every 6 months). The test is usually ordered on a more frequent basis for patients who have difficulty maintaining control of their blood glucose levels. The A_{1c} test is also ordered when the physician makes an adjustment to a patient's diabetic management plan to assess the effectiveness of the change in treatment.

GLUCOSE METERS

In the medical office, a glucose meter is often used to measure the blood glucose level quantitatively. The test most frequently performed using the glucose meter is the FBS, although some offices also perform the GTT and the 2-hour postprandial test. By measuring the blood glucose concentration in the medical office, better patient care can be provided. On-site testing eliminates the time required for an outside laboratory to provide the results, allowing the physician to make decisions immediately regarding diagno-

PATIENT TEACHING   Obtaining a Capillary Blood Specimen

The medical assistant may need to instruct the patient in the procedure for obtaining and testing a capillary blood specimen for blood glucose measurement. Properly educating the patient to perform the procedure is the most important factor in obtaining accurate test results.

1. **Obtaining the capillary blood specimen.** Inform the patient of the sites available for obtaining the blood specimen, including the fingers and the side of the hand where there are no calluses. Most patients prefer to use an automatic lancet to perform the skin puncture. Using such a device makes the puncture less painful, and the preset puncture depth generally ensures a successful stick. For a finger puncture, instruct the patient to obtain the blood specimen from the lateral side of the fingertip because this area contains fewer nerve endings, and less pain results. If the patient's hands are cold, tell him or her to rub them together or place them in warm water, which improves the blood flow to the area. Instruct the patient in the proper procedure for obtaining enough blood to ensure accurate test results.

2. **Performing the blood glucose test.** The patient performs the test with a reagent strip using a glucose meter. Instruct the

patient in the proper procedure for performing the test, making sure he or she understands that accurate test results assist in greater glucose control. Patients should also be given detailed instructions on the proper care and maintenance of the glucose meter.

3. **Recording results.** Instruct the patient to record each test result in a log book to provide a permanent record between office visits. In addition, most glucose meters are equipped with a memory system that stores test results for later retrieval. Keeping track of these factors helps explain a shift in the blood glucose level and provides the basis for sound self-management decisions. The following information should be included with each recording:

- Date and time
- Number of hours since the patient last ate
- Time of the last insulin injection or oral hypoglycemic medication
- Any feeling of physical or emotional stress
- Amount of exercise the patient has had ■

sis, treatment, and follow-up care. Procedure 33-1 describes how to measure blood glucose using the Accu-Chek Advantage glucose meter.

Reagent Strips

A reagent test strip must be used with the glucose meter; it consists of a plastic strip with a reaction pad. The pad contains chemicals that react with the glucose in whole blood to determine the blood glucose level in mg/dL. Through an electronic signal, the glucose results are displayed as a digital readout. The manufacturer's instructions accompanying the glucose meter must be followed exactly to ensure accurate and reliable test results.

It is important to store the container of test strips properly to prevent their deterioration, which affects the test results. The chemical reagents on the strips are sensitive to heat, light, and moisture and must be stored in a cool, dry area at room temperature (less than 90°F [32°C]) with the cap tightly closed. Strips that are discolored or that have darkened should be discarded to prevent inaccurate test results. The container of test strips includes a desiccant. Its purpose is to promote dryness by absorbing moisture.

Care and Maintenance

The glucose meter must be handled carefully. It is a delicate instrument, and a severe physical jar could result in a malfunction. The glucose meter should not be placed in an area of high humidity, such as a bathroom. In addition, the meter should not be exposed to severe variations in environmental temperature, such as leaving it in a closed vehicle on a hot or cold day.

Proper cleaning of the glucose meter is essential for its accurate and reliable operation. On a regular basis, the exterior of the glucose meter, including the display screen, should be cleaned with a soft, clean cloth slightly dampened with a mild cleaning agent, and it should be dried thoroughly. Do not allow water or detergent to run into the glucose meter, which could damage the internal components.

Because glucose meters are battery operated, periodic replacement of the battery is required. The glucose meter alerts the user to low battery voltage by displaying a special notation on the screen. The type of battery required is specified in the operator's manual, along with directions for installation.

Calibration Procedures

Two calibration procedures may be required for a glucose meter. Because the Accu-Chek Advantage glucose meter is presented in Procedure 33-1, the calibration methods discussed here relate specifically to this meter.

The first calibration procedure ensures that the glucose meter is functioning properly. It should be noted that not all meters require this type of calibration procedure; the manufacturer's instructions accompanying the meter indicate whether this procedure is required. This calibration procedure, if needed, requires the insertion of a plastic check strip into the test strip guide of the meter (Figure 33-2). When the plastic strip is inserted, the meter goes through a series of internal checks to ensure the meter is functioning properly. The steps presented should be followed to perform this calibration procedure with the Accu-Chek Advantage glucose meter.

1. Turn the meter on.
2. Wait until the strip symbol flashes on the display screen, and then insert the check strip into the test strip guide.
3. If the meter is functioning properly, the word "OK" and a checkmark appear on the display screen.
4. If the display exhibits the word "error," repeat the calibration procedure. If the error display appears again, the meter is not working properly and is in need of repair.

The second calibration procedure is a coding procedure and is performed to ensure accurate and reliable test results; most glucose meters require this calibration procedure. The coding calibration procedure must be performed each time a new container of test strips is opened. It is performed to compensate for variables that occur in the manufacturing process, which cause one batch of reagent strips to be a little different from another batch. The coding calibration procedure programs the electronics of the glucose meter to

Figure 33-2. Accu-Chek Advantage check strip calibration procedure to ensure the glucose meter is functioning properly. (From Bonewit-West K: *Clinical procedures for medical assistants,* ed 7, St. Louis, 2008, Saunders.)

match the reactivity of the container of strips that are in current use.

The coding calibration procedure for the Accu-Chek Advantage is performed using a plastic code key that accompanies each container of Accu-Chek Advantage reagent strips (Figure 33-3). Accu-Chek requires lot-specific calibration, meaning that the calibration procedure needs to be performed only once per container of test strips. This is possible because the Accu-Chek glucose meter has a built-in memory system that enables it to retain a point of reference after it has been calibrated. This reference point is retained until the glucose meter is reprogrammed for a new container of test strips. The calibration procedure delineated next should be followed when a new container of Accu-Chek test strips is opened.

1. Ensure that the meter is turned off.
2. Turn the meter over so that the back of the meter is facing you.
3. Remove the old code key, if one is installed, and discard it in a waste container.
4. Insert a new code key by sliding it into the code key slot until it snaps into place (see Figure 33-3A).
5. Turn the meter on. A three-digit code number appears on the display screen. This number must match the code number of the vial of reagent strips (see Figure 33-3B). If it does not, repeat steps 1 through 3.

Control Procedure

A control check should be run to ensure the test results are reliable and valid and errors that might interfere with test results are detected and eliminated. A control check is performed on the Accu-Chek Advantage using commercially available glucose control solutions. Two levels of controls should be used (high and low).

The control solution is effective for 3 months from the date it is opened. When the control solution is opened, the medical assistant must write the date on the container label. The control solution can then be used for 3 months from that date or until the manufacturer's expiration date

A, The code key is inserted into the monitor.

B, The code number must match the code number of the vial of reagent strips.

Figure 33-3. Accu-Chek Advantage code key calibration procedure. (From Bonewit-West K: *Clinical procedures for medical assistants,* ed 7, St. Louis, 2008, Saunders.)

(stamped on the container) is reached, whichever comes first. The control solution is sensitive to heat, light, and moisture and must be stored in a cool, dry area at room temperature (less than 90°F [32°C]) with the cap tightly closed.

A control check should be performed under the following circumstances:
1. When the meter is new
2. Daily, before using the meter for the first time
3. When a new container of reagent strips is opened
4. If the cap is left off the vial of reagent strips for any length of time
5. If the meter is dropped
6. If a test has been repeated, and the blood glucose result is still lower or higher than expected

The control procedure outlined next should be followed to run a control check:
1. Turn the meter on. Check that the code number displayed matches the code number on the container of test strips.
2. Gently insert the end of the test strip with the silver-colored bars into the test strip guide with the yellow target area facing up.
3. Roll the Level 1 (low) control solution between your hands to mix it.
4. Wait until the flashing drop appears on the display. Remove the cap of the control solution, and squeeze one drop of the solution onto a paper towel.
5. Apply the control solution to the strip as follows:
   a. Accu-Chek Advantage Test Strip: Invert the container, and hold it over the yellow target area of the test strip. Squeeze the container, and touch and hold the drop of control solution to the center of the yellow target area.
   b. Accu-Chek Comfort Curve Test Strips: Hold the container at an angle to the edge of the yellow target area of the test strip. Squeeze the container, and touch and hold a drop of control solution to the edge (not the top) of the yellow target area.
6. Promptly replace the lid on the control solution.
7. After a short time, the control value is displayed on the screen of the glucose meter.
8. If the control value is within acceptable range, it will fall within the acceptable control ranges listed on the label of the test strip container.
9. Repeat the control check procedure using a Level 2 (high) control solution.

If the Level 1 or Level 2 control results are not within the acceptable range, the following should be performed:
1. Check the expiration dates of the test strips and control solution to make sure they are not outdated.
2. Determine whether the test strips and control solution were stored at room temperature.
3. Make sure the container lids were tight on the test strip container and control solution container.
4. Check to make sure the code on the meter matches the code on the test strip vial.
5. Review the technique used to run the control to make sure it was followed correctly.

Any errors should be corrected and the control should be run again. If the results are still not within acceptable range, the manufacturer of the glucose meter should be contacted.

PROCEDURE 33-1

 PROCEDURE 33-1 **Blood Glucose Measurement Using the Accu-Chek Advantage Glucose Meter**

Outcome Perform an FBS.

Equipment/Supplies

- Disposable gloves
- Accu-Chek Advantage glucose meter
- Accu-Chek Advantage reagent strips
- Check strip
- Code key

- Control solution
- Lancet
- Antiseptic wipe
- Gauze pad
- Biohazard sharps container

1. Procedural Step Sanitize your hands. Assemble the equipment. Check the expiration date on the container of reagent strips.
Principle. Outdated reagent strips can cause inaccurate test results.

2. Procedural Step. If the meter requires calibration with a check strip, calibrate the glucose meter using the check strip (refer to pp. 795-796).

Principle. Calibrating with the Check Strip ensures that the glucose meter is functioning properly.

3. Procedural Step. If necessary, calibrate the glucose meter using the code key that accompanies the container of reagent strips (refer to pp. 795-796).

Principle. Calibrating with the Code Key compensates for variables that occur in the manufacturing

Continued

PROCEDURE **33-1**   **Blood Glucose Measurement Using the Accu-Chek Advantage Glucose Meter—cont'd**

Assemble the equipment. (From Bonewit-West K: *Clinical procedures for medical assistants,* ed 7, St. Louis, 2008, Saunders.)

process of the reagent strips and must be performed before using strips from a new container.

4. **Procedural Step.** Run a Level 1 (low) and Level 2 (high) control check on the glucose meter using Accu-Chek Advantage control solutions (refer to pp. 796-797).
   Principle. Running a low and high control check ensures that the test results are reliable and valid.

5. **Procedural Step.** Greet and identify the patient. Introduce yourself, and explain the procedure.

6. **Procedural Step.** If a fasting specimen is required, ask the patient whether he or she has had anything to eat or drink (besides water) for the past 12 hours.
   Principle. Consumption of food or fluid increases the blood glucose level, leading to inaccurate interpretation of FBS test results.

7. **Procedural Step.** Turn the meter on. Check that the code number displayed matches the code number on the vial of test strips that you are using. When the test strip symbol flashes on the display, the meter is ready to accept a test strip.

Check the code number. (From Bonewit-West K: *Clinical procedures for medical assistants,* ed 7, St. Louis, 2008, Saunders.)

8. **Procedural Step.** Remove a test strip from the container. Promptly replace the lid of the container to prevent the strips from being exposed to moisture.
   Principle. The reagent pads are moisture sensitive and could be affected by environmental moisture, leading to inaccurate test results.

9. **Procedural Step.** Within 30 seconds, gently insert the end of the test strip with the silver-colored bars into the test strip guide with the yellow target area facing up. When the strip is correctly inserted, a blood drop symbol flashes on the display.

Insert the test strip into the meter. (From Bonewit-West K: *Clinical procedures for medical assistants,* ed 7, St. Louis, 2008, Saunders.)

10. **Procedural Step.** Cleanse the puncture site with an antiseptic wipe, and allow it to dry. Apply gloves, and perform a finger puncture. Dispose of the lancet in a biohazard sharps container.
    Principle. The antiseptic must be allowed to dry to prevent it from reacting with the chemicals on the reagent pad, which would lead to inaccurate test results. Gloves provide a barrier against bloodborne pathogens.

11. **Procedural Step.** After the puncture has been made, wipe away the first drop of blood with a gauze pad. Place the hand in a dependent position (palm facing down), and gently squeeze the finger around the puncture site until a large drop of blood forms.
    Principle. The first drop of blood contains a large amount of serum, which dilutes the specimen and leads to inaccurate test results. A large drop of blood is necessary to cover the target area of the reagent strip completely.

12. Procedural Step. Apply the drop of blood to the test strip as follows:

a. Accu-Chek Advantage Test Strip: Touch and hold the drop of blood to the center of the yellow target area.

b. Accu-Chek Comfort Curve Test Strips: Touch and hold a drop of blood to the edge (not the top) of the yellow target area.

Completely fill the yellow target area. If any yellow mesh is visible after you have applied the initial drop of blood, a second drop of blood may be applied to the target area within 15 seconds of the first drop. If more than 15 seconds has passed, the test result may be erroneous, and you should discard the test strip and repeat the test.

When the blood is correctly applied to the strip, a box rotates on the display until the measurement is completed.

Principle. The entire yellow target area must be completely covered with blood to ensure accurate and reliable test results.

Read the glucose value on the display screen. (From Bonewit-West K: *Clinical procedures for medical assistants,* ed 7, St. Louis, 2008, Saunders.)

Touch the blood to the target area. (From Bonewit-West K: *Clinical procedures for medical assistants,* ed 7, St. Louis, 2008, Saunders.)

13. Procedural Step. Have the patient hold a gauze pad over the puncture site and apply pressure until the bleeding stops.

14. Procedural Step. After a short time, the glucose value is displayed in milligrams per deciliter (mg/dL). If the glucose value is higher or lower than expected, or if the screen displays something other than the glucose value, see the Troubleshooting Guide section of the operator's manual to obtain instructions for correcting the problem. (The glucose result indicated on this glucose meter is 89 mg/dL.)

15. Procedural Step. Remove the reagent strip from the meter, and discard it in a biohazard waste container. Turn the meter off.

16. Procedural Step. Remove the gloves, and sanitize your hands. Chart the results. Include the date and time, when the patient last ate, the type of test (e.g., FBS, random), the glucose test result, and your initials. If the patient has diabetes mellitus, also record the time of his or her last insulin injection or last consumption of oral hypoglycemic medication.

17. Procedural Step. Properly store the glucose meter according to the manufacturer's instructions.

CHARTING EXAMPLE	
Date	
9/20/10	8:30 a.m. FBS: 89 mg/dL. Pt last ate on
	5/17 @ 7:00 p.m. ————————
	———————— M. Villers, CMA (AAMA)

PROCEDURE 33-1

SEROLOGY

Serology is the scientific study of the serum of the blood. More specifically, serology deals with the study of antigen and antibody reactions. An **antigen** is a substance that is capable of stimulating the formation of antibodies in an individual. Antigens may consist of protein, glycoprotein, complex polysaccharides, or nucleic acid. Specific examples of antigens include bacteria and viruses, bacterial toxins, allergens, and blood antigens. An **antibody** is a substance that is capable of combining with an antigen, resulting in an antigen-antibody reaction.

Laboratory testing in serology deals with studying antigen-antibody reactions to assess the presence of a substance (e.g., ABO blood typing) or to assist in the diagnosis of disease (e.g., mononucleosis testing). Serologic tests are often used for the early diagnosis of disease and to follow the course of the disease.

SEROLOGIC TESTS

Specific examples of serologic tests are described next.

Hepatitis Tests

Hepatitis testing is performed to detect viral hepatitis. The five types of viral hepatitis—A, B, C, D, and E—are described in detail in Chapter 17. Hepatitis testing not only detects the presence of viral hepatitis but also determines the type of hepatitis present.

Syphilis Test

Syphilis is a sexually transmitted disease (STD) caused by the microorganism *Treponema pallidum.* The most common tests to detect the presence of syphilis are the Venereal Disease Research Laboratories (VDRL) test and the rapid plasma reagin (RPR) test. The test results are reported as nonreactive, weakly reactive, or reactive. Weakly reactive and reactive results are considered positive for the presence of syphilis antibodies. These tests are screening tests, and a positive result warrants more specific testing to arrive at a diagnosis of syphilis.

Mononucleosis Test

The mononucleosis test ("mono test") is used to detect the presence of infectious mononucleosis. The theory and procedure for this test are discussed in detail in this chapter.

Rheumatoid Factor

Rheumatoid arthritis is a chronic inflammatory disease that affects the joints of the body. The blood of patients with rheumatoid arthritis contains a type of antibody called *rheumatoid factor* (RF). This test detects the presence of RF antibodies and assists in the diagnosis of rheumatoid arthritis.

Antistreptolysin O Test

The antistreptolysin O (ASO) test is used to detect ASO antibodies in the serum. It is the most widely used serologic test for the detection of conditions resulting from streptococcal infections and diseases that occur secondary to a streptococcal infection. This test is useful in assisting in the diagnosis of rheumatic fever, glomerulonephritis, bacterial endocarditis, and scarlet fever.

C-Reactive Protein

During inflammation and tissue destruction, an abnormal protein called *C-reactive protein* (CRP) appears in the blood. Patients with inflammatory conditions or disorders accompanied by tissue destruction have positive results to this test. Because of this, the CRP test is used to assist in diagnosing or charting the progress of rheumatoid arthritis, acute rheumatic fever, widespread malignancy, and bacterial infections.

Cold Agglutinins

The cold agglutinins test is used to detect the presence of antibodies called *cold agglutinins.* This test is performed by incubating the patient's serum with erythrocytes at cold temperatures. If cold agglutinins are present, this causes **agglutination** of the erythrocytes. Cold agglutinins are found in patients with infectious mononucleosis, mycoplasmal pneumonia, chronic parasitic infections, and lymphoma.

ABO and Rh Blood Typing

Blood typing is performed to determine an individual's ABO and Rh blood type. Knowledge of blood type helps to prevent transfusion and transplant reactions and to identify problems, such as hemolytic disease of the newborn.

Rh Antibody Titer

The Rh antibody titer test detects the amount of circulating Rh antibodies in the blood. These antibodies can occur in an Rh-negative pregnant woman who is carrying an Rh-positive fetus. This test is most frequently used to detect the presence of an Rh incompatibility problem with a mother and her unborn child.

RAPID MONONUCLEOSIS TESTING

Infectious mononucleosis is an acute infectious disease caused by the Epstein-Barr virus (EBV). Infectious mononucleosis most frequently affects children and young adults. It is transmitted through saliva by direct oral contact, and because of this, it is often called the "kissing disease." Symptoms of infectious mononucleosis include mental and physical fatigue, fever, sore throat, severe weakness, headache, and swollen lymph nodes.

QuickVue+ Infectious Mononucleosis Test

FOR INFORMATIONAL USE ONLY ■ FOR INFORMATIONAL USE ONLY ■ FOR INFORMATIONAL USE ONLY
Not to be used for performing assay. Refer to most current package insert accompanying your test kit.

TEST PROCEDURE – WHOLE BLOOD

Read all of the procedural instructions before running patient samples.

Remove the Reaction Unit from the pouch and place it on a well lit and level surface.
The "Read Result" window contains a horizontal blue line pre-printed on the membrane.

Capillary Tube Procedure

For fingertip blood, fill the capillary tube (50 µL) to line.
Dispense all blood into the "Add" well.

Venipuncture Procedure

For whole blood samples in tubes, use the sample pipette provided.
Place one drop of sample in the "Add" well.

Hold the Developer bottle vertically.
Add 5 drops of Developer to the "Add" well.

Read results at 5 minutes.

"Test Complete" line must be visible by 10 minutes.

INTERPRETATION OF RESULTS
FOR PATIENT SAMPLES, POSITIVE AND NEGATIVE CONTROLS

Positive Result

Any shade of a blue vertical line forming a (+) sign in the "Read Result" window along with the blue "Test Complete" line, is a positive result. **Even a faint blue vertical line should be reported as a positive.**

Negative Result

No blue vertical line in the "Read Result" window along with the blue "Test Complete" line, is a negative result.

Invalid Result

Test results are invalid:
■ If after 10 minutes no signal is observed in the "Test Complete" window. (View #1.)
■ If after 10 minutes a blue color fills the "Read Result" window. (View #2.)

An invalid result indicates either the test was not performed correctly or the reagents are not working properly.

Should an invalid result occur, re-test the sample using a new Reaction Unit.

If the problem continues, contact Technical Support toll-free in the U.S. at (800) 874-1517. Outside the USA, contact your local representative.

LIMITATIONS

1. As is the case of any other diagnostic procedure, the results obtained by this kit yield data that must be used in addition to other information available to the physician.
2. QuickVue+ Infectious Mononucleosis test is a qualitative test for the detection of IM heterophile antibodies.
3. A negative result may be obtained from patients at the onset of the disease due to antibody concentration below the sensitivity of this test kit. If symptoms persist or increase in intensity, the test should be repeated.
4. Some segments of the population who contract Infectious Mononucleosis do not produce measurable levels of heterophile antibodies. Approximately 50% of children under 4 years of age who have IM may test as IM heterophile antibody negative.[4]

Figure 33-4. Procedure for performing the QuickVue+ Infectious Mononucleosis Test. (Courtesy and modified from Quidel Corporation, San Diego.)

The rapid mono test is often performed in the medical office and is used to assist in the diagnosis of infectious mononucleosis. Rapid mono tests are easy to perform and provide reliable results in a short time. Patients with infectious mononucleosis produce an antibody called *heterophile antibody*, usually by 6 to 10 days into the illness. Rapid mono tests detect this antibody. The presence of the heterophile antibody along with patient symptoms can provide the basis for the diagnosis of infectious mononucleosis. Figure 33-4 outlines the procedure for performing a rapid mono test using the QuickVue+ Mononucleosis Test (Quidel Corporation, San Diego).

MEDICAL PRACTICE and the LAW

When running laboratory tests, you must ensure that all equipment is functioning properly. This is done by the periodic calibration or running of controls on each piece of equipment. Know how and how often to calibrate or run controls, and document appropriately. Without these quality controls, results cannot be trusted to be accurate. Inaccurate results can lead to an inaccurate diagnosis and treatment. Use personal protective equipment appropriate to each test to avoid transmission of disease and cross-contamination of specimens. ▪

What Would You Do? What Would You *Not* Do? RESPONSES

Case Study 1
Page 789

What Did Michelle Do?
❏ Tried to calm and reassure Karen.
❏ Explained to Karen that the cholesterol results are not affected by food, so eating before the health fair should not have affected her results.
❏ Told Karen that before a cholesterol analyzer is used, it is usually checked to ensure it is working properly.
❏ Reassured Karen that the physician was checking her cholesterol again and running some additional tests to determine whether she is having any problems.
❏ Told Karen that if she must take medication, the physician will determine what drug is best for her.

What Did Michelle Not *Do?*
❏ Did not tell Karen that her cholesterol is extremely high.
❏ Did not tell Karen that she should be more careful about what she eats because she is overweight.
❏ Did not tell Karen that there was no way to know whether the cholesterol analyzer used at the health fair was calibrated and had controls run on it.

What Would You Do?/What Would You *Not* Do? Review Michelle's response and place a checkmark next to the information you included in your response. List additional information you included in your response.

_____

_____

_____

_____

Case Study 2
Page 790

What Did Michelle Do?
❏ Apologized to Crystal for the inconvenience. Explained to her that it takes 3 to 4 hours to run a GTT because several specimens must be collected over time to see how her body handles sugar.
❏ Explained to Crystal that eating and smoking causes the test results to be inaccurate. Told her that she could eat and smoke as soon as the test was over.
❏ Told Crystal that she needs to sit quietly during the test, so it would not be possible for her to bring her children.
❏ Informed the physician of Crystal's situation to see whether he had any suggestions.

What Did Michelle Not *Do?*
❏ Did not become defensive or intimidated by Crystal's behavior.
❏ Did not tell Crystal that the staff would watch Crystal's children during the test.
❏ Did not tell Crystal that it was not a good idea for her to smoke around her children.

What Would You Do?/What Would You *Not* Do? Review Michelle's response and place a checkmark next to the information you included in your response. List additional information you included in your response.

_____

_____

_____

_____

What Would You Do? What Would You *Not* Do?   RESPONSES—cont'd

Case Study 3
Page 793

What Did Michelle Do?

❏ Told Dave that it would be fine for him to perform his own finger-stick.

❏ Made sure that his finger was cleansed with an antiseptic wipe and that he wiped away the first drop of blood.

❏ Explained to Dave that the air bubbles take up space that the insulin should occupy, and that if he does not get rid of them, he will not get his full dose of insulin.

❏ Demonstrated how to remove air bubbles, and had Dave practice it at the office.

❏ Told Dave he must not reuse his needle and syringe. Explained that a used needle could cause him to get an infection. Asked Dave whether he had checked to see if his insurance would cover the cost of the needles and syringes.

❏ Told Dave that he should put his used needles and syringes in a thick plastic container, such as an empty detergent container.

After the container is full, he should close it tightly with a screw lid, and then it can be thrown out with his regular trash. Explained that this will protect his family and the trash handlers from getting stuck while disposing of the trash.

What Did Michelle Not *Do?*

❏ Did not tell Dave he didn't need to worry about the air bubbles in the syringe.

What Would You Do?/What Would You *Not* Do? Review Michelle's response and place a checkmark next to the information you included in your response. List additional information you included in your response.

_____

_____

_____

_____

TERMINOLOGY REVIEW

Agglutination (as it pertains to blood) Clumping of blood cells.

Antibody A substance that is capable of combining with an antigen, resulting in an antigen-antibody reaction.

Antigen A substance capable of stimulating the formation of antibodies.

Glycogen The form in which carbohydrate is stored in the body.

Glycosylation The process of glucose attaching to hemoglobin.

HDL cholesterol A lipoprotein, consisting of protein and cholesterol, that removes excess cholesterol from the cells.

Hemoglobin A$_{1c}$ Compound formed when glucose attaches or glycosylates to the protein in hemoglobin.

Hyperglycemia An abnormally high level of glucose in the blood.

Hypoglycemia An abnormally low level of glucose in the blood.

LDL cholesterol A lipoprotein, consisting of protein and cholesterol, that picks up cholesterol and delivers it to the cells.

Lipoprotein A complex molecule consisting of protein and a lipid fraction such as cholesterol. Lipoproteins function in transporting lipids in the blood.

ON THE WEB

For Information on Diabetes:

American Diabetes Association: www.diabetes.org

Joslin Diabetes Center: www.joslin.org

National Diabetes Education Initiative: www.ndei.org

The National Institute of Diabetes: www.niddk.nih.gov

 PREPARE FOR CERTIFICATION Visit the Evolve site at http://evolve.elsevier.com/Bonewit/today/ to actively Prepare for your Certification.

 *Check out the **Companion CD** bound with the book to access additional interactive activities.*

34

Medical Microbiology

LEARNING OBJECTIVES

PROCEDURES

Microorganisms and Disease

1. List and explain the stages of an infectious disease.
2. List and describe the three classifications of bacteria based on shape.
3. Give examples of infectious diseases caused by the following types of cocci:
   Staphylococci
   Streptococci
   Diplococci
4. State examples of infectious diseases caused by bacilli, spirilla, and viruses.

Microscope

1. Explain the function of each of the following parts of a compound microscope: base, arm, stage, light source, substage condenser, iris diaphragm, body tube, coarse adjustment, and fine adjustment.

   Use a microscope.

2. Identify the function of each of the following microscope lenses: low power, high power, and oil immersion.

   Properly handle and care for a microscope.

3. List the guidelines for proper care of the microscope.

Microbiologic Specimen Collection

1. Explain the purpose of obtaining a specimen, and identify body areas from which a specimen can be taken for microbiologic examination.

   Collect a specimen for a throat culture.

2. List ways to prevent contamination of a specimen by extraneous microorganisms.
3. Explain the precautions a medical assistant should take to prevent infection from a pathogenic specimen.

Microbiologic Tests

1. Explain the importance of the early diagnosis of streptococcal pharyngitis.

   Perform a streptococcus test using a rapid strep test.

2. Explain the purpose of and describe the procedure for a sensitivity test.

   Prepare a wet mount.

3. Explain the purpose of a microbiologic smear.

   Prepare a microbiologic smear.

4. Explain the purpose of Gram staining.
5. Identify infectious diseases caused by gram-positive bacteria and gram-negative bacteria.
6. Give examples of methods to prevent and control infectious diseases in the community.

CHAPTER OUTLINE

Introduction to Microbiology
Normal Flora
Infection
   Stages of an Infectious Disease
Microorganisms and Disease

Bacteria
Viruses
Microscope
Support System
Optical System

CAAHEP COMPETENCIES

Clinical Competencies
Specimen Collection
- Obtain specimens for microbiologic testing.

Diagnostic Testing
- Perform microbiologic testing.

Patient Care
- Screen and follow up test results.

General Competencies
Patient Instruction
- Provide instruction for health maintenance and disease prevention.

Organizational Functions
- Use methods of quality control.

ABHES COMPETENCIES

Clinical Duties
- Use quality control.
- Collect and process specimens.
- Perform selected CLIA-waived tests that assist with diagnosis and treatment.
- Screen and follow up patient test results.
- Obtain throat specimen for microbiological testing.

- Perform wound collection procedure for microbiological testing.
- Perform microbiology testing.

Instruction
- Teach patients methods of health promotion and disease prevention.

KEY TERMS

bacilli (bah-SILL-ie)
cocci (KOK-sie)
contagious (kon-TAE-jus)
culture
culture medium
false negative
false positive
immunization (im-yoo-ni-ZAY-shun)
incubate (IN-kyoo-bate)
incubation period

infectious disease
inoculate (in-NOK-yoo-late)
microbiology (mie-kroe-bie-OL-oe-jee)
mucous membrane (MYOO-kus MEM-brain)
normal flora
resistance
sequela (SEK-kwe-lah)
smear
specimen (SPESS-ih-men)
spirilla (spa-RILL-ah)

Introduction to Microbiology

Microbiology is the scientific study of microorganisms and their activities. As described in Chapter 17, microorganisms are tiny living plants and animals that cannot be seen by the naked eye, but must be viewed under a microscope. Anton van Leeuwenhoek (1632-1723) designed a magnifying glass strong enough for viewing microorganisms. He was the first individual to observe and describe protozoa and bacteria (Figure 34-1). Leeuwenhoek's magnifying glass was the precursor of modern microscopes used today for studying microorganisms. A microscope allows the observer to see individual microbial cells and to differentiate and identify microorganisms.

For the most part, microbiology deals with unicellular, or one-celled, microscopic organisms. All of the life processes necessary to sustain the microbe are performed by one cell. Among them are the ingestion of food substances

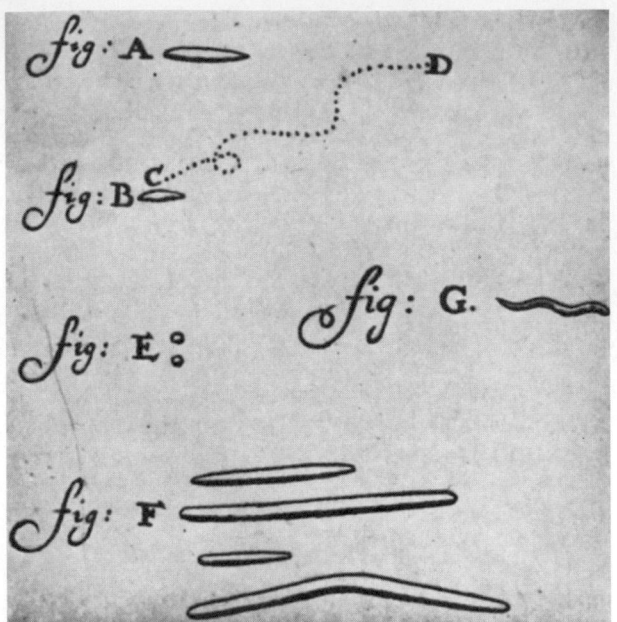

Figure 34-1. Bacteria drawn by van Leeuwenhoek in 1684. (From Fuerst R: *Frobisher and Fuerst's microbiology in health and disease,* ed 15, Philadelphia, 1983, Saunders.)

Coughing to elbow, washing hands

and their use for energy, growth, reproduction, and excretion.

Microorganisms are *ubiquitous;* they are found almost everywhere—in the air, in food and water, in the soil, and in association with plants, animals, and human life. Although there are vast numbers of microorganisms, only a relatively small number are pathogenic and able to cause disease.

When a pathogen infects a host, it often produces a set of symptoms peculiar to that disease. Scarlet fever is characterized by a sore throat, swelling of the lymph nodes in the neck, a red and swollen tongue, and a bright red rash covering the body. These symptoms aid the physician in diagnosing the disease.

Microbiologic laboratory tests are also used to help the physician identify the pathogen causing the disease. Identification of the pathogen leads to the proper treatment of the disease. The medical assistant must be alert to all symptoms the patient describes and relay this information to the physician through careful and concise charting of these symptoms in the patient's medical record.

Although most microbiologic tests are performed in the hospital or medical laboratory, the medical assistant is frequently responsible for the collection of specimens in the medical office. This chapter provides an introduction to microbiology, including a description of techniques that are performed in the medical office. Before undertaking this study, the medical assistant should review Chapter 17, which discusses introductory concepts that are basic to this chapter.

NORMAL FLORA

normal flora in GI tract

Every individual has a **normal flora,** which consists of the harmless microorganisms that normally reside in many parts of the body but do not cause disease. The surface of the skin, the **mucous membrane** of the gastrointestinal tract, and parts of the respiratory and genitourinary tracts all have an abundant normal flora. Some microorganisms that comprise the normal flora are beneficial to the body, such as the microorganisms contained in the intestinal tract that feed on other potentially harmful microscopic organisms. Other examples are microorganisms found in the intestinal tract that synthesize vitamin K, an essential vitamin needed by the body for proper blood clotting. In rare instances, if the opportunity arises (e.g., lowered body resistance), certain microorganisms of the normal flora can become pathogenic and cause disease.

INFECTION

The invasion of the body by pathogenic microorganisms is known as *infection.* Under conditions favorable to the pathogens, they grow and multiply, resulting in an **infectious disease** that produces harmful effects on the host. Not all pathogens that enter a host are able to cause disease, however. When a pathogen enters the body, it attempts to invade the tissues so that it can grow and multiply. The body tries to stop the invasion with its second line of natural defense mechanisms,* which includes inflammation, phagocytosis by white blood cells, and the production of antibodies. These defense mechanisms work to destroy the pathogen and remove it from the body. If the body is successful, the pathogens are destroyed and the individual experiences no adverse effects. If the pathogen is able to overcome the body's natural defense mechanisms, an infectious disease results.

Many infectious diseases are **contagious,** meaning that the pathogen that causes the disease can be spread from one person to another directly or indirectly. Frequently, *droplet infection* is the mode of transmission of pathogens. This is the inhalation of pathogens from a fine spray emitted by a person infected with the disease. When the infected individual exhales, as during breathing, talking, coughing, or sneezing, the pathogens are dispersed into the air on minute liquid particles. Infected individuals should cover their mouths and noses while coughing or sneezing. See Figure 17-1 for examples of other means of pathogen transmission.

mask on

Stages of an Infectious Disease

When a pathogen becomes established in the host, a series of events generally ensues. The stages of an infectious disease are as follows:

*The first line of natural defense mechanisms, which work to prevent the entrance of pathogens into the body (e.g., coughing, sneezing), is described in Chapter 17.

1. The *infection* is the invasion and multiplication of pathogenic microorganisms in the body.
2. The **incubation period** is the interval of time between the invasion by a pathogenic microorganism and the appearance of the first symptoms of the disease. Depending on the type of disease, the incubation period may range from a few days to several months. During this time, the pathogen is growing and multiplying.
3. The *prodromal period* is a short period in which the first symptoms that indicate an approaching disease occur. Headache and a feeling of illness are common prodromal symptoms.
4. The *acute period* is when the disease is at its peak, and symptoms are fully developed. Fever is a common symptom of many infectious diseases.
5. The *decline period* is when the symptoms of the disease begin to subside.
6. The *convalescent period* is the stage in which the patient regains strength and returns to a state of good health. gaining strength

MICROORGANISMS AND DISEASE

The groups of microorganisms known to contain species capable of causing human disease include bacteria, viruses, protozoa, fungi (including yeasts), and animal parasites. Bacteria and viruses are most frequently responsible for causing human diseases and are discussed next.

Bacteria

Bacteria are microscopic single-celled organisms. Of the 1700 species known to dwell in humans, only approximately 100 produce human disease. The discovery of antibiotics has helped immensely in combating and controlling bacterial infections. Antibiotics are not effective against viral infections, however.

Bacteria can be classified according to their shape into three basic groups (Figure 34-2). Round bacteria are known as **cocci**. The cocci can be categorized further as diplococci, streptococci, or staphylococci, depending on their pattern of growth. Rod-shaped bacteria are **bacilli**. Spiral and curve-shaped bacteria are **spirilla,** and they include spirochetes and vibrios.

Cocci

Staphylococci are round bacteria that grow in grapelike clusters (Figure 34-3A). The species *Staphylococcus epidermidis* is widely distributed and is normally present on the surface of the skin and the mucous membranes of the mouth, nose, throat, and intestines. *S. epidermidis* is usually nonpathogenic; however, a cut, abrasion, or other break in the skin can allow invasion of the tissues by the organism, resulting in a mild infection.

Staphylococcus aureus is commonly associated with pathologic conditions such as boils, carbuncles, pimples, impetigo, abscesses, *Staphylococcus* food poisoning, and wound infections. Infections caused by staphylococci usually cause

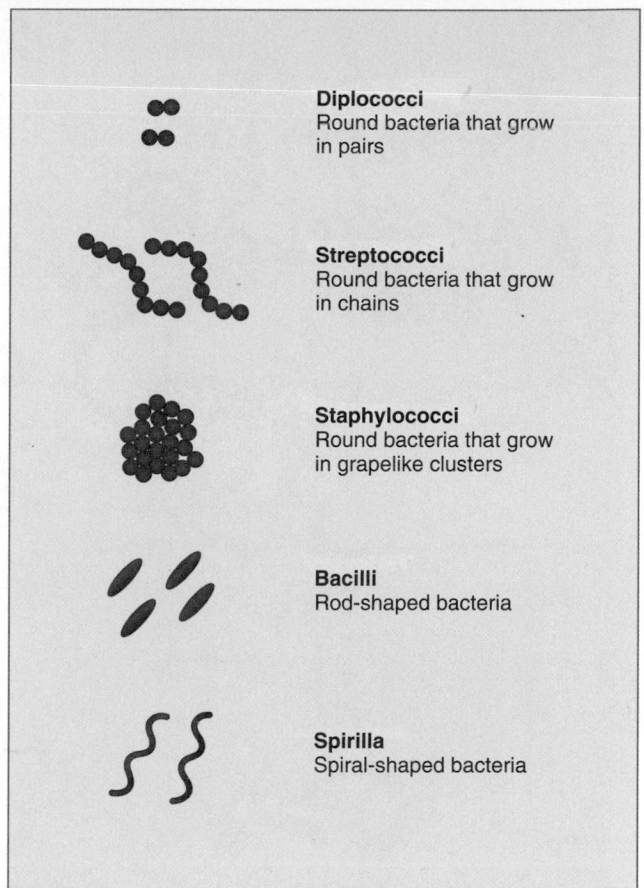

Figure 34-2. Classification of bacteria based on shape. (From Bonewit-West K: *Clinical procedures for medical assistants,* ed 7, St. Louis, 2008, Saunders.)

much pus formation (suppuration) and are termed *pyogenic* infections.

Streptococci are round bacteria that grow in chains (Figure 34-3B). Before the advent of antibiotics, streptococcal infections were a major cause of human death. Diseases caused by streptococci include streptococcal sore throat ("strep throat"), scarlet fever, rheumatic fever, pneumonia, puerperal sepsis, erysipelas, and skin conditions such as carbuncles and impetigo.

Diplococci are round bacteria that grow in pairs. Pneumonia, gonorrhea, and meningitis are infectious diseases caused by diplococci.

Bacilli

Bacilli are rod-shaped bacteria that are frequently found in the soil and air (Figure 34-3C). Some bacilli are able to form spores, a characteristic that enables them to resist adverse conditions such as heat and disinfectants. Diseases caused by bacilli include botulism, tetanus, gas gangrene, gastroenteritis produced by *Salmonella* food poisoning, typhoid fever, pertussis (whooping cough), bacillary dysentery, diphtheria, tuberculosis, leprosy, and plague.

Escherichia coli is a species of bacillus that is found among the normal flora of the large intestine in enormous numbers

Figure 34-3. Types of bacteria. **A,** Staphylococci. **B,** Streptococci. **C,** Bacilli. **D,** Escherichia coli. **E,** Spirilla. (**A, B,** and **D** from Mahon CR, Manuselis G Jr: *Textbook of diagnostic microbiology,* ed 2, Philadelphia, 2000, Saunders; **C** courtesy Cathy Bissonette; **E** courtesy Dr. Andrew G. Smith.)

(Figure 34-3D). It is normally a harmless bacterium; however, if it enters the urinary tract as a result of lowered **resistance,** poor hygiene practices, or both, it may cause a urinary tract infection.

Spirilla

Spirilla are spiral or curve-shaped bacteria. *Treponema pallidum,* a spirochete, is the causative agent of syphilis (Figure 34-3E). This microorganism cannot be grown in commonly available culture media; the diagnosis of syphilis is generally made using serologic tests. A serologic test is performed on the serum of the blood. Cholera is caused by another type of spirillum, *Vibrio cholerae.* **Immunization** and proper methods of sanitation and water purification have all but eliminated cholera in the United States.

Viruses

Viruses are the smallest living organisms. They are so small that an electron microscope must be used to view them. Viruses infect plants, animals, and humans and use nutri-

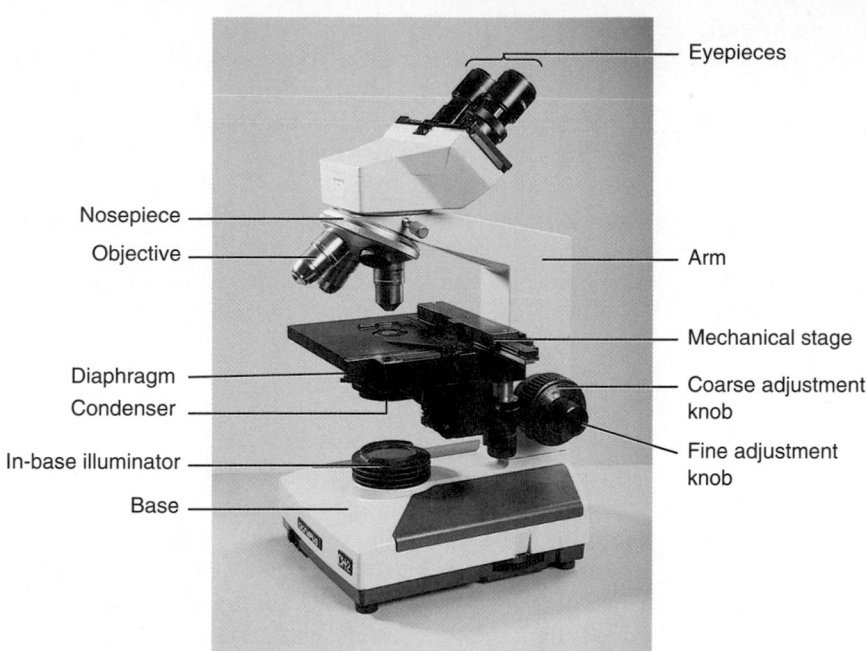

Nosepiece

Objective

Diaphragm

Condenser

In-base illuminator

Base

Eyepieces

Arm

Mechanical stage

Coarse adjustment knob

Fine adjustment knob

Figure 34-4. Parts of the microscope. (From Bonewit-West K: *Clinical procedures for medical assistants,* ed 7, St. Louis, 2008, Saunders.)

Prions cell
mad cow diseases

What Would You Do? What Would You *Not* Do?

Case Study 1

Paula Hutchinson brings her 8-year-old daughter Caitlin to the medical office. Caitlin has had a fever, sore throat, and difficulty eating for the past 2 days. The physician orders a rapid strep test. Caitlin refuses to open her mouth so that the specimen can be collected. She says that she doesn't want that "swab thing" in her mouth because she's afraid it will make her throw up. Paula wants to know why the strep test must be run. She says that Caitlin's throat is very red with white patches and wants to know why the physician does not just prescribe an antibiotic for her without running the test. ◼

ents inside the host's cells for their metabolic and reproductive needs. Infectious diseases caused by viruses include influenza, chickenpox, rubeola (measles), rubella (German measles), mumps, poliomyelitis, smallpox, rabies, herpes simplex, herpes zoster, yellow fever, hepatitis, and most infectious diseases of the upper respiratory tract, including the common cold.

MICROSCOPE

Many kinds of microscope are available, but the type used most often for office laboratory work is the *compound microscope*. The compound microscope consists of a two-lens system, and the magnification of one system is increased by the other. A source of bright light is required for proper illumination of the object to be viewed. This combination of lenses and light permits visualization of structures that cannot be seen with the unaided eye, such as microorganisms and cellular forms. The compound microscope consists of two main components—the support system and the optical system. The medical assistant should be able to identify the parts of a microscope (Figure 34-4) and be able to use and care for it properly. Procedure 34-1 outlines the correct use and care of a microscope.

Support System

Frame

The working parts of the microscope are supported by a sturdy frame consisting of a *base* for support and an *arm* for carrying it without damaging the delicate parts. The arm is also necessary to support the magnifying and adjusting systems.

Stage

The *stage* of a microscope is the flat, horizontal platform on which the microscope slide is placed. It is located directly over the condenser and beneath the objective lenses. The stage has a small round opening in the center that permits light from below to pass through the object being viewed and up into the lenses above. The slide should be placed on the stage; the object to be viewed is positioned over this opening so that it is satisfactorily illuminated by the light source below. Standard microscope stages have metal clips attached to the stage to hold the glass slide securely in place. With this type of stage, the slide must be moved by hand to examine various areas on it.

Other types of microscope have a *mechanical stage* that allows movement of the slide in a vertical or horizontal

Smear used

position by using adjustment knobs. The mechanical stage provides precise positioning of the slide, which is essential for performing certain procedures, such as differential white blood counts and inspection of Gram-stained smears.

Light Source

The light source is at the base of the microscope and consists of a built-in illuminator, along with a switch for turning it on and off. The light is directed to the condenser above it and then through the object to be viewed.

Condenser

Compound microscopes have a lens system between the light source and object, known as the *substage condenser*. A popular condenser is the *Abbé condenser,* which consists of two lenses used to illuminate objects with transmitted light. The condenser collects and concentrates the light rays and directs them up, bringing them to a focus on the object so that it is well illuminated.

Diaphragm

The amount of light focused on the object also can be controlled by the *diaphragm,* located beneath or inside the condenser. The diaphragm consists of a series of horizontally arranged interlocking plates with a central opening, or *aperture.* The diaphragm has a lever that is used to increase or decrease the amount of light admitted by increasing or decreasing the aperture.

Appropriate intensity of light is essential for properly viewing the specimens, especially at a higher magnification. A general rule is that as the desired magnification increases, the more intense the light must be. Increased light intensity is required for good visualization of a specimen with the oil-immersion objective. With the low-power objective, the light must be diminished to produce the appropriate contrast for specimen detail and reduce glare. The degree of illumination is also influenced by the density of the object; stained structures (e.g., a Gram-stained smear of bacteria) usually require more light than do unstained specimens.

Adjustment Knobs

Two adjustment knobs are used to bring the specimen into focus: the coarse adjustment knob and the fine adjustment knob. The *coarse adjustment* is used first to obtain an approximate focus quickly. The *fine adjustment* is then used to obtain the precise focusing necessary to produce a sharp, clear image. On some microscope models, the adjustment knobs are mounted as two separate knobs; on others, they are placed together with the smaller fine adjustment knob extending from a larger coarse adjustment wheel.

Optical System

Compound microscopes have a two-lens magnification system. *Magnification* is defined as the ratio of the apparent size of an object viewed through the microscope to the actual size of the object.

Eyepiece

The first lens system is the eyepiece, or ocular lens, located at the top of the body tube and marked 10×, meaning that it magnifies 10 times. Microscopes that have one eyepiece only are called *monocular* microscopes, and microscopes with two eyepieces are called *binocular.* A binocular microscope is recommended for medical office laboratory work because it causes less eye fatigue than the monocular type. The binocular eyepieces can be adjusted to the individual by moving the eyepieces apart or together as needed.

Objective Lenses

The second lens system consists of three objective lenses located on the revolving *nosepiece,* each with a different degree of magnification. The metal shafts of the objective lenses differ in length and are identified by power of magnification. The short objective is known as the *low-power objective* and has a magnification of 10×. The *high-power objective* is also known as the "high-dry objective" because it does not require the use of immersion oil; it has a magnification of 40×. The *oil-immersion objective* has the highest power of magnification, which is 100×.

The degree of magnification is engraved onto the metal shaft of each objective. In addition, some microscope manufacturers identify each objective lens by colored rings that encircle the metal shaft of the objective. Yellow is used for low power, blue for high power, and white for oil immersion. If the objective is not color coded, it can be identified by the length of the metal shaft; the low-power objective is the shortest, and the oil-immersion objective is the longest.

The objective lens magnifies the specimen, and the ocular lens magnifies the image produced by the objective lens. The *total magnification* of each objective is determined by multiplying the ocular magnification by the objective magnification. The total magnification of the low-power objective is 100 times (100×) the actual size of the object being viewed (10 × 10). The total magnification of the high-power objective is 400× (10 × 40), and the oil-immersion magnification is 1000× (10 × 100).

Focus

Depending on the type of microscope, there are two ways to focus on a specimen. Some microscopes are equipped with a *barrel focus.* With this type of microscope, the body tube (or barrel) moves while the stage remains stationary during focusing. Other microscopes focus on the specimen using *stage focus.* With this type of microscope, the stage moves while the body tube remains stationary during focusing.

Low and High Power

The low-power objective is used for the initial focusing and light adjustment of the microscope. The low-power objective is also used for the initial observation and scanning requirements needed for most microscopic work. Urine sediment is first examined using the low-power objective to scan the specimen for the presence of casts.

The high-power objective is used for a more thorough study, such as observing cells in more detail. The *working distance,* defined as the distance between the tip of the lens and the slide, is short when using this objective. Because of this, care must be taken in focusing the high-power objective to prevent it from striking and breaking the slide or damaging the lens.

Most compound microscopes are *parfocal.* This means that when the specimen is focused with the low-power objective, the nosepiece can be rotated to the high-power objective and focused simply with the fine adjustment knob.

Oil Immersion

The oil-immersion objective provides the highest magnification and is used to view very small structures or the detail of larger structures, such as microorganisms and blood cells. The oil-immersion objective has a very short working distance, and when it is in use, the lens nearly rests on the microscope slide itself. A special grade of oil, known as *immersion oil,* must be used with this lens. Oil has the advantage of not drying out when exposed to air for a long time. A drop of oil is placed on the slide and resides between the oil-immersion objective and the slide. The oil provides a path for the light to travel on between the slide and the lens and prevents the scattering of light rays, which permits clear viewing of very small structures. The oil also improves the resolution of the objective lens (i.e., its ability to provide sharp detail, which is particularly necessary at high magnifications). Procedures that require oil immersion include differential white blood cell counts and examination of Gram-stained smears.

Care of the Microscope

The microscope is a delicate instrument and must be handled carefully. These guidelines should be followed to care for the microscope properly:

1. Always carry the microscope with two hands. Place one hand firmly on the arm and the other hand under the base for support. Place the microscope down gently to prevent jarring it, which could damage delicate parts.
2. Always handle the microscope in such a way that your fingers do not touch the lenses, to avoid leaving fingerprints on them. When using a microscope, avoid wearing mascara because it is difficult to remove from the ocular lens.
3. When it is not in use, keep the microscope covered with its plastic dust cover and stored in a case or cupboard. Store it with the nosepiece rotated to the low-power objective and as close as possible to the stage.
4. Periodically clean the microscope by washing the enameled surfaces with mild soap and water and drying them thoroughly with a soft cloth. Never use alcohol on the enameled surfaces because it might remove the finish.
5. After each use, wipe the metal stage clean with gauze or tissue. If immersion oil comes in contact with the stage, remove it with a piece of gauze that is slightly moistened with xylene.
6. The ocular, objectives, and condenser consist of handground optical lenses, which must be kept spotlessly clean by using clean, dry lens paper. Optical glass is softer than ordinary glass; to prevent scratching the lens, do not use tissues or gauze. If the lenses are especially dirty, use a commercial lens cleaner or xylene in the cleaning process. Apply a small amount of cleaner to the lens paper, followed by thorough drying and polishing with a clean piece of lens paper.
7. Keep the light source free of dust, lint, and dirt by periodic polishing with lens paper.
8. A malfunctioning microscope should be repaired only by a qualified service person. Attempting to fix the microscope yourself may result in further damage.

PROCEDURE 34-1

PROCEDURE 34-1   Using the Microscope

Outcome Use a microscope.

Equipment/Supplies

- Microscope
- Lens paper
- Specimen slide
- Tissue or gauze

- Immersion oil
- Xylene
- Soft cloth

1. Procedural Step. Clean the ocular and objective lenses with lens paper.

2. Procedural Step. Turn on the light source.

3. Procedural Step. Rotate the nosepiece to the low-power objective (10×), clicking it into place. Use the coarse adjustment knob to provide sufficient working

Continued

PROCEDURE 34-1   Using the Microscope—cont'd

Clean the lens. (From Bonewit-West K: *Clinical procedures for medical assistants,* ed 7, St. Louis, 2008, Saunders.)

space for placing the slide on the stage and to avoid damaging the objective lens as follows:
   a. **Barrel focus:** Raise the objective all the way up using the coarse adjustment knob.
   b. **Stage focus:** Lower the stage all the way down using the coarse adjustment knob.
4. Procedural Step. Place the slide on the stage, with the specimen side up, and make sure it is secure.

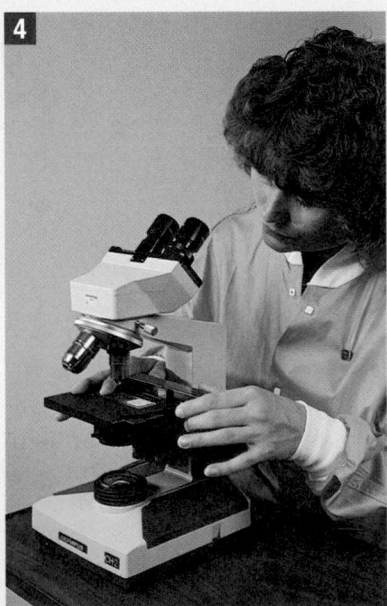

Place the slide on the stage. (From Bonewit-West K: *Clinical procedures for medical assistants,* ed 7, St. Louis, 2008, Saunders.)

5. Procedural Step. Position the low-power objective until it almost touches the slide using the coarse adjustment knob. Be sure to observe this step to prevent the objective from striking the slide.
6. Procedural Step. Look through the ocular. If a monocular microscope is being used, keep both eyes open to prevent eyestrain. With a binocular microscope,

adjust the two oculars to the width between your eyes until a single circular field of vision is obtained.
7. Procedural Step. Bring the specimen into coarse focus as follows:
   a. **Barrel focus:** Slowly raise the objective using the coarse adjustment knob.
   b. **Stage focus:** Slowly lower the stage using the coarse adjustment knob. Observe the specimen through the ocular until it comes into focus.

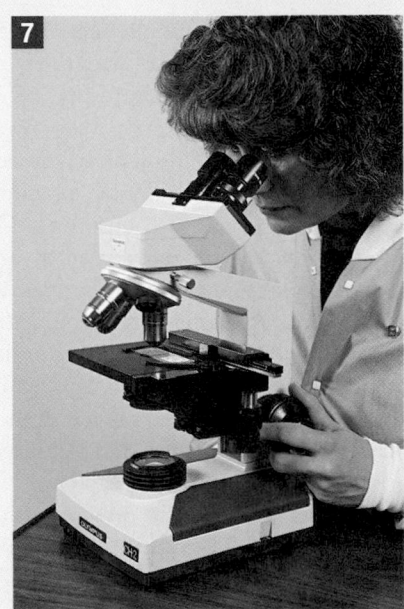

Focus the specimen. (From Bonewit-West K: *Clinical procedures for medical assistants,* ed 7, St. Louis, 2008, Saunders.)

8. Procedural Step. Use the fine adjustment knob to bring the specimen into a sharp, clear focus.
9. Procedural Step. Adjust the light as needed, using the iris diaphragm to provide maximal focus and contrast.
10. Procedural Step. Rotate the nosepiece to the high-power objective, making sure it clicks into place. Proper focusing with the low-power objective ensures that the objective does not hit the slide during this operation. Use the fine adjustment knob to bring the specimen into a precise focus. Do not use the coarse adjustment to focus the high-power objective to prevent the objective from moving too far and striking the slide.
11. Procedural Step. Examine the specimen as required by the test or procedure being performed.
12. Procedural Step. Turn off the light after use, and remove the slide from the stage.
13. Procedural Step. Clean the stage with a tissue or gauze.
14. Procedural Step. Properly care for and store the microscope.

PROCEDURE 34-1

Adjust the light. (From Bonewit-West K: *Clinical procedures for medical assistants,* ed 7, St. Louis, 2008, Saunders.)

Using the Oil-Immersion Objective

1. **Procedural Step.** Rotate the nosepiece to the oil-immersion objective. Do not click it into place, but move it to one side.

2. **Procedural Step.** Place a drop of immersion oil on the slide directly over the center opening in the stage.

Place a drop of oil on the slide. (From Bonewit-West K: *Clinical procedures for medical assistants,* ed 7, St. Louis, 2008, Saunders.)

3. **Procedural Step.** Move the oil-immersion objective into place until a click is heard. Ensure that the objective does not touch the stage or slide.

4. **Procedural Step.** Using the coarse adjustment, slowly position the oil-immersion objective until the tip of the lens touches the oil but does not come in contact with the slide. A "pop" of light is observed. Be sure to observe carefully this step of the procedure.

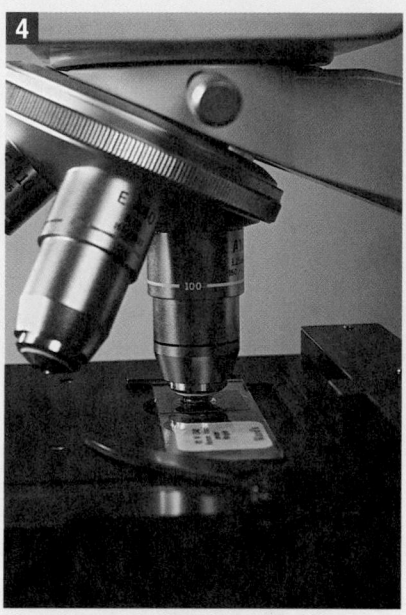

Move the lens until it just touches the oil. (From Bonewit-West K: *Clinical procedures for medical assistants,* ed 7, St. Louis, 2008, Saunders.)

5. **Procedural Step.** Look through the eyepiece, and focus slowly using the coarse adjustment until the object is visible.

6. **Procedural Step.** Use the fine adjustment to bring the object into sharp focus to view fine details.

7. **Procedural Step.** Adjust the light as needed, using the iris diaphragm to provide maximal focus and contrast. Increased light intensity is required for good visualization of the specimen with the oil-immersion objective.

8. **Procedural Step.** Examine the specimen as required by the test or procedure being performed.

9. **Procedural Step.** Turn off the light after use. Remove the slide from the stage, being careful not to get oil on the high-power objective or the stage.

Continued

PROCEDURE **34-1**   Using the Microscope—cont'd

10. Procedural Step. Using a piece of clean, dry lens paper, gently clean the oil-immersion objective. The lens must be cleaned immediately after use to prevent oil from drying on the lens surface. In addition, the oil may seep into the lens and perhaps loosen it.

11. Procedural Step. Clean the oil from the slide by immersing it in xylene and wiping it off with a soft cloth.

Clean the oil from the lens. (From Bonewit-West K: *Clinical procedures for medical assistants,* ed 7, St. Louis, 2008, Saunders.)

MICROBIOLOGIC SPECIMEN COLLECTION

If the physician suspects that a particular disease is caused by a pathogen, he or she may want to obtain a specimen for microbiologic examination. This examination identifies the pathogen causing the disease and aids in the diagnosis. If a urinary tract infection is suspected, a urine specimen is obtained for bacterial examination. In this instance, a clean-catch midstream collection is required to obtain a specimen that excludes the normal flora of the urethra and urinary meatus.

A **specimen** is a small sample or part taken from the body to represent the whole. The medical assistant is often responsible for collecting specimens from certain areas of the body, such as the throat, nose, and wound. The medical assistant may be responsible for assisting the physician in the collection of specimens from other areas, such as the cervix, vagina, urethra, and rectum. In most instances, a sterile swab is used to collect the specimen. A *swab* is a small piece of cotton wrapped around the end of a slender wooden or plastic stick. It is passed across a body surface or opening to obtain a specimen for microbiologic analysis.

To prevent inaccurate test results, good techniques of medical and surgical asepsis must be practiced when a specimen is obtained. The medical assistant must be careful not to contaminate the specimen with *extraneous microorganisms.* These are undesirable microorganisms that can enter the specimen in various ways; they grow and multiply and possibly obscure and prevent identification of pathogens that might be present. To prevent extraneous microorganisms (i.e., normal flora) from contaminating the specimen,

all supplies used to obtain the specimen (e.g., swabs, specimen containers) must be sterile. In addition, the specimen should not contain microorganisms from areas surrounding the collection site. When obtaining a throat specimen, the swab should not be allowed to touch the inside of the mouth.

The OSHA Bloodborne Pathogens Standard presented in Chapter 17 should be carefully followed when performing microbiologic procedures. Specifically, the medical assistant must wear gloves when it is reasonably anticipated that hand contact might occur with blood or other potentially infectious materials. Eating, drinking, smoking, and applying makeup are strictly forbidden when one is working with microorganisms because pathogens can be transmitted to the medical assistant through hand-to-mouth contact. In addition, labels for specimen containers should not be licked, and any break in the skin, such as a cut or scratch, must be covered with a bandage. If the medical assistant accidentally touches some of the material in the specimen, the area of contact should be washed immediately and thoroughly with soap and water. If the specimen comes in contact with the worktable, the table should be cleaned immediately with soap and water, followed by a suitable disinfectant, such as phenol. The worktable should also be cleaned with a disinfectant at the end of each day.

After collection, the specimen must be placed in its proper container with the lid securely fastened. The container must be clearly labeled with the patient's name, date, source of the specimen, medical assistant's initials, and any other required information. Procedure 34-2 outlines the procedure for collecting a specimen for a throat culture.

Putting It All into Practice

My name is **Natalie Moorehead,** and I work for a physician who specializes in family practice. Working as a medical assistant, one can encounter many challenges. One experience that I had involved a 4-year-old boy. The patient came into the office with a very sore throat and a high fever. He did not think that his office visit had gone too badly until he found out that the physician had ordered a rapid strep test to check for strep throat. That's when he decided he did not care for me, my tongue depressor, or my swab. He decided to protest by keeping his mouth tightly shut. Rather than forcing the procedure on the child, I took my time and kept my patience. I managed to convince the child that even though the procedure was uncomfortable and tasted bad, it was the only way we would know if he was really sick or not. I also explained that the test was the only way the doctor would know what kind of medicine to prescribe so he could get well and feel like playing again. It took awhile, but we got our specimen, and the patient received the right antibiotic that he needed to get better. ■

Prepare for Success

Figure 34-5. Starswab II Collection and Transport System (Starplex Scientific, Beverly, Mass.). (From Bonewit-West K: *Clinical procedures for medical assistants,* ed 7, St. Louis, 2008, Saunders.)

Wound Specimens

Wound specimens are collected using many of the techniques described previously. In many cases, two swabs are used to collect the specimen. The specimen is obtained by inserting the swab into the area of the wound that contains the most drainage and gently rotating the swab from side to side to allow it to absorb completely any microorganisms present. The swab is placed in the specimen container, and the process is repeated using a second swab. To obtain accurate and reliable test results, it is important to collect a specimen from within the wound, rather than from the surface.

Collection and Transport Systems

Microbiologic collection and transport systems are available to facilitate the collection of a specimen to be transported to an outside laboratory for analysis; examples include Culturette (Becton Dickinson, Franklin Lakes, N.J.) and the Starswab II (Starplex Scientific, Beverly, Mass.) (Figure 34-5). These systems consist of a sterile swab and a plastic tube that contains a transport medium. The transport medium prevents drying of the specimen and preserves it in its original state until it reaches its destination. The collection and transport system comes packaged in a peel-apart envelope and should be stored at room temperature. The procedure for the use of a microbiologic collection and transport system is outlined next.

1. Complete a laboratory request form.
2. Sanitize your hands, and apply gloves.
3. Check the expiration date on the peel-apart envelope.
4. Peel back the envelope, and remove the cap from the collection tube. Remove the cap/swab unit from the peel-apart envelope. The cap is permanently attached to the sterile swab.
5. Using aseptic technique, collect the specimen. Do not allow the swab to touch any area other than the collection site.
6. Insert the swab into the collection tube.
7. Push the cap/swab in as far as it will go to immerse the swab completely in the transport medium. Make sure the cap is tightly in place.
8. Remove gloves, and sanitize your hands.
9. Label the tube with the patient's name, the date, the source of the specimen (e.g., throat, wound), and your initials. Place the tube in a biohazard specimen transport bag. Place the laboratory request in the outside pocket of the bag.
10. Chart the procedure.
11. Transport the specimen to the laboratory within 24 hours.

Handling and Transporting Microbiologic Specimens

After the microbiologic specimen has been collected, care should be taken in handling and transporting it. Delay in processing the specimen may cause the death of pathogens or the overgrowth of the specimen by microorganisms that are part of the normal flora usually collected along with the pathogen from the specimen site. If the specimen is to be analyzed in the medical office, it should be examined under the microscope or cultured immediately. Otherwise, it should be preserved (if possible) with the method used by the medical office.

Specimens transported to an outside medical laboratory by a courier service are usually placed in a transport medium. The transport medium prevents drying of the specimen and preserves it in its original state until it reaches its destination. Transport media are discussed in more detail in the section on "Collection and Transport Systems."

Outside laboratories provide the medical office with specific instructions on the care and handling of specimens being transported to them. These specimens must be accompanied by a laboratory request that designates the physician's name and address; the patient's name, age, and gender; the date and time of collection; the type of microbiologic examination requested; the source of the specimen (e.g., throat, wound, urine); and the physician's clinical diagnosis. There is usually a space on the form to indicate whether the patient is receiving antibiotic therapy. Antibiotics may suppress the growth of bacteria, a factor that could produce **false-negative** results.

PROCEDURE 34-2

What Would You Do? What Would You *Not* Do?

Case Study 2

Hollie Dolley, age 18, is at the medical office complaining of fatigue, fever, headache, and a terrible sore throat. She just enrolled in a medical assisting program and has been really worried about doing well in her classes. Hollie says that she stays up until midnight every night studying, and she works 30 hours each week at a drugstore. The physician orders a rapid mononucleosis test on Hollie, and it is positive. Hollie says she has never felt so awful in her whole life and wants to know whether she is going to die from this. She says it hurts really bad to swallow and she cannot eat. Hollie says that she has heard one gets mono from kissing, and she does not have a boyfriend, so she does not understand how she could possibly have mono. Hollie wants to know why the physician did not prescribe an antibiotic for her so that she could get well sooner and not have to miss any of her classes. ■

PROCEDURE **34-2** Collecting a Specimen for a Throat Culture

Outcome Collect a specimen for a throat culture.

A specimen for a throat culture is obtained by using a sterile swab. It is commonly used to aid in the diagnosis of infections such as streptococcal sore throat, pharyngitis, and tonsillitis. Less frequently, it is used to diagnose whooping cough and diphtheria. These latter diseases are not prevalent today because of the availability of immunizations against them. This procedure outlines the steps necessary to obtain a throat specimen to perform a rapid streptococcus test, which is discussed later in the chapter.

Equipment/Supplies

- Disposable gloves
- Tongue depressor
- Sterile swab
- Waste container

1. **Procedural Step.** Sanitize your hands, and assemble the equipment.
2. **Procedural Step.** Greet and identify the patient. Introduce yourself, and explain the procedure.
3. **Procedural Step.** Position the patient, and adjust the light to provide clear visualization of the throat.
   Principle. The throat must be clearly visible so that the medical assistant is able to determine the proper area for obtaining the specimen.
4. **Procedural Step.** Apply gloves. Remove the sterile swab from its peel-apart package, being careful not to contaminate it.
   Principle. Contamination of the swab may lead to inaccurate test results.

Remove the swab. (From Bonewit-West K: *Clinical procedures for medical assistants,* ed 7, St. Louis, 2008, Saunders.)

5. **Procedural Step.** Depress the tongue with the tongue depressor.
   Principle. The tongue depressor holds the tongue down and facilitates access to the throat.
6. **Procedural Step.** Place the swab at the back of the throat (posterior pharynx), and firmly rub it over any lesions or white or inflamed areas of the mucous membrane of the tonsillar area and posterior pharyngeal wall. Rotate the swab constantly as you collect the specimen, making sure there is good contact with the tonsillar area. Do not allow the swab to touch any areas other than the throat, such as the inside of the mouth.
   Principle. The swab should be rubbed over suspicious-looking areas where pathogens are likely to be found. A rotating motion is used to deposit the maximal amount of material possible on the swab. Touching it to any areas other than the throat contaminates the specimen with extraneous microorganisms.
7. **Procedural Step.** Keeping the patient's tongue depressed, withdraw the swab and remove the tongue depressor from the patient's mouth.
8. **Procedural Step.** Properly dispose of the tongue depressor in a regular waste container to prevent transmission of microorganisms.
9. **Procedural Step.** Process the swab according to the directions accompanying the rapid strep test.
10. **Procedural Step.** Remove gloves, and sanitize your hands. Chart the test results.

6

Collect the specimen. (From Bonewit-West K: *Clinical procedures for medical assistants,* ed 7, St. Louis, 2008, Saunders.)

CHARTING EXAMPLE	
Date	
9/20/10	10:30 a.m. Throat specimen collected.
	QuickVue Strep Test: Positive.
	—————— N. Moorehead, CMA (AAMA)

PROCEDURE 34-2

Memories *from* Externship

Natalie Moorehead: Terrified and excited at the same time to be experiencing my first externship, I found myself in a busy pediatric office. After a few days of watching and learning, I prepared to work up an infant for a well-child examination. Before entering the room I was told by a staff member that the HIV status of the infant's mother was questionable. Alarmed at first as to how I would feel in this situation, I immediately remembered all the precautions we had talked about in class. As I took the infant from the mother to weigh and measure him, I have to admit many thoughts ran through my mind, but again I was calmed because of all the information we had received in school regarding OSHA precautions. Faced with that situation today, after practicing wisely and safely for 5 years, I would not think twice about it because I know from my education and experience that these types of situations can be handled without alarm. ■

Prepare for Success

STREPTOCOCCUS TESTING

The most common streptococcal condition is streptococcal sore throat, or *streptococcal pharyngitis,* which primarily affects children and young adults. The causative agent of streptococcal pharyngitis is a group A beta-hemolytic streptococcus known as *Streptococcus pyogenes.*

Streptococcal pharyngitis is a potentially serious condition because some patients develop a poststreptococcal sequela. A **sequela** is a morbid secondary condition that occurs as a result of a less serious primary infection. A few patients with streptococcal pharyngitis (primary infection) develop rheumatic fever; the rheumatic fever is considered a poststreptococcal sequela. Owing to the risk of a sequela, early diagnosis and treatment with antibiotics of streptococ-

cal pharyngitis is important. In the medical office, commercially available rapid streptococcus tests are often used for identification of group A beta-hemolytic streptococci.

Rapid Streptococcus Tests

Rapid streptococcus tests directly detect group A streptococcus from a throat swab in a very short time. Most tests require only 4 to 10 minutes to process; diagnosis can often be made and antibiotics prescribed, if necessary, before the patient leaves the office.

The most frequently used rapid streptococcus test is the direct antigen identification test, which confirms the presence of group A streptococcus through an antigen-antibody reaction. The test works by combining particles sensitized to the streptococcus antibody with the throat specimen. If group A streptococcal antigen is in the specimen, it combines with the antibody-sensitized particles to produce a color change that can be observed with the unaided eye. Rapid streptococcus tests also include a control that determines whether the test results are accurate and reliable.

The advantage of the direct antigen identification test is that it provides the physician with immediate test results rather than requiring an overnight culture. Specific instructions are included with every commercially available antigen identification test; examples of these tests include QTest Strep (Becton Dickinson, Franklin Lakes, N.J.), Clearview Strep A (Wampole Laboratories, Princeton, N.J.), and QuickVue In-Line Strep A (Quidel, San Diego) (Figure 34-6).

SENSITIVITY TESTING

The physician may request not only that the laboratory identify the infecting pathogen, but also that a sensitivity test be performed on it to determine the best antibiotic to treat the condition. A sensitivity test determines the susceptibility of pathogenic bacteria to various antibiotics.

If liquid has not moved across the Result Window in 1 minute, completely remove the swab and reinsert.

Figure 34-6. Procedure for performing the QuickVue In-Line One-Step Strep A test. (Courtesy Quidel Corporation, San Diego.)

The most common method for sensitivity testing is the *disc-diffusion method* (Figure 34-7). Commercially prepared discs impregnated with known concentrations of various antibiotics are dropped on the surface of a solid **culture medium** in a Petri plate **inoculated** with the pathogen. The Petri plate is **incubated,** allowing the antibiotics to diffuse into the culture medium. If the pathogen is susceptible or sensitive to an antibiotic, there is a clear zone without bacterial growth around the disc. This indicates that the antibiotic was effective in destroying the pathogen. If the pathogen is unaffected by or resistant to the antibiotic, there is no clear zone around the disc, indicating that the antibiotic was unable to kill the pathogen. Sensitivity testing enables the physician to decide which antibiotics would most likely be effective against the infectious disease in question.

MICROSCOPIC EXAMINATION OF MICROORGANISMS

Microorganisms can be examined under a microscope in the fixed state or in the living state. Examination in the fixed state involves the preparation of a smear through heat fixation, followed by a staining process such as Gram stain (see later). Most microorganisms are examined in the fixed state because it is easier to examine them when they are stained.

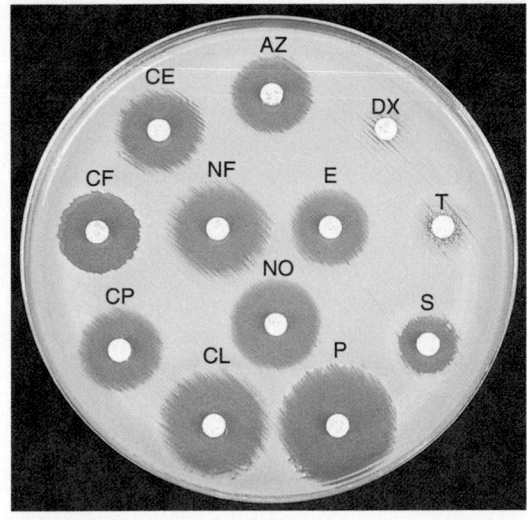

AZ: Azithromycin
CE: Cephalothin
CF: Ciprofloxacin
CL: Clarithromycin
CP: Ciprozil
DX: Doxycycline
E: Erythromycin
NF: Nitrofurantoin
NO: Norfloxacin
P: Penicillin
S: Sulfisoxazole
T: Tetracycline

Figure 34-7. Sensitivity testing. (From Mahon CR, Manuselis G Jr: *Textbook of diagnostic microbiology,* ed 2, Philadelphia, 2000, Saunders.)

Penicillin

PATIENT TEACHING | **Strep Throat**

Answer questions patients have about strep throat.

What is strep throat?

Strep throat is a contagious and acute infection that is medically known as *streptococcal pharyngitis.* It is caused by the bacterium group A streptococcus. Strep throat is transmitted directly from one person to another through droplets of saliva or nasal secretions. It most frequently occurs in children 5 to 10 years old and during the months of October through April. Strep infections are different from most other infectious diseases because having one strep infection does not prevent the development of another at a future date.

What are the symptoms of strep throat?

The symptoms of strep throat are a sore throat with severe pain on swallowing, a bright red pharynx (called "beefy red pharynx"), fever, white patches on the tonsils, swollen glands in the neck, muscular aches and pains, and a feeling of tiredness.

How is strep throat diagnosed and treated?

Strep throat is diagnosed by taking a throat specimen and running a laboratory test on it to determine whether group A streptococcus is present. Strep throat is usually treated by antibiotics taken orally for 10 days. It is important to take all of the antibiotic prescribed by the physician to prevent complications that can occur from strep throat. A patient with strep throat should also rest in bed and avoid contact with others to prevent spreading it.

What are the complications of strep throat?

Severe complications can result from strep throat if it is not adequately treated, including rheumatic fever and glomerulonephritis, which is a kidney disorder. These complications are rare because most patients seek early treatment for strep infections.

- Encourage the patient to complete the entire prescribed course of antibiotics.
- Instruct the patient to notify the physician if new symptoms develop.
- Provide the patient with educational materials about strep throat. ■

Some microorganisms require examination in the living state, however, owing to special circumstances, such as their inability to be readily stained or difficulty in culturing them. The living state also allows visualization of the movement of motile microorganisms. This is especially helpful in the identification of certain motile microorganisms, such as *Trichomonas vaginalis,* which is the causative agent of the vaginal infection trichomoniasis. To observe the motility of microorganisms, they first must be suspended in a liquid medium so that they are free to move about. The most common method of examining microorganisms in the living state is the wet mount method, which is described next.

Wet Mount Method

In the wet mount method, the medical assistant places a drop of fluid containing the organism on a glass slide and covers it with a coverslip (Figure 34-8). The coverslip may be ringed with petroleum jelly to provide a seal between the slide and coverslip. The purpose is to reduce the rate of evaporation through air currents that lead to drying and possible death of the specimen.

The slide is placed under the microscope for examination by the physician using the high-power objective. For satisfactory visualization, the intensity of the light must be diminished by partially closing the diaphragm of the microscope. The slide and coverslip should be properly disposed of in a biohazard sharps container.

Smears

A **smear** consists of material spread on a slide for microscopic examination. It can be prepared directly from the specimen collected on the swab, or the specimen can be grown first on a culture medium and a smear then prepared. Most smears must be stained before they can be viewed under the microscope, using one of many staining techniques. Bacteria contained in a smear are colorless and usually difficult to identify under the microscope unless some type of staining is used.

Smears are often helpful when time is a factor because a smear can be prepared immediately from the specimen. This procedure gives the physician a preliminary clue to the causative agent while other, more time-consuming tests are being performed. Procedure 34-3 outlines the method to prepare a microbiologic smear.

A drop of fluid containing the organism is placed on a glass slide.

The specimen is covered with a coverslip ringed with petroleum jelly.

Figure 34-8. Wet mount method of slide preparation for examining microorganisms in the living state. (From Bonewit-West K: *Clinical procedures for medical assistants,* ed 7, St. Louis, 2008, Saunders.)

Gram Stain

Gram stain is often used in combination with other tests to help in the diagnosis and treatment of infectious diseases. As already discussed, bacteria contained in a smear are colorless and usually difficult to identify under the microscope unless some type of staining is used. Gram stain allows the observer to view directly the size, shape, and growth patterns of the bacteria.

In 1883, Christian Gram, a Danish physician, discovered a way to differentiate bacteria on the basis of their color reactions to various stains. Gram stain is based on the fact that when treated with crystal violet dye, certain bacteria permanently retain this dye after undergoing a decolorization process. These bacteria exhibit a purple color when viewed under the microscope and are known as *gram-positive* bacteria (Figure 34-9A). Other bacteria are unable to retain this dye after being decolorized and become colorless. They must be counterstained with a red dye to become visible under the microscope. These bacteria exhibit a pink or red color and are known as *gram-negative* bacteria (Figure 34-9B). These staining characteristics are due to differences in the chemical composition of the bacterial cell walls.

Gram stain allows for the division of most bacteria into two groups—gram-positive and gram-negative. Infectious diseases caused by gram-positive bacteria include streptococcal sore throat, scarlet fever, rheumatic fever, diphtheria, lobar pneumonia, tetanus, and botulism. Infectious diseases caused by gram-negative bacteria include whooping cough, gonorrhea, meningitis, bacillary dysentery, cholera, typhoid fever, and plague.

Bacteria that are Gram-stained are also observed for their characteristic shape and fall into one of the following categories: gram-positive rods, gram-negative rods, gram-positive cocci, or gram-negative cocci. The causative agent of gonorrhea is a gram-negative diplococcus.

Figure 34-9. Gram-positive and gram-negative bacteria. **A,** Diphtheria is caused by a gram-positive bacillus. **B,** Gonorrhea is caused by a gram-negative diplococcus. (**A** courtesy Cathy Bissonette; **B** from Mahon CR, Manuselis G Jr: *Textbook of diagnostic microbiology,* ed 2, Philadelphia, 2000, Saunders.)

PREVENTION AND CONTROL OF INFECTIOUS DISEASES

Individuals in the community can help prevent and control infectious diseases by practicing good techniques of medical asepsis, obtaining proper nutrition and rest, and using good hygienic measures. In addition, infected individuals should contact their physicians in an effort to ensure early diagnosis and treatment of the infectious disease. Immunizations are available to prevent a wide range of infectious diseases. The medical assistant has a responsibility to help educate community members about practices that reduce the transmission of pathogens and help control and prevent infectious diseases.

What Would You Do? What Would You *Not* Do?

Case Study 3

John Seimer calls the medical office. He says that he is not a patient at the office but would like some assistance. He says that for the past 3 days he has had a headache, fever, chills, and aching muscles. He says that a week ago he pulled a tick off his lower leg, and several days later he found a red rash around the tick bite. He says that he went on the Internet and looked up his symptoms, and he is sure that he has Lyme disease. The Internet site recommended taking doxycycline for 3 weeks to treat Lyme disease. John says that he does not like to go to the doctor and has not been to see a doctor for more than 10 years. He wants to know whether the doctor could call in a prescription for doxycycline for him. He says that he has health insurance and the doctor could bill him for an appointment, just as long as he does not have to come in. ■

PROCEDURE 34-3
PROCEDURE 34-3 Preparing a Smear

Outcome Prepare a microbiology smear.

Equipment/Supplies

- Disposable gloves
- Bunsen burner
- Clean glass slide
- Microbiologic specimen
- Slide forceps
- Sterile swab
- Biohazard waste container

1. **Procedural Step.** Sanitize your hands.
2. **Procedural Step.** Assemble the equipment. Label the slide with the patient's name and the date.
3. **Procedural Step.** Apply gloves. Hold the edges of the slide between your thumb and index finger. Starting at the right side and using a rolling motion, gently and evenly spread the material from the specimen over the slide. The material should cover approximately one half to two thirds of the slide. Do not rub the material vigorously over the slide. Properly dispose of the contaminated swab in a biohazard waste container.

Spread the specimen over the slide. (From Bonewit-West K: *Clinical procedures for medical assistants,* ed 7, St. Louis, 2008, Saunders.)

Principle. The specimen may contain pathogens that are capable of infecting the medical assistant; it is important to wear gloves. A rolling motion is used to deposit the maximal amount of material possible on the slide. Rubbing may disintegrate the cellular structures making up the microorganisms in the specimen.

4. **Procedural Step.** Allow the smear to air dry in a flat position for at least 30 minutes. Heat should not be applied at this time.
Principle. Air-drying allows the bacterial cells to dry slowly. Applying heat at this stage would burst the bacterial cells, resulting in an inappropriate smear.

5. **Procedural Step.** Holding the slide with the slide forceps, heat-fix the smear by quickly passing the slide back and forth (approximately three times) through the flame of a Bunsen burner. The slide has been fixed properly if the back of the slide feels uncomfortable (but not too hot) when touched to the back of your hand. Excessive heat should be avoided. Allow the slide to cool completely. An alternative to heat-fixing the slide is to apply ethyl alcohol to the slide and allow it to air-dry.
Principle. Heat-fixing the slide kills the microorganisms and attaches them firmly to the slide so that they

Continued

PROCEDURE 34-3 Preparing a Smear—cont'd

do not wash off during the staining process. An excessive amount of heat could result in distortion of the bacterial cells.

6. **Procedural Step.** Prepare the slide for examination under the microscope. Inform the physician that the slide is ready for examination.

Heat-fix the smear. (From Bonewit-West K: *Clinical procedures for medical assistants*, ed 7, St. Louis, 2008, Saunders.)

MEDICAL PRACTICE *and the* LAW

This chapter addresses the collection and identification of microorganisms that cause infections. You must maintain standard precautions whenever handling potentially infectious material to protect yourself, your coworkers, and your patients. Microbiology is an exact science—one stray microorganism can contaminate the entire specimen. Sanitize hands thoroughly, and apply new gloves between handling of specimens to avoid cross-contamination. If specimen contamination occurs, immediately discard the specimen, and collect a new one. Be precise in your labeling—a mislabeled specimen can cause unnecessary concern, treatment, or both for the patient.

Maintain confidentiality of information. Certain infectious diseases must be reported to the Centers for Disease Control and Prevention (CDC) or local board of health. Otherwise, do not give information to anyone else but the patient or legal guardian. ∎

What Would You Do? What Would You *Not* Do? RESPONSES

Case Study 1
Page 809

What Did Natalie Do?
❑ Told Paula that it is important that the physician find out whether Caitlin has strep throat because strep can sometimes develop into a more serious infection. Explained that if Caitlin does have strep throat, the doctor would want to prescribe the best antibiotic to treat the infection.
❑ Talked with Caitlin about the reason for the test. Explained that it will help the doctor find the best way to treat her so that she starts feeling better as soon as possible.
❑ Reassured Caitlin that the procedure would be very quick and it would be over before she knew it.
❑ Told Caitlin that after the specimen was obtained, she could choose a prize from the treasure box.

What Did Natalie Not Do?
❑ Did not force the collection swab into Caitlin's mouth.

What Would You Do?/What Would You *Not* Do? Review Natalie's response and place a checkmark next to the information you included in your response. List additional information you included in your response.

_____

_____

_____

_____

Case Study 2
Page 816

What Did Natalie Do?
❑ Told Hollie that mononucleosis is usually transmitted by kissing, but it can sometimes be transmitted by coughs and sneezes from an infected person.
❑ Sympathized with Hollie and told her that it probably feels like she is going to die, but she should start to feel better as her body begins to fight off the disease.

What Would You Do? What Would You *Not* Do? RESPONSES—cont'd

❏ Explained to Hollie that mononucleosis is caused by a virus and that antibiotics do not work against viruses.

❏ Told Hollie to try drinking cold fluids or sucking on a Popsicle until she feels more like eating.

What Did Natalie *Not Do*?

❏ Did not ignore or minimize Hollie's concerns.

What Would You Do?/What Would You *Not* Do? Review Natalie's response and place a checkmark next to the information you included in your response. List additional information you included in your response.

_____

_____

_____

_____

Case Study 3
Page 821

What Did Natalie *Do*?

❏ Empathized with John and told him that a lot of people do not like coming to see the doctor. Told him that the doctor could

not legally or ethically prescribe medication for him without seeing him.

❏ Told John that the office could not bill him for an appointment that he did not have.

❏ Asked John whether he wanted to make an appointment to see the doctor.

What Did Natalie *Not Do*?

❏ Did not tell John he should not be diagnosing himself with information he found on the Internet.

What Would You Do?/What Would You *Not* Do? Review Natalie's response and place a checkmark next to the information you included in your response. List additional information you included in your response.

_____

_____

_____

_____

♻ TERMINOLOGY REVIEW

Bacilli (*sing.* **bacillus**) Bacteria that have a rod shape.

Cocci (*sing.* **coccus**) Bacteria that have a round shape.

Contagious Capable of being transmitted directly or indirectly from one person to another.

Culture The propagation of a mass of microorganisms in a laboratory culture medium.

Culture medium A mixture of nutrients on which microorganisms are grown in the laboratory.

False negative A test result denoting that a condition is absent when it is actually present.

False positive A test result denoting that a condition is present when it is actually absent.

Immunization The process of becoming protected from a disease through vaccination.

Incubate In microbiology, the act of placing a culture in a chamber (incubator) that provides optimal growth requirements for the multiplication of the organisms, such as the proper temperature, humidity, and darkness.

Incubation period The interval of time between the invasion by a pathogenic microorganism and the appearance of first symptoms of the disease.

Infectious disease A disease caused by a pathogen that produces harmful effects on its host.

Inoculate To introduce microorganisms into a culture medium for growth and multiplication.

Microbiology The scientific study of microorganisms and their activities.

Mucous membrane A membrane lining body passages or cavities that open to the outside.

Normal flora Harmless, nonpathogenic microorganisms that normally reside in many parts of the body but do not cause disease.

Resistance The natural ability of an organism to remain unaffected by harmful substances in its environment.

Sequela A morbid (secondary) condition occurring as a result of a less serious primary infection.

Smear Material spread on a slide for microscope examination.

Specimen A small sample or part taken from the body to show the nature of the whole.

Spirilla (*sing.* **spirillum**) Bacteria that have a spiral or curved shape.

ON THE WEB

For Information on Disease and Infection Control:

American Society for Microbiology: www.ams.org

Association for Professionals in Infection Control and Epidemiology: www.apic.org

Centers for Disease Control and Prevention: www.cdc.gov

World Health Organization (WHO): www.who.int/en

Infection Control Today: www.infectioncontroltoday.com

Infectious Diseases Society of America (IDSA): www.idsociety.org

National Multiple Sclerosis Society: www.nmss.org

Cystic Fibrosis Foundation (CFF): www.cff.org

PREPARE FOR CERTIFICATION   Visit the Evolve site at http://evolve.elsevier.com/Bonewit/today/ to actively Prepare for your Certification.

CD   *Check out the **Companion CD** bound with the book to access additional interactive activities.*

35

Emergency Medical Procedures

LEARNING OBJECTIVES

First Aid
1. State the purpose of first aid.
2. Explain the purpose of the emergency medical services (EMS) system.
3. List the OSHA standards for administering first aid.
4. List the guidelines that should be followed when providing emergency care.

Common Emergency Situations
1. List and describe conditions that cause respiratory distress.
2. List the symptoms of a heart attack and a stroke.
3. Explain the causes of each of the following types of shock: cardiogenic, neurogenic, anaphylactic, and psychogenic.
4. Identify and describe the three classifications of external bleeding.
5. Explain the difference between an open wound and a closed wound.
6. Describe the characteristics of each of the following types of fracture: impacted, greenstick, transverse, oblique, comminuted, and spiral.
7. Identify the characteristics of each of the following types of burns: superficial, partial thickness, and full thickness.
8. Explain the difference between a partial seizure and a generalized seizure.
9. List examples of each of the following types of poisoning: ingested, inhaled, absorbed, and injected.
10. Identify factors that place an individual at higher risk for developing heat-related and cold-related injuries.
11. Describe the difference between type 1 and type 2 diabetes mellitus.
12. Explain the causes of insulin shock and diabetic coma.
13. Identify the symptoms and describe the emergency care for each of the following conditions: respiratory distress, heart attack, stroke, shock, bleeding, wounds, musculoskeletal injuries, burns, seizures, poisoning, heat and cold exposure, and diabetic emergencies.

PROCEDURES

Respond to common emergency situations.

CHAPTER OUTLINE

CAAHEP COMPETENCIES

General Competencies
Communication
- Recognize and respond to verbal communications.
- Recognize and respond to nonverbal communications.

ABHES COMPETENCIES

Communication
- Recognize and respond to verbal and nonverbal communications.

Clinical Duties
- Recognize emergencies.
- Perform first aid and CPR.

KEY TERMS

burn
crash cart
crepitus (KREP-it-us)
dislocation
emergency medical services (EMS) system
first aid
fracture (FRAK-shur)
hypothermia (hie-poe-THER-mee-ah)

poison
pressure point
seizure (SEE-zhur)
shock
splint
sprain
strain
wound

Introduction to Emergency Medical Procedures

Medical emergencies often arise inside and outside of the workplace, and they can result in the sudden loss of life or permanent disability. If an emergency situation occurs in the medical office, the physician provides immediate medical care for the patient. Some medical offices maintain a crash cart for this purpose. In these situations, the medical assistant may be required to assist the physician in providing the emergency medical care.

The medical assistant may need to administer first aid for medical emergencies that occur outside of the medical office environment. **First aid** is defined as the immediate care administered before complete medical care can be obtained to an individual who is injured or suddenly becomes ill. The medical assistant is most likely to administer first aid to a family member or friend. The purpose of first aid is to save a life, reduce pain and suffering, prevent further injury, reduce the incidence of permanent disability, and increase the opportunity for an early recovery.

This chapter focuses on common emergency situations that the medical assistant may encounter and the first aid required for each. It is not intended, however, as a substitute for thorough first aid instruction through the American Red Cross, National Safety Council, or American Heart Association.

OFFICE CRASH CART

A **crash cart** is a specially equipped cart for holding and transporting medications, equipment, and supplies needed to perform lifesaving procedures in an emergency. A growing number of physicians are incorporating crash carts into their medical offices. Patients who are injured or suddenly become ill might be brought to the medical office for emergency medical care. In addition, a patient might develop a sudden illness at the medical office that requires emergency medical care. Examples of these situations include life-threatening cardiac dysrhythmias, shock, cardiac arrest, poisoning, and traumatic injury.

The items on an office crash cart vary widely among medical offices depending on the extent of the emergency medical care that is likely to be administered. This is directly related to the time it takes for emergency medical personnel to arrive and the location of the nearest hospital. Table 35-1 is a general list of the medications, equipment, and supplies that may be included on an office crash cart. The medical assistant may be responsible for regularly checking the crash cart to replenish supplies and check the expiration dates on medications.

EMERGENCY MEDICAL SERVICES SYSTEM

The **emergency medical services (EMS) system** is a network of community resources, equipment, and emer-

Table 35-1 Office Crash Cart

Name	Drug Category	Emergency Use
MEDICATIONS USED IN CARDIOVASCULAR EMERGENCIES		
Epinephrine (Adrenalin)	Sympathomimetic*	Helps restore cardiac rhythm in cardiac arrest
Sodium bicarbonate	Alkalinizing agent	To correct metabolic acidosis after cardiac arrest
Lidocaine (Xylocaine)	Antiarrhythmic	For rapid control of acute ventricular arrhythmias after myocardial infarction
Bretylium tosylate	Antiarrhythmic	For treatment of ventricular fibrillation or ventricular tachycardia that fails to respond to lidocaine
Procainamide (Pronestyl)	Antiarrhythmic	Alternative drug when lidocaine fails to suppress ventricular arrhythmias
Atropine	Parasympatholytic†	For treating bradycardia associated with hypotension
Isoproterenol (Isuprel)	Sympathomimetic	To increase heart rate in bradycardia that fails to respond to atropine
Dopamine (Intropin)	Sympathomimetic	For treatment of hypotension associated with cardiogenic shock
Dobutamine (Dobutrex)	Sympathomimetic	To manage congestive heart failure when increase in heart rate is not desired
Nitroprusside (Nitropress)	Antihypertensive-vasodilator	For immediate reduction of blood pressure in hypertensive crisis and cardiogenic shock
Norepinephrine (Levophed)	Sympathomimetic	To increase blood pressure in cardiogenic shock and other hypotensive emergencies
Adenosine (Adenocard)	Antiarrhythmic	To manage complex paroxysmal supraventricular tachycardia
Verapamil (Calan, Isoptin)	Antiarrhythmic	For treatment of supraventricular tachycardia that fails to respond to adenosine
Furosemide (Lasix)	Diuretic	For treatment of congestive heart failure and acute pulmonary edema
Nitroglycerin (Nitrostat)	Coronary vasodilator	For treatment of chest pain associated with angina pectoris and acute myocardial infarction
INTRAVENOUS SOLUTIONS		
5% Dextrose (D-5-W)	Glucose	Solution of 5% glucose in water used to replace fluid and nutrients
Isotonic saline	Electrolyte	Solution of sodium chloride in purified water used to replace lost fluid, sodium, and chloride
Lactated Ringer's solution	Electrolyte	Sterile solution of sodium chloride, potassium chloride, and calcium chloride in purified waters, used to replace fluids and electrolytes
MEDICATIONS USED IN BREATHING EMERGENCIES		
Epinephrine (Adrenalin)	Sympathomimetic	For symptomatic relief in acute attacks of bronchial asthma or bronchospasm associated with chronic bronchitis and emphysema
Terbutaline (Brethine)	Sympathomimetic	For symptomatic relief of bronchial asthma and reversible bronchospasm associated with bronchitis and emphysema
Aminophylline	Bronchodilator	For symptomatic relief in acute attacks of bronchial asthma or reversible bronchospasm associated with chronic bronchitis and emphysema
Albuterol (Proventil, Ventolin)	Sympathomimetic	For symptomatic relief of bronchial asthma and reversible bronchospasm associated with chronic bronchitis and emphysema
MEDICATIONS USED IN ANAPHYLACTIC REACTIONS		
Epinephrine (Adrenalin)	Sympathomimetic	For treatment of hypersensitivity reactions caused by medications, allergens, or insect stings
Diphenhydramine (Benadryl)	Antihistamine	To counteract histamine in treatment of hypersensitivity reactions
Methylprednisolone (Solu-Medrol)	Glucocorticoid	—
MEDICATIONS USED FOR POISONING		
Ipecac syrup	Emetic	To induce vomiting of ingested poisons
Activated charcoal	Antidote, adsorbent	Used as general-purpose antidote to adsorb swallowed poisons; to decrease absorption of poison or drug by binding with any unabsorbed drug from digestive tract
Naloxone (Narcan)	Narcotic antagonist	For treatment of overdoses caused by narcotics or synthetic narcotic agents

Continued

Table 35-1 Office Crash Cart—cont'd

Name	Drug Category	Emergency Use
MEDICATIONS USED IN NEUROLOGIC EMERGENCIES		
Diazepam (Valium)	Anticonvulsant, antianxiety	For treatment of convulsions in major motor seizures, status epilepticus, and acute anxiety states
Phenytoin (Dilantin)	Anticonvulsant	For controlling status epilepticus; for management of generalized tonic-clonic seizures, complex partial seizures, and critical focal seizures
Phenobarbital	Anticonvulsant, sedative-hypnotic	For management of generalized tonic-clonic seizures and partial seizures, and in the control of acute convulsive episodes (status epilepticus, febrile seizures)
MEDICATIONS USED IN METABOLIC EMERGENCIES		
Glucose (e.g., orange juice)	Glucose	To provide glucose for conscious patients with hypoglycemia
50% Dextrose	Glucose	To provide glucose for unconscious patients with hypoglycemia
EQUIPMENT AND SUPPLIES		

Cardiac Equipment
Defibrillator
Defibrillator pads

Intravenous Equipment
Tourniquet
Surgical tape
IV catheters
IV cannulas
IV tubing and needles
Armboard
IV cut-down tray

Surgical Equipment
Scalpel
Curved and straight hemostats
Needle holder
Tissue forceps
Small scissors
Local anesthetic
Gauze squares

Airway Equipment
Suction equipment
Suction pumps
Suction tubing
Suction catheters
Oral and nasal airways
Oxygen equipment
Oxygen
Oxygen facemask
Nasal cannula
Oxygen tubing
Laryngoscope handle and blades
Endotracheal tubes
Lubricant

Table 35-1 Office Crash Cart—cont'd

Name	Drug Category	Emergency Use
Miscellaneous Supplies		
Sterile gloves		
Clean gloves		
Biohazard containers		
Syringes (assorted sizes)		
Needles (assorted sizes)		
Filter needles		
Tubex syringe		
Alcohol swabs		
Betadine (povidone-iodine) swabs		
Sterile dressings		
Roller gauze (various widths)		
Adhesive tape		
Adhesive strip bandages		
Bandage scissors		
Local anesthetic (lidocaine [Xylocaine])		
Lidocaine ointment		
Lidocaine spray		
Lubricant		
Tongue blades		
Flashlight		
Cold packs		
Sphygmomanometer		
Stethoscope		

From Bonewit-West K: *Clinical procedures for medical assistants,* ed 7, St. Louis, 2008, Saunders.

*A drug that stimulates the sympathetic nervous system; also called an *adrenergic.*

†A drug that inhibits the action of the parasympathetic nervous system; also called an *anticholinergic.*

gency medical technicians (EMTs) that provides emergency care to victims of injury or sudden illness. An *EMT-basic* (EMT-B) is a professional provider of prehospital emergency care, which includes care at the scene and during transportation to the hospital. An EMT-B has received formal training and is certified to provide basic life support measures. An *EMT-paramedic* (EMT-P) is qualified to provide advanced life support care, including advanced airway maintenance, starting intravenous drips, administration of medication, cardiac monitoring and interpretation, and cardiac defibrillation.

Activating EMS is often the most important step in an emergency. The rapid arrival of EMTs increases the patient's chances of surviving a life-threatening emergency. In most urban and in some rural areas in the United States, the medical assistant can activate the local EMS by dialing 911 on the telephone. Other areas have a local seven digit number, in which case it is important to keep the number at hand.

When calling local EMS, the medical assistant speaks with an *emergency medical dispatcher* (EMD). An EMD has had formal training in handling emergency situations over the phone. The responsibility of the EMD is to answer the emergency call, listen to the caller, obtain critical information, determine what help is necessary, and send the appropriate personnel and equipment. The EMD is also responsible for relaying instructions to the caller about providing emergency care until the EMTs arrive.

These guidelines should be followed when calling EMS:

- Speak clearly and calmly to the EMD. Identify the problem as accurately and concisely as possible so that proper equipment and personnel can be sent. The EMD needs to know the number of victims, the condition of the victim or victims, and the emergency care that has already been administered.
- The EMD will ask you for your phone number and address. In responding, relay the exact location of the victim to the dispatcher, including the correct street name and house number, and (if applicable) the building name, floor, and room number. With the 911 enhanced emergency system, the address automatically appears on a monitor; however, there is a chance that the address will not show up on the monitor. In addition, the emergency may not be in the same location as the caller. If possible, have someone meet the ambulance personnel and direct them to the scene.
- Do not hang up until the EMD gives you permission to do so. The dispatcher may need additional information or may give you instructions on treating the patient until EMTs arrive.

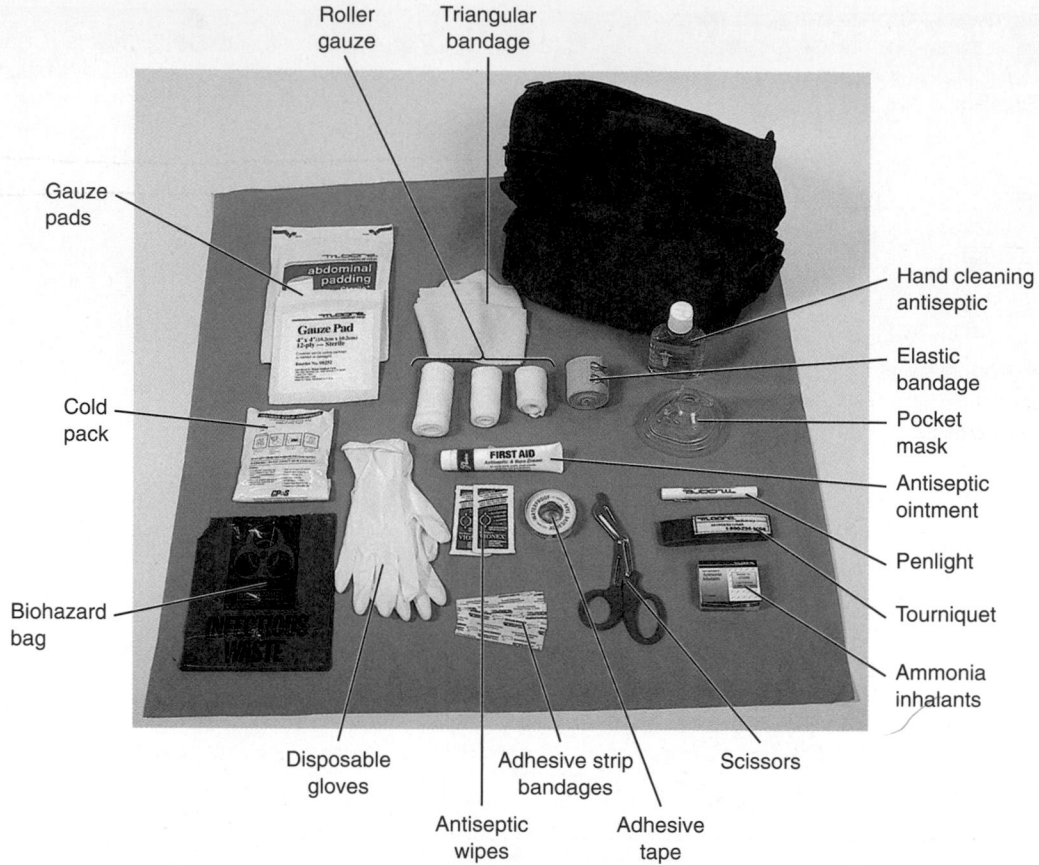

Figure 35-1. First aid kit. (From Bonewit-West K: *Clinical procedures for medical assistants,* ed 7, St. Louis, 2008, Saunders.)

FIRST AID KIT

The medical assistant should acquire and maintain a first aid kit. A first aid kit contains basic supplies to provide emergency care to individuals who have been injured or become suddenly ill (Figure 35-1). It is recommended that a first aid kit be kept at home and in the car.

First aid kits are available at most drug stores. It is also possible to make your own. Along with the items shown in Figure 35-1, the first aid kit should include the phone numbers of the local EMS, poison control center, and police and fire departments. It is important to check the first aid kit regularly and replace supplies as needed.

OSHA SAFETY PRECAUTIONS

To avoid exposure to bloodborne pathogens and other potentially infectious materials, the OSHA Bloodborne Pathogens Standard presented in Chapter 17 should be followed when performing first aid. The following guidelines help reduce or eliminate the risk of infection:

1. Make sure that your first aid kit contains personal protective equipment, such as gloves, a face shield and mask, and a pocket mask.

2. Wear gloves when it is reasonably anticipated that your hand will come into contact with the following: blood and other potentially infectious materials, mucous membranes, nonintact skin, and contaminated articles or surfaces.

3. Perform all first aid procedures involving blood or other potentially infectious materials in a manner that minimizes splashing, spraying, spattering, and generation of droplets of these substances.

4. Wear protective clothing and gloves to cover cuts or other lesions of the skin.

5. Sanitize your hands as soon as possible after removing gloves.

6. Avoid touching objects that may be contaminated with blood or other potentially infectious materials.

7. If your hands or other skin surfaces come in contact with blood or other potentially infectious materials, wash the area as soon as possible with soap and water.

8. If your mucous membranes (in eyes, nose, and mouth) come in contact with blood or other potentially infectious materials, flush them with water as soon as possible.

9. Avoid eating, drinking, and touching your mouth, eyes, and nose while providing emergency care or before you sanitize your hands.

10. If you are exposed to blood or other potentially infectious materials, report the incident as soon as possible to your physician so that postexposure procedures can be instituted.

GUIDELINES FOR PROVIDING EMERGENCY CARE

The remainder of this chapter presents specific emergency situations that may be encountered by the medical assistant and the emergency care for each. These guidelines should be followed when providing emergency care:

1. Remain calm, and speak in a normal tone of voice. These measures help calm and reassure the patient.
2. Make sure that the scene is safe before approaching the patient. It is important that you protect yourself from harm in an emergency situation.
3. Before administering emergency care to a conscious patient, you must first have permission or consent. To obtain consent, you must inform the patient who you are, your level of training, and what you are going to do to help. *Never* administer care to a conscious patient who refuses it. When a life-threatening condition exists, and the patient is unconscious or otherwise unable to give consent, consent is assumed or implied. Under law, it is implied that if the patient could give consent to care, he or she would.
4. Follow the OSHA standards when providing emergency care to reduce or eliminate exposure to bloodborne pathogens or other potentially infectious materials.
5. Know how to activate your local EMS system. Activating the EMS is often the most important step you can take to help a patient who has experienced an injury or sudden illness.
6. Do not move the patient unnecessarily. Unnecessary movement can result in further injury or be life-threatening to a patient with a serious condition.
7. Obtain information as to what happened from the patient, family members, coworkers, or bystanders.
8. Look for a medical alert tag on the patient's wrist or neck. A medical alert tag provides information on a medical condition the patient may have.
9. Continue caring for the patient until more highly trained personnel arrive. On the arrival of emergency medical personnel or a physician, relay the condition in which you found the patient and the emergency care that has been administered.

Respiratory Distress

Respiratory distress indicates that the patient is breathing but is having great difficulty in doing so. Respiratory distress may lead to respiratory arrest. It is important that the medical assistant be alert for the signs and symptoms of respiratory distress, which may include noisy breathing, such as gasping for air or rasping, gurgling, or whistling sounds; breathing that is unusually fast or slow; and breathing that is painful. The general care for respiratory distress is to place the patient in a comfortable position that facili-

Highlight on Good Samaritan Laws

In most states, Good Samaritan laws have been enacted to provide immunity to individuals, such as the medical assistant, who administer first aid at the scene of an emergency. These laws were enacted to encourage individuals to help others in an emergency. They assume that an individual would do her or his best to save a life or prevent further injury.

The legal immunity provided by Good Samaritan laws protects an individual from being sued and found financially responsible for a patient's injury. The individual is immune from liability (except for "gross negligence") if he or she acts in good faith and uses a reasonable level of skill that does not exceed the scope of the individual's training.

Good Samaritan laws do not mean that an individual cannot be sued for administering first aid. An individual is not protected from liability if he or she is grossly careless or reckless in handling the situation. Because the components of Good Samaritan laws vary from state to state, the medical assistant must become familiar with the laws that govern his or her state. ■

tates breathing. Most patients prefer a sitting or semireclining position. Remain calm, and reassure the patient to help reduce anxiety. Calming the patient may help the patient breathe easier. If the patient's condition worsens or does not resolve within a few minutes, activate the local EMS services. Examples of conditions frequently causing respiratory distress are described next.

Asthma

Asthma is a condition characterized by wheezing, coughing, and dyspnea. During an asthmatic attack, the bronchioles constrict and become clogged with mucus, which accounts for many of the symptoms of asthma.

Asthma may occur at any age, but it is more common in children and young adults. If the condition is not treated, it can lead to serious complications, such as permanent lung damage. It is frequently, but not always, associated with a family history of allergies. Any of the common allergens, such as house dust, pollens, molds, or animal danders, may trigger an asthmatic attack. Asthmatic attacks may also be caused by nonspecific factors, such as air pollutants, tobacco smoke, chemical fumes, vigorous exercise, respiratory infections, exposure to cold, and emotional stress. Normally, an individual with asthma easily controls attacks with medications. These medications stop the muscle spasms and open the airway, making breathing easier.

Some patients may develop a severe, prolonged asthmatic attack that is life-threatening, which is known as *status asthmaticus*. These patients can move only a small amount of air. Because so little air is being moved, the typical breathing sounds associated with asthma may not be audible. The patient may have a bluish discoloration of the skin and extremely labored breathing. Status asthmaticus is a true emergency and requires immediate transportation of the patient to an emergency care facility by the fastest way possible.

Emphysema

Emphysema is a progressive lung disorder in which the terminal bronchioles that lead into the alveoli become plugged with mucus. Because of this problem, the alveoli become damaged, resulting in less surface area to diffuse oxygen into the blood. Eventually, this condition results in a loss of elasticity of the alveoli, causing inhaled air to become trapped in the lungs. This makes breathing difficult, particularly during exhalation.

Emphysema usually develops over many years and is found most frequently in heavy smokers. It also occurs in patients with chronic bronchitis and in elderly patients whose lungs have lost their natural elasticity. Chronic emphysema is one of the major causes of death in the United States. As the lungs become progressively less efficient, breathing becomes more and more difficult. Patients with advanced cases may go into respiratory or cardiac arrest.

Hyperventilation

Hyperventilation literally means "overbreathing." Hyperventilation is a manner of breathing in which the respirations become rapid and deep, causing an individual to exhale too much carbon dioxide. The low carbon dioxide levels in the body account for many of the symptoms of hyperventilation. Hyperventilation is often the result of fear or anxiety and is more likely to occur in individuals who are tense and nervous. It is also caused by serious organic conditions, such as diabetic coma, pneumonia, pulmonary edema, pulmonary embolism, head injuries, high fever, and aspirin poisoning.

In addition to rapid and deep respirations, the signs and symptoms of hyperventilation include dizziness, faintness, and lightheadedness; visual disturbances; chest pain; tachycardia; palpitations; fullness in the throat; and numbness and tingling of the fingers, toes, and the area around the mouth. Despite their rapid breathing efforts, patients complain that they cannot get enough air. They often think they are having a heart attack.

Treatment for hyperventilation caused by emotional factors is as follows: Calm and reassure the patient, and encourage him or her to slow the respirations, allowing the carbon dioxide level to return to normal. In the past, breathing into a paper bag was advocated as a remedy for hyperventilation. More recent studies no longer recommend this practice because it could be harmful if an underlying medical condition exists or if the patient is not actually hyperventilating. If the medical assistant suspects that hyperventilation has been caused by an organic problem, EMS should be activated immediately.

Heart Attack

A heart attack, also known as a *myocardial infarction* (MI), is caused by partial or complete obstruction of one or both of the coronary arteries or their branches. In most cases, the severity of the attack depends on the size of the obstructed artery and the amount of myocardial tissue nourished by that artery. If a small branch of a coronary artery is obstructed, the myocardial damage and symptoms may be mild, whereas the damage is usually extensive and the symptoms intense if a coronary artery is completely blocked.

The principal symptom of a heart attack is chest pain or discomfort. Patients describe the chest pain as squeezing or crushing pressure, severe indigestion or burning, heaviness, or aching. Chest discomfort can range in severity from feeling only mildly uncomfortable to being intense and accompanied by a feeling of suffocation and doom. The pain is usually felt behind the sternum and may radiate to the neck, throat, jaw, both shoulders, and both arms. The pain associated with a heart attack is prolonged and is usually not relieved by resting or taking nitroglycerin. Other signs and symptoms of a heart attack include shortness of breath, profuse perspiration, nausea, and fainting.

If the medical assistant suspects that the patient is having a heart attack, EMS should be activated immediately. Meanwhile, loosen tight clothing and have the patient rest in a comfortable position that facilitates breathing. If cardiac arrest occurs, the medical assistant should begin CPR immediately.

Stroke

A stroke, also called a *cerebrovascular accident* (CVA), results when an artery to the brain is blocked or ruptures, causing an interruption of the blood flow to the brain. The signs and symptoms of a stroke include sudden weakness or numbness of the face, arm, or leg on one side of the body; difficulty in speaking; dimmed vision or loss of vision in one eye; double vision; dizziness; confusion; severe headache; and loss of consciousness.

If the medical assistant suspects that the patient is having a stroke, EMS should be activated immediately. Meanwhile, loosen tight clothing and have the patient rest in a comfortable position. If respiratory arrest, cardiac arrest, or both occur, begin rescue breathing CPR as required.

Shock

For the body to function properly, adequate blood flow must be maintained to all of the vital organs. This is accomplished by the three important cardiovascular functions, as follows:

* Adequate pumping action of the heart
* Sufficient blood circulating in the blood vessels
* Blood vessels being able to respond to blood flow

When an individual experiences a severe injury or illness, one or more of these cardiovascular functions may be affected, which can lead to shock.

Shock is defined as the failure of the cardiovascular system to deliver enough blood to all of the body's vital organs. Shock accompanies different types of emergency situations, such as hemorrhaging, an MI, and severe allergic reaction. The five major types of shock are categorized according to cause: hypovolemic, cardiogenic, neurogenic, anaphylactic, and psychogenic. Each type of shock is described in this section. If not treated, most types of shock become life-threatening. This is because shock is progressive—when it reaches a certain point, it becomes irreversible, and the patient's life cannot be saved.

The signs and symptoms of shock are caused by failure of the vital organs to receive enough oxygen and nutrients. The organs most affected are the heart, brain, and lungs, which can be irreparably damaged in 4 to 6 minutes. The general signs and symptoms of shock are weakness, restlessness, anxiety, disorientation, pallor, cold and clammy skin, rapid breathing, and rapid pulse.

If not treated, these symptoms can progress rapidly to a significant drop in blood pressure, cyanosis, loss of consciousness, and death. The signs and symptoms of shock may be subtle or pronounced. In addition, no single sign or symptom determines accurately the presence or severity of the shock. Because of this, it is crucial to consider the nature of the illness or injury in determining whether the patient is a possible victim of shock. If a patient has a traumatic injury to the abdomen, shock should be considered a possibility, even if the patient's signs and symptoms do not suggest shock.

Shock (with the exception of psychogenic shock) requires immediate medical care. The medical assistant should activate EMS without delay so that proper medical care can be obtained as soon as possible.

Hypovolemic Shock

Hypovolemic shock is caused by a loss of blood or other body fluids. Conditions that result in this type of shock include external and internal hemorrhaging; plasma loss from severe burns; and severe dehydration from vomiting, diarrhea, or profuse perspiration. The first priority of hypovolemic shock is to control bleeding. A patient in hypovolemic shock must have the volume of fluid that was lost replaced and must be transported to an emergency care facility immediately.

Cardiogenic Shock

Cardiogenic shock is caused by the failure of the heart to pump blood adequately to all of the body's vital organs. This type of shock occurs when the heart has been injured or damaged. Cardiogenic shock is most frequently seen with MI. Other causes include dysrhythmias, severe congestive heart failure, acute valvular damage, and pulmonary embolism. When a patient develops cardiogenic shock, it is difficult to reverse and has a high fatality rate (80% to 90%).

Neurogenic Shock

Neurogenic shock occurs when the nervous system is unable to control the diameter of the blood vessels. In normal situations, the nervous system instructs the blood vessels to constrict or dilate, which controls blood pressure. In neurogenic shock, that control is lost, and the blood vessels dilate, causing the blood to pool in peripheral areas of the body away from vital organs.

This type of shock is most often seen with brain and spinal injuries. The blood vessels become dilated, and there is not enough blood in the circulatory system to fill the dilated vessels, causing the blood pressure to drop significantly.

Anaphylactic Shock

Anaphylactic shock is a life-threatening reaction of the body to a substance to which an individual is highly allergic. Allergens that are most apt to result in anaphylaxis are drugs (e.g., penicillin), insect venoms, foods, and allergen extracts used in hyposensitization injections.

An anaphylactic reaction causes the release of large amounts of histamine, resulting in dilation of the blood vessels throughout the entire body and a decrease in the blood pressure. The symptoms of anaphylactic shock begin with sneezing, hives, itching, angioedema, erythema, and disorientation and progress to difficulty in breathing, dizziness, faintness, and loss of consciousness. Medical care should be obtained immediately because most fatalities occur within the first 2 hours.

The emergency care for anaphylactic shock is the administration of epinephrine. Because time is a factor, individuals known to have a severe allergy carry an anaphylactic emergency treatment kit that contains injectable epinephrine (Figure 35-2) and oral antihistamines. With the kit, treatment for a severe allergic reaction can be started immediately.

Psychogenic Shock

Psychogenic shock is the least serious type of shock. It is caused by unpleasant physical or emotional stimuli, such as pain, fright, and the sight of blood. With psychogenic shock, a sudden dilation of the blood vessels causes the blood to pool in the abdomen and extremities. This temporarily deprives the brain of blood, causing a temporary loss of consciousness (fainting), usually lasting 1 to 2 minutes. Fainting generally occurs when an individual is in an upright position. Before fainting, the patient usually experiences some warning signals such as sudden lighthead-

Figure 35-2. Anaphylactic emergency epinephrine injector. (From Bonewit-West K: *Clinical procedures for medical assistants,* ed 7, St. Louis, 2008, Saunders.)

edness, pallor, nausea, weakness, yawning, blurred vision, a feeling of warmth, and sweating.

An individual who is about to faint should be placed in a position that facilitates blood flow to the brain and told to breathe deeply. The preferred position is to move the patient into a supine position with the legs elevated approximately 12 inches and the collar and clothing loosened (Figure 35-3). This position is not always possible, such as when a patient is seated; in this case, the patient's head should be lowered between the legs (Figure 35-4). A patient who has fainted should be placed in the supine position with the legs elevated. It is recommended that a patient who has fainted contact her or his physician for further evaluation.

Figure 35-3. Prevention and treatment of fainting. (From Bonewit-West K: *Clinical procedures for medical assistants,* ed 7, St. Louis, 2008, Saunders.)

Figure 35-4. Prevention of fainting. (From Bonewit-West K: *Clinical procedures for medical assistants,* ed 7, St. Louis, 2008, Saunders.)

Bleeding

Bleeding, or hemorrhaging, is the escape of blood from a severed blood vessel. Bleeding can range from very minor to very serious, leading to shock and death. The amount of blood that can be lost before bleeding becomes life-threatening varies according to each individual. In general, a loss of 25% to 40% of an individual's total blood volume can be fatal. This equates to approximately 2 to 4 pints of blood for the average adult.

External Bleeding

External bleeding is bleeding that can be seen coming from a wound. Common examples of external bleeding include bleeding from open fractures, lacerations, and the nose. Individuals with serious external bleeding exhibit the following symptoms: obvious bleeding, restlessness, cold and clammy skin, thirst, increased and thready pulse, rapid and shallow respirations, a drop in the blood pressure (a late symptom), and decreasing levels of consciousness. There are three types of external bleeding, classified according to the type of blood vessel that has been injured: capillary, venous, and arterial.

Capillary Bleeding

Capillary bleeding is the most common type of external bleeding and consists of a slow oozing of bright red blood. This type of bleeding occurs with minor cuts, scratches, and abrasions.

Venous Bleeding

Venous bleeding occurs when a vein has been punctured or severed. This type of bleeding is characterized by a slow and steady flow of dark red blood.

Arterial Bleeding

Arterial bleeding is the most serious type of external bleeding and occurs when an artery is punctured or severed. It is the least common type of bleeding because arteries are situated deeper in the body and are protected by bone. Arterial bleeding is characterized by bright red blood that spurts. The arteries most frequently involved in accidents are the carotid, brachial, radial, and femoral arteries.

Emergency Care for External Bleeding

The most effective way to control bleeding is to apply direct pressure to the bleeding site. The pressure functions by slowing down or stopping the flow of blood. The amount of pressure required depends on the type of bleeding. A small amount of pressure is usually sufficient to control capillary bleeding, whereas significant pressure is often required to control arterial bleeding.

If bleeding cannot be controlled with direct pressure, a pressure point can be used. A **pressure point** is a site on the body where an artery lies close to the surface of the skin and can be compressed against an underlying bone. Figure 35-5 illustrates pressure points. Using a pressure point helps slow or stop the flow of blood from the wound. The pressure points used most often are on the brachial and femoral

Temporal

Carotid

Facial

Brachial

Radial-ulnar

Subclavian

Femoral

Figure 35-5. Location of pressure points. Shaded areas show the regions in which bleeding may be controlled by pressure at the points indicated. (From Miller BF, Keane CB: *Encyclopedia and dictionary of medicine, nursing, and allied health,* ed 7, Philadelphia, 2003, Saunders.)

arteries. The brachial artery is located on the inside of the upper arm midway between the elbow and shoulder. Squeezing the brachial artery helps control severe bleeding in the arm. The femoral artery is located in the groin and helps control severe bleeding in the leg.

The specific steps for controlling bleeding are as follows:

1. Apply direct pressure to the wound with a clean covering such as a large, thick gauze dressing (Figure 35-6A). If gauze is unavailable, a clean material such as a sanitary napkin, washcloth, handkerchief, or sock can be used. If the wound is located on an extremity, elevate the limb while continuing to apply direct pressure.

2. Apply additional dressings if needed. If the dressing soaks through, apply another dressing over the first one and continue to apply pressure (Figure 35-6B). (Never remove a dressing after it has been applied because this could result in more bleeding.) If the bleeding cannot be controlled with direct pressure, apply pressure to the appropriate pressure point while continuing to apply direct local pressure.

3. Apply a pressure bandage. When bleeding has been controlled, apply a bandage snugly over the dressing to maintain pressure on the wound (Figure 35-6C).

4. Transport the patient to an emergency care facility or, if the case is serious enough, activate the local EMS.

Nosebleeds

A nosebleed, or epistaxis, is a common form of external bleeding and is usually not serious but is more of a nuisance. Nosebleeds are usually caused by an upper respiratory infection but can also result from a direct blow from a blunt object, hypertension, strenuous activity, and exposure to high altitudes.

Emergency Care for a Nosebleed

1. Position the patient in a sitting position with the head tilted forward. This prevents the blood from running down the back of the throat, which may result in nausea.

2. Apply direct pressure by pinching the nostrils together (Figure 35-7A). Do not release the pressure too soon because the bleeding may resume. It usually takes about 15 minutes for adequate clot formation. An ice pack can also be applied to the bridge of the nose to help control the bleeding (Figure 35-7B). If these measures do not control the bleeding, apply pressure on the upper lip, just below the nose.

Figure 35-6. Control of bleeding. **A,** Apply direct pressure to the wound with a large, thick gauze dressing. **B,** If blood soaks through the dressing, apply another dressing over the first one, and continue to apply pressure. **C,** When bleeding has been controlled, apply a pressure bandage. (From Bonewit-West K: *Clinical procedures for medical assistants,* ed 7, St. Louis, 2008, Saunders.)

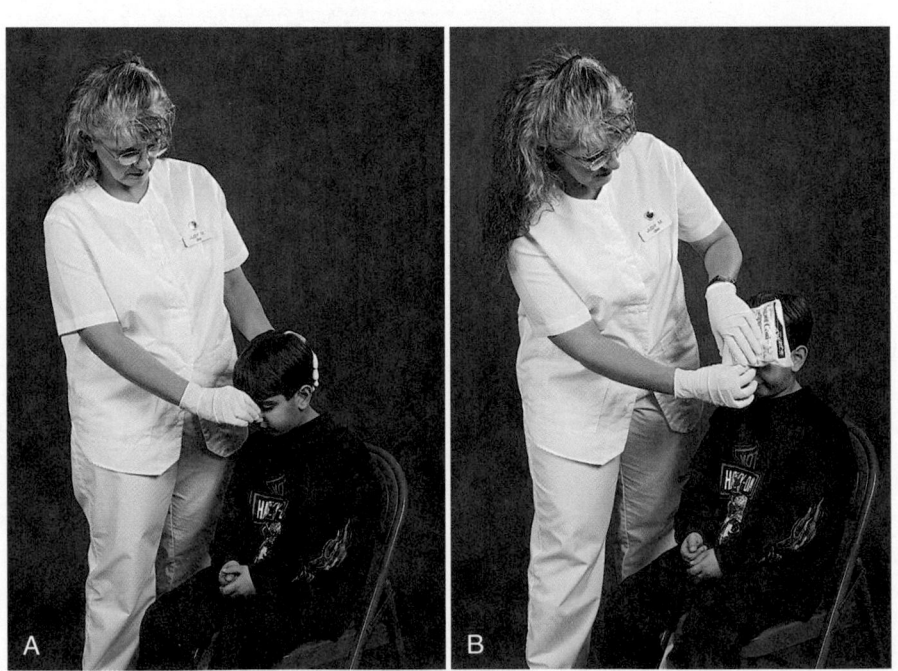

Figure 35-7. Care of a nosebleed. **A,** Apply direct pressure by pinching the nostrils together. **B,** An ice pack can be applied to the bridge of the nose to help control the bleeding. (From Bonewit-West K: *Clinical procedures for medical assistants,* ed 7, St. Louis, 2008, Saunders.)

3. After the bleeding has stopped, tell the patient not to blow the nose for several hours because it could loosen the clot, causing the bleeding to start again.

4. If bleeding cannot be controlled, transport the patient to an emergency care facility for further treatment.

Internal Bleeding

Internal bleeding is bleeding that flows into a body cavity, an organ, or between tissues. It may be minor, as in the case of a contusion, or it may be very serious, such as a severe, blunt blow to the abdomen.

Severe internal bleeding is a life-threatening emergency. Because there is no obvious blood flow, the nature of the injury and the signs and symptoms of bleeding must be used to recognize internal bleeding. Signs and symptoms include bruises, pain, tenderness, or swelling at the site of the injury; rapid, weak pulse; cold, clammy skin; nausea and vomiting; excessive thirst; a drop in the blood pressure; and decreased level of consciousness.

If a patient is suspected to have internal bleeding, the local EMS should be activated immediately. Until emergency medical personnel arrive, the patient should be kept quiet and treated for shock.

Wounds

A **wound** is a break in the continuity of an external or internal surface, caused by physical means. Wounds are either open or closed.

Open Wounds

An open wound is a break in the skin surface or mucous membrane that exposes the underlying tissues. Because the skin is broken, hemorrhaging and wound contamination are primary concerns with open wounds. Open wounds include incisions, lacerations, punctures, and abrasions (Figure 35-8). An individual with an open wound should receive prompt medical attention by a physician if any of the following occur: spurting blood; bleeding that cannot be controlled; a break in the skin that is deeper than just

Putting It All into Practice

My name is Judy Markins, and I work at a large clinic in the family medicine department with 12 physicians. We also have 6 to 10 physicians who do their internships and residency programs with us.

One day as I was performing my usual morning duties of getting the office ready for that day's patients, the office door opened. There stood a mother with her very ill child. I immediately took the patients back to a room. When I took the boy's temperature, it was 104°F. I asked the mother if she had been giving him any type of fever reducer. She said she had, but that it was not helping. Under the direction of our physician I immediately started trying to reduce the fever. The fever started to come down, and the look of relief on the mother's face was beyond words. That was one of the many days that reinforced how satisfied I am with my career choice. ■

Prepare for Success

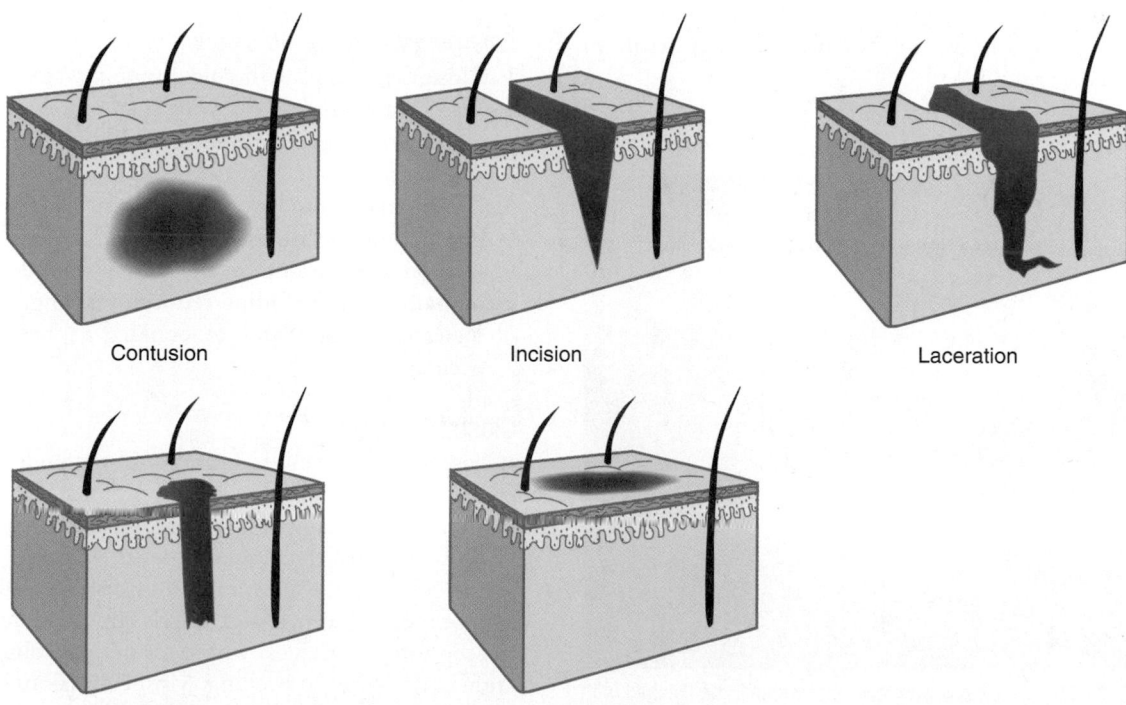

Contusion   Incision   Laceration

Puncture   Abrasion

Figure 35-8. Types of wounds. (From Bonewit-West K: *Clinical procedures for medical assistants,* ed 7, St. Louis, 2008, Saunders.)

the outer skin layers; embedded debris or an embedded object in the wound; involvement of nerves, muscles, or tendons; and occurrence on the mouth, tongue, face, genitals, or other area where scarring would be apparent.

Incisions and Lacerations

An incision is a clean, smooth cut caused by a sharp cutting instrument, such as a knife, razor, or piece of glass. Deep incisions are accompanied by profuse bleeding; in addition, damage to muscles, tendons, and nerves may occur. Because the edges of the wound are smooth and straight, incisions usually heal better than lacerations.

A laceration is a wound in which the tissues are torn apart, rather than cut, leaving ragged and irregular edges. Lacerations are caused by dull knives, large objects that have been driven into the skin, and heavy machinery. Deep lacerations result in profuse bleeding, and a scar often results from the jagged tearing of the tissues.

Emergency Care for Incisions and Lacerations
Minor Incisions and Lacerations
1. Assess the length, depth, and location of the wound.
2. Control bleeding by covering the wound with a dressing and applying firm pressure.
3. Clean the wound with soap and water to remove dirt and other debris (Figure 35-9).
4. Cover the wound with a dry, sterile dressing. Instruct the patient to check the wound for redness, swelling, discharge, or increase in pain and to contact a physician if any of these problems occur.

Serious Incisions and Lacerations
1. Control bleeding by covering the wound with a large, thick gauze dressing and applying firm pressure. Do not clean or probe the wound because this may result in more bleeding.

Figure 35-9. Minor incisions and lacerations should be cleaned with soap and water to remove dirt and other debris. (From Bonewit-West K: *Clinical procedures for medical assistants*, ed 7, St. Louis, 2008, Saunders.)

2. Transport the individual to a physician or, if the wound is serious enough, activate the local EMS.

Punctures

A puncture is a wound made by a sharp, pointed object piercing the skin layers and sometimes the underlying structures. Objects that cause a puncture wound include a nail, splinter, needle, wire, knife, bullet, and animal bite. A puncture wound has a very small external skin opening, and for this reason bleeding is usually minor. A tetanus booster may be administered because the tetanus bacteria grow best in a warm, anaerobic environment, as would be found in a puncture wound.

Emergency Care for Puncture Wounds
1. Allow the wound to bleed freely for a few minutes to help wash out bacteria.
2. Clean the wound with soap and water.
3. Apply a dry, sterile dressing to prevent contamination.
4. Transport the individual to a physician so that medical care can be provided to prevent infection and ensure that the patient's tetanus toxoid immunization is up to date.

Abrasions

An abrasion, or scrape, is a wound in which the outer layers of the skin are scraped or rubbed off. Blood may ooze from ruptured capillaries; however, the bleeding is not usually severe. Abrasions are caused by falls, resulting in floor burns and skinned knees and elbows. Dirt and other debris are frequently rubbed into the wound; it is important to clean scrapes thoroughly to prevent infection.

Emergency Care for Abrasions
1. Rinse the wound with cold running water.
2. Wash the wound gently with soap and water to remove dirt and other debris. A physician should remove embedded debris.
3. Cover large abrasions with a dry, sterile dressing. Small minor abrasions do not require a dressing.
4. Instruct the patient to check the wound for signs of inflammation, including redness, swelling, discharge, or increase in pain, and to contact a physician if they occur.

Closed Wounds

A closed wound involves an injury to the underlying tissues of the body without a break in the skin surface or mucous membrane; an example is a contusion or bruise. A contusion results when the tissues under the skin are injured (see Figure 35-8) and is often caused by a sudden blow or force from a blunt object. Blood vessels rupture, allowing blood to seep into the tissues, which results in a bluish discoloration of the skin and swelling. Most contusions heal without special treatment, but cold compresses may reduce bleeding, reduce swelling and discoloration, and relieve pain. After several days, the color of the contusion turns greenish or yellow, owing to oxidation of blood pigments. Contusions commonly occur with injuries such as fractures, sprains, strains, and black eyes. These injuries, along with the corresponding emergency care, are discussed next.

Musculoskeletal Injuries

The musculoskeletal system comprises all of the bones, muscles, tendons, and ligaments of the body. Injuries that affect the musculoskeletal system include fractures, dislocations, sprains, and strains.

Fracture

A **fracture** is any break in a bone. The break may range in severity from a simple chip or a crack to a complete break or shattering of the bone. Fractures can occur anywhere on the surface of the bone, including across the surface of a joint such as the wrist or ankle. Fractures result from a direct blow, a fall, bone disease, or a twisting force as may occur in a sports injury. Although fractures often cause severe pain, they are seldom life-threatening.

The two basic types of fracture are closed fractures and open fractures (Figure 35-10). A *closed fracture* is the most common type and occurs when there is a break in a bone but no break in the skin over the fracture site. An *open fracture* involves a break in the bone along with a penetration of the overlying skin surface. Open fractures are more serious owing to the risk of blood loss and contamination leading to infection.

The signs and symptoms of a fracture include pain and tenderness, deformity, swelling and discoloration, loss of

Figure 35-10. Fractures. **A,** Open fracture. **B,** Closed fracture. (From Connolly JF: *DePalma's the management of fractures and dislocations: an atlas,* Philadelphia, 1981, Saunders.)

function of the body part, and numbness or tingling. The patient usually guards the injured part and may relay to you that he or she heard the bone break or snap or felt a grating sensation. This grating sensation, known as **crepitus,** is caused by the bone fragments rubbing against each other.

Fractures can also be classified according to the nature of the break: impacted, greenstick, transverse, oblique, comminuted, and spiral. Figure 35-11 illustrates and describes these types of fracture.

Dislocation

A **dislocation** is an injury in which one end of a bone making up a joint is separated or displaced from its normal position. A dislocation is caused by a violent pulling or pushing force that tears the ligaments. Dislocations usually result from falls, sports injuries, and motor vehicle accidents. The signs and symptoms of a dislocation include significant deformity of the joint, pain and swelling, and loss of function.

Sprain

A **sprain** is a tearing of ligaments at a joint. Sprains may result from a fall, a sports injury, or a motor vehicle accident. The joints most often sprained are the ankle, knee, wrist, and fingers. The signs and symptoms of a sprain include pain, swelling, and discoloration. Sprains can vary in seriousness from mild to severe, depending on the amount of damage to the ligaments.

Strain

A **strain** is a stretching and tearing of muscles or tendons. Strains are most likely to occur when an individual lifts a heavy object or overworks a muscle, as during exercise. The muscles most commonly strained are those of the neck, back, thigh, and calf. The signs and symptoms of a strain are pain and swelling. Strains do not usually cause the intense symptoms associated with fractures, dislocations, and sprains.

Emergency Care for a Fracture

Determining whether a patient has a fracture, dislocation, or sprain is often difficult because the symptoms of these injuries are similar. Because of this, any serious musculoskeletal injury to an extremity should be treated as though it were a fracture.

The primary goal of emergency care for a fracture is to immobilize the body part. Immobilization reduces pain and prevents further damage. A **splint** is any item that immobilizes a body part. In an emergency situation, items such as a length of wood, cardboard, or rolled newspapers or magazines can be used for splinting. The splint should be padded with a soft material such as a rolled-up towel.

The body part should be splinted in the position in which you found it. Severely angulated fractures may have to be straightened before splinting, however. If you attempt to straighten an angulated fracture, be careful not to force the affected part. A dislocated bone end can become "locked"

Impacted Fracture
The broken ends of the bones are forcefully jammed together.

Greenstick Fracture
The bone remains intact on one side, but broken on the other, in much the same way a that a "green stick" bends; common in children, whose bones are more flexible than those of adults.

Transverse Fracture
The break occurs perpendicular to the long axis of the bone.

Oblique Fracture
The break occurs diagonally across the bone; generally the result of a twisting force.

Comminuted Fracture
The bone is splintered or shattered into three or more fragments; usually caused by an extremely traumatic direct force.

Spiral Fracture
The bone is broken into a spiral or S-shape; caused by a twisting force.

Figure 35-11. Types of fractures. (From Bonewit-West K: *Clinical procedures for medical assistants,* ed 7, St. Louis, 2008, Saunders.)

and would have to be realigned at the hospital. If you straighten an angulated bone and encounter pain, stop and splint it in the position in which you found it. The splint should also immobilize the area above and below the injury. When splinting an injury to the wrist, the hand and forearm should also be immobilized (Figure 35-12A). When splinting an injury to the shaft of the bone, the joints above and below the injury should be immobilized. When splinting the forearm, the elbow joint and the wrist joint should be immobilized.

The splint should be held in place with a roller gauze bandage or other suitable material, such as neckties, scarves, or strips of cloth (Figure 35-12B). The splint should be applied snugly, but not so tightly that it interferes with proper circulation. After applying the splint, check the pulse below the splint to ensure the splint has not been applied too tightly. If you cannot detect a pulse, immediately loosen the splint until you can feel the pulse (Figure 35-12C).

Whenever possible, elevate an injured extremity after it has been immobilized to reduce swelling (Figure 35-12D). An ice pack can also be applied to the injured part. The cold limits the accumulation of fluid in the body tissues by constricting blood vessels and reducing leakage of fluid into the tissues. In addition, cold temporarily relieves pain

because of its anesthetic or numbing effect, which reduces stimulation of nerve receptors.

After you have properly immobilized the injury, transport the patient to an emergency care facility or, if the injury is serious enough, activate the local EMS. In any situation in which an injury to the spine is suspected, activate EMS.

Burns

A **burn** is an injury to the tissues caused by exposure to thermal, chemical, electrical, or radioactive agents. The severity of a burn depends on the depth of the burn, the percentage of the body involved, the type of agent causing the burn, the duration and intensity of the agent, and the part of the body. Burns are classified according to the depth of tissue injury, as illustrated in Figure 35-13.

Superficial (First-Degree) Burn

A superficial burn is the most common type of burn. It involves only the top layer of skin, the epidermis. With this type of burn, the skin appears red, is warm and dry to the touch, and is usually painful. Sunburn is a common example of a superficial burn. A superficial burn heals in 2 to 5 days of its own accord and does not cause scarring.

Figure 35-12. Emergency care of a fracture. **A,** The splint should immobilize the area above and below the injury. **B,** The splint is held in place with a gauze roller bandage. **C,** After the splint is applied, the pulse below the splint should be checked to ensure the splint has not been applied too tightly. **D,** A sling can be used to elevate the extremity to reduce swelling. (From Henry M, Stapleton E: *EMT prehospital care,* ed 2, Philadelphia, 1997, Saunders.)

Partial-Thickness (Second-Degree) Burn

A partial-thickness burn involves the epidermis and extends into the dermis but does not pass through the dermis to the underlying tissues. The burned area usually appears red, mottled, and blistered. In most cases, the blisters should not be broken because they provide a protective barrier against infection. Partial-thickness burns are usually very painful, and the area often swells. This type of burn usually heals within 3 to 4 weeks and may result in some scarring.

Full-Thickness (Third-Degree) Burn

A full-thickness burn completely destroys the epidermis and the dermis and extends into the underlying tissues, such as fat, muscle, bone, and nerves. The affected area appears charred black, brown, and cherry red, with the damaged tissues underneath often pearly white. The patient may experience intense pain; however, if there has been substantial damage to the nerve endings, the patient may feel no pain at all. During the healing process, dense scars typically result. Infection is a major concern, and the patient must be carefully monitored.

Thermal Burns

Thermal burns usually occur in the home, often as a result of fire, scalding water, or coming into contact with a hot object, such as a stove or curling iron.

Emergency Care for Major Thermal Burns

1. Stop the burning process to prevent further injury. If the individual is on fire, wrap him or her in a blanket, rug, or heavy coat and push him or her to the ground to help smother the flames. If a covering is unavailable, shout at the individual to drop to the ground and roll around to smother the flames.

2. Cool the burn, using large amounts of cool water from a faucet or garden hose. Do not use ice or ice water because this may result in further tissue damage; it also causes heat loss from the body. If the burn covers a large surface area (greater than 20%), do not use water. The loss of a large amount of skin surface places the patient at risk for hypothermia (generalized body cooling). With large surface area burns, you may cool the most painful areas, but not an area greater than 20% of the body (i.e., two arms, one leg).

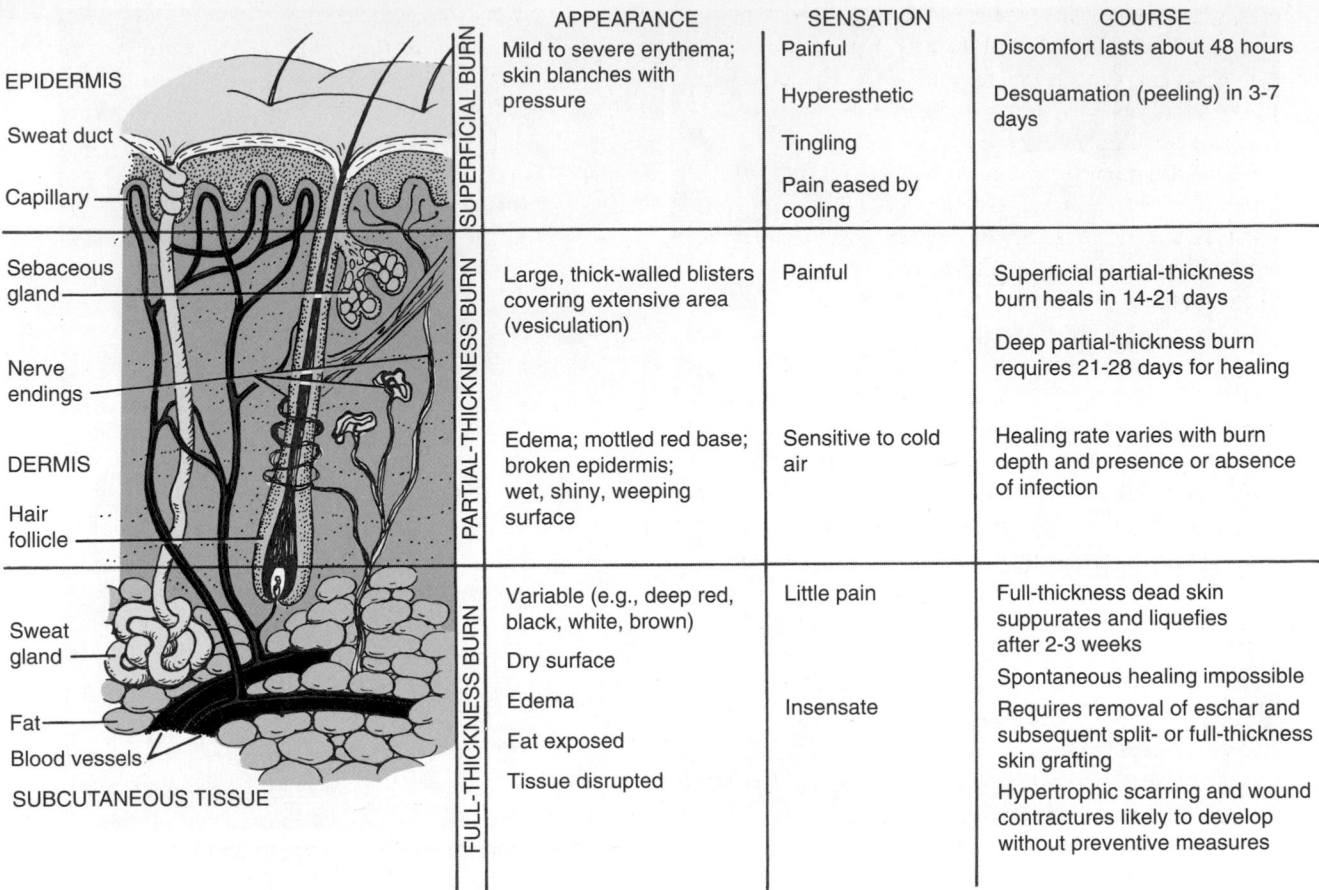

		APPEARANCE	SENSATION	COURSE
	SUPERFICIAL BURN	Mild to severe erythema; skin blanches with pressure	Painful Hyperesthetic Tingling Pain eased by cooling	Discomfort lasts about 48 hours Desquamation (peeling) in 3-7 days
	PARTIAL-THICKNESS BURN	Large, thick-walled blisters covering extensive area (vesiculation) Edema; mottled red base; broken epidermis; wet, shiny, weeping surface	Painful Sensitive to cold air	Superficial partial-thickness burn heals in 14-21 days Deep partial-thickness burn requires 21-28 days for healing Healing rate varies with burn depth and presence or absence of infection
	FULL-THICKNESS BURN	Variable (e.g., deep red, black, white, brown) Dry surface Edema Fat exposed Tissue disrupted	Little pain Insensate	Full-thickness dead skin suppurates and liquefies after 2-3 weeks Spontaneous healing impossible Requires removal of eschar and subsequent split- or full-thickness skin grafting Hypertrophic scarring and wound contractures likely to develop without preventive measures

Figure 35-13. Types of burns. (From Polaski AL, Tatro SE: *Luckmann's core principles and practice of medical-surgical nursing,* Philadelphia, 1996, Saunders.)

3. Activate the local EMS.
4. Cover the patient with a clean, nonfuzzy material such as a tablecloth or sheet. The cover maintains warmth, reduces pain, and reduces the risk of contamination. Do not apply any type of ointment, antiseptic, or other substance to the burned area.

Emergency Care for Minor Thermal Burns
1. Immerse the affected area in cold water for 2 to 5 minutes. Be careful not to break any blisters because they provide a protective barrier against infection.
2. Cover the burn with a dry sterile dressing.

Chemical Burns
Chemical burns occur in the workplace and at home. The severity of the burn depends on the type and strength of the chemical and the duration of exposure to the chemical. The main difference between a chemical burn and a thermal burn is that the chemical continues to burn the patient's tissues as long as it is on the skin. Because of this factor, it is important to remove the chemical from the skin as quickly as possible and then to activate the local EMS.

Liquid chemical burns should be treated by flooding the area with large amounts of cool running water until emergency personnel arrive. If a solid substance such as lime has been spilled on the patient, it should be brushed off before flooding the area with water. This is because a dry chemical may be activated by contact with water.

Seizures
A **seizure** is a sudden episode of involuntary muscular contractions and relaxation, often accompanied by a change in sensation, behavior, and level of consciousness. A seizure results when the normal electrical activity of the brain is disturbed, causing the brain cells to become irritated and overactive. Specific conditions that trigger a seizure include epilepsy, encephalitis, a recent or old head injury, high fever in infants and young children, drug and alcohol abuse or withdrawal, eclampsia associated with toxemia of pregnancy, diabetic conditions, and heatstroke.

Seizures are classified as partial or generalized according to the location of the abnormal electrical activity in the brain. *Partial seizures* are the most common type, occurring in approximately 80% of individuals who have seizures. With a partial seizure, the abnormal electrical activity is localized into specific areas of the brain; only the brain functions in those areas are affected.

Partial seizures are classified further as simple or complex, depending on whether the patient's level of consciousness is affected. The symptoms of a *simple partial seizure* include twitching or jerking in just one part of the body. This type of seizure lasts less than 1 minute, and the patient remains awake and alert during the seizure. With a *complex partial seizure,* the patient's level of consciousness is affected, and the patient has little or no memory of the seizure afterward. The symptoms of this type of seizure include abnormal behavior such as confusion, a glassy stare, aimless wandering, lip smacking or chewing, or fidgeting with clothing, which lasts from a few seconds to a minute or two. Both simple and complex partial seizures can progress to generalized seizures.

With a *generalized seizure,* the abnormal electrical activity spreads through the entire brain. The best-known type of generalized seizure is a *tonic-clonic seizure* (formerly known as a "grand mal seizure"). With this type of seizure, the patient exhibits tonic-clonic activity followed by a postictal state. During the tonic phase, the patient suddenly loses consciousness and exhibits rigid muscular contractions, which result in odd posturing of the body. Respirations are inhibited, which may cause cyanosis around the mouth and lips. The patient may lose control of the bladder or bowels, resulting in involuntary urination and defecation. The tonic phase lasts 30 seconds, followed by the clonic phase. During the clonic phase, the patient's body jerks about violently. The patient's jaw muscles contract, which may cause the patient to bite the tongue or lips. The final phase of the seizure is the postictal state, lasting 10 to 30 minutes, in which the patient exhibits a depressed level of consciousness, is disoriented, and often has a headache. The patient generally has little or no memory of the seizure and feels confused and exhausted for several hours after the seizure.

In some instances of seizures, particularly in patients with epilepsy, an aura precedes the seizure. An *aura* is a sensation perceived by the patient that something is about to happen; examples include a strange taste, smell, or sound; a twitch; or a feeling of dizziness or anxiety. An aura provides the patient with a warning signal that a seizure is about to begin.

Although seizures are frightening to observe, they are usually not as bad as they look. Most patients fully recover within a few minutes after the seizure begins. An exception to this is *status epilepticus,* in which seizures are prolonged or come in rapid succession without full recovery of consciousness between them. Status epilepticus is a potentially life-threatening situation that requires immediate medical care.

Emergency Care for Seizures

The most important criterion in caring for a patient in a seizure is to protect the patient from harm. Remove hazards from the immediate area to prevent the patient from injury by striking a surrounding object. Do not restrain the patient. Loosen restrictive clothing that may interfere with breathing, such as collars, neckties, scarves, and jewelry. The seizure will occur no matter what you do; restraining the patient could seriously injure the patient's muscles, bones,

or joints. Do not insert anything into the patient's mouth during the seizure because this could damage the teeth or mouth or interfere with breathing. In addition, it could trigger the gag reflex, causing the patient to vomit and possibly aspirate the vomitus into the lungs. If the patient vomits, roll him or her onto one side so that the vomitus can drain from the mouth.

If you are uncertain as to the cause of the seizure, or if you suspect that the patient is having status epilepticus, activate your local EMS immediately. Otherwise, transport the patient to an emergency medical care facility for further evaluation and treatment after the seizure is over.

Poisoning

A **poison** is any substance that causes illness, injury, or death if it enters the body. Most poisoning episodes occur in the home, are accidental, and occur in children younger than 5 years old. Poisoning usually involves common substances, such as cleaning agents, medications, and pesticides. For most poisonous substances, the reaction is more serious in children and the elderly than in adults. A poison can enter the body in four ways: ingestion, inhalation, absorption, or injection.

Poison control centers are valuable resources that are easily accessible to medical personnel and the community. More than 500 regional poison control centers exist across the United States; most are located in the emergency departments of large hospitals. These centers are staffed by personnel who have access to information about almost all poisonous substances. Most of the centers are staffed 24 hours a day, and calls are toll-free. In addition, a National Poison Control Hotline number (1-800-222-1222) can be called 24 hours a day.

Ingested Poisons

Poisons that are ingested enter the body by being swallowed. Ingestion is the most common route of entry for poisons.

Memories *from* Externship

Judy Markins: As it turned out, one of my most terrible moments during my externship was a great learning experience. I was drawing blood (which was not my favorite procedure) and missed the vein—not once, but twice. You could see the sweat under my gloves. My stomach was in my throat, and I did not want to try again. Thank goodness my patient was understanding, and I had an excellent externship supervisor. She insisted that I try again, encouraging me that I could do it and suggesting some techniques that she had learned from her many years of experience. I got the blood specimen along with some newfound confidence.

In most situations, someone can help you if you have questions. Use your resources when you need to. Be honest, know your procedure, and have confidence in yourself. ▪

Prepare for Success

Examples of poisons that are often ingested include cleaning products, pesticides, contaminated food, petroleum products (e.g., gasoline, kerosene), and poisonous plants. The abuse of drugs, alcohol, or both can also result in poisoning from an accidental or intentional overdose. The signs and symptoms of poisoning by ingestion are based on the specific substance that has been consumed but often include strange odors, burns or stains around the mouth, nausea, vomiting, abdominal pain, diarrhea, difficulty in breathing, profuse perspiration, excessive salivation, dilated or constricted pupils, unconsciousness, and convulsions.

Emergency Care for Poisoning by Ingestion

1. Acquire as much information as possible about the type of poison, the amount ingested, and when it was ingested.
2. Call your poison control center or local EMS. *Never induce vomiting unless directed to do so by a medical authority.* Vomiting is often contraindicated—when an individual is unconscious, has swallowed a petroleum product, or has swallowed a corrosive poison such as a strong acid or base. Corrosive poisons may cause more injury to the esophagus, throat, and mouth if they are vomited back up. If it is available, you may be directed by the poison control center to administer activated charcoal. Activated charcoal is used to absorb the poison that remains in the stomach and prevents absorption by the intestine.
3. If the individual vomits, collect some of the vomitus for transport with the patient to the hospital for analysis by a toxicologist, if necessary. In addition, bring along containers of any substances ingested, such as empty medication bottles and household cleaner containers, because the label of the container often lists the ingredients in the product.

Inhaled Poisons

A poison that is inhaled is breathed into the body in the form of gas, vapor, or spray. The most commonly inhaled poison is carbon monoxide, such as from car exhausts, malfunctioning furnaces, and fires. Other inhaled poisons include carbon dioxide from wells and sewers and fumes from household products such as glues, paints, insect sprays, and cleaners (e.g., ammonia, chlorine). The signs and symptoms of inhaled poisoning often include severe headache; nausea and vomiting; coughing or wheezing; shortness of breath; chest pain or tightness; facial burns; burning of the mouth, nose, eyes, throat, or chest; cyanosis; confusion; dizziness; and unconsciousness.

Emergency Care for Inhaled Poisons

1. Determine whether it is safe to approach the patient. Toxic gases and fumes can also be dangerous to individuals helping the patient.
2. Remove the individual from the source of the poison and into fresh air as quickly as possible.
3. Call your poison control center or local EMS.
4. If oxygen is available, you may be directed to administer it under the supervision of a physician. Oxygen is the primary antidote for carbon monoxide poisoning.

Absorbed Poisons

A poison that is absorbed enters the body through the skin. Examples of absorbed poisons include fertilizers and pesticides used for lawn and garden care. The signs and symptoms of absorbed poisoning are irritation, burning and itching, burning of the skin or eyes, headache, and abnormal pulse or respiration or both.

Emergency Care for Absorbed Poisons

1. Remove the patient from the source of the poison. Avoid contact with the toxic substance.
2. Call your poison control center or local EMS. In most cases, you will be instructed to flood the area that has been exposed to the poison with water. Dry chemicals should be brushed from the skin before flooding with water.

Injected Poisons

An injected poison enters the body through bites, through stings, or by a needle. Examples of injected poisons include the venom of insects, spiders, snakes, and marine creatures, such as jellyfish and the bite of rabid animals. The poison may also be a drug that is self-administered with a hypodermic needle, such as heroin. The general signs and symptoms of injected poisoning include an altered state of awareness; evidence of stings, bites, or puncture marks on the skin; mottled skin; localized pain or itching; burning, swelling, or blistering at the site; difficulty in breathing; abnormal pulse rate; nausea and vomiting; and anaphylactic shock.

Insect Stings

It is estimated that 1 of every 125 Americans is allergic to insect stings. Approximately 40 people in the United States die every year from a severe allergic reaction to insect stings. The incidence of deaths is low because most people know they need to obtain medical attention immediately if an allergic reaction begins.

What Would You Do? What Would You *Not* Do?

Case Study 1

Beth Eaton calls the office. She says that she thinks her 3-year-old daughter, Olivia, has eaten some chewable vitamins. Beth was taking a shower and when she came out, Olivia was holding an empty vitamin bottle and saying "Good candy." Beth says she does not know how Olivia got the child-proof top off. She thinks the bottle was about a third of the way full. Beth says that Olivia is complaining that her tummy hurts. Beth says she has syrup of ipecac and wants to know whether she should give some to Olivia. ■

Almost all of the insects whose venom can cause allergic reactions belong to a group called *Hymenoptera,* which includes honeybees and bumblebees, wasps, yellow jackets, and hornets. When a honeybee stings, its stinger remains embedded in the victim's skin, causing the bee to die as it tries to tear itself away. Wasps, yellow jackets, and hornets are more aggressive than bees and can sting repeatedly. Hornets are the most aggressive of the group and may sting even when not provoked. Yellow jackets are close behind in aggressiveness, and wasps usually sting only if someone interferes with them near their nest.

If an insect sting does not cause an allergic reaction within 30 minutes, chances are excellent that no problem will occur. A normal reaction to an insect sting includes localized pain, redness, swelling, and itching lasting 1 to 2 days. Any generalized reaction not arising directly from the area of the sting is almost certain to be an allergic reaction, which begins with symptoms such as sneezing, hives, itching, angioedema, erythema, and disorientation and progresses to difficulty in breathing, dizziness, faintness, and loss of consciousness.

Medical care should be sought immediately because these are the symptoms of an anaphylactic reaction, and most fatalities occur within 2 hours of the sting. Because time is a factor, individuals known to have a severe allergy to insect stings carry an anaphylactic emergency treatment kit containing injectable epinephrine and oral antihistamines (see Figure 35-2). With this kit, treatment for a severe allergic reaction can be started immediately.

Emergency Care for Insect Stings

1. Remove the stinger and attached venom sac. Scrape the stinger off the patient's skin with your fingernail or a plastic card such as a credit card (Figure 35-14). Do not use tweezers or forceps because squeezing the venom sac may cause more venom to be injected into the patient's tissues.
2. Wash the site with soap and water.
3. Apply a cold pack to the affected area to reduce pain and swelling.
4. Observe the patient for the signs of an anaphylactic reaction.

Spider Bites

Although spiders are numerous throughout the United States, most do not cause injuries or serious complications. Only two spiders have bites that cause serious or life-threatening reactions: the black widow spider and the brown recluse spider. Both of these spiders prefer dark, out-of-the-way places, such as in woodpiles, in brush piles, under rocks, and in dark garages and attics. Because of this, bites usually occur on the hands and arms of individuals reaching into places where the spiders are hiding. Often the individual does not know that he or she has been bitten until he or she begins to feel ill or notices swelling and a bite mark on the skin.

The black widow spider is approximately 1 inch long and is black with a distinctive bright-red hourglass shape on

Figure 35-14. Removing a honeybee stinger and venom sac using the edge of a credit card. (From Bonewit-West K: *Clinical procedures for medical assistants,* ed 7, St. Louis, 2008, Saunders.)

What Would You Do? What Would You *Not* Do?

Case Study 2

Anita Alland calls the office and says that her son, Garon, was stung by a yellow jacket about an hour ago while mowing the grass. She says that his entire arm and back are red and swollen and he has a lot of redness and swelling around his eyes. Garon is itching all over and seems fuzzy headed. Anita says she has never seen anyone do this after being stung. She says she had Garon take a cold shower to see if it would help. After the shower he started feeling faint and dizzy, and now he is having trouble breathing. Anita wants to know whether she can bring him to the office so that he can be seen by the physician. ■

its abdomen. The venom injected when this spider bites an individual is toxic to the central nervous system. The signs and symptoms of a black widow bite are swelling and a dull pain at the injection site; nausea and vomiting; a rigid, boardlike abdomen; fever; rash; and difficulty in breathing or swallowing. Although the symptoms are severe, they are not usually fatal. An antivenin is available; however, because of its undesirable and frequent side effects, it is generally administered only to individuals with severe bites and to individuals who may have a heightened reaction, such as elderly individuals and children younger than 5 years old.

The brown recluse spider is light brown with a dark-brown violin-shaped mark on its back. The bite of a brown recluse causes severe local effects, including tenderness, redness, and swelling at the injection site. Systemic effects, such as difficulty in breathing or swallowing, seldom occur.

Emergency Care for Spider Bites

1. Wash the wound.
2. Apply a cold pack to the affected area to reduce pain and swelling.
3. Obtain medical help immediately if you suspect the individual has been bitten by a black widow spider or a brown recluse spider, or if a severe reaction begins to occur.

Snakebites

Snakebites kill very few people in the United States. Every year, approximately 45,000 persons are bitten by a snake; however, only 7000 of these bites involve a poisonous snake, and fewer than 15 of the individuals die. The species of snakes that are poisonous in the United States include rattlesnakes, copperheads, cottonmouths (water moccasins), and coral snakes. Individuals, zoos, or laboratories may own other poisonous species, however. Rattlesnakes account for most snakebites and nearly all fatalities from snakebites. Most snakebites occur near the home, as opposed to in the wild. Because it is often difficult to identify a snake, any unidentified snake should be considered poisonous. The general signs and symptoms of a bite from a poisonous snake include puncture marks on the skin, pain and swelling at the puncture site, rapid pulse, nausea, vomiting, unconsciousness, and convulsions.

Emergency Care for Snakebites

1. Wash the bite area gently with soap and water.
2. Immobilize the injured part, and position it below the level of the heart.
3. Call emergency personnel. Do not apply ice to a snakebite. Do not apply a tourniquet, and do not cut or suction the wound.
4. If the snake is dead, inform emergency personnel of its location so that it can be transported to the hospital for identification.

Animal Bites

Bites and other injuries from animals range in severity from minor to serious and fatal. Most people who are bitten by animals do not report the bite to a physician. Because of this factor, the incidence of animal bites in the United States each year is unknown but has been estimated at approximately 1 to 2 million for dog bites and 400,000 for cat bites.

The most serious type of bite is one from an animal with rabies. Rabies is a viral infection transmitted through the saliva of an infected animal. If the condition is not treated, rabies is generally fatal. Certain animals tend to have a higher incidence of rabies than others. These include skunks, bats, raccoons, cats, dogs, cattle, and foxes. Hamsters, gerbils, guinea pigs, chipmunks, rats, mice, gophers, and rabbits are rarely infected with the rabies virus.

An individual who has been bitten by an animal that has rabies or is suspected of having rabies must obtain medical care. To prevent rabies, a rabies vaccine, which produces antibodies to fight the rabies virus, is administered to the individual.

Emergency Care for Animal Bites

Minor Animal Bites. Wash the wound with soap and water. Apply an antibiotic ointment and a dry sterile dressing. Transport the individual to a physician so that medical care can be provided to prevent infection and to ensure that the patient's tetanus toxoid immunization is up to date.

Serious Bites. If the wound is bleeding heavily, first control the bleeding with direct pressure. Do not clean the wound because this may result in more bleeding. Transport the patient to a physician or, if the bite is serious enough, call the local EMS.

All Animal Bites. If you suspect that the animal has rabies, relay this information to the appropriate authorities, such as medical personnel, the police, or animal control personnel. If possible, try to remember what the animal looked like and the area in which you last saw it.

Heat and Cold Exposure

Exposure to excessive environmental heat or cold can result in injury to the body ranging in severity from minor to life-threatening. Heat-related injuries are most apt to occur on very hot days that are accompanied by high humidity with little or no air movement. The three conditions caused by overexposure to heat are heat cramps, heat exhaustion, and heatstroke.

The two major types of cold-related injury are frostbite and hypothermia. Although cold-related injuries are most apt to occur in the winter months, they can also occur at other times of the year, such as when an individual is exposed to cold water in a near-drowning incident.

Certain individuals are at higher risk for developing heat-related and cold-related injuries, as follows:

- Elderly individuals
- Young children, particularly infants
- Individuals who work or exercise outdoors
- Individuals with medical conditions that cause poor blood circulation, such as diabetes mellitus and cardiovascular disease
- Individuals who have had heat-related or cold-related injuries in the past
- Individuals under the influence of drugs or alcohol

Heat Cramps

Heat cramps are the least serious of the three types of heat-related injury. Heat cramps are most apt to occur when an individual is exercising or working in a hot environment and fails to replace lost fluids and electrolytes. Lost electrolytes can be replaced with a commercial sports drink (e.g., Gatorade).

The signs and symptoms of heat cramps include painful muscle spasms, particularly of the legs, calves, and abdomen; hot, sweaty skin; weakness; and a rapid pulse. These symptoms are a warning that an individual is having a problem with the heat. If the problem is ignored, heat cramps may

Figure 35-15. Treatment of heat exhaustion consists of removing the patient to a cool environment, replacing fluids and electrolytes, and applying a cold compress to the forehead; the patient should then rest. (From Bonewit-West K: *Clinical procedures for medical assistants,* ed 7, St. Louis, 2008, Saunders.)

progress to a more serious condition, such as heat exhaustion or heatstroke.

Treatment of heat cramps consists of removal of the patient to a cool environment, rest, and replacement of fluids and electrolytes. If the patient's condition does not improve, he or she should be transported to an emergency care facility for further treatment.

Heat Exhaustion

Heat exhaustion is the most common heat-related injury. It occurs most often in individuals involved in vigorous physical activity on a hot and humid day, such as athletes and construction workers. It can also occur in people who are wearing too much clothing on a hot and humid day. The signs and symptoms of heat exhaustion are similar to those of influenza: cold and clammy skin that is pale or gray, profuse sweating, headache, nausea, dizziness, weakness, and diarrhea.

Treatment of heat exhaustion consists of removal of the patient to a cool environment, replacement of fluids and electrolytes, application of a cold compress to the forehead, and rest (Figure 35-15). Tight clothing should be loosened, and excessive layers of clothing should be removed. In most cases, these measures improve the patient's condition in approximately 30 minutes. If the patient's condition does not improve, however, he or she should be transported to an emergency care facility.

What Would You Do? What Would You *Not* Do?

Case Study 3

David Brently has come to the medical office. He is a member of Kiwanis, and this year it was his turn to deliver Easter candy and flowers to patients at the local hospital and nursing home while wearing a bunny costume. It is a very warm day, and David says that he got really hot and sweaty in his costume and then started feeling dizzy and nauseous. He got a little worried and decided to drive himself to the medical office. David says he cannot get his costume off because the zipper is stuck. He does not want to cut it off because that would ruin it and Kiwanis would not be able to use it next year. He is hoping the physician can fix him up well enough so that he can drive home. David says he is sure his wife can get the costume off without damaging it. ■

Heatstroke

Heatstroke is the least common, but most serious, of the three heat-related injuries. Heatstroke is most apt to occur in elderly people during a heat wave and in athletes who overexert themselves in a hot and humid environment. Heatstroke can occur in a very short time, as when a child has been left to wait in a closed car on a hot day.

During heatstroke, the body becomes so overheated that the heat-regulating mechanism breaks down and is unable to cool the body. The body temperature increases to a dangerous level, causing the destruction of tissues. The signs and symptoms of heatstroke include a body temperature of 105°F (40°C) or greater; red, hot, dry skin; a rapid, weak pulse; dizziness and weakness; rapid, shallow breathing; decreased levels of consciousness; and seizures.

Heatstroke is a life-threatening emergency and requires immediate transport of the patient to an emergency care facility by the fastest way possible. If not treated, heatstroke is always fatal. During transport, every attempt should be made to lower the body temperature, such as setting the air conditioner to its maximal capacity; covering the victim with cool, wet sheets; or fanning the victim.

Frostbite

Frostbite is the localized freezing of body tissue as a result of exposure to cold. The severity of the frostbite depends on the environmental temperature, the duration of exposure, and the wind-chill factor. Frostbite most commonly affects the hands, fingers, feet, toes, ears, nose, and cheeks. Although frostbite is not life-threatening, it can cause severe tissue damage that may require amputation of the affected body part. The signs and symptoms of frostbite include loss of feeling in the affected area; cold and waxy skin; and white, yellow, or blue discoloration of the skin.

Treatment of frostbite requires rewarming of the affected body part to prevent permanent damage. This is best accomplished in an emergency care facility because improper rewarming can result in further tissue damage. To transport the patient, loosely wrap warm clothing or blankets around the affected body part. The frozen area can also be placed in contact with another body part that is warm. It is important to handle the affected area gently. Do not rub or massage the affected area because this can damage frozen tissue further.

Hypothermia

Hypothermia is a life-threatening emergency in which the temperature of the entire body falls to a dangerously low level. Hypothermia can occur rapidly, such as when an individual falls through the ice on a frozen lake. It also can occur slowly when an individual is exposed to a cold environment for a long time, such as a hiker lost in the woods.

When the core body temperature decreases too much, the body loses its ability to regulate its temperature and to generate body heat. The signs and symptoms of hypothermia are shivering, numbness, drowsiness, apathy, a glassy stare, and decreased levels of consciousness.

Treatment of hypothermia should focus on preventing further heat loss. Remove the patient from the cold or, if this is impossible, wrap him or her in blankets. Do not attempt to rewarm the patient such as through immersion in warm water. Rapid rewarming can result in serious respiratory and cardiac problems. The patient should be transported immediately to an emergency care facility.

Diabetic Emergencies

Glucose is the end product of carbohydrate metabolism. It serves as the chief source of energy to perform normal body functions and to assist in maintaining body temperature. The body maintains a constant blood glucose level to ensure a continuous source of energy for the body. Glucose that is not necessary for energy can be stored in the form of glycogen in muscle and liver tissue for later use. When no more tissue storage is possible, excess glucose is converted to fat and stored as adipose tissue.

Insulin is a hormone secreted by the beta cells of the pancreas and is required for normal use of glucose in the body. Insulin enables glucose to enter the body's cells and be converted to energy. Insulin also is necessary for the proper storage of glycogen in liver and muscle cells.

Diabetes mellitus is a disease in which the body is unable to use glucose for energy because of a lack of insulin in the body. There are two types of diabetes—a severe form, usually appearing in childhood, known as *type 1 diabetes*, and a mild form, usually appearing in adulthood, known as *type 2 diabetes.* Most individuals with diabetes (90%) have type 2 diabetes. There is no cure for diabetes mellitus, but significant advances have been made in controlling the disease through a combination of drug therapy, diet therapy, and activity. The goal for the diabetic patient is to balance food intake and level of activity with the body's insulin.

A diabetic patient can experience two types of emergency: *hypoglycemia,* commonly referred to as "insulin shock," and *diabetic ketoacidosis,* commonly known as "diabetic coma." Insulin shock (hypoglycemia) occurs when there is too much insulin in the body and not enough glucose. Insulin shock can be caused by administration of too much insulin, skipping meals, and unexpected or unusual exercise. The symptoms of insulin shock are normal or rapid respirations; pale, cold, and clammy skin; sweating; dizziness and headache; full, rapid pulse; normal or high blood pressure; extreme hunger; aggressive or unusual behavior; fainting; and seizure or coma. The onset of insulin shock occurs rapidly, usually over 5 to 20 minutes, after the blood glucose level begins to decrease. Because the brain requires a constant supply of glucose for proper functioning, permanent brain damage or death can result from severe hypoglycemia.

Diabetic coma (diabetic ketoacidosis) occurs when there is not enough insulin in the body. This causes the blood glucose level to increase, resulting in hyperglycemia. When glucose cannot be used for energy, fat is broken down. This results in a buildup of acid waste products in the blood, known as *ketoacidosis.* The combined effect of the hyperglycemia and ketoacidosis causes the following symptoms: polyuria; excessive thirst and hunger; vomiting; abdominal pain; dry, warm skin; rapid, deep sighing respirations; a sweet or fruity (acetone) odor to the breath; and a rapid, weak pulse.

If the condition is not treated, diabetic coma can progress to dehydration, hypotension, coma, and death. In contrast to insulin shock, however, the onset of diabetic coma is gradual, usually developing over 12 to 48 hours. Diabetic coma can be caused by illness and infection, overeating, forgetting to administer an insulin injection, or administering an insufficient amount of insulin.

Most individuals with diabetes have a thorough knowledge of their disease and manage it effectively. Because of this, diabetic emergencies are most apt to occur when there is an unusual upset in the insulin/glucose balance in the body, such as might be caused by illness or infection. An emergency situation may also arise in an individual who has diabetes but in whom the condition has not yet been diagnosed.

It may be difficult to tell the difference between insulin shock and diabetic coma because the symptoms are similar. Often a patient with either of these conditions seems to be intoxicated. If he or she is conscious, the diabetic patient usually knows what the trouble is; you should listen carefully to the patient to determine what may have caused the problem (e.g., not eating, forgetting to administer an insulin injection). If the patient is unconscious and unable to communicate, you should observe the patient's respirations. A patient in insulin shock has normal or rapid respirations, whereas a patient in diabetic coma has deep, labored respirations. Most diabetic patients carry an emergency medical identification, such as a medical alert bracelet or necklace and a wallet card (Figure 35-16), to alert others to their condition when they cannot.

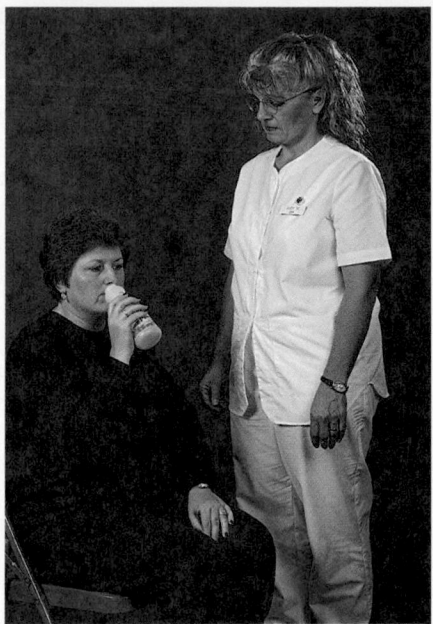

Figure 35-17. Orange juice is administered to a diabetic patient showing signs and symptoms of insulin shock. (From Bonewit-West K: *Clinical procedures for medical assistants,* ed 7, St. Louis, 2008, Saunders.)

Figure 35-16. Diabetic medical identification. **A,** Diabetic medical alert bracelet. **B,** Diabetic wallet card. (From Bonewit-West K: *Clinical procedures for medical assistants,* ed 7, St. Louis, 2008, Saunders.)

Emergency Care in Diabetes

Insulin Shock (Hypoglycemia)

A patient in insulin shock needs sugar immediately. For a conscious patient, glucose should be administered by mouth in the form of fruit juice (e.g., orange juice), nondiet soft drinks, candy, honey, or table sugar dissolved in water (Figure 35-17). Improvement is usually rapid after the glucose has been consumed. If the patient is unconscious, do not give anything by mouth because it may be aspirated into the lungs. Instead, provide the fastest possible transportation of the patient to an emergency care facility.

Diabetic Coma (Diabetic Ketoacidosis)

A patient in diabetic coma needs insulin and must be transported as soon as possible to an emergency care facility.

Doubtful Situations

If you are ever in doubt as to whether a patient is developing insulin shock or diabetic coma, give sugar, even though the final diagnosis may be diabetic coma. This is because insulin shock develops much more rapidly than diabetic coma and can quickly cause permanent brain damage or death. If you give sugar to a patient in diabetic coma, there is little risk of making the condition worse because a patient can withstand a high blood glucose level longer than he or she can tolerate a low blood glucose level.

MEDICAL PRACTICE and the LAW

Emergency medicine is one of the most litigious (lawsuit-prone) areas of health care. Owing to the nature of emergencies, there is little time to plan your actions, and one misstep could cause damage. Keep in mind that your actions would be compared in court with those of a "reasonably prudent medical assistant with similar education and experience." Do not perform procedures you are not comfortable performing.

Whenever possible, obtain written consent for all procedures. In a life-or-death situation, this is not usually possible. In this case, you are held accountable to try to save the life of the patient, even without consent.

Patients or families often become hysterical during emergencies. As a health care professional, you are expected to keep a cool head and calm the patient and family while attending to the emergency situation.

If you are out of the office and encounter an emergency situation, many states have a "Good Samaritan" law that protects you from legal action if you perform only procedures with which you are familiar, such as emergency first aid or CPR. ■

What Would You Do? What Would You *Not* Do? RESPONSES

Case Study 1
Page 844

What Did Judy Do?

❑ Gave Beth the National Poison Control hotline number (1-800-222-1222) and told her to call it immediately. Explained that was the fastest way to obtain information on what to do.

❑ Told Beth not to give the syrup of ipecac to Olivia unless she was told to do so by the poison control center.

❑ Told Beth to have the vitamin bottle in her hand when she calls. Told her that the poison control center would want to know information from the label and would especially want to know whether the vitamins contained iron.

❑ Told Beth to call the office back if she needs any more help after talking with the poison control center.

What Did Judy Not *Do?*

❑ Did not tell Beth she should give Olivia syrup of ipecac because some poisons can cause additional problems if they are brought back up.

What Would You Do?/What Would You *Not* Do? Review Judy's response and place a checkmark next to the information you included in your response. List additional information you included in your response.

_____

_____

_____

_____

Case Study 2
Page 845

What Did Judy Do?

❑ Told Anita that Garon needs to get to the hospital as soon as possible. Explained that he is having a very serious allergic reaction that could be life-threatening.

❑ Told her to stay calm and call 911 immediately.

❑ Notified the physician of the situation.

What Did Judy Not *Do?*

❑ Did not tell her to bring Garon to the office because he may need special life-support equipment available at the hospital.

What Would You Do?/What Would You *Not* Do? Review Judy's response and place a checkmark next to the information you included in your response. List additional information you included in your response.

_____

_____

_____

_____

Case Study 3
Page 847

What Did Judy Do?

❑ Took David to an examining room that was cool and gave him a glass of water.

❑ Told David she needed to get his costume off as soon as possible. Explained that if his condition gets worse, it could become life-threatening.

❑ Helped David out of the costume and gave him another glass of water.

What Did Judy Not *Do?*

❑ Did not let David keep the costume on.

What Would You Do?/What Would You *Not* Do? Review Judy's response and place a checkmark next to the information you included in your response. List additional information you included in your response.

_____

_____

_____

_____

TERMINOLOGY REVIEW

Burn An injury to the tissues caused by exposure to thermal, chemical, electrical, or radioactive agents.

Crash cart A specially equipped cart for holding and transporting medications, equipment, and supplies needed for lifesaving procedures in an emergency.

Crepitus A grating sensation caused by fractured bone fragments rubbing against each other.

Dislocation An injury in which one end of a bone making up a joint is separated or displaced from its normal anatomic position.

Emergency medical services (EMS) system A network of community resources, equipment, and personnel that provides care to victims of injury or sudden illness.

First aid The immediate care administered before complete medical care can be obtained to an individual who is injured or suddenly becomes ill.

Fracture Any break in a bone.

Hypothermia A life-threatening condition in which the temperature of the entire body falls to a dangerously low level.

TERMINOLOGY REVIEW—cont'd

Poison Any substance that causes illness, injury, or death if it enters the body.

Pressure point A site on the body where an artery lies close to the surface of the skin and can be compressed against an underlying bone to control bleeding.

Seizure A sudden episode of involuntary muscular contractions and relaxation, often accompanied by a change in sensation, behavior, and level of consciousness.

Shock The failure of the cardiovascular system to deliver enough blood to all of the vital organs of the body.

Splint Any device that immobilizes a body part.

Sprain Trauma to a joint, which causes tearing of ligaments.

Strain A stretching or tearing of muscles or tendons caused by trauma.

Wound A break in the continuity of an external or internal surface, caused by physical means.

 ON THE WEB

For Information on Emergency Medicine:

American Red Cross: www.redcross.org

Federal Emergency Management Agency: www.fema.gov

 PREPARE FOR CERTIFICATION | Visit the Evolve site at http://evolve.elsevier.com/Bonewit/today/ to actively Prepare for your Certification.

CD *Check out the* **Companion CD** *bound with the book to access additional interactive activities.*

36

The Medical Record

LEARNING OBJECTIVES

Components of the Medical Record
1. List and describe the functions served by the medical record.
2. Identify the information contained in each of the following medical office administrative documents: patient registration record and correspondence.
3. Identify the information contained in each of the following medical office clinical documents: health history report, physical examination report, progress notes, medication record, consultation report, and home health care report.
4. List and describe the information included in each of the following diagnostic procedure documents: electrocardiogram report, Holter monitor report, sigmoidoscopy report, colonoscopy report, spirometry report, radiology report, and diagnostic imaging report.
5. State the purpose of each of the following therapeutic services: physical therapy, occupational therapy, and speech therapy.
6. Identify the information contained in each of the following hospital documents: history and physical report, operative report, discharge summary report, pathology report, and emergency department report.

Consent Documents
1. Identify the information contained in each of the following consent documents: consent to treatment form and release of medical information form.

Medical Record Formats
1. Describe the organization of a source-oriented medical record and a problem-oriented medical record (POMR).
2. List and define the four subcategories included in the progress notes of a problem-oriented record (POR).
3. Explain the difference between a paper-based patient record (PPR) and an electronic medical record (EMR).

Health History
1. List and describe the seven parts of the health history.

2. List the guidelines that should be followed in recording the chief complaint (CC).

Charting
1. List and describe the guidelines to follow to ensure accurate and concise charting.

PROCEDURES

Prepare a medical record for a new patient.

Obtain patient consent for treatment.
Assist a patient in completing a release of medical information form.
Release information according to a completed release of medical information form.

Identify the parts of a source-oriented medical record and a POMR.

Complete or assist the patient in completing a health history form.

Chart the following:
Procedures

2. List and describe the types of progress notes that are charted by the medical assistant.
3. List examples of subjective symptoms and objective symptoms.
4. List and describe common symptoms.

Administration of medication
Specimen collection
Laboratory tests
Progress notes
Instructions given to the patient
Obtain and record patient symptoms.

CHAPTER OUTLINE

CAAHEP COMPETENCIES

Clinical Competencies
Perform Clerical Functions
- Organize a patient's medical record.

Patient Care
- Perform telephone and in-person screening.
- Obtain and record patient history.
- Maintain medication and immunization records

General Competencies
Professional Communications
- Respond to and initiate written communications.
- Recognize and respond to verbal communications.
- Recognize and respond to nonverbal communications.
- Demonstrate telephone techniques.

Legal Concepts
- Identify and respond to issues of confidentiality.
- Perform within legal and ethical boundaries.
- Establish and maintain the medical record.
- Document appropriately.
- Demonstrate knowledge of federal and state health care legislation and regulations.

Patient Instruction
- Explain general office policies.

Operational Functions
- Utilize computer software to maintain office systems.

ABHES COMPETENCIES

Professionalism
- Project positive attitude.
- Maintain confidentiality at all times.

Communication
- Use proper telephone techniques.
- Interview effectively.
- Receive, organize, prioritize, and transmit information expediently.
- Recognize and respond to verbal and nonverbal communication.
- Principles of verbal and nonverbal communication.
- Recognition and response to verbal and nonverbal communication.

Administrative Duties
- Prepare and maintain medical records.
- Apply computer concepts for office procedures.

Clinical Duties
- Interview and record patient history.
- Maintain medication and immunization records.
- Perform telephone and in-person screening.

Legal Concepts
- Document accurately.
- Use appropriate guidelines when releasing records or information.
- Follow established policy in initiating or terminating medical treatment.
- Monitor legislation related to current health care issues and practices.

Instruction
- Orient patients to office policies and procedures.

KEY TERMS

attending physician
charting
consultation report
diagnosis (dye-ag-NOE-sis)
diagnostic procedure
discharge summary report
electronic medical record (EMR)
familial (fah-MIL-yul)
health history report
home health care
informed consent
inpatient
medical impressions

medical record
medical record format
objective symptom
paper-based patient record (PPR)
patient
physical examination
physical examination report
problem
prognosis (prog-NOE-sis)
reverse chronological order
SOAP
subjective symptom
symptom (SIMP-tum)

Introduction to the Medical Record

Medical records are a crucial part of a medical practice. A **medical record** is a written record of the important information regarding a **patient** including the care of that individual and the progress of his or her condition. A patient is defined as an individual receiving medical care.

The patient's medical record serves many important functions. The physician uses the information in the medical record as a basis for decisions regarding the patient's care and treatment. The medical record documents the results of treatment and the patient's progress. The medical record provides an efficient and effective method by which information can be communicated to authorized personnel in the medical office.

The medical record also serves as a legal document. The law requires that a record be maintained to document the care and treatment being received by a patient. If something goes wrong, good documentation works to protect the physician and the medical staff legally. Incomplete records could be used as evidence in court to show that a patient did not receive the quality of care that meets generally accepted standards.

The medical assistant must always keep in mind that the information contained in a patient's medical record is strictly confidential and must not be read by or discussed with anyone except the physician or medical staff involved with the care of the patient (see the box titled *Highlight on the HIPAA Privacy Rule*).

COMPONENTS OF THE MEDICAL RECORD

A medical record consists of numerous documents. Each document in the medical record has a specific function or purpose. Most of these documents are preprinted forms that contain specific information entered by a physician or other health professionals. A large variety of forms are available; the type of form used is based on the specific requirements of each medical office.

Medical record documents can be classified into categories. Each of these categories is outlined in Box 36-1 along with the specific documents included in each.

It is important that the medical assistant be familiar with each type of document in the medical record. A description of the function or purpose of each type of medical record document follows (by category), along with the specific information that each contains.

Highlight on the HIPAA Privacy Rule

What Is the HIPAA Privacy Rule?

The acronym *HIPAA* stands for the *Health Insurance Portability and Accountability Act.* HIPAA is a federal law consisting of several components, one of which contains provisions to protect a patient's privacy, known as the HIPAA Privacy Rule.

The HIPAA Privacy Rule went into effect on April 14, 2003. The primary purpose of this rule is to provide patients with more control over the use and disclosure of their health information. All health care providers, health plans, and health care clearinghouses (e.g., billing services) that use, store, maintain, or transmit health information must comply with this rule.

What Is Included in the HIPAA Privacy Rule?

The HIPAA Privacy Rule is outlined here as it relates to the medical office:

1. The medical office must develop a written document known as a Notice of Privacy Practices (NPP). The NPP must explain to patients how their protected health information (PHI) will be used and protected by the medical office. *Protected health information* includes health information in any form (written, electronic, or oral) that contains patient-identifiable information (e.g., name, Social Security number, telephone number). The medical office must make a reasonable effort to provide an NPP to each patient and to obtain a signed acknowledgment from the patient that he or she has received an NPP.

2. A patient's written consent is not required for the use or disclosure of PHI for the following:
   - Medical treatment: *Examples:*
     (1) Patient referral to a specialist
     (2) Emergency care at a hospital
     (3) Laboratory performing tests on a patient
   - Payment: *Examples:*
     (1) Determination of eligibility for insurance benefits
     (2) Reviewing services provided for medical necessity
     (3) Utilization review activities
   - Health care operations: *Examples:*
     (1) Quality assessment activities
     (2) Contacting patients with information about care or treatment
     (3) Employee review activities
     (4) Training health care students

3. Patients have the right to access their medical records and to request changes to the records if they believe them to be inaccurate.

4. To prevent unnecessary or inappropriate access to PHI, the medical office must make an effort to limit the use of, disclosure of, and requests for PHI to the minimum necessary to accomplish the intended purpose (e.g., a request from an insurance company for procedures performed on a patient). This requirement does not apply, however, to the use of PHI for the routine practice of medicine within the medical office.

5. Patients have a right to request an accounting of the transfer of their information for purposes other than treatment, payment, or health care operations.

6. Business associates to whom the medical office may disclose PHI must respect the HIPAA Privacy Rule. The medical office must execute a written agreement with each business associate to handle PHI in accordance with HIPAA. Business associates may include the following organizations and firms:
   - Medical laboratories
   - Transcription services
   - Law firms
   - Accounting firms
   - Software and hardware consultants
   - Billing services

7. The medical office must implement a basic training program in privacy and security of PHI for all employees.

8. The medical office is required to put in place appropriate administrative, physical, and technical security safeguards to protect the privacy of PHI from accidental use or disclosure or violation of the previously listed requirements.

What if a Medical Office Does Not Comply with the HIPAA Privacy Rule?

Severe penalties, which can include civil and criminal penalties, apply if a medical office fails to comply with the HIPAA Privacy Rule.

Where Can More Information on the HIPAA Privacy Rule Be Found?

The following website contains current information on HIPAA: www.hhs.gov/ocr/hipaa ■

MEDICAL OFFICE ADMINISTRATIVE DOCUMENTS

Administrative documents contain information necessary for the efficient (record-keeping) management of the medical office. Medical office administrative documents include the patient registration record and patient-related correspondence.

Patient Registration Record

The patient registration record (Figure 36-1) consists of demographic and billing information. All new patients must complete a patient registration record form. After the patient completes the registration record, the medical assistant enters the information into a computer. This allows the demographic and billing information to be used for numerous computerized functions, such as scheduling appointments, posting patient transactions, and processing patient statements and insurance claims. The original patient registration record is placed in the front of the patient's medical record.

Demographic Information

Demographic information required on a patient registration form includes the following:

BOX 36-1 Categories of Medical Record Documents

Medical Office Administrative Documents
- Patient registration record
- Correspondence

Medical Office Clinical Documents
- Health history report
- Physical examination report
- Progress notes
- Medication record
- Consultation report
- Home health care report

Laboratory Documents
- Hematology report
- Clinical chemistry report

Laboratory Documents—cont'd
- Serology report
- Urinalysis report
- Microbiology report
- Parasitology report
- Cytology report
- Histology report

Diagnostic Procedure Documents
- Electrocardiogram report
- Holter monitor report
- Sigmoidoscopy report
- Colonoscopy report
- Spirometry report
- Radiology report
- Diagnostic imaging report

Therapeutic Service Documents
- Physical therapy report
- Occupational therapy report
- Speech therapy report

Hospital Documents
- History and physical report
- Operative report
- Discharge summary report
- Pathology report
- Emergency department report

Consent Documents
- Consent to treatment form
- Release of medical information form

From Bonewit-West K: *Clinical procedures for medical assistants,* ed 7, St. Louis, 2008, Saunders.

- Full name
- Address
- Telephone number (home and work)
- Date of birth
- Gender
- Marital status
- Employer

Billing Information

Billing information is required to bill charges to the patient or an insurance company. Billing information required on a patient registration form includes the following:
- Name of responsible party (person responsible for the account)
- Social Security number
- Address of responsible party
- Name of insured (policyholder)
- Insurance company
- Policy number and group number

Correspondence

Correspondence is an important part of the medical record. Correspondence regarding a patient may be received from various individuals or facilities, such as the patient's insurance company, the patient's attorney, and the patient himself or herself. Insurance correspondence includes such documents as a precertification authorization for a hospital admission and a request for additional information from the insurance company. Correspondence also includes copies of letters concerning the patient that are sent out of the office; examples are a copy of a letter referring the patient to a specialist and a copy of a collection letter sent to the patient.

What Would You Do? What Would You *Not* Do?

Case Study 1

Moira Celeste, an account executive for a large insurance company, comes to the office complaining of insomnia and depression. Three months ago her husband of 27 years left, and now they are legally separated. Since then, Moira has had a lot of trouble sleeping at night. She also feels lethargic during the day and hasn't been eating much. Moira says that she's been having some problems with alcohol. She wants to know of any community agencies that could help her with her problem but that would be sure to keep the information confidential. She has a very responsible job with her firm and does not want anyone to know about her alcohol problem. She also does not want any information about her problem put in her chart, and she especially does not want the physician to know about it because he is friends with many of her colleagues at work. ■

MEDICAL OFFICE CLINICAL DOCUMENTS

Medical office clinical documents include a variety of records and reports that assist the physician in the care and treatment of the patient. Common medical office clinical documents are listed and described next.

Health History Report

A **health history report** is a collection of subjective data about the patient. Most of this information is obtained by having the patient complete a preprinted form that is then reviewed for completeness by the medical assistant. Some of the information included in the health history is obtained by the physician or medical assistant by interviewing the patient.

PATIENT INFORMATION   CONFIDENTIAL

File no. 10140
Date 11-21-10

(PLEASE PRINT)

Name: Carol   H   Jones   Birth date 1-20-68   Home phone 740-555-1248
First   Middle   Last

Address: 743 Evergreen Terrace   City Springfield   State OH   ZIP 12345

Check appropriate box: ☐ Minor ☐ Single ☒ Married ☐ Divorced ☐ Widowed ☐ Separated   Gender: ☐ Male ☒ Female

Employer: Rockford, Inc.   Work phone 740-555-1234

Business Address: 1 Rockford Place   City Shelbyville   State OH   ZIP 21346

Spouse or parent's name: John Jones   Employer Self-emp.   Work phone 740-555-8654

If patient is a student, name of school/college: N/A   City _____ State _____

Whom may we thank for referring you? Henry Peterson, MD

Person to contact in case of emergency: John Jones   Phone 740-555-1248

RESPONSIBLE PARTY

Name of person responsible for this account: Carol Jones   Relationship to patient Self

Address: 743 Evergreen Terrace   City Springfield   State OH   ZIP 12345   Home phone 740-555-1248

Employer: Rockford, Inc.   Work phone 740-555-1234

Is this person currently a patient in our office? ☒ Yes   ☐ No

INSURANCE INFORMATION

Name of insured: Carol Jones   Relationship to patient Self

Birth date 1-20-68   Social Security number 123-45-6789   Date Employed 5-1-93

Name of Employer: Rockford, Inc.   Work phone 740-555-1234

Address of Employer: 1 Rockford Place   City Shelbyville   State OH   ZIP 21346

Insurance company: Anthem BC/BS   Group number 51045

Insurance company address: 521 Anthem Drive   City New Haberville   State OH   ZIP 21436

DO YOU HAVE ANY ADDITIONAL INSURANCE? ☐ YES ☒ NO   **IF YES, COMPLETE THE FOLLOWING:**

Name of insured _____   Relationship to patient _____

Birth date _____   Social Security number _____   Date Employed _____

Name of Employer _____   Work phone _____

Address of Employer _____   City _____ State _____ ZIP _____

Insurance company _____   Group number _____

Insurance company address _____   City _____ State _____ ZIP _____

X *Carol Jones*
SIGNATURE OF PATIENT OR PARENT IF MINOR

Figure 36-1. Patient registration record. (Courtesy and modified from Patterson Office Supplies, Champaign, Ill.)

Along with the physical examination and laboratory and diagnostic tests, the health history is used for the following reasons: to determine the patient's general state of health, to arrive at a diagnosis and to prescribe treatment, and to document any change in a patient's illness after treatment has been instituted. The term **diagnosis** refers to the scientific method of determining and identifying a patient's condition.

A thorough history of personal health is obtained for each new patient, and subsequent office visits provide additional information regarding changes in the patient's condition or treatment. A complete discussion of the health history report is presented later in this chapter.

Physical Examination Report

A **physical examination** is an assessment of each part of the patient's body. The purpose of the physical examination is to provide objective data about the patient, which assists the physician in determining the patient's state of health. (The physical examination is described in detail in Chapter 20.)

The **physical examination report** is a summary of the physician's findings from the assessment of each part of the patient's body and includes the following:
- General appearance
- Head and neck

Putting It All into Practice

My name is Dawn Bennett, and I work for an orthopedic surgeon. I work in the front area of the office as an administrative supervisor in billing and collections.

Working in billing and collections is very challenging and sometimes stressful. It can even be embarrassing. We are a new practice, and when we opened, there was no collection system. When it came time to review our accounts, we realized that, like every other business, we needed a collection system. We immediately jumped in and took charge.

The primary physician at our office is from New York, and we were unfamiliar with his family members. One day he walked into our office with a very puzzled look. I asked him what was wrong. He replied, "You guys are doing a great job with our collection rate. I asked you to be stern, but thoughtful, when sending out patient collection letters, but did you have to send one to my mother-in-law?!" Needless to say, we fixed the error immediately. This incident prompted us to restructure our collection system, and we added a comment screen to our computer system on all of our patients' accounts. Going into a medical office that already has a system in place may be easier, but you can learn a lot more by setting up an office system yourself. ∎

Prepare for Success

- Eyes
- Ears
- Nose
- Mouth and pharynx
- Arms and hands
- Chest and lungs
- Heart
- Breasts
- Abdomen
- Genitalia and rectum
- Legs and feet

Progress Notes

Progress notes involve updating the medical record with new information each time the patient visits or telephones the medical office. Progress notes serve to document the patient's health status from one visit to the next. It is important that the date and time be included with each progress note, along with the signature and credentials of the individual making the entry. A thorough discussion of charting progress notes is presented later in this chapter.

Medication Record

A medication record consists of detailed information related to a patient's medications. The record may include one or more of the following categories: prescription medications, over-the-counter (OTC) medications, and medications administered at the medical office. Most medical offices use one form to record prescription and OTC medications and another form to record medications administered to the patient at the medical office.

Prescription and Over-the-Counter Medication Record Form

A medication record form for recording the patient's prescription and OTC medications includes the following:

- Patient's name and date of birth
- Drug allergies
- Date the patient began taking the medication
- Name of the medication
- Dosage
- Frequency of administration of the medication
- Route of administration
- Refills (prescription medications only)
- Date the patient stopped taking the medication

Medication Administration Record Form

A form for recording medications administered to the patient at the medical office (Figure 36-2) includes the following:

- Patient's name and date of birth
- Drug allergies
- Name of the medication
- Dosage administered
- Route of administration
- Injection site
- Date of administration
- Manufacturer, lot number, and expiration date of the medication
- Signature and credentials of the individual administering the medication

Consultation Report

A **consultation report** is a narrative report of a clinical opinion about a patient's condition by a practitioner other than the primary physician, known as a *consultant* (Figure 36-3). The consultant is usually a specialist in a certain field of medicine (e.g., cardiology, endocrinology, urology). The consultant's opinion of the patient's condition is based on a review of the patient's record and an examination of the patient. The consultation report must include the following:

- Documentation that the consultant reviewed the patient's health history
- Documentation that the consultant examined the patient
- A report of the consultant's impressions
- Any care or treatment provided by the consultant
- A report of the consultant's recommendations

Home Health Care Report

Home health care is the provision of medical and non-medical care in a patient's home or place of residence. The purpose of home health care is to minimize the effect of

MEDICATION ADMINISTRATION RECORD

PATIENT NAME _Kristen Antle_   BIRTH DATE _1/9/76_

ALLERGIES _Ø_

SITE ABBREVIATIONS:

| RD: Right deltoid | RDG: Right dorsogluteal | RVL: Right vastus lateralis |
| LD: Left deltoid | LDG: Left dorsogluteal | LVL: Left vastus lateralis |

MEDICATION AND DOSAGE	ROUTE	DATE	MANUFACTURER	LOT#	EXP DATE	SITE	ADMIN BY
Rocephin 500 mg	IM	2/5/10	Roche	1053	10/5/11	RDG	D. Bennett, CMA (AAMA)
Depo-Provera 150 mg	IM	8/14/10	Pharmacia & Upjohn	68FUF	12/5/10	LDG	D. Bennett, CMA (AAMA)
Fluzone 0.5 ml	IM	11/4/10	Aventis Pasteur	OF1120	6/10/11	RD	D. Bennett, CMA (AAMA)
Depo-Provera 150 mg	IM	11/4/10	Pharmacia & Upjohn	87FUF	12/7/11	RDG	D. Bennett, CMA (AAMA)

Figure 36-2. Medication record. (From Bonewit-West K: *Clinical procedures for medical assistants,* ed 7, St. Louis, 2008, Saunders.)

disease or disability by promoting, maintaining, and restoring the patient's health. There is a growing preference for home health care over equivalent health care options. Research shows that familiar surroundings contribute positively to a patient's emotional and physical well-being.

Home health care must be ordered by the patient's physician and is provided by skilled professionals. Home health care professionals include nurses, home health aides, dietitians, physical therapists, occupational therapists, speech therapists, and social workers. Examples of specialized services available through home health care include cardiac home care, intravenous (IV) therapy, respiratory therapy, pain management, diabetes management, rehabilitation, and maternal-child care. Home health care providers must periodically provide a summary report (Figure 36-4) to the patient's physician that includes the following:

- Observations and evaluations
- Type of care or service provided
- Instructions given to the patient on medications
- Safety measures recommended for the home
- Diet
- Activities permitted

LABORATORY DOCUMENTS

A laboratory report is a report of the analysis or examination of body specimens. Its purpose is to relay the results of laboratory tests to the physician to assist in diagnosing and treating disease. A thorough discussion of laboratory documents is presented in Chapter 29. The specific categories of laboratory tests follow.

Hematology

Laboratory analysis in hematology deals with the examination and analysis of blood for the detection of abnormalities and includes areas such as blood cell counts, cellular morphology, clotting ability of the blood, and identification of cell types.

Clinical Chemistry

Laboratory analysis in clinical chemistry involves detecting the presence of chemical substances and determining the amount of substances in body fluids, excreta, and tissues (e.g., blood, urine, cerebrospinal fluid). The largest area in clinical chemistry is blood chemistry.

Serology

Laboratory analysis in serology deals with studying antigen-antibody reactions to assess the presence of a substance or to determine the presence of disease.

Urinalysis

Laboratory analysis in urinalysis involves the physical, chemical, and microscopic analysis of urine.

HAROLD B. COOPER, M.D.
6000 MAIN STREET
VENTURA, CA 93003

June 15, 2008

John F. Millstone, M.D.
5302 Main Street
Ventura, CA 93003

Dear Dr. Millstone:

RE: Elaine J. Silverman

This 69-year-old woman was seen at your request. The patient was admitted to the hospital yesterday because of chills, fever, and abdominal and back pain.

REVIEW OF HEALTH HISTORY: The history has been reviewed. A prominent feature of the history is the presence of intermittent, severe, shaking chills for four days with associated left lower back pain, left lower quadrant abdominal pain, and fever to as high as 103 or 104 degrees. The patient has had hypertension for a number of years and has been managed quite well with Aldomet 250 mg twice a day.

PHYSICAL EXAMINATION: On examination her temperature at this time is 100.6 degrees. The pulse is 110 and regular. Blood pressure is 190/100. The patient has partial bilateral iridectomies, the result of previous cataract surgery. Otherwise, the head and neck are not remarkable. Lung fields are clear throughout. The heart reveals a regular tachycardia, and heart sounds are of good quality. No murmurs are heard, and there is no gallop rhythm present. The abdomen is soft. There is no spasm or guarding. A well-healed surgical scar is present in the right flank area. There is considerable tenderness in the left lower quadrant of the left mid abdomen, but as noted, there is no spasm or guarding present. Bowel sounds are present. Peristaltic rushes are noted, and the bowel sounds are slightly high pitched. The extremities are unremarkable.

IMPRESSIONS: I believe the patient has acute diverticulitis. She may have some irritation of the left ureter in view of the findings on the urinalysis. She appears to be responding to therapy at this time in that her temperature is coming down and there has been a slight reduction in the leukocytosis from yesterday.

RECOMMENDATIONS: I agree with the present program of therapy, and the only suggestion would be to possibly increase the dose of gentamicin to 60 mg q8h, rather than the 40 mg q8h that she is now receiving.

Thank you for asking me to see this patient in consultation.

Sincerely,

Harold B. Cooper

Harold B. Cooper, M.D.

mtf

Figure 36-3. Consultation report. (Modified from Diehl MO, Fordney MT: *Medical transcription: techniques and procedures,* ed 5, Philadelphia, 2003, Saunders.)

Figure 36-4. Home health care report. (Form Number 3514. Courtesy Briggs, Des Moines.)

Microbiology

Laboratory analysis in microbiology deals with the identification of pathogens in specimens taken from the body (e.g., urine, blood, throat, sputum, wound, urethral, vaginal, cerebrospinal).

Parasitology

Laboratory analysis in parasitology deals with the detection of disease-producing human parasites or eggs in specimens taken from the body (e.g., stool, vagina, blood).

Cytology

Laboratory analysis in cytology deals with the detection of abnormal cells.

Histology

Laboratory analysis in histology deals with the detection of diseased tissues.

DIAGNOSTIC PROCEDURE DOCUMENTS

A diagnostic procedure report consists of a narrative description and interpretation of a diagnostic procedure. A **diagnostic procedure** is a type of procedure performed to assist in the diagnosis, management, or treatment of a patient's condition. The procedure may be performed by a physician, the medical assistant, or a technician specially trained in the procedure. A physician is responsible for interpreting the results

of the diagnostic procedure and completing the written report. Examples of diagnostic procedure reports follow.

Electrocardiogram Report

An electrocardiogram (ECG) report is a narrative description of a cardiologist's interpretation of an ECG, including the implications for the patient. The graphic tracing is usually included with the report.

Holter Monitor Report

A Holter monitor report is a narrative description of the interpretation of a 24-hour ambulatory ECG, including the evaluator's impressions. Portions of the graphic tracing are usually included with the report.

Sigmoidoscopy Report

A sigmoidoscopy report is a narrative description of the interpretation of a sigmoidoscopic examination, including the practitioner's impressions.

Colonoscopy Report

A colonoscopy report is a narrative description of a colonoscopic examination, including the practitioner's impressions.

Spirometry Report

A spirometry report is a narrative and graphic description of the interpretation of a patient's breathing capacity using a spirometer.

Radiology Report

A radiology report is a narrative description of a diagnostic or therapeutic radiologic procedure (Figure 36-5). A radiologist examines the radiograph and provides a written report, which includes a detailed interpretation of the radiograph and his or her impressions. The patient's physician receives a copy of the radiology report; the actual radiographic film or digital images are kept on file in the hospital's radiology department but are available for review by the patient's physician.

Diagnostic Imaging Report

A diagnostic imaging report is a narrative description of a diagnostic imaging procedure (Figure 36-6). The report includes a detailed interpretation of the diagnostic image, along with the practitioner's impressions. Examples of common diagnostic imaging procedures include ultrasonography, computed tomography (CT) scan, and magnetic resonance imaging (MRI). The diagnostic computer image is kept on file at the hospital but is available for review by the patient's physician.

THERAPEUTIC SERVICE DOCUMENTS

A therapeutic service report documents the assessments and treatments designed to restore a patient's ability to function.

Examples of therapeutic services that the physician may order follow.

Physical Therapy

Physical therapy involves the use of therapeutic exercise, thermal modalities, cold, hydrotherapy, electrical stimulation, massage, and other physical agents to restore function and promote healing after an illness or injury. A physical therapist might help a football player with a knee injury to regain normal functioning of the knee or assist a patient recovering from a stroke to use his or her legs to walk again. Figure 36-7 shows an example of a physical therapy report.

Occupational Therapy

Occupational therapy helps a patient learn new skills to adapt to a physically, developmentally, emotionally, or mentally disabling condition. This enables the patient to perform the activities of daily living and to achieve as much independence as possible. An occupational therapist might help an individual with a physical disability learn how to get dressed and how to prepare meals.

Speech Therapy

Speech therapy refers to treatment for the correction of a speech impairment resulting from birth, disease, injury, or prior medical treatment.

COLLEGE HOSPITAL
4567 BROAD AVENUE
WOODLAND HILLS, MD 21532

RADIOLOGY REPORT

Examination Date:	June 14, 2008	Patient:	Rose Baker
Date Reported:	June 14, 2008	X-ray No.:	43200
Physician:	Harold B. Cooper	Age:	19
Examination:	PA Chest, Abdomen	Hospital No.:	80-32-11

FINDINGS

PA CHEST: Upright PA view of chest shows the lung fields are clear, without evidence of an active process. Heart size is normal. There is no evidence of pneumoperitoneum.

IMPRESSION: NEGATIVE CHEST

ABDOMEN: Flat and upright views of the abdomen show a normal gas pattern without evidence of obstruction or ileus. There are no calcifications or abnormal masses noted.

IMPRESSION: NEGATIVE STUDY

RADIOLOGIST: _Marian B. Skinner_
Marian B. Skinner, MD

Figure 36-5. Radiology report. (Modified from Diehl MO, Fordney MT: *Medical keyboarding, typing, and transcribing*, ed 4, Philadelphia, 1997, Saunders.)

DIAGNOSTIC IMAGING REPORT			
Mt. Carmel Hospital, **Columbus, OH 43201**			
DATE REQUESTED 6/6/2008	DATE TO BE DONE 6/10/2008	TODAY'S DATE 6/10/2008	DATE OF BIRTH 8/19/1943
☐ WHEELCHAIR	☐ PORTABLE	☒ AMBULATORY	☐ CART

PATIENT:	INSURANCE:
Vera Ruth	Industrial

SEX F	ROOM NO. OP	RESPONSIBLE PERSON OR EMPLOYER J.B. Warren, Inc.	RADIOLOGIST Richard W. Adams, MD
CLINICAL INFORMATION AND PROVISIONAL DIAGNOSIS			ATTENDING PHYSICIAN Christopher Robb, MD
Back injury			NURSE

EXAMINATION REQUESTED (PINPOINT AREA OF CONCERN IF POSSIBLE)
CT LUMBAR SPINE

TECHNIQUE:

CT of the lumbar spine without contrast was performed from L-3 through S-1.

FINDINGS:

The L3-4 level appears satisfactory without evidence of osseous proliferation or disc protrusion.

At the L4-5 level there is some increased density at the disc level, which may be more prominent on the left. This is partially obscured due to facet artifact crossing obliquely.

There does appear to be some retention of epidural fat plane. This, however, may represent left-sided disc bulge or protrusion with the appropriate corresponding clinical appearance. Osseous variation at this level is not identified.

At the L5-S1 level, significant variation is not apparent.

IMPRESSION:

Variation at the L4-5 level on the left, which may represent annular disc bulge or perhaps protrusion on the left. However, confirmation with myelography and/or Ampaque enhanced computed tomography of the lumbar spine should be suggested prior to any surgical intervention.

Richard W. Adams, MD

Richard W. Adams, MD

Figure 36-6. Diagnostic imaging (CT scan) report. (From Bonewit-West K: *Clinical procedures for medical assistants,* ed 7, St. Louis, 2008, Saunders.)

HOSPITAL DOCUMENTS

Hospital documents are prepared by the physician responsible for the care of a patient while at the hospital; this physician is known as the **attending physician.** The attending physician may be the patient's regular physician or a different physician. An example of the latter is a physician attending a patient at an urgent care center or the emergency department of a hospital.

Hospital documents are dictated by the attending physician and transcribed at the hospital. The original document is filed in the patient's hospital medical record, and a copy is sent to the patient's regular physician. Hospital documents assist the patient's physician in reviewing the patient's hospital visit and in providing follow-up care.

History and Physical Report

The term **inpatient** refers to a patient who has been admitted to the hospital for at least one overnight stay. A health history must be obtained and a physical examination performed on all inpatients. There is one exception to this: If a patient history and physical examination are performed at the medical office within 1 week before admission, a copy of these documents may be used. In the event that a reliable health history cannot be obtained from the patient, it must be obtained from the person best able to relay the facts.

The history and physical report is a physician's narrative report of the patient's history and physical examination, along with the physician's medical impressions (Figure 36-8). The purpose of the history is to document the patient's current complaints and symptoms, whereas the purpose of

PHYSICAL THERAPY EVALUATION

OBJECTIVE DATA TESTS AND SCALES PRINTED ON REVERSE.

DATE OF SERVICE_____/_____/_____

HOMEBOUND REASON: ❑ Needs assistance for all activities   ❑ Residual weakness
❑ Requires assistance to ambulate   ❑ Confusion, unable to go out of home alone
❑ Unable to safely leave home unassisted   ❑ Severe SOB, SOB upon exertion
❑ Dependent upon adaptive device(s)   ❑ Medical restrictions
❑ Other (specify)_____

SOC DATE_____/_____/_____

(If Initial Evaluation, complete Physical Therapy Care Plan)

PERTINENT BACKGROUND INFORMATION

OTHER DISCIPLINES PROVIDING CARE: ❑ SN ❑ OT ❑ ST ❑ MSW ❑ Aide

MEDICAL HISTORY

❑ Hypertension   ❑ Cancer
❑ Cardiac   ❑ Infection
❑ Diabetes   ❑ Immunosuppressed
❑ Respiratory   ❑ Open wound
❑ Osteoporosis   ❑ Falls with injury
❑ Fractures   ❑ Falls without injury
❑ Other (specify)_____

REASON FOR EVALUATION (Diagnosis/Problem)

_____
_____
_____
_____
_____
_____
_____

LIVING SITUATION

❑ Capable ❑ Able ❑ Willing caregiver available
❑ Limited caregiver support (ability/willingness)
❑ No caregiver available

HOME SAFETY BARRIERS:
❑ Clutter ❑ Throw rugs ❑ Bath bench/equipment ❑ Needs grab bar
❑ Needs railings ❑ Steps (number/condition) _____
❑ Other (specify)_____

PRIOR LEVEL OF FUNCTION

ADLs:
❑ Independent ❑ Needed assistance ❑ Unable
Equipment used: _____

IN-HOME MOBILITY (gait or wheelchair/scooter):
❑ Independent ❑ Needed assistance ❑ Unable
Equipment used: _____

COMMUNITY MOBILITY (gait or wheelchair/scooter):
❑ Independent ❑ Needed assistance ❑ Unable
Equipment used: _____

BEHAVIOR/MENTAL STATUS

❑ Alert ❑ Oriented ❑ Cooperative ❑ Confused ❑ Memory deficits
❑ Impaired judgement ❑ Other (specify)_____
_____

VITAL SIGNS/CURRENT STATUS

Blood Pressure:_____
Temperature:_____
Pulse:_____
Respirations:_____
O_2 saturation _____% (when ordered): ❑ at rest ❑ with activity
Skin:_____
Edema:_____
Vision:_____
Sensation:_____
Communication:_____
Hearing:_____
Posture:_____
Endurance:_____

PAIN

INTENSITY: 0 1 2 3 4 5 6 7 8 9 10
LOCATION: _____
AGGRAVATING FACTORS: _____
_____
_____
RELIEVING FACTORS: _____
_____
_____
BEST PAIN GETS:_____ **WORST PAIN GETS:**_____
ACCEPTABLE LEVEL OF PAIN: _____
CURRENT LEVEL OF PAIN: _____
IMPACT ON THERAPY POC? ❑ None ❑ (describe) _____
_____
_____

PATIENT NAME – Last, First, Middle Initial

ID#

Form 3507P © BRIGGS, Des Moines, IA 50306 (800) 247-2343 www.BriggsCorp.com
305   PRINTED IN U.S.A.

PHYSICAL THERAPY EVALUATION
❑ Continued on Reverse

Figure 36-7. Physical therapy report. (Form Number 3507P. Courtesy Briggs, Des Moines.)

PHYSICAL THERAPY EVALUATION (Cont'd.)

MUSCLE STRENGTH/FUNCTIONAL ROM EVAL

AREA	STRENGTH Right	STRENGTH Left	ACTION	ROM Right	ROM Left
UPPER EXTREM. Shoulder			Flex/Extend		
			Abd./Add.		
			Int. Rot./Ext. Rot.		
Elbow			Flex/Extend		
Forearm			Sup./Pron.		
Wrist			Flex/Extend		
Fingers			Flex/Extend		
LOWER EXTREM. Hip			Flex/Extend		
			Abd./Add.		
			Int. Rot./Ext. Rot.		
Knee			Flex/Extend		
Ankle			Plant./Dors.		
Foot			Inver./Ever.		
SPINE AREA	STRENGTH		ACTION	ROM	

MANUAL MUSCLE TEST (MMT) MUSCLE STRENGTH

GRADE	DESCRIPTION
5	Normal functional strength - against gravity - full resistance.
4	Good strength - against gravity with some resistance.
3	Fair strength - against gravity - no resistance - safety compromise.
2	Poor strength - unable to move against gravity.
1	Trace strength - slight muscle contraction - no motion.
0	Zero - no active muscle contraction.

FUNCTIONAL RANGE OF MOTION (ROM) SCALE

GRADE	DESCRIPTION	GRADE	DESCRIPTION
5	100% active functional motion.	2	25% active functional motion.
4	75% active functional motion.	1	Less than 25%.
3	50% active functional motion.		

FUNCTIONAL INDEPENDENCE/BALANCE EVAL

	TASKS	ASSIST SCORE	ASSISTIVE DEVICES/COMMENTS
BED MOBILITY	Roll/Turn		
	Sit/Supine		
	Scoot/Bridge		
TRANSFERS	Sit/Stand		
	Bed/Wheelchair		
	Toilet		
	Floor		
	Auto		
BALANCE	Static Sitting		
	Dynamic Sitting		
	Static Standing		
	Dynamic Standing		
W/C SKILLS	Propulsion		
	Pressure Reliefs		
	Foot Rests		
	Locks		

FUNCTIONAL INDEPENDENCE SCALE (bed mobility, transfers, balance, W/C skills)

GRADE	DESCRIPTION
5	Independent - physically able and independent.
4	Verbal cue (VC) only needed.
3	Stand-by assist (SBA) - 100% patient/client effort.
2	Minimum assist (Min A) - 75% patient/client effort.
1	Maximum assist (Max A) - 25% - 50% patient/client effort.
0	Totally dependent - total care/support.

GAIT

ASSISTANCE: ❑ Independent ❑ SBA ❑ Min. assist ❑ Mod. assist ❑ Max. assist ❑ Unable

SURFACES: ❑ Level ❑ Uneven ❑ Stairs (number/condition)_____ **DISTANCE/TIME:**_____

WEIGHT BEARING STATUS: ❑ FWB ❑ WBAT ❑ PWB ❑ TDWB ❑ NWB

ASSISTIVE DEVICE(S): ❑ Cane ❑ Quad Cane ❑ Crutches ❑ Hemi Walker ❑ Walker ❑ Wheeled Walker

❑ Other (specify)_____

QUALITY/DEVIATIONS/POSTURES: _____

SUMMARY

Instruction provided: ❑ Safety ❑ Exercise ❑ Other (describe)_____

Equipment needed (describe) _____

❑ PT Evaluation only. No further indications for PT services.

❑ Orders for PT evaluation only. Needs additional PT services. See PT Care Plan for recommendations.

  ❑ Need to obtain orders.

❑ Orders for PT services with specific treatments, frequency and duration. See PT Care Plan/485.

DISCHARGE DISCUSSED WITH: ❑ Patient/Family

  ❑ Care Manager ❑ Physician ❑ Other (specify)_____

CARE COORDINATION: ❑ Physician ❑ SN ❑ PT ❑ OT ❑ ST ❑ MSW

  ❑ Aide ❑ Other (specify)_____

APPROXIMATE NEXT VISIT DATE_____/_____/_____

PLAN FOR NEXT VISIT_____

_____

_____

PATIENT SIGNATURE (if applicable)_____

THERAPIST'S SIGNATURE/TITLE_____

DATE_____/_____/_____ **TIME IN**_____ **TIME OUT**_____

Figure 36-7, cont'd.

HISTORY AND PHYSICAL
ST. MERCY HOSPITAL

Patient Name: ___Carol Jacobs___   Room #: ___215___

Physician: ___Charles Thomas, MD___   Hospital #: ___5422___

Admission Date: ___12/14/08___

CHIEF COMPLAINT: Chest pain

HISTORY OF PRESENT ILLNESS: Patient is an 85-year-old female complaining of chest pain. Patient was found to have abnormal cardiac enzymes in the Emergency Room consistent with acute myocardial infarction. Patient denied any pain radiating; however, she did complain of left-sided chest pain and lower back pain. Patient did not admit to any shortness of breath, nausea, or diaphoresis.

MEDICATIONS: Lasix, Darvocet-N 100, Lisinopril, Lopressor, Glynase, Relafen, Cytotec, and Micro K.

ALLERGIES: No drug allergies known.

PAST MEDICAL HISTORY: Significant for congestive heart failure, chronic obstructive pulmonary disease, diabetes mellitus type 2, coronary atherosclerosis, hypertension, and osteoporosis.

SOCIAL HISTORY: Not a drinker and not a smoker. Patient resides in a nursing home.

PHYSICAL EXAMINATION:

General: Patient is in acute distress. She is obese.

HEENT: She has 2 centimeters jugular venous distention. Pupils are equal and reactive to light and accommodation. No evidence of scleral or conjunctival icterus.

Chest: +2 bibasilar rales.

Heart: Regular rate and rhythm. +2/6 systolic ejection murmur in the left sternal border.

Abdomen: Soft, nontender, no splenomegaly and no hepatomegaly and positive bowel sounds.

Extremities: No evidence of edema or deep venous thrombosis.

Neurological: Cranial nerves II through XII grossly intact.

IMPRESSIONS: Congestive heart failure
                      Rule out myocardial infarction

Charles Thomas, MD

Charles Thomas, MD

Figure 36-8. Hospital history and physical examination report. (From Bonewit-West K: *Clinical procedures for medical assistants,* ed 7, St. Louis, 2008, Saunders.)

the physical examination is to assess the patient's current health status. **Medical impressions,** or simply impressions, are conclusions drawn from an interpretation of data. In this case, the physician interprets the data from the health history and physical examination and draws conclusions as to the patient's state of health. Other terms for impressions include *provisional diagnosis* and *tentative diagnosis.*

Operative Report

An operative report (Figure 36-9) must be completed for all patients who have had a surgical procedure. This report describes the surgical procedure and must be completed and signed by the surgeon who performed the operation. The operative report must include the following:

- Patient identification information
- Date of the surgery
- Preoperative diagnosis
- Name of the surgical procedure
- Full description of the findings at surgery (normal and abnormal)
- Description of the technique and procedures used during surgery

Figure 36-9. Operative report. (From Bonewit-West K: *Clinical procedures for medical assistants,* ed 7, St. Louis, 2008, Saunders.)

- Ligatures and sutures used
- Number of packs, drains, and sponges used
- Description of any specimens removed
- Condition of the patient at the completion of surgery
- Postoperative diagnosis
- Name of the surgeon

Discharge Summary Report

The **discharge summary report** is a brief (usually one page) summary of the significant events of a patient's hospitalization (Figure 36-10). The report must be completed and signed by the attending physician. The discharge summary report includes a concise account of the patient's illness, course of treatment, and response to treatment, as well as the condition of the patient at the time of discharge from the hospital. The purpose of this report is to document information needed by the patient's physician to provide for the continuity of future care. It is also used to respond to authorized requests for information regarding the patient's

hospitalization. The discharge summary report must include the following:

- Patient identification information
- Dates of hospitalization
- Reason for the hospitalization (provisional diagnosis)
- Brief health history
- Significant findings from examinations and tests
- Course of treatment
- Response to treatment
- Condition of the patient at discharge
- Discharge diagnosis (final diagnosis)
- Prognosis
- Discharge instructions
- Recommendations and arrangements for follow-up care

Pathology Report

A pathology report consists of a macroscopic (gross) and a microscopic description of tissue removed from a patient

DISCHARGE SUMMARY

Brennan, Susan
97-32-11
June 18, 2008

ADMISSION DATE: June 14, 2008   **DISCHARGE DATE:**   June 16, 2008

HISTORY OF PRESENT ILLNESS:
This 19-year-old female, nulligravida, was admitted to the hospital on June 14, 2008, with fever of 102°, left lower quadrant pain, vaginal discharge, constipation, and a tender left adnexal mass. Her past history and family history were unremarkable. Present pain had started two to three weeks prior to admission. Her periods were irregular, with latest period starting on May 30, 2008, and lasting for six days. She had taken contraceptive pills in the past but had stopped because she was not sexually active.

PHYSICAL EXAMINATION:
She appeared well developed and well nourished, and in mild distress. The only positive physical findings were limited to the abdomen and pelvis. Her abdomen was mildly distended, and it was tender, especially in the left lower quadrant. At pelvic examination, her cervix was tender on motion, and the uterus was of normal size, retroverted, and somewhat fixed. There was a tender cystic mass about 4-5 cm in the left adnexa. Rectal examination was negative.

PROVISIONAL DIAGNOSIS:
1. Probable pelvic inflammatory disease (PID).
2. Rule out ectopic pregnancy.

LABORATORY DATA ON ADMISSION:
Hgb 10.8, Hct 36.5, WBC 8,100 with 80 segs and 18 lymphs. Sedimentation rate 100 mm in one hour. Sickle cell prep+ (turned out to be a trait). Urinalysis normal. Electrolytes normal. SMA-12 normal. Chest x-ray negative, 2-hour UCG negative.

HOSPITAL COURSE AND TREATMENT:
Initially, she was given cephalothin 2 gm IV q6h, and kanamycin 0.5 gm IM bid. Over the next two days the patient's condition improved. Her pain decreased and her temperature came down to normal in the morning and spiked to 101° in the evening. Repeat CBC showed Hgb 9.8, Hct 33.5. The pregnancy test was negative. She was discharged on June 16, 2008 in good condition. She will be seen in the office in one week.

DISCHARGE DIAGNOSIS:
Pelvic inflammatory disease.

Harold B. Cooper, MD
Harold B. Cooper, MD

Figure 36-10. Discharge summary report. (Modified from Diehl MO, Fordney MT: *Medical transcription: techniques and procedures,* ed 5, Philadelphia, 2003, Saunders.)

during surgery or a diagnostic procedure. The report also includes a diagnosis of the patient's condition (Figure 36-11). A pathologist is required to examine the tissue specimen, complete the report, and sign it.

Emergency Department Report

The emergency department report is a record of the significant information obtained during an emergency depart-

ment visit (Figure 36-12). The report is prepared and signed by the emergency department physician, and a copy is sent to the patient's family physician for the purpose of providing follow-up care. The emergency department report includes the following:
- Date of service
- Patient identification information
- Nature of the illness or injury

COLLEGE HOSPITAL
4567 BROAD AVENUE
WOODLAND HILLS, MD 21532

PATHOLOGY REPORT

Date:	June 20, 2008	Pathology No.:	430211
Patient:	Molly Ramsdale	Room No.:	1308
Physician:	Harold B. Cooper, M.D.		
Specimen Submitted:	Tumor, right axilla		

FINDINGS

GROSS DESCRIPTION: Specimen A consists of an oval mass of yellow fibroadipose tissue measuring 4 x 3 x 2 cm. On cut section, there are some small, soft, pliable areas of gray apparent lymph node alternating with adipose tissue. A frozen section consultation at time of surgery was delivered as NO EVIDENCE OF MALIGNANCY on frozen section, to await permanent section for final diagnosis. Majority of the specimen will be submitted for microscopic examination.

Specimen B consists of an oval mass of yellow soft tissue measuring 2.5 x 2.5 x 1.5 cm. On cut section, there is a thin rim of pink to tan-brown lymphatic tissue and the mid portion appears to be adipose tissue. A pathological consultation at time of surgery was delivered as no suspicious areas noted and to await permanent sections for final diagnosis. The entire specimen will be submitted for microscopic examination.

MICROSCOPIC DESCRIPTION: Specimen A sections show fibroadipose tissue and nine fragments of lymph nodes. The lymph nodes show areas with prominent germinal centers and moderate sinus histiocytosis. There appears to be some increased vascularity and reactive endothelial cells seen. There is no evidence of malignancy.

Specimen B sections show adipose tissue and 5 lymph node fragments. These 5 portions of lymph nodes show reactive changes including sinus histiocytosis. There is no evidence of malignancy.

DIAGNOSIS: A & B: TUMOR, RIGHT AXILLA: SHOWING 14 LYMPH NODE FRAGMENTS WITH REACTIVE CHANGES AND NO EVIDENCE OF MALIGNANCY.

Stanley T. Nason, MD

Stanley T. Nason, MD

Figure 36-11. Pathology report. (Modified from Diehl MO, Fordney MT: *Medical transcription: techniques and procedures,* ed 5, Philadelphia, 2003, Saunders.)

EMERGENCY DEPARTMENT REPORT
CAMDEN CLARK HOSPITAL

Name: _____ John Larimer _____   DOB: _____ 2/2/68 _____

ER Physician: __ John Parsons, MD ____   Date: _____ 7/7/08 _____

ER Number: _____ 07398 _____

Physician: _____ James Woods, MD ____

NATURE OF ILLNESS/INJURY: This 40-year-old male presents to the Emergency Department complaining of a laceration of the sole of his right foot. Patient cut his foot on a rock 2 days ago and thinks he might have an infection now. Patient also complains of coughing over the past several days.

PHYSICAL EXAMINATION: Temperature 97.4, Pulse 76, Respirations 20, Blood Pressure 120/70. Patient is alert and oriented and is in no acute distress. ENT is normal. Lungs show diffuse rhonchi without crackles or wheezing. Heart has a regular rate and rhythm. Right great toe with marked tenderness with edema and erythema and heat.

DIAGNOSIS: Asthmatic Bronchitis
                Cellulitis, right foot first MTP

TREATMENT: PCMX scrub to right foot. Bacitracin dressing. Tetanus Diphtheria 0.5 cc IM. Biaxin 500 mg bid x 10 days. Guaifenesin with codeine 2 tsp q4h prn. Entex LA,1 bid prn. Debridement of skin flap.

PATIENT INSTRUCTIONS: Patient to follow up with family doctor in 7 days. Discussed bronchospasms with the patient.

James Woods, MD

_____
James Woods, MD

Figure 36-12. Emergency department report. (From Bonewit-West K: *Clinical procedures for medical assistants,* ed 7, St. Louis, 2008, Saunders.)

- Laboratory or diagnostic test results
- Procedures performed
- Treatment rendered
- Diagnosis
- Condition of the patient at discharge
- Instructions regarding follow-up care

CONSENT DOCUMENTS

Consent forms are legal documents required to perform certain procedures or to release information contained in the patient's medical record.

Consent to Treatment Form

The completion of a consent to treatment form (Procedure 36-1) is required for all surgical operations and nonroutine therapeutic and diagnostic procedures (e.g., sigmoidoscopy) performed in the medical office. The form must be signed by the patient or his or her legally authorized representative and must provide written evidence that the patient agrees to the procedure or procedures listed on the form (Figure 36-13).

For the patient's consent to be valid, it must be informed consent. **Informed consent** means that the patient has received the following information before giving consent:
- The nature of the patient's condition
- The nature and purpose of the recommended procedure
- An explanation of risks involved with the procedure
- Alternative treatments or procedures available
- The likely outcome (**prognosis**) of the procedure
- The risks of declining or delaying the procedure

The explanation must be in terms the patient can understand, and the patient should be given an opportunity to ask questions regarding the information.

The consent to treatment form should not be signed until the patient has been provided with all necessary information related to the procedure. The patient's signature must be witnessed; this is usually the responsibility of the medical assistant. *Witnessing a signature* means only that the medical assistant verified the patient's identity and watched the patient sign the form; it *does not* mean that the medical assistant is attesting to the accuracy of the information provided.

The consent to treatment form outlines the details of the discussion with the patient and includes the following information:

(Attach label or complete blanks.)

First name: _____ Last name: _____

Date of Birth: _____ Month _____ Day _____ Year

Account Number: _____

Procedure Consent Form

I, _____ , hereby consent to have

Dr. _____ perform _____ .

I have been fully informed of the following by my physician:

1. The nature of my condition
2. The nature and purpose of the procedure
3. An explanation of risks involved with the procedure
4. Alternative treatments or procedures available
5. The likely results of the procedure
6. The risks involved with declining or delaying the procedure

My physician has offered to answer all questions concerning the proposed procedure.

I am aware that the practice of medicine and surgery is not an exact science, and I acknowledge that no guarantees have been made to me about the results of the procedure.

Patient _____   Date _____
          (or guardian and relationship)

Witnessed _____   Date _____

Figure 36-13. Consent to treatment form. (From Bonewit-West K: *Clinical procedures for medical assistants,* ed 7, St. Louis, 2008, Saunders.)

- The patient's full name
- Name of the procedure to be performed
- Name of the surgeon
- A statement indicating the patient agrees to receive the procedure
- Acknowledgment that a disclosure of information has been made
- Acknowledgment that all questions were answered in a satisfactory manner
- A statement that no guarantee as to the outcome has been made
- Signature of the patient or his or her legal representative
- Signature of the witness

Release of Medical Information Form

As previously explained in the box titled *Highlight on the HIPAA Privacy Rule,* a patient's written consent is not required for the use or disclosure of protected health information (PHI) for the purpose of medical treatment, payment, and health care operations (TPO). If a request for PHI is required for purposes that are not part of TPO,

however, a detailed form must be completed, known as a *release of medical information form* (Figure 36-14). If a patient is moving to another state and wants to transfer his or her medical record to a new physician, a release of medical information form must be completed.

The release of medical information form must be signed by the patient authorizing the disclosure of his or her PHI (Procedure 36-2). If the patient is a minor, the form must be signed by the parent or legal guardian of the minor. The release of medical information form must stipulate the following:

- The patient's full name and address
- Name of the medical practice releasing the information
- Name of the individual or facility to receive the information
- Specific information to be released
- The purpose of or the need for the information
- Method of release of the information
- Signature of the patient or his or her legal representative
- Date that the consent was signed
- The expiration date of the consent form

RELEASE OF MEDICAL INFORMATION

All information contained in the medical record is confidential, and the release of information is closely controlled. A properly completed and signed authorization form is required for the release of the following information.

PATIENT INFORMATION

Patient Name _____

Address _____ Social Security # _____

City _____ State _____ ZIP _____ Birth date _____/_____/_____

Phone (Home) _____ Work _____

RELEASE FROM:

Name _____

Address _____

City _____ State _____ ZIP _____

RELEASE TO:

Name _____

Address _____

City _____ State _____ ZIP _____

INFORMATION TO BE RELEASED:

1. GENERAL RELEASE:

____Entire Medical Record (excluding protected information)

____Hospital Records only (specify)_____

____Lab Results only (specify) _____

____X-ray Reports only (specify)_____

____Other Records (specify) _____

2. INFORMATION PROTECTED BY STATE/FEDERAL LAW: If indicated below, I hereby authorize the disclosure and release of information regarding:

____Drug Abuse Diagnosis/Treatment

____Alcoholism Diagnosis/Treatment

____Mental Health Diagnosis/Treatment

____Sexually Transmitted Disease

PURPOSE/NEED FOR INFORMATION:

____Taking records to another doctor

____Moving

____Legal purposes

____Insurance purposes

____Worker's Compensation

____Other/Explain:_____

METHOD OF RELEASE:

____ US Mail

____ Fax

____ Telephone

____ To Patient

PATIENT AUTHORIZATION TO RELEASE INFORMATION:

Authorization is valid for 60 days only from the date of my signature. I reserve the right to revoke this authorization at any time prior to 60 days (except for action that has already been taken) by notifying the medical office in writing.

I understand that my records are protected under HIPAA (Health Insurance Portability and Accountability Act) Standards for Privacy of Individually Identifiable Information (45 CFR Parts 160 and 164) unless otherwise permitted by federal law. Any information released or received shall not be further relayed to any other facility or person without my written authorization. I also understand that such information will not be given, sold, transferred, or in any way relayed to any other person or party not specified above without my further written authorization.

I hereby grant authorization to release the information listed above. I certify that this request has been made voluntarily and that the information given above is accurate to the best of my knowledge.

_____   _____

Signature of Patient/Legally Responsible Party   Date

_____   _____

Witness Signature   Date

OFFICE USE ONLY

Information indicated above released on _____
                                          Date

Explanation of information released: _____

_____

Signature and credentials of individual releasing information: _____

Figure 36-14. Release of medical information form. (From Bonewit-West K: *Clinical procedures for medical assistants,* ed 7, St. Louis, 2008, Saunders.)

Mailed or Faxed Requests for Release of Medical Information

Most medical offices require that the patient come to the office to sign the release of medical information form; however, this may not always be possible. An example is a patient who has moved away and is requesting the transfer of his or her medical records to a new physician. In this instance, a completed and signed release of medical information form may be mailed or faxed to the medical office. The procedure for processing this type of request is outlined at the end of Procedure 36-2.

PROCEDURE 36-1 Completion of a Consent to Treatment Form

Outcome Complete a consent to treatment form.

Equipment/Supplies

• Consent to treatment form

1. **Procedural Step.** Type or print all required information on the consent to treatment form in the spaces provided (e.g., patient's full name, name of the procedure to be performed).
2. **Procedural Step.** Ensure that the physician has had a discussion to give the patient complete information about the procedure to be performed.
   Principle. For the patient's consent to be valid, it must be informed consent.
3. **Procedural Step.** Greet the patient and introduce yourself. Identify the patient by his or her full name and date of birth. Explain the purpose of the consent form to the patient.
4. **Procedural Step.** Give the consent form to the patient, and ask him or her to read it. Ask the patient whether he or she has any questions.
5. **Procedural Step.** Ask the patient to sign the consent form. Witness the patient's signature by signing your name in the appropriate space on the form. Include today's date.
   Principle. Witnessing a signature means only that the medical assistant verified the identity of the patient and watched the patient sign the form; it does not mean that the medical assistant is attesting to the accuracy of the information provided.
6. **Procedural Step.** Provide the patient with a copy of the completed consent form for his or her files.
7. **Procedural Step.** File the original consent to treatment form in the patient's medical record.
   Principle. Maintaining the form provides legal documentation that the patient gave permission for treatment.

Ask the patient to read the consent form. (From Bonewit-West K: *Clinical procedures for medical assistants,* ed 7, St. Louis, 2008, Saunders.)

Ask the patient to sign the consent form. (From Bonewit-West K: *Clinical procedures for medical assistants,* ed 7, St. Louis, 2008, Saunders.)

PROCEDURE 36-1

PROCEDURE 36-2   Release of Medical Information

Outcome (1) Assist a patient in the completion of a release of medical information form. (2) Release medical information according to a completed release of medical information form.

Equipment/Supplies

- Release of medical information form

1. **Procedural Step.** Greet the patient and introduce yourself. Identify the patient by his or her full name and date of birth. Explain the purpose of the release of medical information form. (*Note:* If you do not recognize the patient, ask him or her to provide photo identification, such as a driver's license.)

2. **Procedural Step.** Provide the patient with a release of medical information form, and ask the patient to complete the form. Provide assistance if needed.
   Principle. Information from a patient's medical record can be released only on written authorization of the patient (except when permitted by law).

3. **Procedural Step.** Check to ensure all the requested information on the form has been completed by the patient.

4. **Procedural Step.** Ask the patient to sign the form. Witness the patient's signature by signing your name in the appropriate space on the form. Include today's date. If required by your medical office policy, ask the physician to initial the completed release of medical information form.
   Principle. To release information, the form must be signed by the patient authorizing the disclosure of medical information.

5. **Procedural Step.** Provide the patient with a copy of the release of medical information form for his or her files.

6. **Procedural Step.** Copy the information requested on the form. Release only the information requested. Include a copy of the completed release form with the medical information.

7. **Procedural Step.** Document what information is being released and the date of its release. Sign the document with your name and credentials.

8. **Procedural Step.** File the original document and the release of medical information form in the patient's medical record.
   Principle. Maintaining the release form provides legal documentation that the patient gave permission for the release of his or her medical information.

9. **Procedural Step.** Send the medical information to the appropriate site according to your medical office policy.

Mailed or Faxed Requests for Release of Medical Information

These steps should be followed when a completed release of medical information form has been mailed or faxed to the medical office:

1. **Procedural Step.** Check the expiration date on the release of medical information form. If the authorization is outdated, a new release form needs to be completed.

2. **Procedural Step.** Verify the authenticity of the signature on the form. This can be accomplished by comparing the patient's signature on the form with the patient's signature in his or her medical record. If you have any doubt as to the authenticity of the signature, do not release the records.

3. **Procedural Step.** Copy the information requested on the form. Release only the information requested. Include a copy of the completed release form with the medical information.

4. **Procedural Step.** Document what information is being released and the date of its release. Sign the document with your name and credentials.

5. **Procedural Step.** File the original document and the release of medical information form in the patient's medical record.

6. **Procedural Step.** Send the medical information according to your medical office policy.

Witness the patient's signature. (From Bonewit-West K: *Clinical procedures for medical assistants,* ed 7, St. Louis, 2008, Saunders.)

MEDICAL RECORD FORMATS

Most medical offices rely on the use of paper medical records, known as **paper-based patient records (PPRs).** Although most of the medical record is paper based, some patient data is maintained on the computer; this includes patient registration information and patient charges and payments. As technology advances, some offices are converting to an **electronic medical record (EMR)** for maintaining patient health information. With an EMR, the entire record is stored in a database on the computer, including the health history report and physical examination report, progress notes, laboratory and diagnostic reports, and hospital reports. Because most offices currently use paper-based records, this chapter focuses on the PPR.

The way a PPR is organized is known as its *format.* The two main types of **medical record formats** are the source-oriented record and the problem-oriented record. Each of these formats is described.

Source-Oriented Record

The source-oriented format is used most often in the medical office for organizing a medical record. The documents in a source-oriented record are organized into sections based on the department, facility, or other source that generated the information (e.g., laboratory, hospital, consultant). Because documents from each source are filed together, it is easier to compare information from laboratory and diagnostic test results, assessments, and treatments.

Each section in a source-oriented record is separated from the other sections by a chart divider. Attached to each divider is a color-coded tab labeled with the title of its section (Figure 36-15). Within each of these sections, the documents are arranged according to date. Most offices use the reverse chronological order to arrange the documents. **Reverse chronological order** means that the most recent document is placed on top or in front of the others, and thus the oldest document is on the bottom or at the end of that section.

The titles that identify each section vary depending on the medical office's preference; however, typical examples include the following:
- History and Physical
- Progress Notes
- Medications
- Laboratory Reports
- ECG
- X-ray Reports
- Consultations
- Rehabilitation Therapy
- Home Health Care
- Hospital Reports
- Insurance
- Consents
- Correspondence
- Miscellaneous

Problem-Oriented Record

The documents in a problem-oriented record (POR), or problem-oriented medical record (POMR), are organized according to the patient's health problems. The advantage of using the POR is that each of the patient's problems can be defined and followed individually. The POR is developed in four stages:
1. Establishing a *database*
2. Compiling a *problem list*
3. Devising a *plan* of action for each problem
4. Following each problem with *progress notes*

Database

The first step in developing a POR is to establish a database. The database consists of a collection of subjective and objective data. These data include the health history report, physical examination report, and results of baseline laboratory and diagnostic tests. The information in the database is used to identify and compile a problem list.

Problem List

The problem list is developed shortly after the database is completed and consists of a list of all of the patient's prob-

---

What Would You Do? What Would You *Not* Do?

Case Study 2

Tessa Walsh, her husband, and their two children are moving to another state. They will be leaving in 2 days. Tessa calls the office to have their medical records transferred to their new physician. Tessa's daughter has type 1 diabetes, so it is important that this be done as soon as possible. Tessa is quite annoyed to learn that she has to come in and sign a special form. She says that their medical records belong to them. Tessa says that the whole family has been coming there for the past 8 years and is well known by the physician and staff. She says that they have been good patients, have followed the physician's advice, and have always paid their bills on time. Tessa thinks that verbal permission should be enough. She's extremely busy packing and taking care of other moving details and doesn't have a minute to spare. ■

Figure 36-15. Chart dividers in a source-oriented record. (From Bonewit-West K: *Clinical procedures for medical assistants,* ed 7, St. Louis, 2008, Saunders.)

lems (Figure 36-16). A **problem** is defined as any patient condition that requires observation, diagnosis, management, or patient education. This includes not only medical problems but also psychological and social problems. The problem list is a crucial part of the POR and is always located in the front of the medical record.

The problem list should be thought of as a table of contents for the record. Each problem in the list is numbered and titled. The problem title is stated as a diagnosis, a physiologic finding, a symptom, or an abnormal test result. All subsequent data (plans and progress notes) added to the medical record are cross-referenced to these numbered problems.

The problem list is modified as needed. If a new problem is identified, it is added to the list and dated accordingly. When a problem is resolved, it is marked as such, and the date is recorded.

Plan

After examining the problem list, the physician develops the third section of the POR. This involves devising a plan of action for further evaluation and treatment of each problem. Each plan begins with a heading that identifies the number of the problem, followed by the plan of action for the problem. This may include plans for laboratory and diagnostic tests, medical or surgical treatment, therapy, and patient education.

Progress Notes

The last stage in the development of the POR is the follow-up for each problem, or the progress notes (Figure 36-17). The progress notes begin with the number of a problem and include the following four categories:

PATIENT RECORD

Name: Morani, Betty

Number: ____   Blood Type: A+

ALLERGIES/SENSITIVITY: Codeine, Sulfa

Prob. No.	Date	PROBLEM DESCRIPTION	Date Resolved	Index	Prob. No.	Date	PROBLEM DESCRIPTION	Date Resolved	Index
1	10/01	Hypertension - essential		✓					
2	10/01	Diabetes mellitus (mild)		✓					
3	1/04	L. Retinopathy	see below						
4	4/2008	Atherosclerosis with cerebral vascular insuffic.							
5	4/2008	Hearing loss							
6	1/2008	HBP Non-compliance	2/04						
3	1/2008	Bilat. Grade II Retinopathy							

Prob. No.	CONTINUING MEDICATIONS	Start	Stop	Prob. No.	CONTINUING MEDICATIONS	Start	Stop
1	Sinoserp 1 mg. b.i.d.	10/01	10/05				
2	Orinase 0.5 gm. daily	10/01	10/05				
1	Hydrodiuril 50 mg. A.M.	10/05					
2	1500 cal. diet low Na hi K	2/2008					

| Periodic Health Examination | Dates | 1/04 | 4/2006 | | | | | | | | | |

Figure 36-16. Problem-oriented record problem list. (From Bonewit-West K: *Clinical procedures for medical assistants,* ed 7, St. Louis, 2008, Saunders.)

PROBLEM ORIENTED - PROGRESS NOTES

Date	Time	Problem Number	FORMAT: Problem Number and TITLE: S = Subjective O = Objective A = Assessment P = Plan
11/15/10	9:30 AM	1	S: Mother states that her child has had a runny nose and her throat has been
			sore for 2 days.
			O: Vital signs: T 98.8 P 96 R 24
			Weight: 42 lb.
			General: alert and active. HEENT: sclera clear. TMs negative. Positive clear
			rhinorrhea. Pharynx benign. Heart: regular without murmur.
			Lungs: clear to auscultation and percussion. Abdomen: negative tenderness.
			Positive bowel x 4. GU: negative. Neuro: good tone.
			A: Upper respiratory tract infection.
			P: 1. A prescription for Rondec DM, 1/2 tsp q6h prn cough and congestion.
			2. Instructed mother to contact office if child does not improve.

NAME–Last	First	Middle	Attending Physician	Record No.	Room/Bed
Michaels	Jessica	L	Frank Edwards, MD	1	24

Form 653/2S © BRIGGS, Des Moines, IA 50306 (800) 247-2343 www.BriggsCorp.com
R404   PRINTED IN U.S.A.

PROBLEM ORIENTED - PROGRESS NOTES

Figure 36-17. Problem-oriented record SOAP progress notes. (Form Number 653/2S. Courtesy Briggs, Des Moines.)

Continued

PROBLEM ORIENTED - PROGRESS NOTES

Date	Time	Problem Number	FORMAT: Problem Number and TITLE: S = Subjective O = Objective A = Assessment P = Plan

NAME–Last	First	Middle	Attending Physician	Record No.	Room/Bed
Michaels	Jessica	L	Frank Edwards, MD	1	24

PROBLEM ORIENTED - PROGRESS NOTES

Figure 36-17, cont'd.

Subjective data: Subjective data obtained from the patient

Objective data: Objective data obtained by observation, physical examination, and laboratory and diagnostic tests

Assessment: The physician's interpretation of the current condition based on an analysis of the subjective and objective data

Plan: Proposed treatment for the patient

The acronym for this process is **SOAP,** and the writing of progress notes in this format is called *soaping.* Some physicians who use the source-oriented format have found it advantageous to record progress notes in SOAP format. This structured type of note increases the physician's ability to deal with each problem clearly and to analyze data in an orderly, systematic manner.

PREPARING A MEDICAL RECORD FOR A NEW PATIENT

When a patient comes to the medical office for his or her first visit, a medical record must be prepared for that patient (Procedure 36-3). The method used to prepare the record depends on the following criteria: the format used to organize the record, the filing system, and the type of storage equipment. Most medical offices use the source-oriented format to organize their medical records, the alphabetic filing system to arrange the records, and shelf filing units to store the medical records. Methods used to prepare a medical record are described in the following sections and are based on these criteria.

Medical Record Supplies

Certain supplies are required to prepare a medical record. These supplies are categorized and described next.

File Folders

A file folder is a protective cover made of a heavy material, such as manila card stock. A file folder is used to hold medical record documents in an organized format. Flexible metal fasteners are typically used to hold documents in the folder. Folders are available with fasteners located on the top or left side of the folder.

Folders are available with tabs. A tab is a projection extending from a folder and is used to identify its contents. The tab is located on either the side or top of the folder. A folder with a tab extending across its entire side or top is called a *full cut tab.*

In the medical office, a file folder with a full cut side tab is typically used to prepare a new patient's chart. There are indentations at intervals along the full cut tab to indicate the placement of adhesive labels. This ensures that the labels on all the medical records are affixed at the same place on the file folders.

Folder Labels

Labels to identify the medical record are commercially available in rolls or continuous folded strips for typewriter use. Labels also are available on 8½-× 11-inch sheets for use with a computer and printer. The most common types of labels used in the medical office include name labels, alphabetic color-coded labels, color-coded year labels, and miscellaneous chart labels.

Chart Dividers

Chart dividers are used to identify each section of the medical record by subject (see Figure 36-15). Chart dividers consist of a heavy material, such as manila card stock. Attached to each divider is a color-coded tab labeled with a subject title; the most frequently used subject titles are illustrated in Box 36-2 along with the documents typically filed under each title.

BOX 36-2 Chart Divider Subject Titles and Documents Typically Filed under Each Title

History and Physical
- Health history
- Physical examination report

Progress Notes
- Progress notes
- Medication record

Laboratory/X-ray
- Hematology report
- Clinical chemistry report
- Serology report
- Urinalysis report
- Microbiology report
- Parasitology report
- Cytology report
- Histology report
- Electrocardiogram report

Laboratory/X-ray—cont'd
- Holter monitor report
- Sigmoidoscopy report
- Colonoscopy report
- Spirometry report
- Radiology report
- Diagnostic imaging report

Hospital
- History and physical report
- Operative report
- Pathology report
- Discharge summary report
- Emergency department report

Correspondence
- Consultation report
- Letter from patient

Correspondence—cont'd
- Letter from patient's attorney
- Referral letter

Insurance
- Copy of patient's insurance card
- Precertification authorization for hospital admission
- Request for additional information from insurance company

Miscellaneous
- Consent to treatment form
- Release of medical information form
- Home health care report
- Physical therapy report
- Occupational therapy report
- Speech therapy report

From Bonewit-West K: *Clinical procedures for medical assistants,* ed 7, St. Louis, 2008, Saunders.

PROCEDURE 36-3 Preparing a Medical Record

Outcome Prepare a medical record.

The following procedure outlines the method for preparing a medical record for a new patient using the following organization: a source-oriented format stored in shelf files using a color-coded alphabetic filing system.

Equipment/Supplies

- Patient registration form
- Notice of Privacy Practices (NPP)
- NPP acknowledgment form
- File folder with a full cut side tab
- Metal fasteners
- Name labels

- Color-coded alphabetic bar labels
- Miscellaneous chart labels
- Set of chart dividers
- Blank preprinted forms
- Two-hole punch

1. **Procedural Step.** Greet the patient when he or she arrives at the medical office. Introduce yourself and identify the patient. Verify that the patient is a new patient.

2. **Procedural Step.** Ask the patient to do the following:
   a. Complete a patient registration form.
   b. Read a Notice of Privacy Practices (NPP).
   c. Sign an NPP acknowledgment form.

3. **Procedural Step.** When the patient returns the completed forms, check the patient registration form for accuracy and make sure that you can read the patient's handwriting. If you have any questions regarding the information on the form, ask the patient for clarification. If required by the medical office policy, ask the patient for his or her insurance card and make a copy of it.
   Principle. A copy of the patient's insurance card is used for third-party billing.

4. **Procedural Step.** Enter the data on the completed registration record into the computer.

5. **Procedural Step.** Assemble supplies needed to prepare the medical record. Type the patient's full name on a name label following these guidelines:
   a. Type the patient's name in transposed order as follows: last name, first name, middle name (or initial).
   b. Type the patient's name two or three typewritten spaces from the left edge of the label and one line down from the top of the label.
   c. Ensure the patient's name is spelled correctly.
   Principle. Following these guidelines facilitates the accurate and efficient filing of the patient's medical record.

6. **Procedural Step.** Determine the first two letters of the patient's last name and select the appropriate alphabetic color-coded labels. Attach the color-coded labels to the (full cut) side tab. The labels should be affixed to the folder using the label placement indentations on the tab.

Principle. Using the label placement indentations ensures that all labels on medical records are affixed at the same place.

7. **Procedural Step.** Affix the name label immediately above the first color-coded alphabetic label.

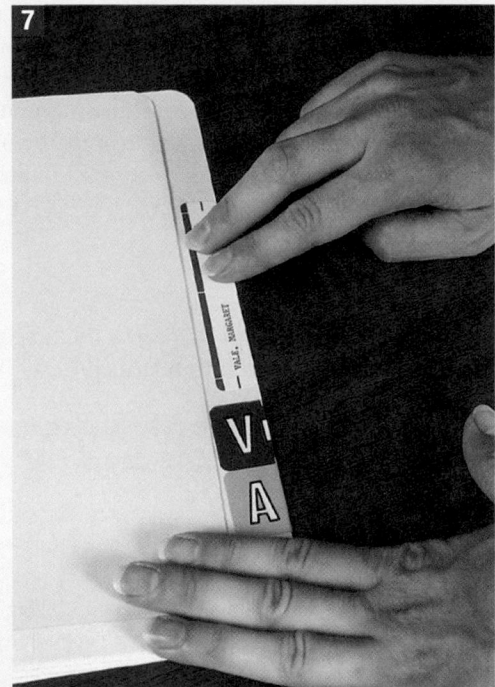

Affix the name label. (From Bonewit-West K: *Clinical procedures for medical assistants,* ed 7, St. Louis, 2008, Saunders.)

8. **Procedural Step.** Attach any additional chart labels, such as a year label and miscellaneous chart labels (e.g., allergy, insurance), to the folder according to the office policy.

9. **Procedural Step.** Insert the chart dividers onto the metal fasteners of the file folder.

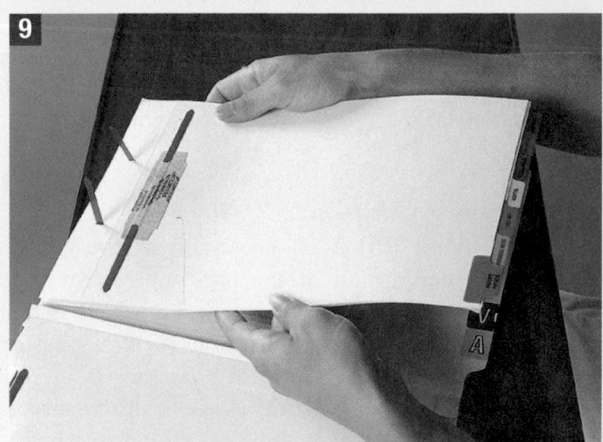

Insert the chart dividers into the metal fasteners. (From Bonewit-West K: *Clinical procedures for medical assistants,* ed 7, St. Louis, 2008, Saunders.)

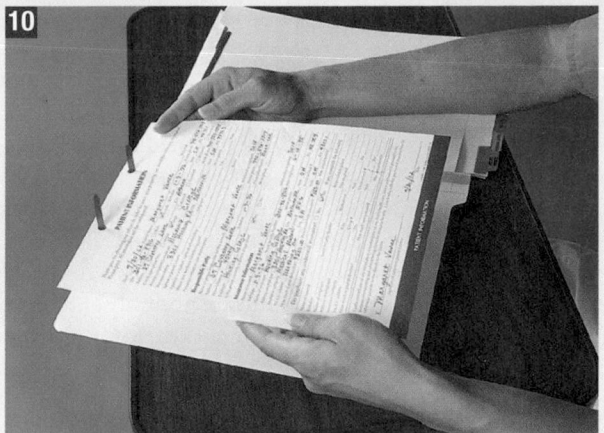

Place the patient registration form in the front of the medical record. (From Bonewit-West K: *Clinical procedures for medical assistants,* ed 7, St. Louis, 2008, Saunders.)

10. Procedural Step. Place the original patient registration form in the front of the medical record. Place the signed NPP acknowledgment form and the copy of the patient's insurance card in the appropriate section of the record.

11. Procedural Step. Label preprinted forms to be placed in the record with required information such as the patient's name and date. These forms typically include the medical history form, physical examination form, progress note sheets, and a medication record form.

If the forms are not prepunched, the medical assistant must use a two-hole punch to insert two holes into the top or side of the form.

12. Procedural Step. Insert each form under its proper chart divider. Refer to the box on p. 879 for a list of chart divider subject titles and documents typically filed under each title.

13. Procedural Step. Check the medical record to ensure that it has been prepared properly.

PROCEDURE 36-3

Memories *from* Externship

Dawn Bennett: During my externship as a medical assisting student, I was placed in a family practice clinic. I was very nervous my first day, wondering how in the world I would be able to remember everything I had learned in school. My first patients were an elderly couple. The wife was there for some test results for cancer. I looked at the results, and they were positive. After the physician relayed the results, the husband broke down. He had just lost his granddaughter to a heart attack and his son-in-law to a stroke. You could tell that he just could not bear losing his wife, too.

One week later, the elderly man's wife was placed in a nursing home. He came into our office for an appointment. As I was working him up, he was telling me stories about himself and his wife when they were first married. He looked so sad. I sat with him for a few minutes after completing his workup and gave his stories my full attention. As I was leaving the room, a smile came across his face, and he thanked me for listening to him. I realized that working in a physician's office is more than just knowing what I learned in school. Compassion and showing the patients you really do care about them is just as important. I felt good about myself that day. ■

Prepare for Success

What Would You Do? What Would You *Not* Do?

Case Study 3

Brett Oberlin is 21 years old and lives at home. He commutes to a local college and is a junior majoring in art education. His mother and father have come to the medical office and ask to see his medical record. The physician is attending a medical conference and will not return for another 4 days. Mr. and Mrs. Oberlin found some medications in Brett's room and looked them up on the Internet. They found out that they are used to treat HIV infection. Brett would not talk to them about the medications and told them he is an adult and it is none of their business. Mr. and Mrs. Oberlin are very concerned about Brett. They also are worried about other members of the family being exposed to HIV. They say that because they are supporting him, they should be allowed to see his record. ■

TAKING A HEALTH HISTORY

The health history is a collection of subjective health data obtained by interviewing the patient and by having the patient complete a preprinted health history form that is then reviewed for completeness by the medical assistant. A thorough history is taken for each new patient, and subsequent office visits (in the form of progress notes) provide information regarding changes in the patient's illness or treatment. A quiet, comfortable room that allows for privacy encourages the patient to communicate honestly and openly. Showing genuine interest in and concern for the patient reduces apprehension and facilitates the collection of data.

Components of the Health History

The health history is taken before the physical examination, providing the physician the opportunity to compare findings. The health history consists of seven parts or sections.

Identification Data

The identification data section is included at the beginning of the health history form to obtain basic demographic data on the patient (Figure 36-18A). The patient completes the identification data section.

Chief Complaint

The chief complaint (CC) identifies the patient's reason for seeking care—that is, the symptom causing the patient the most trouble. The CC is used as a foundation for the more detailed information obtained for the present illness and review of systems sections of the health history. The medical assistant is usually responsible for obtaining the CC from the patient and recording it in the patient's chart. In most offices, this information is recorded on a preprinted, lined form (Figure 36-18F). Certain guidelines must be followed in obtaining and recording the CC, as follows:

- An open-ended question should be used to elicit the CC from the patient: What seems to be the problem? How can we help you today? What can we do for you today?
- The CC should be limited to one or two symptoms and should refer to a specific, rather than vague, symptom.
- The CC should be recorded concisely and briefly, using the patient's own words as much as possible.
- The duration of the symptom (onset) should be included in the CC.
- The medical assistant should avoid using names of diseases or diagnostic terms to record the CC.

Recording Chief Complaints

The following are correct and incorrect examples of recording CCs.

    Correct Examples
- Burning during urination that has lasted for 2 days
- Pain in the shoulder that started 2 weeks ago
- Shortness of breath for the past month

    Incorrect Examples
- Has not felt well for the past 2 weeks (This statement refers to a vague, rather than a specific, complaint.)

- Ear pain and fever (The duration of the symptoms is not listed.)
- Pain on urination indicative of a urinary tract infection (Names of diseases should not be used to record the CC; the duration of the symptom is not listed.)

Present Illness

The present illness (PI) is an expansion of the CC and includes a full description of the patient's current illness from the time of its onset. The medical assistant is often responsible for completing this section of the health history, which is recorded on the same form as the CC (Figure 36-18F). To complete this section of the health history, the medical assistant asks the patient questions to obtain a detailed description of the symptom causing the greatest problem. Much skill and practice in asking the proper questions are required to elicit detailed information. A general guide for obtaining further information on symptoms is presented in Procedure 36-4, and a more thorough study for analyzing a symptom is included in the *Study Guide* for students (Chapter 36).

Past History

The past medical history is a review of the patient's past medical status (Figure 36-18B). Obtaining information on past medical care assists the physician in providing optimal care for the current problem. Most medical offices ask the patient to complete this section of the health history through a checklist type of form. The medical assistant should assist the patient with this section as needed by offering to answer any questions regarding the information required. The past history includes the following areas:

- Major illnesses
- Childhood diseases
- Unusual infections
- Accidents and injuries
- Hospitalizations and operations
- Previous medical tests
- Immunizations
- Allergies
- Current medications

Family History

The family history is a review of the health status of the patient's blood relatives (Figure 36-18C). This section of the health history focuses on diseases that tend to be familial. A **familial** disease is one that occurs in or affects blood relatives more frequently than would be expected by chance. Examples of familial diseases include hypertension, heart disease, allergies, and diabetes mellitus. The patient usually completes this section of the health history and is asked to provide the following information about each blood relative:

- State of health
- Presence of any significant disease
- If deceased, cause of death

PATIENT HEALTH HISTORY

A **IDENTIFICATION DATA**   Please print the following information.

Today's date _____

Name _____

_____ Male _____ Female

Address _____

_____ Married _____ Separated _____ Divorced _____ Widowed _____ Single

_____

Date of Birth _____

Telephone _____   _____
Home number   Work number

B **PAST HISTORY**

Have you ever had the following: (Circle "no" or "yes", leave blank if uncertain)

Measles _____ no yes	Heart Disease _____ no yes	Diabetes _____ no yes	Hemorrhoids _____ no yes
Mumps _____ no yes	Arthritis _____ no yes	Cancer _____ no yes	Asthma _____ no yes
Chickenpox _____ no yes	Sexually Transmitted Disease _____ no yes	Polio _____ no yes	Allergies _____ no yes
Whooping Cough _____ no yes	Anemia _____ no yes	Glaucoma _____ no yes	Eczema _____ no yes
Scarlet Fever _____ no yes	Bladder Infections _____ no yes	Hernia _____ no yes	AIDS or HIV+ _____ no yes
Diphtheria _____ no yes	Epilepsy _____ no yes	Blood or Plasma Transfusions _____ no yes	Infectious Mono _____ no yes
Pneumonia _____ no yes	Migraine Headaches _____ no yes	Back Trouble _____ no yes	Bronchitis _____ no yes
Rheumatic Fever _____ no yes	Tuberculosis _____ no yes	High Blood Pressure _____ no yes	Mitral Valve Prolapse no yes
Stroke _____ no yes	Ulcer _____ no yes	Thyroid Disease _____ no yes	Any other disease _____ no yes
Hepatitis _____ no yes	Kidney Disease _____ no yes	Bleeding Tendency _____ no yes	Please list: _____

MAJOR HOSPITALIZATIONS: If you have ever been hospitalized for any major medical illness or operation, write in your most recent hospitalizations below.

Hospitalizations	Year	Operation or illness	Name of hospital	City and state
1st Hospitalization				
2nd Hospitalization				
3rd Hospitalization				
4th Hospitalization				

TESTS AND IMMUNIZATIONS: Mark an X next to those that you have had.

Tests:
- [ ] TB Test
- [ ] Rectal/Hemoccult
- [ ] Sigmoidoscopy
- [ ] Colonoscopy
- [ ] Electrocardiogram
- [ ] Chest x-ray
- [ ] Mammogram
- [ ] Pap Test

Immunizations:
- [ ] Influenza
- [ ] Hepatitis B
- [ ] Tetanus
- [ ] MMR
- [ ] Polio

ALLERGIES: List all allergies (foods, drugs, environment). [ ] None

_____
_____
_____
_____

CURRENT MEDICATIONS: List the following that you are currently taking: Prescription medications, over-the-counter (OTC) medications, vitamin supplements, and herbal supplements. [ ] None

Medication	Frequency

ACCIDENTS/ INJURIES: Describe all serious accidents, severe injuries, head injury, or fractures. Include the date each occurred. [ ] None

Accident/Injury: Date:

_____
_____
_____
_____

Figure 36-18. Health history form. (From Bonewit-West K: *Clinical procedures for medical assistants,* ed 7, St. Louis, 2008, Saunders.)

Continued

C FAMILY HISTORY

For each member of your family, follow the purple or blue line across the page and check boxes for:
1. His or her present state of health
2. Any illnesses he or she has had

	Good Health	Poor Health	Deceased	If deceased, write in age and cause of death.	Allergies or Asthma	Diabetes	Heart Disease	Stroke	Cancer	High Blood Pressure	Glaucoma	Arthritis	Ulcer	Kidney Disease	Mental Health Problems	Alcohol/Drug Abuse	Obesity	High Cholesterol	Thyroid Disease
Father:																			
Mother:																			
Brothers/Sisters:																			

D SOCIAL HISTORY

EDUCATION _____ High school _____ College _____ Postgraduate

Occupation _____ Years _____

Previous occupations _____ Years _____

_____ Years _____

Have you ever been exposed to any of the following in your environment?

☐ Excess dust (coal, lime, rock)   ☐ Cleaning fluids/solvents   ☐ Radiation   ☐ Other toxic materials

☐ Sand   ☐ Hair spray   ☐ Insecticides

☐ Chemicals   ☐ Smoke or auto exhaust fumes   ☐ Paints

Please answer the follwing questions by placing an X in the box in front of the word Yes or No, except where you are asked for specific information. This information is obviously highly confidential and will be released to other healthcare professionals or insurance carriers ONLY with your consent.

DIET:

Do you eat a good breakfast? ☐ Yes ☐ No

Do you snack between meals (soft drinks, chips, candy bars)? ☐ Yes ☐ No

Do you eat fresh fruits and vegetables each day? ☐ Yes ☐ No

Do you eat whole grain breads and cereals? ☐ Yes ☐ No

Is your diet high in fat content? ☐ Yes ☐ No

Is your diet high in cholesterol content? ☐ Yes ☐ No

Is your diet high in salt content? ☐ Yes ☐ No

Are you allergic to any foods? ☐ Yes ☐ No

How many glasses of water do you drink each day? _____

How would you describe your overall eating habits? ☐ Excellent ☐ Good ☐ Fair ☐ Poor

PERSONAL HISTORY:

Do you find it hard to make decisions? ☐ Yes ☐ No

Do you find it hard to concentrate or remember? ☐ Yes ☐ No

Do you feel depressed? ☐ Yes ☐ No

Do you have difficulty relaxing? ☐ Yes ☐ No

Do you have a tendency to worry a lot? ☐ Yes ☐ No

Have you gained or lost much weight recently? ☐ Yes ☐ No

Do you lose your temper often? ☐ Yes ☐ No

Are you disturbed by any work or family problems? ☐ Yes ☐ No

Are you having sexual difficulties? ☐ Yes ☐ No

Have you ever considered committing suicide? ☐ Yes ☐ No

Have you ever desired or sought psychiatric help? ☐ Yes ☐ No

EXERCISE:

Do you exercise on a regular basis? ☐ Yes ☐ No

Does your job require strenuous, sustained physical work? ☐ Yes ☐ No

SLEEP PATTERNS:

Do you seem to feel exhausted or fatigued most of the time? ☐ Yes ☐ No

Do you have difficulty either falling asleep or staying asleep? ☐ Yes ☐ No

USE OF TOBACCO/ALCOHOL/CAFFEINE/DRUGS: Amt:

How much do you smoke per day? ☐ Cigarettes __

☐ Don't smoke ☐ Cigars/pipes __

Do you take two or more alcoholic drinks per day? ☐ Yes ☐ No

Do you drink six or more cups of coffee or tea per day? ☐ Yes ☐ No

Are you a regular user of sleeping pills, marijuana, tranquilizers, pain killers, etc? ☐ Yes ☐ No

Have you ever used heroin, cocaine, LSD, PCP, etc? ☐ Yes ☐ No

List any country outside the USA you have visited in the past six months. _____

When did you have your last physical examination? _____

Figure 36-18, cont'd.

Patient's Name_____

E | **REVIEW OF SYSTEMS**

HEAD AND NECK
_____ Frequent headaches
_____ Neck pain
_____ Neck lumps or swelling

EYES
_____ Wears glasses
_____ Blurry vision
_____ Eyesight worsening
_____ Sees double
_____ Sees halo
_____ Eye pain or itching
_____ Watery eyes
_____ Eye trouble

EARS
_____ Hearing difficulties
_____ Earaches
_____ Running ears
_____ Buzzing in ears
_____ Motion sickness

MOUTH
_____ Dental problems
_____ Swellings on gums or jaws
_____ Sore tongue
_____ Taste changes

NOSE AND THROAT
_____ Congested nose
_____ Running nose
_____ Sneezing spells
_____ Head colds
_____ Nosebleeds
_____ Sore throat
_____ Enlarged tonsils
_____ Hoarse voice

RESPIRATORY
_____ Wheezes or gasps
_____ Coughing spells
_____ Coughs up phlegm
_____ Coughed up blood
_____ Chest colds
_____ Excessive sweating,
      night sweats

CARDIOVASCULAR
_____ High blood pressure
_____ Racing heart
_____ Chest pains
_____ Dizzy spells
_____ Shortness of breath
_____ Shortness of breath at night
_____ More pillows to breathe
_____ Swollen feet or ankles
_____ Leg cramps
_____ Heart murmur

DIGESTIVE
_____ Heartburn
_____ Bloated stomach
_____ Belching
_____ Stomach pains
_____ Nausea
_____ Vomited blood
_____ Difficulty swallowing
_____ Constipation
_____ Loose bowels
_____ Black stools
_____ Gray stools
_____ Pain in rectum
_____ Rectal bleeding

URINARY
_____ Night frequency
_____ Day frequency
_____ Wets pants or bed
_____ Burning on urination
_____ Brown, black, or bloody urine
_____ Difficulty starting urine
_____ Urgency

MALE GENITAL
_____ Weak urine stream
_____ Prostate trouble
_____ Burning or discharge
_____ Lumps on testicles
_____ Painful testicles

FEMALE GENITAL
_/_/_ Last menstrual period
_/_/_ Last Pap test
_____ Postmenopausal or hysterectomy
_____ Noticed vaginal bleeding
_____ Abnormal LMP
_____ Heavy bleeding during periods
_____ Bleeding between periods
_____ Bleeding after intercourse
_____ Recent vaginal itching/discharge
_____ No monthly breast exam
_____ Lump or pain in breasts
_____ Complications with birth control

OBSTETRIC HISTORY
_____ Gravida
_____ Para
_____ Preterm
_____ Miscarriages
_____ Stillbirths
_____ Has had an abortion

MUSCULOSKELETAL
_____ Aching muscles
_____ Swollen joints
_____ Back or shoulder pains
_____ Painful feet
_____ Disability

SKIN
_____ Skin problems
_____ Itching or burning skin
_____ Bleeds easily
_____ Bruises easily

NEUROLOGICAL
_____ Faintness
_____ Numbness
_____ Convulsions
_____ Change in handwriting
_____ Trembles

F | **PROGRESS NOTES**

Date	

Figure 36-18, cont'd.

Social History

The social history section of the health history includes information on the patient's lifestyle, such as health habits and living environment (Figure 36-18D). The social history is important because the patient's lifestyle may affect his or her condition and may influence the course of treatment chosen by the physician. The social history also provides the physician with information regarding the effect that the illness may have on the patient's daily living pattern. If it is necessary for the individual to make a major lifestyle adjustment (e.g., stop smoking, reduce working hours), the physician may recommend support services to assist in this transition. This section of the history is usually completed by the patient and includes the following areas:

- Education
- Occupation (past and present)
- Living environment
- Diet
- Personal history
- Exercise

Review of Systems

A review of systems (ROS) is a systematic review of each body system to detect any symptoms that have not yet been revealed. The importance of the ROS is that it assists in identifying symptoms that might otherwise remain undetected. The physician usually completes the ROS by asking a series of detailed and direct questions related to each body system; the results of this section of the health history assist the physician in a preliminary assessment of the type and extent of physical examination required. Figure 36-18E shows an example of an ROS form.

CHARTING IN THE MEDICAL RECORD

Charting is the process of making written entries about a patient in the medical record and is performed by medical office personnel who are directly involved with the health care of the patient. The medical record is considered a legal document; the information must be charted as completely and accurately as possible. Developing good charting skills requires a thorough knowledge of charting guidelines combined with much repeated practice. To provide guidance in attaining this important skill, charting guidelines are presented in this section, followed by examples of proper charting entries.

Charting Guidelines

To ensure accurate and concise charting, specific guidelines must be followed. These are listed and described as follows:

1. *Check the name on the chart before making an entry to ensure you have the correct chart.* If the medical assistant records in the wrong patient's chart by mistake, information such as a procedure that was performed on a patient may be excluded from the correct patient's record. As previously stated, from a legal standpoint, a procedure not documented was not performed.

2. *Use black ink to make entries in the patient's chart.* Black ink must be used to provide a permanent record. In addition, entries made in black ink are easier to reproduce when a record must be duplicated for insurance company purposes and patient referral.

3. *Write in legible handwriting.* For the medical record to be meaningful to others, the medical assistant must chart information legibly. If the medical assistant's cursive script is not legible, the information should be printed.

4. *Chart information accurately, using clear and concise phrases.*
   - The medical assistant should be brief but thorough and should avoid vagueness and duplication of information.
   - It is not necessary to include the patient's name in the entry because the entire medical record centers on one patient; it is assumed the information refers to that patient.
   - Each phrase should begin with a capital letter and end with a period.
   - Each new entry should begin on a separate line and be dated with the month, day, year, and time (either AM/PM or military time).
   - Standard abbreviations, medical terms, and symbols can be used to help save time and space. It is *crucial* that the medical assistant first check the office policy to determine the abbreviations, medical terms, and symbols that are commonly used in that office. Using commonly accepted terminology avoids confusing others who read the chart. A list of abbreviations and symbols commonly used in medical offices is presented in Table 36-1.
   - *Spell correctly.* Correct spelling is essential for accuracy in charting. If you are in doubt about the spelling of a word, consult a dictionary.

5. *Chart immediately after performing a procedure.* When a procedure has been performed, it should be charted without delay. If a time lapse occurs between performing the procedure and charting it, the medical assistant may not remember certain aspects of the procedure, such as the results of the treatment or the patient's reaction. Procedures should never be charted in advance. The individual performing the procedure should be the one to chart it; in other words, never chart for someone else.

6. *Each charting entry should be signed by the person making it.* The signature should include the medical assistant's first initial, full last name, and title (e.g., D. Bennett, CMA [AAMA]). The following title abbreviations are often used for medical assistants:
   - **CMA (AAMA):** certified medical assistant
   - **RMA:** registered medical assistant
   - **MA:** medical assistant
   - **SMA:** student medical assistant

Table 36-1 Abbreviations and Symbols Commonly Used in the Medical Office

Abbreviations Used to Chart Symptoms and Procedures			
āā	of each	Fe	iron
Ab	abortion	flex sig	flexible sigmoidoscopy
abd	abdomen	freq	frequent
abs	absent	F/U	follow-up
ac	before meals	Fx	fracture
ad lib	as desired	GYN	gynecology
admin	administer	h or hr	hour
AM or a.m.	before noon	H/A	headache
amt	amount	HBP	high blood pressure
AP	apical pulse	HC	head circumference
approx	approximately	Hep B	hepatitis B vaccine
appt	appointment	Hg	mercury
ASA	acetylsalicylic acid (aspirin)	H_2O	water
ASAP	as soon as possible	HR	heart rate
BA	backache	HRT	hormone replacement therapy
b/c	because	hs	at bedtime
BC	birth control	ht	height
bid	twice a day	ID	intradermal
BM	bowel movement	IM	intramuscular
BP	blood pressure	IPV	inactivated polio vaccine
BPM	beats per minute	IV	intravenous
BS	blood sugar	lab	laboratory
BSE	breast self-examination	lac	laceration
c̄	with	lat	lateral
caps	capsules	lax	laxative
cath	catheter, catheterize	LB	lower back
CC	chief complaint	LBP	lower back pain
chemo	chemotherapy	liq	liquid
CMA (AAMA)	certified medical assistant	LMP	last menstrual period
c/o	complains of	med, meds	medication, medications
CS	cesarean section	min	minute
Cx	cervix	MMR	measles, mumps, and rubella
d	day	mod	moderate
/d	per day	N/A	not applicable
d/c	discontinue	NB	newborn
D&I	dry and intact	N/C	no complaints
dil	dilute	neg	negative
disch	discharge	NH	nursing home
DNKA	did not keep appointment	NICU	newborn intensive care unit
DOB	date of birth	NKA	no known allergies
DOI	date of injury	NKDA	no known drug allergies
DRE	digital rectal examination	NMP	normal menstrual period
DSD	dry, sterile dressing	noct	nocturnal
DTaP	diphtheria and tetanus toxoids and acellular pertussis vaccine	NS	normal saline
		N&V	nausea and vomiting
D&V	diarrhea and vomiting	NVA	near visual acuity
DVA	distance visual acuity	NVD	nausea, vomiting, and diarrhea
ea	each	OB	obstetrics
ED	emergency department	occ	occasionally
EDD	expected date of delivery	oint	ointment
		op	operation

Continued

Table 36-1 Abbreviations and Symbols Commonly Used in the Medical Office—cont'd

Abbreviations Used to Chart Symptoms and Procedures—cont'd

OR	operating room
OT	occupational therapy
OTC	over-the-counter (nonprescription medication)
OV	office visit
P	pulse
Pap	Pap test
path	pathology
pc	after meals
peds	pediatrics
PEN	penicillin
per	by or through
pharm	pharmacy
PM or p.m.	afternoon
PMS	premenstrual syndrome
po or PO	by mouth
pos	positive
postop	postoperative (after surgery)
preop	preoperative (before surgery)
prep	preparation
prn	as needed
PT	physical therapy
Pt or pt	patient
qd	every day
qh	every hour
q(2,3,4)h	every (2,3,4) hours
qid	four times a day
qn	every night
QNS	quantity not sufficient
qod	every other day
QS	quantity sufficient
quad	quadriplegic
R	respiration
RE	rectal examination
reg	regular
rehab	rehabilitation
RMA	registered medical assistant
Rx	prescription
s̄	without
SC or SQ	subcutaneous
S/E	side effects
sec	second
sigmoid	sigmoidoscopy
sl	slight
sm	small
SOB	shortness of breath
sol	solution
spec	specimen
STAT	immediately
surg	surgery

T	temperature
tab, tabs	tablet, tablets
temp	temperature
ther	therapy
tid	three times a day
TLC	total lung capacity, tender loving care
TPR	temperature, pulse, and respiration
tr	trace
TSE	testicular self-examination
vag	vagina, vaginal
VE	vaginal examination
vit	vitamin
VO	verbal order
VS	vital signs
wk	week
WNL	within normal limits
WO	written order
w/o	without
wt	weight
W/U	workup

Abbreviations Used to Chart Body Parts and Locations

abd	abdomen
AD	right ear
AS	left ear
AU	in each ear, both ears
EENT	eye, ear, nose, and throat
GI	gastrointestinal
GU	genitourinary
Ⓛ or lt	left
ⓁA	left arm
ⓁL	left leg
LLQ	lower left quadrant
LRQ	lower right quadrant
LUQ	left upper quadrant
OD	right eye
OS	left eye
OU	in each eye, both eyes
Ⓡ or rt	right
ⓇA	right arm
ⓇL	right leg
RLQ	right lower quadrant
RUQ	right upper quadrant

Abbreviations Used to Chart Measurement

C	Celsius
cc	cubic centimeter
cm	centimeter
dL	deciliter
F	Fahrenheit
G	gram

Table 36-1 Abbreviations and Symbols Commonly Used in the Medical Office—cont'd

Abbreviations Used to Chart Measurement—cont'd		URI	upper respiratory infection
kg	kilogram	USI	urinary stress incontinence
L	liter	UTI	urinary tract infection
L	length	**Diagnostic Procedures**	
Lb	pound	CT, CAT	computed axial tomography
M	meter	CXR	chest x-ray
mcg	microgram	ECG	electrocardiogram
mg	milligram	Echo	echocardiogram
ml	milliliter	EEG	electroencephalogram
mm	millimeter	FOBT	fecal occult blood test
oz	ounce	IVP	intravenous pyelogram
pt	pint	LP	lumbar puncture
qt	quart	MRI	magnetic resonance imaging
ss	one half	NST	nonstress test
T	tablespoon	PFT	pulmonary function test
tsp	teaspoon	TRUS	transrectal ultrasound
Miscellaneous Abbreviations		US	ultrasound
Patient Examination		**Laboratory Tests**	
Dx	diagnosis	BG	blood glucose
H/O	history of	Bx	Biopsy
H&P	history and physical	CBC	complete blood count
Hx	history	C&S	culture and sensitivity
MHx	medical history	diff	differential
PE or Px	physical examination	ESR	erythrocyte sedimentation rate
prog	prognosis	FBS	fasting blood sugar
Sx	symptoms	GCT	glucose challenge test
Tx	treatment	GTT	glucose tolerance test
Conditions		Hct	hematocrit
BPH	benign prostatic hypertrophy	Hgb	hemoglobin
CA	cancer	PPBS	postprandial blood sugar
CAD	coronary artery disease	PSA	prostate-specific antigen
CHF	congestive heart failure	PT	prothrombin time
COPD	chronic obstructive pulmonary disease	RBC	red blood count
CRC	colorectal cancer	RBS	random blood sugar
CVA	cerebrovascular accident	SG	specific gravity
DM	diabetes mellitus	trig	triglycerides
Fe def	iron deficiency	UA	urinalysis
GC	gonorrhea	U/C	urine culture
GDM	gestational diabetes mellitus	WBC	white blood count
HTN	hypertension	**Symbols**	
IBS	irritable bowel syndrome	Ø	none, no
MI	myocardial infarction	✓	check
MS	multiple sclerosis	>	greater than
OA	osteoarthritis	<	less than
OM	otitis media	↑	increase
PID	pelvic inflammatory disease	↓	decrease
RA	rheumatoid arthritis	♀	female
RF	rheumatic fever	♂	male
STD	sexually transmitted disease	°	degree
TB	tuberculosis	@	at

Continued

Table 36-1 Abbreviations and Symbols Commonly Used in the Medical Office—cont'd

×	times	+		positive
x̄	except	–		negative
p̄	after	Ⓡ		rectal temperature
#	number	Ⓐ		axillary temperature
1°	primary	"		inches
2°	secondary	'		prime

From Bonewit-West K: *Clinical procedures for medical assistants,* ed 7, St. Louis, 2008, Saunders.

Figure 36-19. Proper method for correcting an error in a patient's medical record. (From Bonewit-West K: *Clinical procedures for medical assistants,* ed 7, St. Louis, 2008, Saunders.)

7. *Never erase or obliterate an entry.* If an error is made in charting, the medical assistant must never erase or obliterate it. Should the physician or medical staff be involved in litigation, erased or obliterated entries tend to reduce credibility. If incorrect information is charted, the medical assistant should draw a single line through the incorrect information, permitting it to remain legible. The word *error* is then written above the incorrect data, including the date and the medical assistant's first initial, last name, and credentials. Some medical offices may request that the reason for the change also be recorded. The correct information is then inserted next to the error (Figure 36-19).

The medical assistant should always take the time to chart properly in the patient's medical record. Good charting helps coordinate efforts in the medical office and leads to high-quality health care.

Charting Progress Notes

After completion of the initial health history, a system is necessary to update the medical record with new information each time the patient visits the medical office. Most offices use progress notes to fulfill this function. Progress notes document the patient's health status and the care and treatment being received by the patient in chronological order. Progress notes provide effective communication among medical office personnel and serve as a legal document.

The medical assistant is frequently responsible for charting progress notes in the medical record. They are usually charted on special preprinted lined sheets known as *progress note sheets.* These sheets have a column for the date and a column for charting information (Figure 36-18F). Types

of progress notes that are often charted by the medical assistant are presented next, along with a charting example of each.

Charting Patient Symptoms

The medical assistant takes patient symptoms during office visits and telephone conversations. Information conveyed during a telephone conversation helps determine whether the patient needs to be seen and the immediacy of the situation.

A **symptom** is any change in the body or its functioning that indicates the presence of disease. Symptoms can be classified as subjective or objective. A **subjective symptom** is one that is felt by the patient and cannot be observed by another person. Pain, pruritus, vertigo, and nausea are examples of subjective symptoms. An **objective symptom** is one that can be observed by another person and by the patient. Rash, coughing, and cyanosis are objective symptoms. The medical assistant should have a thorough knowledge of common symptoms and should be able to recognize them. Table 36-2 lists and describes common symptoms.

Taking patient symptoms during an office visit consists of the following:
1. Obtaining a CC (see earlier discussion)
2. Obtaining additional information about the CC

If the patient complains of pain in the abdomen that has lasted for 2 days (CC), additional information is necessary to describe the pain, including the type, specific location, onset, intensity, precipitating factors, and duration of the pain. The procedure for taking patient symptoms during an office visit is outlined in Procedure 36-4. Additional skill and practice on taking patient symptoms is included in Chapter 36 of the *Study Guide* for students.

Table 36-2 Common Symptoms

Integumentary System

Diaphoresis	Excessive perspiration
Flushing	A red appearance to the skin, which generally affects the face and neck. A flushed appearance is commonly present with a fever
Jaundice	A yellow appearance to the skin, first evident in the whites of the eyes
Rash	An eruption on the skin

Circulatory System

Bradycardia	An abnormally slow pulse rate
Dehydration	A decrease in the amount of water in the body. A patient has a flushed appearance, dry skin, and a decreased output of urine
Edema	The retention of fluid in the tissues, resulting in swelling. Skin over the area is tight. Edema is most easily observed in the extremities
Tachycardia	An abnormally fast pulse rate

Gastrointestinal System

Anorexia	A loss of appetite and a lack of interest in food
Constipation	A condition in which the stool becomes hard and dry, resulting in difficult passage from the rectum. The consistency of the stool, rather than the frequency of defecation, is used as a guide in determining the presence of constipation. (Frequency of bowel movements varies with the individual; some people have a bowel movement only every 2-3 days but are not constipated.) Other symptoms of constipation include headache, nausea, and general malaise
Diarrhea	The passage of an increased number of loose, watery stools. The fecal material moves rapidly through the intestinal tract, resulting in decreased absorption by the body of water, electrolytes, and nutrients. Other symptoms usually associated with diarrhea are intestinal cramping and general weakness
Flatulence	The presence of excessive gas in the stomach or intestines
Nausea and vomiting	Nausea is a sensation of discomfort in the stomach with a feeling that vomiting may occur. Vomiting is the ejection of the stomach contents through the mouth, also known as *emesis*. The ejected content is known as *vomitus*

Respiratory System

Cough	An involuntary and forceful exhalation of air followed by a deep inhalation. A cough may be productive (meaning a discharge is produced) or nonproductive (no discharge is present)
Cyanosis	A bluish discoloration of the skin due to a lack of oxygen
Dyspnea	Labored or difficult breathing
Epistaxis	Hemorrhaging from the nose (nosebleed)

Nervous System

Chills	A feeling of coldness accompanied by shivering. Chills are generally present with a fever
Convulsions	Involuntary contractions of the muscles
Fever, or pyrexia	A body temperature that is higher than normal
Headache	A feeling of pain or aching in the head. It is a common symptom that accompanies many illnesses. Tension, fatigue, and eyestrain can result in a headache
Malaise	A vague sense of body discomfort, weakness, and fatigue, often marking the onset of a disease and continuing through the course of the illness
Pain	Irritation of pain receptors, resulting in a feeling of distress or suffering. Pain is an important indication that a part of the body is not working properly
Pruritus	Severe itching
Vertigo	A feeling of dizziness or lightheadedness

From Bonewit-West K: *Clinical procedures for medical assistants*, ed 7, St. Louis, 2008, Saunders.

PROCEDURE 36-4   Obtaining and Recording Patient Symptoms

Outcome Obtain and record patient symptoms.

Equipment/Supplies

- Medical record of the patient to be interviewed
- Black ink pen

1. **Procedural Step.** Assemble the equipment. Ensure that you have the correct patient's record and a black ink pen for charting patient symptoms.
   Principle. Black ink must be used to provide a permanent record.
2. **Procedural Step.** Go to the waiting room and ask the patient to come back.
3. **Procedural Step.** Escort the patient to a quiet, comfortable room, such as an examination room, that allows for privacy.
   Principle. Patient symptoms should be taken in a room that encourages communication.
4. **Procedural Step.** In a calm and friendly manner, greet the patient and introduce yourself. Identify the patient by his or her full name and date of birth.
   Principle. A warm introduction sets a positive tone for the remainder of the interview.
5. **Procedural Step.** Ask the patient to be seated. You should seat yourself so that you face the patient at a distance of 3 to 4 feet.
   Principle. This type of seating arrangement facilitates open communication.
6. **Procedural Step.** Use good communication skills to interact with the patient. These include the following:
   a. Use the patient's name of choice.
   b. Show genuine interest and concern for the patient.
   c. Maintain appropriate eye contact.
   d. Use terminology the patient can understand.
   e. Listen carefully and attentively to the patient.
   f. Pay attention to the patient's nonverbal messages.
   g. Avoid judgmental comments.
   h. Avoid rushing the patient.
7. **Procedural Step.** Locate the progress note sheet in the patient's medical record. Chart the date and time and the abbreviation for chief complaint (CC).
8. **Procedural Step.** Use an open-ended question to elicit the CC, such as "What seems to be the problem?"
   Principle. An open-ended question allows the patient to verbalize freely.
9. **Procedural Step.** Chart the CC following the charting guidelines outlined on pp. 886 and 890 and pp. 893-894. In addition, these guidelines should be followed:
   a. Limit the CC to one or two symptoms, and refer to a specific rather than a vague symptom.
   b. Chart the CC concisely and briefly, using the patient's own words as much as possible.

   c. Include the duration of the symptom (onset) in the CC.
   d. Avoid using names of diseases or diagnostic terms to record the CC.
10. **Procedural Step.** Obtain additional information regarding the CC using *what, when,* and *where* questions. Following proper charting guidelines, chart this information after the CC.

What Questions:

- What exactly have you been experiencing?
- Does the symptom occur suddenly or gradually?
- Does anything make it worse?

Where Question:

- Where is the symptom located?

When Questions:

- When did the symptom first occur?
- How long does it last?
- Does anything cause it to occur?
   Principle. This information provides a complete description of the CC.
11. **Procedural Step.** Thank the patient and proceed to the next step in the patient workup. (This usually includes measuring vital signs and height and weight and preparing the patient as needed for the physical examination [see Chapters 19 and 20].)
12. **Procedural Step.** Inform the patient the physician will be with him or her soon.
13. **Procedural Step.** Place the patient's medical record where it can be reviewed by the physician (as designated by the medical office policy).
    Principle. The physician will want to review the patient's medical record before examining the patient.

CHARTING EXAMPLE	
Date	
6/30/10	3:15 p.m. CC: Intense pain in the ⓛ ear for the past 2 days. Pt states pain is sharp and continuous. Pt noted sl yellow discharge from ⓛ ear. Fever of 101° F began last night about 9 p.m. Took Tylenol 2 tabs @ 8 a.m. ———————————— D. Bennett, CMA (AAMA)

Other Activities That Need to Be Charted

Procedures

The medical assistant frequently charts procedures performed on the patient, including vital signs, weight and height, visual acuity, and ear irrigations. Procedures should be charted immediately after being performed; from a legal standpoint, a procedure that is not documented was not performed. In general, the following information should be included: the date and time, the type of procedure, the outcome, and the patient reaction. The specific information to be charted is included with each procedure presented in this text.

CHARTING EXAMPLE

Date	
6/30/10	9:15 a.m. Irrigated ®ₑₐᵣ ear c̄ 200 ml of
	normal saline @ 98.6° F. Mod amt of
	cerumen in returned solution. Pt states can
	hear better. —— D. Bennett, CMA (AAMA)

Procedure. (From Bonewit-West K: *Clinical procedures for medical assistants*, ed 7, St. Louis, 2008, Saunders.)

Administration of Medication

Charting medications administered to the patient is an important responsibility in the medical office. The recording should include the date and time, the name of the medication, the dosage given, the route of administration, the injection site used (for parenteral medication), and any significant observations or patient reactions.

CHARTING EXAMPLE

Date	
6/30/10	10:15 a.m. Bicillin 900,00 units IM, Ⓛ
	dorsogluteal. —— D. Bennett, CMA (AAMA)

Administration of medication. (From Bonewit-West K: *Clinical procedures for medical assistants*, ed 7, St. Louis, 2008, Saunders.)

Specimen Collection

Each time a specimen is collected from a patient, the medical assistant should chart the date and time of the collection, the type of specimen, and the area of the body from which the specimen was obtained. If the specimen is to be sent to an outside laboratory for testing, this information should also be charted, including the tests requested, the date the specimen was sent, and where it was sent. In this way, the physician would know that the specimen was collected and sent to the laboratory when test results are not back yet.

CHARTING EXAMPLE

Date	
6/30/10	1:30 p.m. Venous blood spec collected from Ⓡ
	arm. Sent to Ross Lab for CBC and diff on
	6/30/10. —— D. Bennett, CMA (AAMA)
Date	
6/30/10	2:00 p.m. Throat spec collected. Sent to
	Ross Lab for C&S on 6/30/10.——
	—— D. Bennett, CMA (AAMA)

Specimen collection. (From Bonewit-West K: *Clinical procedures for medical assistants*, ed 7, St. Louis, 2008, Saunders.)

Diagnostic Procedures and Laboratory Tests

Diagnostic procedures and laboratory tests ordered for a patient should always be charted in the medical record. If the patient does not undergo the test, documented proof exists that the test was ordered. Charting diagnostic procedures and laboratory tests protects the physician legally and refreshes the physician's memory of the procedures and tests being run on the patient when results are not yet back from the testing facility. Information in the charting entry includes the date and time, type of procedure or test ordered, scheduling date, and where it is being performed.

CHARTING EXAMPLE

Date	
6/30/10	10:15 a.m. Mammography scheduled for
	7/5/10 at Grant Hospital. ——
	—— D. Bennett, CMA (AAMA)
Date	
6/30/10	11:30 a.m. Pt given lab request for GTT at
	Ross Lab. —— D. Bennett, CMA (AAMA)

Diagnostic/laboratory tests. (From Bonewit-West K: *Clinical procedures for medical assistants*, ed 7, St. Louis, 2008, Saunders.)

Results of Laboratory Tests

It is usually unnecessary to chart results from laboratory reports returned from outside laboratories because the report itself is filed in the patient's record. In case of a STAT request or critical findings, the test results may be telephoned to the medical office, requiring the medical assistant to record the results on a report form. Careful recording is essential to avoid errors, which could affect the patient's diagnosis. Results of laboratory tests performed by the medical assistant in the office should be charted in the medical record and must include the date and time, name of the test, and test results.

CHARTING EXAMPLE

Date	
6/30/10	8:00 a.m. FBS: 82 mg/dL.————————
	———————————— D. Bennett, CMA (AAMA)
Date	
6/30/10	4:15 p.m. Quick Vue+ Mono Test: neg. ————
	———————————— D. Bennett, CMA (AAMA)

Laboratory test results. (From Bonewit-West K: *Clinical procedures for medical assistants,* ed 7, St. Louis, 2008, Saunders.)

Patient Instructions

The medical assistant must often relay instructions to a patient regarding medical care (e.g., wound care, cast care, care of sutures). The medical assistant should chart this information, taking care to include the date and time and the type of instructions relayed to the patient. Many medical offices have printed instruction sheets that are given to the patient. The patient is asked to sign a form, which is filed in the patient's record, indicating that he or she has read and understands the instructions (Figure 36-20). The form should also be signed by the medical assistant, who functions as a signature witness. This protects the physician legally in the event that the patient fails to follow the instructions and causes further harm or damage to a body part.

Other areas in which the medical assistant is responsible for charting in the medical record include missed or canceled appointments, telephone calls from patients, medication refills, and changes in medication or dosage by the physician.

CHARTING EXAMPLE

Date	
6/30/10	9:30 a.m. Instructions provided for BSE. Pt
	given a BSE educational brochure. ————
	———————————— D. Bennett, CMA (AAMA)
Date	
6/30/10	10:00 a.m. Explained wound care. Written
	instructions provided. Signed copy in chart.
	To return in 2 days for suture removal. ——
	———————————— D. Bennett, CMA (AAMA)
Date	
6/30/10	10:25 a.m. Provided instructions for applying
	a heating pad to the lower back. ————
	———————————— D. Bennett, CMA (AAMA)

Patient instructions. (From Bonewit-West K: *Clinical procedures for medical assistants,* ed 7, St. Louis, 2008, Saunders.)

CHARTING EXAMPLE

Date	
6/30/10	11:15 a.m. Phoned office. States that
	swelling in the Ⓡ ankle is almost gone.
	———————————— D. Bennett, CMA (AAMA)
Date	
6/30/10	1:15 p.m. Missed appointment scheduled for
	6/30/10 @ 1:00 p.m. ————————
	———————————— D. Bennett, CMA (AAMA)

Telephone call and missed appointment. (From Bonewit-West K: *Clinical procedures for medical assistants,* ed 7, St. Louis, 2008, Saunders.)

Figure 36-20. Instruction sheet for patients. (From Bonewit-West K: *Clinical procedures for medical assistants,* ed 7, St. Louis, 2008, Saunders.)

PATIENT INSTRUCTIONS FOR WOUND CARE

Name of patient: _____

Follow the instructions indicated below for care of your wound:

1. Use ice bag and elevate to reduce swelling and pain. Elevate higher than your heart.
2. You may take aspirin/Tylenol for pain.
3. Keep the dressing clean and dry.
4. Replace the dressing within _____ days.
5. Discard the dressing within _____ days.
6. Cleanse the wound daily as instructed.
7. Stitches should be removed in _____ days.
8. Despite the greatest of care, any wound can become infected. If your wound becomes red or swollen, shows pus or red streaks, or feels more sore instead of less sore, contact the physician **immediately**.

I have received and understand the above instructions:

Patient (or representative): _____

Relationship to patient: _____

Witness: _____   Time and date: _____

MEDICAL PRACTICE and the LAW

Documentation can be a deciding factor in a legal case. Everything you do for a patient should be documented in a factual manner in the medical record, or "chart." When a legal issue arises, often several years pass before it comes to trial. If you are involved, you will be asked detailed questions as to your actions on a particular day for a particular patient. Few people have accurate memories for that long. Juries give more credibility to documentation performed at the time of the action than to a memory of years ago.

Ethically, you owe the patient thorough documentation to provide optimal continuity of care. Remember that all patient information is confidential.

Proper charting is a crucial skill for a medical assistant to master. Although proper documentation would not prevent a lawsuit, it might determine the outcome. Pay particular attention to the rules for consents and charting guidelines outlined in this chapter, and follow them to the letter. ■

What Would You Do? What Would You *Not* Do? RESPONSES

Case Study 1
Page 856

What Did Dawn Do?
❑ Listened carefully to Mrs. Celeste and relayed concern through both verbal and nonverbal behavior.
❑ Reassured Mrs. Celeste that her information would be kept completely confidential. Explained to Mrs. Celeste that health care professionals are required by law to keep all patient information confidential.
❑ Told Mrs. Celeste how important it is to chart information that relates to her health. Explained that the physician must have accurate data to diagnose and treat her. Stressed that certain medications can be harmful to a patient if consumed with alcohol.
❑ Gave Mrs. Celeste information (including brochures) on community agencies that could help her. Explained that these agencies are required to maintain confidentiality and encouraged her to contact them.

What Did Dawn Not *Do?*
❑ Did not tell Mrs. Celeste to go to a different physician to ensure her information remained private.
❑ Did not tell Mrs. Celeste that she needed to stop drinking before it affected her health.

What Would You Do/What Would You *Not* Do? Review Dawn's response and place a checkmark next to the information you included in your response. List the additional information you included in your response.

_____

_____

_____

_____

Case Study 2
Page 875

What Did Dawn Do?
❑ Reassured Tessa that she and her family have been good patients and apologized for the inconvenience.
❑ Told Tessa that it is against the law to transfer medical records without the patient's written authorization. Explained that the reason for the law is to safeguard a patient's privacy.
❑ Asked Tessa if she has a fax machine because the forms could be faxed to her for signing and then faxed back to the office.

If not, explained that Tessa and her husband would need to come to the office to sign release forms.

What Did Dawn Not *Do?*
❑ Did not get defensive about Tessa being so annoyed.
❑ Did not send their medical records to the new physician without the signed release forms.

What Would You Do/What Would You *Not* Do? Review Dawn's response and place a checkmark next to the information you included in your response. List the additional information you included in your response.

_____

_____

_____

_____

Case Study 3
Page 881

What Did Dawn Do?
❑ Listened to and empathized with Mr. and Mrs. Oberlin's concerns.
❑ Told Mr. and Mrs. Oberlin that because Brett is of adult age, it would be against the law to let them see his medical record without his written authorization. Explained that the law is there to protect a patient's right to privacy and just as it protects Brett's right, the law also protects the parents' rights so that no one can obtain information from their medical records without their authorization.
❑ Suggested that they talk with Brett again regarding the situation.

What Did Dawn Not *Do?*
❑ Did not give them any information from Brett's medical record

What Would You Do/What Would You *Not* Do? Review Dawn's response and place a checkmark next to the information you included in your response. List the additional information you included in your response.

_____

_____

_____

TERMINOLOGY REVIEW

Attending physician The physician responsible for the care of a hospitalized patient.

Charting The process of making written entries about a patient in the medical record.

Consultation report A narrative report of an opinion about a patient's condition by a practitioner other than the attending physician.

Diagnosis The scientific method of determining and identifying a patient's condition.

Diagnostic procedure A procedure performed to assist in the diagnosis, management, or treatment of a patient's condition.

Discharge summary report A brief summary of the significant events of a patient's hospitalization.

Electronic medical record (EMR) A medical record that is stored on a computer.

Familial Occurring or affecting members of a family more frequently than would be expected by chance.

Health history report A collection of subjective data about a patient.

Home health care The provision of medical and nonmedical care in a patient's home or place of residence.

Informed consent Consent given by a patient for a medical procedure after being informed of the nature of his or her condition, the purpose of the procedure, an explanation of risks involved with the procedure, alternative treatments or procedures available, the likely outcome of the procedure, and the risks involved with declining or delaying the procedure.

Inpatient A patient who has been admitted to a hospital for at least one overnight stay.

Medical impressions Conclusions drawn by the physician from an interpretation of data. Other terms for impressions include *provisional diagnosis* and *tentative diagnosis*.

Medical record A written record of the important information regarding a patient, including the care of that individual and the progress of the patient's condition.

Medical record format The way a medical record is organized. The two main types of medical record formats are the source-oriented record and the problem-oriented record.

Objective symptom A symptom that can be observed by an examiner.

Paper-based patient record (PPR) A medical record in paper form.

Patient An individual receiving medical care.

Physical examination An assessment of each part of the patient's body to obtain objective data about the patient that assists in determining the patient's state of health.

Physical examination report A report of the objective findings from the physician's assessment of each body system.

Problem Any condition that requires further observation, diagnosis, management, or patient education.

Prognosis The probable course and outcome of a disease and the prospects for a patient's recovery.

Reverse chronological order Arranging documents with the most recent document on top or in the front, which means that the oldest document is on the bottom or at the back of a section or file.

SOAP format A method of organization for recording progress notes. The SOAP format includes the following categories: subjective data, objective data, assessment, and plan.

Subjective symptom A symptom that is felt by the patient, but is not observable by an examiner.

Symptom Any change in the body or its functioning that indicates the presence of disease.

ON THE WEB

For Information on Cultural Diversity:

National Geographic Society: www.nationalgeographic.com

Generations United: www.gu.org

For Information on Communication Assistance:

AT&T Toll-Free Directory: www.tollfree.att.net

United Parcel Service: www.ups.com

Federal Express: www.fedex.com

DHL: www.dhl-usa.com

PREPARE FOR CERTIFICATION
Visit the Evolve site at http://evolve.elsevier.com/Bonewit/today/ to actively Prepare for your Certification.

*Check out the **Companion CD** bound with the book to access additional interactive activities.*

37

Patient Reception

assignment (ah-SIGN-ment) of benefits
call-in times
copayment

Medicaid (MEH-dih-kayed)
tickler file

Introduction to Patient Reception

The medical assistant may be responsible for opening the office, preparing for patients, and processing patients as they arrive for appointments. It is important to be sure that all parts of the office are prepared for patients because there is little time to pick up or arrange facilities once patient appointments begin. There are several forms that new patients must fill out, and the patient signature must be kept on file as permission to provide treatment, bill insurance, and verify that the patient has been given an opportunity to read the office's Notice of Privacy Practices. At the end of the day, the medical assistant must prepare for the next day and close the medical office.

PREPARING FOR PATIENTS

Opening the Medical Office

Office staff need to arrive at the medical office early enough to make sure the office is prepared for the patients. The medical assistant is often responsible for opening the office (Procedure 37-1). Several activities must be performed immediately:

- Disarming the alarm system (if the office has one)
- Turning on the lights
- Unlocking the door through which patients enter
- Unlocking file cabinets, medical record files, and medication cabinets
- Turning on all of the office equipment that will be used during the day, such as computers and copy machines

Depending on the way the medical office is organized, several other tasks should be completed before the first patient arrives.

Checking for Messages and/or Faxes

Someone must review messages and prepare the telephone system for the day's activities. The telephone message must be switched from the night/weekend message to the telephone system used during the day. Usually the night/weekend message states that the office is closed, gives an emergency telephone number, or directs the caller to leave a message if the matter is not urgent. During the day, the medical assistant may answer the telephone directly or the caller may have to select an option from a menu before being connected to a member of the office staff.

If the medical office uses an answering service, the medical assistant must call the service to indicate that the office is open. The medical assistant must also obtain any messages that have come in within the past hour or nonurgent messages left during the night. For calls relating to illness, the answering service would have contacted the physician on call overnight.

After checking the message mailbox or answering machine, the medical assistant usually checks for faxes that have arrived overnight and routes the messages and faxes to the appropriate person.

A separate mailbox or answering machine may be used for prescription refill requests. If this is the case, the medical assistant should retrieve the messages from this mailbox before the physician arrives.

Preparing for the Day's Activities

It is helpful to take a minute at the beginning of the day to organize the day's tasks. This includes reviewing the appointment schedule and noting deviations from the routine schedule, such as physicians who are out of the office for all or part of the day. If the medical office uses a manual day sheet, it must be dated and prepared for use. (This is discussed in detail in Chapter 44.) Reminders about the day's activities may be stored using an electronic task system and/or a physical **tickler file.** A tickler file is a set of 43 file folders, one for each month (for a total of 12 folders) and an additional set of 31 folders for the days of the current month. Written notes, bills to be paid, receipts, or other items are filed in these folders to "tickle" the memory at the time when they must be handled. (Tickler files are also discussed in Chapter 41.)

Making Sure Patient Charts Are Prepared

Patient charts are usually pulled the evening before the next appointment day or are prepared in the morning before the patients arrive. The charts must be arranged for each physician in order of the arrival of the patient. A separate appointment schedule is usually prepared for each physician. A charge slip may be created for each person before the visit and placed with the medical record, or it may be printed when the patient arrives for the appointment.

Copies of the appointment schedule(s) are printed and placed at designated locations. The medical assistant usually places a schedule in each physician's office, at the reception desk, and at the medical assistant's desk. Because the appointment schedule is usually updated with new appointments in the early morning, this may be the last thing done before patients begin to arrive.

Charts for the day are usually kept at the front desk. Some physicians prefer to have all medical records for their scheduled patients on their private desk when they start to see patients.

Checking the Office and Waiting Room

The waiting room, reception area, and examination/treatment rooms all need to be checked for the following: cleanliness, neatness, correct temperature, and appropriate reading material. The medical assistant should make sure that the cleaning service has cleaned all parts of the office and emptied the trash. The medical assistant may need to turn on a television, radio, and/or DVD player in the patient waiting room. Magazines should be stored neatly and replaced with current issues as needed. If there are toys in the waiting room, they should be cleaned regularly and stored neatly. Holders in the waiting room that contain information brochures for patients should be restocked and arranged neatly (Figure 37-1).

Checking Equipment and Supplies

The medical assistant should perform a visual safety check of the medical office daily. This includes removing any hazards that might block hallways or exits and making sure that all equipment is performing correctly. It is helpful to fill the paper trays of the copier, printer, and fax machine every morning.

The reception area and examination rooms should be tidied and restocked daily, either in the morning or at closing and sometimes again at a specified time during the day. Biohazard waste containers should be checked and discarded properly if necessary. The medical assistant may need to turn on or set up equipment used for clinical

procedures, run controls in the laboratory, and/or remove items from a battery charger. It may also be necessary to unload the autoclave and put away items that were sterilized the evening before.

Closing the Medical Office

At the end of the day, the activities of the morning are reversed. Many medical offices run the autoclave in the afternoon so that items can dry overnight. Medical records for the following day may be created for new patients and removed from the files for established patients. This is often done in the afternoon because it leaves more time in the morning. Before leaving the office, the medical assistant must perform the following tasks (Procedure 37-2):

- Make a backup copy of the main computer hard drive if the office does not subscribe to an online computer backup service.
- Turn off computers, printers, copiers, and other equipment (with the exception of the fax machine).

Putting It All into Practice

My name is Keisha White, and I work in a small office with two internists. We are the primary care providers for most of our patients. I am responsible for opening the office every day, and I usually arrive at about 8:00 AM. I leave before the office closes every day except Friday. Gerri, another medical assistant, is responsible for closing the office. We had an alarm system put in about 5 years ago, so as soon as I enter the office, I go to the keypad and enter the code so that the alarm won't go off. Then I have a look around as I turn on the lights. Sometimes the air seems a little stale, so I either open a window or turn up the air conditioning, depending on how hot it is outside. After I turn on the copier and the computers, I call the answering service to tell them that I have arrived. I take down any messages and handle them. Then I make sure the telephones are set so that patients can call. Next I turn on the lights in the patient waiting area, make sure everything is tidy, and unlock the door for patients. We like to have music in the waiting room, so I make sure there are six CDs in the player and turn it on. I usually change the selection every day because we get tired of hearing the same music all the time. We have shifted over to an electronic medical record, but we haven't scanned in all our old records yet. Gerri pulls the old medical records for the next day before she leaves in the afternoon. Once the computers are warmed up, I check the electronic calendar to see if there is anything special to do that day, and I print appointment schedules. We keep one schedule at the front desk, and I put one on each physician's desk. When each patient arrives, we print a charge slip and place it with the paper record. Then we call the patient to escort him or her to the examination room. The first appointment is scheduled for 8:30, so I really have to keep moving in order to be ready for the day. ■

Prepare for Success

Figure 37-1. The waiting area should be kept tidy for patients. (From Klieger D: *Saunders textbook of medical assisting,* St. Louis, 2005, Saunders.)

- Change the telephone to the night message or call the answering service to tell them the office is closing.
- Lock the door through which patients enter.
- Lock file cabinets, medical record files, and medication cabinets.
- Make sure the coffee machine or other kitchen equipment is turned off.
- Unplug equipment, such as a toaster, that might be a fire hazard.
- Turn off the lights.

  The last person to leave the medical office makes sure the door is locked and sets the alarm system.

PROCEDURE 37-1   Opening the Medical Office

Outcome Open the medical office.

Equipment/Supplies

- Medical office

1. **Procedural Step.** Enter the office and disarm any alarm system immediately.
2. **Procedural Step.** Turn on the lights.
3. **Procedural Step.** Adjust heat or air conditioning to a comfortable setting.
4. **Procedural Step.** Unlock the door through which patients and visitors will enter the office.
   Principle. Medical office staff usually enter the office through a different door than patients and visitors.
5. **Procedural Step.** Turn on machines that will be used all day, including computers, printers, and copier.
6. **Procedural Step.** Set the telephone system to the day setting and get messages, either from an electronic mailbox, telephone answering machine, or answering service.
   Principle. Callers to a business expect calls to be picked up as soon as the business opens. An important telephone message may need attention.
7. **Procedural Step.** Listen to any messages in order, writing down the pertinent information for each message on a message pad. (See Chapter 39, Procedure 39-2, Taking a Telephone Message.) Fill in the information, including the name of the caller, business affiliation (if any), date, time of the call, telephone number including area code, and the information the caller wishes to leave about the reason for the call. Place your initials on the message in case there are questions.
   Principle. Complete information is necessary to return a call.

8. **Procedural Step.** Arrange the messages in order of importance. Deal with any urgent calls at once, then work through other calls. Pull medical records for calls from patients and place the messages in the appropriate locations for various office staff to review.
9. **Procedural Step.** Review the day's activities and note any special tasks that must be completed that day.
10. **Procedural Step.** Check the office for safety hazards including frayed wires, items blocking corridors or walkways, or other hazards.
11. **Procedural Step.** Straighten up the waiting room, including reading material; clean childrens' toys as needed; turn on radio, television, and/or DVD player; and restock patient information brochures.
12. **Procedural Step.** Print appointment lists as needed and make sure all patient medical records have been pulled and arranged in order. Print or stamp today's date on the progress notes and place the medical records in the designated location.
13. **Procedural Step.** If it is office policy, prepare charge slips and clip to each patient's medical record.
14. **Procedural Step.** Check biohazard waste containers and discard properly.
15. **Procedural Step.** Check examination rooms to be sure they are clean and contain all needed supplies and equipment.
16. **Procedural Step.** Run the autoclave as needed, or empty the autoclave if it was run the evening before.

PROCEDURE 37-2   Closing the Medical Office

Outcome Close the medical office.

Equipment/Supplies

- Medical office

1. **Procedural Step.** Make sure examination rooms are clean and contain all necessary supplies.
2. **Procedural Step.** Run the autoclave if needed.
   Principle. If the autoclave is run at the end of the day, supplies can dry overnight.
3. **Procedural Step.** Print a patient schedule for the next day, and pull the medical records. Print charge slips and clip to each patient's medical record if it is office policy.
4. **Procedural Step.** Make sure all cabinets or rooms containing medical records are locked.
5. **Procedural Step.** Place money collected during the day in the office safe or take it to the bank to be deposited.
   Principle. Cash and checks should not be left unattended in the office overnight.
6. **Procedural Step.** Make sure the night system for the telephones is activated. Switch the message on the electronic telephone system or answering machine, and call the answering service as needed.
7. **Procedural Step.** Turn off all machines throughout the medical office that are only used during the day. Exceptions include the fax machine and telephone system. Unplug machines like the coffee maker or toaster oven that might pose a fire hazard.
   Principle. Machines that generate heat like coffee makers can pose a fire hazard. Unplugging these machines is also an extra reminder to make sure they do not remain on overnight.
8. **Procedural Step.** Lock the door through which patients and visitors enter the medical office.
9. **Procedural Step.** Turn the heat or air conditioning to the night setting.
10. **Procedural Step.** Turn off the lights.
11. **Procedural Step.** Arm the security system and make sure the door is securely locked as you leave the medical office.

PROCEDURE 37-2

PATIENT CHECK-IN

It is important to acknowledge each person who enters the office as soon as possible to prevent that person from feeling awkward. The medical assistant or a receptionist usually sits at the reception desk. This person should greet everyone who enters the office. If a sign-in sheet is used, it is recommended that this sign-in sheet have adhesive peel-off strips for each line so that the medical assistant can remove the patient's name immediately after check-in.

Maintaining Confidentiality

Many offices have a sliding glass window. This prevents people in the waiting room from hearing telephone conversations or other discussions in the reception area. In some facilities, the medical assistant sits behind a reception desk that is recessed but open (Figure 37-2). Because patients standing near the desk can hear any conversation behind the desk, these offices usually have a separate room for scheduling appointments. When a patient is at the desk, the medical assistant should not carry on a telephone conversation with another patient. Only one patient should be at the desk or window at a time. The medical assistant can instruct other patients and/or family members to have a seat in the waiting room.

If it is necessary to discuss sensitive or personal information, the patient should be taken to a private area.

New Patients

The office must obtain several types of information about new patients. Personal and insurance information is either obtained when the appointment is made or at the first visit.

The patient is usually asked to sign a statement that allows the office to release information to the insurance

Figure 37-2. If an open desk is used for reception, the waiting room should be large enough to prevent other patients from overhearing the conversation at the desk.

company for billing purposes. This consent may be part of the patient information form or may be a separate sheet. If the office accepts payments directly from the insurance company (called accepting **assignment of benefits**), the patient must also sign a form authorizing this. The assignment of benefits statement is usually included with the consent to release information to insurance companies. Figure 37-3 shows an example of a new patient information form. By signing the bottom section, the patient authorizes

REGISTRATION
(PLEASE PRINT)

Home Phone: _____ Today's Date: _____

PATIENT INFORMATION

Name_____ Soc. Sec.# _____
       Last Name   First Name   Initial

Address_____

City _____ State _____ Zip _____

Single ____ Married ____ Widowed ____ Separated ____ Divorced ____ Sex M____ F____ Age____ Birthdate _____

Patient Employed by_____ Occupation _____

Business Address _____ Business Phone _____

By whom were you referred?_____

In case of emergency who should be notified? _____ Phone _____
                                              Last Name   Relationship to Patient

PRIMARY INSURANCE

Person Responsible for Account _____
                               Last Name   First Name   Initial

Relation to Patient _____ Birthdate _____ Soc. Sec.# _____

Address (if different from patient's) _____ Phone _____

City_____ State _____ Zip _____

Person Responsible Employed by_____ Occupation _____

Business Address _____ Business Phone _____

Insurance Company_____

Contract # _____ Group # _____ Subscriber # _____

Name of other dependents covered under this plan _____

ADDITIONAL INSURANCE

Is patient covered by additional insurance?   ____Yes ____ No

Subscriber Name _____ Relationship to Patient _____ Birthdate _____

Address (if different from patient's) _____ Phone _____

City _____ State _____ Zip _____

Subscriber Employed by_____ Business Phone _____

Insurance Company _____

Contract #_____ Group # _____ Subscriber # _____

Name of other dependents covered under this plan _____

ASSIGNMENT AND RELEASE

I, the undersigned, certify that I (or my dependent) have insurance coverage with _____
                                                                          Name of Insurance Company(ies)

and assign directly to Dr. _____ insurance benefits, if any, otherwise payable to me for services rendered. I understand that I am financially responsible for all charges whether or not paid by insurance. I hereby authorize the doctor to release all information necessary to secure the payment of benefits. I authorize the use of this signature on all insurance submissions.

_____   _____   _____
     Responsible Party Signature   Relationship   Date

ORDER# 58-8426 • © 1996 BIBBERO SYSTEMS, INC. • PETALUMA, CALIFORNIA • TO REORDER CALL TOLL FREE: (800) 242-9330

Figure 37-3. New patient information form. (Courtesy Bibbero Systems, Inc., Petaluma, Calif., [800] 242-2376; Fax [800] 242-9330; www.bibbero.com.)

the physician or medical practice to release information to the insurance company and authorizes the insurance company to pay the medical practice directly. In addition, the patient has agreed to be responsible for charges not covered by insurance. In addition to the new patient information form, the medical office may use a more extensive form authorizing the release of protected health information. This form is optional, but it does allow the office to obtain consent to leave voicemail messages at the patient's home and mail laboratory reports or appointment reminders (Figure 37-4).

Acknowledgement of Receipt of HIPAA Privacy Practices

The Health Insurance Portability and Accountability Act (HIPAA) requires that patients sign a form acknowledging that they were given the opportunity to read or given a copy of the office privacy practices (Figure 37-5). The Notice of Privacy Practices itself is usually very detailed.

Patient History Form

Most offices also have a history form for the patient to fill out before being seen by the physician. It may be mailed to the new patient before the first appointment, or the patient may fill it out in the waiting room. The medical assistant

What Would You Do? What Would You *Not* Do?

Case Study 1

Angela Harris is a 62-year-old new patient. When she comes to the reception desk to check in, she gives Keisha the completed patient history form that had been mailed to her. Keisha hands her a Notice of Privacy Practices and a clipboard and pen. She asks her to fill out a new patient information form and sign the form, acknowledging the receipt of the Notice of Privacy Practices to sign. Ms. Harris seems reluctant to take the clipboard. She says, "I'm sorry, I don't have my reading glasses with me. I didn't know I would need them. Besides, I gave you all that information on the telephone, didn't I?" ∎

Patient Consent for Use and Disclosure of Protected Health Information

I hereby give my consent for [**Practice Name**] to use and disclose protected health information (PHI) about me to carry out treatment, payment and health care operations. (The *Notice of Privacy Practices* describes such uses and disclosures more completely.)

I have the right to review the *Notice of Privacy Practices* before signing this consent. I understand that the *Notice of Privacy Practices* can be revised at any time, and I can obtain a copy of any revision upon written request.

I authorize [**Practice Name**] to call my home or other alternative location and leave a message on voice mail or in person in reference to any items related to treatment, payment and health care operations. This includes appointment reminders, questions about insurance and any calls pertaining to my clinical care, including laboratory test results, among others.

I authorize [**Practice Name**] to mail to my home or other alternative location any items that assist in my care such as appointment reminder cards and patient statements as long as they are marked "Personal and Confidential."

I have the right to request that [**Practice Name**] restrict how it uses or discloses my PHI to carry out treatment, payment and health care operations. The practice is not required to agree to my requested restrictions, but if it does, it is bound by this agreement.

By signing this form, I am consenting to allow [**Practice Name**] to use and disclose my PHI as required in the course of treatment and obtaining payment for services to me.

I may revoke my consent in writing except to the extent that the practice has already made disclosures in reliance upon my prior consent.

_____   _____   _____
Patient or Legal Guardian's Signature   Date   Relationship to Patient

_____   _____
Print Patient's Name   Print Name of Legal Guardian (if any)

Figure 37-4. The office may use an optional consent for disclosure of personal health information.

Acknowledgement of Receipt of the Notice of Privacy Practices

Please Review Carefully

The Notice of Privacy Practices tells you how [**Practice Name**] uses and discloses information about you. Not all situations will be described. We are required to give you a notice of our privacy practices for the information we collect and keep about you. We reserve the right to revise this notice, and you can obtain a copy of any revision upon written request.

I, _____, have been given a copy of the **Notice of**
Privacy Practices.

_____ _____ _____
Patient or Legal Guardian's Signature   Date   Relationship to Patient

_____   _____
Print Patient's Name   Print Name of Legal Guardian (if any)

_____   _____
Signature of Witness (If signed with an "X" or mark)   Date

Effective Date: April 14, 2003

Figure 37-5. HIPAA requires new patients to sign a form acknowledging receipt of a medical office's privacy practices.

---

goes over this form with the patient in the examination room to be sure that all of the relevant information has been included. Medical information should not be discussed at the front desk.

Verifying Insurance and Obtaining Authorizations

After a new patient has filled out the patient information sheet, the medical assistant should ask for his or her insurance card. After making a photocopy of both sides or scanning the card, the copy is stored with the patient's medical record. It verifies the information given by the patient and sometimes gives additional information needed for billing. An insurance card scanner at the front desk may be used to read both sides of the insurance card and scan it into the computer. Information from the card can be transferred to the practice management software, and an image of the card can be saved to the patient's electronic medical record.

Some types of insurance require authorization every time the patient visits the primary care physician. Patients with Medicaid must usually have their coverage verified and/or must receive prior authorization for each visit. **Medicaid** is an insurance program established by the federal government that pays for low-income patients' medical needs. Each state administers Medicaid, and the program has a different name in each state. The cost is split between the state and the federal government. In some states, some patients on Medicaid receive new identification cards each month; in other states patients can be verified by telephone, fax, or an

electronic card reader. An electronic card reader is a small machine in the physician's office that is connected via telephone to the insurance company's database and can verify insurance benefits while the patient is in the office. Many offices use a card reader that can not only read the patient's insurance card, but also several types of credit cards (Figure 37-6).

For other types of insurance, it may be necessary to call the patient's insurance company to obtain authorization for treatment (especially if the patient needs minor surgery or a special treatment). This may be done when the patient makes the appointment, when the patient checks in, or after the first visit, when the physician has identified what treatment is necessary and how many visits are anticipated.

Each office has its own procedure for verifying insurance. In general, if there is a question whether the patient has insurance coverage, or whether the service will be covered, the medical assistant should contact the insurance company before the service is provided (Procedure 37-3).

Verifying a Managed Care Referral

If the patient has been referred by another physician through a managed care plan, it is important to validate that the patient has a completed referral form from the primary care physician. This may be a paper form. Sometimes the referring physician has sent it in advance, but the patient may bring it personally to the visit. For some managed care plans, it will be possible to access the referral using the

Figure 37-6. Card reader used to validate insurance coverage for Medicaid and other insurance plans.

Internet. If there is no valid referral, the insurance company may not pay for the visit.

The referral will state how many visits are allowed (how many will be paid for by the managed care plan) and the problem for which the patient is being referred. Depending on the patient's insurance or managed care plan, the patient may also be required to sign a statement promising to pay any charges that the insurance does not cover.

Managed care plans usually do not allow physicians who accept referrals to bill for excess charges to the patient (a practice known as *balance billing*). Medicare also does not allow balance billing from providers who agree to accept Medicare patients. The medical office is allowed to bill for services that the patient's insurance plan does not cover.

If the patient has not yet obtained a referral form, or if it is uncertain that the insurance will cover the services, the patient must be informed that he or she will be responsible for payment of the bill before any service is provided.

Established Patients

If the patient has been seen in the office before, it is still necessary to verify that the billing information is still correct. When checking a patient in, the medical assistant should ask if the address and telephone number are still the same. The patient should also be asked for his or her insurance card. If any information has changed, the updated information should be entered into the computer billing system and into the medical record, whether paper or electronic.

Accepting Copayments

A **copayment** is a fixed amount of money that the patient is required to pay each time he or she receives medical treat-

What Would You Do? What Would You *Not* Do?

Case Study 2
Joseph Ritano is a 38-year-old new patient. While filling out the new patient information form, he comes to the desk and says, "I don't seem to have my insurance card with me today. I must have forgotten to put it back in my wallet when I gave you the information over the telephone last week. I know that the company is Bristol Medical Care, but I don't know my ID number. Do you have it in the computer? I know that my copayment is $10.00." ∎

Memories *from* Externship

Keisha White: One of my duties during my externship was to prepare the medical records and charge slips each day. In the afternoon, I was given an appointment schedule for each physician, and I pulled the medical record for each patient on the schedule. Sometimes I had to hunt for one. Occasionally it was misfiled, but usually I found it on the desk of the physician, office manager, or insurance specialist. Then I prepared a charge slip for each patient. This was about 8 years ago, and at that time we were doing them by hand. Now we print the charge slips when the patient arrives. I wrote in the patient's name and address, date of birth, telephone number, insurance information, and the date on the top of the form. Then I clipped the form to the front of the medical record. I opened the record to be sure that there was room for the physician to write on the top sheet, and I stamped tomorrow's date after the last note. I arranged the medical records in order and placed the records for each physician in a neat pile with the appointment list on top. The next day, I would check the list about once an hour. If any patients had been added to the schedule, I would find the medical record for those patients and prepare a charge slip. Once or twice I couldn't find a medical record, even after I had looked everywhere. For those patients, we would make up a temporary progress note sheet and clip it to the charge slip. The first time this happened, it took us a week to find the medical record. It had slipped behind the others in the vertical file cabinet and gotten wedged in the back. The other time, the physician found the medical record in his office that afternoon. Everyone was relieved when all the records were accounted for. ∎

Prepare for Success

ment. The amount of the copayment is printed on the patient's insurance card. Many offices collect the copayment before the visit because it is a fixed fee, although it can also be done at the end of the visit. The amount paid is entered on the patient's charge slip. A receipt should be given to the patient at the time the copayment is made.

Indicating That the Patient Is in the Waiting Room

After the patient has been checked in at the front desk, the medical record is placed in the designated space for patients who are ready to be seen. If a computerized record is used, a routing slip is generated.

The forms that the patient filled out are inserted in the medical record. The charge slip is usually attached to the front of the record for the physician to fill in. If an electronic medical record is used, any forms must be scanned into the medical record. The patient information must either be entered into the computer system or updated (if it was obtained by telephone at the time the visit was scheduled).

PROCEDURE 37-3   Obtaining New Patient Information

Outcome Obtain information from a new patient, obtain consents, and validate insurance coverage.

Equipment/Supplies

- Clipboard
- Pen
- New patient information form containing consent to treatment and assignment of benefits consents
- Notice of Privacy Practices
- Receipt of Notice of Privacy form
- Consent for release of protected health information (optional)

- Photocopier
- Insurance card reader (optional)
- Telephone
- Medical record
- Computer
- Scanner

1. **Procedural Step.** Place a new patient information form on a clipboard with a pen, and ask a new patient to complete the form and return it to you.
   Principle. Complete information about the patient facilitates the billing and insurance process.

2. **Procedural Step.** Make sure the form is complete and the patient or authorized representative has signed the form as needed.
   Principle. The patient must consent to treatment, consent for the office to bill the insurance company, and consent to allow the insurance company to pay the physician in writing.

3. **Procedural Step.** Ask to see the insurance card of the patient or other insured person.

4. **Procedural Step.** Photocopy both sides of the insurance card and place the copy in the patient's medical record.
   Principle. The insurance card contains information about the patient's copayment amount, as well as the address and telephone number of the insurance company.

5. **Procedural Step.** Confirm patient eligibility for insurance coverage using a card reader, computer, or telephone if required by the patient's insurance, and confirm that there is a complete referral form if necessary. If the visit will not be completely covered by insurance, discuss the patient's financial responsibility. If personal information is discussed, take the patient to a private area.
   Principle. The patient has a right to know what his or her financial obligation will be before receiving service.

6. **Procedural Step.** Give the patient a copy of the Notice of Privacy Practices and ask the patient to sign the form acknowledging the receipt of the Notice of Privacy Practices. Sign the form as a witness to the patient's signature.
   Principle. HIPAA requires that the patient acknowledge the receipt of the Notice of Privacy Practices in writing.

7. **Procedural Step.** Ask the patient to read and sign any consent for release of protected health information used by the office.
   Principle. A general consent for release of personal health information enables the office to obtain written consent to leave messages on the patient's answering machine, to send laboratory results to the patient's home address, etc.

8. **Procedural Step.** Insert any new forms into the medical record and place it with the charge slip to indicate that the patient is ready to be examined. Ask the patient to have a seat and tell him or her the approximate waiting time for the examination.
   Principle. When the paperwork is complete, it will help the patient feel more in control to know how long he or she can expect to wait before the examination.

9. **Procedural Step.** Transfer the information from the new patient information form to the patient's computer account, or validate that information obtained by telephone is correct.
   Principle. Billing is almost always performed using the computer.

10. **Procedural Step.** Scan the new patient information form, insurance card, and other consent forms if it is office policy (usually if the office uses an electronic medical record).
    Principle. If the office stores a patient's medical record electronically in addition to billing records, all paper records must be scanned into the computer.

ORIENTING PATIENTS TO THE MEDICAL OFFICE
Information for New or Prospective Patients

The medical assistant may be responsible for informing new patients and prospective patients about the medical office and its policies and procedures (Procedure 37-4). The medical assistant should be familiar with all of the following information:

- A brief description of the physicians, how long each has been in practice, each physician's credentials, and if each physician is accepting new patients
- Specialties of the physicians in the practice, types of patients seen, and basic philosophy of the physician(s)
- Information about languages spoken by staff, if the physician practices alternative therapies (e.g., acupuncture), or if the physician insists that patients stop smoking
- Location of the main office and satellite offices, directions to each office, and a description of available parking and access to public transportation, if applicable
- The types of insurance that the practice accepts, if the patient's insurance will be accepted, and if payment is required at each visit
- How to make appointments and the policy regarding canceling appointments. Patients are normally asked to give 24 hours' notice if possible for a cancellation
- The telephone procedure and if the physician has **call-in times** (when the physician takes telephone calls)
- What hospital(s) each physician is affiliated with; some patients might also want to know if the physician makes nursing home visits
- How medication refills are handled

A physician might not be accepting new patients for a few reasons:

1. A physician may have so many patients that he or she cannot in all fairness accept new patients. If the patient load decreases, the physician may begin again to accept new patients.
2. The physician may be returning from a maternity, family, or personal disability leave and be working a reduced schedule.
3. The physician may be easing back before retiring.

PROCEDURE 37-4

What Would You Do? What Would You *Not* Do?

Case Study 3

Donna Pohl calls the office to ask about the medical practice. An acquaintance has recommended Dr. Sylvia Lawrence. She says that she prefers a female physician. She asks for information about her and her specialty. Dr. Lawrence specializes in general internal medicine. At the current time she is pregnant, and her due date is 1 month away. Although Dr. Lawrence is still seeing established patients, she has instructed Keisha not to make any appointments for her with new patients for the next 3 months. The other physician in the practice, Dr. William Rudner, also specializes in general internal medicine. ■

The medical assistant should also be able to tell prospective patients how much time to allow for a first (new patient) visit. Most physicians only see new patients on certain days and times. Medical assistants should be sure to remind new patients to bring all of their medications to the initial appointment, as well as a written list of concerns.

Patient Information Booklet

An increasing number of practices today have a booklet or brochure that contains the previously mentioned information. If a medical office puts out a first-time booklet or a new booklet, each patient should be encouraged to take one at the end of a visit. New patients should be given one at the beginning of the first visit, when they are given their new patient forms to fill out.

The patient information booklet must be kept up to date to include any changes in location or practitioners.

Patient information booklets are very successful marketing and public relations tools. They are greatly appreciated by patients. However, they often receive low priority on the list of things to do in the crush of day-to-day patient care.

PROCEDURE 37-4   Explaining Office Policies and Procedures

Outcome   Orient a new or prospective patient to the medical office.

Equipment/Supplies

- Patient information booklet (if available)
- Map
- List of points to cover

1. Procedural Step. Offer to give or send the patient a patient information booklet if one is available.

Principle. A patient information booklet provides a handy resource to answer questions about a medical practice.

Continued

PROCEDURE **37-4** Explaining Office Policies and Procedures—cont'd

2. **Procedural Step.** Identify the name, credentials, and specialties of physicians who are accepting patients in the medical office.
   Principle. Some physicians may not currently be accepting patients.
3. **Procedural Step.** Offer information as required about languages spoken by staff in the medical office and additional services or specialized complementary practices.
4. **Procedural Step.** Identify the location of the office and/or satellite offices and give directions as needed. Identify where the patient can park if necessary.
5. **Procedural Step.** Tell the patient if the office accepts his or her medical insurance plan and discuss expectations for payment of the patient's bill.
   Principle. The patient has a right to know what his or her financial obligation will be before receiving service.

6. **Procedural Step.** Describe how far in advance to make appointments and the office policy on canceling appointments.
   Principle. Most offices reserve the right to charge the patient if the appointment is not cancelled at least 24 hours in advance.
7. **Procedural Step.** Tell the patient when and how to contact the office, and notify the patient if the physician has specific call-in times (times when he or she takes telephone calls.)
8. **Procedural Step.** Explain how prescriptions and prescription refills are handled as needed.
9. **Procedural Step.** Identify the hospital(s) that each physician is affiliated with. Answer any questions about other services (e.g., nursing home visits) that each physician may provide.

MEDICAL PRACTICE and the LAW

One function of the medical office that has been affected by HIPAA is patient check-in. The Privacy Rule is not specific about sign-in lists, but medical offices need to take all possible measures to protect patient privacy. Not all offices use sign-in sheets, but if they are used, they should have adhesive peel-off strips for each line so that patients who come later cannot read the names of patients who arrived earlier. The Privacy Rule does permit incidental disclosures of certain information as long as the health care facility has reasonable safeguards to protect against disclosure of protected health information. Silent wireless paging systems are available but are usually too expensive for medical offices. Generally, it is considered acceptable to have patients say their names at the reception desk and call them by name from the waiting room unless patients have asked specifically for the staff not to do this.

In some offices, however, patients may check in at the window by signing a sheet with a map of the waiting room that indicates their seat location. They do not have to say their name out loud, and they can be located without calling their names.

It is important to protect information on paper and computer screens at the information desk from being seen by others. The computer screen should be turned so that it cannot be read from the patient side of the reception desk. If medical assistants leave the reception desk for any reason, they should log off from their computer account. In addition, all patient records and information should be stored so that names and other information are not visible to patients who approach the desk. A shredder is usually available at the front desk so that any information that will not be filed in the patient's medical record can be destroyed. ■

What Would You Do? What Would You *Not* Do? RESPONSES

Case Study 1
Page 903

What Did Keisha Do?
- ❏ Checked to see if there were other patients in the waiting room. Because there were, she took Ms. Harris to a private area.
- ❏ Asked Ms. Harris for each piece of information on the new patient information form and filled it in for her.
- ❏ Read each statement at the bottom of the form out loud and showed Ms. Harris where to sign the form.
- ❏ Explained that Ms. Harris could read the Notice of Privacy Practices at a later time when she had her glasses, but Keisha asked her to sign the form acknowledging receipt of the Notice of Privacy Practices.

What Did Keisha Not Do?
- ❏ Did not tell the patient that she should have realized she might need her reading glasses.
- ❏ Did not tell the patient to sign any of the consents without reading them to her.
- ❏ Did not ask for protected health information where another patient could hear the conversation.

What Would You Do/What Would You *Not* Do? Review Keisha's response and place a checkmark next to the information you included in your response. List the additional information you included in your response.

What Would You Do? What Would You *Not* Do?   RESPONSES—cont'd

Case Study 2
Page 905

What Did Keisha Do?

- ❏ Looked up the policy number for Mr. Ritano in the computer and handed it to him in writing so that he could write it on the form.
- ❏ Attempted to call the insurance company to verify his coverage.
- ❏ Explained that she needed to take a photocopy of his insurance card and asked him to bring it in as soon as possible.
- ❏ Accepted his check for $10.00 for his copayment.
- ❏ Explained that if it turned out that his insurance did not cover this visit or if he needed an authorization or referral, he would be responsible to pay the charges for the visit.
- ❏ Gave him an estimate of the cost of the visit.
- ❏ Allowed him to reschedule if he wanted to wait until he had his insurance card.

What Did Keisha Not *Do?*

- ❏ Did not refuse to let Mr. Ritano see the physician until he brought his insurance card.
- ❏ Did not make negative comments about forgetting the insurance card or imply that she didn't believe he had insurance.
- ❏ Did not discuss his protected health information in front of other patients.
- ❏ Did not talk to other staff members about the forgotten insurance card to other staff members unless he stated he would bring the card when she did not expect to be in the office.

What Would You Do/What Would You *Not* Do? Review Keisha's response and place a checkmark next to the information you included in your response. List the additional information you included in your response.

Case Study 3
Page 907

What Did Keisha Do?

- ❏ Explained that Dr. Sylvia Lawrence would be out on leave and could not accept appointments for 3 months.
- ❏ Offered to make an appointment with Dr. Lawrence after the 3-month period.
- ❏ Offered to make an appointment with Dr. William Rudner as soon as he had one available.
- ❏ Listened sympathetically if Ms. Pohl was displeased about not being able to be seen more promptly by a female physician.
- ❏ Responded calmly and in a normal speaking voice if the patient became irritated or upset.
- ❏ Made a recommendation about another female physician only if specifically instructed to do so by Dr. Lawrence.

What Did Keisha Not *Do?*

- ❏ Did not agree to make an appointment with Dr. Sylvia Lawrence before the end of the 3-month period just this once.
- ❏ Did not become defensive or imply that Ms. Pohl's preference for a female physician was silly.
- ❏ Did not become irritated or upset with Ms. Pohl.
- ❏ Did not talk about the telephone conversation later to other office staff.

What Would You Do/What Would You *Not* Do? Review Keisha's response and place a checkmark next to the information you included in your response. List the additional information you included in your response.

⟲ TERMINOLOGY REVIEW

Assignment of benefits Authorization given by the patient to allow the insurance company to make payments directly to the health care provider instead of to the patient.

Call-in times Blocks of time when a physician accepts telephone calls from patients.

Copayment A fixed amount of money that the patient is responsible to pay at each visit.

Medicaid A federal and state insurance program for low-income patients. The Medicaid program has a different name in each state.

Tickler file A chronological file containing reminders of things to be done.

ON THE WEB

For Information on HIPAA:

U.S. Department of Health and Human Services, Office for Civil Rights—HIPAA: www.hhs.gov/ocr/hipaa

Sample Notice of Privacy Practices at Medicare.gov: www.medicare.gov/privacypractices.asp

 PREPARE FOR CERTIFICATION   Visit the Evolve site at http://evolve.elsevier.com/Bonewit/today/ to actively Prepare for your Certification.

 *Check out the **Companion CD** bound with the book to access additional interactive activities.*

38

Medical Office Computerization

LEARNING OBJECTIVES

Computer Concepts

1. Explain the difference between data and a program.
2. Explain the purpose of each of the following parts of the data processing cycle: input, processing, and output.
3. List examples of input and output devices.
4. Explain the difference between software and hardware.
5. Explain the function of an operating system.
6. State the function of application software.
7. List and state the function of the following components of the main computer unit: mainboard, CPU, main computer memory, video card, sound card, hard drive, optical drive, and power supply.
8. Explain the difference between random access and sequential access.
9. Describe the care and maintenance of the main computer unit.
10. List and describe the two types of monitors used with a microcomputer.
11. Describe the care, maintenance, and ergonomics of the computer monitor.
12. List and describe the function of the special keys on a computer keyboard.
13. Describe the care, maintenance, and ergonomics of a computer keyboard.
14. Identify the guidelines to follow in the care and maintenance of a printer.
15. List and describe the storage devices used with microcomputer systems.
16. Describe the method of organization that a hard disk uses to store and retrieve information.
17. Explain the difference between read and write.

Medical Office Computerization

1. Explain why it is important to have a foundation in computer concepts before engaging in hands-on computer operations.
2. List and explain the advantages and disadvantages of medical office computerization.
3. List and describe measures that can be taken to promote the efficient running of a computerized medical office.
4. Explain the purpose of a medical practice management software program.
5. Explain the function performed by each of the following medical practice management systems: patient registration, appointments, posting transactions, patient billing, insurance billing, reports, and file maintenance.

Electronic Medical Record

1. List the general functions of electronic medical record (EMR) software.
2. Explain the advantages and disadvantages of EMRs.
3. Describe the modifications required to produce or convert each administrative and clinical document in a medical record into a digital format.
4. Describe the functions performed by an EMR prescription program.
5. List the procedures performed by the physician and medical assistant using an EMR.
6. Describe the methods used to maintain security of the EMR.
7. List and describe methods used to back up computer data in the medical office.
8. State the various types of system maintenance that should be performed on a computer system.
9. List the various types of service agreements available for a computer system.

CAAHEP COMPETENCIES

Operational Functions

- Utilize computer software to maintain office systems.

ABHES COMPETENCIES

Communication

- Application of electronic technology

Administrative Duties

- Apply computer concepts for office procedures.

KEY TERMS

ALU (arithmetic/logic unit)

application software

backup

byte

computer

computer system

control unit

CPU (central processing unit)

data

data processing

digital image

documentation

electronic medical record (EMR)
firewall
floppy disk
gigabyte (GB)
hard disk
hardcopy
hardware
information
input
input device
kilobyte (KB)
mainboard
main computer memory
medical practice management program
megabyte (MB)
microcomputer
operating system
optical disc
optical drive
output

output device
pixels
printing speed
processing
program
RAM (random-access memory)
read
resolution
sequential-access memory
softcopy
software
sound card
special keys
storage capacity
storage device
system software
user
video card
write

Introduction to Medical Office Computerization

The computer is the most frequently used piece of equipment in today's medical office. It is essential that the medical assistant be familiar with the computer system used in his or her office and the programs (e.g., medical practice management program, electronic medical record program) being run on that computer system.

This chapter presents an overview of the parts of the medical office computer system, as well as its uses, which range from scheduling appointments and processing patient statements and insurance claims to maintaining computerized medical records.

COMPUTER CONCEPTS

A **computer** is a device consisting of electronic components, which has the ability to process data according to a program in order to produce a desired result. The primary advantage of using a computer to perform administrative procedures in the medical office is that these tasks are performed with greater speed and accuracy than with other types of devices (e.g., typewriter, pegboard system, calculator). In addition, computers are versatile: Rather than performing only one function (e.g., typing, posting a payment, math calculations), a computer can perform a wide variety of administrative procedures.

Computers are useful tools because they can perform the same tasks repeatedly while maintaining the same level of efficiency. It should always be remembered, however, that the computer does not have a mind of its own. You are always in charge, and the computer will never do anything without your direction.

Most medical offices use **microcomputers** (also known as *personal computers* or *desktop computers*). The microcomputers in a medical office are linked together to form a *network*. This allows the computers in the network to communicate with each other and share data and resources. The number of computers in a network varies based on the size of the medical practice and the type and number of tasks performed on the computer. For example, a two-physician medical office using a practice management program typically has between four and eight networked computers.

This section on computer concepts has been designed to provide you with the theoretical foundation necessary to effectively use computers in the medical office. Because the microcomputer is typically used in the medical office, it focuses on the theory and techniques of microcomputer systems.

DATA PROCESSING CYCLE

As previously described, computers function by processing data. **Data processing** is the term applied to changing raw facts or data into usable **information.** To fully comprehend data processing, it is important to have a thorough understanding of the terms *data* and *program*. **Data** is a general term used to describe the raw, unorganized facts presented to the computer for processing. Patients' names, addresses, and telephone numbers are examples of data frequently entered into the computer in the medical office.

A **program** is defined as a set of instructions organized in a logical step-by-step sequence that tells the computer how to perform a specific function. In order to process data, you must have a program to tell the computer what to do with the data. As in cooking, when a recipe is required to tell you how to mix ingredients, a computer requires a program to tell it how to process data.

Computers process data in a logical three-part sequence known as the *data processing cycle* (Figure 38-1). The data processing cycle includes the following phases: input, processing, and output. Each phase of the data processing cycle contributes to the desired result and involves a specific activity, which is described as follows.

Of note is that the terms *input* and *output* have slightly different meanings depending on how they are used. When referring to the data processing cycle, they are used from the "computer's point of view" as verbs to describe the transfer of information. Input and output are also used as nouns to describe the data that have been entered into the computer (input) and the information that has been generated by the computer (output). As these terms appear throughout this chapter, you will become familiar with their different meanings.

Input

The **input** of data is the transfer of data to the computer for processing. Input includes both the entering of data into the computer and the conversion of it into an electronic form that can be understood by the computer. Because computers cannot understand the "written word" in the form used in communication by humans, that data must first be translated into an electronic code that can then be processed by the computer. Once the computer is finished working on the "electronic" data, it must be converted back into a form that can be understood by the user. A **user** is defined as the individual using the computer.

Data must be entered into the computer through an **input device** (see Figure 38-1). The most common example of an input device is the computer keyboard. The computer keyboard converts data into the electronic code that can be understood and processed very quickly by the computer. Other examples of input devices include a mouse, scanner, and microphone.

Processing

The **processing** of data is the computer's handling and arranging of the electronic data according to a program; in other words, the data undergo some type of manipulation or change to produce useful information. Depending on the result, the processing phase may include one or more of the following: classifying, sorting, calculating, summarizing, or listing of the data (see Figure 38-1).

Output

The final phase of the data processing sequence is the output of the processed data. **Output** is the transfer of usable information back to the user. Because the computer works with an electronic code, an output device must be used to communicate with the user. The **output device** converts the electronic code into a form that can be understood by the user. The most common output devices are the monitor and the printer (see Figure 38-1).

COMPONENTS OF THE COMPUTER SYSTEM

All of the components making up the computer are collectively known as the **computer system** (Figure 38-2). Computer systems include two major divisions: software and hardware.

Software

Software is a general term for the programs or instructions that tell a computer what to do. Software tells the computer how to perform specific tasks in a series of step-by-step instructions organized in a logical sequence. Two categories of software exist: system software and application software. System software assists the computer in carrying out its tasks, whereas application software assists the user in carrying out his or her computer tasks. Each software category is described in more detail next.

Figure 38-1. Data processing cycle.

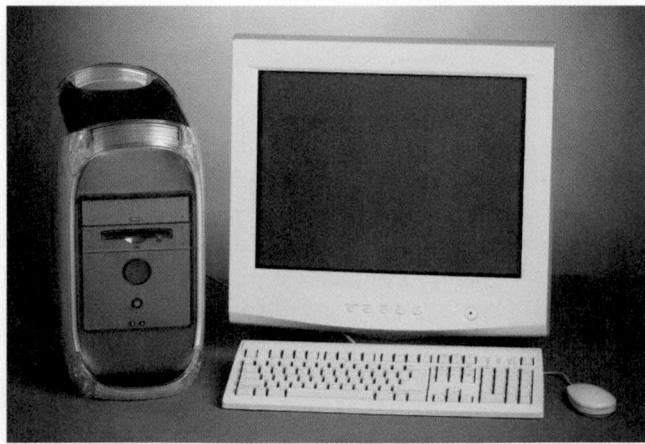

Figure 38-2. Computer system.

System Software

System software is made up of a group of special programs that control or maintain the operations of a computer. The most important type of system software is the **operating system.** The operating system is installed on the hard disk of the computer and is automatically loaded into the computer's main memory (RAM) when the computer is turned on. An example of an operating system frequently used in the medical office is Windows (Microsoft Corporation). The operating system performs "housekeeping" chores required by the computer system to operate itself. The most important function performed by an operating system is to serve as an intermediary to tell the hardware how to run an application program. Hence, application programs are useless without an operating system.

Highlight on Operating Systems

Almost all of today's medical office computers run on a Windows operating system. The Windows operating system was designed in the early 1990s to mimic the Apple Macintosh operating system (Mac OS) designed for Macintosh computers. An operating system allows interactions between the computer and the user, between the computer and peripheral equipment, and between computer and computer. The interaction may occur using a direct connection, wireless network, telephone line, and the Internet. Each time a new operating system is developed, it allows for ever-more complex computer system interactions.

Windows and Mac OS are based on the concept of the graphical user interface (GUI, pronounced "gooey"). The theory behind this type of operating system is that it operates the way people think—it is intuitive. When the computer is turned on, a desktop appears. The desktop is the computer analogy of all the items needed to open and view programs and files, to perform operations, and to create and store files.

An individual item, such as a patient record, a daily appointment list, or a medical record, is called a *file.* A file is a set of computer data that has been saved to disk. Files are collected in folders, indicated by an icon of a file folder. Folders can be displayed individually either within a window or on the desktop. When a folder is opened, it appears as a window, and all the files that reside in the folder are in the window. Files can be moved from one folder to another, just as they might be at a desk with papers, folders, and files.

Arranged on the desktop screen are icons. Icons are small graphics that provide a link to files, folders, or applications. With a Windows operating system, these icons include a small computer (My Computer), a recycle bin, and icons for application programs. At the bottom left of the screen is a start button. One click on the start button causes a list of options to rise from it. Many of the options have small arrows pointing to the right; highlighting one of these items causes submenus to appear. By clicking again, an application can be opened. ▪

Application Software

Software designed to allow a user to accomplish a specific task is known as **application software,** also known as an *application program* or *software program.* Application software constitutes the greatest proportion of the software available for use with a computer.

Four types of application programs are combined to make up a medical practice management program. These include a word processing program, a spreadsheet program, a telecommunication program, and a database management program. These application programs are discussed in more detail as follows.

Word processing Word processing software allows the user to enter, edit, format, and file (store) text. Microsoft Word is an example of a commercially available word processing application program. A medical practice management program uses a word processing application to produce letters (e.g., referral letter) and reports (e.g., health history report).

Spreadsheet A spreadsheet is an electronic ledger designed to perform mathematic calculations quickly. Spreadsheet programs are used to produce financial reports and to analyze and process statistics. An example of a commercially available spreadsheet application program is Microsoft Excel. A medical practice management program uses a spreadsheet application to generate financial reports for the office.

Telecommunications A telecommunications application provides the means for one computer to "talk" with another computer. Electronic communication between computers greatly reduces the time it takes to send information. A medical practice management program uses a telecommunications application for the electronic submission of insurance claims. In addition, telecommunications software is used to send letters and messages as electronic mail (e-mail).

Database management Database management is the storing and retrieving of data in and from a database. Database management allows the user to store large amounts of data on a storage device (e.g., hard disk). The data can then be easily retrieved and manipulated. An example of a commercially available database management software program is Microsoft Access. A medical practice management program uses a database management program to perform the majority of the administrative procedures in the medical office. Database management increases efficiency in recordkeeping and eliminates numerous time-consuming repetitive tasks. The database for a medical practice consists of patient records, patient transactions, diagnosis codes, procedure codes, insurance carriers, and so on. This information is stored on the hard disk of the computer for later retrieval and use as needed. A database also provides the ability to add new information, modify existing information, and delete unneeded information. The most significant aspect of a database is that the computer can cross-reference all of the information stored in its database.

The medical practice database can be thought of as a large pool of information that the computer can access in a multitude of ways according to the task being performed.

Documentation

Documentation is a written set of instructions designed to assist the user in understanding how to operate an application program. Clear, concise, and easy-to-understand documentation makes it much easier to learn and use the program. Documentation includes the following: (1) the program user manual, which contains complete instructions for learning and using the program; (2) on-line help screens displayed on the computer monitor; and (3) reference cards containing frequently needed details for quick reference. It is important to learn to seek out and rely on the documentation that comes with the medical practice management program you are using. This results in more efficient operation of the computer system and less frustration in solving computer problems when they arise.

Putting It All into Practice

My name is Emma Hayes, and I am a certified medical assistant. Since I graduated, I have been working at the main office of an internal medicine practice. Our office manager is very interested in computers, and we have been using integrated practice management and EMR software for the past 4 years. When a new patient calls for an appointment, we obtain all their personal and insurance information and enter it into the computer during that first conversation. When they first come to the office, we have them sit at a computer terminal in a private room next to the waiting room and enter their medical history. If the patient is not comfortable with the computer, we have the patient complete a paper form, and then I enter the data from the form into the computer. We have a scanner at the front desk to scan the patients' insurance cards and all the forms they sign at the first visit. We keep a folder for our patients with forms that they have signed, but everything is also available in electronic form.

One of the things our patients really like is that our physicians send all prescriptions to the pharmacy electronically. At the first visit, we ask patients for the name, address, and telephone number of the pharmacy they want to use. I also ask the patient what medications they are taking and enter them into the computer. After that, the physician can go to the patient's EMR, enter the information about the medication he wants to prescribe, and automatically send the prescription directly to the patient's pharmacy. The EMR program checks for drug interactions with all the medications that the patient is taking. Our physicians believe that this saves time and is actually more accurate, because the pharmacist doesn't have to read their handwritten prescriptions. ■

Prepare for Success

Hardware

Hardware is the term for the physical equipment making up the computer system; that is, the tangible computer parts. Although a computer system may include a variety of hardware, the following hardware devices are necessary to perform administrative procedures in the medical office: main computer unit, monitor, computer keyboard and mouse, and printer.

MAIN COMPUTER UNIT

The main computer unit, or simply the main unit, consists of a hard plastic case that is usually rectangular in shape. The main unit houses all the components that make the computer work and consists of the following eight major components: mainboard, central processing unit (CPU), main computer memory (RAM), video card, sound card, hard disk, optical drive, and power supply. The eight major components of the main computer unit are discussed next.

Mainboard

The **mainboard** (also known as the "motherboard") is the primary circuit board of the main computer unit. Each of the other components of the main computer unit either sit on the mainboard itself (e.g., CPU) or are connected to it in some way (e.g., hard disk). Electrical circuits the width of human hairs are etched onto the mainboard; the electrical impulses that carry messages to and from the computer travel through these circuits. The mainboard provides a means for all of the components making up the main unit to communicate with each other and can be thought of as the "nervous system" of the computer.

Central Processing Unit

The **central processing unit (CPU)** is the functional core or "brain" of the computer and is the most complex computer component. The CPU interprets and executes the instructions that operate the computer. The CPU consists of a microprocessor chip, and therefore the CPU is often referred to as a *microprocessor*. The CPU resides on the mainboard housed in the main unit of the computer. More so than any other computer component, the CPU determines how fast a computer can process information. The speed of the CPU is expressed in gigahertz (abbreviated GHz) and the higher the value, the faster the computer. For example, a computer with a 3 GHz microprocessor chip can process information approximately twice as fast as a computer with a 1.5 GHz chip. The leading manufacturers of these microprocessor chips are Intel and AMD.

The CPU consists of two separate parts: (1) the control unit and (2) the arithmetic/logic unit. Each of these performs a specific function, described as follows.

Control Unit

The **control unit** coordinates the entire computer system functioning as a "traffic patrolman" to direct the step-by-step operation of all the processing functions. Specifically, the control unit reads and interprets the preset instructions of a program and tells the other components of the computer system what to do. During the processing phase, it keeps track of which steps of the program have been performed and which remain. Finally, the control unit collects the output and directs it to the designated output device (e.g., the printer). It is important to note that the control unit does not execute instructions or process any data itself, but directs the computer in how to carry out these functions.

Arithmetic/Logic Unit

The **arithmetic/logic unit** (abbreviated **ALU**) actually executes the program's instructions by performing mathematic computations and logical operations. Mathematic computations include addition, subtraction, multiplication, and division. Logical operations involve making comparisons between items and performing a function based on the results. Items are compared by the ALU to determine if they are equal or if one has a greater or lesser value than the other. These compared values may be either numeric or alphabetic. An example of an alphabetic operation would be alphabetizing a list of patient's names. All processing of data performed by a computer relies on either arithmetic computations, logical comparisons, or a combination of the two. Thus, computers would not be able to perform most of the tasks we find useful without the ALU.

Main Computer Memory

Main computer memory (or simply **main memory**) consists of computer chips mounted on a small board that connects the mainboard. Main memory is responsible for temporarily storing information until ready for use by the CPU. Main memory can be compared to a holding tank for the CPU in which items are placed for immediate access and use when needed for processing. Among those items commonly held in main memory are the operating system, the application program in current use, data waiting to be processed, and information ready for output.

In a microcomputer, main computer memory has a special name known as *RAM.*

RAM is an acronym for **random-access memory** and, as you have just learned, is the main memory of a microcomputer. It is called *random access* because the computer can get to any part of the information stored in its memory directly, rather than having to look through all the rest of its stored information. This is in contrast to **sequential-access memory** in which all stored data must be searched sequentially from beginning to end to locate the desired information. Much less time is involved in locating information using random access, and it is one of the factors that allows computers to perform tasks very quickly.

As previously described, the purpose of RAM is to temporarily store items until they are needed by the computer. When you first turn on the computer, RAM is empty; therefore, you must first place the items you want to work

with in RAM. A copy of the application program is transferred into RAM from the hard disk (by using the mouse to click on the appropriate program icon the desktop of the computer. Data is transferred into RAM through an input device, such as a keyboard. To run the application program, a copy of the operating system needs to be transferred from the hard disk into RAM; this is accomplished automatically by the computer when you turn on the computer. Once these items are in RAM, they are easily accessible and can be quickly retrieved when needed by the CPU for processing. After the data have been processed according to the instructions in the program, the resulting usable information is then placed back in RAM for temporary storage.

One very important aspect of RAM is that it provides only *temporary* storage, not permanent storage. When the computer is turned off, all of the items stored in RAM are "dumped out"; in other words, RAM will be empty when the computer is turned back on and therefore ready to accept more storage items. Because of this, you *must be sure* to permanently store information that you do not want to lose before turning off the computer. In the medical office, this information is stored on the hard disk of the computer. Other common storage devices include USB flash drives and compact discs, which are described later in this chapter.

Storage Capacity of Random-Access Memory

RAM has a **storage capacity,** which refers to the maximum amount of information that RAM can hold at any one time. The capacity of RAM is measured in units of storage known as **bytes.** One byte is approximately equal to one character, such as a letter or number. Stating the capacity of RAM in bytes, however, results in astronomically high numbers. Therefore, it is more convenient to use larger units, such as kilobytes, megabytes, and gigabytes. A **kilobyte (KB)** is equal to 1024 bytes, which is usually rounded off to 1000 bytes. A **megabyte (MB)** is equal to a little more than 1 million bytes; in terms of kilobytes, 1 MB is equal to 1000 KB. An even larger measure than a megabyte is a **gigabyte (GB);** 1 GB is equal to 1 billion bytes or 1000 MB.

As you would imagine, the larger the capacity of RAM, the more information it can hold at one time. For example, a computer with 2 GB of RAM has the ability to hold more than 2 billion bytes. Most microcomputers now come with a main memory of 1 GB or more.

The capacity of a computer's memory (RAM) correlates directly to the level of complexity of the programs it can run. A program takes up a certain amount of space in RAM. A small and simple application program that performs a limited number of tasks occupies much less space in RAM than a large, complex, and powerful program that performs numerous complicated tasks, such as a medical practice management program. The capacity of RAM is an important criterion to consider when working with or purchasing a computer or an application program. A computer with less than the required memory for a particular program would not have enough storage space to hold that program.

Hence, that program could not be run on that particular computer. The packaging of the application program is labeled with information on *computer system requirements*. System requirements tell you what requirements your computer system must have (e.g., type of operating system, microprocessor speed amount of memory, hard disk space) in order to run the program.

Video Card

The **video card** (also known as a *graphics card*) connects to the mainboard through a video card slot. A video card converts video output into electronic signals. These electronic signals are then sent to the monitor, where they are converted into text and images that are displayed on the screen of the monitor.

Sound Card

The **sound card** is a small circuit board that is connected to the mainboard. A sound card converts audio output into electronic signals. The electronic signals are then sent to speakers that convert them into sound, such as sound effects, music, and narration.

Hard Disk

A **hard disk** is housed in a hard disk drive. A hard disk permanently stores information and (unlike RAM) retains this information when the power is off. Hard disks are discussed in more detail later in this chapter under Storage Devices.

Optical Drive

An **optical drive** uses a laser to read or write optical discs, such as CDs and DVDs. Optical discs are discussed in more detail later in this chapter under Storage Devices.

Power Supply

The power supply provides the power needed by the computer to run itself.

Care and Maintenance of the Main Computer Unit

The main computer unit should be placed on a flat, stable surface, such as a computer desk. This prevents excessive vibration during operation, which could loosen the electronic circuit boards. Most main units are now designed (e.g., a tower) to be placed in a vertical position. Information on proper positioning is always indicated in the instruction manual accompanying the computer.

Computers operate best in a moderately cool temperature environment. Extreme heat and inadequate ventilation increases the chance of malfunction. As a precautionary measure, the main unit should not be placed near a window or other areas that receive direct sunlight. In addition, to prevent overheating, the ventilation slots on the main unit should not be obstructed.

The primary cause of improper functioning of the computer is exposure to environmental contaminants, such as dust, dirt, and smoke. For this reason, rooms with computers should be kept clean with no smoking permitted. The casing of the main unit should be periodically wiped with a slightly damp, lint-free cloth to remove dust and dirt. Aerosol sprays, solvents, and abrasives should never be used to clean the casing because they can damage the finish. The interior of the main computer unit should be cleaned occasionally according to the instructions outlined in the computer's user manual.

Liquids should be kept away from the computer. A liquid spilled into the main unit can cause irreparable damage to the electronic circuit boards. In addition, an electrical short may occur and could result in a fire or small explosion.

The main unit is attached by cables to the other computer components (i.e., monitor, keyboard, printer). The cables should be checked on a regular basis to ascertain that they are secure. A loose or disengaged cable can result in temporary malfunctioning of the computer system.

COMPUTER MONITOR

A computer monitor is a piece of electrical equipment that displays images generated by a computer. The monitor permits the user to view both **input,** or more specifically, the data entered into the computer, and **output,** or the information produced by the computer as a result of processing.

Viewing the input displayed on the monitor allows the user to check the data for accuracy as it is entered. As an output device, the monitor is often used to review information that needs to be viewed briefly and for which a printed copy (hardcopy) is not necessary. For example, if a patient calls your office to inquire when his next appointment is scheduled, you can quickly call up this information, view it on the display screen, and relay it to the patient. The term used to describe the visual display of information on the screen of the monitor is **softcopy.** In summary, softcopy is useful when information is necessary immediately and a permanent printed record is not required.

Types of Monitors

The two main types of monitors used with a microcomputer include CRT monitors and LCD flat panel monitors. These are discussed in more detail below.

CRT monitor   A CRT monitor is a big, bulky, and heavy visual display device similar to most television sets (Figure 38-3). CRT is an abbreviation for *cathode-ray tube*. A cathode-ray tube works by spraying electrons onto a viewing screen under the direction of a magnetic field, to form characters on the screen. In the past, this was the type of monitor used most often with a microcomputer system because it produced a quality image at a reasonable cost. However, LCD monitors are increasing in popularity as their costs decrease in price.

LCD flat panel monitor   An LCD flat panel desktop monitor (Figure 38-4) is small, lightweight, and compact, and therefore takes up much less desk space than a CRT monitor. LCD monitors consume very little power and

Figure 38-3. CRT monitor.

Figure 38-4. LCD flat panel monitor.

are therefore more energy efficient than CRT monitors. LCD is an abbreviation for *liquid crystal display.* An LCD monitor creates a visual image on the screen by manipulating light within a layer of liquid crystal cells. With an LCD monitor, it is sometimes difficult to view the image on the screen from an angle.

Screen Size

Screen size refers to the measurement of a computer screen in inches from one corner of the screen diagonally across to the opposite corner. (*Note:* Computer manufacturers usually include the plastic casing around the screen when stating the size of a CRT monitor. This means that the actual screen size would not be as big as is stated by the manufacturer. When stating the size of an LCD monitor, the plastic casing is not included in the measurement, which gives you the actual size of the screen.) The typical desktop monitor used in a medical office has a screen size from 17 to 20 inches

across measured diagonally, with the range of available screen sizes falling between 14 and 23 inches.

Monitor Resolution

An important area of consideration when working with a computer system is the resolution of the monitor. The term **resolution** refers to the sharpness of the image displayed on the screen. A computer monitor with a high resolution produces a sharp image with crisp, clear, easy-to-read characters that works to prevent eyestrain and headaches. High resolutions also allow the computer to display a larger work area.

Resolution is measured in units called *picture elements* or *pixels.* **Pixels** are "dot" locations on the screen that can be lit up as needed to display characters and other images. The more dots present, the sharper the image. A monitor with a resolution of 1280 × 1024 can display 1280 pixels horizontally and 1024 pixels vertically on the screen. Screen resolutions typically range from 640 × 480 to 1600 × 1200 or more. High-resolution monitors display 1280 × 1024 pixels or more and are usually preferred for use in the medical office.

Dot Pitch

Dot pitch (abbreviated DP) is a measure of the clarity of the images on the display screen. *Dot pitch* refers to the amount of space between the dots or pixels that make up the images on the screen. DP is measured in millimeters and the less space between the pixels, the better the image quality. Currently, computers come with a DP between 0.26 mm and 0.23 mm.

Monitor Controls

Located on either the front or side of the monitor are three important controls that are used to operate and adjust the display screen. The first of these is a push-button *on/off button.* When the monitor is turned on, an indicator light comes on denoting the monitor is receiving power and ready for use.

Two controls exist for adjusting the resolution of the viewing screen: the *brightness* control and the *contrast* control. These controls work much like the same controls on a television set. The brightness control allows you to increase or decrease the intensity of the images on the screen. This control should be adjusted until the background just disappears, which provides a good balance between the screen and character brightness.

The contrast control is used to adjust the screen for comfortable viewing. *Contrast* refers to the degree of difference between the light and dark areas on the display screen. For example, if you work on a monitor that displays black text on a white background, the contrast would be the amount of difference that exists between the text characters (dark area) and the background (light area). Too much contrast makes it uncomfortable to look at the characters on the screen, whereas not enough contrast results in difficulty in viewing the characters. Because of individual viewing preferences, you should adjust both the brightness and contrast control when first beginning work on the computer to find the setting that works best for your viewing comfort.

Other controls typically found on a computer monitor include vertical and horizontal size and position controls. As their names suggest, these controls adjust both the size and position of the screen image.

Monitor Ergonomics

The monitor should be placed directly in front of the user and at an arm's length distance when sitting back in a chair. This position provides the most comfortable viewing distance. The monitor should be positioned so that the top of the monitor is approximately 2 to 3 inches above eye level. This position helps to prevent back and neck tension. It is known that eye muscles must work harder to focus on near objects. Therefore, when working on the computer for a prolonged period of time, occasionally focus your eyes on a distant object (more than 20 feet away) to prevent eye strain. It is also important to blink frequently while you work to lubricate and moisten the eyes to prevent them from drying out.

To avoid glare, the monitor should be positioned so that the screen does not reflect bright light, which could result in eye strain. For example, positioning the monitor directly in front of a bright window causes a distracting reflection on the screen. Subdued overhead lighting is considered best for computer use because it causes the least amount of glare. Glare filters are available to help reduce unavoidable reflections, such as from bright overhead fluorescent lights. A glare filter is a tinted transparent covering that fits over the front of the computer screen similar to placing a camera filter over the lens of a camera.

Monitor Care and Maintenance

The monitor should rest on a flat, stable surface, such as a computer desk. A number of ventilation slots on the monitor allow heat to escape. To prevent overheating of the monitor, do not stack items around the monitor and never place anything on top of the monitor (not even a piece of paper).

Monitors collect dust and dirt, and therefore must be properly maintained. The screen should be cleaned regularly. Microfiber cloths used to clean eyeglasses can be used to clean the screen of a monitor. The screen can also be cleaned with a commercially available computer screen cleaner applied with a clean, lint-free cloth. The cleaner should not be applied directly to the screen as it may run down into the inside of the case and damage the electrical circuits. Keeping the screen clean helps prevent distracting reflections.

The outside casing of the monitor should periodically be wiped with a damp, lint-free cloth to remove dust and dirt. Dust and dirt act like insulation and cause heat to build up in the monitor. This heat causes the electronic components within the monitor to wear out much faster than they normally would. Aerosol sprays, solvents, and abrasives should not be used to clean the casing because they can damage the finish.

COMPUTER KEYBOARD

The computer keyboard is the most common input device. It contains keys that are pressed to enter data and instructions into the computer. Different brands of computer keyboards vary in size, shape, and layout, but all contain the same basic elements (Figure 38-5).

Computer keyboards include all the keys normally found on a typewriter keyboard. The composition of the keyboard is alphanumeric; that is, it consists of both alphabetic and numeric keys. The keys are located in the same place as on the standard typewriter keyboard and are used for the same purpose. Computer keyboards produce both upper and lowercase letters and have the standard typewriter "QWERTY" layout, named for the first row of letters. Many desktop computer keyboards also have a numeric keypad on the right side of the keyboard, which is used for entering numbers quickly.

As previously explained, computers can only work with electronic data. When a key is pressed on a computer keyboard, an electronic code is generated, which is passed along to the computer for processing. At the same time, the electronic code is sent to the video card, which then allows that computer to display the input as words and symbols on the monitor.

The keyboard of a desktop computer is typically attached by a cable to the main computer unit. This allows the user to position the keyboard according to his or her preference and comfort. Cordless, wireless keyboards are also available. A wireless keyboard communicates with the computer through radio waves or infrared light waves.

Special Keys

The most significant difference between a computer keyboard and a typewriter keyboard is the presence of additional keys known as **special keys.** Special keys issue commands to the computer to perform specific functions on the information displayed on the screen. Pressing a special key does not cause a character to be typed on the screen, nor does the command appear on printed copy. Instead these keys allow the user to perform such tasks as

Figure 38-5. Computer keyboard.

saving text, printing text, capitalizing text, deleting and inserting text, and moving the cursor.

An example of a special key that functions the same regardless of the type of computer or program being used is the Enter key. The Enter key (also called the *return key*) is the most frequently used special key. Pressing the Enter key tells the computer to act on the instructions that have been given to it. In simple terms, it gives the computer the "okay" to go ahead with a function. For example, if you have given the computer the Print command, the Enter key can be pressed to tell the computer to go ahead with this instruction.

Special keys can be divided into categories and include modifier keys, lock keys, and navigation keys. *Modifier keys* are used in conjunction with another key to enter commands into the computer and include the following: control key, shift key, alternate key, and the command key. For example, with most application programs, control-P can be used to print a document. *Lock keys* are used to lock a key in position and include the following: caps lock, numeric lock, and scroll lock. *Navigation keys* are used to control the movement of the cursor on the screen and include the following: arrow keys, home/end key, page scroll key, enter key, backspace key, insert key, delete key, and tab key.

Most keyboards have *function keys* that can be programmed to perform certain tasks that will assist the user, such as saving text or printing a document. The number of such keys varies but is now usually 12 or more. Function keys are usually located above the top row of alphanumeric keys on the keyboard. These keys are usually preprogrammed by the application software package that makes use of them, but some computers permit these keys to be user programmed directly from the keyboard.

Mouse

After the keyboard, the mouse is the second most commonly used input device. A mouse is a pointing device that fits comfortably under the palm of your hand. The mouse is used to move the pointer on the screen to an object on the screen, such as a menu item, an icon, or a line of text. The mouse must then be "clicked" to perform a certain action associated with that object.

Keyboard Ergonomics

To prevent muscle fatigue of the upper extremities, the computer keyboard should be placed at a level that is lower than that of a conventional desk or table. The feet should be flat on the floor and the hands should rest comfortably at the keyboard with the shoulders relaxed and the elbows flexed at a 90-degree angle or tilted slightly upward. An adjustable chair with good back support is recommended to attain the proper typing height for each individual working with the computer (Figure 38-6).

When entering data, a light touch should be used and the hands and fingers should be kept as relaxed as possible. If using a mouse, position it at the same height as the keyboard. Be sure to allow adequate workspace to use both the keyboard and mouse comfortably. These measures help to prevent strain on the wrists and hands.

An adequate working space should be available to position the material being entered into the computer. The material should be placed so that it can be viewed easily either by placing it lying flat on the work surface or being held vertically in a copy holder.

Keyboard Care and Maintenance

With extended use, a residue may build up on the surface of the keyboard. This residue, often referred to as *grime,* should be cleaned with an antiseptic wipe or a slightly damp, lint-free cloth. Aerosol sprays should never be used to clean the keyboard because liquid may drip down into the keyboard, damaging its electrical components. The keyboard interior can be "dusted" by using a compressed inert gas that comes in a pressurized can and is available from

Figure 38-6. Keyboard ergonomics.

computer supply stores. Alternatively, a vacuum cleaner with a small brush attachment may be used to clean the keyboard interior.

The following steps should be followed when cleaning the computer keyboard:

1. Shut down the computer.
2. Disconnect the keyboard cable.
3. Hold the keyboard upside down and shake it to remove any dust, dirt, or crumbs that may be stuck in the keyboard.
4. Clean the keyboard using a can of compressed air following the manufacturer's instructions.
5. Clean the top and side of the keys with an antiseptic wipe or a damp, lint-free cloth to remove grime. A cotton swab moistened with alcohol can be used to clean between the spaces of the keys.
6. Allow the keyboard to dry completely (about 30 minutes) before reconnecting it to the computer.

Because of their electronic components, computer keyboards can be damaged if liquids spill into them, particularly those that are sweet or sticky, such as soft drinks. Therefore, it is best not to place beverages close to the keyboard. If a liquid is accidentally spilled into the keyboard, the computer should immediately be turned off. If the liquid spilled is thin and clear, such as water, unplug the keyboard, turn it upside down and shake it gently to get as much liquid out as possible. Keep the keyboard inverted to allow additional liquid to drain out and use a paper towel or cloth to wipe off the top of the keyboard. Let the keyboard dry in an inverted position for 24 hours at room temperature. If, after taking these steps, the keyboard does not work, it should be replaced. A greasy, sweet, or sticky liquid such as a soft drink spilled into the keyboard often causes permanent damage and the keyboard must be replaced.

PRINTER

A printer is an output device capable of printing text and graphics on paper. Printers convert processed data from a combination of electronic impulses into a printed form called **hardcopy.** In the medical office, a hardcopy of the computer input is frequently required; examples include patient reminders, patient receipts, prescriptions, patient statements, and office reports.

Some printers can also double as fax machines and photocopiers, but this is only practical when there is only a small volume of work. A printer can be dedicated to one computer or can be networked to a number of computers.

The printers most commonly used in the medical office are inkjet and laser printers. At one time, dot-matrix printers were frequently used in the medical office (Figure 38-7). Dot-matrix printers use an impact printing method that allows them to print multiple-copy documents using carbonless copy paper (e.g., encounter forms). Today, most offices prefer to use inkjet and laser printers due to their faster printing speed and quieter mode of operation.

Figure 38-7. Dot matrix printer.

Figure 38-8. Inkjet printer.

Inkjet Printer

An inkjet printer (Figure 38-8) uses droplets of ink to form text characters and graphics. This type of printer contains nozzles that spray tiny drops of ink onto the paper to create an image. Inkjet printers are lightweight and inexpensive and can produce text and graphics in both black and white and color on a variety of paper types.

Printing speed refers to the number of pages per minute (ppm) generated by the printer. Printing speed for an inkjet printer ranges from 8 to 36 ppm. Pages that contain text print at a faster rate than pages that are in color or contain graphics.

Although the initial cost of an inkjet printer is low, operating costs are higher than those of a laser printer. The ink used by an inkjet printer is contained in cartridges, which are expensive and must be replaced frequently. Most inkjet printers have at least two ink cartridges—one containing black ink, and one or more containing colored ink.

Laser Printer

The most significant feature of a laser printer (Figure 38-9) is that it has a "computer of its own" to direct its functioning. Laser printers use a micro-thin beam of light (laser beam), electric charges, and a toner powder to produce each page of text. Under direction of the printer's computer, the laser beam is bounced off a series of mirrors onto a positively charged rotating drum. The pulses of the beam correspond to the characters making up the document being printed. The areas where the laser beam hits the drum become neutral, which enables the toner powder to stick to them and form characters. Finally, the characters are transferred from the rotating drum to paper with the use of pressure and heat to solidify the toner powder on the paper. This process is similar to that of a photocopy machine.

The toner powder used with a laser printer is housed in a plastic cartridge and must be replaced when it runs out. Most laser printers have an operating panel on the printer that displays the level of toner remaining in the cartridge. Although the initial cost of a laser printer is more than an inkjet printer, the operating cost is less than an inkjet. This is because the cost per page of using toner powder (laser printer) is less than the cost per page of using ink cartridges (inkjet printer).

The print quality of laser printers is superb, nearly attaining the quality of typesetting seen in textbooks. Laser printers are available in both black-and-white and color models. Other advantages of laser printers include their fast printing speed and quiet mode of operation. The printing speed of laser printers is faster than that of inkjet printers. Depending on the model of laser printer, the printing speed ranges from 12 to 35 or more ppm. Text prints at a faster rate and color and graphics print at a slower rate. Laser printers do not have as many mechanical moving parts as other types of printers, which usually reduces their frequency of repair.

Printer Care and Maintenance

Proper maintenance keeps the printer operating at its best and prolongs its life. Some general guidelines that should be followed to properly care for and maintain an inkjet and laser printer are as follows:

1. Place the printer on a flat, stable surface.
2. Avoid placing the printer in a location that would expose it to direct sunlight, excessive heat, moisture, or dust.
3. Sufficient room should be left around the printer to allow for easy access for such tasks as adding paper and replacing ink or toner cartridges.
4. Add paper when needed following the manufacturer's instructions. Inkjet and laser printers use individual sheets of paper stored in a tray in the printer's casing.
5. Replace ink cartridges in inkjet printers and toner cartridges in laser printers as required following the manufacturer's instructions.
6. After turning off the printer, wait at least 5 seconds before turning it back on. Rapid switching of the power off and on can damage the printer.
7. The printer should be cleaned regularly to remove accumulated dust and dirt. The outside case should be cleaned with a soft clean cloth dampened with a mild detergent solution. Never use strong detergents or solvents on the casing because they could damage the finish. The inside of the printer should be cleaned according to the instructions in the printer's user manual.

STORAGE DEVICES

A **storage device** consists of a storage medium that permanently stores information for later retrieval by the computer. A storage device retains its information after the power has been removed and is used to store both programs and data. Examples of storage devices available for microcomputer systems include hard disks, floppy disks, CDs, DVDs, and USB flash drives, which are discussed on the following pages.

The **storage capacity** of a storage device is the maximum amount of information that the device can hold. Storage capacity is measured in bytes, such as kilobytes, megabytes, and gigabytes. Storage capacity varies widely based on the type of storage device. For example, a floppy disk can only hold 1.4 MB, whereas a typical hard disk has a storage capacity of 250 GB.

Hard Disks

A **hard disk** derives its name from the fact that it consists of thin, rigid platters made of metal or glass (Figure 38-10). The composition of a hard disk is designed to maximize its

Figure 38-9. Laser printer.

Figure 38-10. Hard disk drive.

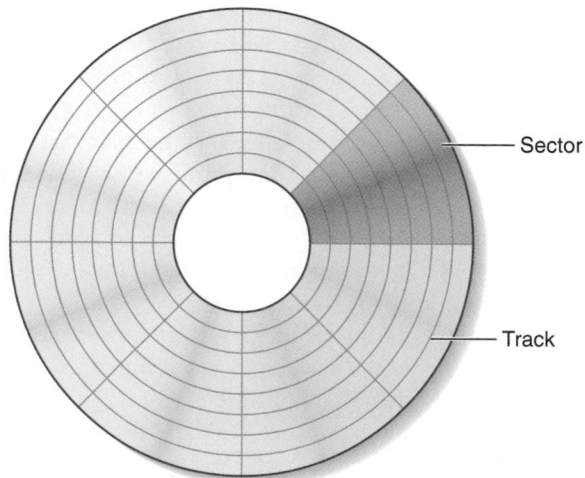

Figure 38-11. Tracks and sectors.

important functions: the storage and retrieval of information. To accommodate the storage of information, hard disks are coated with a magnetically sensitive material. Data are stored on the disk as magnetic particles.

To store and retrieve the information on the disk as quickly as possible, a method or organization that divides the disk into designated areas similar to the division of a piece of property into housing lots is used. The disk surface is divided into a set of concentric circles; each of these circles is called a *track* (Figure 38-11). Data are stored on these tracks in the form of magnetized particles. Tracks are further divided into *sectors* that resemble the wedge-shaped pieces of a pie (see Figure 38-11). Through a process called *formatting,* the tracks and sectors are numerically marked to facilitate the location of information stored on the disk.

The following example provides a comparison of how the arrangement of tracks and sectors and formatting assists in locating information stored on the disk. Let's say that a friend invites you to her house at 102 Sunnyside Drive in Greenfield Village. You arrive at Greenfield Village and first locate the proper street and then you look for the house number. But just think how difficult and time consuming it would be to locate your friend's house without a street name or a house number. Comparing this example to the

organization of hard disks, tracks and sectors are comparable to the division of Greenfield Village into streets and housing lots, and the formatting process (which numerically marks each track and sector) is comparable to the street names and house numbers.

Hard Disk Drive

Information is stored on a hard disk and retrieved from a hard disk within a device known as a *hard disk drive.* A hard disk drive is a mechanical device that rotates a hard disk at a high rate of speed. A read/write head mounted on an arm (see Figure 38-10) floats on a layer of air above the spinning disk and has instant access to all the tracks and sectors on the disk. All computers have an internal hard disk drive, meaning it is located inside the main computer unit. Because a hard disk is very sensitive to dirt, dust, and smoke, the entire disk unit is encased in a permanently sealed, air-tight container to protect it from these contaminants. The entire disk unit (consisting of the hard disks and read/write heads) makes up the hard disk drive.

The purpose of the read/write head is to (1) store information onto and (2) retrieve information from the hard disk. The term used to describe the storage of information onto a storage device is **write,** and the term used to describe the retrieval of information from a storage device is **read.** When information is written from a hard disk, it is transferred from RAM to the hard disk. On the other hand, when information is read, it is transferred from the hard disk and into RAM.

To increase storage capacity, a hard disk consists of two or more platters stacked on top of one another. Both sides of the disk are used to store information and each side of the disk has its own read/write head. Hard disks come in a variety of storage sizes beginning at about 80 GB and ranging up to 750 GB or more depending on the computer.

Floppy Disks

Floppy disks (also known as "floppies") were once commonly used storage devices for microcomputers. They are now being phased out and have been replaced by USB flash drives and compact discs. In fact, new computers do not include a floppy disk drive as a standard feature. If desired by the buyer, it must be requested as a customized add-on feature to the main computer unit or an external floppy disk drive must be purchased separately and attached to the main unit through a cable.

A **floppy disk** is a circular, thin, platter-like storage medium with a flexible, bending quality that gives rise to the term "floppy." A floppy disk is made of Mylar plastic that has been coated with a magnetically sensitive material. Information is stored on and retrieved from a floppy disk using tracks and sectors in a similar manner to a hard disk. It is not possible to view the actual floppy disk first-hand because it is almost entirely enclosed and sealed in a permanent protective plastic covering known as the *disk jacket* (Figure 38-12). Thus, the round disk appears square because

Figure 38-12. Permanent storage devices.

of its enclosure in the disk jacket. The disk must be placed in a floppy disk drive in order to store or retrieve information.

Advantages of floppy disks include their low cost and portability. Disadvantages include low storage capacity and their sensitivity to damage by environmental factors. Even a floppy disk with the highest storage capacity only has a maximum capacity of 1.4 MB. Therefore, to accommodate a large amount of information, numerous floppy disks would be required. In addition, environmental factors, such as heat, magnets, dust, dirt, smoke, food, and liquids, can cause destruction of the magnetic material of the disk, resulting in loss of data.

Optical Discs

Optical discs are storage devices that store data using laser technology. Optical discs are used to store system software, application software, data, photographs, music, and movies. An optical disc consists of a flat, round portable disc made of metal, plastic, and lacquer (see Figure 38-12). It is usually 4.75 inches in diameter and less than 1/20 of an inch thick.

An optical disc may be *read-only,* which means that data can only be read (retrieved) from the disc; data cannot be written (saved) on the disc. An example of a read-only disc is a CD-ROM. The data on a CD-ROM are stored as microscopic pits along a spiral groove that runs along the surface of the disc. Data are read from a CD-ROM with a beam of laser light known as a *laser diode.*

Most application software today comes on CD-ROMs and is installed onto a computer's hard drive to operate. CD-ROMs hold about 650 MB of information. Sometimes, only a portion of the application program is installed into the computer's hard drive; the rest remains on the CD-ROM so as not to fill up the hard drive storage capacity. In this case, the CD must be in the CD-ROM optical drive to successfully run the program.

Optical discs may also be *read/write,* which means that data can be read from the disc and written onto the disc. Writing on an optical disc is often termed "burning" a disc.

An example of a read/write disc is a CD-RW (compact disc rewritable).

A DVD (digital versatile disc or digital video disc) uses another type of optical disc technology. This type of disc can hold about six times as much information as a CD-ROM, and therefore it has become popular as a means of storing music and movies, both of which require large amounts of storage space.

An optical drive uses a laser to read an optical disc or write onto an optical disc. Today's computers include one or more optical drives that are installed in drive bays on the main computer unit. To use an optical drive, a button is pushed to slide out a tray, the optical disc is then inserted into the tray (label-side up), and the same button is pushed to close the tray.

USB Flash Drive

A USB flash drive is a portable storage device that consists of a small circuit board in a plastic case (see Figure 38-12). Other terms for a flash drive include a *jump drive* and a *thumb drive.* A flash drive stores information using flash memory, which is a type of electrical computer memory. To use a flash drive, it must be inserted into a USB port on the main unit. A USB flash drive has a storage capacity that ranges between 1 GB and 64 GB or more. Since the development of flash drives, floppy disks have become much less popular as a portable storage device. This is because a flash drive has a much greater storage capacity and is easier to carry around than a floppy disk.

MEDICAL OFFICE COMPUTERIZATION

Medical office computerization is the use of the computer to perform medical office administrative procedures. With the advent of the microcomputer, medical offices now use a computer to perform administrative procedures that were previously performed manually. This, in turn, has increased the demand for qualified individuals trained in medical office computerization not only to perform the administrative tasks on the computer, but also to instruct other staff members in computer operations.

Prerequisite Computer Concepts

Before beginning to work with a medical practice management program, it is important to first acquire a thorough knowledge of computer concepts. Just as medical terminology is a necessary prerequisite to clinical procedure courses, a knowledge of computer concepts is necessary to effectively operate a computer system in the front office.

The benefits of understanding computer concepts include increased confidence and ease when working on the computer and the ability to understand the computer terminology presented in the program user manual. Furthermore, a computer concepts base helps you to communicate with computer software specialists, such as the technical support staff for your medical practice management program. Working with technical support is often necessary when first learning the medical practice management program or when a problem is encountered with the program. To acquire this foundation, the beginning of this chapter provides a presentation of computer concepts.

Impact of Medical Office Computerization

Computers are often promoted as being the solution to all medical office management problems. Although there are distinct advantages to using a computer, it should be realized that there are also some disadvantages that can lead to difficulties. It is important to be aware of these problem areas so that steps can be taken to either prevent them altogether or be better prepared for them if they occur. Adequate preparation will result in the least amount of disruption to the efficient running of a computerized front office. The following discussion outlines both advantages and disadvantages of medical management computerization.

Advantages of Computerization

The advantages of computerizing the front office include the following:

Speed and productivity   One of the principal advantages of a computer is that it can process a large amount of data quickly. For example, if your physician asks you to compile a list of all patients with a diagnosis of hypertension, accomplishing this task by hand would require considerable time and effort. However, with a computer an inquiry search can be performed in which the computer searches all the patient files and automatically generates a list of patients with hypertension. Billing and health insurance requirements have placed a tremendous burden on the medical office of today. In addition, the completion of insurance claims becomes ever more complicated. Thus, a large portion of front office responsibility is often devoted to preparing and submitting patient statements and insurance claims. Because they can prepare and process items in a short period of time, computers provide much assistance in this area. In addition, faster computer processing of these items often leads to better collections for the medical office.

Efficiency   Computers are particularly good at performing repetitive tasks in which information is used over and over again but in a different format. For example, once a patient's name and address have been entered into the computer's database, they can be used on a number of different forms without having to reenter them. The computer automatically transfers this information where needed, based on the task being performed. The patient's name and address can be automatically transferred by the computer to a patient statement, insurance form, and mailing label depending on the task being performed. Medical practice management programs also keep track of the status of functions that have been executed in the office, such as the submission of insurance claims.

Accessibility   Information that has been entered into the computer system is easy to retrieve when needed. For example, after a patient registration record has been entered, it is quite simple to request information on that patient and have it instantly displayed on the screen of the monitor. This avoids having to perform the much more time-consuming task of manually hunting through a filing system to locate the patient's chart.

Audit trail   The computer can keep track of data entry. When new information is entered or existing information is changed, a log is created to record the time and date of the entry, as well as the name of the computer operator. This log is stored and can be retrieved by the practice manager to detect irregularities. If an error was made, the program lists the name of the operator and date the information was entered.

Reduced costs   After the initial cost of purchasing the hardware and software, computerization of the front office helps to decrease operating costs by reducing the amount of time required to perform front office procedures.

Disadvantages of Computerization

The disadvantages presented by computers in the medical office include the following:

Initial cost   An initial investment is required for the purchase of hardware and software. Hardware is defined as the physical devices making up a computer system (e.g., main computer unit, keyboard, monitor, printer), whereas software is a general term for the programs or instructions that tell a computer what to do. The cost of software (e.g., medical practice management program) varies considerably from vendor to vendor, and the hardware expense depends on the complexity of the software, number of computers, and type and number of printers. The combined expense of these items can easily fall into thousands of dollars. In addition, an office may periodically upgrade its computer system or even purchase an entirely new system altogether, leading to further expenses.

Time investment   Because medical management programs perform highly sophisticated tasks, it takes considerable time to learn a program and use it with ease. Most software vendors provide on-site training of staff for a newly purchased program, as well as technical support when problems are encountered with the program. Even with all of this assistance, however, learning a medical management program can easily last a month or more. During this time, the medical assistant may experience much frustration when difficulty is encountered in executing a task. However, once the initial training period is completed, most individuals agree the time and patience expended are worth the outcome.

Start-up tasks   Certain tasks must be performed before a medical practice management program becomes operational, or in other words, before it can be used to perform medical office administrative procedures. Fortunately, most offices are already computerized and these start-up tasks have previously been performed. However, if an office is just opening, or if an office purchases a new practice management program, start-up tasks will be required. Examples of start-up tasks include (1) all of the diagnoses and procedures used in the office must be entered into the computer system and (2) patient registration records must be set up, which includes entering demographic and insurance data on each patient. All start-up tasks must be performed before the program can be used to operate the front office. The start-up data only need to be entered once. Later, additional information can be added as needed and the length of input time is greatly diminished.

Computer System Malfunctions

Even the best hardware and software systems can and will occasionally fail, and one or more of the front office procedures will come to an abrupt halt. Some problems have no explanations, whereas others are directly related to a specific event, such as operator error, a software "bug," or a hardware malfunction.

Measures to Promote Efficient Computer Operation

The challenges presented by computerizing the front office can for the most part be overcome by implementing the following preventative measures. These measures work to reduce computer frustration and promote the efficient running of a computerized medical office.

1. *Selection of hardware and software:* Hardware and software should be selected from experienced and established vendors. Some medical offices use a consultant to assist with this process.
2. *Qualified personnel:* Individuals working on the computer should be well trained in computer concepts and hands-on computer operation. This can be accomplished by employing office staff who have graduated from a formal educational program or by having the front office staff attend computer workshops and seminars. Untrained staff can adversely affect the efficient operation of a computer system.
3. *Proper care and maintenance of the computer system:* Proper care and maintenance of the computer system are undoubtedly directly related to reliable operation of the system. The beginning of this chapter presents the proper care and maintenance for each component in the computer system. Make sure you thoroughly review this information before working with a computer system. In addition to providing many years of reliable service, a well-cared-for system is much less likely to malfunction.

MEDICAL PRACTICE MANAGEMENT PROGRAM

A **medical practice management program** provides instructions to the computer for performing front office procedures. Practice management programs consist of a number of areas of specialization. Each area of specialization

is known as a *system,* and each system performs procedures related to its particular area of specialization. Practice management programs include the following: patient registration system, posting transactions system, appointment system, patient billing system, insurance billing system, reports system, and file maintenance system. Each system is described in detail next.

Patient Registration System

The patient registration system is used to set up a registration record for each patient in the medical practice. The patient registration record includes demographic and medical insurance information, such as the patient's name and address, telephone number, gender, date of birth, Social Security number, the patient's insurance carrier, policy number, and group number. This system is also used to review and update information on existing registration records. For example, if the patient's address changes, this system is used to delete the old address and enter the new address. Information entered into the patient registration system is used for a number of procedures, such as preparing a new patient's chart, posting transactions, and processing patient statements and insurance claims.

Appointment System

The appointment system handles all procedures related to appointment scheduling. These include making an appointment, canceling an appointment, rescheduling an appointment, finding an appointment, printing an appointment log, and printing a patient reminder card. Occasionally a medical office prefers to use an appointment book for patient scheduling rather than the computer. Even though the computer is faster, some medical offices prefer to have a written record of appointments rather than storing this information in the computer system. They reason that in the event of a computer breakdown, a written record of appointments is still accessible.

Computerized appointment scheduling accomplishes three important goals. First, it is easier to change an appointment on a computer than with pencil and paper. Using a computer, the patient's name can simply be deleted and the space in the schedule template left open. Second, at the beginning of the day, the day's schedule can be printed out and does not have to be generated manually from the appointment book. Third, if a patient needs to make regular weekly or monthly visits, a time of day and day of week can be chosen and the computer will automatically record the patient's name in that time slot for as many visits as are needed.

Posting Transactions System

When a patient has been seen by the physician, the medical assistant must post the charges of the office visit and any payments made by the patient. The posting transactions system is responsible for performing this task.

The posting transactions system lets you post charges for all the services and procedures performed on a patient. The medical assistant enters the services and procedures provided to the patient from the encounter form. The encounter form lists all of the services and procedures that were performed during the visit. The computer has codes for all services and procedures in its database and knows how much should be charged for each service and procedure.

In addition, the posting transactions system also permits you to post payments made by the patient (e.g., copayment) or a third-party payer. This system conveniently allows you to print out a patient receipt of the time-of-service (TOS) charges and payments.

Patient Billing System

One of the most important tasks required for the effective functioning of a medical office is to ensure prompt payment of patient bills. The function of the patient billing system is to prepare bills and print billing statements. When patient charges, payments, and adjustments are posted, this information is stored in the computer and is available when needed by the patient billing system. This system is responsible for searching the medical practice database to obtain the information necessary to generate bills for patients with outstanding balances.

Insurance Billing System

The function of the insurance billing system is to prepare and generate insurance claims. As procedures and diagnoses are entered into the computer during posting transactions, they are stored in the medical practice database. Later, this information is available when needed to prepare insurance claims. From the information stored in the database, the computer can automatically fill out every portion of the insurance claim form.

Insurance claims can be submitted to insurance companies either by mailing paper claim forms or sending them electronically. Medical practices are moving to electronic filing of insurance claims. With electronic filing, the insurance claim is sent using a computer protocol called *electronic data interchange.* Issues of data security in electronic transactions and their effect on patient confidentiality have been the biggest barriers to more rapid implementation of electronic claim submission. With electronic claim filing comes electronic payment, which means that insurance companies transfer payment electronically into the medical practice's bank account rather than issuing paper checks.

Reports System

The function of the reports system is to generate a variety of reports for the medical practice. The information contained in the reports is accessed by the computer from the medical practice database. These reports allow the physician to review and analyze many business and practice activities.

File Maintenance System

Before a medical practice management program becomes operational or, in other words, before you can start performing front office procedures on the computer, a number of start-up tasks must be performed. These tasks are performed using the file maintenance system and are required in order to customize the practice management program to meet the specific requirements of a medical office. Start-up tasks include the following: entering practice information, assigning user passwords, entering provider information, entering diagnosis and procedure codes, entering insurance carriers, entering place of service information, and entering referring physicians into the computer system.

Fortunately, most offices are already computerized and these start-up tasks have previously been performed. However, if an office is just opening, or if an office purchases a new practice management program, start-up tasks will be required. Once a practice management program is operational, the file maintenance system continues to be used to add additional information as required and to review, edit, and delete information previously entered into the system.

ELECTRONIC MEDICAL RECORD

An **electronic medical record (EMR)** or *electronic health record (EHR)* is a computerized record of the important health information regarding a patient including the care of that individual and the progress of the patient's condition.

Memories *from* Externship

Emma Hayes: When I did my externship, it was the first time I really realized how much a modern medical office relies on its computer system. At that time, the office where I was placed was using a computer program to schedule appointments and manage the patient billing, but they were using a traditional paper medical record. There were four computers in the office, and they were networked together with two laser printers. The night before, we printed a list of patients scheduled for the next day, and we used that list to pull the medical records. In the evening, we also backed up all the computer files from that day. We were using a magnetic tape drive at that time to make a copy of all the files from the financial management software and appointment program. Individuals who did word processing or used a spreadsheet program had to back up their own files. I think that there wouldn't be enough storage space for most offices to do backups this way today. One day, the office computer system was not working, and we couldn't look anything up. It was very frustrating because we didn't know how much the patient's copayment was and we couldn't enter information about the visit. We did have the paper charge slips that the physicians had filled out, and by the next day everything was working again. I think it would be even more difficult now because we are using an electronic medical record as well. ∎

Prepare for Success

Making the transition to an EMR is a major undertaking for a medical office. Medical offices are slowly moving toward the EMR. Approximately 25% of the medical offices in the United States have converted to an EMR and the percentage is expected to gradually increase over time. The biggest deterrent is the financial and time investment required for a medical office to make the conversion to the EMR.

EMR software allows for the creation, storage, organization, editing, and retrieval of medical records on a computer. The EMR software is usually linked to the practice management software. This allows the EMR to communicate with the practice management software and facilitates certain administrative tasks, such as billing and insurance.

As previously discussed in Chapter 36, a medical record consists of numerous documents. Each document in the medical record has a specific function. In a paper-based patient record (PPR), some of these documents consist of preprinted forms that contain specific information entered by a physician or other health professional (e.g., patient registration form, health history form, laboratory report form). With an EMR, the preprinted forms of a PPR are displayed on a computer screen and each form (known as a *template*) is filled out in much the same way as a paper form. A familiar example of an on-screen form is the form an individual completes when purchasing an item on the Internet; in this case, the form includes spaces (known as *fields*) for the individual to enter shipping and billing information.

Advantages of the Electronic Medical Record

The incorporation of an EMR in the medical office typically leads to better quality patient care through improved communication, faster access to data, and clearer and better documentation. These advantages are accomplished in the following ways:

Speed and productivity   One of the principal advantages of an EMR is that the computer can retrieve requested documents from a patient's record very quickly. This avoids having to perform the much more time-consuming task of manually hunting through the record to locate this information. In addition, documents received from outside facilities, such as laboratory reports, can be stored very quickly in the EMR. EMRs do not need to be filed as with a paper-based medical record. This saves considerable time and frees up the office space required to store paper records. Paper costs are also reduced and time is saved in not having to look for lost charts.

Efficiency   EMR software facilitates the entry of data into the patient's medical record. To assist in entering data, EMR programs use point and click technology, such as check-boxes and drop-down lists. A familiar example of this is the drop-down list of states often used when an individual must indicate his or her state on an on-line address form. EMR programs also have the capability to print customized patient education instructions and handouts. For example, if a patient has been diagnosed

with strep throat, patient education on strep throat can be printed and given to the patient. One of the principle advantages of an EMR is the ability to generate prescriptions, which is described in detail later in this chapter.

Accessibility   The EMR provides ready access to the patient's medical record. A patient's EMR is available at any EMR computer workstation, allowing more than one person to view the chart at the same time. The EMR is also readily accessible if a patient telephones the office. This avoids having to find the patient's record and calling the patient back.

Disadvantages of the Electronic Medical Record

The disadvantages presented by the EMR in the medical office include the following:

Initial cost   An initial investment is required for the purchase of hardware and EMR software. Because computer access is required to use an EMR, the office must have a sufficient number of desktop computers, laptop computers, or tablet computers to accommodate the number of health care providers in the medical office. The combined expense of the hardware and software can easily fall into thousands of dollars. In addition, an office must periodically upgrade the EMR software, leading to further expenses.

Time investment   It takes considerable time to learn an EMR program and use it with ease. Most software vendors provide on-site training of staff for a newly purchased program, as well as technical support when problems are encountered with the program. Even with all of this assistance, however, learning an EMR program and using it with ease can take up to several months or more.

Operational tasks   Certain tasks must be performed before an EMR program becomes operational. To be effective, older records should be incorporated into a patient's EMR.

This can be accomplished by manually scanning the records into a digital format using an input device known as a *scanner*. An application program known as an *optical character recognition* (OCR) program can also assist in this process. Once the record has been scanned into the computer, the OCR program converts typed text into text that can be manipulated by the computer. An OCR program can also convert a handwritten document into text, but it has a difficult time converting illegible handwriting into text.

Once a document has been scanned into the computer, the medical assistant must follow the medical office policy on what to do with the paper document. Most offices shred the paper documents, but some offices may want to keep certain documents such as consent to treatment forms.

Electronic Medical Record Documents

The documents included in an EMR come from many locations and sources. These documents fall into two categories: administrative documents and clinical documents.

What Would You Do? What Would You *Not* Do?

Case Study 1

Olivia Young has moved to the community and has come to the medical office for a new patient appointment for her chronic asthma. Olivia is leaving the office and is quite upset. She says that she doesn't like having computers in the examining rooms—that it's not natural. She feels like the physician and medical assistant are ignoring her and interacting more with the computer than with her. Olivia says it's like there's a barrier between her and the doctor. She says that the medical office she used to go to didn't have computers in the examination rooms and the doctor really paid attention to her and listened to what she had to say. She says she's thinking of looking for another doctor so that she doesn't have to play second fiddle to a computer. ■

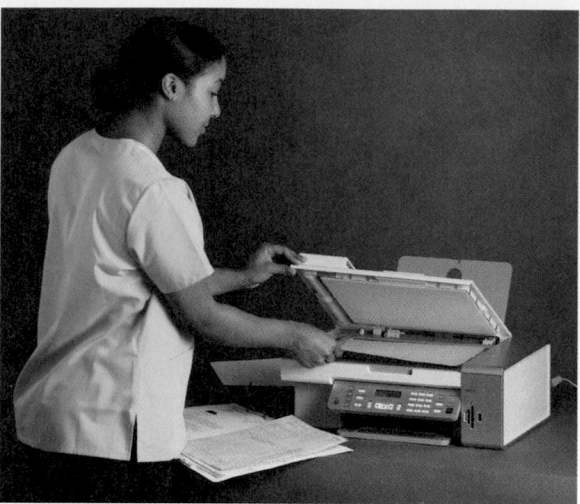

Figure 38-13. Medical assistant scanning information into the computer.

The type of administrative and clinical documents included in an EMR are identical to those included in a paper-based record (refer to Chapter 36 for a review of paper-based record documents). The difference is that the EMR documents are in a digital format rather than a paper format. These documents are described here in terms of the modifications that are necessary to produce them in a digital format or convert them into a digital format.

Electronic Medical Record Administrative Documents

Administrative documents in the EMR contain information necessary for efficient management of the medical office. They include the patient registration record and patient-related correspondence.

Patient registration record The patient registration record consists of demographic and billing information. In most EMR medical offices, the patient completes a paper-and-pencil patient registration form. The medical assistant then enters the data into a form on the screen of the computer and then (if office policy dictates) shreds the paper form. In some offices, the patient may be asked to enter this information directly into the computer. A private area must be provided for this task, and the medical assistant must be available to answer any patient questions related to this task.

NPP acknowledgement form A Notice of Privacy Practices (NPP) is a written document that explains to patients how their protected health information will be used and protected by the medical office. The patient must sign a form acknowledging that he or she has received the NPP. Most medical offices give the patient a paper consent form to sign and then the form is scanned into the computer and filed in the patient's EMR.

Correspondence Correspondence regarding a patient may be received from a number of individuals or facilities. Examples include the patient's insurance company, the patient's attorney, or the patient himself or herself. If the correspondence is transmitted electronically to the medical office, it will already be in a digital format and

can be transferred to the patient's EMR. An example of this is a letter from an insurance company sent as an attachment to an e-mail. If the correspondence is received in a paper format, the medical assistant must first convert the correspondence into a digital format by scanning it into the computer (Figure 38-13). The medical assistant then transfers the correspondence to the patient's EMR and (if office policy dictates) then shreds the paper document. Correspondence also includes copies of letters concerning the patient that are sent out of the office; examples are a copy of a letter referring the patient to a specialist and a copy of a collection letter sent to the patient. Because this correspondence is generated by the office in an electronic format through word processing, it can easily be transferred to the patient's EMR.

Electronic Medical Record Clinical Documents

Clinical documents in the EMR include a variety of records and reports that assist the physician in the care and treatment of the patient. Common EMR clinical documents are listed and described next.

Health history report A health history report is a collection of subjective data about the patient. In an office with an EMR, the patient may complete a health history paper-and-pencil form and the medical assistant then enters the data into the computer and (if office policy dictates) then shreds the paper form. An alternative is for the medical assistant to enter the information directly into the computer while asking the patient questions related to his or her health status. Although not yet in widespread use, computer-guided questionnaires are available for some patients to complete their own health histories. The medical office must provide a private area for the patient to complete the questionnaire and the medical assistant must be available to answer questions.

Physical examination report A physical examination is an assessment by the physician of each part of the patient's body. With an EMR, the physician can use free-text entry, drop-down lists, and check-boxes on an on-screen form to record findings. The EMR program uses this information to generate the physical examination report. This means that by the end of the examination, the physical examination report is complete and the physician does not need to dictate his or her findings at a later time. This alleviates the need for transcribing the physician's dictation into a written report.

Progress notes   Progress notes update the medical record with new information each time the patient visits or telephones the medical office. With an EMR, the physician or medical assistant enters this information directly into the computer using free-text entry, drop-down lists, and check-boxes.

Medication record   A medication record consists of detailed information related to the patient's medications. The medical assistant enters this information into a digital form on the screen of the monitor using free-text entry, drop-down lists, fill-in boxes, and check-boxes.

EMR software includes a prescription program, which greatly reduces the amount of time needed to prescribe and refill medication. The prescription program generates and prints a prescription(s) on a regular sheet of 8½ by 11 inch paper, which is then signed by the physician and given to the patient. The program can also transmit the prescription electronically (by e-fax or e-mail) to the patient's pharmacy. Both of these features eliminate the need of the pharmacist to decipher the physician's handwriting. If the medical office uses a paper medical record, physicians may still have the ability to send prescriptions directly to the patient's pharmacy using a hand-held device, such as a smartphone (see Chapter 39).

To use an EMR, the physician first selects the medication. The program displays a list of the available dosage strengths and preparation forms (e.g., tablets, oral solution, parenteral solution, suppository) for that medication. The physician highlights the dosage strength and preparation desired and enters the information into the computer. Next, the physician selects additional information related to the prescription, such as dosage frequency and number of refills using fill-in boxes, drop-down lists, and check-boxes. The program automatically checks the prescription against any drug allergies the patient may have. It also checks for potential interactions with other medications being taken by the patient. Once the physician has entered the prescription into the computer, the medication is recorded in the patient's medication list. The prescription is then printed out, signed by the physician, and given to the patient or sent electronically to the pharmacy. The prescription program usually provides access to extensive and current product information on all FDA-approved medications.

The EMR prescription program usually has the capability to compare the prescription to the formulary or list of drugs covered by the patient's insurance plan. If the prescription is not in the patient's formulary, the physician is advised of alternate drugs that are covered by the patient's insurance plan.

The EMR prescription program also has the capability to quickly refill a prescription and print a list of prescriptions being taken by the patient. The patient can use this list to keep track of the medications he or she is taking.

Consultation report   A consultation report is a narrative report of a clinical opinion about a patient's condition other than the primary physician. If the consultation report is received by the office as an electronic letter, the medical assistant transfers it to the patient's EMR. If the correspondence is received in a paper format, the medical assistant is responsible for scanning the report into the computer and transferring it to the patient's EMR and (if office policy dictates) then shredding the paper document.

Home health care report   Home health care is the provisions of medical and nonmedical care in a patient's home or place of residence. The purpose of home health care is to minimize the effect of disease or disability by promoting, maintaining, and restoring the patient's health. Currently, most home health care reports are in a paper format and must be scanned into the computer and transferred to the patient's EMR, and (if office policy dictates) then the paper report is shredded. As technology advances, the outside facility providing the service will be able to complete this report on a computer and transmit it electronically to the medical office for inclusion in the EMR.

Laboratory documents   A laboratory document is a report of the analysis or examination of body specimens. Many medical offices already communicate with outside laboratories electronically using a computer system that interfaces with the computer of the outside laboratory. This provides distinct advantages for the medical office using an EMR. Laboratory requisition forms can be completed on a request form displayed on the computer screen using fill-in boxes, drop-down lists, and

---

What Would You Do? What Would You *Not* Do?

Case Study 2

Kacy Ervin comes to the medical office and is diagnosed with strep throat. The physician gives her a prescription for an antibiotic, instructions for taking the medication, and patient information on strep throat printed on two regular sheets of paper that have been generated by the computer. The next day Kacy calls the office to say that she drove to her pharmacy on the way home from the doctor's appointment. When she pulled the papers out of her purse from the doctor's office, she found a sheet of paper with information about her prescription that was signed by the physician, but could not find the prescription form to give to the pharmacist. She says she must have lost the prescription and wants to know if the office could call in the prescription to her pharmacy. ■

check-boxes. The form can then be transmitted electronically to the medical laboratory. Once the patient's tests have been completed, the laboratory test results can be sent electronically to the medical office. The EMR program receives this electronic information and files it in the appropriate patient's EMR. At the same time, a copy of the laboratory report is placed in the physician's "electronic review bin" for his or her review and electronic signature. Abnormal values are highlighted on the report; for example, a high value may be highlighted in red and a low value in green. If a critical result appears on the laboratory report, an urgent message is e-mailed to the physician.

Other advantages of the EMR include the ability to quickly view laboratory results in a chronological order. In addition, the results of a laboratory test performed on a routine basis (e.g., blood glucose) can be accessed by the computer and graphed. This permits an abnormal trend to be identified early so that appropriate action can be taken.

If the medical office is not networked through computers with an outside laboratory, the laboratory reports received by the office must be scanned into the computer and filed in the patient's EMR, and (if office policy dictates) then the paper report is shredded. A scanned report has some limitations. The computer can display the report, but the data on the report cannot be accessed or manipulated. Because of this, the laboratory data cannot be used for many of the functions available with an electronic report. For example, the data on a scanned report cannot be accessed and incorporated into a graph for trend analysis.

Diagnostic procedure documents A diagnostic procedure report consists of a narrative description and interpretation of a diagnostic procedure. Diagnostic procedure reports completed by an outside facility may be sent electronically to the medical office. This makes it easy to store the report in the patient's EMR. If the report is in the form of a paper report, the medical assistant must first convert it to a digital format by scanning it into the computer. The medical assistant must then transfer the report to the patient's EMR and (if office policy dictates) shred the paper report.

The image of the diagnostic procedure (e.g., x-ray, CAT scan, MRI, ECG) can also be stored in the EMR as a digital image. A **digital image** is a picture stored in the computer in the form of pixels. EMR software can then display the digital image on the screen of the computer. If the diagnostic procedure is performed at an outside facility (e.g., an x-ray department of a hospital), the outside facility must have the capability to produce and transmit digital images. If the procedure is performed in the medical office (e.g., ECG, spirometry), the diagnostic equipment must be linked with the office's computer system. This enables a digital image of the procedure to be sent from the diagnostic equipment to the computer.

Therapeutic service documents A therapeutic service report documents the assessments and treatments designed to restore a patient's ability to function. They include physical therapy report, occupational therapy report, and speech therapy report. Currently, most of these reports are in a paper format and must be scanned into the computer and transferred to the patient's EMR, and (if office policy dictates) then the paper report is shredded. As technology advances, the outside facility providing the service will be able to complete this report on a computer and transmit it electronically to the medical office for inclusion in the EMR.

Hospital documents Hospital documents are prepared by the physician responsible for the care of a patient while at the hospital. These reports include a history and physical report, operative reports, discharge summary report, pathology report, and emergency department report. If a hospital document is received by the office in an electronic format, the medical assistant can file it in the patient's EMR without any further processing. If the report is received in a paper format, however, the medical assistant must first scan the document into the computer and file it in the patient's EMR. The medical assistant must then (if office policy dictates) shred the paper report.

Consent forms Consent forms are legal documents required to perform certain procedures or to release information contained in the patient's medical record. Most medical offices give the patient a paper consent form to sign, and then the form is scanned into the computer and filed in the patient's EMR.

Medical Assistant's Use of the Electronic Medical Record

EMR programs include an index that allows the medical assistant to access the various areas of information in the EMR program. The medical assistant must first select the patient who is being seen and enter information about the visit (Figure 38-14). Once the medical assistant begins working with the patient, there is a mechanism within the EMR program to select an activity or topic. The selection

Figure 38-14. Medical assistant taking patient symptoms using a computer and an electronic medical record program.

may be made through a set of tabs on the screen or through a drop-down list. Selecting a tab such as *Medical History* moves the user to a screen containing information about the patient's medical history and the ability to move to other screens with more specific information. The EMR combines areas where data can be entered (e.g., blood pressure) and lists from which the user chooses an option (e.g., sitting, standing, lying).

Functions Performed by the Medical Assistant

The following functions are typically performed by the medical assistant using an EMR:

- Access the daily schedule
- Select a patient
- Enter the time that the patient has checked in
- Enter the examination room number (Figure 38-15)
- Enter the patient's chief complaint
- Enter or review the patient history
- Enter or review patient allergies
- Enter or review the patient's current medications
- Enter vital signs
- Enter measurements such as height and weight
- Enter results of tests, such as vision screening or hearing screening
- Enter results of laboratory tests performed at the office (e.g., urinalysis, hemoglobin, strep testing) (Figure 38-16)

Physician's Use of the Electronic Medical Record

The physician enters data into the EMR about the examination, assessments, and plan for the patient. The physician can also review and update all information entered by the medical assistant. If the program is linked to the practice management software, the physician can specify the type of visit and patient diagnosis. This assists in billing as part of the check-out procedure. The physician can also print a summary of the visit for the patient by selecting information from a list on the screen to include in the summary. Examples include physical examination findings, laboratory test results, vital signs, and treatment recommendations. The physician can also enter notes and reminders. Often there is a capacity to electronically send messages to other physicians or staff members within the system in a manner similar to e-mail. For example, the physician may send an electronic message to the medical assistant to schedule a patient for a particular test or to call in a prescription refill for a patient.

COMPUTER NETWORK SECURITY

Because all HIPAA regulations apply to the EMR, the medical office must provide secure access to patient health information stored in the computer's database. If there is a centralized system used in several office locations, there may be more extensive security controls. Security of the computer network is accomplished through the methods described as follows.

Authentification

Each health care worker with permission to use the computer network must have a password and must log in to access the network. Passwords should be changed at regular

Figure 38-15. Electronic medical record screen. (Courtesy AltaPoint Data Systems, LLC.)

Figure 38-16. Electronic medical record screen. (Courtesy AltaPoint Data Systems, LLC.)

intervals, and in fact there may be a system function that requires this. The medical assistant should not share his or her password with anyone else. Effective passwords include random series of digits, letters, and symbols rather than English words, telephone numbers, or other combinations that have meaning.

Levels of Authorization

A computer network has specific levels of authorization so that certain screens and certain functions are only available to users with the correct level of authorization. For example, at the end of a patient visit that has been recorded in the EMR, the physician must electronically sign the record. This closes the visit so that information about that visit cannot be changed at a later date. A medical assistant would not be authorized to perform this function.

Automatic Logoff

All users should log out of the computer network when their workstations are unattended. If the user forgets to do this, the software has a feature that automatically logs a user off after a predetermined period of inactivity.

Audit Controls

Practice management programs and EMR programs have the ability to track the activity of individuals using the computer system. This can be used to determine if security violations have occurred and to identify the individual with whom those violations may be associated.

Antivirus Software

Antivirus software is a type of system software known as a *utility program.* Antivirus software should be installed on the computer system to scan for computer viruses. The term *computer virus* refers to software designed to penetrate a computer or network without consent. A computer virus can access information and/or cause damage. Once installed, antivirus software operates in the background and monitors all files for viruses. It also updates itself regularly because new computer viruses are developed constantly and can be spread quickly through the Internet.

Firewall

A **firewall** is a system that protects a computer network from unauthorized access by users on its own network or another network, such as the Internet. A firewall takes its name from a wall in a building that is made of a material that will prevent a fire from spreading from one part of a building to another. A firewall may be in the form of a utility software program, or it may be more complex and consist of a firewall hardware device that connects to the computer.

All inquiries and messages entering or leaving the computer system must pass through the firewall, which examines each inquiry or message and blocks those that do not meet the firewall's specified security criteria. If the firewall is unsure about whether or not to grant access, it will display a screen message for the user regarding the access. The computer user is given the following choices: to refuse access, to permit access once, or to permit unlimited access. The firewall does not substitute for antivirus software because it cannot protect against viruses received as e-mail attachments.

BACKUPS

In the medical office, information is permanently stored on the computer's internal hard disk. A copy of this information, known as a *backup,* should be made each day. A **backup** is a duplicate copy of a program or data kept for reference in case the original is damaged, lost, or destroyed.

Many medical offices contract with an online backup service that provides secure backups of all files used in the office for a monthly fee. These backups may be performed every few hours or at scheduled times. The information is encrypted using methods similar to those used by banks and financial institutions. Although this service may seem expensive, it ensures that data will not be lost or destroyed.

Large health care facilities may be able to back up information from individual computers using their own network system. These backups may occur automatically, or it may be necessary for a staff member to initiate the backup.

Using external hard drives, CD-RWs, and DVD-RWs to create physical backup copies is also possible. When a physical copy is used for backup, it should be stored in a safe place that is physically remote from the computer system. Many offices accomplish this by having the physician or medical assistant take the backup home. Another option is to store the backup in a fireproof safe in the medical office.

SYSTEM MAINTENANCE

The medical office must assign an individual to be responsible for system maintenance. System maintenance involves setting up and overseeing the computer system. System maintenance consists of three aspects:
1. Disk cleanup
2. Disk defragmentation
3. System administration

What Would You Do? What Would You *Not* Do?

Case Study 3

John Gurnsey comes to the medical office for a check-up for his psoriasis and clinical depression. John says he likes the computer system used in the office but worries about the security of his medical record. He says that he doesn't want any of his friends or coworkers to know that he has psoriasis or that he is on an antidepressant. John wants to know how the office protects his medical record from people like computer hackers. He says since there is a computer in every room, how is a patient left alone in a room prevented from looking up patient records on the computer? John says that viruses keep getting into his computer at home and that data on his hard drive have been destroyed three different times. He wants to know if this ever happens at the medical office. ∎

Disk Cleanup

Unneeded files stored on the hard drive slow down system performance and should be removed periodically. This is especially important if the Internet is being used frequently by the medical office. In addition, outgoing e-mail messages and incoming messages that have been read and deleted continue to reside in the system and should be eliminated. Disk cleanup is accomplished through a utility program that may come with the computer or can be purchased separately. Disk cleanup frees up significant amounts of hard drive space and can significantly improve system performance.

Disk Defragmentation

Disk defragmentation rearranges information on the hard disk so that files and programs are stored closer. This allows the computer to locate information on the hard disk in a shorter period of time, which results in improved system performance. Disk defragmentation can take a long time, particularly with a hard disk that has a large storage capacity, such as those being used in a medical office. To avoid interfering with the office routine, disk defragmentation is usually performed at night or on a weekend.

System Administration

The system administrator is the person designated to maintain the computer system, especially a large network system. He or she is responsible for overall system/network function. The system administrator is usually a computer specialist known as an *information technologist* (IT). Small offices often use a consultant, sometimes from the company that provided the practice management software. Practices with several sites, health maintenance organizations, and community health centers often have an IT specialist, or even an IT department, that handles both administration of the current system and planning for future computer needs.

SERVICE AGREEMENTS

The medical assistant is usually responsible for maintaining the service agreements for the office's computer systems. These agreements include maintenance agreements for the hardware, system support agreements for the software, and training of personnel on the software.

The medical assistant should designate an area in the medical office for the storage of the user manuals that come with the hardware and software. Examples of user manuals include the computer manuals, printer and scanner manuals, and application program manuals. One individual in the office should be designated to be responsible for all the computers. This person is responsible for being the liaison with any companies providing service for the hardware and software, such as maintenance, software upgrades, and software consultations.

MEDICAL PRACTICE and the LAW

As more patient information is stored on computers, shared on computer networks that can often be accessed from a doctor's home, and sent electronically to third-party payers, security and privacy has become a national priority. Several legal and regulatory measures can have an impact on health care organizations and the way they maintain security of electronically recorded and stored patient information. These include federal regulations, as well as guidelines from professional organizations and accrediting agencies, such as the Joint Commission. The most comprehensive regulation is provided by the Health Insurance Portability and Accountability Act of 1996 (HIPAA).

The Transaction and Code Set Rule prescribes electronic data interchange standards for structuring information that must be used for Medicare and Medicaid insurance claims.

The Security Rule complements the Privacy Rule by setting standards to maintain security of personal health information that is transmitted electronically. It identifies administrative, physical, and technical security safeguards for electronic protected health information (EPHI).

In addition, within a medical office, each individual who uses the computer should have a unique password, which should be changed on a regular basis. The password is a set of alphanumeric characters that allow the user to log on (enter) the system or specific parts of the computer system. Individuals should not share their passwords with others.

Each individual should have access to only the types of information and applications that fall within his or her scope of work and responsibility. System security should be designed in such a way that each security level permits access to only the applications and databases each individual needs to perform his or her tasks. Each specific application should know which individuals are authorized to use it.

If a practice uses a service bureau to prepare documents, at the end of the contractual period, all documents, in paper or electronic media, should be returned to the practice. ■

What Would You Do? What Would You *Not* Do? RESPONSES

Case Study 1
Page 930

What Did Emma Do?
- ❑ Listened carefully to what Olivia was saying and agreed that sometimes patients feel like the computer seems to place a barrier between the patient and the doctor.
- ❑ Reassured Olivia that the doctor and staff always pay attention and listen very closely to what she has to relay about her health.
- ❑ Explained that the staff is still getting used to the computer system and that it takes more of their attention now than it will when everyone becomes familiar with the system.
- ❑ Stressed to Olivia that computerized medical records provide better patient care through improved communication, faster access to data, and clearer and better documentation.
- ❑ Relayed Olivia's concern at the next medical office staff meeting.

What Did Emma Not Do?
- ❑ Did not minimize or ignore Olivia's concerns.
- ❑ Did not tell Olivia that she is outdated and needs to adjust to the twenty-first century.

What Would You Do/What Would You *Not* Do? Review Emma's response and place a checkmark next to the information you included in your response. List the additional information you included in your response.

_____

_____

Case Study 2
Page 931

What Did Emma Do?
- ❑ Explained that the physician is now using an ordinary sheet of paper to print prescriptions from the computer and even though it doesn't look like a traditional prescription form, it really is a prescription with all the proper information on it signed by the physician.
- ❑ Reassured Kacy that many patients are confused about this until they get used to the new system. Told Kacy that the pharmacies are very familiar with these types of prescriptions and that she won't have any trouble getting it filled.
- ❑ Instructed Kacy to locate the prescription sheet she was given at the office and to take this sheet to the pharmacy so that her prescription can be filled.

What Did Emma Not Do?
- ❑ To help Kacy get used to the new system, did not call in another prescription unless Kacy says that she has thrown the paper away.
- ❑ Did not tell Kacy that if she would have shown her prescription sheet to the pharmacist, she wouldn't have to drive all the way back to the pharmacy again.

What Would You Do/What Would You *Not* Do? Review Emma's response and place a checkmark next to the information you

What Would You Do? What Would You *Not* Do? RESPONSES—cont'd

included in your response. List the additional information you included in your response.

_____

_____

_____

_____

Case Study 3
Page 935

What Did Emma Do?
❑ Reassured John that it is a legitimate concern to want to make sure his medical information is kept confidential.
❑ Explained to John that something called a "firewall" protects the office computers from unauthorized access by computer hackers.
❑ Told John that each staff member has to enter a password to log into the computer and that a patient would not have a password and not be able to log into the computer.

❑ Explained to John that the office places a lot of emphasis on maintaining security of the computer system and preventing loss of data. Told John that the office has antivirus software running all the time to protect the computer from viruses and that the office also has a backup system so that even if data were lost, there would be a backup of the data.

What Did Emma Not *Do?*
❑ Did not minimize John's concerns.
❑ Did not criticize John for not having an antivirus program on his home computer.

What Would You Do/What Would You *Not* Do? Review Emma's response and place a checkmark next to the information you included in your response. List the additional information you included in your response.

_____

_____

_____

_____

TERMINOLOGY REVIEW

ALU (arithmetic/logic unit) The part of the CPU that executes the program's instructions by performing mathematic computations and logical operations.

Application software Software designed to accomplish a specific task (e.g., word processing); also called *application program* and *software program.*

Backup A duplicate copy of a program or data kept for reference in case the original is damaged, lost, or destroyed.

Byte A unit of computer storage capacity. One byte is approximately equal to one character.

Computer An electronic machine that has the ability to process data according to a program in order to produce a desired result.

Computer system All of the hardware and software components making up the computer.

Control unit The part of the CPU that directs and coordinates the processing functions of the computer.

CPU (central processing unit) The "brain" of the computer housed in the main unit that interprets and executes the instructions that operate the computer. The CPU consists of the control unit and the ALU.

Data Raw, unorganized facts about subject matter presented to the computer for processing.

Data processing The changing of raw facts or data into usable information following a three-part sequence: input, processing, output.

Digital image A picture stored in the computer in the form of pixels.

Documentation A written set of instructions accompanying an application program, designed to assist the user in understanding how to operate the program. Examples include the user manual, help screens, and reference cards.

Electronic medical record (EMR) A computerized record of the important health information regarding a patient including the care of that individual and the progress of the patient's condition.

Firewall A system that protects a computer network from unauthorized access by users on its own network or another network, such as the Internet.

Floppy disk A portable storage device consisting of a flexible Mylar plastic disk coated with a magnetically sensitive material. The disk is encased in a square plastic jacket that protects it from damage.

Gigabyte (GB) A unit of computer storage capacity. One gigabyte is equal to a little more than 1 billion bytes or 1000 megabytes.

Hard disk A storage device consisting of one or more rigid, nonflexible platters coated with a magnetically sensitive material and encased in a permanently sealed, air-tight container.

Hardcopy Printed output from a computer.

Hardware The physical devices making up a computer system (e.g., main computer unit, keyboard, monitor, printer).

Information Data that has been processed into a usable form by the computer.

Input 1. (noun) Data that has been entered into the computer. 2. (verb) The transfer of data to the computer for processing.

Continued

TERMINOLOGY REVIEW—cont'd

Input device A device for entering data into the computer (e.g., keyboard, mouse, scanner).

Kilobyte (KB) A unit of computer storage capacity. One kilobyte is equal to 1024 bytes (characters).

Mainboard The primary circuit board of the main computer unit, which allows all of the computer components to communicate with each other.

Main computer memory The part of the CPU that is responsible for temporarily storing information until it is needed for processing by the computer. Main memory in a microcomputer is known as *RAM*.

Medical practice management program A program that provides instructions to the computer for performing medical practice management procedures.

Megabyte (MB) A unit of computer storage capacity. One megabyte is equal to a little more than 1 million bytes or 1000 kilobytes.

Microcomputer A small general purpose computer that relies on a tiny microprocessor chip to perform its processing functions.

Operating system A type of system software that performs tasks required by the computer to operate itself.

Optical disc A storage device consisting of a flat, round portable disk that stores data using laser technology.

Optical drive A device installed in a drive bay on the main computer unit that uses a laser to read an optical disc or write onto (burn) an optical disc.

Output 1. (noun) Information that has been generated by the computer. 2. (verb) The transfer of processed data back to the user.

Output device A device that transfers processed data to the user (e.g., computer monitor, printer).

Pixels (picture elements) Dot locations on a computer screen that can be lit up as needed to display images.

Printing speed The number of pages per minute (ppm) generated by a printer.

Processing The manipulation and reorganization of data according to the instructions in a program.

Program A set of instructions organized in a logical step-by-step sequence, which tells the computer how to perform a specific function.

RAM (random-access memory) The main computer memory of a microcomputer, which is used to temporarily store items until needed by the computer for processing. Also known as *main computer memory*.

Read The transfer of information from a storage device, such as a hard disk, to computer memory.

Resolution The number of horizontal and vertical pixels in a display device, such as a computer screen.

Sequential-access memory Computer memory in which all stored data must be searched sequentially from beginning to end to locate the desired information.

Softcopy The visual display of information on the display screen of a computer monitor.

Software A general term for the programs or instructions that tell a computer what to do.

Sound card A circuit board connected to the mainboard that converts computer audio output into electronic signals. The electronic signals are then sent to speakers that convert them into sound.

Special keys Keys that issue commands to the computer to perform specific functions on the information displayed on the screen.

Storage capacity The maximum amount of information that a device can hold, measured in bytes.

Storage device A device that permanently stores information for later retrieval by the computer.

System software A group of programs that control or maintain the operations of a computer.

User The individual using the computer.

Video card A circuit board connected to the mainboard that converts computer video output into electronic signals. The electronic signals are then sent to the monitor, where they are converted into text and images that can be viewed by the user.

Write The transfer of information from computer memory to a storage device, such as a hard disk.

ON THE WEB

For Information on Medical Office Computerization:

American Health Information Management Association (AHIMA): www.ahima.org

Computer-Based Patient Record Institute: www.cpri.org

Computer Security Institute: www.gocsi.com

Department of Health and Human Services HIPAA website: www.hhs.gov/ocr/hipaa

Microsoft Windows: www.microsoft.com/windows

Microsoft Office: www.microsoft.com/office

 PREPARE FOR CERTIFICATION   Visit the Evolve site at http://evolve.elsevier.com/Bonewit/today/ to actively Prepare for your Certification.

 *Check out the **Companion CD** bound with the book to access additional interactive activities.*

39

Telephone Techniques

LEARNING OBJECTIVES

1. Describe the importance of effective telephone courtesy and a pleasing telephone personality for the medical assistant.
2. Explain the use multiline telephones, fax machines, cell phones, smartphones, and pagers in the medical office.
3. Differentiate between incoming telephone calls the medical assistant can handle and other incoming calls.
4. Describe the correct procedure for screening incoming calls.
5. Describe the correct procedure for taking messages and transcribing messages recorded on an answering machine or voice mail.
6. Identify the correct steps to respond to a telephone call regarding an emergency or urgent medical problem.
7. Describe how to deal with problem calls.
8. Explain how the medical assistant should make outgoing telephone calls.

PROCEDURES

Perform telephone screening.
Take a telephone message.
Take requests for medication or prescription refills.

Telephone a patient for follow-up.

CHAPTER OUTLINE

Introduction to Telephone Techniques
Using the Telephone Effectively
  Telephone Courtesy
  Telephone Personality
  Effective Telephone Communication
Telephone Technology
  Multiline Phones
  Answering Machines and Voice Mail
  Electronic Information Transfer
  Cell Phones and Smartphones
  Pagers

Incoming Calls
  Centralized or Electronic Routing
  Managing Incoming Calls
  Urgent or Emergency Calls
  Dealing with Problem Calls
Outgoing Calls
  Local Calls
  Long-Distance Calls
  Conference Calls

CAAHEP COMPETENCIES

Clinical Competencies
Patient Care
- Perform telephone screening.

General Competencies
Professional Communications
- Recognize and respond to verbal communication.
- Demonstrate telephone techniques.

Legal Concepts
- Identify and respond to issues of confidentiality.

Communication
- Serve as liaison between physician and others.
- Use proper telephone techniques.
- Receive, organize, prioritize, and transmit information expediently.

- Recognition and response to verbal and nonverbal communication
- Application of electronic technology

DSL (digital subscriber line)
enunciation (ee-nun-see-AY-shun)
pager
PDA (personal digital assistant)

smartphone
SSL (Secure Sockets Layer)
voice mail

Introduction to Telephone Techniques

Contact with a patient takes many forms. In addition to face-to-face contact, medical assistants often speak to patients and other callers over the telephone. The telephone is often the first contact between the medical office and a patient. In addition, the telephone is used throughout the day to make and receive referrals, request laboratory results, call in prescriptions for patients, and respond to patient questions.

Managing the phone is one of the most important jobs in the office. It is the first chance the medical assistant has to project a positive attitude and image to a patient. One never has a second chance to make a first impression.

USING THE TELEPHONE EFFECTIVELY

Telephone Courtesy

The telephone in a medical office should always be answered promptly. Some offices have a policy that every phone call should be answered within three rings. The medical assistant identifies the office, gives his or her name, then finds out who is calling. If the call will be transferred, the staff member needs to know who will be on the other end of the call.

The medical assistant should always speak before putting someone on hold. It is not courteous to place a call to hold immediately before speaking to the caller. The caller cannot even be sure that they have reached the correct telephone number. It is far more polite to obtain the caller's name and purpose for calling before putting the caller on hold. It is helpful to keep a written record of each caller's name, with the number of the line where he or she is holding. A physician should not be placed on hold if it can be avoided. The medical assistant should check back about every 30 seconds

or so with a person who is on hold. This reassures the caller that the medical assistant is aware of the call. The medical assistant should also try to give an idea of how long it will take before the call will be answered.

When handling a call, the medical assistant should not chew gum or eat. Paying close attention during the telephone call is also important. A caller can tell if the medical assistant is distracted.

Telephone Personality

In addition to words, many nonverbal cues are given in the quality of a medical assistant's voice on the telephone. The "telephone personality" is important. It is important to stay focused on the call and smile. The medical assistant should use the same volume as when speaking in person and speak naturally. An artificial telephone voice may be perceived as cold and unreal.

All words should be spoken clearly so that they are easy to understand. Good **enunciation** is the act of speaking so that the message can be easily understood. It may be necessary to speak a little more slowly on the telephone, and it is very important to avoid mumbling. It may be helpful for a medical assistant to record a telephone greeting and analyze the quality of his or her voice and the personality that is projected.

Qualities such as interest, friendliness, concern, and understanding are clearly communicated over the telephone. So too are boredom, anxiety, and indifference.

Effective Telephone Communication

When speaking on the telephone, the medical assistant should try to complete the call without interruption. If it is necessary to put someone on hold, the medical assistant should give a reason and apologize to the caller when the call is resumed. Information and materials should be readily available to handle calls and take messages. These include message slips, pen, the office appointment book or computer appointment screen, and a list of frequently used telephone numbers. A desk clock, computer clock, or wristwatch should be visible to note the time when taking messages.

The medical assistant begins the conversation by identifying the practice; for example, "Primary Care Associates, Channa speaking." If the caller asks a question or asks for a staff member without identifying himself or herself, the medical assistant asks politely for the caller's name: "With whom am I speaking?" or "Whom shall I say is calling?" Using complete sentences is important because the medical assistant does not want to sound abrupt or rude.

The medical assistant should sit with the back supported and the head in a neutral position (not forward or to one side). The feet should be flat on the floor or supported on a foot stool. Figure 39-1 shows proper body position for answering the telephone. If the receiver is tucked between the head and shoulder, it places strain on the shoulder muscles and may change the voice quality, so this should be avoided. A headset, which consists of an earpiece that fits over the ear and a mouthpiece in front of the mouth, allows for good body posture and leaves the hands free. This is recommended if the medical assistant spends a lot of time on the telephone. Figure 39-2 shows such a headset.

The medical assistant should be clear with callers who leave messages about when they can expect their calls to be returned. Many physicians have specific times when they return nonurgent telephone calls, such as late morning, lunch time, or the end of the day.

One should avoid cutting into a person's replies, even if he or she rambles on and repeats information. When the medical assistant gets the chance to speak, he or she should try to give a focused answer that lets the caller know what can be done and what the medical assistant is going to do.

TELEPHONE TECHNOLOGY

Advances in telephone technology have given medical offices many options to maintain contact with patients, physicians, pharmacies, laboratories, and hospitals.

Multiline Phones

Most offices have a multiline phone, with several extensions. It is important for the medical assistant to learn how to determine which line is ringing, how to place calls on hold, and how to transfer calls to all parts of the medical office. Figure 39-3 illustrates a multiline telephone with many extensions.

A flashing light usually identifies a line that is ringing; it flashes at a different rate on a line where a person is on hold.

Figure 39-2. A telephone headset leaves the hands free and facilitates good body posture.

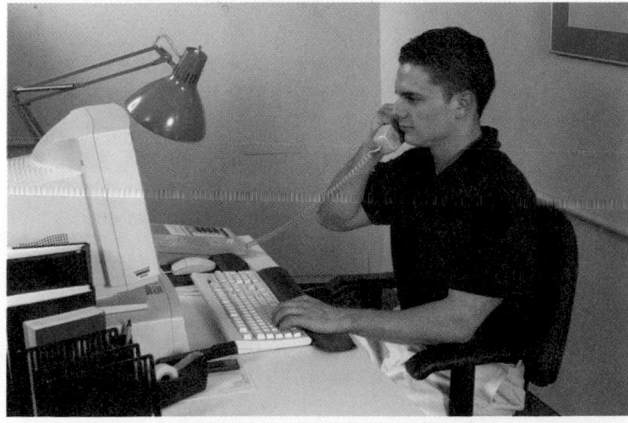

Figure 39-1. Good posture when answering the telephone improves voice quality and prevents muscle strain.

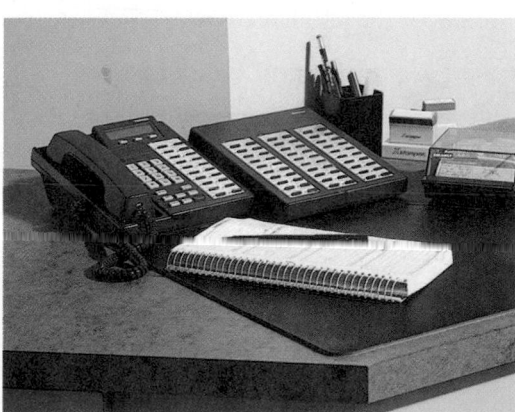

Figure 39-3. A multiline telephone is commonly used in a medical office. (From Young AP, Proctor DB: *Kinn's the medical assistant,* ed 10, St. Louis, 2007, Saunders.)

The medical assistant answers a call by pressing the button on the telephone that corresponds to the line that is ringing. If a second call comes in while the medical assistant is speaking to a caller, the medical assistant should tell the first caller that he or she needs to place the caller on hold by pressing the hold button. The medical assistant answers the second call, identifies the caller, and usually places that caller on hold before returning to the first caller and apologizing for the interruption. The calls are then handled in order.

If the caller asks to be connected to another extension or person, the medical assistant should first obtain the caller's name. To transfer a call, the medical assistant may need to press another button and/or dial an extension number, depending on the type of telephone system. Knowing the caller's name allows the medical assistant to announce the caller when the call is connected, and it is also helpful if the call is disconnected for some reason.

While a caller is on hold, the light on that line will flash. If the light continues to flash, the medical assistant should pick up that line about every 30 seconds and ask if the person would like to continue holding or leave a message. Sometimes transfers do not go through or the call is not picked up.

Special Features

Multiline telephone systems come with many other features, including speed dialing, call forwarding, call park, and caller ID.

Speed dialing allows storage of frequently called telephone numbers in the telephone system's memory. These numbers can be called by pressing a button or a one- or two-digit code.

Call forwarding allows forwarding of incoming calls to another telephone number. This service is turned on and off by dialing a sequence of numbers and activity keys.

Call park allows a call to be placed on hold and retrieved from another telephone.

Caller ID identifies the caller's telephone number before the telephone is answered. This feature may be available on some, but not all, telephones within a telephone system.

The medical assistant must learn how to use these and other features of the telephone system efficiently.

Answering Machines and Voice Mail

Physicians have always needed to be available at all times. Most physicians' offices still use an answering service for getting messages to physicians during hours when the office is normally closed. This is an independent company that answers telephones for a number of clients. Some offices also have an answering machine or voice mail system, which has a message with a number to call outside of office hours and gives people the option to leave a nonurgent message. **Voice mail** is a method for message delivery, storage, and retrieval that is built into the telephone system. Answering services and answering machines are activated whenever the office is closed, including during lunch break if no one is assigned to take phone calls during that time. The answer-

Putting It All into Practice

My name is Channa Eng, and I am a certified medical assistant. I work for an internal medical practice with two physicians and two nurse practitioners in an urban area. We have many Asian and Hispanic patients. I don't speak much Spanish, but I do speak Cambodian and some Vietnamese. Another medical assistant speaks Spanish, and we both help with translating telephone calls from a patient who has difficulty in English. When patients call our office, they get three choices right away. They can hear the message in English, Spanish, or Cambodian. Most patients like this because they can hear the instructions in a language they are comfortable with. On Tuesdays and Thursdays, I spend most of the day on the telephone making appointments and responding to patients with medical problems. I don't usually sit at the front desk. Instead, we have a telephone room with three telephones. When it is very busy, there are usually two of us. I can tell if a patient wants a routine appointment or has medical questions depending on which line the call comes in on. When patients are sick, I have to ask a lot of questions to find out how urgent their problem is. Last year I worked with the office manager to revise our procedure manual, so I am very familiar with what questions to ask. My goal is to handle each call as quickly and efficiently as possible while still making the patients feel that their needs were met. Every time I take a message, I put it on the corner of my desk, and a file clerk takes it to get the patient's medical record. In our office we think that telephone conversations are very important. We try very hard to answer all telephone calls promptly and to avoid putting patients on hold. ■

Prepare for Success

ing service should be notified if the office is closed, although they usually pick up phones after a predetermined number of rings.

Increasingly, physicians' offices are going to voice mail systems. Voice mail is a system provided by the office's telephone carrier that allows for messages to be left in a number of "mailboxes" for different people. Each physician might have his or her own voice mail box, as well as each medical assistant, the business manager, and so on.

The message will have a number to call for urgent messages outside of office hours, but will also offer the caller the option of leaving a message in any voice mail box. Each box has a two- to four-number extension. Many voice mail systems have a directory by which people can find voice mail box numbers by using their touch-tone phone to type in some or all of the letters of the last name of the person with whom they would like to speak.

Even if an office has a voice mail system, most medical offices will still need to have a contract with an answering service. The answering service provides a medical office with coverage outside of normal business hours. The service either answers all of the office's telephone calls or takes calls that are forwarded to it by individuals who listen to the voice mail system message and press the appropriate message code for an urgent message. The answering service must be informed how to deal with urgent calls.

Electronic Information Transfer

Fax Machine

Telephone lines are also used to send data rapidly. Paper copies can be sent quickly from one location to another using a fax machine. The original document is fed into the fax machine, which encodes the images on the paper into signals to be sent over the phone. At the other end, a second fax machine prints black dots on a piece of paper that correspond to the information received. There should be a dedicated telephone line and telephone number for the fax machine, which is shown in Figure 39-4. The phone number for the fax machine should be listed next to each telephone so that any caller can be told how to fax information to the office.

The fax is useful for doing business (e.g., ordering supplies) and for sending out meeting agendas or receiving resumés when hiring. To protect confidentiality, fax transmissions of patient health information should only be made when patient consent has been obtained or in an emergency situation when prompt information transfer is required. A cover sheet should be used for privacy, and the recipient should be notified by telephone when the fax is being sent so that he or she can remove it from the receiving fax machine promptly. The cover sheet should contain a confidentiality statement similar to the one in Figure 39-5.

Electronic Data Transmission

Information from the office computer system, including e-mail, billing, and insurance information, can be transmitted using telephone lines. Various technologies exist for electronic data transmission, but some are considerably faster than others. A modem carries signals via a conventional telephone line and must make a connection with an Internet provider. The resulting transmission is usually slow. **DSL (digital subscriber line)** technologies allow for continuous digital connection over the telephone line, which can still be used for voice calls. This type of connection provides much faster transmission. Telephone companies are also providing fiberoptic cables with a glass core that transmit electronic information as light impulses. A method of transmitting electronic information that does not use a telephone line is a cable modem. This type of modem hooks up to a cable television connection. *smartphone*

E-mail

E-mail (electronic mail) is a method of composing, sending, receiving, and storing messages that are sent over the Internet. Files, such as documents, spreadsheets, and images, can be attached. Security and confidentiality are issues when using e-mail. The medical assistant should assume that an e-mail message may be read by someone else (e.g., a member of the recipient's family). It is also likely that the organization the medical assistant works for may have access to e-mail messages, even if they have been deleted. In the medical office, e-mail should not be used for private messages or information.

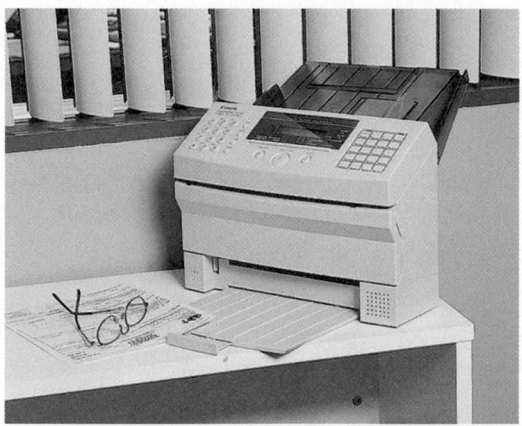

Figure 39-4. A fax machine allows transmission of images from one location to another using a telephone line. (From Young AP, Proctor DB: *Kinn's the medical assistant,* ed 10, St. Louis, 2007, Saunders.)

CONFIDENTIALITY STATEMENT:

The documents accompanying this transmission may contain confidential information that is protected under the Privacy Act of 1974. It is being faxed to you after appropriate patient authorization or under circumstances that do not require patient authorization. This information is intended only for the use of the intended recipient(s). The authorized recipient(s) of this information is/are prohibited from disclosing this information to any other party unless permitted to do so by law or regulation.

If the reader of this message is not the intended recipient(s) or the employee or agent responsible for delivering the attached information to the intended recipient(s), please note that any dissemination, distribution or copying of this information is strictly prohibited. **Anyone who receives this information in error should notify the sender immediately and arrange for the return or destruction of the transmitted information.**

Figure 39-5. A medical office should include a confidentiality statement on the cover sheet for fax transmissions.

Electronic Transmission of Billing and Insurance Information

Insurance and billing information is often transmitted electronically via telephone lines to billing departments, billing affiliates, and/or insurance companies. The HIPAA Security Rule sets standards to safeguard the transmission of patient health information electronically, and each medical office must comply with these standards. This includes maintaining secure networks and using an encryption system, such as **SSL (Secure Sockets Layer),** a protocol for managing data transmission over the Internet.

Cell Phones and Smartphones

A cell phone allows two individuals to speak to each other like a regular telephone, but it uses radio signals instead of telephone wires. A **smartphone** is a device that adds computer capabilities to the cell phone, such as a **PDA (personal digital assistant)** with a drug reference, address book, and other tools, Internet connection, the ability to send and receive e-mails, and sometimes even access to the electronic medical record system used by the health care facility. Many physicians use cell phones or smartphones to remain in contact with the medical office when they are in other locations. The telephone numbers of the physicians' cell phone should never be given to patients, but they should be available to office staff so that physicians can be contacted as needed.

Pagers

Pagers are used in areas with unreliable cell phone service and sometimes in large institutions like hospitals. A **pager** (also called a *beeper*) is like a radio that is always tuned in to a single station. When it "hears" its unique access code signal, it lights up, beeps, or vibrates to indicate that a message is being received. Some pagers are also linked to voice mail. Pagers used by physicians or other health professionals are either numeric or alphanumeric. A numeric pager's message is a telephone number (e.g., the answering service, the office, the emergency department, home, a colleague). The physician then returns the call to the number on the display. An alphanumeric pager displays an entire message, so the physician can return a phone call or act on the information that is relayed to the pager. Some pagers also include e-mail so that a return message can be sent. If the physicians use pagers, the office staff should have the pager numbers for each physician in the practice.

A simple type of pager may also be used for patients in ambulatory care areas of hospitals or clinics. It is similar to pagers used in restaurants and lights up and/or vibrates to notify patients when it is their turn. Patients can leave the waiting area and be notified when to return. This type of pager provides patient confidentiality because it eliminates the need to call the patient by name.

Highlight on Analog versus Digital Technology

Until the middle of the 1980s, telephone service used only analog technology, which translates the audio signals from a telephone into electronic pulses. These pulses are usually transmitted along wires that link all telephones together physically. In cordless telephones analog signals are transmitted from the telephone base to the receiver using radio waves. The advantage of analog technology was, and still is, high sound quality with minimal distortion. Analog telephones are also relatively inexpensive. The disadvantage is that analog signals can only carry a limited amount of information. Also, analog signals cannot be encrypted, so the information being transmitted is not secure, especially when using a cordless telephone or cell phone.

Digital technology converts analog signals from a microphone in the telephone into binary code (consisting of 0s and 1s). The message is transmitted to the receiver through wires or radio signals, where it is converted back into its original signal. Because of the conversion, quality of the signal may be lost, although modern digital equipment has improved in this area. Digital technology is also more expensive. The main advantage of digital technology for the medical office is the ability to transfer electronic data securely using telephone lines. Both voice and computer transmissions can be encrypted in such a way that they cannot be intercepted and decoded. The encryption key is necessary at the receiving end in order to decode the information.

Digital and analog equipment cannot be connected together without using an adapter. Modern multiline telephone systems are digital. If an analog telephone, modem, or fax machine is connected to a digital system without using a digital-to-analog adapter, it can draw too much current and damage itself or even the entire telephone system. ∎

INCOMING CALLS

An incoming telephone call sounds like a routine event. But breaking down the process, it becomes clear that a number of different elements go into answering a routine call.

Centralized or Electronic Routing

Many offices use an electronic routing system to direct calls. At each extension, the telephone may be answered or the call will go to voice mail, and the caller can leave a message for office staff members who are not available. By offering the caller several options (e.g., scheduling an appointment, being connected to the medical assistant, if there is a billing question), the electronic routing system directs the call to the appropriate part of the office, saving the expense of a staff person who would otherwise be answering the call. It also keeps patients from being put on hold, which some people appreciate.

However, other patients find electronic routing of messages confusing and frustrating, especially if the person they need to speak with is not available and does not return calls promptly.

If electronic routing is used, the message should be kept up to date and should be as clear and concise as possible.

In other offices, incoming calls are answered directly by the medical assistant. Although the personal touch is appreciated by many patients, when several calls come in at the same time, some callers end up on hold. If the office has several staff members, many of the calls end up being transferred anyway.

Managing Incoming Calls

Performing Telephone Screening

The first step in handling telephone calls is to find out how urgent the call is and what is necessary to handle the call.

Most calls are routine and can be taken in the order in which they come. In most cases, a new call is placed on hold while the previous call is handled. However, there are some exceptions:

- Calls from other physicians are put through at once.
- Emergency calls are treated as urgent and receive top priority. They will be discussed in detail later in this chapter.
- If the caller is a relative of the physician, the medical assistant either puts the caller through or speaks to the physician via intercom to determine how to handle the call.

When answering calls, it is polite to obtain the caller's name and ask permission to place the caller on hold. This gives the caller the opportunity to identify if it is an urgent call.

After obtaining a caller's name, the caller usually states the reason for the call or asks for a staff member or department. When the caller asks for a staff member by name, the medical assistant usually transfers the call. If that staff member is with a patient, the medical assistant may offer to take a message or transfer the call to voice mail. Often the caller asks for the physician. Most physicians do not take calls while they are seeing patients. Additional questions may show that the medical assistant can handle the call, or it may be necessary to take a message for the physician (Procedure 39-1).

Calls the Medical Assistant Usually Handles

The medical assistant usually handles four kinds of calls.

1. Requests to Schedule Appointments—The medical assistant will usually schedule appointments and tests, either in the office or at an outside laboratory or the hospital. This topic is discussed in the next chapter.

What Would You Do? What Would You *Not* Do?

Case Study 1

Channa has answered a telephone call from Jane Weston, who has called to make a routine appointment. Although the patient has been offered several different appointment days and times, none of the choices has been satisfactory. A low buzz indicates a call on another telephone line. Channa is the only person available to take the call. She tells Mrs. Weston that she will need to put her on hold for a minute. Mrs. Weston says, "Please don't put me on hold. I'll take that last appointment. What time was it for?" ■

2. Billing Inquiries—The medical assistant may handle inquiries about a patient bill or insurance. For this type of call, the medical assistant refers to the patient account in the computer and gives the caller the information requested. If the caller's question is complicated, the call may be referred to a billing specialist or the office manager.

3. Receiving Diagnostic Test and Lab Results—The medical assistant can also take calls regarding diagnostic test and lab results. Many lab results today are sent to physicians' offices by fax or directly on the computer system. But if a laboratory calls in test results, the medical assistant needs to have a blank laboratory slip so that the results can be filled in, along with the patient's name and the date the tests were taken. After taking the results, the medical assistant pulls the patient's medical record, clips the results to the front, and places the medical record where the physician can review it. Taking all results accurately is very important.

4. Requests for Information—Finally, the medical assistant can handle calls requesting information, such as directions to get to the office, office hours, and the office's medical specialty.

Taking Messages

The medical assistant takes messages using a message form. Some forms are pressure sensitive so that a copy is created with the original message. The originals stay in the message book and form a telephone log. If the message form does not create a copy, it is helpful to keep a separate telephone log for future reference. In some offices a form is used that has a space for the physician to write orders or desired follow-up on the bottom of the form. The medical assistant should not write in this space when taking the message. If telephone messages are filed in the patient's medical record after the physician or other recipient has responded to the message, a form with a peel-off backing is preferable.

When taking a message about a patient, the message should include the following information:

- Date and time
- Name of the physician or staff member
- Patient's full name and date of birth (or age)
- Name of the caller (if not the patient)

- Message or question that indicates clearly what the patient wants (e.g., prescription, laboratory results, medical advice)
- Additional information to clarify the message, such as symptoms, medication and pharmacy information, and actions that have already been taken
- If the patient is ill or requests medication, any medication allergies should be noted
- Telephone number
- Initials of the person taking the message

When a medical assistant transcribes messages from an answering machine or from voice mail, the same message form should be used. The time the call was recorded should be used. The medical assistant may need to play the message more than once in order to record all information (Procedure 39-2).

Patients Requesting Test Results

When a patient calls requesting test results, the medical assistant should find out when and where the test was done and take a message for the physician. Following the call, the medical assistant should locate the medical record, be sure the results of the laboratory or diagnostic test in question are in the record, and leave the message and medical record for the physician. It may be office policy to use a sticky paper flag to identify the report in the medical record.

Some offices choose to send patients letters about laboratory results, which cuts down on the number of telephone calls requesting information, especially for routine tests.

After reviewing the laboratory or diagnostic test results, the physician may instruct the medical assistant to call the patient back to give the results, to schedule follow-up testing, and/or to ask the patient to schedule an appointment to discuss the results.

Patients Reporting Satisfactory or Unsatisfactory Progress

Physicians often tell a patient to call and check at a specified interval after a visit, to report on how a condition is resolving after treatment.

If the patient reports satisfactory progress, the medical assistant should take a brief message, clip it to the chart, and leave it for the physician. An unsatisfactory report should generate a more complete message, and the chart should be pulled and the message clipped to it so that the physician can call the patient. When a patient gives a progress report on the telephone, either the original message should be filed in the patient record or the medical assistant should document the telephone conversation in the record.

Requests for Medication or Prescription Refills

Often patients or pharmacies call with requests to have prescriptions refilled or renewed. When the pharmacy calls, it is important to get the patient's name and date of birth, name of the medication, dosage, and amount of medication prescribed. When the patient calls, it is important to get the pharmacy name, location, and phone number, in addition to the name of the medication, dosage, and how often the

patient takes it. If the patient usually obtains the medication by mail order, this should be noted on the message with the complete address so that a written prescription can be sent to the patient. If the medication is an antibiotic or a controlled substance used for pain relief, the medical assistant should ask about symptoms that would require a refill. The medical assistant should tell patients to check with the pharmacy the next day unless they hear from the physician or office. A message to request medication is also clipped to the patient's medical record. Physicians often follow up directly with the pharmacy, especially if they are using an electronic prescription routing service, but in some offices the physician writes the prescribing information on the bottom of the message for the medical assistant to call in to the pharmacy. When medical assistants call in prescriptions, they should always note this in the progress notes and/or medication record (Procedure 39-3).

Calls for Referrals or Requesting Laboratory or Diagnostic Tests

A patient may call to say he or she needs a referral (because of a particular insurance company's policy) to see a specialist outside the medical group or to have a laboratory test or diagnostic procedure done.

The medical assistant takes the necessary information (what type of referral, for what, to whom) on a message form for the physician. If a referral is appropriate—or necessary because of an insurance company or health maintenance organization policy—the medical assistant fills out a referral form as completely as possible and gives it to the physician to complete and sign. If the patient is asking for a laboratory test, such as a throat culture, the medical assistant should fill out the laboratory form for the patient to pick up or enter the information into the computer, after verifying with the physician that the requested test is appropriate. The physician may ask the medical assistant to call the patient and schedule an appointment before authorizing the referral.

Patients with Medical Questions

For patients with medical questions, the medical assistant takes a message for a physician or refers the call to another staff member designated by the office to handle such calls. The office should have written guidelines to follow if a

---

What Would You Do? What Would You _Not_ Do?

Case Study 2

Mary Woodward, a 62-year-old woman with hypertension, has called because she has run out of her blood pressure medication. Mrs. Woodward tells Channa that the medication is atenolol and she is pretty sure that the dose is 50 mg every morning. When Channa asks for the pharmacy telephone number, Mrs. Woodward says, "It's the Best Buy Pharmacy in Whittier. You must have the telephone number. I don't know what it is off hand." ∎

medical assistant screens medical questions. The medical assistant should follow the written guidelines closely and take a message for the physician about any concern or question that falls outside the preset guidelines.

Calls from Other Physicians

Calls from other physicians are usually put through right away, even if the physician is examining a patient. If the medical assistant has to find the physician, this may be given as a reason to place the caller on hold briefly, but the medical assistant should locate the physician as quickly as possible and explain which physician is calling. The physician may ask the medical assistant to transfer the call to another extension to avoid talking in front of a patient.

Calls from Salespeople

Often a sales representative from a pharmaceutical company or equipment company calls before visiting the physician's office. Salespeople are usually seen by the office manager, who gives the information to the physician. Drug representatives sometimes drop by, but if they hope to talk to the physician they usually must call and ask for an appointment. Physicians usually schedule sales representatives during lunch. The physician has to agree to see the representative before a medical assistant makes an appointment.

Urgent or Emergency Calls

If a patient calls with a medical problem, the medical assistant asks questions to determine how urgent the problem is. After obtaining the caller's name and telephone number and identifying who has the problem (the patient's name, age, and relationship to the caller), the medical assistant should obtain the patient's symptoms and current condition. In most offices there is a guide to telephone screening in the office procedure manual. This helps the medical assistant identify which questions to ask in order to determine how urgent the problem is. In the next chapter, there is a more complete discussion on the kind of appointment to offer a patient based on the symptoms the patient reports.

If the medical assistant determines that the call represents an urgent problem or emergency, he or she should follow office policy. The call should be referred to a physician if one is in the office; in a group practice, one physician may be assigned at all times to take urgent calls. If there is no physician in the office, a nurse practitioner or physician's assistant may be assigned to take urgent calls. If no licensed professional is present in the office, the medical assistant must advise the caller or contact the on-call physician. The following are the guidelines for dealing with such a call:

1. If the emergency is serious or life threatening, the caller should be instructed to call an ambulance by dialing 911. This activates the emergency medical services (EMS) system. If the caller is a child, or seems upset or confused, the medical assistant can offer to call an ambulance for the caller.

2. If the emergency is a case of poisoning, the caller should be instructed to call the local poison control center. The telephone number of the poison control center (1-800-222-1222) should be placed next to every telephone in the medical office. Even if it is a case of poisoning, if the patient is unconscious or not breathing, the caller should be instructed to call an ambulance.

3. If the patient has a problem that requires treatment in an emergency department but is conscious and able to walk (e.g., a fractured arm), the caller should be instructed to take the patient to the nearest emergency department or call an ambulance. If the patient is alone, an ambulance should be called.

4. If the patient's problem is usually treated in the office, the patient should be given an appointment for that day.

5. If the condition of the patient is not life threatening and the medical assistant is unsure how urgent the problem is, the physician should be contacted for instructions either by cell phone or pager. If there is any doubt about how serious the patient's condition is, it is safer to instruct the patient to call an ambulance and/or go to the hospital emergency department.

Whenever an urgent call is handled, the medical assistant should fill out a message form to be sure that the information has been written down. Either the message form or the instructions given to the patient should later be documented in the medical record. If a patient has been instructed to go to the emergency department, the physician should be notified promptly.

Dealing with Problem Calls

The Caller Who Refuses to Give Information

When callers ask for a physician and refuse to identify themselves, it is probably because they want to speak to the physician but suspect that if they give a name, they will be asked to leave a message. The medical assistant should explain politely that the physician is not available and offer to take a message. If the caller still refuses to give information, the medical assistant can instruct the caller to write a letter to the physician and mark it "personal."

Complaints

The medical assistant should listen carefully to callers with complaints, avoid getting defensive or angry, and ask for specific information. It is important to remain calm so that a professional demeanor is maintained. The medical assistant should state clearly what he or she can and will do. It may be necessary to refer the matter to the office manager or the physician, but the medical assistant should get as much information as possible at the initial contact.

It is important to avoid hanging up on an angry caller. It is usually possible to calm a caller down as long as the medical assistant does not raise his or her voice and does not become defensive. The caller should be told a specific time when he or she can expect to hear back from someone in the office.

Patients with Special Problems

If a patient calls who is confused or has difficulty with English, the medical assistant should listen carefully and try as hard as possible to understand. The medical assistant may speak more slowly than usual but should not speak louder. If it is impossible to communicate, even using simple language, the medical assistant should try to at least obtain the caller's name and telephone number. Then it may be possible to find out from the medical record if the patient speaks a different language or if there is an emergency contact number. If the person seems confused, the medical assistant should ask if there is another person with whom he or she can speak because this may be a medical emergency. The medical assistant may need to ask for guidance from the physician or office manager.

PROCEDURE 39-1   **Performing Telephone Screening**

Outcome Screen incoming telephone calls.

Equipment/Supplies

- Telephone
- Message pad
- Pen or pencil

- Appointment book or computer terminal
- Clock or watch

---

1. **Procedural Step.** Answer the telephone each time it rings within the first three rings.
   Principle. Callers become annoyed when their calls are not answered promptly.

2. **Procedural Step.** Identify the medical office and give your name. Each practice will have a preferred way for all employees to answer the telephone. Example: "Primary Care Associates, this is Channa speaking." Do not rush through the greeting. The caller needs to hear this first sentence clearly.
   Principle. Callers need to know whom they have reached and with whom they are speaking. Otherwise they will have to ask if this is Primary Care Associates.

3. **Procedural Step.** Listen carefully to what the caller says and decide as soon as possible if this is a call you can handle, if you need to take a message, or if the call should be transferred to someone else in the office.
   Principle. The caller does not want to have to repeat all the details if the call must be transferred. If you need to take a message, begin writing.

4. **Procedural Step.** Ask for the caller's name. "May I ask who is calling?"
   Principle. You will need the caller's name either to address the caller by name, to take a message, or to identify the caller before transferring the call.

5. **Procedural Step.** If you can handle the call, such as a call for an appointment, do so promptly.

6. **Procedural Step.** If you need to take a message see Procedure 39-2, Taking a Telephone Message.

7. **Procedural Step.** If you need to transfer the call to someone else in the office, place the caller on hold, noting the caller's name and the extension. Tell the person you are transferring the call to who is calling and what extension the call is on.
   Principle. It is a courtesy to tell the person you transfer a call to who is calling; he or she must be able to locate the call if more than one line has a call on hold.

8. **Procedural Step.** If the caller describes symptoms that require immediate care, ask questions to assess the problem following guidelines in the office procedure manual. If there is a physician or other licensed professional in the office, transfer the call immediately. Otherwise, assess the urgency of the problem and follow up according to office guidelines. If the patient's health is at risk, instruct the caller to call 911.
   Principle. Patients expect correct medical advice from a health care facility when they have urgent medical problems.

9. **Procedural Step.** If your telephone has more than two lines, it is helpful to keep a list of the names of callers and extensions. When a call is on hold, the light for that telephone line blinks. If you have transferred a call, but the call remains on hold, within 30 to 45 seconds you should determine if the caller is still holding; if so, you should try to transfer the call again or take a message.
   Principle. Sometimes a transfer does not go through or the call is not picked up. The caller has no way to

get back in contact with you to leave a message or ask to speak to someone else.

10. **Procedural Step.** If the telephone rings for another call, ask if you may put the caller you are speaking to on hold and wait for the caller to agree. After pressing the hold button, answer the other call and explain that you are speaking to a caller on another line. Give the second caller the option to hold and wait for you or take their number and offer to call back as soon as you are finished.

    Principle. In general calls are handled in the order they are received. By asking for permission to put the caller on hold, you give the caller a chance to tell you

if it is an emergency. Some callers prefer to hold; others prefer to be called back. Time passes slowly when a caller is on hold, and the caller may become tired of waiting and wish to leave a message.

11. **Procedural Step.** At the end of the call, repeat any information you have discussed (such as the date and time of an appointment). End the call politely by thanking the caller (if appropriate) and saying "good-bye."

    Principle. Confirmation helps avoid misunderstandings. Thanking the caller and closing the conversation demonstrates telephone courtesy.

PROCEDURE 39-2

PROCEDURE 39-2 Taking a Telephone Message

Outcome Take a telephone message.

Equipment/Supplies

- Telephone
- Message pad
- Pen or pencil
- Clock or watch

---

1. **Procedural Step.** If you determine that the person a telephone caller wants to speak to is not available, offer to take a message.

    Principle. A message is a way of communicating to a person who is not available to speak on the telephone.

2. **Procedural Step.** Give the caller a reason why the person cannot take the call. Acceptable reasons are as follows: busy with a patient, not at his or her desk, not in the office, on another line. Generally physicians do not take calls except possibly during specified hours. Patients who ask for the physician are told that the physician is not in the office or that the physician is busy with patients.

    Principle. Most callers are willing to leave a message if they understand why their call is not being answered.

3. **Procedural Step.** Fill in the information on the message form, including the name of the caller, business affiliation (if any), date, time of the call, telephone number including area code, and information the caller wishes to leave about the reason for the call. Place your initials on the message in case there are questions. If there is a

section at the bottom for a response to the message, leave that area blank.

    Principle. Complete information is necessary to return a call.

4. **Procedural Step.** Verify the information. If possible, give a time when the call might be returned. If the message recipient does not have a scheduled time to return messages, say, "I will give him (or her) the message."

    Principle. Callers like to know when to expect a return call.

5. **Procedural Step.** End the call politely.

6. **Procedural Step.** If the call is from a patient or concerns a patient, pull the medical record and clip the message to it.

    Principle. This ensures that information about the patient is available and the action taken on the call can be charted if necessary.

7. **Procedural Step.** Place the message (with the patient record, if needed) where the person for whom it is intended expects to find messages. This may be on a desk or in a mailbox.

Continued

PROCEDURE 39-2   Taking a Telephone Message—cont'd

4

MESSAGE FROM								
For Dr. *Lawler*	Name of Caller *Anne Richards*	Ref. to pt. *mother*	Patient *Janice*	Pt. Age. *4*	Pt. Temp. *101°*	Message Date *10/13/xx*	Message Time *9:00* ⊙AM ☐PM	Urgent ☐ Yes ☐ No

Message: *Child has been on antibiotic for two days — still has fever. Should she come in again?*   Allergies *∅*

Respond to Phone # *814-322-6570*	Best Time to Call *any* AM PM	Pharmacy Name / # *West Side* *814-754-9817*	Patient's Chart Attached ☒Yes ☐No	Patient's chart #	Initials *KJ*

DOCTOR - STAFF RESPONSE

Doctor's / Staff Orders / Follow-up Action

	Call Back ☐ Yes ☐ No	Chart. Mes. ☐ Yes ☐ No	Follow-up Date / /	Follow-up Completed-Date/Time / /	AM PM	Response By:

Product # 78-9156-Pkg, #78-9157-Pads, Bibbero Systems, Inc., Petaluma, CA. To order, call toll free 800-BIBBERO (800 242-2376) OR FAX 800-242-9330.

Fill in the information on the message form. (From Hunt SA: *Saunders fundamentals of medical assisting,* St. Louis, 2007, Saunders.)

PROCEDURE 39-3   Taking Requests for Medication or Prescription Refills

Outcome Take a message requesting medication or a prescription refill.

Equipment/Supplies

- Telephone
- Message pad
- Pen or pencil
- Medical record
- Clock or watch

1. **Procedural Step.** Identify the caller and telephone number.
2. **Procedural Step.** Identify if the caller is a patient or a pharmacy.
3. **Procedural Step.** If the caller is a patient, take the information about the medication requested, dose, and number of times a day the patient takes the medication. Write down the name and telephone number of the patient's preferred pharmacy.
4. **Procedural Step.** If the caller is a pharmacy, usually the medical assistant takes a message, including the name and address of the patient, the medication requested, and the dosage and amount of medication to be prescribed. Inform the pharmacy when the physician is likely to approve the refill so that the pharmacy can tell the patient.

Principle. Usually physicians have specific times when they review and respond to messages.

5. **Procedural Step.** End the call politely.
6. **Procedural Step.** Pull the patient's medical record and place with the message where the physician can review it. If the physician responds directly to pharmacy calls, put the pharmacist on hold, pull the patient's medical record, and give it to the physician before transferring the call.

Principle. The physician will need to review information about the patient before agreeing to refill or prescribe medication.

7. **Procedural Step.** Usually the physician indicates on the message slip if the prescription may be refilled or writes a new prescription on the message slip. The medical assistant can then call the pharmacy with the informa-

MESSAGE FROM									
For Dr. Hughes	**Name of Caller**	**Ref. to pt.**	**Patient** Roland Aiken	**Pt. Age** 40+	**Pt. Temp.**	**Message Date** 10/13/XX	**Message Time** 3:00 AM/PM	**Urgent** ☐ Yes ☒ No	

Message: needs more Aldactazide (25mg tabs) — takes ⊤ dose daily **Allergies** ∅

Respond to Phone # 814-798-2010	**Best Time to Call** AM PM	**Pharmacy Name / #** Westside 814-754-9817	**Patient's Chart Attached** ☒ Yes ☐ No	**Patient's chart #**	**Initials** KJ

DOCTOR - STAFF RESPONSE

Doctor's / Staff Orders / Follow-up Action

OK – call to pharmacy JH
#30
12 refills
Sig: ⊤ po qam

Call Back ☐ Yes ☐ No	**Chart. Mes.** ☐ Yes ☐ No	**Follow-up Date** / /	**Follow-up Completed-Date/Time** / / AM PM	**Response By:**

Product # 78-9156-Pkg, #78-9157-Pads, Bibbero Systems, Inc., Petaluma, CA. To order, call toll free 800-BIBBERO (800 242-2376) OR FAX 800-242-9330.

The physician may write prescription information on the message form. (From Hunt SA: *Saunders fundamentals of medical assisting*, St. Louis, 2007, Saunders.)

tion. Read the prescription from the message slip exactly as the physician has written it.

Principle. The medical assistant functions as an agent of the physician in this case. He or she must give the exact information the physician has indicated.

8. **Procedural Step.** Document the refill or prescription in the patient's medical record. In some offices the message itself is filed in the medical record, and in others the medical assistant writes the information in the progress notes of the medical record.

Principle. Any treatment of the patient must be documented in the medical record as part of the continuous record of care given. See Chapter 26 for specifics on documenting medications.

CHARTING EXAMPLE

Date	
10/13/10	4:30 p.m. Prescription called to Westside Pharmacy for Aldactazide 25 mg tabs, #30, Sig: i po q am, 12 refills. ———————— ———————— K. Anderson, CMA (AAMA)

OUTGOING CALLS

More calls come into the office than go out. But there are certainly enough outgoing calls. Medical assistants make many of them. Outgoing calls a medical assistant may make include calls to patients, suppliers, insurance companies, other medical offices, laboratories, pharmacies, and hospitals. In some systems it is necessary to dial the number "9" before the telephone number in order to get an outside line. Local telephone books are still provided by the telephone service provider, although it is also possible to look up telephone numbers using the Internet.

Local Calls

Calls to patients, whether the matter is medical or financial, should not be made from the front desk unless a privacy window is closed. The medical assistant must prepare information and supplies before making the call. If calling a patient, the patient's medical record should be at hand with any notes from the physician. If the call is picked up by an answering machine, it is permissible to leave your name, practice name, and telephone number for the patient to call back. Because the patient's family members may have access to the answering machine or voice mail, no medical information should be included in the message (Procedure 39-4).

It may be necessary to call a patient about an overdue account. The medical assistant should not call the patient at work for this type of call or discuss billing information with anyone other than the person responsible for the bill.

For calls to laboratories, hospitals, or suppliers, the medical assistant should be sure to have organized the information necessary to complete the call before dialing the telephone number.

What Would You Do? What Would You *Not* Do?

Case Study 3

The physician asks Channa to schedule an appointment for Andrew Page, a 35-year-old man whose recent lipid profile shows an elevated cholesterol and triglyceride level. This is a change from previous laboratory work. The physician says to tell the patient that he wants to discuss the recent blood work in person. When Channa calls the patient, his wife answers the telephone. Channa identifies herself and the medical office and asks to leave a message for Mr. Page to return her call. Mrs. Page says, "He's away on a business trip until Thursday. What is this about? Is it really important?" ■

If the medical assistant places a call for one of the office's physicians, the physician must be ready to talk before the call is placed. As soon as the physician being called is located, the medical assistant connects the physician placing the call.

Medical assistants and other office staff should not make or receive personal calls using the office telephone system except for emergencies, both to avoid tying up the telephone and because telephone calls take time away from work. The medical assistant can check messages and make outgoing calls during breaks or at lunchtime using a pay phone or personal cell phone. Although permission may be given to make an urgent call using the office telephone, a personal long-distance call is never appropriate.

Long-Distance Calls

Long-distance calls are almost always dialed directly. The telephone number for a long-distance call can be obtained from directory assistance (411). It is less expensive to use one of the free 411 services that can be found by searching the Internet using the search term "free 411."

The medical assistant should know what kind of calling plan the office has because the time of a call can make a difference in the rate for long-distance calls. When calling distant locations, it is important to be aware of the different time zones.

To make international calls, the medical assistant should dial 1, then the country code, then the telephone number.

In order to prevent unauthorized long-distance calls, most offices have a code that must be used to access the long-distance system. Long-distance services may also be limited to one or two extensions.

Conference Calls

Some phone systems allow conference calls among three parties, such as a physician and two individuals who are being called at two different telephone numbers. If the telephone system allows this, the medical assistant should learn how to set up such calls for the physicians.

Memories *from* Externship

Channa Eng: I was terrified of the telephone when I first started my externship. It was a busy clinic, and I started out in adult medicine. In the morning, I sat at the front desk to check patients in, take copayments, and answer the telephone. I was always afraid that I wouldn't know what to say. We got the callers who wanted to speak to someone in person, so you never knew what to expect. My supervisor told me to answer each call with the name of the clinic and my own name, and then ask how I could help the caller. If I didn't know how to handle the call, I was supposed to put the caller on hold and ask Mary Lynn, the other medical assistant, for guidance. One call that I remember particularly was from an older woman who seemed lonely and confused. She asked for her physician, but she was willing to leave a message when I told her that the physician didn't take calls while he was seeing patients. She said that she couldn't remember if she was supposed to take her blood pressure medication once a day or twice a day and she wasn't sure if it was one pill or two pills. She told me that her daughter set up her pills in a pill container every week but she had forgotten if she should take them both in the morning or one in the morning and one at night. I told her to get the bottle of medication and read the label to me. From the label we determined that she was supposed to take two pills every morning. She thanked me, and I indicated on the message form that we had clarified the problem. After the call, Mary Lynn complimented me for being so helpful and for handling the call by myself. After that I began to feel more confident about taking telephone calls. ■

Prepare for Success

For conference calls where there will be many parties, most of the large long-distance carriers will set up conference calls for several participants. Usually all parties to the call will be asked to dial the same 1-800 number. The host, who is managing the call, will get a "host code." Other participants on the call will get a "participant code."

At the appointed time for the call, the host and participants all dial the 1-800 number, enter their codes, and are connected to the call. When the medical assistant is responsible for putting such a call together, he or she needs to work with the long-distance carrier to obtain the time, the 1-800 number to be dialed, and all of the host and participant codes. Then all of the participants must be informed of the time, the 1-800 number, and their particular participant code. This is usually done by e-mail so that each participant has a written record. If participants are notified by telephone, a follow-up fax with the written information should be sent to each participant. The instructions for each participant and for the host should be written as follows:

Date and time:

Dial-in: 1-800-XXX-XXXX

Host or Participant Code: YYYYYYYYY

PROCEDURE 39-4   Telephoning a Patient for Follow-up

Outcome Place an outgoing telephone call to a patient for follow-up.

Equipment/Supplies

- Telephone
- Scratch paper
- Pen or pencil

- Material necessary to place the call, such as a telephone book, instructions from physician, and/or patient medical record

1. **Procedural Step.** Organize all materials that may be necessary during the telephone call. Schedule calls during business hours.
   Principle. Preparation allows calls to be made more efficiently.

2. **Procedural Step.** Write the telephone number on a piece of paper. Include the area code and a country code, if necessary.
   Principle. It may be difficult to remember the number, especially if you do not reach the number on the first attempt.

3. **Procedural Step.** Place the call. When it is answered, ask for your party. Identify yourself with your practice name and your name ("This is Channa from Primary Care Associates").

4. **Procedural Step.** If you reach an answering machine, identify yourself with your practice name and your

name and ask the intended recipient to call you back. Leave your telephone number with area code.
   Principle. The subject of the telephone call should not be left on an answering machine to protect patient confidentiality.

5. **Procedural Step.** If you are speaking to the patient, give the information requested by the physician. This may be an instruction to make an appointment or may include laboratory results. Do not give more information than the physician has authorized.
   Principle. As an agent of the physician, you have limited authorization to provide information.

6. **Procedural Step.** If the patient has additional questions, offer to take a message for the physician.

7. **Procedural Step.** Close the call politely. Repeat instructions if any were given.

PROCEDURE 39-4

MEDICAL PRACTICE *and the* LAW

Recognizing and responding to medical emergencies

When a telephone call concerns a life-threatening or serious emergency, the medical assistant becomes legally responsible to provide appropriate assistance, even if the medical office is not equipped to provide the actual care needed. Once the medical assistant identifies an emergency, he or she must maintain contact with the caller, help the caller get assistance, and follow up to be sure that care was received.

Good Samaritan laws generally do not apply to the medical office because people expect to receive medical care and/or medical advice from physicians and medical offices.

The most desirable response is to refer an emergency or urgent call to a physician or other licensed health care provider in the office (nurse practitioner, physician's assistant, or licensed nurse). However, if no licensed professional is able to take the call, the medical assistant should assist the caller. The medical assistant should assess the situation and instruct the caller to arrange transportation to an emergency department if the patient's health will be harmed by delayed treatment.

The following guidelines describe an appropriate response to an emergency call:

- Medical assistants should always ask if they may put the caller on hold and wait for a response. This gives the caller an opportunity to state that the call is truly urgent or an emergency.
- Every medical office should keep an updated procedure manual near the telephone. The manual should list specific urgent problems and situations, specific questions to ask, and responses to the caller's questions. A list of emergency numbers should be placed near all telephones; these include the numbers for the EMS system (usually 911); the number for the poison control center; and the pager numbers or cell phone numbers for all the physicians in the practice.
- Medical assistants should write down a caller's name and telephone number as early in the call as possible, in case the call is interrupted. Keeping a telephone log provides documentation of how calls were handled.
- If the medical assistant believes delay in treatment poses a threat to the health of the ill or injured person, the caller should be instructed to call an ambulance. If the caller is a child or

Continued

MEDICAL PRACTICE *and the* LAW—cont'd

seems too confused or anxious to make the call, the medical assistant can call 911. The location of the emergency should be determined before making the call. It is preferable to use a different line to place a call to an ambulance so that contact can be maintained with the caller.

After instructing a caller to call an ambulance, there are several steps to follow up. The medical assistant should notify the physi-cian (if this has not already been done) and call the emergency department at the local hospital to inform them that one of the practice's patients will be coming in. If the injured or ill person is a patient of the practice, this should be noted in the patient's medical record. If the injured or ill person is not a patient of the practice, an incident report should always be completed. See Chapter 48 to learn how to fill out an incident report. ■

What Would You Do? What Would You *Not* Do?   RESPONSES

Case Study 1
Page 945

What Did Channa Do?
❑ Spoke politely, and told Mrs. Weston that she needed to pick up the other call.
❑ Gave Mrs. Weston the choice of being placed on hold or being called back.
❑ Assured Mrs. Weston that she would get back to the telephone call with her as soon as possible.
❑ Kept her voice calm and friendly.

What Did Channa Not Do?
❑ Did not let the second telephone call ring more than three times.
❑ Did not promise Mrs. Weston that she would put the other call on hold immediately.
❑ Did not try to rush through the call with Mrs. Weston without making sure that she was clear about the appointment date and time.

What Would You Do/What Would You *Not* Do? Review Channa's response and place a checkmark next to the information you included in your response. List the additional information you included in your response.

_____
_____
_____
_____

Case Study 2
Page 946

What Did Channa Do?
❑ Told Mrs. Woodward to get the bottle of pills that has a record of the dose and the pharmacy telephone number.
❑ Told Mrs. Woodward she would place her on hold. She instructed Mrs. Woodward to stay on the line after finding the medication bottle.

❑ Gave Mrs. Woodward the option of calling back when she had found the bottle of pills.
❑ If Mrs. Woodward seemed confused or distressed, Channa could verify the medication dose from the patient's medical record and look up the telephone number of the pharmacy.
❑ Remained calm and friendly.
❑ Made sure to follow up and complete the message.

What Did Channa Not Do?
❑ Did not become impatient or tell Mrs. Woodward that she should know she needed her bottle of medication ready when she called to ask for a refill.
❑ Did not pass on the message without confirming that Mrs. Woodward had asked for the correct dose of medication.
❑ Did not pass on the message without a pharmacy telephone number.

What Would You Do/What Would You *Not* Do? Review Channa's response and place a checkmark next to the information you included in your response. List the additional information you included in your response.

_____
_____
_____
_____

Case Study 3
Page 952

What Did Channa Do?
❑ Reassured Mrs. Page that it was not an urgent matter, but said she hoped Mr. Page would return her call after his trip.
❑ Told Mrs. Page politely that she could not discuss the matter with anyone but Mr. Page.

What Did Channa Not Do?
❑ Did not tell Mrs. Page exactly why she was calling her husband.
❑ Did not tell Mrs. Page that the matter was not important.

What Would You Do? What Would You *Not* Do? RESPONSES—cont'd

❑ Did not ask Mrs. Page to contact her husband before he returned from his business trip.

❑ Did not tell Mrs. Page that the physician could give her more information about the matter.

What Would You Do/What Would You *Not* Do? Review Channa's response and place a checkmark next to the information

you included in your response. List the additional information you included in your response.

_____
_____
_____
_____

TERMINOLOGY REVIEW

DSL (digital subscriber line) Technology that allows digital signals to be transmitted over telephone lines at high speed even if the telephone line is also being used for voice transmission.

Enunciation The act of speaking clearly and concisely.

Pager An electronic device that notifies the recipient to receive a message or return a telephone call.

PDA (personal digital assistant) A portable handheld computing device with access to various reference tools,

such as a drug reference, calculator, and address book.

Smartphone A cell phone with computer capabilities.

SSL (Secure Sockets Layer) A protocol for managing secure transmission of data over the Internet by means of encryption.

Voice mail A method for delivery, storage, and retrieval of telephone messages that is built into the telephone system.

ON THE WEB

For Information on Poison Control Centers:

American Association of Poison Control Centers: www. aapcc.org

For Information on Time Zones:

The Official U.S. Time: www.time.gov

PREPARE FOR CERTIFICATION Visit the Evolve site at http://evolve.elsevier.com/Bonewit/today/ to actively Prepare for your Certification.

CD *Check out the **Companion CD** bound with the book to access additional interactive activities.*

40

Scheduling Appointments

LEARNING OBJECTIVES	PROCEDURES
Methods of Scheduling	
1. Explain why scheduling appointments efficiently is crucial to the smooth operation of the medical office.	
2. Describe the correct use of appointment books and computer scheduling to make appointments.	
3. Describe the legal implications of the daily appointment schedule.	
Types of Scheduling	
1. Describe several types of scheduling including stream scheduling, double booking, wave, modified wave, and open booking.	
2. Identify types of patient appointments that may be clustered in the appointment schedule.	
Setting Up the Appointment Matrix	
1. Identify factors to be considered when setting up the appointment matrix.	Set up the appointment matrix.
2. List the steps in setting up the appointment matrix.	
Making an Appointment	
1. Differentiate between the information needed to make an appointment for a new patient and an established patient.	Make an appointment.
2. Differentiate between medical conditions that require emergency care, urgent care, and routine care.	
3. Describe how to schedule appointments for individuals who are not patients.	
Managing the Appointment Schedule	
1. Describe the method for changing or canceling appointments.	Manage the appointment schedule.
2. Describe how to update the schedule on the day of the appointment and document changes.	
3. Identify three methods to remind patients to make or keep appointments.	
4. Describe how to store appointment books and daily schedules.	
Scheduling Referral Appointments, Diagnostic Tests, Procedures, and Admissions	
1. Describe how to complete referral forms and obtain preauthorizations.	Complete a referral form for managed care.
2. Identify how to schedule outpatient and outpatient diagnostic tests and procedures.	Schedule inpatient or outpatient diagnostic tests or procedures.
3. Identify how to schedule hospital admissions and surgery.	Schedule inpatient or outpatient surgery.

CAAHEP COMPETENCIES

Administrative Competencies
Perform Clerical Functions
- Schedule and manage appointments.
- Schedule inpatient and outpatient admissions and procedures.

Clinical Competencies
Patient Care
- Perform telephone and in-person screening.

General Competencies
Professional Communication
- Respond to and initiate written communications.
- Recognize and respond to verbal communications.
- Demonstrate telephone techniques.

Legal Concepts
- Identify and respond to issues of confidentiality.
- Perform within legal and ethical boundaries.
- Document appropriately.
- Demonstrate knowledge of federal and state health care legislation and regulations.

Patient Instruction
- Explain general office policies.

Operational Functions
- Use computer software to maintain office systems.

ABHES COMPETENCIES

Professionalism
- Maintain confidentiality at all times.
- Be courteous and diplomatic.

Communication
- Use proper telephone techniques.
- Recognition and response to verbal and nonverbal communication.
- Application of electronic technology.
- Fundamental writing skills.

Administrative Duties
- Perform basic secretarial skills.
- Schedule and monitor appointments.
- Apply computer concepts for office procedures.
- Schedule inpatient and outpatient admissions.
- Obtain managed care referrals and precertification.

Legal Concepts
- Document accurately.
- Follow established policy in initiating or terminating treatment.

Instruction
- Orient patients to office policies and procedures.

blocked
clustering
double booking
established patient
fixed appointment scheduling
hospice
matrix (MAY-trix)
modified wave scheduling
new patient

no-show
preadmission testing (PAT)
preauthorization (PREE-awe-thur-eye-zay-shun)
referral
single booking
stream scheduling
time-specified scheduling
triage (TREE-ahzh)
wave scheduling

Some doctor are going for home visits

Introduction to Appointment Scheduling

Scheduling appointments is one of the most important administrative responsibilities performed in the medical office. Until the 1970s, people went to a medical office expecting to wait as long as an hour or more. Most physicians liked to see a full waiting room; it reassured them that their practice was healthy.

Going into the new century, people have little tolerance for waiting in a medical office. Lifestyles have changed and people have busy lives. Many have to take personal time away from work to go to the medical office, and they feel that their time is as valuable as the physician's time.

Scheduling appointments correctly and efficiently is crucial to the smooth operation of the medical office. Many factors must be taken into consideration when scheduling appointments. The patient who has made an appointment weeks or even months in advance wants to be seen within 15 to 20 minutes after arriving at the medical office. The physician wants a smooth flow of patients during the time scheduled for seeing patients. Patients who are ill or have accidents want to be able to see their physician on the day of the illness or injury. They prefer to be given a specific time, even if it is later in the day, rather than come into the office and wait for an open moment.

GUIDELINES FOR APPOINTMENT SCHEDULING

The most important criteria the medical assistant must take into consideration when scheduling appointments are exhibiting good interpersonal skills and reducing the amount of time a patient has to wait to see the physician. To meet these criteria, the medical assistant should follow seven guidelines:

1. Maintain the confidentiality of the patient. For example, do not discuss protected health information within hearing distance of other patients.

2. Speak clearly and do not appear rushed. Make sure the tone of your voice is friendly and courteous.

3. Concentrate only on the person to whom you are speaking.

4. Obtain all of the necessary information from the patient. Make sure the information is both correct and complete.

5. Repeat the information relayed to you by the patient. This avoids errors.

6. Schedule the proper amount of time for the type of appointment you are scheduling. For example, a new patient requires more time than an established patient.

7. Document all of the necessary information correctly in the appointment book or in the computer appointment scheduling system.

METHODS OF SCHEDULING

Two methods are used to schedule appointments. Appointments can be scheduled manually, using an appointment book. They can also be scheduled electronically using a computer. These methods are described in more detail next.

Appointment Book Scheduling

Appointment books are usually spiral-bound, so they will lie flat when opened (Figure 40-1). Each physician in the practice may have a separate book, or one book may serve the needs of two or more physicians. Appointment books are available in the following formats: pages for a single day, pages that display a week when open (over two pages), or pages with two or three physicians' schedules for a single day. The pages are further divided into time intervals. The pages are typically divided into 10- or 15-minute intervals. The medical assistant should choose the appointment book format that meets the needs of the practice.

The appointment book is usually maintained in pencil so that information can be changed if needed (e.g., when rescheduling a patient's appointment). In preparing for a day's visits, a typed or hand-printed list of patients, known as a *daily appointment schedule,* must be created. This list or the appointment book itself (if kept in ink) must be retained as a permanent record. The daily appointment schedule is discussed in more detail later in the chapter.

Computer Scheduling

Using a computer to schedule appointments offers advantages. The computer allows the medical assistant to designate appointment intervals. The appointment interval can be adjusted to 10, 15, or 20 minutes depending on the needs of the practice. The computer makes it easy to add, delete, or change appointments; set up repeating appointments; and set up a recall system. A recall system identifies patients that need to be contacted when it is time for them to schedule another appointment.

The medical assistant enters the patient's appointment into a data entry screen. This screen requires the entry of the same information as an appointment book. The computer also allows the medical assistant to print out a daily appointment schedule of patients to be seen for the day (Figure 40-2).

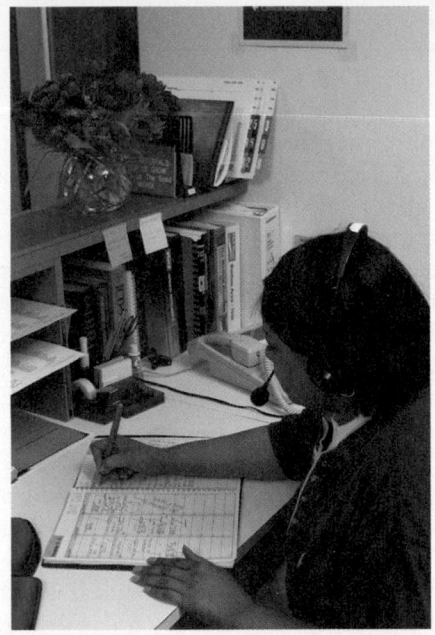

Figure 40-1. Medical assistant with appointment book.

Western Medical Center

(handwritten: 30 to 45 minutes)

Richard Warner, MD
Schedule for May 30, 2010

Time	Name	Reason	Home Phone	Work Phone
9:00 AM	ROBERT RICIGLIANO	Physical exam	(490) 459-2811	(490) 459-6217
9:10 AM	*			
9:20 AM	*			
9:30 AM	JUNE ST. JAMES	BP & ECG	(490) 459-5807	(490) 459-9222
9:40 AM	*			
9:50 AM	DARLA SISSLE	Influenza vaccine	(490) 220-1156	
10:00 AM	Catch-up			
10:10 AM	*			
10:20 AM	LLOYD RIDLON	Recheck	(490) 459-4242	(490) 459-0419
10:30 AM	ESTELLE JORDAN	New patient	(490) 459-8249	(490) 459-1062
10:40 AM	*			
10:50 AM	*			
11:00 AM	MARIA SANTOS	Physical exam	(490) 459-0022	
11:10 AM	*			
11:20 AM	THOMAS MAXWELL	Recheck	(490) 459-4123	(490) 459-9201
11:30 AM	*			
11:40 AM	ROBIN SOTO	Well baby	(490) 459-1349	
11:50 AM	*			
12:00 PM	LUNCH			
12:10 PM	*			
12:20 PM	*			
12:30 PM	*			
12:40 PM	*			
12:50 PM	*			
1:00 PM	LUCILLE MORENA	Chem screen	(490) 459-6677	(490) 459-1566
1:10 PM	*			
1:20 PM	*			
1:30 PM	*			

Figure 40-2. Computer appointment schedule.

DAILY APPOINTMENT SCHEDULE

Each day a list of the patients to be seen for that day must be created. This is called a *daily appointment schedule*. The daily appointment schedule serves several functions. It is used as a guide for pulling the patient's medical records for that day. It also is used as an office reference sheet of patients with appointments for that day. Usually the daily appointment schedule contains the patient's name, telephone number, and reason for the visit (e.g., new patient, physical examination, recheck). A separate schedule is created for each physician.

If the medical office uses an appointment book, the daily appointment schedule must be typed or hand-printed by the medical assistant. If a computer is used to schedule appointments, the list is printed out in hardcopy form. When additions need to be made to the daily appointment schedule, they must be made in dark-blue or black ink. This is because the daily appointment schedule is an official legal record of the patients seen on a given day. It may be used to verify tax returns and insurance claims.

Following the HIPAA requirements, the daily appointment schedule must be posted in an office area not accessible to patients. If this is not possible, a blank sheet of paper should be taped in front of the schedule to maintain confidentiality of patient information.

TYPES OF SCHEDULING

A number of different methods are available to schedule appointments in the medical office. They include the following: time-specified, wave, modified wave, double booking, and open booking. In addition, appointments may be clustered or categorized depending on the type of patient or type of examination or treatment. The method an office uses to schedule appointments is based on the needs of the practice and physician preference.

Time-Specified (Stream) Scheduling

Time-specified scheduling, also known as **stream scheduling,** involves scheduling appointments at a specific time. Most offices use this method for scheduling appointments. The goal of time-specified appointments is to minimize the waiting time for the patient and, at the same time, to keep a steady flow of patients moving through the office (like a stream of water). The amount of time allotted for a time-specified appointment depends on the reason for the visit. In general, the following times are allotted:

- New patient: 30 to 45 minutes
- Complete physical examination: 30 to 45 minutes
- Established patient: 10 to 20 minutes

When using the time-specified method, the medical assistant needs to make sure to allow time in the schedule to accommodate urgent visits, such as ill or injured patients. There are two other terms that may be used for this type of scheduling: **fixed appointment scheduling** or **single booking.**

Wave Scheduling

With **wave scheduling,** three or four patients are scheduled every half hour and are seen in the order in which they arrive at the office. The goal is for patients to arrive in "waves" so that there is always a patient waiting to be seen. Sometimes, ill patients are seen before those with routine appointments.

This scheduling system assumes that some patients will need to be worked into the schedule. Sometimes patients become uncomfortable when they realize that another patient was given the same appointment time, but a simple explanation can usually reassure the patient. The medical assistant might say, "We schedule all our patients on the hour, and then they are seen in the order they arrive. There is always a patient to be seen, and we find that waiting time is often shorter."

Modified Wave Scheduling

The wave system can be changed in several ways to create a **modified wave schedule.** The office may schedule patients at specific times during the first half of each hour, and keep the second half hour open for special circumstances. This may include working in patients, seeing patients who arrived late, or finishing up with patients from the first half hour.

Another modification to the wave system is to schedule one appointment that is expected to take longer on the hour (e.g., physical examination), and to schedule three or four rechecks (follow-up appointments) on the half hour (Figure 40-3).

Double Booking

When two patients are given the same appointment time, the practice is called **double booking.** Double booking means that two patients are scheduled into a single time slot. Double booking may be used when a patient can be fitted in around a patient undergoing a diagnostic procedure such as an electrocardiogram (ECG). It is also used when a patient with an injury or acute illness must be added to an already-full schedule.

Open Booking

Sometimes patients are not given a specific appointment time but are told to come in during a time range, such as between 9:00 AM and 11:00 AM. The patients are then seen in the order in which they arrive. In an open-booking system, patients with an injury or an acute illness are usually seen ahead of patients with less significant complaints.

Sometimes medical offices and clinics have walk-in hours designated for acute conditions before regular office hours. In this situation, patients are seen in the order of arrival.

Open booking works best when there is a constant stream of patients or when a practice is not busy. Because patient flow is unpredictable, patients often have to wait a long time.

Time	Single Booking	Time	Wave Scheduling	Time	Modified Wave Scheduling
9:00	Robert Ricigliano (490) 459-1111	9:00	Robert Ricigliano (490) 459-1111	9:00	Robert Ricigliano (490) 459-1111
9:10	*Physical exam*		*Physical exam*		*Physical exam*
			June St. James *Re* √		
9:20			(490) 459-1000		
			Robin Soto		
9:30	June St. James *Re* √ (490) 459-1000		(490) 297-1349	9:30	June St. James *Re* √ (490) 459-1000
9:40	Robin Soto (490) 297-1349		*Well-child visit*		Robin Soto (490) 297-1349
9:50	*Well-child visit*				*Well-child visit*

Figure 40-3. Comparison of single booking, wave scheduling, and modified wave scheduling.

Clustering or Categorization

Clustering involves scheduling patients with similar problems or conditions into groups. Each group is seen on a certain day or within a certain time block during the day. This scheduling method is also called *categorization.* Examples of conditions that can easily be clustered into a day or portion of a day are:

- Physical examinations
- Prenatal patients in an OB/GYN practice
- Diagnostic procedures

Multiple Offices

Some physicians see patients in more than one office. Appointments may be scheduled in each office or through a central system. In this case, it is important to clarify which office the patient wants to visit. It may be necessary to transport the medical record from office to office if an electronic medical record system is not in place.

SETTING UP THE APPOINTMENT MATRIX

Appointments are usually scheduled up to 6 months in advance. Before scheduling can begin, the appointment book or computer software must be set up to indicate the times when the physician will see patients. Times when the physician is not available to see patients must be **blocked out.** The resulting page is known as an appointment **matrix** (Procedure 40-1).

How the times are blocked out depends on the scheduling method used by the office. If the office uses an appointment book, the times are blocked out by drawing lines through the blocked times. If a computer is used to schedule appointments, the times are blocked out by setting aside blocks of time. A colored background is usually used for blocked times in a computer scheduling program (Figure 40-4).

The appointment matrix must take three variables into consideration: the scheduling system, the physician's preferences and needs, and the facilities and equipment requirements. Each of these is discussed later.

Appointment Intervals

Appointments are usually scheduled at intervals of 10 minutes, 15 minutes, or 20 minutes in either a manual or computer system. An appointment may be scheduled for more than one block, depending on the type of appointment. For example, if a 10-minute interval is used, an established patient coming to have his blood pressure checked might be scheduled for one 10-minute interval and a new patient might be scheduled for three 10-minute intervals. In this case, a 10-minute interval uses one line and a new patient uses three lines in the appointment book or on the computer schedule. If a 15-minute interval is used, all appointments are scheduled in multiples of 15 minutes. In general, more time must be allotted for new patients, physical examinations, and special procedures than for routine follow-up visits.

Physician's Preference and Needs

The second variable influencing the appointment matrix is the physician's preferences and needs. At times during the day, the physician is not able to see patients and therefore these times must be blocked out on the schedule. Time must be blocked out when the physician has another obligation, such as hospital rounds and nursing-home visits. Time may also need to be blocked out for lunch, pharmaceutical representatives, and catch-up. Days are also blocked out of the schedule for vacation, days off, attendance at conferences, giving lectures, or other professional activities.

Facilities and Equipment Requirements

The third variable affecting the appointment matrix is the availability of facilities and equipment. The appointment matrix must be set up so that examination rooms and rooms with equipment required for certain procedures are available to all physicians who are seeing patients. For optimal use of resources, one or more physicians should be available to see patients whenever the office is open.

Physicians like to have at least two examination rooms available for seeing patients, preferably side by side. This improves efficiency and time management for examining patients.

PROCEDURE 40-1   Setting Up the Appointment Matrix

Outcome Set up an appointment matrix.

Equipment/Supplies

- Appointment book or computer program
- Pen
- Physician schedule
- Office calendar

---

1. **Procedural Step.** Block times when the office is not open to see patients. This includes times in the book before office hours begin, lunch and/or breaks, afternoons or days when the office is closed, and holidays when the office will be closed. Some offices set up the appointment matrix 6 months in advance, whereas others do it for a year in advance. In an appointment book, draw an **X** through times that the office is closed. If the office uses a computer program, set up times when the office is open and set the appointment interval (10, 15, or 20 minutes).

   Principle. In an effective appointment schedule, only available appointment times are blank.

2. **Procedural Step.** Block times when each individual physician is NOT available to see patients, including lunch and hospital rounds. In addition, block days each physician will be away from the office for vacations, conferences, or other anticipated absences. If the physician has regular meetings or other regular commitments (such as nursing home visits), mark these also. In an appointment book, draw an **X** through the times the physician is not available. If the office uses a computer program, schedule the meeting, vacation, or such like an appointment using a colored background to show that the times are unavailable.

3. **Procedural Step.** For each physician, mark times when the physician does certain types of examinations, procedures (e.g., physical examinations, obstetric visits), or surgery. In an appointment book these are often highlighted with a marker or given a written title at the beginning of the time block. In a computer program these times may be set up as if for a separate physician (e.g., Dr. Gomez and Dr. Gomez-OB visits).

4. **Procedural Step.** Depending on office policy, block out as much time as is anticipated for same-day appointments, catch-up time, and unexpected needs. Depending on the practice, catch-up time may be 15 minutes in the morning and afternoon for each doctor and time for same-day appointments may be an hour or longer for all physicians or one particular physician on a rotat-

ing basis. These times can be marked in various ways as long as office staff understand that they must be saved until the scheduled day.

Example: On this day, the office will be open from 9-5, but Dr. Warner will only be available to see patients from 9-1 because he plans to attend a conference in the afternoon. The appointment interval is 15 minutes. Dr. Warner likes to have 15 minutes set aside for catch-up time at 10:30 in the morning.

Block times when the physician is not available using a colored background. (Screenshot used by permission of MCKESSON Corporation. All Rights Reserved. © MCKESSON Corporation 2008.)

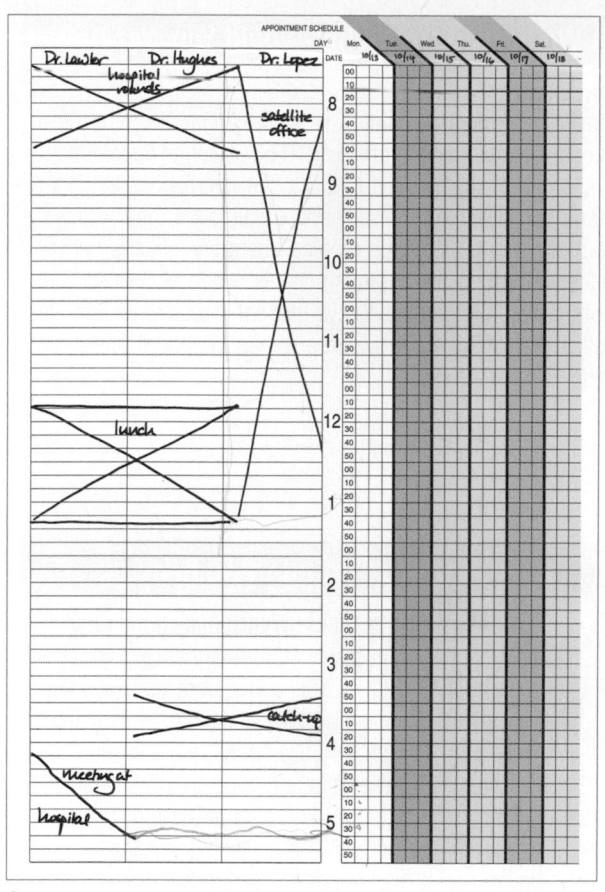

Time	Dr. Warner	Dr. Gomez
8:30 AM		
8:40 AM		
8:50 AM		
9:00 AM		
9:10 AM		
9:20 AM		
9:30 AM		
9:40 AM		
9:50 AM		
10:00 AM		
10:10 AM	Catch-up	
10:20 AM		
10:30 AM		
10:40 AM		Catch-up
10:50 AM		
11:00 AM		
11:10 AM		
11:20 AM		
11:30 AM		
11:40 AM		
11:50 AM	Lunch meeting – Memorial Hospital	
12:00 PM		
12:10 PM		
12:20 PM		
12:30 PM		Lunch
12:40 PM		
12:50 PM		
1:00 PM		
1:10 PM		
1:20 PM		
1:30 PM		

A   B

Figure 40-4. A, Appointment matrix from appointment book. **B,** Computer appointment matrix. (**A** from Hunt SA: *Saunders fundamentals of medical assisting,* St. Louis, 2007, Saunders.)

GUIDELINES FOR SCHEDULING

When scheduling an appointment, the medical assistant needs to obtain the proper information from the patient, document it accurately, and confirm it with the patient. The procedure for scheduling appointments varies depending on whether the patient is an established patient or a new patient.

Established Patients

For insurance billing, an **established patient** is defined as a patient who has been seen in the medical office within the past 3 years and has a current medical record. Patients who have not been seen within the past 3 years are typically treated as new patients, although their old medical records will be found if possible.

If an established patient is scheduling a return appointment, the physician usually specifies a time period on the patient's encounter form for the return visit (e.g., 1 week, 2 weeks, 1 month, 6 months). The appointment should be scheduled as close as possible to the date specified by the physician. The appointment must also be scheduled for the length of time preferred by the physician, which is

usually 10 to 15 minutes. Before locating available appointment times to offer the patient, the medical assistant should ask what day of the week and what time of day are convenient for the patient. For an established patient, it is necessary to obtain the patient's name, date of birth, and physician. If an appointment book is being used, it may be easier to ask the patient for a home and work telephone number than to look up this information. When a computer system is used, telephone numbers appear in the appointment window when the correct patient is selected.

If the patient is at the office, the medical assistant should complete an appointment reminder card and give it to the patient. The medical assistant enters the patient's name, the name of the physician, and the date and time of the new appointment on the card.

Special Situations

Some situations require special attention when scheduling an appointment for an established patient. The most common situation is when a patient visits the medical office and the physician orders laboratory tests to be performed at a medical laboratory. The physician will want to review the results of these tests before the patient comes in for a return visit. When scheduling the patient's return visit, the medical assistant must be sure to allow enough time for the patient to have these tests performed and the results to be returned to the office.

Patients who must undergo a laboratory test at the medical office that requires fasting (e.g., fasting blood sugar) should be scheduled early in the morning. This provides the least amount of inconvenience for the patient who must abstain from food and fluids until the specimen has been collected.

Sometimes the patient needs to be scheduled for an appointment for a date later than can be accommodated by the appointment book. In this situation, the medical assistant can either ask the patient to call later to schedule the appointment or the patient's name can be put on a list and scheduled later. In the latter instance, the medical assistant must make sure to call the patient when the appointment is scheduled.

New Patients and Referrals

Specific information needs to be obtained when scheduling an appointment for a **new patient.** This includes the patient's full name, daytime telephone number, and the reason for the visit or type of visit (e.g., sick visit, physical examination, diagnostic procedure). The medical assistant should ask the patient if he or she has been referred by another physician. Usually managed care referrals are made directly by a physician's office, but for some types of insurance, the patient may bring the referral form at the time of the visit.

Most offices schedule new patients for 30 to 45 minutes. The medical assistant should set aside the correct amount of time for the appointment depending on the physician's preference.

The medical assistant may need to relay directions to the patient on the office location. Some offices mail the health history form to new patients and instruct them to bring the completed form to the first appointment. An office brochure containing information about the practice may also be mailed to the patient or given to the patient at the first appointment.

When the patient has been referred by another physician, the patient should be given an appointment as soon as possible, especially if the patient has urgent symptoms or if the patient's primary physician's office is calling to make the appointment (Procedure 40-2).

Same-Day Appointments

The following problems are usually treated in the medical office and are usually scheduled the same day as the patient calls. The medical assistant should be familiar with office policy because each office varies in the degree of complexity of care it offers.
- Wounds without fracture or dislocation
- Sprains and strains
- Nausea, vomiting, or diarrhea that persists for more than 2 or 3 days

What Would You Do? **What Would You *Not* Do?**

Case Study 1

Sandra Meyers has been sitting in the waiting room for several minutes. She arrived at the office at 10:50 AM for an appointment scheduled at 11:00 AM. At 11:15 AM she approaches the front desk and asks how long she will have to wait to see the physician. On this day, the physician is running about 25 minutes behind schedule, and there are still two patients ahead of Sandra. She appears to be upset, and she says that she needs to be back in her office by 12:30 PM to prepare for an important afternoon meeting. ■

Putting It All into Practice

My name is Elaine Wyatt, and I am a certified medical assistant. My primary responsibility is to schedule routine and urgent care appointments, although sometimes I sit at the front desk and check patients in. I work in an office with five internists and two nurse practitioners. Calls from patients who select "Make an Appointment" from our telephone menu will end up with me or another medical assistant, or the receptionist may transfer a call to me. I also check patients out after they have been seen and make follow-up appointments using our computer system. Sometimes the telephone is ringing off the hook, and I really have to concentrate to keep track of each call. Our office has a procedure manual with guidelines for handling urgent calls, and we try very hard to give patients appointments the same day if they are sick. We leave several open appointments for this, but even if we have to double book, we will fit them in because our physicians want to be sure that everyone receives the care they need. All of our physicians and nurse practitioners are accepting new patients, and we always ask new patients to arrive at the office about 15 minutes early to fill out a patient history form. Usually our appointment system works pretty well and patients do not have to wait more than 10 or 15 minutes—at least, that is our goal. There are days, of course, when the physicians get behind, but through trial and error, we have developed a system that works pretty well for us. ■

Prepare for Success

- High fever (over 101°F for children and over 102-103° for adults)
- Sudden illness or severe pain without bleeding, fainting, or loss of consciousness
- Sore throat, especially with fever
- Burning, frequency or urgency on urination, especially if accompanied by fever or blood in the urine

- Vaginal bleeding in a pregnant woman (who may also be sent to the emergency department)

If a patient's primary physician's schedule is booked, patients with these types of conditions may need to be scheduled with a practitioner who has a more flexible schedule. In many multipractitioner offices, a period of time is blocked off in one physician's schedule to accommodate same-day appointments.

Urgent Care and Emergencies

The majority of appointments are made well in advance of the date a patient will see the physician, but there are times when urgent or emergency situations occur. A patient calling the office with an emergency presents a challenging situation for the medical assistant. It is important to give a caller a chance to tell you that it is an urgent situation before putting the call on hold. A life-threatening or serious medical problem should be immediately referred to the physician. The physician will make the decision about the appropriate course of action to take. If the physician is not present, the caller should be referred to emergency medical services, usually by calling 911 (Box 40-1). The office procedure manual should be used when responding to emergencies.

Walk-in Patients

Sometimes patients come to the office without an appointment and ask to be seen. If the patient is experiencing an emergency or urgent problem, the physician may ask the medical assistant to work the patient into the schedule. In routine situations, however, the patient is asked to return at a later date and offered an appointment. In these situations, the medical assistant should tactfully inform the patient of the medical office policy with respect to scheduling appointments.

Individuals Who Are Not Patients

The physician may see various individuals who are not patients during office hours. Time should be blocked from

---

BOX 40-1 Medical Conditions Referred to Emergency Medical Services (911)

1. Conditions that may result in damage to body structures. This is especially important for problems that can cause a significant decrease in oxygen to the body because of breathing or circulation disorders:
   - Breathing problems, or respiratory arrest
   - Severe chest pain, or cardiac arrest
   - Bleeding that cannot be controlled
   - Large open wounds
   - Any suspicion of internal bleeding
   - Potential poisoning or overdose
   - Bleeding in, or injury to, a pregnant woman
2. Conditions that result in very low blood pressure:
   - Shock
   - Serious burns
   - Severe bleeding
3. Conditions that result in a change in the level of consciousness (loss of consciousness, disorientation, confusion, loss of alertness)
4. Fractures or large wounds that require the equipment found in an emergency department

---

Highlight on Triage

Triage is the process of sorting patients according to their need for care. When a disaster occurs, health care workers choose which patients to treat first, depending both on the severity of their injuries and the likelihood the person will survive.

Victims are sorted into three groups—hence the word *triage*—from a French word meaning "sort." Some victims' injuries are minor and can wait for treatment; some have injuries so severe they will probably not survive no matter what effort is put into their treatment; and some have severe injuries but will probably survive if prompt treatment is given.

This system has been adapted to the office and appointment scheduling to decide if a patient can wait for the next available appointment, if the patient should be seen immediately, or if the patient should be sent to the emergency department. Triage in the medical office setting is rarely a case of life or death, and the term *triage* is usually reserved for screening performed by licensed health care personnel with the education needed to assess the medical needs of ill patients.

The medical assistant does screen calls and make decisions on the basis of guidelines established by the physicians where he or she works. The medical assistant must remember that if there is any question about a patient needing immediate care, either the telephone call should be referred to a qualified person in the office or the patient should be directed to an emergency department or other facility where care can be obtained. The medical assistant should be familiar with the policies of his or her employer and work within them both to avoid injuring the patient and to protect against liability in a potential lawsuit. ■

What Would You Do? What Would You *Not* Do?

Case Study 2

On a winter afternoon, there is only one physician in the office. He must leave promptly at 3:45 because he is scheduled to give a lecture to medical students at a nearby hospital shortly after 4:00. The physician has been running behind because two extra patients have been worked into the schedule. At 2:30, in addition to three patients in the waiting room, he still has four established patients scheduled, as well as one new patient scheduled for 3:15, the last appointment of the day. ■

the schedule to accommodate these appointments. Many offices have a specific time slot, often during the lunch hour, to schedule representatives of pharmaceutical companies or representatives of companies with medical equipment or computer equipment that the office may be thinking of purchasing. There is usually a maximum of one or two appointments set aside for each physician for this type of appointment each day. Some physicians may have only one day a week for this type of appointment.

PROCEDURE 40-2   Making an Appointment

Outcome Make an appointment for a patient.

Equipment/Supplies

- Appointment book or computer program
- Pencil

1. Procedural Step. Obtain information from the patient: which physician to book the appointment with, the purpose of the appointment, and any scheduling preference. Referrals are usually offered the first available appointment. If you do not recognize the patient's name, ask if the patient has been seen before. New patients may be encouraged to choose a physician who has joined the practice recently and is not as busy as the more established physicians. Established patients are usually booked with their primary physician, but if it is an urgent problem they may accept an appointment with another provider in the practice.

2. Procedural Step. Offer the patient a date and time for the appointment. Keep locating appointments until an acceptable date and time has been found. The more urgent the appointment, the more the patient must adapt to the office schedule.

3. Procedural Step. For a new patient, obtain the patient's demographic data (e.g., address, telephone number, date of birth), the name of the patient's insurance company, the name of the insured, the patient's insurance group number and ID number, a referral number, or other information related to insurance. Be sure to discuss the cost of the visit if the patient does not have insurance. Inform the patient if a referral form from the primary physician is necessary. Enter this informa-

tion directly into the computer as you obtain it from the patient.

Principle. Before making an appointment for a new patient, it is important to be sure that the patient can pay the bill. Information about insurance and referral provides a basis to inform the patient what his or her personal financial liability is likely to be.

4. Procedural Step. For an established patient, obtain the information to make the appointment. This includes the patient's name, date of birth, reason for the visit, and daytime telephone number.

5. Procedural Step. If using an appointment book, enter the information in pencil and block out the correct amount of time. If using a computer program, enter the patient's name, the correct amount of time for the appointment, and the reason for the visit.

6. Procedural Step. Repeat the information to the patient before ending the call. Offer a new patient directions to the office.

Example: The appointment schedule shows a 30-minute appointment for the new patient Estelle Jordan, a 10-minute appointment for the established patient Thomas Maxwell, and a 20-minute appointment for a well-child visit for Robin Soto (also an established patient).

6				
10:30 AM	ESTELLE JORDAN	New Patient	(490) 459-8249	(490) 459-1062
10:40 AM	*			
10:50 AM	*			
11:00 AM	MARIA SANTOS	Physical Exam	(490) 459-0022	
11:10 AM	*			
11:20 AM	THOMAS MAXWELL	Recheck	(490) 459-4123	(490) 459-9201
11:30 AM	*			

Schedule appointment times for the correct amount of time.

MANAGING THE APPOINTMENT SCHEDULE

Changing Appointments

The most frequent modification required in the appointment schedule is to change an appointment from one time slot to another. The way in which this is done is based on the method used by the medical office to schedule appointments. If the manual method is used, the original appointment is erased and the information is written into the new time slot. If a computer is used to schedule appointments, the original appointment is deleted and then inserted into the new time slot. Usually the computer program has a feature that does this with one operation.

Occasionally an entire block of patients has to be rescheduled. This occurs when the physician is unexpectedly absent or delayed during office hours. The absence or delay may be due to an emergency, being delayed at the hospital, or personal illness. Every effort must be made to accommodate scheduled patients by giving them a new appointment as quickly as possible. If there are patients in the office when a physician is severely delayed or must leave, it is important to tell patients how long they can expect to wait. The patients should be given the option of waiting or rescheduling their appointments.

If the physician is running seriously behind schedule, patients often become impatient. Some may wish to reschedule, and this should be done willingly. Usually the physician is willing to stay late to finish the day's appointments, but if the physician must leave at a particular time, appointments set for late in the day may need to be rescheduled.

No-shows are patients who simply do not show up for their appointment. No-shows and cancellations on the day of the appointment should be marked in red ink on the daily appointment schedule. The information should also be documented in the patient's medical record. This provides a permanent record if the patient's condition becomes worse and the patient claims that the physician would not see him or her.

Most offices have a policy of reviewing records of patients after three consecutively missed appointments. If the patient is not motivated to adhere to the treatment plan, the physician may wish to terminate the relationship with the patient (Procedure 40-3).

Late Patients

The office should have a policy regarding late patients. Traffic problems or other incidents can delay even the most punctual person, and usually the office attempts to work the patient into the schedule. If a patient telephones to say that he will be unexpectedly delayed, the schedule can either be adjusted or the patient can be offered a new appointment. Patients who habitually arrive late can cause delays in the appointment schedule. They may be given the last appointment of the day when the physician is most likely to be running late. In some practices habitual latecomers are told that their appointment time is 15 to

Memories *from* Externship

Elaine Wyatt: The office where I did my externship was always very busy. I remember one afternoon when one of the physicians had to leave suddenly. She was expected to be gone about 2 hours. I was told to call the list of afternoon patients and tell them that the physician had been called away from the office and would be delayed about 2 hours. If the patient wanted to reschedule, I had to put him or her on hold and transfer the call to the appointment scheduler. If the patient wanted to be seen that day, I had to give him or her a time from the revised list. I was surprised that about half of the patients were completely willing to reschedule, so there did end up being enough appointment times for the patients who still wanted to be seen. The major problems occurred when we could not reach the patients by telephone. There were about five of them, and they all came. Two of them were during the 2-hour delay, and both of them decided to reschedule. The other three had appointments after the physician returned. We managed to fit them in close to their original appointment time, and they never even knew that the physician had been out of the office unexpectedly. ∎

Prepare for Success

30 minutes earlier than the appointment is actually scheduled.

Appointment Reminders

Patients who make appointments while in the office are usually given an appointment reminder card. Appointment cards help patients remember the exact date and time of their next appointment (Figure 40-5).

Most offices also call patients 1 or 2 days before the appointment. The medical assistant uses the information that was documented when the appointment was made (manually or by computer) to call each patient scheduled for an appointment.

Patients have a right to confidentiality regarding their appointment. Patients should be asked if it is acceptable to leave an appointment reminder message on an answering machine or voice mail system.

Computer programs have the capability to identify patients who need periodic routine examinations, such as a physical examination or a gynecologic examination. Many offices send out reminders to patients who need to make an appointment for a routine examination. These reminders may be in the form of letters generated by the computer, or they may be e-mails generated by the computer.

Storing Appointment Books and Daily Schedules

In some offices, the appointment book is maintained in ink and used as the office record of appointments. The official book or all daily schedules are updated as described earlier in this chapter and should be stored in a secure area.

PROCEDURE 40-3

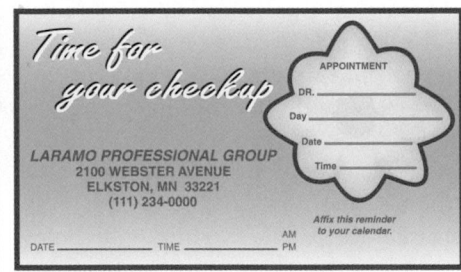

Figure 40-5. Appointment reminder cards. (From Young AP, Proctor DB: *Kinn's the medical assistant,* ed 10, St. Louis, 2007, Saunders.)

PROCEDURE 40-3   Managing the Appointment Schedule

Outcomes

1. Review the daily appointment schedule.
2. Cancel a patient appointment.
3. Change a patient appointment.
4. Indicate a missed appointment.
5. Document cancellations and missed appointments on the day of the appointment.

Equipment/Supplies

- Appointment book or computer program
- Printed appointment schedule
- Red pen

1. **Procedural Step.** Review the daily appointment schedule and be sure that all medical records and other necessary paperwork are prepared.
2. **Procedural Step.** Check patients in on the official daily schedule as they arrive. Depending on office procedure, you may also check them in using the computer program.
3. **Procedural Step.** If a patient calls to cancel an appointment, locate the appointment on the appointment schedule, in the appointment book, and/or in the computer appointment program.
4. **Procedural Step.** To cancel an appointment (except on the day of the appointment), erase the appointment in the appointment book or delete the appointment in the computer program. To cancel an appointment on the day of the appointment, draw a line through the appointment on the official schedule in red and note that the appointment was canceled.
   Principle. The official schedule is a legal document. Changes are made in red to indicate that they occurred on the day of the appointment.
5. **Procedural Step.** If the patient cancels an appointment, offer to make another appointment for the patient.
6. **Procedural Step.** If the patient cancels an appointment and declines or postpones making a new appointment, document the cancellation in the patient's medical record.
   Principle. Documentation of cancelled or missed appointments makes it readily apparent if this behavior is a common pattern for the patient.

7. **Procedural Step.** If the patient wants to change or reschedule an appointment, after canceling the old appointment, find an acceptable time to reschedule.
8. **Procedural Step.** Enter the patient's name and contact information into the new time in the appointment book or computer program.
9. **Procedural Step.** Repeat the information to the patient before ending the call or fill out an appointment card if the patient is present in the office.
10. **Procedural Step.** If the patient misses an appointment without canceling, draw a red line through the appointment on the daily appointment sheet and label the appointment "No Show."
11. **Procedural Step.** It may be office policy to telephone the patient to determine why the appointment was missed and offer another appointment.
12. **Procedural Step.** Document the missed appointment in the medical record, and indicate whether the patient has rescheduled.

PROCEDURE 40-3

CHARTING EXAMPLE

Date	
6/07/10	11:45 a.m. Patient did not keep appointment
	at 9:30 a.m. Unable to reach the patient at
	11:30 a.m. Telephone disconnected. No other
	contact information. ———————————
	——————————— Elaine Wyatt, CMA (AAMA)

10

Western Medical Center

Richard Warner, MD
Schedule for May 30, 2010

Time	Name	Reason	Home Phone	Work Phone
9:00 AM	ROBERT RICIGLIANO	Physical exam	(490) 459-2811	(490) 459-6217
9:10 AM	*			
9:20 AM	* NO SHOW			
9:30 AM	JUNE ST. JAMES	BP & ECG	(490) 459-5807	(490) 459-9222
9:40 AM	*			
9:50 AM	DARLA SISSLE	Influenza vaccine	(490) 220-1156	
10:00 AM	Catch-up			
10:10 AM	*			

Draw a red line through appointments that the patient fails to keep.

SCHEDULING REFERRAL APPOINTMENTS, DIAGNOSTIC TESTS, PROCEDURES, AND ADMISSIONS

Referrals and Preauthorizations

A referral is an authorization for a visit to another physician, usually a specialist. A referral is also an authorization for a treatment. A **referral** is made by the patient's primary care physician. It is an authorization for a specific number of visits to or treatments by a specialist or other health care practitioner. Usually, the primary care provider can initiate a referral to a physician who participates in the patient's managed care plan without **preauthorization** (official permission from the patient's insurance company). This is consistent with the primary physician's role as "gatekeeper," or person responsible for deciding what care is medically necessary for the patient. For patients covered by Medicaid, however, all care other than visits to the primary care provider must be authorized. (The Medicaid program has a different name in every state.)

Preauthorization may be required for certain medical procedures, therapy (e.g., physical therapy, occupational therapy, speech therapy), certain diagnostic procedures, and consultations by a physician who does not participate in the insurance plan, surgery, and hospitalization. If preauthorization is required, the medical assistant usually calls the insurance company to obtain a preauthorization number. Written follow-up or computer entry may be required by the insurance company.

Three types of referrals are common:
1. To a specialist physician for a consultation on a particular disease, condition, or injury
2. To a provider of ongoing therapy, such as physical therapy, occupational therapy, or psychological therapy
3. To a provider of community-based services, such as home health care, visiting nurses, or respite care for a caregiver

The physician determines the type and amount of service needed, but the medical assistant usually completes the referral form(s).

After obtaining all necessary information to make the referral, the medical assistant either instructs the patient to make the appointment himself or calls to make the appointment for the patient. Some managed care plans require the referring provider's office to make the appointment. If the medical assistant calls from the office, the patient may be able to obtain an earlier appointment, but it is important to verify the date and time with the patient. Figure 40-6 is an example of a referral form.

For a referral to a community resource, the medical assistant must know the patient's name, address, and telephone number, as well as the particular resource needed, the diagnosis, and the reason for the service. Community services include home health care and **hospice** care (a range of services provided to an individual with a terminal illness). Most community agencies do an intake evaluation of the patient, but others depend on the primary care or other physician and staff to tell them what resources the patient needs.

Especially for patients who have managed-care insurance, every referral must be documented closely and often justified to the insurance company's utilization review personnel. Medical assistants play an important role in facilitating the referral process (Procedure 40-4).

Scheduling Diagnostic Procedures and Hospital Admissions

It is often easier for a physician's office to schedule a diagnostic procedure or laboratory test for a patient than to have the patient schedule it. Hospital admissions are always scheduled by the physician's office. Scheduling procedures and admissions can be performed while the patient is at the office or when the patient is at home. If the patient is at home, the details of the appointment and any special patient instructions must be mailed to the patient and followed up with a telephone call.

Scheduling a Diagnostic Procedure

Before scheduling a diagnostic procedure for a patient with an outside facility, the medical assistant should compile all of the information that needs to be relayed to the facility. This includes the patient's name, telephone number, the type of procedure being performed, the reason for the procedure, the time frame within which the procedure must be performed, and insurance information including any need for a preauthorization number or written referral.

After an appointment has been made, the medical assistant must contact the patient to relay when and where the procedure will be performed. The medical assistant may also need to provide directions to the facility. Patients are often required to prepare for a diagnostic procedure. For example, a patient undergoing a colonoscopy needs to perform procedures at home to cleanse the colon of gas and fecal material. These instructions must be relayed to the patient by the medical assistant. If written instructions are available, they should be given or sent to the patient. The medical assistant should document in the patient chart the type of verbal and written instructions provided to the patient. Following the procedure, the medical assistant should document when and how the patient was notified

---

What Would You Do? What Would You *Not* Do?

Case Study 3

Anna Greene, a 17-year-old girl, came to see the physician for a physical examination. On the basis of her history and physical examination, the physician has ordered her to have an echocardiogram (ultrasound of the heart). Anna's mother says that the physician did not really explain why Anna needs this test, and she expresses concern that her insurance will not cover the total cost of the test. She appears to be reluctant to allow the test to be scheduled and says that she will call and schedule it herself in a few days. ■

Health Plan
Referral Form

REFERRAL NUMBER: A06

WRITTEN REFERRALS ARE REQUIRED FOR ALL SERVICES, EXCEPT FOR ROUTINE YEARLY EYE EXAMS, ORAL SURGERY, LAB, DIAGNOSTIC & RADIOLOGICAL SERVICES.

(1) Patient Name: _____

(2) Date of Referral: _____ / _____ / _____

(3) Patient Identification Number: _____ (4) SUFFIX # REQUIRED _____

(5) Date of Birth: _____ / _____ / _____

(6) Referred From: _____
NAME OF PERSONAL CARE PHYSICIAN   Provider ID #

(7) I.P.A. No. _____

(8) _____
ADDRESS OF PERSONAL CARE PHYSICIAN

Referred To: _____
NAME OF SPECIALTY CARE PHYSICIAN/PROVIDER/EMERGENCY   Provider ID #

(10) _____
ADDRESS OF SPECIALTY CARE PHYSICIAN/PROVIDER/EMERGENCY

REFERRAL STATUS:
(CHECK ONE)

In I.P.A.
☐   ☐   ☐   ☐

REASON FOR REFERRAL (STATE DIAGNOSIS): _____

SERVICES REQUESTED (CHECK ONE)

REFERRAL VALID FOR TWELVE MONTHS FROM DATE OF REFERRAL.

☐ Consultative OPINION. (One (1) visit only) CONTACT PCP PRIOR TO INITIATING TREATMENT.

☐ SECOND SURGICAL OPINION ONLY (Surgery is not to be performed by this provider)

☐ Consultative OPINION and NECESSARY DIAGNOSTIC STUDIES. (Not to exceed three (3) visits)

☐ Consultative OPINION and NECESSARY DIAGNOSTIC STUDY AND TREATMENT. **Indicate number of visits** _____

☐ Mental Health EVALUATION: Circle one (1) or two (2) visits only. (FOR PCP USE ONLY)

☐ Substance Abuse Outpatient EVALUATION: Circle one (1) or two (2) visits only. (FOR PCP USE ONLY)

☐ Mental Health/Substance Abuse Treatment (PSYCHIATRIC REVIEWER USE ONLY) subsequent visits, indicate number _____

AUTHORIZATION FOR MENTAL HEALTH OR SUBSTANCE ABUSE OUTPATIENT SERVICES DOES NOT OVERRIDE BENEFIT MAXIMUMS.

☐ Therapies (type of therapy: _____). **Indicate number of visits** _____ (PT not to exceed six (6) visits per referral)

☐ Obstetrical Treatment. Designate duration of care: _____

☐ Emergency Room Treatment. Date of service: _____ / _____ / _____
SEPARATE REFERRAL FORM REQUIRED FOR EACH EMERGENCY ROOM DATE OF SERVICE

Note: Only those services included in the Health Plan Description of Benefits will be covered. If you have any questions contact your Professional Relations Coordinator.

I have enclosed a clinical document summary, have performed the following diagnostic studies, and am supplying the information to assist you.

DIAGNOSTIC PROCEDURES	DATE OF SERVICE	RESULTS

INSTRUCTIONS

PCP:	SPECIALIST:	ER AUTHORIZATION
• Complete Form	• For Referrals to another Specialist Consult W/ PCP	• Send Health Plan Copy to Appropriate Address (see above)
• Send Health Plan Copy and Specialist Copy to Specialist	• Send Health Plan Copy to Appropriate Address (see above)	• Retain Copy for your file
• Retain PCP Copy for your file		• Be sure to notify

X _____
SIGNATURE OF PERSONAL CARE PHYSICIAN

_____ / _____ / _____
AUTHORIZATION DATE

X _____
SIGNATURE OF PHYSICIAN REVIEWER*

_____ / _____ / _____
AUTHORIZATION DATE

*ALL OUT OF PLAN REFERRALS REQUIRE PHYSICIAN REVIEWER SIGNATURE

Figure 40-6. Referral form. (From Hunt SA: *Saunders fundamentals of medical assisting*, St. Louis, 2007, Saunders.)

of the results of the diagnostic procedure. Precise documentation in patient charts is necessary to avoid later claims of malpractice or abandonment (Procedure 40-5).

Scheduling an Inpatient Admission

The medical assistant has several tasks that must be performed when a patient is admitted to the hospital. The medical assistant must contact the patient's insurance company to obtain preauthorization. The next step is to call the hospital's admitting department to schedule the admission.

The medical assistant must provide the admitting department with the patient's name, address, date of birth, admitting diagnosis, and the patient's insurance information and preauthorization number. A patient must be seen by his or her physician within the first 24 hours after admission. Because of this, the hospital may ask when the physician is coming to see the patient. In addition, admitting orders must be sent or faxed before the patient is admitted to the hospital.

The procedure for admitting a patient to the hospital is modified somewhat if the patient is first seen in the emergency department and then admitted to the hospital. In this situation, the hospital obtains the information from the patient and then contacts the physician to obtain admitting orders (Procedure 40-6).

(Give the pt Instructed)

Scheduling Surgery

Scheduling a surgery is similar to scheduling a diagnostic procedure; however, more information is necessary to schedule a patient for surgery. In addition to the patient's name, date of birth, and telephone number, the medical assistant must also know the type of surgery to be performed, the time frame within which the surgery is to be performed, who the surgeon and any assistant surgeons will be, who the anesthesiologist will be, and the name of the hospital or outpatient center at which the surgery will be performed.

Before scheduling the surgery, the medical assistant must call the patient's insurance company and obtain preauthorization (prior approval by the insurance company). The preauthorization number must be relayed when scheduling surgery. This number facilitates payment by the insurance company for the procedure. The patient's insurance may require the patient to undergo the surgery at specific hospitals or outpatient facilities.

Before a patient undergoes a surgical procedure, **preadmission testing (PAT)** is performed. PAT includes blood tests, an ECG, and a chest x-ray. The purposes of PAT are to obtain data about the patient's health before surgery, to be sure that the patient can tolerate the proposed surgical procedure and anesthesia, and to obtain baseline data for comparison during and after the surgical procedure. The medical assistant helps the patient to schedule this testing.

In some communities the hospital performs the PAT, whereas in other communities the PAT is performed in the medical office. If performed in the medical office, the PAT is done at either the surgeon's office or at the office of the patient's primary care physician.

A patient may also need to be scheduled to donate one or more units of his or her own blood. This blood would then be available if a patient needs a transfusion during or after surgery.

Giving a Patient Instructions before Surgery

The medical assistant is often responsible for providing the patient with specific instructions before the surgery. If the patient is receiving a general anesthetic, he or she must fast for a period of time before the surgery. Fasting requires that the patient have nothing to eat or drink for approximately 12 hours before the surgery. If the patient takes medication for hypertension or heart problems, the surgeon may allow the patient to take his or her morning medication with a sip of water. Other examples of preparation that may be required before a surgical operation include washing with an antibiotic soap and taking antibiotics for 1 to 2 days. Patients should be instructed not to bring valuables with them to the hospital. If they are having outpatient surgery, they need to have someone available to drive them home following the surgery.

Documenting an Appointment for Surgery

It is important for the medical assistant to carefully document all information relayed to the patient regarding the surgery. Other information that should be documented includes the interactions with the surgical team members, patient, and facilities.

PROCEDURE 40-4 Completing a Referral Form for Managed Care

Outcome Complete a referral form for managed care.

Equipment/Supplies

- The patient's medical record and insurance information
- Physician's directions about the service to be provided
- Referral form
- Telephone

1. Procedural Step. Assemble information to complete the referral form, including the patient's name, address, telephone number, and insurance information.

2. Procedural Step. From the patient's medical record or the physician, determine the service for which the patient will be referred, including the specialist or service provider, the reason for the referral, and the number of visits.

3. **Procedural Step.** Obtain preauthorization from the patient's insurance if necessary by calling the toll-free number provided by the insurance company. Describe the service requested, reason for the referral, and number of visits requested.

   Principle. The patient's medical condition must justify the service requested. Failure to obtain preauthorization required by the insurance company will result in denial of the patient's insurance claim.

4. **Procedural Step.** Complete a referral form, including the requested information about the patient, referring physician, specialist or facility to which the patient is being referred, reason for the referral, preauthorization number (if verbal preauthorization was obtained), and amount of service authorized.

5. **Procedural Step.** If preauthorization is required, submit the form to the patient's insurance company for approval. In some cases the patient will not be able to obtain service until written preauthorization is received from the insurance company.

6. **Procedural Step.** Retain a copy of the referral for the patient's medical record, and give the remaining copies to the patient to submit when service is received. You may also choose to send the referral forms directly to

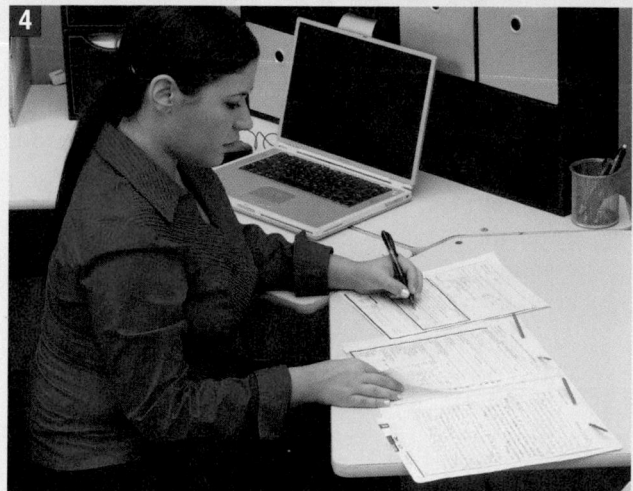

Complete the referral form required by the patient's insurance.

the specialist or facility to whom the patient has been referred.

7. **Procedural Step.** Instruct the patient how to make the appointment (or assist the patient to make the first appointment).

8. **Procedural Step.** File the referral form in the patient's medical record.

PROCEDURE **40-5** Scheduling Inpatient or Outpatient Diagnostic Tests or Procedures

Outcome Schedule an inpatient or outpatient diagnostic test or procedure.

Equipment/Supplies

- The patient's medical record and insurance information
- Name of the test or procedure to be scheduled
- Telephone

- Telephone number of the facility and name of the appropriate department to schedule the test or procedure

1. **Procedural Step.** Assemble necessary information about the patient, including the patient's demographic and insurance information.

2. **Procedural Step.** From the patient's medical record and/or a diagnostic test or procedure requisition filled out by the physician, determine the facility and department to call for scheduling. If the office uses a computerized system, be sure the test, procedure, or hospital admission has been ordered in the computer.

   Principle. Any admission, diagnostic test, or diagnostic procedure must have a valid physician order. For insurance reimbursement, a facility that participates in the patient's insurance plan must be used.

3. **Procedural Step.** Determine the time frame for scheduling and, if possible, discuss with the patient preferred days and times.

4. **Procedural Step.** Obtain preauthorization from the patient's insurance, if necessary, by calling the toll-free number provided by the insurance company.

   Principle. The patient's medical condition must justify the service requested. Failure to obtain preauthorization required by the insurance company will result in denial of the patient's insurance claim.

5. **Procedural Step.** Call the department of the facility where the procedure will be performed.

6. **Procedural Step.** Provide the patient's name, demographic, and insurance information as needed and

Continued

PROCEDURE 40-5   Scheduling Inpatient or Outpatient Diagnostic Tests or Procedures—cont'd

preauthorization number if needed. Identify the test or procedure to be scheduled and set up a specific day and time.

7. Procedural Step. Inform the patient of the date and time for the test or procedure and provide verbal and written instructions, including preparation for the test, special instructions, and dietary restrictions.

Go over any instructions with the patient before the test.

Principle. The patient must know how to prepare for the test or procedure. Written instructions reinforce verbal explanations.

8. Procedural Step. Send a computer or paper requisition to the facility or give a paper requisition to the patient to take to the test.

9. Procedural Step. Document the scheduled diagnostic test or procedure and instructions given to the patient in the patient's medical record.

CHARTING EXAMPLE

Date	
9/22/10	3:45 p.m. Barium swallow scheduled at
	Memorial Hospital for 9/28/10 at 9:15 a.m. Pt.
	instructed to remain NPO after midnight and
	given directions to Memorial Hospital x-ray
	department. Pt. verbalizes understanding
	that she cannot eat or drink anything
	(including water) after midnight. ————
	———————— Elaine Wyatt, CMA (AAMA)

PROCEDURE 40-6   Scheduling Inpatient or Outpatient Admissions

Outcome Schedule an inpatient or outpatient admission for a patient.

Equipment/Supplies

- The patient's medical record and insurance information
- Name of the procedure to be scheduled or reason for the hospital admission

- Telephone
- Telephone number of the facility and the admitting department

1. Procedural Step. Assemble necessary information about the patient, including the patient's demographic and insurance information.

2. Procedural Step. From the patient's medical record and/or directions from the physician, determine the reason for the inpatient or outpatient admission.

Principle. Any admission must have a valid physician order. For insurance reimbursement, a facility that participates in the patient's insurance plan must be used.

3. Procedural Step. Determine the time frame for the admission. If it is for an elective procedure or surgery, discuss with the patient preferred days and times.

4. Procedural Step. Obtain preauthorization from the patient's insurance by calling the toll-free number provided by the insurance company.

Principle. The patient's medical condition must justify the service requested. Failure to obtain preauthorization required by the insurance company will result in denial of the patient's insurance claim.

5. Procedural Step. Call the admissions department to schedule the admission.

Principle. The patient must be entered into the facility's computer system with all demographic and insurance information for an inpatient or outpatient hospital admission.

6. **Procedural Step.** Provide all necessary information including demographic and insurance information about the patient, preauthorization number (if any), diagnosis or reason for the admission, and date of the admission.

7. **Procedural Step.** For an inpatient admission, provide admitting orders as needed or fill out admitting orders according to the patient's medical record and fax to the department or nursing floor.

8. **Procedural Step.** If the patient is to be admitted to the hospital directly from the physician's office, assist the patient to notify a family member, prepare a patient transfer form, obtain consent forms to release information, and make arrangements for the patient to be transported to the hospital.

9. **Procedural Step.** If the patient is to be admitted for a procedure or surgery in the future, inform the patient of the date and time for the test or procedure and provide verbal and written instructions, including preparation, special instructions, and dietary restrictions.

Principle. The patient must know how to prepare for the procedure or surgery. Written instructions reinforce verbal explanations.

10. **Procedural Step.** Document the admission or scheduled procedure or diagnostic test and instructions given to the patient in the patient's medical record. For a hospital admission, identify any documents sent with the patient.

CHARTING EXAMPLE

Date	
6/15/10	1:30 p.m. Patient to be admitted to Memorial Hospital, Room 802 by ambulance for shortness of breath and dyspnea. Admitting orders and copy of medical record will be sent with the patient. Patient's son notified and states he will meet his mother at the hospital.
	———————— Elaine Wyatt, CMA (AAMA)

PROCEDURE 40-6

MEDICAL PRACTICE *and the* LAW

The office is required to keep a permanent list of patients seen. This is a legal record. Because the appointment book is usually maintained in pencil, the daily appointment sheet is usually maintained as the legal record, which is why additions and corrections must be done in ink. If the office has a computerized appointment system, there is an electronic record of the appointment schedule, which should be backed up daily. A single red line is usually drawn through the names of patients on the list who cancelled their appointments or did not come for their appointments. The Internal Revenue Service (IRS) can ask for records to validate tax returns. Government insurance programs may also require these records as proof that services were provided. The daily schedules should be kept for a minimum of 5 years, but most practices keep them indefinitely.

If a physician wishes to terminate the relationship with a patient, such as a patient who consistently breaks appointments or does not follow up on treatment, it is recommended that the patient be sent a letter explaining the reasons for terminating care and giving the patient time to arrange for other medical care. This protects the physician if the patient initiates a lawsuit for abandonment. Without proper notification, the patient may still consider himself or herself the physician's patient, even if he or she does not follow the physician's treatment plan or keep scheduled appointments. In order to be sure that the patient has received the letter, it should be sent certified mail with return receipt requested. ∎

What Would You Do? What Would You *Not* Do? RESPONSES

Case Study 1
Page 964

What Did Elaine Do?
❏ Listened to Sandra's concerns without interrupting.
❏ Apologized for the delay and agreed that it is difficult to wait when you have other obligations.
❏ Informed Sandra that the physician was running behind schedule and that there were two patients ahead of her. Gave her a realistic estimate of when she would be taken to an examination room.

❏ Offered to reschedule the appointment if Sandra said that she really could not wait to see the physician that day.

What Did Elaine Not Do?
❏ Did not tell Julia that she would be taken to an examination room in just a minute.
❏ Did not give a long explanation about why the physician was delayed.
❏ Did not give exaggerated or made-up excuses to imply that this was a one-time crisis.
❏ Did not become defensive or interrupt Julia.

Continued

What Would You Do? What Would You *Not* Do? RESPONSES—cont'd

What Would You Do/What Would You *Not* Do? Review Elaine's response and place a checkmark next to the information you included in your response. List the additional information you included in your response.

_____

_____

_____

_____

Case Study 2
Page 965

What Did Elaine Do?

❑ Asked the physician if it would be a good idea to reschedule the new patient or some of the other patients for another appointment in the next few days.

❑ If instructed to do so, called patients, explained that the physician was going to have to leave the office early, and asked if they would be willing to reschedule.

❑ If instructed to do so, explained to the patients in the waiting room that the physician was delayed and asked if they would like to reschedule.

❑ Evaluated all patients carefully to be sure that everything was prepared to make their examinations go smoothly.

What Did Elaine Not *Do?*

❑ Did not reschedule patients without discussing it with the physician.

❑ Did not tell the patients specific information about the physician's commitments.

What Would You Do/What Would You *Not* Do? Review Elaine's response and place a checkmark next to the information you included in your response. List the additional information you included in your response.

_____

_____

Case Study 3
Page 970

What Did Elaine Do?

❑ Made a general statement that the physician thought the test was important, and it would help the physician to provide the best care for Anna.

❑ Asked Mrs. Greene and Anna to wait to see if the physician could give them more information about the reason for and need for the test.

❑ Offered to call the insurance company to determine whether Mrs. Greene's insurance would cover the cost of the test.

❑ Explained that the office preferred to schedule this type of test to be sure that the testing facility had all necessary information from the physician.

❑ Documented the interaction with the patient in detail.

What Did Elaine Not *Do?*

❑ Did not give a reason for the test unless authorized by the physician.

❑ Did not imply that the mother cared more about the money than her daughter.

❑ Did not say that the physician knows what he is doing.

❑ Did not insist on scheduling the test even if Mrs. Greene did not agree to it.

What Would You Do/What Would You *Not* Do? Review Elaine's response and place a checkmark next to the information you included in your response. List the additional information you included in your response.

_____

_____

_____

_____

TERMINOLOGY REVIEW

Blocked Times in the appointment matrix when physicians are not available to see patients.

Clustering Scheduling similar types of patients or examinations on the same day or part of the day.

Double booking Scheduling two patients for the same appointment time.

Established patient A patient who has been receiving services from the same medical practice on a regular basis.

Fixed appointment scheduling An appointment scheduling method in which each patient is given a different, specific appointment time. Also called *stream scheduling, time-specified scheduling,* or *single booking.*

Hospice Palliative service provided for patients whose life expectancy is less than 6 months. Services may be provided in the patient's home, nursing home, or special hospice facility.

Matrix A rectangular or linear arrangement of numbers or information.

Modified wave scheduling An appointment system that has some fixed appointments and some appointment times during which patients are seen in order of arrival.

New patient For billing purposes, a patient who has not received services during the previous 3 years from any physician in a medical practice.

TERMINOLOGY REVIEW—cont'd

No-show A patient who does not keep a scheduled appointment.

Preadmission testing (PAT) A series of diagnostic tests done before surgery to establish the patient's health status and identify any potential problems that may occur during surgery.

Preauthorization Permission from a patient's insurance company for a test, procedure, or surgery. Usually the insurance company issues a preauthorization number, which must be communicated to the laboratory or hospital that will be billing for the test or procedure.

Referral Recommendation that a patient receive additional medical services. For patients with managed care insurance, a referral must be accompanied by a written form that specifies the nature of the service and the number of visits that have been authorized.

Single booking An appointment scheduling method in which each patient is given a different, specific appoint-ment time. Also called *stream scheduling* or *fixed appointment scheduling.*

Stream scheduling An appointment scheduling method in which each patient is given a different, specific appointment time. Also called *fixed appointment scheduling, time-specified scheduling,* or *single booking.*

Time-specified scheduling An appointment scheduling method in which each patient is given a different, specific appointment time. Also called *stream scheduling, fixed appointment scheduling,* or *single booking.*

Triage The process of separating patients by the urgency of their need for care.

Wave scheduling A method of scheduling appointments in which several patients are given the same appointment time and seen in the order in which they arrive.

ON THE WEB

For Information on HIPAA Regulations:

United States Department of Health and Human Services HIPAA website: aspe.hhs.gov/admnsimp

Center for Medicare and Medicaid Services HIPAA website: www.cms.hhs.gov/HIPAAGenInfo

For Information on Organizations with Information on Practice Management:

American Academy of Family Physicians: www.aafp.org/online/en/home.html

PREPARE FOR CERTIFICATION Visit the Evolve site at http://evolve.elsevier.com/Bonewit/today/ to actively Prepare for your Certification.

CD Check out the *Companion CD* bound with the book to access additional interactive activities.

41

Medical Records Management

CAAHEP COMPETENCIES

Administrative Competencies
Perform Clerical Functions
- Organize a patient's medical record.
- File medical records.

General Competencies
Legal Concepts
- Establish and maintain the medical record.
- Identify and respond to issues of confidentiality.

ABHES COMPETENCIES

Administrative Duties
- Perform basic secretarial skills.
- Prepare and maintain medical records.
- Apply computer concepts for office procedures.

acronym (AK-row-nim)
active record
cross-index
electronic health record (EHR)
electronic medical record (EMR)
filing system
inactive record

indexing units
medical records management
out guide
sorter
surname (SIR-name)
tab
terminal digit filing

Introduction to Medical Records

A medical record (also known as a *patient chart*) contains the important information related to an individual patient in written or electronic form. It includes the care given to that patient and the progress of the patient's condition. **Medical records management** is the process of controlling and handling medical records from the time a record is created until it is placed in permanent storage or destroyed. In addition to recording the care given to patients, medical records may also be used to review quality of care and for recording statistical information.

It is impossible for a physician or other professional to remember every detail of care, such as the results of a physical examination or doses of particular medications. Many people in the primary care physician's office have contact with a patient, as well as consulting professionals, laboratories, and hospitals. It is important that each interaction is recorded in the patient's medical record. This provides an ongoing record of both the patient's state of health and the service provided by the medical office.

Medical records are also legal documents, if there are questions about the care given. If a patient sues a physician, the court will require documentary evidence, such as a medical record, to be presented in court. The court will take the position that whatever is documented in the record is the care that was given. If something is not documented, officially it never happened. To protect the legal interests of the physician's office, it is therefore important to keep complete medical records.

PAPER-BASED MEDICAL RECORDS

Many medical records still rely on paper-based medical records to document care. A manila file folder is created for each patient containing all documents related to the care of that patient. These records are maintained in files to be available each time the patient is seen at the office.

ELECTRONIC MEDICAL RECORDS

In many medical offices, part or all of the medical record is maintained on computer. This is usually called an **electronic health record (EHR)** or **electronic medical record (EMR)**. Information is entered directly into the computer system, using computer terminals, hand-held devices, and/or voice recognition systems. The computer terminals may be located in each examination room or at selected areas within the office. Entry of information is necessary whenever care is provided or information is obtained from the patient. The EMR is usually linked to the computer appointment and billing systems.

This type of system offers a number of advantages:
- Medical information is always legible.
- Information is easy to retrieve.
- Medical offices can be linked to laboratories, hospitals, and insurance companies. Access to laboratory data and test results is also easy and quick.
- The EMR can be linked to medical information such as information about medications or treatment protocols for specific medical conditions.
- Less time is spent filing.
- Less storage space is required.

The change from a paper system to an electronic system often seems overwhelming. In addition to the important issues related to data security (and hence patient confidentiality), there are several other challenges to overcome:
- Cost of computer hardware, software maintenance, and staff training
- Orienting new or temporary staff to the EMR system
- Difficulty in adding older records to an EMR system
- Difficulty preventing unauthorized alterations and authenticating digital signatures
- Structuring data so that it can be transferred between different digital systems

Some facilities print a full or partial record for office visits and then enter new information during the visit or immediately after the patient has been seen. Old records are usually gradually scanned into the system, but until this process is complete, established patients often have an old paper record in addition to the new electronic record. Even with high-quality scanning systems, handwritten originals may not be legible after scanning.

Despite the challenges, many hospitals have made or are in the process of making the transition to a paperless system. This encourages physicians who are affiliated with those hospitals to do the same.

EQUIPMENT AND SUPPLIES

Storage Equipment

Medical records may be kept in various types of file cabinets or on open shelves. The choice of equipment depends on the following: the number of people that need to access the medical records, the office layout, and the amount of floor space available. Usually they are stored with the files side to side. The files may take up part or all of a room. In a rotary system, the medical assistant can move sections of shelving to access other shelves behind. Large offices may even use an automated system, which stores more records and brings the record to the medical assistant.

File Cabinets

Cabinets or shelves used to store medical records should always be of heavy construction, with proper weighting on the bottom so that they will not tip over, especially if the drawers or shelves pull out. File cabinets should have a locking system. Lateral drawer file cabinets are more common than vertical file cabinets for medical records, although vertical file cabinets may be used for storing other types of information. Lateral drawer file cabinets have drawers that open from the long side, resembling a chest of drawers.

Shelf Filing Units

Shelf filing units consist of shelves arranged horizontally similar to bookshelves. Shelf units are often used to store medical records because the records can be accessed without having to open and close drawers. Adjustable metal shelf dividers that interlock at the back of the shelves come with the units. Their function is to keep the records in an upright position, thus preventing the records from slumping or sliding under one another.

File folders with side tabs (described later in this chapter) must be used with shelf units to permit the patient's name to be visible on the shelf. A record is placed on the shelf with the bottom edges of the folder down and the side tabs facing outwards. This means that the record is accessed from the side, rather than the top, as with drawer filing cabinets.

Shelf files are preferred because they allow easier access to records, and a number of people can have access to the shelves at the same time. For example, a medical assistant may need to retrieve the medical records of patients to be seen that day, while at the same time, another medical assistant may need to look up information for an insurance company or to document a patient telephone call.

Shelf units are available in two styles: open-shelf units or pull-down front units. As the name suggests, open-shelf units are open to the environment and cannot be closed. They must be in a room that can be locked separately from other parts of the office. The pull-down front units have lids that can be pulled over the front of the shelves and locked. This protects the records from environmental factors and allows the each part of the file to be locked (Figure

Putting It All into Practice

My name is Ellen McDonald, and I am a certified medical assistant. I have been working for a group practice specializing in internal medicine and cardiology for about a year. Although our office uses a computer-based billing and appointment system, our patient medical records are still in paper-based format. We file our records alphabetically. The physicians are hoping to change to an electronic system within the next few years, but the process is still in the planning stage. There is always a big stack of reports, correspondence, and other paperwork to be filed. We are not allowed to file any report unless the physician has seen it. In addition, our physicians dictate their progress notes, which are sent electronically to a transcription service. Every day we print the dictation that the transcription service has returned to us electronically, and we stamp them for the physicians to initial after they read them and make any corrections. I am responsible for making sure the files of medical records are kept in good order. In addition to pulling records and putting them away, I sometimes have to look for a misplaced record. If I can't find a patient's medical record, I begin to look for it. First I check the piles of records for patients who will be seen that day or the next day. Sometimes a medical record gets caught on another record, so it is important to check through the piles thoroughly. Next I check the computer to find out when the patient was last seen. I check on and behind the desks of the physician the patient last saw, as well as the billing desk. I also check through the files looking for a record that has been misfiled. We use color-coded labels, so it is usually easy to see when a record is out of place. These measures are usually enough to find the record, although sometimes it may take as long as a week before the record turns up. One time we looked for a record for 3 weeks before we found it. Whenever I am filing, I am very careful, because I remember how much work it is to find a record that has been misfiled. ∎

Prepare for Success

41-1). It must always be possible to lock either the entire medical record room or individual shelving units.

Filing Supplies

File Folders

A file folder is a protective cover used to hold medical record documents in an organized format. Usually file folders are made of manila card stock. Flexible metal fasteners at the top of the inside of the folder hold documents in place. Although the folders expand as the number of documents increase, it is recommended that the folder be broken down into two folders after attaining a width of ¾ inch.

Folders are available with tabs. A **tab** is a projection of a folder that extends beyond the top or side edge of the folder. Folders for a file cabinet with drawers have tabs on the top, whereas folders for shelf units have tabs at the side of the file folder. In the medical office with shelf filing cabinets, a folder with a full cut side tab is used. Indentations at intervals along the tab indicate the placement of adhesive labels. This ensures that all the labels on all the medical records are affixed at the same place on the file folders (Figure 41-2).

Folder Labels

Labels are used to identify the medical record and are commercially available in rolls or continuous folded strips. Most

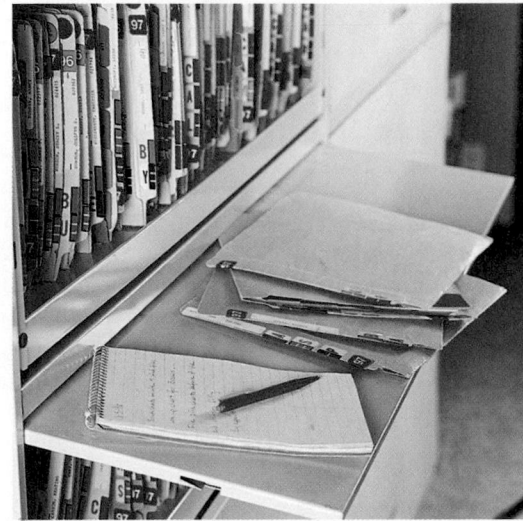

Figure 41-1. The pull-down front of a shelf storage unit may function as a work space. (From Young AP, Proctor DB: *Kinn's the medical assistant,* ed 10, St. Louis, 2007, Saunders.)

offices use pressure-sensitive self-adhesive labels. The labels for an alphabetic system assign colors to letters in either the first third or first half of the alphabet, while the remaining letters are assigned the same colors along with some type of distinguishing mark, such as one or two white stripes. If the office uses a numeric filing system, each digit from zero to nine is assigned a specific color. Color-coded year labels are often used to identify the last year a patient was seen at the office. The current year label is placed on a new record and updated the first time a patient has an office visit each year. This allows the records of patients who have not been seen for some time to be removed from the active files and placed in inactive storage.

Chart Dividers

Chart dividers are used to identify each section of the medical record by subject. Chart dividers are made of a heavy material such as manila card stock. Each divider has a tab for identification. Common categories include Progress Notes, History/Physical, Lab Reports, Diagnostic Testing, Hospital Reports, Immunizations/Medications, and Correspondence, but this varies according to medical office requirements.

Mounting Sheets

Laboratory reports, copies of prescriptions, and telephone messages are often filed on mounting sheets with adhesive strips. Usually several items can be filed on the same sheet. The medical assistant files the first item at the bottom with each succeeding item shingled up the mounting sheet. With

Figure 41-2. File folders for shelf units have a full-cut side tab. Color labels are affixed in the same position on each folder. (Modified from Hunt SA: *Saunders fundamentals of medical assisting,* St. Louis, 2007, Saunders.)

Figure 41-3. Laboratory reports are often mounted one above the other so that the most recent is visible on top. (Courtesy Bibbero Systems, Inc., Petaluma, Calif., [800] 242-2376; Fax [800] 242-9330; www.bibbero.com.)

Figure 41-4. Out guides. (Courtesy Bibbero Systems, Inc., Petaluma, Calif., [800] 242-2376; Fax [800] 242-9330.)

this system, the most recent item is always on top. Figure 41-3 shows this type of mounting sheet.

Other Supplies

Out guides, shown in Figure 41-4, are placed in the file to mark the place where a folder has been removed. Each guide has a pocket for a card indicating who removed the record and/or items that accumulate while the record is out of its storage area. Another type of out guide is made of heavy cardboard and has lines to write the name of the individual removing the record.

A **sorter** is a device that facilitates placing documents in alphabetic or numeric order. It has pockets or dividers for each letter or number.

What Would You Do? What Would You *Not* Do?

Case Study 1

A patient has come to the office to request that a copy of her medical record be sent to another physician. She says that her name is Anna Soubrette and her birth date is 4/25/52. She says that she has not been seen for 4 years, but her current physician had asked about various medications she had taken for a heart problem in the past. Ellen looks the patient up in the computer under Soubrette in the computer, but she does not find the patient listed. ∎

FILING SYSTEMS

The way in which records are arranged is referred to as a **filing system.** The primary purpose of a filing system is to facilitate the storage and retrieval of records, while a secondary function is to allow for expansion of the records with a minimum of disruption. The two systems used to arrange medical records are alphabetic and numeric. In addition, records can be arranged in chronological order, by subject, or by geographic location.

Alphabetic Filing

The alphabetic system is considered a direct system, which means that the patient's name is used directly to locate the medical record. It is commonly used in medical offices with fewer than 5000 records. Alphabetic filing uses parts of the legal name as indexing units. **Indexing units** are pieces of information used to identify the correct filing location. The records are arranged alphabetically based on the first unit.

All names that have exactly the same first unit are then arranged by the second unit, the third unit, etc. If the name is unusual, if the patient uses more than one name, or if it is unclear which name is the last name, the record may be cross-indexed. To **cross-index** means to file under one unit and to file a guide or card referring to the primary filing location under another unit.

Following consistent rules when filing alphabetically is important. One resource for guidelines is ARMA International, an association for records and information management personnel. The medical assistant must always clarify the procedures followed by any given medical office (Procedure 41-1).

Rule 1: Individual Names

In a patient's name, the **surname** (last name) is the first indexing unit, the given name (first name) is the second unit, and the middle name or middle initial is the third unit. A name with only two units is filed before a name with three units. (Nothing always comes before something.) A unit with only an initial is filed before a unit with a full name beginning with that initial. Business names are indexed in the order of the names in the business (excluding "a," "an," and "the"). Examples are as follows:

Name	Unit 1	Unit 2	Unit 3
Mary Ann Stede	Stede	Mary	Ann
Alan Stone	Stone	Alan	
Alan C. Stone	Stone	Alan	C.
Alan Charles Stone	Stone	Alan	Charles
Stoneham Medical Supply	Stoneham	Medical	Supply
Peter H. Stones	Stones	Peter	H.

Rule 2: Prefixes

If the last name has a prefix, such as Mc, Mac, Van, de, Des, or D', the prefix is considered part of the last name. Therefore, it begins the first indexing unit. Traditionally these prefixes were lowercase, but today they may be uppercase or lowercase. The prefixes Mc and Mac are usually filed in regular order. In some medical offices, however, they may all be filed as Mc, often as a separate group from other names beginning with "M." Examples are as follows:

Name	Unit 1	Unit 2	Unit 3
Lyndon A. De Larosa	Delarosa	Lyndon	A.
Stephen P. Dennis	Dennis	Stephen	P.
Mary Ann d'Entremont	Dentremont	Mary	Ann
Joanne McCarthy	Mccarthy	Joanne	
John Vanderbilt	Vanderbilt	John	
Joel P. van Twisk	Vantwisk	Joel	P.

Rule 3: Abbreviations and Nicknames

It is recommended that abbreviated first and last names be filed as written. If the patient commonly uses an abbreviated first name, the abbreviation is used as an indexing unit. If a nickname is used on the record, it is indexed as if it were the legal name (often it is). If an abbreviation is part of the last name (such as St.), it is part of the first indexing unit. (In some offices, abbreviations such as St. are filed as though they are written out.) Acronyms or initials in business names are indexed as one unit. Examples are as follows:

Name	Unit 1	Unit 2	Unit 3
Dottie A. Settland	Settland	Dottie	A.
SSI Transport Service	SSI	Transport	Service
Alex M. St. Croix	Stcroix	Alex	M.
E. V. Thomas	Thomas	E.	V.
Bill van der Post	Vanderpost	Bill	
Wm. T. Vanderpost	Vanderpost	Wm.	T.

Rule 4: Hyphenation

Hyphenated names are indexed as one unit, whether first names, last names, or names of children using both parents' last names. Examples are as follows:

Name	Unit 1	Unit 2	Unit 3
Eustace F. Brightfellow	Brightfellow	Eustace	F.
Claire Bryant-Litson	Bryantlitson	Claire	
Ann Marie Smith	Smith	Ann	Marie
Annabelle Smith	Smith	Annabelle	
Ann-Marie Smith	Smith	Annmarie	

Rule 5: Titles and Seniority Terms

Disregard titles unless the complete name is not given or unless they are necessary to distinguish between two individuals with the exact same name. Seniority terms, such as Jr., may be indexed as the last unit. Numeric seniority terms are indexed in numeric order before alphabetic terms. If a male child has exactly the same name as his father, he is called "Jr." until his father dies. He is a "III" if his father is a "Jr." In this case, he has the exact same name as his father and his grandfather. If he is named exactly for his grandfather, who is still living, but not for his father, he is called "II." Examples are as follows:

Name	Unit 1	Unit 2	Unit 3
Samuel Molson Jr.	Molson	Samuel	Jr.
Samuel Molson Sr.	Molson	Samuel	Sr.
Dr. Patricia A. Moy	Moy	Patricia	A.

Rule 6: Names of Married Women

A married woman may take her husband's surname, but she retains her own first and middle names. She may also retain her original name or use both her original name and her husband's name. If two last names are used, they may or may not be hyphenated.

A woman's married name may take several forms. The examples assume that Helen Ann Thurman marries James M. Walker.

- She may keep her own first and middle names, and take her husband's surname (Helen Ann Walker).
- She may keep her own first name, use her family's surname as a middle name (her maiden name), and take her husband's surname (Helen Thurman Walker).
- She may keep her own first and middle name and use a hyphenated last name consisting of her original name and her husband's surname (Helen Ann Thurman-Walker).
- She may keep her own first name, middle name, and her original (family) surname (Helen Ann Thurman).

Sometimes the hyphenated surname is used only for the couple's children with the woman using one of the other options. It would not be correct to use the husband's first name as a filing unit of a married woman unless her given name is unknown. Examples are as follows:

Name	Unit 1	Unit 2	Unit 3
Mrs. Arlene Sandra Trim	Trim	Arlene	Sandra
Mrs. Joan Walker Trim	Trim	Joan	Walker
Mrs. John (Sandra A.) Trim	Trim	Sandra	A.
Mrs. Ann Walker	Walker	Ann	
Mrs. Ann R. Walker	Walker	Ann	R.
Mrs. Diane A. Walker-Trim	Walkertrim	Diane	A.

Rule 7: Companies and Businesses

The names of companies and businesses are indexed in the same order as written. These are not used for medical records, but the medical assistant may use an alphabetic file for telephone numbers. Disregard punctuation, such as commas, apostrophes, or hyphens. Disregard articles such as *a, an,* and *the.* When indexing an **acronym** (a word formed using the first letters of all the words in a name, such as NYNEX), the acronym is indexed as one word. Examples are as follows:

Company Name	Unit 1	Unit 2	Unit 3
Edson's Pharmacy	Edsons	Pharmacy	
The Redline Supply Company	Redline	Supply	Company
Rent-A-Computer Service	Rentacomputer	Service	

Rule 8: Identical Names

If two names are exactly the same, index them first under the name, and then under the location, beginning with the city as the first unit, state as second unit, street as third unit, and street number from lowest to highest. This applies to names of patients and businesses.

Numeric Filing

In many practices, each new patient is assigned a number. This number is used to identify the patient and file the medical record (Procedure 41-2). The patient's number can be accessed with other data in the computer, although the patient may also be given a plastic card with the medical ID number. A numeric system has two major advantages:
1. It is easier to preserve confidentiality.
2. In a large practice, it is easier to identify a patient by number when several patients have the same last name.

The main disadvantage of using a numeric system for medical records management is that it is an indirect system. This means a cross-referenced index must be maintained to link the patient's name with the record identification number. Computers can cross-reference information without difficulty, so the EMR is usually linked to a patient identification number.

Terminal Digit Filing Systems

The most common numeric filing system used in medical offices and hospitals uses a six-digit number with a hyphen between each group of two digits (e.g., 01-22-19). The filing system is called **terminal digit filing,** a indexing system that uses the final group of digits as the first indexing unit.

With terminal digit filing, the numbers are indexed by group, working back from the final to the first group. Within each group the numbers are arranged from lowest to highest. To file the record with the number 01-22-19, the medical assistant would first locate the position of charts that end in 19 (first indexing unit). Assuming that there would be several records that end in -19, the medical assistant would then locate the position of charts that end in -22-19. Finally, the medical assistant would file the record between 00-22-19 and 02-22-19.

A terminal digit filing system mixes up active and inactive records in the files, so the numbers of the newest (and usually most active) patients are not all located in the same section of the file shelves.

Examples using two-digit groups are as follows:

Number	Unit 1	Unit 2	Unit 3
89-25-68	68	25	89
48-31-69	69	31	48
48-35-69	69	35	48

Another way to provide nonconsecutive filing is to assign each patient a combination of both letters and numbers. The records are then filed under the letters alphabetically, followed by the numbers.

Consecutive Filing Systems

In consecutive filing systems, numbers are arranged and filed from the lowest to the highest. In such a system, zeroes are assigned or assumed as the first unit, so each number has the same number of digits. This type of filing system may be used in a small medical office. Libraries often use this system for library cards. Examples are as follows:

Number	Unit 1	Unit 2	Unit 3	Unit 4	Unit 5	Unit 6
000642	0	0	0	6	4	2
000853	0	0	0	8	5	3

Subject Filing

Filing systems for documents (e.g., preprinted forms, invoices, purchase orders, service agreements) are often arranged according to subject. Within the subject category, documents may be arranged alphabetically or by date. In the medical office, subject filing is often used for insurance, bills, research, or other documents related to running the practice rather than the patient records.

Chronological Filing

A tickler file, which is used to "tickle" the memory by serving as a reminder that a specific action must be taken on a specific date, is a type of chronological system. It may consist of cards or folders. A card or folder is used for each day of the month, with file guides for each of the 12 months and each day of the month. As each month passes, the day guides are added to items for the current months. A manual system may be useful to identify bills to pay or other activities related to paper documents, but a computer reminder system is often used for daily tasks and/or patient reminders.

What Would You Do? What Would You *Not* Do?

Case Study 2
Lorna Bennett, a 45-year-old woman with hypertension, has come to the office for a physical examination. When Ellen takes her to the examination room, the patient says: "I'm glad I had an appointment today because I can take care of two things at once. My husband and I are moving out of state next month, so I guess I will just take my medical record with me today so that I can give it to my new physician out there. That will give me a chance to read it, too. I've always wondered what was in there." ■

PROCEDURE 41-1   Filing Patient Records: Alphabetic

Outcome File patient records correctly using an alphabetic filing system.

Equipment/Supplies

- Patient records with patient names
- Alphabetic sorter
- File cabinet or shelves
- Out guides
- Index cards

1. Procedural Step. Gather the records that are ready to be filed and remove any elastic bands or paper clips. *Principle.* Paper clips, elastic bands, and so on prevent the record from sliding easily in and out of the file.

2. Procedural Step. Check the records to be sure that no loose sheets of paper are present. If loose sheets are found, insert them in the record.

3. Procedural Step. Sort the records alphabetically by last name using the alphabetic sorter if available.

4. Procedural Step. Find the correct location in the file for the first record, pull the out guide halfway out, slide the record in front of the out guide in the correct location in the file, and finish removing the out guide. If your office does not use out guides, use your hand to make a space between the record before and the record after the one you are filing.

5. Procedural Step. If there is an index card in the out guide showing who had the record from the out guide, remove it. Place the out guide with other unused out guides. Some offices keep index cards for the physicians in separate boxes so that new cards do not need to be written; some offices cross out the name and reuse the index cards; some offices use slips of paper that are discarded after each use.

6. Procedural Step. File each record in the same way until all records have been filed.

Slide the record in front of the out guide.

PROCEDURE 41-2

PROCEDURE 41-2   Filing Patient Records: Numeric

Outcome File patient records correctly using a terminal digit filing system.

Equipment/Supplies

- Patient records with terminal digit labels
- File cabinet or shelves
- Numeric sorter
- Out guides
- Index cards

1. Procedural Step. Gather the records that are ready to be filed and remove any elastic bands or paper clips. *Principle.* Paper clips, elastic bands, and so on prevent the record from sliding easily in and out of the file.

2. Procedural Step. Check the records to be sure that no loose sheets of paper are present. If loose sheets are found, insert them in the record.

3. Procedural Step. Sort the records according to the terminal digit indexing units using the sorter if available.

4. Procedural Step. Find the correct location in the file for the first record based on the final group of numbers. Refine your search based on the middle group of numbers and then the first group of numbers. At the correct location for the record, pull the out guide halfway out, slide the record in front of the out guide,

and finish removing the out guide. If your office does not use out guides, use your hand to make a space between the record before and the record after the one you are filing.

5. Procedural Step. If there is an index card in the out guide showing who had the record from the out guide, remove it. Place the out guide with other unused out guides. Some offices keep index cards for the physicians in separate boxes so that new cards do not need to be written; some offices cross out the name and reuse the index cards; some offices use slips of paper that are discarded after each use.

6. Procedural Step. File each record in the same way until all records have been filed.

RETRIEVING OR FILING A PAPER MEDICAL RECORD

Retrieving Patient Records

A patient record has to be removed from its proper location in the file whenever someone in the office wants to look at it (i.e., for an appointment, when a patient leaves a message).

The record is located using the filing guidelines of the particular office. Medical records needed for patients with appointments on a particular day are usually pulled the afternoon before the appointments using the printed appointment list. Then they are arranged by appointment time, with the record of the patient with the earliest appointment on top. Each time a record is taken from storage, an out guide is placed exactly where the record was removed, as illustrated in Figure 41-5.

The person removing the record fills in a card with the name or number on the record and the name of the person who will have the record. Although it seems cumbersome to fill in a card for every record removed, in the long run it is much less frustrating than searching the entire office for a record when the patient is in the waiting room.

Filing Records

Each day, several records need to be returned to the file. In most offices, records ready for filing are placed in one location.

Before filing records or documents, the medical assistant should be sure that the records are ready to file. To condition a record, the medical assistant takes several steps:

- All clips, pins, or other extraneous material should be removed.
- Any tears or broken punch holes should be repaired with tape.
- Any sticky notes or other loose papers should either be removed or filed in the record in the correct location.

A sorter is used to arrange the records so that they can be filed efficiently according to name or medical record number. It is important to locate the correct position to replace the record and remove the out guide. Any items to be filed in the pocket of the out guide should be filed in the record at this time.

Filing Reports and Correspondence

All reports, letters, and other materials that come into the office should be reviewed by the physician, initialed, and then filed in the patient record. A date stamp is often used to identify exactly when a report or letter was received. If the physician dictates progress notes, these must also be reviewed and initialed before filing. With the paper medical record, there is no end to the number of papers that the physician must review. Sometimes physicians even come into the office on the weekend to catch up with all their paperwork. Because of this, there is often a stack of material to be filed on Monday. The physician may indicate an action for the medical assistant to take on a message form or sticky note. These actions can range from arranging laboratory or diagnostic follow-up to notifying the patient of results of laboratory or diagnostic tests to calling a pharmacy with a prescription. The medical assistant must complete any follow-up before filing the report (or record) (Procedure 41-3).

Several steps facilitate filing reports or other items in the medical record:

- Each report or note to be filed should be initialed by the physician and any required action should be complete.
- Reports should be sorted before filing according to name or medical record number.
- Once the correct record has been located, the report is filed at the front of the appropriate section. It may be necessary to remove a section of the record to insert the new item.
- The record should be reassembled before being replaced in the file.
- Reports for items that are not in their correct locations should be set aside. After all other reports have been filed, if time permits, the medical assistant can locate the missing records.

Measures to Ensure Accuracy or Locate Misplaced Records

Seven steps can ensure accuracy in filing or locating a misplaced record. A missing record creates multiple problems. Working carefully can help avoid lost records.

1. The medical assistant should work slowly and carefully when filing records.
2. It is recommended to use out guides to keep track of the record.
3. Medical records should be returned to storage after use and not just handed on to others in the medical office. If it is necessary to give a record to the physician, the out guide should be updated.
4. Physicians and other personnel should be discouraged from hoarding records. The medical assistant should encourage the physician(s) to finish all dictation each day, review laboratory reports, and sign off on them.

Figure 41-5. Placing an out guide.

5. Records should be kept in orderly piles when they are out of the files. This makes it easier to scan for one particular record.

6. If the medical assistant notices a misfiled record from the files, it should be removed and filed correctly without delay.

7. Hunting for "missing" records and being alert to find them in unexpected places are important. After all possible measures fail to locate a missing record, it may be necessary to create a second record for a patient until the record can be found.

What Would You Do? What Would You *Not* Do?

Case Study 3

When Ellen is pulling medical records for the next day's appointments, she does not find the medical record for Alan DuBois under "Dubois." The file also has no out guide. Ellen remembers that the patient was seen within the past week or two. She also checks under "Bois," but the record is not filed there, either. ■

PROCEDURE 41-3 Filing Reports

Outcome File reports, correspondence, and other material in a patient record.

Equipment/Supplies

- Medical records
- Assorted reports
- Letters or other material to be filed
- Hole punch
- Tape
- Stapler
- Sorter

1. **Procedural Step.** Assemble materials to be filed and necessary supplies to assist in the filing process.

2. **Procedural Step.** Remove extraneous materials, such as paper clips or pins; mend any tears with tape; and staple related pages together. Punch holes if necessary.
   Principle. Preparation before filing allows all materials in the record to be maintained in good condition.

3. **Procedural Step.** Verify that each report is ready to be filed. In most offices the physicians initial reports after they have seen them. If the initials are missing, the report should go back to him or her.
   Principle. The physician must see each report that comes to the medical office. A procedure verifying that the physician has seen it before filing prevents reports from being accidentally overlooked.

4. **Procedural Step.** Sort the reports using the sorter alphabetically or numerically, depending on the filing system. Sort by letters, numbers, or number groups first, then sort within each letter or number group.
   Principle. Even in a small office, large numbers of reports need to be filed in patient records if a paper record system is used. It is more efficient to file in order, especially when patients have more than one report to be filed.

5. **Procedural Step.** Gather all reports for a particular patient, find the correct record, and insert the report(s) into the record in the correct location. In any section, reports are filed chronologically with the most recent reports at the front of the section. When several reports are shingled on a page, the oldest report goes at the bottom with newer reports progressing up the page and in front of the older reports. You may need to place a divider in the record if you are filing the first report in a given section.

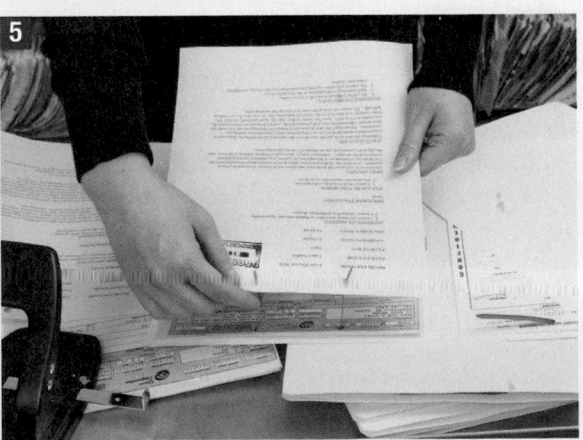

Insert the report(s) into the medical record.

Continued

Principle. The record usually contains several sections in a specific order. Reports need to be in the correct section to be easily located.

6. **Procedural Step.** Put the record back together if necessary and file with other medical records.

Principle. It is easier to file records in the wrong record when several records are out.

7. **Procedural Step.** If the record is not in the file, place the report back in the sorter or in the pocket of the out guide.

Principle. It is more efficient to file reports in records you can find easily than to hunt for records just to file reports.

ELECTRONIC MEDICAL RECORD

The EMR has many of the same sections as the paper medical record. The health information is usually linked to the demographic, billing, and insurance information for the patient. There are sections for the patient's medical history, previous visits, medications, allergies, problem list, and so on. Information is entered during or immediately after each patient interaction, which reduces the need for filing. Paper reports, correspondence, and consent forms are usually scanned into the record as soon as possible. The originals may be shredded or stored in a paper record depending on the office.

EMRs are password protected, and patient data are compartmentalized so that access can be limited to the information that any given staff member needs to view. A system administrator should authorize users and remove them from the system as appropriate. Data should be encrypted between the server and the user, and the infrastructure for access should be secure. The medical assistant should never allow other personnel to access patient information with his or her password.

STORING MEDICAL RECORDS

The storage area for medical records should be well-lighted and climate controlled. It is important to maintain the relative humidity between 48% and 52% to prevent deterioration of the records. Basement storage is not recommended unless the humidity is well controlled. The records should also be protected from dust, insects, rodents, fires, and floods. As discussed earlier, records should be secure when the office is closed so that unauthorized personnel do not have access to them. The Occupational Health and Safety Administration (OSHA) requires that main aisles leading out of a room or to a fire exit must be a minimum of 5 feet wide, and secondary aisles, such as between shelving units, must be a minimum of 3 feet wide.

The shelf files should be full enough to allow the folders to stand upright but loose enough to allow folders to be easily stored and retrieved.

Highlight on Electronic Signatures

When talking about electronic signatures, it is important to distinguish between actual signatures that are captured electronically and an electronic entry specific to one individual that authenticates identity and can be linked to a specific date and time.

When a medical office uses an electronic medical record (EMR), the staff can use two ways to handle actual patient signatures. In the first method, the patient signs a paper consent form and the paper consent form is then scanned into the electronic record. In the second method, the patient reads the consent form, either in a paper version or on a computer screen, and then the patient signs an electronic signature pad that captures an image of the actual signature and inserts it into an electronic version of the form being signed.

Physicians and other staff in the medical office usually use an *electronic signature,* an electronic sound, symbol, or process added to an electronic record that indicates intent to sign. These processes are built into the software with safeguards to validate the time of the entry and the identity of the individual making the entry. Electronic signatures are also used for transmitting insurance claims and for validating entries to the EMR. Electronic signatures are valid in all states and are accepted by HIPAA provided that the software program being used validates identity, validates that the document has not been altered later, and provides that the user cannot later repudiate the electronic signature.

The term *digital signature* is used for a form of encryption that binds electronic records to an "electronic fingerprint." Digital signatures require validation by private companies called *certification authorities.* The entire document is encrypted and decrypted using public and private keys (mathematic formulas). Digital signatures are used for transferring money and signing legal documents electronically. This level of security is currently not required for EMRs. ■

Memories *from* Externship

Ellen McDonald: I did my externship in a clinic affiliated with a large hospital that had made the transition from paper medical records to an EMR. When a patient checked in, we entered the data from the patient information sheet into the computer immediately, and we used a signature pad at the front desk to obtain electronic signatures from the patient for consent to treatment, authorization to disclose information for billing, and acknowledgement of receipt of HIPAA confidentiality information.

Each medical assistant had to log in to the system in order to enter information in the medical record. Even as a student, I was given a password so that I could check patients in, enter vital signs, and enter other information. For example, the machine for electrocardiograms (ECGs) looked like a laptop computer attached to the ECG cables. It was also connected to the EMR. We entered patient information using a computer keyboard. I learned how to print the ECG as a hard copy, but the physician could also view the tracing on the computer.

When the clinic made the transition to the EMR, the records of active patients were scanned into the system, but they kept the paper records for inactive patients. I remember one time when a patient who had not been seen for about 6 years made an appointment. He was experiencing medical problems that he thought might be connected to earlier radiation therapy. I was instructed to create a new electronic record for him, and then I was sent to find the old record. Several rooms were full of paper medical records, arranged in order by clinic number. I found it confusing because I was not that familiar with the terminal digit method of filing, but one of the staff members helped me to find the record. After the appointment, I had to return the record to storage. ∎

Prepare for Success

Active Records

Active records—belonging to patients who have been seen within the past 2 to 5 years, depending on the practice—are stored in the medical office as described earlier.

Inactive Records

Records of patients who have not been seen within a time period specified by the practice (**inactive records**) are usually kept in the office in closed storage. If there is not enough space in the office to store inactive records, they are sometimes stored in a storage room elsewhere in the office building, or in rented storage space. If a patient has not been seen for several years, a new medical record may be created. However, the old record may still need to be consulted.

At regular intervals inactive records are removed from the active record area. Most offices place a sticker for the current year on a patient's medical record at the first visit in a new year to show that the record is active for that year. For example, an office that uses an alphabetic filing system might consider the record of any patient who has not been seen in the office for the past 4 years inactive. At the end of 2015, the medical assistant would remove any record that did not have a sticker for 2015, 2014, 2013, or 2012. The old records would then be placed in storage. They would be filed there in alphabetic order with the other inactive records so that they could be located if needed.

Retention of Records

The length of time that a medical record must be retained is difficult to determine. Each state has a law limiting the time period for beginning a lawsuit for malpractice. This is known as the *statute of limitations* for medical malpractice. A state may also have a minimum requirement for retaining medical records. In the absence of state regulations, a medical office can review retention guidelines established by the American Medical Association (AMA) in 1994. The AMA recommends that records be retained primarily based on the health needs of the patient, but at least as long as the state requires or the length of time as the statute of limitations for malpractice claims. For a minor, the time period should be considered to begin at the age of majority. Records of Medicare and Medicaid patients should be retained for at least 5 years after the last contact.

At the end of the retention period, the inactive medical record may be destroyed (by shredding or burning) or put in a final storage place to be kept permanently. The AMA recommends that the patient have an opportunity to claim the record before it is destroyed, if possible. Records that are closed (it is known that the patient will not return) may be transferred to microfilm or microfiche. They can also be copied using a laser beam and stored on laser disks. These options are expensive and time consuming, but may be worthwhile for larger practices.

Other records that should be kept indefinitely are insurance policies, licenses, and Drug Enforcement Administration (DEA) controlled-substance records. All tax records should also be kept for 7 years; after that, background records used to determine taxes can be destroyed, but copies of tax forms should be kept indefinitely.

Storing Computerized Records

EMRs should be backed up regularly and securely. The system manager is usually responsible for ensuring that the backup system is implemented according to plan. Backups may be done to network storage and/or storage devices, such as hard drives, DVDs, or other devices. It is important to maintain some kind of backup off-site in case of fire or disaster. Inactive electronic records can be transferred to separate storage if the system capacity becomes strained. The system administrator must also be sure that program updates are compatible with previously stored data.

MEDICAL PRACTICE *and the* LAW

Legal implications of the medical record

The medical record is initiated by the medical office and belongs to the person or group who produced it. The physician or office owns the physical record whether its form is paper or electronic.

The information in the record belongs to the patient, however, and the patient controls access to the information. Any request to release copies of records must come from the patient or someone who is authorized to act for the patient.

The original record must never be released. If the original record is subpoenaed by a court, an employee of the office should travel with the record to safeguard it and be sure that no part is lost or tampered with. A copy of the record should be left at the office.

The office should have a form for patients to sign that gives permission to release the medical record or information about specific conditions, like HIV or AIDS, that require separate consent forms. The release must be signed by the patient or by a guardian if the patient is a minor.

When a patient begins a new relationship with a physician's office, the patient routinely signs a release form allowing the physician to send necessary information to an insurance company. One of the standards being developed under the Health Insurance Portability and Accountability Act legislation concerns a standard format for electronic signatures.

Another time that records are usually released is when a patient moves away or begins a relationship with another physician. If the purpose of copying records is for such continuity of care, offices do not charge. However, sometimes they do charge a copying fee, a handling fee, and postage, especially if the record is requested by a lawyer for litigation. ■

What Would You Do? What Would You *Not* Do? RESPONSES

Case Study 1
Page 982

What Did Ellen Do?
❑ Made every possible attempt to find the patient's record.
❑ Asked the patient if she could have been seen under another last name.
❑ Tried to locate the patient under her maiden name.
❑ Attempted to locate the patient in the computer using the birth date and/or the first name.
❑ Attempted to locate the record in the storage area for inactive patients under Soubrette.
❑ Even if Ellen was not able to locate the record, she asked Ms. Soubrette to fill out a release of information sheet, took her telephone number, and said she would contact her to let her know if she had been able to locate the record.
❑ Asked the office manager for other ideas to locate the record.

What Did Ellen Not Do?
❑ Did not tell the patient that she must have been thinking about a different practice.
❑ Did not assume that the record had been lost or destroyed.
❑ Did not tell the patient that after such a long time, the information probably would not be useful anyway.

What Would You Do/What Would You *Not* Do? Review Ellen's response and place a checkmark next to the information you included in your response. List the additional information you included in your response.

Case Study 2
Page 984

What Did Ellen Do?
❑ Explained that the office would be glad to send a copy of the medical record to the new physician as soon as Ms. Bennett provided a physician name and address.
❑ Encouraged the patient to take a release of information sheet to mail back when she had selected a new physician.
❑ Explained that Ms. Bennett was in charge of the information in the medical record, but the record itself belonged to her physician.
❑ Encouraged Ms. Bennett to ask the physician for permission to view the record.

What Did Ellen Not *Do*?
❑ Did not allow the patient to take the original medical record.
❑ Did not allow Ms. Bennett to read her medical record without authorization from the patient's physician.

What Would You Do/What Would You *Not* Do? Review Ellen's response and place a checkmark next to the information you included in your response. List the additional information you included in your response.

What Would You Do? What Would You *Not* Do? RESPONSES—cont'd

Case Study 3
Page 987

What Did Ellen Do?
❑ Looked up Allan DuBois in the computer to identify the date of his last appointment and who saw him.
❑ Checked the physician's office, as well as the billing desk.
❑ Looked behind furniture, especially in the physician's office.
❑ Asked other staff members if they had seen this medical record.

What Did Ellen *Not* Do?
❑ Did not give up looking for the record until she had made an extensive search.

❑ Did not accuse any staff member of hiding the medical record.
❑ Did not call the patient and change his appointment in case the record could not be located.

What Would You Do/What Would You *Not* Do? Review Ellen's response and place a checkmark next to the information you included in your response. List the additional information you included in your response.

_____
_____
_____
_____

TERMINOLOGY REVIEW

Acronym A word formed from the first letters in a name.

Active record The medical record of a patient who has been seen within a time frame specified by the office (usually 2 to 3 years).

Cross-index To file under one unit and use a guide or card filed under another unit that refers to the primary filing location.

Electronic health record (EHR) An individual patient's health record in digital format. Also called an *electronic medical record.*

Electronic medical record (EMR) An individual's medical record in digital format. Also called an *electronic health record.*

Filing system The way in which records are arranged. Common filing systems in the medical office include alphabetic, numeric, subject, or chronological.

Inactive record The medical record of a patient who has not been seen within the past 2 to 3 years, or some other time frame specified by a given medical office.

Indexing units Pieces of information used to identify a correct filing location.

Medical records management Activities related to the creation, management, use, and disposition of patient medical records.

Out guide A cardboard or plastic card to insert in a file when a medical record is removed.

Sorter A device that facilitates putting papers or records in alphabetic or numeric order.

Surname Last name or family name of an individual terminal digit filing.

Tab A projection of a folder that extends beyond the top or side of the folder.

Terminal digit filing A chronological filing system that uses the last number or number group as the first indexing unit.

ON THE WEB

For Information on Records Management:

American Health Information Management Association: www.ahima.org

ARMA International: www.arma.org

Medical Records Institute: www.medrecinst.com

National Information Standards Organization: www.niso.org

U.S. Department of Health and Human Services—Health Information Technology: www.hhs.gov/healthit

PREPARE FOR CERTIFICATION Visit the Evolve site at http://evolve.elsevier.com/Bonewit/today/ to actively Prepare for your Certification.

*Check out the **Companion CD** bound with the book to access additional interactive activities.*

42

Written Communications

CAAHEP COMPETENCIES

General Competencies
Professional Communication
- Respond to and initiate written communications.
- Recognize and respond to verbal communications.

Operational Functions
- Utilize computer software to maintain office systems.

Communication

- Receive, organize, prioritize, and transmit information expediently.
- Recognize and respond to verbal and nonverbal communication.
- Use correct grammar, spelling, and formatting techniques in written works.

- Application of electronic technology
- Fundamental writing skills

Administrative Duties

- Perform basic secretarial skills.

KEY TERMS

collate (CALL-ate)
duplex
e-mail
fax
full block style
grammar
left justified
letterhead

memo (memorandum)
modified block style
proofread
right justified
semiblock style
simplified letter style
template
transcription

Introduction to Written Communication

Until 20 years ago, almost all written communication between the medical office and other parties was managed by letters or forms and mailed through the U.S. Postal Service. Today, it is also common to transmit data electronically or by fax, and these data can be viewed and/or printed in written form. Regardless of how the written material is transmitted, however, written communication must still adhere to professional standards. The medical assistant is often responsible for preparing letters, memoranda, reports, and other types of written communication. To do this professionally requires thorough knowledge of grammar, spelling, format, and the technology that supports modern methods of producing written documents. In addition, the medical assistant must be familiar with the implications of HIPAA regulations regulating access to patient health information. These regulations were covered in detail in Chapter 3. The procedure for obtaining consent to release information from the medical record was discussed in Chapter 36.

BUSINESS LETTERS

Letters leaving the medical office—whether sent to a referring physician, an attorney, another business or an insurance company—require proper formatting. Some letters may be dictated by the physician and transcribed by the medical assistant. The medical assistant may also compose and send letters independently. The medical office may also use form letters and/or templates for routine matters. A **template** is a standard form to which additional data can be added as needed.

Equipment and Supplies

Business letters are usually created using a computer and printer. A word processing program is used to create the letter so that formatting can easily be adjusted and any necessary corrections can be made. The process of dictation and transcription is described later in the chapter.

The medical office orders stationery and envelopes preprinted with the practice name, address, telephone number, and business logo. Individual physician names are also often included. A sheet of this type of stationery is called **letterhead.** Blank sheets of the paper of exactly the same type and weight must be purchased for letters that are longer than one page.

Copies of letters (for the medical record or other recipients) are usually photocopied so that the letterhead appears, but letterhead stationery can be conserved.

Parts of a Business Letter

Heading

The heading includes the return address and the date line. The return address is composed of the name and address of the business sending the letter. If office letterhead is used, no return address needs to be added. The date line is the date the letter is mailed in month, day, year order. The month is written out in full on the date line. It is usually entered on the second line below the return address. On letterhead stationery, it is placed to fall a few spaces below the bottom of the letterhead.

Inside Address

The inside address includes the name and address of the party to whom the letter is being sent. Beginning with the inside address, information is single spaced with a blank space between sections. The inside address should be located in a position so that the body of the letter is centered top to bottom on the page. If the letter is long enough to require two pages, the inside address begins on the second or third space below the date line.

Salutation or Greeting

Because a business letter is formal, the recipient's last name and title (e.g., Mr., Ms., Miss, Dr.) should be used. The greeting is punctuated with a colon. Correct examples include the following: Dear Ms. Wilson:, Dear Dr. Taylor:, Dear Mrs. Porto:. The following are *incorrect:* Dear Amy, Dear Amy Wilson:, Dear William Taylor, MD:. If the recipient's name is not known, it is permissible to use "Dear Sir," "Dear Madam," "Dear Sir or Madam," or "To Whom It May Concern." One space is left blank after the salutation.

Body of the Letter

The body of the letter contains the substance, which should be presented clearly and concisely. A subject line may be used to begin this section. Within a paragraph, the letter is single-spaced, but a blank line should separate each new paragraph.

Complimentary Close or Closing

The complimentary close is the line with which the letter's personal communication to the party receiving the letter is ended. It is a sign of respect and can be adjusted depending on how well the letter's author and the party being addressed know each other. "Sincerely" is the standard close. A more formal closing is "Yours truly" or "Very truly yours." It is followed by a comma and separated from the body of the letter by a blank line.

Signature, Printed Signature, and Title

The signature is the actual written signature of the individual sending the letter. It is added after the letter has been printed. The printed signature is the name of the individual sending the letter, with credentials (e.g., M.D.). It is entered four to five lines below the complimentary close to leave room for the written signature. A business title (e.g., Office Manager) is capitalized and entered on the line below the printed signature.

The medical assistant uses his or her own name and signature for a letter to a supplier or a letter to a patient responding to a billing question. Any letter dictated or composed by a physician will be signed by the physician.

End Notations

Various pieces of information may be given in notations at the bottom of the letter, generally with a blank space between each item. The order of the end notations may vary according to the preference of the office. A reference notation notes the initials of the person who composed the letter (in uppercase) followed by the initials of the person who typed or keyed the letter (in lowercase). If the letter contains enclosures, such as a log of visits and/or billing records, this is noted in the enclosure notation, on the second line below the title. "Enclosure" or "Enc." may be used for one enclo-

sure. "Enclosures" followed by the number in parentheses is used for more than one enclosure. This alerts the recipient to make sure that everything the sender intended to include actually accompanies the letter. A copy notation (distribution notation) identifies the recipient(s). The letters "cc" are used, followed by a colon and the name(s) of those who are receiving copies. Figure 42-1 shows a business letter with the parts of the letter identified.

Format of Business Letters

Setting Up a Letter

When preparing letters using a word processing program, the medical assistant should first set the margins. The top margin of the letter should be large enough to accommodate the letterhead (usually 2 to 2½ inches). The side margins may be 1 to 2 inches. Wider margins are used for a short letter. The body of the letter is single spaced.

When writing a business letter, the generally accepted font is Times New Roman 12 point. The entire letter should be created in the same font. The word processing program may include a letter wizard, which formats the letter automatically. It is also possible to use or create a letter template so that all letters from the office have the same format.

If the letter has two pages, a header should be placed at the left top margin of the second page with the name of the recipient, the page number, and the date.

Letter Styles

1. **Full block style:** The letterhead may be centered, but all other lines are **left justified,** which means that they start at the left margin on the page. This allows rapid entry of information and easy formatting. A double space is left between the end of one paragraph and the beginning of the next (Figure 42-2).
2. **Modified block style:** All lines in the inside address, salutation, and body of the letter and reference lines are left justified, and there are double spaces between paragraphs. However, the date line, complimentary close, and signature lines begin in the center of the letter or are sometimes **right justified** (aligned with the right margin) (Figure 42-3).
3. **Semiblock style (also called *modified block with indented paragraphs*):** All lines in the inside address, salutation, and body of the letter and reference lines are left justified. Paragraphs are indented five to eight spaces, and there are double spaces between paragraphs. The date line, complimentary close, and signature lines begin in the center of the letter or are sometimes right justified. Semiblock style is the same as modified block style, except that the first sentence of each new paragraph is indented (Figure 42-4).
4. **Simplified letter style:** This style resembles a memorandum. Instead of a salutation, a subject line typed all in capital letters is placed three lines below the inside address, and the complimentary close and signature lines are replaced by an all-capital-letter signature five lines below the letter's body (Figure 42-5).

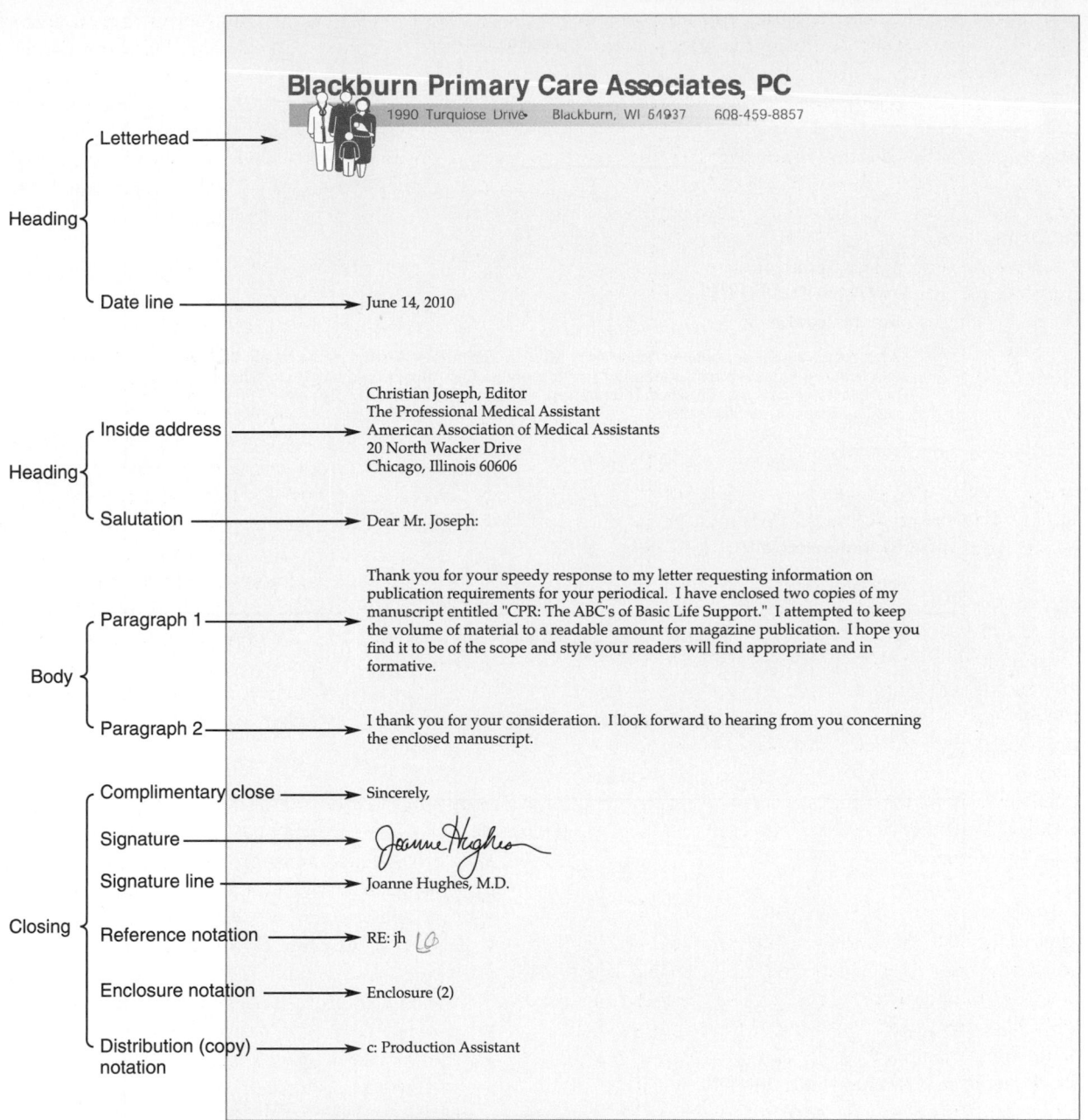

Figure 42-1. Sample business letter with the parts of the letter identified. (Modified from Hunt SA: *Saunders fundamentals of medical assisting,* St. Louis, 2007, Saunders.)

Composing a Business Letter

A medical assistant may be asked to create a form letter to send to patients or compose a business letter to order supplies, request information, or handle a problem. In addition to using a professional tone, it is important to use correct grammar and spelling to convey the desired information.

Before beginning the letter, the medical assistant should jot down the important points to cover in the letter and check to make sure they are presented in a logical order. If the office sends similar letters fairly often, it is helpful to review the wording of old letters. Once the content has been established, the medical assistant should enter the letter into the word processing program using the letter style preferred by the medical office. If the medical assistant is unsure about the wording of the letter, a draft letter can be printed for the office manager and/or physician to review.

The letter should be proofread for accuracy, grammar, and spelling before the final version is printed. Because letters represent the medical practice, they must be as accurate and professional as possible (Procedure 42-1).

[Letterhead]

July 21, 2010

Edith Fowler
222 Signal Hill Drive
Western Ridge, OH 44770

Dear Ms. Fowler:

After reviewing the consultation report from Morgan Nephrology Associates, we would like you to schedule a follow-up renal ultrasound in two months. Our office would be glad to schedule this test for you, or you can schedule it yourself. Please call our office at (216) 444-1100 if you need assistance with this matter.

Sincerely yours,

Richard Warner, MD

RW/mt

Figure 42-2. Sample letter—full block style.

[Letterhead]

July 21, 2010

Edith Fowler
222 Signal Hill Drive
Western Ridge, OH 44770

Dear Ms. Fowler:

After reviewing the consultation report from Morgan Nephrology Associates, we would like you to schedule a follow-up renal ultrasound in two months. Our office would be glad to schedule this test for you, or you can schedule it yourself. Please call our office at (216) 444-1100 if you need assistance with this matter.

Sincerely yours,

Richard Warner, MD

RW/mt

Figure 42-3. Sample letter—modified block style.

[Letterhead]

July 21, 2010

Edith Fowler
222 Signal Hill Drive
Western Ridge, OH 44770

Dear Ms. Fowler:

After reviewing the consultation report from Morgan Nephrology Associates, we would like you to schedule a follow-up renal ultrasound in two months. Our office would be glad to schedule this test for you, or you can schedule it yourself. Please call our office at (216) 444-1100 if you need assistance with this matter.

Sincerely yours,

Richard Warner, MD

RW/mt

Figure 42-4. Sample letter—semiblock style (also called *modified block with indented paragraphs*).

[Letterhead]

July 21, 2010

Edith Fowler
222 Signal Hill Drive
Western Ridge, OH 44770

FOLLOW-UP RENAL ULTRASOUND

After reviewing the consultation report from Morgan Nephrology Associates, we would like you to schedule a follow-up renal ultrasound in two months. Our office would be glad to schedule this test for you, or you can schedule it yourself. Please call our office at (216) 444-1100 if you need assistance with this matter.

RICHARD WARNER, MD

RW/mt

Figure 42-5. Sample letter—simplified style.

Highlight on Letters to Inform Patients of Test Results

Although medical offices use many different methods to inform patients of results of laboratory and diagnostic test results, notifying patients by letter is a method that preserves patient confidentiality and provides consistent and reliable information to the patient about follow-up. Studies have shown that patients prefer to receive all results, whether or not they are normal.

Many medical practices use templates or form letters that allow the medical assistant or physician to fill in the appropriate values and add comments. The final letter may include the actual results or a statement describing generally if the results are normal, slightly elevated (or low), or very elevated (or low). A specific time frame for follow-up testing or instructions to make a follow-up appointment is also included.

If the practice uses an electronic medical record, test results can be tracked in the system to be sure that results have been received from the laboratory or testing facility. It is also possible to track that the patient has been notified and follow-up testing has been performed. The system can also post an alert when follow-up testing is overdue. If the office uses a paper-based medical record, the medical assistant often keeps a separate log book for laboratory and diagnostic tests to track receipt of results, review by physicians, and follow-up to patients.

As a means of managing physician time efficiently while maintaining the personal touch, the medical assistant may prepare the letter, enter the information about the laboratory results, and place the letter with the test results for the physician to verify accuracy, sign the letter, and add any comments. ∎

PROCEDURE 42-1   Composing a Business Letter

Outcome Compose and key a business letter.

Equipment/Supplies

- Letterhead stationery
- Blank stationery
- Typewriter
- Computer and printer

1. **Procedural Step.** Assemble materials, determine the address of the recipient, and decide on a format for the letter.

2. **Procedural Step.** Formulate the content for the business letter. List and organize the essential content to be sure all necessary information is included.

3. **Procedural Step.** Insert the date on the second or third line below the letterhead. For block style, the date is at the left margin. For modified block style and semiblock style, the date begins at the center of the line.

4. **Procedural Step.** Place the inside address 4 to 10 lines below the date at the left margin. If using a computer, adjust the number of spaces below the date line after the letter has been keyed so that the body of the letter is centered on the page.

5. **Procedural Step.** Place the salutation two lines below the inside address. The salutation should include a title and the person's last name (e.g., Dear Dr. Gordon, Dear Mrs. Wilson, Dear Rev. Meyers). It is followed by a colon.
   Principle. A business letter is more formal than personal correspondence.

6. **Procedural Step.** If desired, place a subject line two lines below the salutation. A subject line begins with the Latin abbreviation "re" (meaning about) followed by a colon. The abbreviation is usually capitalized (e.g., RE: Annual meeting on Thursday, June 12, 2010.).
   Principle. Although optional, a subject line helps the recipient identify the subject of the letter before reading it.

7. **Procedural Step.** Begin the body of the letter two lines below the salutation (or subject line, if used). The body of the letter is single-spaced with two spaces between paragraphs. In block and modified block letter styles, the paragraphs begin at the left margin. If semiblock style is used, indent the first line of each paragraph five to eight spaces.

8. **Procedural Step.** The final paragraph of the letter should summarize the contents and/or most important ideas.

9. **Procedural Step.** Place the complimentary close two spaces below the final paragraph of the body of the letter. For the block letter style, the complimentary close begins at the left margin. For the modified block

letter style, it begins at a tab directly below the date line. The complimentary close is followed by a comma.

10. Procedural Step. Drop down four lines and insert the first and last name of the sender followed by his or her credentials. Begin the typed signature at the same place as the complimentary close. Place a job title, if appropriate, on the next line.

Principle. Typing the name under the handwritten signature facilitates a response because the signature may be difficult to read.

11. Procedural Step. If necessary, add a reference line, enclosure notation, and/or distribution notation, placing each two lines below the others at the left margin. If you compose and key your own letter, a reference line is unnecessary. If you compose and key a letter for someone else, place your initials in lowercase letters. If you key a letter that was dictated by the person signing the letter, place his or her initials (uppercase) followed by your initials (lowercase) separated by a colon. The enclosure notation may be written out or abbreviated "Enc." The number of enclosures is placed in parentheses if there is more than one. The distribution notation identifies individuals who receive a copy of the letter. The letters "cc" followed by a colon are used with the name of the individual receiving a copy.

Principle. The person who receives the letter is entitled to know who prepared the letter and who received copies. If the number of enclosures is indicated, it is easier to tell if all intended material is enclosed with the letter.

12. Procedural Step. If the letter is longer than one page, the second page should be printed or typed on stationery of the same quality and weight as the letterhead stationery, beginning 1 inch from the top. Include the name of the recipient, the date, and the page number in the top left corner. Space the letter so that at least two lines of the body of the letter continue to the second page.

13. Procedural Step. Spell check the letter and proofread it carefully. If using a computer, print the letter.

Principle. A business letter should not contain errors. If errors are present, the credibility and professionalism of the sender may be doubted.

14. Procedural Step. Obtain the appropriate signature or sign the letter below the complimentary close.

15. Procedural Step. Make a photocopy of the letter for your files and for any individual who will receive a copy of the letter.

Principle. Copies of all business letters are retained in case there are questions or further correspondence is necessary.

16. Procedural Step. Prepare an envelope (see Chapter 43, Procedure 43-3) and place the letter in the designated area to be prepared for mailing. If the letter concerns a patient, a copy of the letter is filed in the patient's medical record. Other letters are usually filed in folders by subject (e.g., letters to suppliers).

RESPONDING TO WRITTEN COMMUNICATION

The medical office receives letters and/or e-mails on a daily basis that require follow-up. Unless letters are marked "personal" or "private," the medical assistant usually screens correspondence. The medical assistant may respond personally to correspondence related to supply orders, billing questions, insurance-related questions, and requests for information about the practice. If an urgent response appears necessary, the medical assistant may use the telephone, but in most cases, the response will be in the same format as the original communication (Procedure 42-2).

Correspondence relating to patient care is referred to the physician, and the medical assistant may clip the letter to the patient's medical record if a paper-based medical record system is used in the office. If the physician dictates a reply to a letter, the medical assistant transcribes the letter as described later in this chapter.

Grammar and Sentence Structure

It is important to respond in a timely manner to written communication using proper grammar and spelling. **Grammar** is a term for the accepted rules to create meaningful sentences in a language.

Parts of Speech

In English, words are classified as one of eight different parts of speech, a set of categories that describe how words are used. Many words can be used in more than one way.

1. **Nouns:** A noun is the name of a person, place, or thing. It can also be a word used to identify a concept or idea. *Common nouns* refer to general things or categories (e.g., *tree, house*). *Proper nouns* are names of specific individuals or places (e.g., *John Stanton, Philadelphia*).

2. **Pronouns:** A pronoun is used in place of a noun. Examples include *I, me, you, he, she, it,* and *they*. Possessive pronouns show ownership (e.g., *mine, yours, hers, its*). None of the possessive pronouns are written with an apostrophe.

3. **Verbs:** A verb either shows action or a state of being. Every sentence requires a verb in order to be complete. Verbs that show a state of being are also called *linking verbs*. Action verbs include *talk, sing, help,* and *communicate*. Verbs that show a state of being include *is, are, feel,* and *seem*.

4. **Adjectives and Articles:** An adjective modifies or qualifies a noun. It is a describing word. Examples include *white, pretty, little,* and *thin*. When two or more words are used together as an adjective to modify or qualify a

Putting It All into Practice

My name is Christine Walters, and I am a registered medical assistant. I have been working for a nephrology practice for the past 3 years. This practice was started by two doctors about 15 years ago, and their office is in a building located next to the local hospital. About a year ago a third nephrologist joined the practice, and it is surprising how much more paperwork this has created. Because the physicians specialize in diseases of the kidney, our patients are usually referred by other physicians. This means that our physicians must communicate with the patient's primary care physician for almost every patient they see. Our physicians use hand-held digital recorders that are connected to our computer network. One of the physicians prefers to have his reports formatted as a consultation report, which is sent with a cover letter to the referring physician. We use a template for the cover letter so that he doesn't have to dictate it each time. The other two physicians usually include their findings in a dictated letter. I am responsible for transcribing these letters and reports, but it really isn't difficult because they follow a fairly regular pattern. I use headphones and a foot pedal that connects to the computer with a USB cable. We have a program installed on our computers that plays the dictated files and allows us to start and stop them with the foot pedal. Usually this takes me a few hours a day, but when the office is busy, sometimes I do get behind and I may even have to stay late to finish. I have been able to personalize the spell checker on the computer I use, so even proofreading isn't that difficult. ■

Prepare for Success

noun, they are often connected by a hyphen *(a 20-year-old female)*. English has three articles: *a, an,* and *the.* They may be included as adjectives or sometimes a separate part of speech.

5. **Adverbs:** An adverb modifies a verb, adjective, or other adverb. Adverbs include words that question *(how?, where?)* and words that end in *-ly (slowly, perfectly).*

6. **Prepositions:** A preposition shows the connection of a noun or pronoun to some other word, especially in relation to space, time, or possession. Examples include *on, in, of,* and *to.*

7. **Conjunctions:** A conjunction joins words, phrases, or clauses in a sentence. The common conjunctions include *and, but, or,* and *because.*

8. **Interjections:** An interjection is a word that expresses feelings. It is often followed by an exclamation point. Examples include *oh! yeah!* and *ouch!* Interjections are rarely used in correspondence or reports.

Sentence Structure

Sentences are composed of various combinations of independent and dependent clauses. A clause contains a subject (noun or pronoun) and a verb. If it can stand alone, it is called an *independent clause.* If it requires an additional

What Would You Do? What Would You *Not* Do?

Case Study 1
The physician asks Christine to obtain brochures with information about different types of electrocardiograph machines. He gives her the name of two manufacturers in which he is interested. The physician said, "I don't want to talk to anyone yet. I just want to see some brochures." ■

clause in order to be meaningful, it is called a *dependent* or *subordinate clause.* Sentence classifications are as follows:

1. **Simple Sentence:** A sentence composed of one independent clause. Example: *The dog was very hungry.*

2. **Compound Sentence:** A sentence composed of two independent clauses connected by a conjunction. A comma separates the two clauses. Example: *The dog returned from its walk, and it drank all the water in its bowl.*

3. **Complex Sentence:** A sentence composed of one independent clause and one or more dependent clauses. If the dependent clause begins the sentence, it is followed by a comma. Example: *When it returned from its walk, the dog drank all the water in its bowl.* If the dependent clause comes after the independent clause, the dependent clause is not separated by a comma. Example: *The dog drank all the water in its bowl when it returned from its walk.*

Sentence Errors

1. **Sentence Fragment:** A sentence fragment is a dependent clause used to stand alone as a sentence. In this case, an additional independent clause is necessary for meaning. Sentence fragment: *When I arrive for my appointment.* Correct sentence: *When I arrive for my appointment, I will bring my insurance card.*

2. **Run-on Sentence:** A run-on sentence is a sentence in which two or more independent clauses are joined without a conjunction. Run-on sentence: *My appointment is on Thursday I will bring my insurance card.* Correct sentence: *My appointment is on Thursday, and I will bring my insurance card.*

3. **Comma Splice:** A comma splice is the incorrect use of a comma to separate two sentences. The sentences should be separated either with a period and a new sentence or with a semicolon. It is also permitted to separate the sentences with a comma and a conjunction.

Comma Rules

1. Use a comma to separate the elements in a series of three or more things. The comma before the conjunction "and" is optional.
   Example: The patient complained of abdominal pain, difficulty breathing, and headache.
   Example: This 40-year-old, well-nourished, Caucasian female was seen on 12/22/10.

2. Use a comma before a conjunction, such as "and," "but," "for," etc. when the conjunction connects two

independent clauses. An independent clause could be used as a complete sentence.

Example: The patient called an ambulance, and the ambulance brought her to Memorial Hospital.

Example: We gave the patient furosemide intravenously, but after an hour her urine output was still poor.

3. Use a comma to set off introductory elements such as prepositional phrases or dependent clauses.

Example: After the upper GI, the patient continued to experience epigastric pain.

Example: Because we were planning surgery for next week, I did not want to prescribe any new medications.

4. Use a comma to set off information that could be omitted or placed in parentheses without changing the meaning of the sentence.

Example: The patient, who was referred by Dr. Jenkins, is a 40-year-old woman in good health.

Example: We will follow this patient closely in the clinic, which is open on Tuesdays and Thursdays.

5. Use a comma before quotation marks except at the end of the sentence where a period precedes the close quotation marks. Do not use a comma to introduce quoted elements introduced by the word *that*.

Example: The patient said, "My incision burns like fire."

Example: "My incision burns like fire," said the patient.

Example: The patient states that her incision burns like fire.

6. Use a comma to avoid confusion.

Example: For most the year is already finished.

Example: For most, the year is already finished.

7. Use a comma between the city and the state, the date and the year, a name and a title, in long numbers, etc.

No comma is necessary when only the month and year are used.

Example: The patient was admitted to Memorial Hospital, Westford, Massachusetts in late July 2002.

Example: On July 5, 2002 the patient was burned severely in a fire in Las Vegas, Nevada.

8. Use commas with terms like *not, however,* and *but* to express contrast.

Example: The wound was large, but healing well.

Example: I had not prescribed antibiotics for the patient before, however she had obtained them from another physician.

9. Use a comma to separate appositives, nouns of direct address, titles that follow a person's name, and introductory words from the rest of the sentence.

Example: We will make an appointment with Dr. Cannon, a gynecologist, sometime next week.

Example: Doctor, there is something else I wanted to ask you.

10. Separate parenthetical expressions from the rest of the sentence using commas. These expressions include the following: *I believe, I am sure, on the contrary, indeed, of course, nevertheless, in my opinion,* and *in fact.*

Example: The report, I hope, will give you more information about multiple sclerosis.

Example: An inadequate supply of oxygen to the myocardium, for example, is caused by narrowing of the coronary arteries.

Spelling

Although word processing programs usually provide a spell-check feature, the medical assistant must still proofread all documents for spelling. The spell check function verifies the spelling of a given word but cannot confirm that it is the intended word or that it is used correctly in context. See Box 42-1 for a list of pairs of words that are commonly confused.

BOX 42-1 Confusing Pairs of Words

Nouns and Adjectives

affect (mood) and effect (result)

councilor (member of a council) and counselor (someone who gives guidance)

ileum (last part of the small intestine) and ilium (part of the pelvis)

principal (head of a school; most important) and principle (basis of a system of belief)

stationary (fixed in place) and stationery (paper and other writing materials)

Verbs, Adjectives, and Adverbs

accept (agree or believe in) and except (verb: object; adverb: left out)

adverse (unfavorable or bad) and averse (strongly disliking)

affect (to make a difference to) and effect (to bring about a difference)

complement (to contribute extra features) and compliment (to praise)

continual (happening frequently) and continuous (without interruption)

eminent (distinguished) and imminent (about to occur)

fewer (not as many) and less (not as much)

imply (to suggest) and infer (to deduce)

loose (to set free; not tight) and lose (to be unable to find)

precede (to go before) and proceed (to continue)

Pronouns

whose (shows possession) and who's (contraction of who is)

your (shows possession) and you're (contraction of you are)

its (shows possession) and it's (contraction of it is)

their (shows possession) and there (shows location)

PROCEDURE **42-2** Responding to Written Communication

Outcome Respond to written communication in an appropriate manner.

Equipment/Supplies

- Received correspondence
- Letterhead stationery
- Blank stationery
- Typewriter
- Computer and printer

1. **Procedural Step.** Review received correspondence to determine an appropriate response.
2. **Procedural Step.** Look up necessary information as needed to respond to the received correspondence.
3. **Procedural Step.** Make notes and/or compose a rough draft if a written response is indicated.
4. **Procedural Step.** Create a business letter following steps in Procedure 42-1 or an e-mail as appropriate. In general, a letter is a correct response to a letter received and an e-mail is a correct response to an e-mail received.

5. **Procedural Step.** Proofread the communication and correct any errors.
6. **Procedural Step.** Save a copy of the letter or e-mail on the computer.
7. **Procedural Step.** Make a copy of a letter, and sign or obtain a signature for a letter.
8. **Procedural Step.** Prepare a letter for mailing as described in Procedure 42-1 or send an e-mail.
9. **Procedural Step.** File the original letter with a copy of the response as indicated.

In order to improve spelling, the medical assistant should keep a personal list of words that cause difficulty, make an effort to learn these words, and remember to check these words in the dictionary every time they are used. The medical office may purchase a medical dictionary program that can be installed on office computers for reference.

TRANSCRIPTION

The purpose of **transcription** is to change dictated notes into a printed format. Although some physicians still hand-write their notes about the patient encounter, most use either some form of dictation and transcription system or an electronic medical record.

A traditional transcription system included a small, hand-held dictation recorder to record the physician's notes and a desktop unit with a foot pedal that the transcriber uses to listen to the dictation tape. Both recorder and transcriber had to use the same size tape (either standard size or microcassette).

Today the physician usually dictates his or her notes into a small digital recorder that is placed into a docking station to transfer the files to a computer. This allows easy transmission of files to the medical assistant or other location. Although letters may be produced in the office, progress notes are usually sent to a transcription service. The actual transcription is done using a foot pedal with a computer and transcription program.

The transcription program allows the speed of dictation to be increased or decreased. The foot pedal allows for easy starting, stopping, backing up, or fast forwarding during the transcription process (Figure 42-6). The completed

Figure 42-6. A foot pedal is used to start and stop the dictation during transcription.

document file is then returned to the office, where it is printed, reviewed, and filed. Some physicians are using voice-recognition software, which translates the physician's voice into a written document automatically. Although voice recognition programs can "learn" to recognize the speech patterns of one individual, the final document still requires extensive editing. This includes changing incorrect words, writing out abbreviations, putting in proper punctuation and paragraph breaks, and making any other necessary changes. The editing may be done by the physician, medical assistant, or transcription service (Procedure 42-3).

Letters

The medical assistant should transcribe letters using one of the standard letter formats as described earlier in the chapter. A dictated letter always requires a reference line with the initials of the individual who dictated the letter in capital letters followed by a colon or slash and the initials of the individual who transcribed the letter. A letter dictated by the physician is prepared for his or her signature. If changes are necessary, a revised copy can be printed easily. Instructions for preparing and mailing the letter are included in Chapter 43.

Memoranda

A common way to communicate within the office is through the use of a **memo (memorandum),** a document used within a company that is usually short and limited to one subject. Although a printed form can be used, it is not difficult to produce a template that can be used frequently in a given office. The title "Memorandum" or "Interoffice Memorandum" should appear at the top of the page.

Four headings commonly appear at the top of the memo:

TO:
FROM:
DATE:
SUBJECT:

The headings may be separated from the body of the memorandum by a line that extends from 2 inches to completely across the page. The message should be informative but succinct. The body of the memo is single spaced. A memo may be printed and circulated to all individuals included in the distribution list, or it may be sent as an e-mail attachment. If the memo is written to all staff members, a copy may be posted on a central bulletin board (Figure 42-7).

Medical Reports

The reports physicians most often dictate in an office setting are progress notes, history and physical examination, and consultation reports. Word processing software allows the transcriber to create a template with the correct format for various reports.

Progress Notes

Progress notes may be set up in SOAP format or using other headings, such as CC (Chief Complaint), PE (Physical Examination), Impression, and Plan. Each note should include the patient's name, clinic number or date of birth, and the date of the office visit. Progress notes are single-spaced, with two spaces between paragraphs or headings. Entries under Impression and Plan are usually numbered. A signature line is usually included for the physician to sign the note.

Each office has a preferred format for progress notes. The progress note for each visit may be printed on a separate piece of paper, or paper with adhesive backing may be used so that each note can be mounted in chronological order in the medical record. When a physician dictates progress notes, the findings of tests and interviews done by the medical assistant are often incorporated into the dictated notes (Figure 42-8).

History and Physical Examination Reports

Several standard formats for dictated history and physical examination reports are available, so the medical assistant

---

INTEROFFICE MEMORANDUM

TO: All Staff

FROM: Howard Lawler, MD

DATE: 6/18/10

SUBJECT: Introduction of new office manager

- -

It is my pleasure to announce that effective July 1, Diane Janes, CMA (AAMA), will join our staff as office manager. Ms. Janes has had extensive experience in a variety of medical settings. Most recently she has been employed as office manager in a family care practice in Minnesota. With the relocation of her family to Wisconsin, Ms. Janes has become available to join our practice. I hope that you will join me in welcoming Ms. Janes over lunch in the office on Friday, June 28.

Figure 42-7. A memo is used for communication within a business. (From Hunt SA: *Saunders fundamentals of medical assisting,* St. Louis, 2007, Saunders.)

PATIENT NAME: Diane Wells

DATE OF BIRTH: 2/26/2002

DATE OF VISIT: 6/18/2010

CHIEF COMPLAINT: This is an 8-year-old female who came to the office complaining of blurred vision in her right eye following a fall from a bicycle two days ago. She states that the right side of her forehead struck the handlebar when she fell. She did not lose consciousness. She has not experienced headaches, but the vision in the right eye remains blurry.

PHYSICAL EXAMINATION: Physical exam was routine except for moderate bruising of the right forehead. Visual examination of the right eye by direct ophthalmoscope is essentially normal and no visual field deficits were noted. Neurological examination is essentially normal.

IMPRESSION: Blurred vision following a fall

PLAN: Refer to ophthalmologist for appointment today.

Richard Warner, MD

Figure 42-8. Sample transcription of a progress note.

should determine the preferred format for the office where he or she is working. Usually, the report is divided into identifying information (patient, clinic number or date of birth, physician, and date of examination), the sections of the history, and sections of the physical examination, with each heading keyed in all capital letters followed by a colon. The text of each section may be lined up flush with the left margin, or to a tab placed to make a separate column beside the headings. The physical examination usually includes a section for each body system examined. The final section of the physical examination usually includes the impression (diagnosis) and any plan for treatment.

Consultation Reports

A consultation report may be dictated as a letter or in a format similar to the history and physical examination report. Medical assistants who work for specialists are more likely to transcribe consultation reports than those who work for primary care practitioners.

Proofreading

While transcribing the report, the medical assistant should look up any unfamiliar words in order to spell them correctly. Abbreviations for medical conditions should be written out, but abbreviations for medication times, measurements, and vital signs are usually acceptable (Table 42-1).

What Would You Do? What Would You *Not* Do?

Case Study 2

Christine is transcribing a letter related to the examination of a patient with hematuria (blood in the urine). She transcribes the patient's history and presenting symptoms, but in the section related to diagnostic testing, the physician uses an abbreviation that she cannot hear clearly. She also does not understand the sentence in which the unknown abbreviation occurs. She transcribes the rest of the report and then returns to the section that caused difficulty. She is still unable to make any sense of the abbreviation and the rest of the sentence. ▪

It is helpful to use medical spell-check software, which is available from several companies. An ordinary spell-check program can also be personalized over time by adding medical words and abbreviations that the program does not recognize; however, additions should always be checked for correctness. After the report has been keyed, the medical assistant should print a copy, **proofread** it (read it carefully and make corrections), and then correct it and print out a final copy. If there is an unintelligible word, a space can be left and marked in pencil for the physician to fill in before signing the report. Figure 42-9 is a list of proofreader's marks.

Figure 42-9. Standard proofreader's marks. (From Diehl MO, Fordney, MT: *Medical typing and transcription: techniques and procedures,* ed 3, Philadelphia, 1991, Saunders.)

Memories *from* Externship

Christine Walters: I did my externship in the office of a family practitioner. I really enjoyed seeing patients of all ages because it gave me different kinds of experiences. In that office they used several different kinds of form letters. For example, their computer system kept a record of infants who were due for immunizations until the child was 2 years old. If the immunizations were more than 1 month overdue, the office sent a letter reminding the parents which immunizations were due and asking them to make an appointment. Twice while I was on my externship, they gave me a computer printout of the children who were overdue for immunizations to prepare letters for. First I had to check the computer system for each child to see if an appointment was scheduled in the next month. If there was an appointment, we didn't send a letter. Then I had to prepare a letter for each child still on the list. It was a form letter, and I filled in the parent's name and address on blank lines for the return address. Then I filled in the name of the child and the overdue immunization(s). When all the letters were prepared, I made copies for the medical records. I folded the letters and placed them in window envelopes so that the address was visible. I remember one patient's mother who kept apologizing for forgetting to make an appointment for her son. She said she had not been able to make the appointment when the child was in the office because she wasn't sure of her schedule, and then she just forgot about it. She thanked us for sending the reminder because she didn't want her son to get behind on his immunizations. ∎

Prepare for Success

Table 42-1 Common Abbreviations Used in Transcription

ABBREVIATIONS FOR DISEASES OR CONDITIONS		ABBREVIATIONS USED IN THE HISTORY & PHYSICAL EXAMINATION	
Abbreviation	Transcribed as	Dictated as	Transcribed as
CAD	coronary artery disease	HEENT	HEENT (head, eyes, ears, nose, throat)
CHF	congestive heart failure	DTRs	deep tendon reflexes
COPD	chronic obstructive pulmonary disease	EOMs	external eye movements
CVA	cerebrovascular accident	P & A	percussion and auscultation
DOB	date of birth	TMs	tympanic membranes
IDDM	insulin dependent diabetes mellitus	GI	gastrointestinal
LMP	last menstrual period	GU	genitourinary
MI	myocardial infarction	PERRLA	PERRLA (pupils equal, round, react to light and accommodation)
STD	sexually transmitted disease		
TB	tuberculosis	SOB	shortness of breath
URI	upper respiratory infection	NKA	NKA (no known allergies)
UTI	urinary tract infection		

PROCEDURE 42-3 Transcribing a Dictated Letter or Report

Outcome Transcribe a dictated letter or report.

Equipment/Supplies

- Letterhead stationery
- Blank stationery or paper
- Transcription machine or computer with foot pedal
- Headphones
- Dictation tape or file
- Computer and printer

1. **Procedural Step.** Assemble materials and decide on a format for the letter or report.
2. **Procedural Step.** Set up the transcription equipment and plug headphones into the transcriber or computer.
3. **Procedural Step.** While listening to the dictation, key the letter following the guidelines given in Procedure 42-1 or key the report.
4. **Procedural Step.** For a letter, be sure to include a reference line using the initials of the person who dictated the letter (uppercase) followed by your initials (lowercase) separated by a colon.
Principle. The person who receives a letter is entitled to know who keyed the letter.

5. **Procedural Step.** Spell check the letter or report and print a copy for proofreading.
6. **Procedural Step.** Check the letter or report for correct grammar and spelling, consistency of style, and overall appearance.
7. **Procedural Step.** Make corrections as needed and print a final copy.
8. **Procedural Step.** Place the letter or report in the designated area for physician review and signature.
Principle. Any dictated document must be reviewed and signed or initialed by the individual responsible for the dictation.

ELECTRONC DATA TRANSMISSION

E-mail

E-mail (electronic mail) has become an accepted means of communication throughout the business world. **E-mail** is the exchange of information from one computer to another. As described in Chapter 39, a computer with an Internet connection is used to send e-mail. Medical assistants usually use e-mail to communicate with business contacts, not patients. These may include other medical assistants, vendors, and insurance companies. It is usually faster and more efficient to send an e-mail for a short message.

An e-mail message should contain an informative subject line. Successive e-mails relating to the same subject are usually created as a reply so that the recipient can read the previous correspondence related to the subject. It is polite to acknowledge receipt of an e-mail, even if there is no reply, so the sender knows that the e-mail has been received.

The tone of an e-mail is somewhat less formal than a letter, but correct grammar and spelling should be used without any of the abbreviated forms that are sometimes used in personal e-mails. Humor should be avoided because the recipient does not have the nonverbal cues to know when a message is meant to be humorous. The medical assistant should also avoid sending an e-mail containing criticism or other negative content because it is easier to be more negative than intended in writing than when speaking directly to an individual.

E-mails usually use plain text. At the foot of the message, the medical assistant should include the business name, contact information, and e-mail address and telephone number. Most e-mail programs allow the medical assistant to create a signature with the contact information to be included at the bottom of every e-mail.

The medical assistant should remember that e-mails are not private. Even after messages have been deleted, they can often be recovered from the computer or network used to create them. The medical assistant should use e-mail only for business communications that are straightforward and not confidential. It is also always important to be sure that the e-mail is being sent to the correct recipient. It is a good policy to review the recipient name(s) before hitting the send button. The account should be set up so that sent messages are saved, but the medical assistant may also want to create printed copies of e-mails related to orders or billing problems.

E-mail Attachments

Programs for sending e-mail allow documents, images, and other types of files to be attached and transmitted with the e-mail. Unfortunately, many computer viruses are spread through e-mail attachments, so a medical assistant should not open attachments unless they are from a trusted source and/or are expected. If an attachment does contain a virus, opening the attachment launches the virus. Any e-mail with an attachment from an unknown recipient should be deleted immediately. If a medical assistant sends a file as an attachment, the recipient may also be hesitant to open the file for the same reason.

The format of an attachment may also pose a problem. The recipient may be able to open the attachment without the software that was used to create the file in the attach-

What Would You Do? **What Would You *Not* Do?**

Case Study 3
An order for clinical supplies has been delivered to the office, and Christine is putting the supplies away. While checking the received items against the packing list, she notices that although there are 10 boxes of urine test strips listed, only 9 boxes have been shipped. In addition, the packing slip states that only one package of five rolls of paper for the Clinitek machine was shipped, but five packages were ordered. As an experiment, the office has placed this order with an Internet supplier. No telephone number is given for the supplier on its home page. On the company's invoice (bill), which has arrived separately, the medical office has been charged for 10 boxes of urine test strips and one package of paper for the Clinitek machine. ■

ment. Document files can always be saved in text format if there is any question about compatible software. Most files can also be saved as web pages, which the recipient can view with his or her web browser.

Fax Transmissions

When a **fax** is being sent, a cover sheet is attached. The cover sheet has information about the sender, such as the office address, the name of the individual sending the fax, the total number of pages in the fax, a return fax number, and a return voice phone number in case the fax does not come through clearly. It may be created on office letterhead. A fax cover sheet for a medical office should identify that the transmission might contain confidential information. This cover sheet is usually used for all fax transmissions, even if they do not contain patient information (Figure 42-10). Like e-mail, fax transmissions are not a secure means of communication. Information that can be compromising to a patient should not be faxed (Procedure 42-4).

PROCEDURE **42-4**   Sending a Fax

Outcome Send a fax.

Equipment/Supplies

- Fax machine
- Cover sheet
- Document to be faxed

1. **Procedural Step.** Prepare the cover sheet including the name, address, and fax number of the recipient; fax number of the sender; and number of pages (including the cover sheet). If there is a message to the sender, include it on the bottom of the cover sheet.

2. **Procedural Step.** Organize all pages to be faxed with the cover sheet first.
   Principle. Pages should be in order and all facing the same direction.

Continued

PROCEDURE 42-4 Sending a Fax—cont'd

3. Procedural Step. Place pages in the fax machine, face up or face down as is correct for the machine being used.

4. Procedural Step. Enter the fax number. Include any extra digits as required, such as a "9" to obtain an outside line, a "1" for long-distance, and/or an area code if required.
Principle. Some areas of the country have introduced so-called overlay area codes requiring all telephone numbers to be dialed with an area code.

5. Procedural Step. Verify the fax number as it appears in the window or on the computer screen to be sure the number is correct.
Principle. To maintain confidentiality, always be sure the fax number has been entered correctly.

6. Procedural Step. Press the correct button to send the fax.

7. Procedural Step. If the fax contains patient health information, place a telephone call to the recipient so that the fax can be removed from the recipient's fax machine as soon as it is received.

8. Procedural Step. Check back to be sure the fax has been sent. Some machines print a confirmation for every fax, and some only print a written report if the fax does not go through.

9. Procedural Step. File the original document appropriately.

Figure 42-10. A fax cover sheet is often created on office letterhead. (Modified from Hunt SA: *Saunders fundamentals of medical assisting,* St. Louis, 2007, Saunders.)

Blackburn Primary Care Associates, PC

1990 Turquiose Drive • Blackburn, WI 54937 • 608-459-8857

DATE: _____ TIME: _____ NUMBER OF PAGES: _____

TO: _____
(name of authorized receiver)

_____
(name of authorized receiver's facility)

TELEPHONE: _____ FAX: _____
(of receiver) (of receiver)

FROM: BLACKBURN PRIMARY CARE ASSOCIATES - DR. _____
(name of sender)

TELEPHONE: 608-459-8857 FAX: 608-459-8342
(of sender) (of sender)

Comments:

******CONFIDENTIALITY NOTICE******

The documents accompanying this telecopy transmission contain confidential information, belonging to the sender that is legally privileged. This information is intended only for the use of the individual or entity named above. The authorized recipient of this information is prohibited from disclosing this information to any other party and is required to destroy the information after its stated need has been fulfilled, unless otherwise required by state law.

If you are not the intended recipient, you are hereby notified that any disclosure, copying, distribution, or action taken in reliance on the contents of these documents is strictly prohibited. If you have received this telecopy in error, please notifiy the sender immediately to arrange for return of these documents.

PHOTOCOPYING

The medical assistant may need to copy documents using a copy machine. It may be necessary to copy documents of several pages (e.g., an article or paper written by a physician) or to make several copies of a document (e.g., a report to be discussed at a staff meeting).

In order to copy efficiently, the medical assistant should become familiar with special features of the available copy machine. Before copying, staples should be removed from the document to be copied, the pages should be arranged in order, and the copy machine should be checked to be sure it has enough paper.

When several copies of a multiple-page document are needed, the machine should be preset to **collate** (arrange each copy in sequence) or sort the pages if the machine has this feature. Some machines will also staple documents.

For a machine that copies only single pages, the desired number of copies of each page must be copied, arranged in order, and stapled manually. The medical assistant should avoid distractions when copying and should be careful to copy each page correctly and place pages in the correct order (Procedure 42-5).

Another feature of many photocopiers is the ability to **duplex,** or store images from both sides of a page in memory to produce two-sided copies.

When copying a patient's medical record, the medical assistant must preserve the confidentiality of the information. Before beginning to make a copy, the medical assistant should verify that the patient has signed an authorization for the release of information. After copying, it is important for the medical assistant to double-check that no originals or copies were left at the machine. The medical assistant is responsible for shredding any spoiled copies.

PROCEDURE 42-5   Preparing Copies of Multiple-Page Documents

Outcome   Prepare copies of documents with multiple pages.

Equipment/Supplies

- Photocopy machine
- Paper
- Document to be copied
- Stapler
- Staples
- Staple remover

---

1. **Procedural Step.** Assemble all pages of the document or report. If it is stapled, remove all staples.
   Principle. Staples may damage the glass or the feeder of the copier.
2. **Procedural Step.** Be sure that the copy machine is on and warmed up.
3. **Procedural Step.** If the report to be copied includes all or part of a patient's medical record, verify that there is a signed release of information.
4. **Procedural Step.** Place the originals in the machine according to the directions for the individual machine.
   Principle. Depending on the size and complexity of the machine and the type of document to be copied, it may be necessary to copy one page at a time or the machine may accept the entire document. The original

may have to be placed face down on the glass (single-sheet copying) or the document may be loaded face down or face up into a feeder.
5. **Procedural Step.** Set the size, number of copies, and if the machine allows, press buttons so that copies will be collated and/or stapled.
6. **Procedural Step.** Press the "start" button.
7. **Procedural Step.** After the copies have been made, if necessary, arrange the pages in the correct order and staple.
8. **Procedural Step.** If the patient will be charged for copying large sections of the medical record (which is common when the patient requests personal copies or an attorney requests copies), verify the number of pages and submit to the person responsible for billing.

MEDICAL PRACTICE *and the* LAW

When a patient's protected health information (PHI) must be communicated in writing, it is always preferable to send the information in a letter instead of writing an e-mail or sending a fax. Although it is possible for a letter to be read by someone other than the addressee, the sender has made every reasonable effort to protect a patient's confidentiality as required by HIPAA (Health Insurance Portability and Accountability Act).

If a medical office has a secure electronic messaging system with approved encryption, it may be acceptable to send e-mail messages containing PHI. Before any communication with patients via e-mail relating to PHI, the patient should be required to provide consent, recognizing that e-mail is not a secure form of communication. Care should be taken to ensure that an e-mail containing PHI is sent only to the intended recipient.

Fax transmissions should be used only if it is necessary to transmit information without the delay inherent in sending a letter. A cover sheet containing a confidentiality statement should be used, and the transmission should be confirmed by telephone if possible. Neither the sending nor receiving fax machine should be located in an area that is accessible to unauthorized personnel (to prevent interception of incoming faxes). If a fax that contains PHI is received in error, the sender should be notified immediately and the fax should either be returned to the sender by mail or destroyed. ∎

What Would You Do? What Would You *Not* Do?   RESPONSES

Case Study 1
Page 1000

What Did Christine Do?

❑ Looked up the two companies mentioned by the physician using the Internet to obtain the exact business names and addresses and model numbers of machines in which the physician might be interested.

❑ Also looked for other companies that might manufacture similar machines.

❑ Prepared letters to each company requesting information using the usual format for office letters.

❑ Used the salutation "Dear Sir or Madam."

❑ Proofread and signed the letters before mailing.

❑ Made a note to herself to follow up after a week.

What Did Christine Not *Do?*

❑ Did not ask the physician how to find the addresses.

❑ Did not initiate a contact that would result in a call by a salesperson.

❑ Did not send the letters out with an incomplete address or with errors.

What Would You Do/What Would You *Not* Do? Review Christine's response and place a checkmark next to the information you included in your response. List the additional information you included in your response.

_____

_____

_____

_____

Case Study 2
Page 1004

What Did Christine Do?

❑ Asked another medical assistant in the office to listen to the section she could not understand.

❑ If she is able to hear the first letter of the abbreviation, Christine tried to look it up in a dictionary of abbreviations to make sense of the sentence.

❑ If still unable to understand one sentence, left a blank line in the letter and indicated on a sticky note that the physician should fill in the blank.

❑ After the letter was reviewed by the physician, corrected the letter and printed a new copy for the physician to sign.

What Did Christine Not *Do?*

❑ Did not write down exactly what she heard if it did not make sense, hoping that the physician would not notice.

❑ Did not mail the letter without correcting and reprinting it.

❑ Did not interrupt the physician to ask about the confusing abbreviation and sentence.

❑ Did not complain to other office staff about the physician's pronunciation.

What Would You Do/What Would You *Not* Do? Review Christine's response and place a checkmark next to the information you included in your response. List the additional information you included in your response.

_____

_____

_____

_____

Case Study 3
Page 1007

What Did Christine Do?

❑ Used either office e-mail or the contact button on the website to send an e-mail about the missing box of test strips.

❑ Used the same professional tone in the e-mail that she would have used in a letter or telephone call.

❑ In the e-mail, included the order number, billing name and address, number of boxes of test strips ordered, and number of boxes of test strips received.

❑ In the e-mail, stated clearly that the company should send an additional box of test strips.

❑ Because the bill only charged for the one package of paper that was shipped, decided to order the other four packages of paper for the Clinitek machine from a more reliable company.

What Did Christine Not Do?

❑ Did not cross out the charge for 10 boxes and test strips and change it to 9 boxes when approving the bill for payment without contacting the company.

❑ Did not ignore the missing box of strips when approving the bill for payment, assuming that the company would send another box automatically.

❑ Did not use casual, critical, or hostile language in the e-mail.

What Would You Do/What Would You *Not* Do? Review Christine's response and place a checkmark next to the information you included in your response. List the additional information you included in your response.

_____

_____

_____

_____

TERMINOLOGY REVIEW

Collate To assemble the pages of a document in numeric order.

Duplex To produce double-sided copies by storing images from both sides of the original in the memory of a photocopier.

E-mail The exchange of information from one computer to another using telecommunication.

Fax Transmission of scanned, printed material by telephone.

Full block style A letter format in which all parts of the letter are left justified.

Grammar The study of accepted rules used to create meaning in a language.

Left justified Lines of type that begin at the left margin of a document.

Letterhead A sheet of stationery preprinted with information about a business, including name, address, telephone number, and other information.

Memo (memorandum) A form of communication within a company that is usually short and limited to one subject.

Modified block style A format for business letters where the date line, complimentary close, and printed signature line are on a tab at the center or right justified and all other parts of the letter are left justified.

Proofread To identify and correct errors in a document.

Right justified Type that is aligned with the right margin of a document.

Semiblock style A letter format in which the date line, complimentary close, and printed signature line are on a tab at the center or right justified, all paragraphs are indented five to eight spaces, and the other parts of the letter are left justified.

Simplified letter style A letter format in which all elements are left justified. The greeting is replaced by a subject line in all capital letters. The complimentary close and typed signature are replaced by a typed signature in all capital letters.

Template A standard form to which additional information can be added as needed.

Transcription The process of changing verbal dictation to typed or printed form.

ON THE WEB

For Information on Improving Written Communication:

Grammar and Spelling—The Purdue Online Writing Lab (OWL): owl.english.purdue.edu

University of Wisconsin Writing Center—Writer's Handbook: www.wisc.edu/writing/Handbook

For Information on Medical Transcription:

Association for Healthcare Documentation Integrity (formerly American Association of Medical Transcriptionists): www.ahdionline.org

For Information on Patient Confidentiality in Written Communication:

Centers for Medicare and Medicaid Services—HIPAA Privacy Rule: www.hhs.gov/ocr/hipaa

PREPARE FOR CERTIFICATION   Visit the Evolve site at http://evolve.elsevier.com/Bonewit/today/ to actively Prepare for your Certification.

Check out the Companion CD bound with the book to access additional interactive activities.

43

Mail

CAAHEP COMPETENCIES

General Competencies
Professional Communication
- Respond to and initiate written communications.

Operational Functions
- Utilize computer software to maintain office systems.

ABHES COMPETENCIES

Communication
- Receive, organize, prioritize, and transmit information expediently.
- Recognize and respond to verbal and nonverbal communication.

- Use correct grammar, spelling, and formatting techniques in written works.
- Application of electronic technology

KEY TERMS

annotate (ANN-oh-tate)
barcode clear zone
Metered Mail
postage meter

postal bar code
ZIP code
ZIP + 4 code

Introduction to Mail and Shipping

Mail communication is an important aspect of the efficient operation of the medical office. Every day the medical assistant processes incoming mail to facilitate delivery to physicians and other employees in the medical office. Preparing outgoing mail is also important. Most of this chapter is devoted to the services and postal addressing standards of the U.S. Postal Service (USPS), which is used to send the bulk of outgoing mail.

U.S. POSTAL SYSTEM

The USPS is an independent agency with an official monopoly on the delivery of mail within the United States. It is financed primarily through the sale of postage and postage stamps. The postal service processes more than 703 million pieces of mail daily and is the second-largest employer in the United States. The USPS provides a variety of ways for mail to be transported from sender to receiver. The cost of these various services depends on the urgency with which mail must be received, as well as any special handling services provided.

ZIP Code and Barcode Systems

In 1963 the USPS introduced the Zone Improvement Plan (ZIP) code system. This system enables the postal service to process mail more accurately, quickly, and economically with automated equipment. A **ZIP code** consists of a five-digit code that identifies the post office to which a piece of mail is to be delivered. In 1967 it became mandatory to use the ZIP code for second- and third-class bulk mailing.

The **ZIP + 4 code,** which was introduced in 1983, consists of the original five-digit code followed by a hyphen and four additional digits. These digits identify a specific geographic segment within the five-digit delivery area, such as a city block, an office building, or a group of post office boxes. The plus-four code is required for certain presorted mailings. The USPS maintains a ZIP code lookup service that makes it easy to use the Internet to look up the ZIP + 4 code for any address in the United States.

For bulk mailing, the ZIP code is translated into a postal bar code that is printed on the piece of mail, by the sender. A computer program is used to add the barcode to pieces of mail, mailing labels, and mailing lists. For ordinary letters, the postal service may add the postal barcode because it makes the mail easier to sort. Unlike supermarket bar codes, which consist of wide and narrow bars, the **postal bar code** consists of long and short bars. Each individual digit in the ZIP code is represented by five bars, and a check digit is used after the ZIP code or ZIP + 4 code. The postal bar code may be printed in the address block above or below the mailing address. When not included in the address block, the postal bar code is placed in the **barcode clear zone,** a blank rectangular area at the lower right of the card or envelope (Figure 43-1).

Classifications of Domestic Mail

Domestic Mail includes mail that is collected and distributed within, among, and between the United States, its territories and possession, the military service, and the United Nations. Classifications are based on speed of delivery, weight of individual pieces of mail, and number of pieces of mail in the mailing.

Express Mail

Express Mail received by the post office before 5 PM is delivered within 24 hours, and by noon to most major cities, including weekends and holidays. It includes letters and packages weighing up to 70 pounds. Envelopes and packing materials are available from the post office. Medical offices may use Express Mail to send laboratory specimens to an outside laboratory for testing. The postage rates for Express Mail are considerably higher than other rates, but they do include insurance against loss or damage.

First-Class Mail

First-Class Mail is used for letters or other lightweight items up to 13 ounces. The postage is based on weight, with a base rate for one ounce and additional postage for each additional ounce. The medical office uses this mail classification to send letters, post cards, patient statements, and some insurance claim forms.

Sending an item First-Class usually results in overnight service to local cities and second-day service nationwide. Delivery by the third day can be anticipated for some outlying areas. All First-Class Mail should be sealed, and it may not be opened for postal inspection without a federal search warrant.

Additional extra mailing services can be purchased for First-Class Mail, such as Certificates of Mailing, Certified

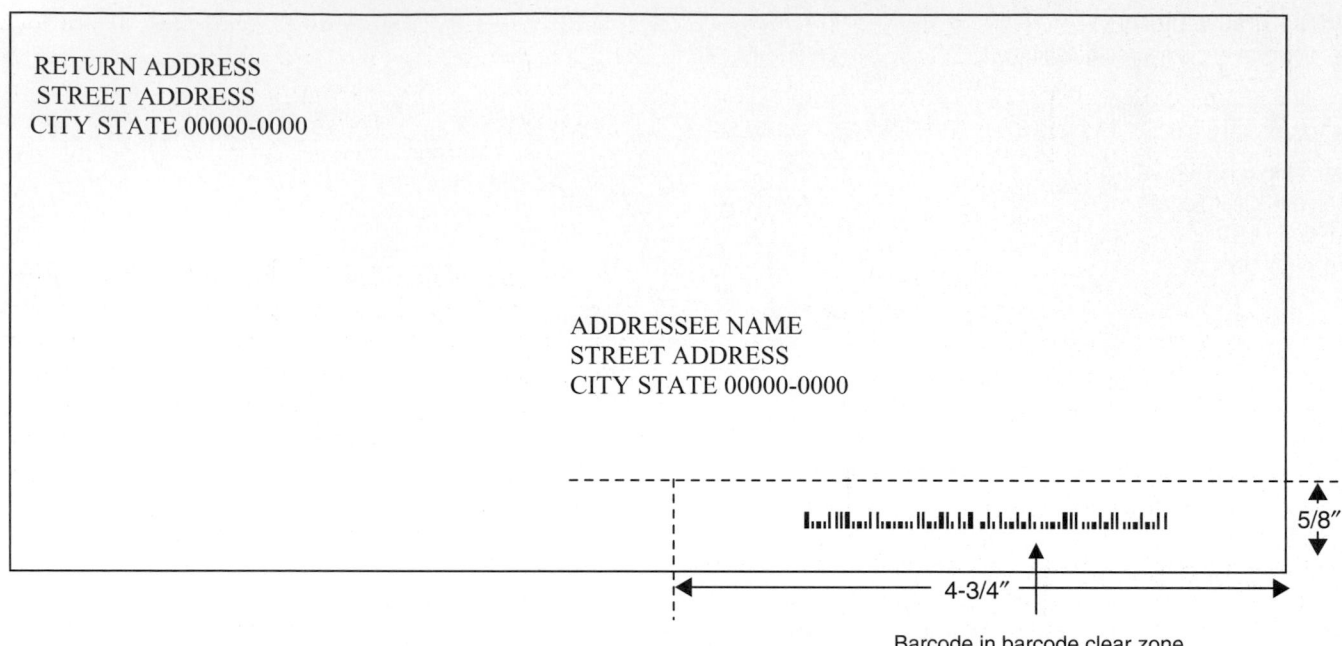

RETURN ADDRESS
STREET ADDRESS
CITY STATE 00000-0000

ADDRESSEE NAME
STREET ADDRESS
CITY STATE 00000-0000

5/8″

4-3/4″

Barcode in barcode clear zone

Figure 43-1. The postal bar code is a series of long and short lines that is either printed by the sender above or below the address or added by the post office in the barcode clear zone at the lower right of the envelope.

Mail, Registered Mail, Collect on Delivery (COD), and Restricted Delivery. If the item that is being sent First-Class is letter size, no additional designation is required on the letter. However, if the item is not letter size, it must be clearly marked "First-Class."

Priority Mail

Priority Mail is used for mail weighing more than 13 ounces that is to be treated as First-Class Mail. It will be delivered anywhere in the United States within 2 to 3 days. The USPS has a set rate for items up to 1 pound, and flat rate envelopes and boxes are available. For an item over 1 pound in ordinary packaging, the rate depends on both the weight of the item and the distance it must be transported. For an additional charge Priority Mail can be combined with Insured Mail, Registered Mail, or Certified Mail or sent COD. Some examples of items that might be sent from the medical office using Priority Mail include copies of medical records.

Standard Mail

This classification of mail is used by newspapers and periodical publishers to send newspapers, journals, magazines, and other periodicals. Periodical mailings must not be sealed and handwritten messages are not permitted. Standard Mail is also used to send large mailings of newsletters and bulletins. The medical office usually does not obtain the special permit to send items at this rate, but it may receive newspapers, magazines for the waiting room, and medical journals. Standard Mail requires a minimum of 200 pieces or 50 pounds per mailing.

Parcel Post and Other Packages

If time is not a significant factor, packages may be sent using one of the ground mail classifications. Parcel Post is used to send merchandise and other items that weigh up to 70 pounds and measure up to 108 inches in length and girth. Instruction slips, packing slips, sales slips, or invoices can be enclosed in a package sent Parcel Post without additional postage. However, in order to send a letter with a package, the letter must be attached to the outside of the package and paid for at the first-class rate. The medical office rarely sends items by Parcel Post, although it may receive supplies sent by this method. Media Mail is a special classification for packages containing books, sound recordings, film, manuscripts, and computer media but not advertising. Bound Printed Matter is a classification for packages containing permanently bound catalogs and other volumes containing advertising (e.g., telephone books).

Insurance and Delivery Confirmation Services

The USPS offers a number of extra mailing services. These services must be purchased in addition to the regular postage required to send an item. The medical assistant must understand these extra services, particularly those that are used most frequently in the medical office, such as Certified Mail and Return Receipt.

Certified Mail

Certified Mail is available for First-Class Mail and Priority Mail. It serves as legal evidence that an item was mailed by providing the sender with a mailing receipt. In addition, a

Putting It All into Practice

My name is Diane Waters, and I am a certified medical assistant. I have been working for an internal medicine practice with three general surgeons for the past 6 years. Our physicians usually have office hours three times a week, either in the morning or the afternoon. They usually operate two to three times a week, and they have to make hospital rounds every day. Two of them also work with residents at a large hospital located near our practice. In the past, each surgeon received an operative report and discharge summary for each patient he or she had operated on in hard copy. When I opened the mail, I had to date stamp each report, find the patient's medical record, and place it for the physician to review before it could be filed. Last year the hospital went to an electronic medical record. The operative reports and discharge summaries are now entered into the electronic medical record automatically, and the physicians review them online. That means that we get significantly less mail because not only those reports but also laboratory reports, pathology reports, and other types of reports no longer come to the office. Of course, we don't have as much filing, either. Our office still gets piles of journals, magazines, and other printed matter, however. Every day when I am sorting the mail, I have to separate the professional journals that our physicians want to read from magazines, catalogs, circulars, and other items that they would only look at if we found some item of special interest to them. One physician likes to look through this material if it comes with his name on it, but the others don't even want it to show up on their desks. ■

Prepare for Success

record of delivery of the certified item is maintained for 2 years. A green certified mail sticker affixed to the envelope identifies the envelope as Certified Mail. The recipient must sign on delivery of a piece of Certified Mail. This service can also be combined with a Return Receipt for an additional fee (Figure 43-2).

Return Receipt

A Return Receipt provides the sender with proof of delivery of a piece of mail and the signature of the person receiving the mail. This may be done through a post card signed by the recipient and returned to the sender or by an e-mail with an attachment containing the recipient's signature. The sender then has a copy of the signature of the person who signed for the piece of mail. This service can be combined with other services. It is often used with Certified Mail to establish proof of mailing, as well as proof of receipt (Figure 43-3).

Signature Confirmation

Signature Confirmation provides a record of the date and time an item was delivered, as well as the name of the person who signed for the item. A delivery record, including the signature of the recipient, is available by fax or mail on request. The medical office usually uses Return Receipt instead of Signature Confirmation for evidence of delivery because the return post card or e-mail will be sent automatically.

Certificate of Mailing

A Certificate of Mailing provides evidence of the date and time an item was mailed, but there is no legal proof that

Figure 43-2. A receipt for Certified Mail form must be filled out by the sender and signed by the recipient. (Modified from Young AP, Proctor DB: *Kinn's the medical assistant,* ed 10, St. Louis, 2007, Saunders.)

UNITED STATES POSTAL SERVICE

First-Class Mail
Postage & Fees Paid
USPS
Permit No. G-10

• Sender: Please print your name, address, and ZIP+4 in this box •

SENDER: *COMPLETE THIS SECTION*

■ Complete items 1, 2, and 3. Also complete item 4 if Restricted Delivery is desired.
■ Print your name and address on the reverse so that we can return the card to you.
■ Attach this card to the back of the mailpiece, or on the front if space permits.

1. Article Addressed to:

COMPLETE THIS SECTION ON DELIVERY

A. Signature

X

☐ Agent
☐ Addressee

B. Received by (*Printed Name*)

C. Date of Delivery

D. Is delivery address different from item 1?　☐ Yes
　　If YES, enter delivery address below:　☐ No

3. Service Type
　☐ Certified Mail　　☐ Express Mail
　☐ Registered　　　☐ Return Receipt for Merchandise
　☐ Insured Mail　　☐ C.O.D.

4. Restricted Delivery? *(Extra Fee)*　☐ Yes

2. Article Number
　(Transfer from service label)

PS Form 3811, February 2004　　　Domestic Return Receipt　　　102595-02-M-1540

Figure 43-3. The sender must fill out a Return Receipt form. (From Young AP, Proctor DB: *Kinn's the medical assistant,* ed 10, St. Louis, 2007, Saunders.)

the item was actually delivered to the recipient. A certificate of mailing might be used when proof of timely mailing is required, such as a tax return. No record is maintained at the post office, so the sender is responsible for keeping the form.

Restricted Delivery

If an item is strictly confidential, Restricted Delivery limits delivery to the addressee, the individual authorized in writing to sign for the addressee, or a parent or guardian. It is not generally necessary to use this service for letters

from the medical office, but if a legal case is pending, it might be advisable.

Registered Mail

Registered Mail is available for First-Class and Priority Mail, to insure the contents up to $25,000.00. Registered Mail is used when the contents of the item mailed are valuable. The items are tracked, and the date and time of delivery or delivery attempts can be verified online. The cost depends on the value of the item being sent. The sender receives a receipt that is kept until the recipient receives the item. The recipient must sign a form acknowledging receipt. For an additional fee, the sender can receive a Return Receipt.

Insured Mail

Insurance can be purchased on the contents of mail up to $5,000.00. The cost depends on the declared value of the contents. If the mail is lost or damaged, the sender presents the receipt to make a claim for reimbursement of the declared value.

Special Handling

Special Handling is used for unusual items that require special treatment, such as a shipment of live bees. Ordinary packages with breakable items can be marked "FRAGILE" and do not require Special Handling provided they are packed with adequate packing material to protect the contents. This service is not usually used by the medical office.

Collect on Delivery

COD is a special mailing service that allows a sender to collect for merchandise and postage on delivery. The amount due is collected by the postal carrier and returned to the sender by a postal money order. This service is rarely used by the medical office.

Postal Money Orders

Postal money orders are a safe way to send money through the mail within the United States. They may be purchased in an amount up to $1,000.00. The sender is given a customer receipt. If the money order is lost or stolen, the sender presents the receipt to the post office for replacement. Some patients may pay bills with postal money orders.

OTHER PACKAGE DELIVERY SERVICES

Private carriers compete with the USPS to provide delivery service of letters and packages. Many companies use DHL, FedEx, or United Parcel Service (UPS) for next-day and 2-day delivery service. Larger packages that are not time sensitive can be shipped via UPS or FedEx Ground service. A shipping service company will pick items up from an office and offer continuous item tracking over the company's website. Each company also provides mailing envelopes and small boxes at no cost to the customer. Once an account has been established, shipping can be arranged and paid for using the Internet.

Private carriers often deliver packages to the medical office. Examples include business supplies and laboratory reagents requiring refrigeration. The medical office may use a private delivery service to send some laboratory specimens to a laboratory for testing if the specimen must go to a special laboratory or cannot wait for the regular laboratory pick-up service.

PROCESSING INCOMING MAIL

Mail is delivered to the medical office in various ways. The postal carrier may deliver the mail directly to the office, or it may be placed in an outside mailbox. Some medical offices use a post office box. In this case, the medical assistant must go to the post office to collect the mail each day. In a large clinic, the mail may be delivered to a central mailroom, where it is sorted and distributed to each department or individual mailbox.

Once the mail is received by the medical office, it must be processed according to the preferences of individual physicians. One physician may want to see all the incoming mail, whereas another physician may want the medical assistant to screen the mail and remove circulars, patient and insurance payments, and magazines for the waiting room (Procedure 43-1).

Incoming mail should be sorted in the following way. If the mail is addressed to a particular physician, it goes into that physician's mailbox or pile. Mail from another physician's office that is not addressed to a particular physician should go into the box or pile of the managing partner, medical director, or office manager.

The medical assistant handles patient and insurance payments, mail from insurance companies, and catalogs from business and medical supply companies. Table 43-1 provides a guide for sorting incoming mail.

Opening Mail

Once the mail is sorted, it must be opened. The medical assistant must know which mail he or she is to open, and which is to go to the individual who must deal with it unopened. Some physicians like to open their own mail, whereas others like to have the mail opened, organized, and ready for them to read and respond to. Clearly, any mail marked "personal" or "confidential" should not be opened.

If the physician or physicians prefer mail to be opened, the medical assistant should use a letter opener to open each piece carefully at the top edge. Each letter or report is stamped with the receipt date and then alphabetized by the patient's last name. The pages of each report should be stapled together, if they are not already that way. A letter or report containing patient information should be attached to the patient's medical record with a paper clip. Some offices use a cover sheet on the top of each report, on which

What Would You Do? What Would You *Not* Do?

Case Study 1

Jerome Stone, a 68-year-old man who has had two laparoscopic surgeries in the past, has called the office and asked to have a copy of his medical record sent to his new surgeon in another state because he needs to have another surgery for the same condition. He tells Diane that the surgery is scheduled for the day after tomorrow and asks if she can send the copy of the record immediately. He gives her the name, address, and telephone number of the new physician. ■

PROCEDURE 43-1

Table 43-1 Sorting Incoming Mail

Mail Category	Recipient
First-Class Mail	
Correspondence addressed to the physician marked "Confidential" or "Personal"	Physician
Correspondence from an attorney	Physician
Laboratory reports	Physician (attach laboratory report to patient's medical record)
Patient records	Physician
Patient payments	Medical assistant
Insurance payments	Medical assistant
Bills for office supplies and equipment	Medical assistant
Bank statements	Medical assistant
Letters from insurance companies	Medical assistant
Resumés for employment	Medical assistant
Periodicals, Circulars, Catalogs	
Professional journals	Physician
Medical conventions and seminars	Physician
Pharmaceutical advertising	Physician
Advertisements for equipment and supplies	Physician
Magazines for the waiting room	Medical assistant
Catalogs for equipment and supplies	Medical assistant
Drug Samples and Packages	
Overnight packages	Screen appropriately
Administrative and clinical office supplies	Medical assistant
Drug samples	Medical assistant (place in drug sample storage area)

Figure 43-4. In a large office, each staff member may have a mailbox at a central location.

What Would You Do? What Would You *Not* Do?

Case Study 2

Diane is preparing an envelope in order to mail a letter that the physician has dictated to a colleague named Dr. Leonie. She uses the USPS website to look up the ZIP code. Although a five-digit ZIP code is displayed, it is accompanied by a message that says: "This address may be nondeliverable." ■

the physician can check off the action he or she wishes to occur with regard to the report (e.g., file, respond, call the patient).

Non–patient-related items are stacked together to be dealt with by the medical assistant or another member of the staff. Medical journals addressed to a particular physician can be put in his or her mail pile; those addressed to

the practice can be put into the medical library or staff lounge. If the office is large, each staff member may have a cubicle in a central location, as shown in Figure 43-4.

Some physicians may instruct the medical assistant to annotate letters. To **annotate** means to underline or highlight important words or phrases in the correspondence. This saves the physician time when reading and responding to the mail. The medical assistant may also be instructed to underline or highlight abnormal values on laboratory reports or diagnostic tests.

When a physician is on vacation, someone on the office staff is delegated to review his or her mail and refer any urgent mail either to the physician by telephone or e-mail at the vacation location, or to a covering physician. Arrange nonurgent mail by date received for the physician to review when he or she returns to the office.

PROCEDURE 43-1 Processing Incoming Mail

Outcome Process incoming mail.

Equipment/Supplies

- Letter opener
- Date stamp
- Paper clips

- Stapler
- Pen or highlighter
- Transparent tape

1. **Procedural Step.** Assemble supplies in a work area large enough to make several piles of mail.
2. **Procedural Step.** Stack all the envelopes so that they face in the same direction. Place any envelopes marked "personal" or "confidential" to the side.
   Principle. Letters marked "personal" or "confidential" should only be opened by the person to whom they are addressed.
3. **Procedural Step.** Tap the lower edge of the first envelope on the desk so that the contents fall to the bottom.
   Principle. Tapping the envelope prevents cutting the contents when the envelope is opened.
4. **Procedural Step.** Using a letter opener, open the envelope along its top edge.
   Principle. Using a letter opener makes it easier to open the envelope neatly and preserves the return address should it be needed.

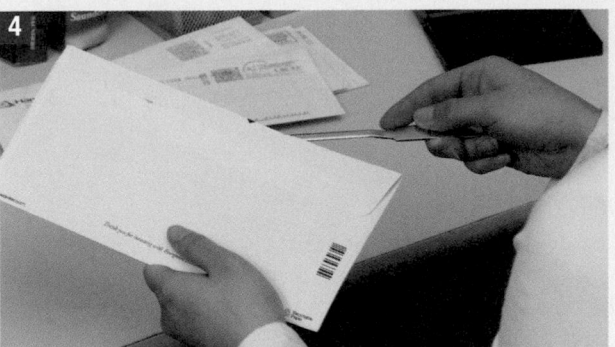

Use a letter opener to open the envelope.

5. **Procedural Step.** Remove the contents of the envelope. Check to be sure the envelope is empty.
6. **Procedural Step.** Unfold and flatten letters. Date stamp each letter, preferably in the upper right-hand corner of the letter.
   Principle. A date stamp provides a record of when the letter was received.
7. **Procedural Step.** Check to make sure that the letter contains an inside address. If not, staple the envelope to the letter. Discard the envelope if it is not needed, unless office policy states otherwise.

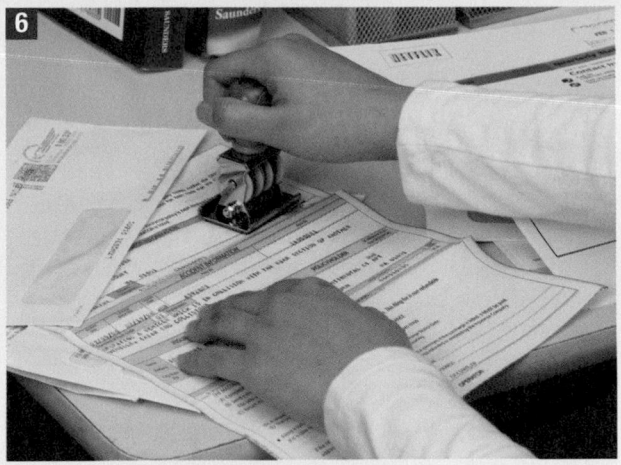

Date stamp each letter.

8. **Procedural Step.** Fasten enclosures to the letter with a paper clip. If a letter indicates an enclosure, but it is missing, write "No" next to the enclosure notation and circle or highlight it.
9. **Procedural Step.** Mend any torn paper with transparent tape to prevent further damage.
10. **Procedural Step.** If directed by the physician, annotate the correspondence by underlining or highlighting important words and phrases in the correspondence. Attach a sticky note indicating any action that should be taken in response to the correspondence.
    Principle. Annotating saves the physician time in reading and responding to incoming mail.
11. **Procedural Step.** Follow the same steps to open each piece of mail as described earlier and separate the pieces of mail into categories: urgent or very important, other letters, letters or reports containing patient information or results, medical journals, and circulars or advertising.
12. **Procedural Step.** Arrange letters and reports containing patient information in alphabetic order, find the appropriate medical record, and attach each letter or report to the medical record with a paper clip.
13. **Procedural Step.** Arrange the mail for each physician with the most important mail on top and the least important on the bottom.
14. **Procedural Step.** Distribute each stack of mail to the appropriate individual.

PROCEDURE 43-1

AUTOMATED MAIL PROCESSING

Since the early 1980s, the methods used to process the mail have evolved from manual and mechanized processing to automated processing. Automated equipment can read and sort mail at a rate of 36,000 letters an hour, more than six times faster than sorting mail manually. Machine-addressed letters are processed using optical character recognition (OCR), the mechanical or electronic recognition and interpretation of text.

Mail that is prepared for automated processing facilitates the sorting process. As an incentive, the USPS offers lower rates to high-volume mailers who prepare their mail for automation by adding postal barcodes and presorting mail. Most medical offices do not qualify for the lower rates because they are not high-volume mailers. To qualify for a

Highlight on Automated Postal Equipment

Automated postal equipment can handle most letters and process them without human intervention. At a Processing and Distribution Center, packages and large pieces of mail are diverted from the stream of mail. All other mail enters the Advanced Facer-Canceller System (AFCS), which rotates the mail so that it faces in the proper direction to postmark and cancel the postage stamp. If a piece of mail has a printed address, it goes to the Multiline Optical Character Reader (MLOCR), which reads the delivery address, translates this information into a barcode, and prints the barcode in the lower right hand corner of the envelope. If the MCLOCR cannot read the address, the piece of mail is separated out of the stream to go to a more sensitive address reader or a postal worker. Once a barcode has been added to the piece of mail, it goes to a Delivery Barcode Sorter (DBCS) that reads and interprets the barcode and sorts it accordingly. Items for local delivery are retained, but other mail is shipped either by air or truck to a destination station, where it is passed through another Delivery Barcode Sorter. At the local destination station the mail is sorted right down to arranging the mail in the order of a carrier's delivery route. Automated equipment is continuously updated and improved by the U.S. Postal Service. ∎

lower rate on First-Class Mail, the mailer must send out 500 letters in one mailing.

POSTAL ADDRESSING STANDARDS

Specific addressing standards must be met to prepare a piece of mail so that it can be processed by automated equipment. The medical assistant should be familiar with these standards and put them into practice to ensure the most efficient and timely delivery of outgoing mail.

Letters and Large Envelopes

To be mailed as a letter, an envelope must be between 3½ and 6⅛ inches in height and 5 inches and 11½ inches in length. The two most common sizes for business envelopes are the #10 envelope (4⅛ × 9½ inches) and the smaller #6¾ envelope (3⅝ × 6½ inches), but other sizes may be used. Square letters and letters that are too thick to pass through automated equipment require additional postage. The address may be printed directly on an envelope or on a label that will be attached to the envelope.

A large envelope requires more postage. It may be 6½ to 12 inches in height and 11½ to 15 inches in length. Large manila or white envelopes may be used to send patient medical records or other documents that have too many pages to fold.

Complete Address

The USPS defines a complete address as one that includes all elements necessary for OCR. To be complete, the address block must include all of the following elements in correct order:

> RECIPIENT LINE
> DELIVERY ADDRESS LINE
> CITY STATE & ZIP LINE

The post office recommends that the address be printed using all uppercase letters without punctuation except for the hyphen after the first five digits in the ZIP + 4.

Recipient Line

The name of the intended recipient must appear on the recipient line, which is the first line of the address. The recipient may be either the name of an individual (e.g., Andrew Davis) or the name of a company (e.g., Riverside Laboratory).

Optional Attention Line

If the name of a company is listed on the recipient line and the mail needs to be directed to a specific individual within the company, an optional attention line containing the name of the recipient is placed above the recipient line.

Example:

GERALDINE KAUFMAN	attention line
BROADVIEW HEALTH CLINIC	recipient line
242 SOUTH STREET	
BLACKBURN WI 54937-0012	

Delivery Address Line

The delivery address specifies the street address, post office box, rural route, or highway contract and is located above the bottom line (city, state, and ZIP) (Box 43-1).

Examples:

100 MAIN ST	Street Address
PO BOX 277	Post Office Box
RR1 BOX 75	Rural Route
HC 55 BOX 32	Highway Contract

City, State, and ZIP Code Line

The city, state, and ZIP code should appear in that order on the bottom line of the address block. There should be at least one space between the city name and the state abbreviation. Two spaces are recommended between the state abbreviation and the ZIP code. The ZIP + 4 code should be used if known (Procedure 43-2). The only punctuation in this line is the hyphen before the final 4 digits of the ZIP + 4 code (Table 43-2).

Address Format

Address format refers to how the various address elements appear on an envelope. The following standards must be followed to format an envelope for automation:

1. The address must be machine-printed for OCR.
2. The automated character reader performs best with black ink on a white background.
3. The address should be printed using plain block letters. A typeface without serifs (cross strokes at the end of the

BOX 43-1 Specific Delivery Address Standards

1. Use common Postal Service standard abbreviations as much as possible.

AVE	Avenuc
BLVD	Boulevard
CTR	Center
CIR	Circle
DR	Drive
EXT	Extension
HWY	Highway
IS	Island
JCT	Junction
LN	Lane
MTN	Mountain
PARK	Park
PKWY	Parkway
RIV	River
RD	Road
SQ	Square
ST	Street
TER	Terrace
VLG	Village
VLY	Valley

2. Use secondary address directional abbreviations (e.g., N, S, NE, SW).

3. Include secondary address locators, such as apartment numbers, suite numbers, and room numbers at the end of the delivery address line (up to a total of 30 spaces). If an additional line is required, the secondary address locator should be placed on the line above the delivery address line.

APT	Apartment
BLDG	Building
STE	Suite
UNIT	Unit

Examples:

RECIPIENT LINE	RECIPIENT LINE
100 MAIN ST APT 54	STE 45
CITY STATE ZIP	2500 GRANDVIEW LEVINE BLVD
	CITY STATE ZIP

4. Dual addressing is not recommended. Dual addressing means that two delivery addresses (e.g., both a street address and a post office box) are included on the piece of mail. If dual addressing is used, the post office delivers according to the information on the delivery address line (i.e., the line immediately above the city, state, and ZIP).

Table 43-2 Two-Letter State and Territory Abbreviations

AL	Alabama	MT	Montana
AK	Alaska	NE	Nebraska
AZ	Arizona	NV	Nevada
AR	Arkansas	NH	New Hampshire
CA	California	NM	New Mexico
CO	Colorado	NY	New York
CT	Connecticut	NC	North Carolina
DE	Delaware	ND	North Dakota
DC	District of Columbia	OH	Ohio
FL	Florida	OK	Oklahoma
GA	Georgia	OR	Oregon
GU	Guam	PA	Pennsylvania
HI	Hawaii	PR	Puerto Rico
ID	Idaho	RI	Rhode Island
IL	Illinois	SC	South Carolina
IN	Indiana	SD	South Dakota
IA	Iowa	TN	Tennessee
KS	Kansas	TX	Texas
KY	Kentucky	UT	Utah
LA	Louisiana	VT	Vermont
ME	Maine	VI	Virgin Islands
MD	Maryland	VA	Virginia
MA	Massachusetts	WA	Washington
MI	Michigan	WV	West Virginia
MN	Minnesota	WI	Wisconsin
MS	Mississippi	WY	Wyoming
MO	Missouri		

main strokes of the letter) is preferred, such as Helvetica or Arial. Script and italic styles should be avoided because they cannot be read by the automated equipment.

4. All lines of the address are formatted with a uniform left margin.

5. All letters in the address should be capitalized.

6. All lines of the address should be parallel to the bottom of the envelope.

7. No punctuation should be used in the address except the hyphen in the ZIP + 4 code.

8. If using a window envelope, the entire address must be visible through the window. At least 1/8-inch clearance (1/4 inch is preferred) must be maintained between the address and the edges of the window to distinguish the address from the edge of the window. No other print should show through the window.

9. Delivery instructions (e.g., personal, confidential) must be placed immediately below the return address. Special services (e.g., registered, certified, insured) must be placed above the address and to the right of the return address below the area where stamps or postage will be affixed.

10. Address labels should be applied using methods and materials that prevent them from becoming damaged or removed during high-speed automated processing.

11. The address should be placed within an area that extends from 5/8 inch to 2¾ inch from the bottom edge of the envelope with a ½-inch margin on each side. This is called the *OCR read area* (Figure 43-5).

12. The barcode clear zone is the area on an envelope where a barcode is printed by the automated equipment. It represents an area that is 5/8 inch high × 4¾ inches long. It must remain free of all printing, markings, or colored borders.

Return Address

The return address identifies the location to which a piece of mail should be returned if it cannot be delivered. It must be located in the upper left corner of the envelope and must not extend into the OCR read area. The return address should include the following elements:

SENDER'S NAME (OPTIONAL)
SENDER'S DELIVERY ADDRESS
SENDER'S CITY, STATE, ZIP

Letterhead envelopes or envelopes preprinted with the return address are usually used.

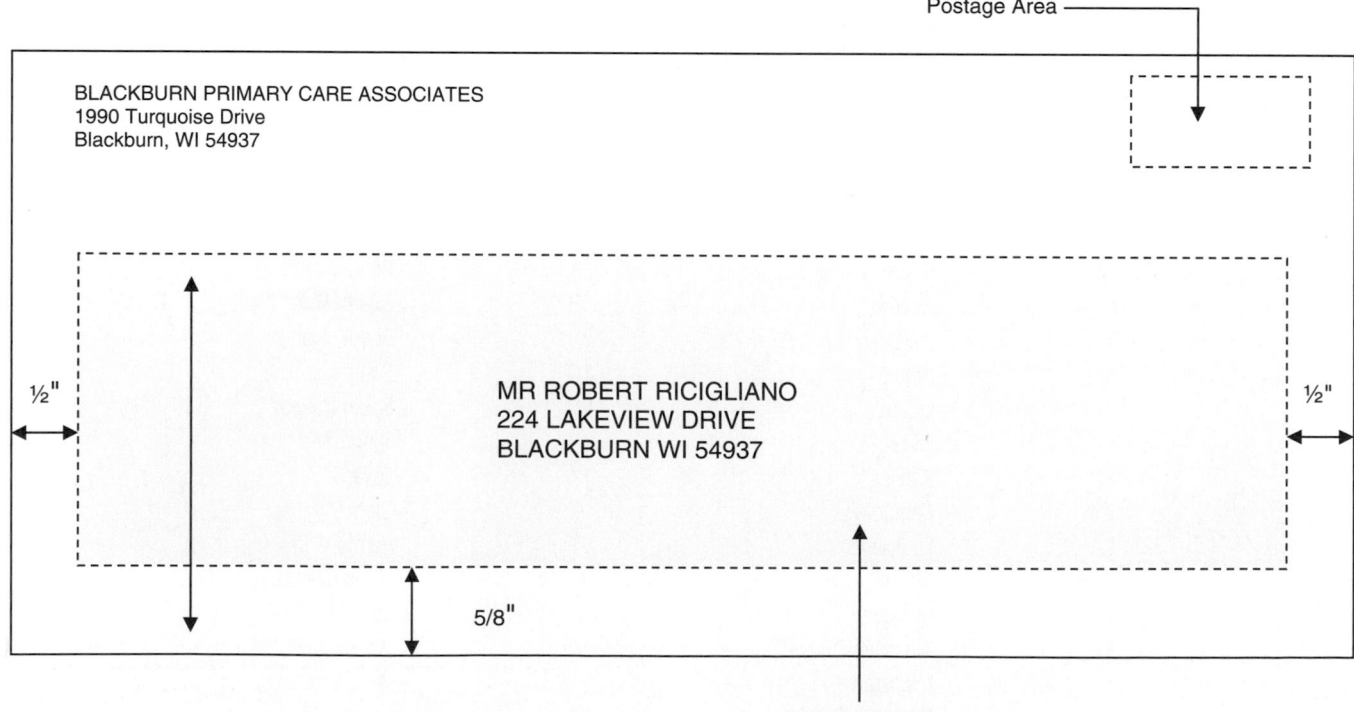

Postage Area

BLACKBURN PRIMARY CARE ASSOCIATES
1990 Turquoise Drive
Blackburn, WI 54937

½"   ½"

MR ROBERT RICIGLIANO
224 LAKEVIEW DRIVE
BLACKBURN WI 54937

5/8"

OCR Read Area

Figure 43-5. Envelope showing address in the optical character recognition *(OCR)* read area.

PROCEDURE 43-2   Looking Up a ZIP Code

Outcome Find the correct ZIP + 4 code for a given address.

Equipment/Supplies

- Computer with Internet access
- Pen and pencil
- Address with incorrect and/or incomplete ZIP code

1. **Procedural Step.** Open the computer's web browser and enter the web address for the USPS.
2. **Procedural Step.** From the USPS Home Page, click on the link labeled "Find a ZIP code."
3. **Procedural Step.** On the "Search by Address" tab, enter the delivery address, city, and state abbreviation of the address for which a ZIP code is sought. (It is also pos-sible to search for a ZIP code if only the city and state are known by clicking on the tab labeled "Search by City.")
4. **Procedural Step.** Copy the ZIP + 4 code on a piece of paper to use in preparing a label or envelope or use the computer "copy" function to copy and paste into a computer file.

OUTGOING MAIL

The process of preparing items for mailing may include addressing envelopes, preparing mailing labels, folding letters or statements to place into envelopes, calculating and adding postage, and mailing items either in mailboxes or at the post office.

Preparing Envelopes or Mailing Labels

Most word processing programs have a feature that creates and prints an address (and return address if desired) on various sizes of envelope. The medical assistant selects the envelope function and enters the delivery address (and return address if not preprinted on the envelope). A single envelope can then be placed in the manual feed tray for printing. Some printers have an optional envelope feed tray for processing several envelopes. When several addresses must be printed, it is more common to use labels. These come in pages and can be printed from lists using the mail merge feature.

Folding and Inserting Letters into Envelopes

The medical assistant should fold letters so that they can be inserted into envelopes easily. It is also important to use standard methods of folding so that letters are not damaged during opening.

Number 10 Envelope

To fold a letter in thirds, bring the bottom third of the letter up and form a crease. Then fold the top third down and make a crease. The second crease of the letter is inserted into the envelope first.

Number 6¾ Envelope

For a smaller envelope, fold the letter in half and make a crease. Then fold the right third in and make a crease. Fold the left third over the right and make another crease. The final crease of the letter is inserted into the envelope first.

Window Envelope

A letter for a window envelope must be folded so that the delivery address is visible through the window. The bottom third of the envelope is folded up to make a crease. The top third of the envelope is then folded back from the previous crease so that the delivery address shows on the outside of the letter. Patient statements are often mailed in window envelopes, and the format of the statement must be adjusted to the specific envelopes that the office uses (Figure 43-6).

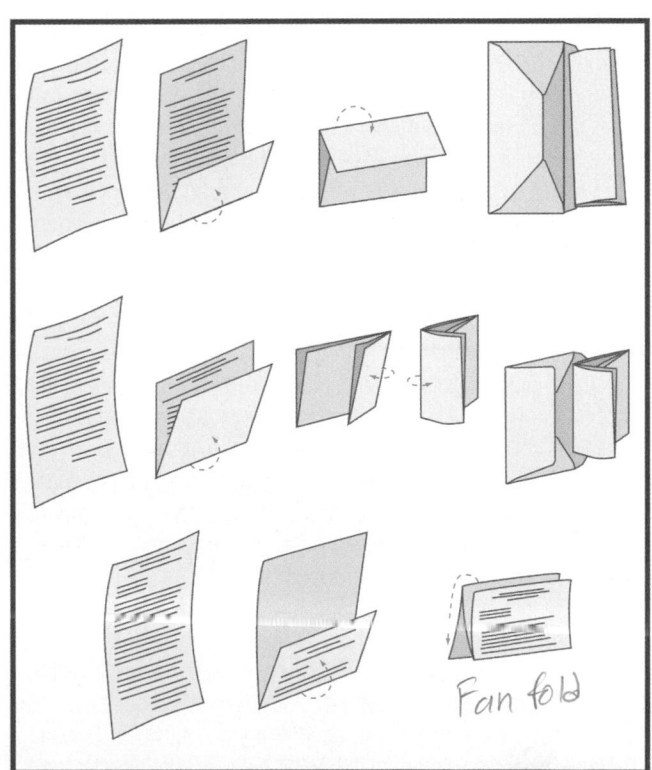

Figure 43-6. Correct methods of folding envelopes. (From Young AP, Proctor DB: *Kinn's the medical assistant*, ed 10, St. Louis, 2007, Saunders.)

Adding Postage

The medical assistant may add postage using stamps or postage meters or by printing postage from the computer (Procedure 43-3).

Postage stamps can be purchased at the post office or by telephone or mail from the USPS. Stamps can also be printed from the computer using a software program and stamp labels. The postage for a stamp printer is purchased online. Patient statements, which are usually sent First-Class, require one First-Class stamp. Letters that weigh more than 1 ounce and envelopes that are larger than 6⅛ × 11½ inches require additional postage. For these letters, an office would either require stamps of various values or a stamp printer, as well as a postage scale, to calculate postage accurately. It is not difficult to look up the correct amount of postage using the USPS website once the weight of an item has been established. Offices that send out a steady volume of mail regularly often use a mechanical postage meter or an online postage service.

Memories *from* Externship

Diane Waters: My externship was at a large clinic with many departments. I spent the majority of the time in the Internal Medicine department, but in order to get experience with all the aspects of medical assisting, I spent time in other departments, including the mailroom. In the morning the mail was sorted. There were usually one or two bags of mail, and we sorted it into small storage crates using one crate for two departments. If the department was indicated on the piece of mail, it was easy to place in the correct crate, but if there was only a name, I had to use a list to identify which department the person worked in. After the mail was sorted, we placed the crates on a mail cart and delivered the mail to the separate departments. In the administration area, we also placed the mail into mailboxes for the staff in that department, but in the clinical areas, we just gave all the mail for the department to the secretary at the front window. In the afternoon, we prepared the outgoing mail. We collected the crates of outgoing mail from all of the departments. In the mailroom, we separated letters in standard envelopes from any large envelopes and packages. I was taught to use the postage meter to print the postage directly on envelopes. The postage meter had a built-in scale, so we could run any letter in a standard envelope through the meter. The large envelopes were weighed and correct postage was printed using strips from the postage meter. John, who was in charge of the mailroom, took the mail to the post office every afternoon because there were always items that needed special services. He said that the other mail would go out faster if it was sent directly from the post office. ∎

Prepare for Success

Postage Meters

A **postage meter** is a machine that automatically stamps outgoing mail with the proper postage. Postage meters may be used for all classes of mail and for any denomination of postage. The postage can be printed directly onto an envelope or onto an adhesive tape strip that is affixed to an envelope or package. Mail that has been stamped by a postage meter is known as **Metered Mail.**

Postage meters cannot be purchased. Instead, they must be rented from one of the postal service's approved vendors. The amount of postage that can be stamped with the meter is predetermined and prepaid either on a regular basis, such as monthly, or when the amount remaining is getting low. Postage can be purchased by telephone or from the post office. In order to use a postage meter for bulk mailings, the medical office must apply for a bulk mailing permit and pay an annual fee.

Many different types of postage meters are available, ranging from simple to complex models. The simplest model has only the ability to stamp the mail. More complex models, on the other hand, have security features and may automatically weigh the mail, fold and insert letters into envelopes, seal the envelopes, and catch envelopes in a stacker tray. Complex models typically consist of two separate components: the meter that adds the postage and a base that performs the other functions. A base that is compatible with the chosen model of postage meter can be purchased outright by the medical office.

Safety Precautions

Certain safety precautions should be followed when using a postage meter:

1. Read the operating guide carefully before operating the postage meter.
2. Do not touch any moving parts of the postage meter when it is in operation.
3. Make sure to keep loose clothing, jewelry, and long hair away from all moving parts of the postage meter.
4. Do not cover the ventilation slots on the machine to prevent overheating.
5. If a paper jam occurs, unplug the machine and make sure all machine mechanisms have come to a stop before clearing the jam.
6. Never attempt to disassemble the machine for repair. If service is required, contact the manufacturer's service representative.

To view simple and more complex postage meters, see Figure 43-7.

Online Postage Services

The medical office may also subscribe to a service that allows the medical assistant to purchase, calculate, and print postage directly from the computer. These services usually allow the client to print stamps, print shipping labels, print postage directly on envelopes, and add special services (e.g., insurance, delivery confirmation, Return Receipt requested). The computer program can also check the accuracy of the address. Postal scales can be integrated with the computer software to calculate postage automatically. Online postage services offer increased versatility with respect to printing and personalizing labels, but if an office has a large volume of First-Class envelopes, a postage meter with envelope handling features may provide more efficient mail handling.

30 question

Figure 43-7. Simple postage meters only apply postage **(A)**; more complex models also weigh, seal, and stack envelopes **(B)**. **(B,** From Young AP, Proctor DB: *Kinn's the medical assistant,* ed 10, St. Louis, 2007, Saunders.)

What Would You Do? What Would You *Not* Do?

Case Study 3

The medical office where Diane works has been using the same postage meter to prepare the mail for several years, and most of the staff is familiar with it. It usually works well when operated by someone who is familiar with it, but new staff members complain that it is "difficult." Diane is familiar with this postage meter and has used another model of postage meter, but she does not know anything specific about online postage services. At a staff meeting, the office manager suggests that it may be time to update the postage meter to a newer model. One of the physicians says that he has heard that the office could save money and handle the mail more efficiently using an online postage service. He asks Diane for her opinion. ■

PROCEDURE **43-3**   Preparing Envelopes for Mailing

Outcome Address an envelope, and process envelopes to be mailed.

Equipment/Supplies

- Envelope
- Other items to be mailed
- Pen
- Typewriter

- Computer and printer
- Postal scale
- Postage meter (optional)
- Stamps

Continued

PROCEDURE **43-3** Preparing Envelopes for Mailing—cont'd

1. **Procedural Step.** Determine the exact address to be used to address the envelope. Addresses may be kept in a computer file or manually in an index card box or circular card file (e.g., Rolodex).

Look up the address in a rotary file.

2. Procedural Step. Select an envelope of the appropriate size. For business letters a #10 envelope is most commonly used. A large manila envelope may be used for documents containing several pages.

3. Procedural Step. Decide on a means to address the envelope (e.g., typewriter, computer, label printer). The address may be printed directly on the envelope or on a label. Avoid addressing ordinary correspondence by hand.

Principle. Standard business correspondence appears more professional if addressed using a typewriter or computer.

4. Procedural Step. Key the address in capital letters near the center of the envelope in the OCR read area with the name of the recipient on the first line, the apartment number or suite (if any) on the second line, the street address on the next line, and the city, state, and nine-number ZIP code on the bottom line. Do not use punctuation except for a hyphen after the first five numbers of the ZIP + 4 code. If using an envelope without letterhead, key the return address in the upper left corner using the same guidelines.

Principle. These are guidelines recommended by the USPS.

5. Procedural Step. Add any special notations, such as "Personal" or "Confidential," below the return address and above the address at the left side of the envelope.

Principle. Nothing must be placed below the address in order for post office equipment to read the envelope correctly.

6. Procedural Step. Add any mailing instructions (e.g., "Via Air Mail" or "First-Class" for a manila envelope) on the right side of the envelope above the address, leaving room for a postage label above them.

7. Procedural Step. Place the item to be mailed in the envelope, folding it as needed, and seal the envelope (unless a postage meter with a sealer will be used).

8. Procedural Step. Weigh the piece of mail if it contains more than two sheets of paper or if an envelope larger than $6\frac{1}{8} \times 11\frac{1}{2}$ is used.

Principle. Large envelopes, rigid envelopes, and envelopes that are not rectangular require more postage than First-Class letters weighing less than 1 ounce.

9. Procedural Step. Calculate and apply the correct amount of postage. One First-Class stamp or equivalent is required for First-Class letters weighing less than 1 ounce. Postage for other items may be calculated from the USPS website, using a postage meter, or using a online postage service. If a postage meter is used, all envelopes to be mailed in one day may be processed together.

10. Procedural Step. Assemble all letters and other items to be mailed.

11. Procedural Step. Sort envelopes according to size.

12. Procedural Step. Separate any items with special mailing instructions that must be taken to the post office. If necessary, add instructions to the envelopes. If the office does not have a postal scale, include any letters that may need extra postage.

13. Procedural Step. Place items with postage in a mailbox or request a pick-up from the postal service.

14. Procedural Step. Take special items to the post office. This may include items that are to be sent Return Receipt, Certified Mail, Registered Mail, or Insured Mail and stamped items weighing more than 1 pound. Items to be sent priority mail (up to 1 pound) can be mailed from the office if appropriate postage is placed on them.

Principle. Stamped mail and priority mail weighing more than 1 pound will not be accepted from a mailbox even if proper postage is attached.

MEDICAL PRACTICE *and the* LAW

Certain hazardous and perishable items may be mailed through the USPS but are subject to specific packaging and labeling requirements.

- Diagnostic clinical specimens that are liquid or contained in liquid must be mailed in a sturdy, securely sealed watertight primary container cushioned in a secondary container. There must be enough cushioning to absorb all the material if the primary container were to break. If the material is or potentially may be infectious, both primary and secondary containers must be marked with the biohazard symbol.
- Noninfectious specimens (e.g., stool specimens for occult blood, newborn blood spots, slides for Pap tests, liquid Pap test bottles) may be mailed in a leakproof envelope or box without any special marking. In the case of a liquid sample, the outer packaging should be sufficient to absorb all material if the inner container were to leak.
- Sharps and regulated medical waste can only be mailed in approved shipping containers marked as containing regulated medical waste and bearing a properly prepared merchandise return service label held in the name of the authorized medical waste manufacturer. The container must be marked with the biohazard symbol, and there must be markings designating the normal upright position of the container. A shipping manifest (which should be provided by the medical waste company) must be affixed to the outside of the container. ■

What Would You Do? What Would You *Not* Do? RESPONSES

Case Study 1
Page 1017

What Did Diane Do?
❏ Took Mr. Stone's telephone number and told him that she would ask his surgeon how he wanted to handle the matter.
❏ Asked Mr. Stone's surgeon for authorization to fax the record or copy it and send it by Express Mail because written consent is not necessary if medical information is shared to provide continuity of medical care.
❏ With the surgeon's permission, made a copy of the medical record, placed it in an Express Mail envelope, prepared a label, applied appropriate postage, and either called for an Express Mail pickup or took the envelope to an Express Mail mailbox or the post office before 5 PM.
❏ With the surgeon's permission, might also send the package using a private carrier, such as FedEx or UPS Next Day Air.
❏ If the physician decided to handle the matter in a different way (e.g., by asking Diane to fax the record, by telephoning the surgeon), accepted the physician's decision.
❏ Called Mr. Stone to inform him how the physician had decided to handle the matter.
❏ Sent Mr. Stone a Consent to Release Information Form as a follow-up, either as an e-mail attachment or in a letter.

What Did Diane Not *Do?*
❏ Did not tell Mr. Stone that his request could not be granted because there wasn't enough time.
❏ Did not make any promise to Mr. Stone about how the matter would be handled before speaking to the surgeon.
❏ Did not criticize Mr. Stone for making an unreasonable request.
❏ Did not fail to follow up on this request.

What Would You Do/What Would You *Not* Do? Review Diane's response and place a checkmark next to the information you included in your response. List the additional information you included in your response.

_____

_____

_____

_____

Case Study 2
Page 1018

What Did Diane Do?
❏ Searched for the correct (or complete) address of Dr. Leonie using other methods, such as looking up the address in the office's address file, looking at previous correspondence, looking up the address using the Internet, or calling Dr. Leonie's office.
❏ After locating the correct (or complete address), looked up the ZIP code again until she received a complete ZIP + 4 code.
❏ Finished preparing the envelope using the correct address and ZIP + 4 code.

What Did Diane Not *Do?*
❏ Did not ask the physician to find Dr. Leonie's address for her.
❏ Did not send the letter using the five-digit ZIP she found from the first search.

What Would You Do/What Would You *Not* Do? Review Diane's response and place a checkmark next to the information you included in your response. List the additional information you included in your response.

_____

_____

_____

_____

Continued

What Would You Do? What Would You *Not* Do? RESPONSES—cont'd

Case Study 3
Page 1025

What Did Diane Do?
❑ Stated that she was familiar with postage meters, but that she did not know about online postage services.
❑ Gave her honest opinion about the ease of using the current postage meter.
❑ Offered to research the benefits and costs of an online postage service versus updating the postage meter.
❑ Offered to try to find out how much time it would take to orient staff to a new method of preparing the mail.

What Did Diane Not *Do?*
❑ Did not give a negative opinion of online postage services just because she did not want to cope with a system change.

❑ Did not automatically agree with the physician that changing to an online postage system would be a good idea.
❑ Did not say that the current postage meter worked very well if a person just took the time to try to understand it.

What Would You Do/What Would You *Not* Do? Review Diane's response and place a checkmark next to the information you included in your response. List the additional information you included in your response.

_____
_____
_____
_____

 ## TERMINOLOGY REVIEW

Annotate To underline or highlight important words and phrases in correspondence.
Barcode clear zone The area on the lower right-hand corner of a card or letter that is left clear for the postal barcode to be printed.
Metered Mail Mail for which the postage has been applied using a postage meter.
Postage meter A machine that automatically stamps a piece of mail with the correct postage.

Postal bar code A series of vertical bars of two lengths, which represent the delivery address of a piece of mail. The barcode facilitates automated sorting of mail.
ZIP code A five-digit code that identifies the post office to which a given piece of mail is to be delivered.
ZIP + 4 code A more detailed mailing code consisting of the original five-digit ZIP code followed by a hyphen and four additional digits. These digits identify a specific geographic segment within the delivery area.

 ## ON THE WEB

For Information on the U.S. Postal Service:

Calculate postage and look up ZIP codes: www.usps.com

Domestic mail manual and postal addressing standards: pe.usps.gov

Online postage: www.usps.com/onlinepostage

Postage meters: www.usps.com/postagesolutions/post_mtr.htm

 PREPARE FOR CERTIFICATION Visit the Evolve site at http://evolve.elsevier.com/Bonewit/today/ to actively Prepare for your Certification.

CD *Check out the **Companion CD** bound with the book to access additional interactive activities.*

44

Managing Practice Finances

1. Compare and contrast manual and computerized methods of maintaining patient accounts.
2. Differentiate between a simple charge slip and a charge slip with diagnosis and procedure codes (superbill).
3. Describe how a charge slip is completed.

Complete a patient charge slip.

4. Identify the information contained on a fee schedule, and describe how it is used.
5. Describe the information contained in a patient account ledger.
6. List the steps to post charges, payments, and/or adjustments to the patient account.

Post charges to the patient ledger.
Post payments and/or adjustments.

7. List the information recorded on a day sheet.

Record a patient's visit on the day sheet.
Balance a day sheet.

8. Identify various types of bank accounts.
9. Discuss the information printed on a check.
10. Describe various methods to write checks.

Write a check.

11. Describe how a bank deposit is prepared and made.

Prepare a bank deposit.

12. Identify reasons why it is important to reconcile every bank statement.

Reconcile a bank statement.

13. Describe the components of accounts payable.
14. Describe how entries are made in the cash disbursement journal.

CHAPTER OUTLINE

Introduction to Patient Accounts
Methods of Maintaining Patient Accounts
Components of a Patient Account
   Charge Slip
   Fee Schedule
   Patient Account Ledger
   Day Sheet

Banking Activities
   Types of Accounts
   Checks
   Bank Deposits
   Reconciling a Bank Statement
Other Financial Accounts
   Accounts Payable or Record of Cash Disbursements
   Petty Cash

CAAHEP COMPETENCIES

Administrative Competencies
Perform Bookkeeping Procedures
- Prepare a bank deposit.
- Post entries on a day sheet.
- Perform accounts receivable procedures.
- Post adjustments.

Operational Functions
- Utilize computer software to maintain office systems.

ABHES COMPETENCIES

Administrative Duties
- Apply computer concepts for office procedures.
- Prepare a bank statement and deposit record.
- Reconcile a bank statement.
- Post entries on a day sheet.
- Prepare a check.
- Establish and maintain a petty cash fund.

- Post adjustments.
- Use a physician fee schedule.

Financial Management
- Use manual and computerized bookkeeping systems.
- Maintain records for accounting and banking purposes.

KEY TERMS

ABA routing number
accounting
accounts payable
accounts receivable
accrual (ah-KREW-ul) basis of accounting
adjustment
assets
bookkeeping
cash basis of accounting
cashier's check
certified check
charge slip
credit

day sheet
debit
disbursements
fee schedule
ledger
liabilities
MICR line
payee (pay-EE)
petty cash
proof of posting
reconciling
superbill

Introduction to Patient Accounts

A medical office is a business. The business of a medical office is providing medical services—one of the most important services in the entire economy. Because the medical office is a business, daily management of the practice's finances is key to the physicians' ability to provide the best services possible for patients. If the practice's bills are not paid and fees are not collected, the practice will cease to be a viable business and the patients will suffer.

Accounting is the term for systematic recording and reporting of financial transactions. The **cash basis of accounting,** which is generally used by medical offices, enters income when payment is received for services. This contrasts with the **accrual basis of accounting,** in which income is entered at the time of sale, even if payment has not yet been received. Companies that sell merchandise usually use the accrual basis of accounting. In both systems, expenses are entered when they are incurred, even if they have not yet been paid.

Bookkeeping refers to the process of recording financial transactions and keeping financial records. Managing the daily finances is a task that often falls to a medical assistant. Professional accountants are usually responsible for general aspects of financial management, such as preparing detailed financial reports, financial planning, and preparing tax returns.

This chapter focuses on the parts of the daily financial activities involved in charging patients for the services provided each day, maintaining patient accounts and other **accounts receivable** (money owed to the practice), and managing the **accounts payable** (money the practice owes).

METHODS OF MAINTAINING PATIENT ACCOUNTS

Patient accounts make up the bulk of the medical practice's income. Some income might come from rental of space—for instance, to a particular laboratory for a blood-draw station or to a social worker, psychologist, or other specialist who consults to the practice. Other income may come from royalties—on a particular medical instrument that one or more of the physicians developed, for instance, or for a book written by the professionals in the practice. But the bulk of the practice's income will be earned on a daily basis from the charges for services to patients.

Patient accounts may be recorded manually or using a computer. Most medical offices use a computerized medical billing system, although they may maintain some manual records, such as a day sheet. A manual system uses:

1. A daily journal, called a *day sheet,* to record all transactions that occurred on that day
2. An accounts receivable ledger card for each patient, to keep a record of transactions related to that patient
3. A cumulative record of financial activity for the month, both for the practice as a whole and for each individual

Highlight on Bookkeeping Systems

The three most common systems for keeping records of accounts in the medical office are single-entry, double-entry, and pegboard or "write-it-once" systems. Historically, financial transactions were recorded in a book called a **ledger** with separate pages for individual accounts. In medical offices, separate cards began to be used for individual accounts (instead of pages of a book). These cards came to be called *ledger cards,* and in medical billing programs, a screen showing cumulative charges and payments for a single patient is called a *patient ledger.*

Patient Accounts and Accounting Systems
Single-Entry Bookkeeping System
This is the simplest system; it requires at least three records:

1. A chronological journal that keeps track of all charges, such as a daily journal
2. A journal that keeps track of payments, such as a checkbook
3. A method to keep track of individual patient accounts; these may be recorded on pages of a book, index cards, or ledger cards

Although the single-entry system is simple, it lacks methods for cross-checking to prevent and/or detect errors. Each entry is made separately, and bills to patients and insurance companies are generated manually.

Double-Entry Bookkeeping System
This is the most complete type of bookkeeping system. However, it usually requires a trained bookkeeper or accountant in order to be used effectively.

Every transaction is posted into two different records, as a credit in one and a debit in the other. A **credit** is a posting that is subtracted from the balance and a **debit** is a posting that is added. Records of **assets**—money and property owned by the business and money owed to the business—are balanced against records of **liabilities**—money owed to others by the business.

A charge for service to a patient, for example, is a credit (added to the balance) in the records of assets because it increases the total assets; but it is a debit (subtracted from the balance) in the records of liabilities because it decreases the amount owed by the business.

A common formulation of the accounting principle is as follows:

$$\text{Assets} = \text{liabilities} + \text{owner's equity}$$

where assets are property owned by the business, liabilities are debts, and owner's equity is the amount by which the owner's assets exceed liabilities.

When a double-entry bookkeeping system is used by a medical practice, the medical assistant is usually responsible only for keeping the daily journal and/or entering charges in the computer. The actual records of assets and liabilities are kept by an accountant.

Pegboard or "Write-It-Once" System
The pegboard system is similar to the single-entry system. The daily journal, which is called a **day sheet,** contains sections at the bottom to facilitate checking the totals in a section called the *proof of posting.* In addition, fewer entries are made manually because the pegboard system uses a duplicating system. The charge slip and patient ledger card are positioned above the day sheet. The entry on the charge slip is duplicated on the patient ledger card and the day sheet. When used to write checks, one entry is posted to the daily journal, payable ledger, and check.

Most computer billing systems are based on the pegboard system because this was the most common bookkeeping system used in medical offices when computerized accounting systems were developed. ∎

Putting It All into Practice

My name is Maria Hernandez, and I am a registered medical assistant. I work at the office of three physicians who specialize in internal medicine. One of my duties is to manage patient accounts. The charges and payments from our charge slips are entered either by myself or one of the other medical assistants, but I enter almost all of the payments we receive in the mail including checks from patients, as well as insurance payments. I am also responsible for paying the bills for the practice. We use two different computer software programs, one for patient billing and another to manage our patient accounts and pay bills. We also use online banking, and we have set up automatic bill payment for those bills that occur every month including our mortgage, condominium fee, electricity, telephone, and answering service bills. We usually pay our other bills by check. The computer accounting program tracks all payments and prints checks. All of the physicians are authorized to sign checks under $500.00. If we purchase an item that costs more than $500.00, it must be signed by any two physicians. When I was in school, I didn't appreciate what a big job it is to manage the patient financial accounts. I really enjoy this part of my job now, and I have come to understand that it always saves time to work carefully and avoid mistakes. ∎

Prepare for Success

physician; this information is recorded on the day sheet, and cumulative totals are carried forward throughout the month

In a computerized billing system, the same types of records are maintained. When procedures are performed, charges for individual patients are entered into the medical billing program and automatically posted to the patient's account and the daily record of charges. In a similar way, payments made by the patient (or an insurance company) are posted to both the patient account and the daily record of charges. The computer program can access data to generate patient bills, insurance claims, and a variety of reports, including monthly statements, activity of individual physicians, and number of specific procedures billed.

COMPONENTS OF A PATIENT ACCOUNT

Four components are used to maintain a patient account whether a manual or computer accounting system is used:
1. Charge slip
2. Fee schedule
3. Patient account ledger
4. Day sheet

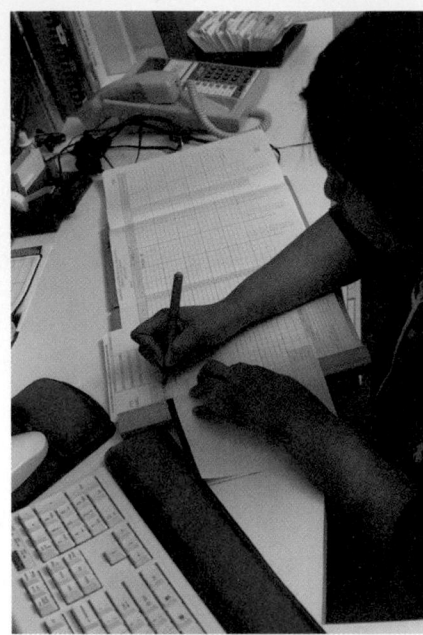

Figure 44-1. Medical assistant using a pegboard system.

Charge Slip

A **charge slip** is a means of keeping track of charges for services and payments made at the time of the patient visit. The charge slip is usually prepared before the patient visit and completed after the patient is seen. In its simplest form, the charge slip contains the patient's name, the date of the service rendered, any procedures performed (including the visit itself), the total charges, and the amount the patient paid.

In the traditional medical office manual accounting systems, a "one-write" or "write-it-once" system (also called a *pegboard system*) was used. All necessary forms were held in place on a metal or plastic board with a row of pegs across the left side to hold the forms in place. In this type of system, information from the top form is transferred to the forms below. Entering information once generates a charge slip and receipt, an entry on the patient's ledger card, and an entry on the daily journal (day sheet) (Figure 44-1).

Many offices continue to use a pegboard mounted day sheet as a manual record of daily transactions and to create a bank deposit slip. Pegboard charge slips and paper ledger cards are rarely used today because most offices use a medical billing program to keep track of individual patient accounts. The format of medical billing programs is based on the old pegboard system, however. A pegboard system may also be used to write checks and keep a check register.

When insurance companies began requiring numerical codes for procedures and diagnoses, a new type of charge slip was developed so that these codes could be identified at the time of service. A **superbill** (sometimes called a

billing encounter form) is a form containing both diagnosis and procedure codes in addition to charges and payments.

Although simple charge slips are sometimes used (especially by providers of limited services such as chiropractors and podiatrists), most medical offices use a customized superbill as a charge slip. The top section of the form is filled out with patient information either by using a printed label, filling it out manually or printing the information on the form from the computer. Figure 44-2 shows an example of a completed superbill.

When the patient is seen, the physician or other provider who sees the patient checks off the boxes next to the correct code for the type of visit (problem-focused/straightforward, detailed/low-complexity, comprehensive/moderately complex, and so forth), as well as any other procedures performed, and also fills in the patient's diagnosis.

Using the fee schedule, charges are added and any payments made by the patient are entered. The completed superbill is used to enter billing information into the computer. For this reason, it is extremely important to be sure that the superbill is filled out accurately.

Fee Schedule

A **fee schedule** is a list of charges for the various procedures a physician performs. Years ago, a physician had one set of fees that he or she charged patients for office visits, procedures, and/or treatments. Today, however, a medical practice may have to accept different amounts as payment for each service it performs, depending on which insurance

Western Medical Center
109 River Street
Western, OH 44770-0421
(490) 555-6464

Richard Warner, MD
Maria Gomez, MD
TAX ID 52-XX63777

PATIENT NAME AND ADDRESS	BIRTHDATE	SUBSCRIBER NAME	MD NAME	TODAY'S DATE
DARLA SISSLE 10 MAPLE STREET WESTERN, OH 44770	2 / 17 / 52	DARLA SISSLE	WARNER	6 / 26 / 08
	ACCOUNT #	INSURANCE COMPANY	INSURANCE PHONE #	TIME
	1015	SHHMO	(490) 565-2000	10:00 AM
TELEPHONE NO.		INSURANCE ID #	GROUP/PLAN #	SEX
(490) 220-1156		21-58624	8300099	MALE ☐ FEMALE X

√	DESCRIPTION	CPT	FEE	√	DESCRIPTION	CPT	FEE	√	DESCRIPTION	CPT	FEE
	OFFICE VISIT				**IMMUNIZATIONS**				**PROCEDURES**		
	NEW PATIENT				Imm. admin, one	90471		√	EKG w// interpretation	93000	65--
	Problem Focused	99201			Imm. admin, each add'l	90472			Spirometry	94010	
	Exp. Prob. Focused	99202			Influenza < 3	90657			Inhalation treatment	94640	
	Detailed	99203			Influenza 3 and >	90658			Remove skin tag < 15	11200	
	Comp/ Mod MDM	99204			Medicare code	G0008			Cerumen removal	69210	
	Comp./ High MDM	99205			Varicella	90716			Wart destruction < 14	17110	
	ESTABLISHED PATIENT				DTaP	90700			I & D abscess	10060	
	Minimal / Nurse Visit	99211			Td adult	90718					
	Problem Focused	99212			Rubella	90706					
√	Exp. Problem Focused	99213	65--		MMR	90707			**OTHER**		
	Detailed	99214			Hep B Child	90744					
	Comprehensive	99215			Hep B Adult	90746					
	Post-op Exam	99024	0.00		IPV	90713					
	WELL VISIT				**WELL VISIT**				**LABORATORY**		
	NEW PATIENT				ESTABLISHED PATIENT				Blood collection Vein	36415	
	Infant – 1 year	99381			Infant – 1 year	99391			Blood collection capillary	36416	
	1yr – 4 yr	99382			1yr – 4 yr	99392			Blood glucose, monitoring dev.	52912	
	5 yr – 11 yr	99383			5 yr – 11 yr	99393			Hemoccult, guaiac	82270	
	12 yr – 17 yr	99384			12 yr – 17 yr	99394			Strep, rapid	87880	
	18 yr – 39 yr	99385			18 yr – 39 yr	99395			UA, dipstick	81000	
	40 yr – 64 yr	99386			40 yr – 64 yr	99396			Urine pregnancy	81025	
	65 yr and over	99387			65 yr and over	99397			Microhematocrit	85013	

DIAGNOSTIC CODES (ICD-9-CM)

☐ 789.0 Abdominal Pain	☐ 562.11 Diverticulitis	☐ 724.2 Low Back Pain	☐ 034.0 Streptococcal Sore Throat
☐ 795.0 Abnormal Pap Smear	☐ 562.10 Diverticulosis	☐ 424.0 Mitral Valve Prolapse	☐ 785.6 Swollen Glands
☐ 706.1 Acne	☐ 782.3 Edema	☐ 715.90 Osteoarthritis, Unspec	☐ 598.0 Urinary Tract Infection
☐ 477.9 Allergic Rhinitis	☐ 492.8 Emphysema	☐ 733.00 Osteoporosis, Unspec	☐ V06.8 Vaccination, Combination
☐ 285.9 Anemia, NOS	☐ V18.0 Family History of Diabetes	☐ 627.1 Postmenopausal Bleeding	☐ V04.8 Vaccination, Influenza
☐ 281.0 Anemia, Pernicious	☐ 780.6 Fever of Undetermined Origin	☐ 625.4 Premenstrual Tension	☐ 787.0 Vomiting, Nausea
☐ 280.9 Anemia, Iron Deficiency	☐ 535.0 Gastritis, Acute	☐ 782.1 Rash	☐ 078.10 Warts, All Sites
☐ 282.6 Anemia, Sickle Cell	☐ 744.0 Headache	☐ 569.3 Rectal Bleeding	☐ V20.2 Well Child Check
■ 413.9 Angina Pectoris	☐ 070.1 Hepatits, type A	☐ 714.0 Rheumatoid Arthritis	☐ V70.0 Well Adult
☐ 427.9 Arrhythmia, NOS	☐ 054.9 Herpes Simplex	☐ 706.2 Sebaceous Cyst	☐ _____ _____
☐ 440.9 Arteriosclerosis	☐ 708.9 Hives/Urticaria	☐ 431.9 Sinusitis, Acute, NOS	☐ _____ _____
☐ 414.0 ASHD	☐ 401.1 Hypertension, Benign	☐ 701.9 Skin Tag(s)	☐ _____ _____
☐ 493.9 Asthma, Unspecified	☐ 401.0 Hypertension, Malignant	☐ 707.9 Skin Ulcer	☐ _____ _____
☐ 466.0 Bronchitis, Acute	☐ 244.9 Hypothyroidism, Primary	☐ 845.00 Sprain, Ankle	☐ _____ _____
☐ 491.2 Bronchitis, chronic obstr.	☐ 380.4 Impacted Cerumen	☐ 848.9 Sprain, Muscle, Unspec.	☐ _____ _____
☐ 786.50 Chest Pain	☐ 487.1 Influenza		

RETURN APPOINTMENT		BALANCE DUE	
_____ Days		Total Charge	$ 130.00
1 Weeks		Amount Paid	$ 20.00
_____ Months		Previous Bal	$ 35.00
_____ PRN		Balance Due	$ 145.00

(Additional diagnostic code column continued:)
☐ 250.01 Diabetes I   Uncomplicated
☐ 250.00 Diabetes II   Uncomplicated
☐ 564.1 Irritable Bowel Syndrome
☐ 464.0 Laryngitis, Acute
☐ Laryngopharyngitis, acute
☐ 454.9 Leg Varicose Veins

Figure 44-2. Completed charge slip (superbill) containing procedure and diagnosis codes.

WESTERN MEDICAL CENTER
Patient Account Ledger
As of 4/19/2008

Entry	Date	POS	Description	Procedure	Document	Provider	Amount
00001015	DARLA SISSLE				(490)220-1156		
	Last Payment: -55.00		On: 3/30/2008				
1	3/21/2008	11		99213	0804190000	RW	65.00
2	3/21/2008	11		80051	0804190000	RW	25.00
6	3/30/2008	11	Ins payment	INS	0804190000	RW	-55.00
	Patient Totals						35.00
	Ledger Totals						35.00

Figure 44-3. Patient account ledger. (Screenshot used by permission of MCKESSON Corporation. All Rights Reserved. © MCKESSON Corporation 2008.)

What Would You Do? What Would You *Not* Do?

Case Study 1
In the afternoon, Maria is entering charges and payments into the patient computer accounts. She is using itemized charge slips (superbills) to do this. In Maria's office the superbills are numbered consecutively, and Maria notices that there are two gaps in the numbers of the superbills. The office records all transactions using a manual day sheet, and Maria verifies that one of the physicians saw two patients for whom she does not have charge slips. ■

provider is paying for the service. The reimbursement varies from a fixed percentage of the physician's charges to a set amount for a given service. Insurance is discussed in detail in Chapter 46.

The medical office usually has a basic fee schedule, listing the usual charges for office visits and procedures. The fee schedule is used to fill out charges on the charge slip or superbill. When a computer billing program is used, the amount charged for each procedure is linked to the procedure and usually comes up automatically when the correct procedure is selected. Most computer billing programs can link a patient's fees to his or her specific insurance fee schedules, such as Medicare and Medicaid (Procedure 44-1).

Patient Account Ledger

Each patient has his or her own account. A cumulative record of charges and patients is kept, usually using a computer program. It is also possible to keep account records manually. This record of charges and payments is called the patient account **ledger.** In a computer billing program, the patient account ledger is linked to the patient demographic and insurance information so that periodic bills and insurance claims can be generated. Information about services provided to an individual patient and payments received for

that patient show up in chronological order on the patient ledger (Figure 44-3).

After the charge slip has been completed, the charges are posted to the patient ledger (Procedure 44-2).

Posting Payments to the Patient Account

Payment for services performed can be received in four ways:

1. The patient pays at the time of service, in full, or in part (e.g., a copayment for a health maintenance organization). The office will accept cash and checks, and many offices also accept credit and debit cards.
2. The patient may make a payment through the mail in response to a bill.
3. The patient may make an online payment using a credit or debit card through the medical practice website.
4. An insurance company may make a payment either by mail or, increasingly, by electronic transfer.

All payments must be posted to the account of the patient for whom they are made. Most computer programs have different codes for each method of payment. Cash and checks must match daily bank deposits. Payments using credit cards, online banking, or electronic transfer must later be matched to bank statements or online banking records.

Posting Adjustments to the Patient Account

A change to the patient account that is neither a charge for services nor a payment is called an **adjustment. Credit** (negative) adjustments are subtracted from the patient balance. Examples of credit adjustments include discounts for payment at the time of service, professional courtesy, and discounts given to insurance companies (also called *insurance write-offs*). Credit adjustments are usually discounts that are given in specific circumstances. (See Box 44-1 for common terminology used in relation to entering charges and payments.)

Debit (positive) adjustments are added to the patient balance. If a patient's check is returned by the bank, the amount of the check must be added back to the amount the patient owes. Because this is not a new charge, it is entered as a debit adjustment. In other words, when the patient's check was returned, it became necessary to make an entry to adjust the patient's balance (Procedure 44-3).

Day Sheet

The day sheet keeps a running tally of the practice's income for that day. Even if a computer billing program is used, a manual day sheet is often kept as a control for data entry into the computer (Figure 44-4). A manual day sheet is also useful if the computer system is temporarily unavailable.

For each individual patient seen, the day sheet records:
1. Charges
2. Payments

3. Previous balance
4. Adjustments
5. New balance

A new sheet is used for each day. Each transaction is recorded on the day sheet in the order it occurs. This includes not only patient visits but also all checks received in the mail that day. Even though the checks pay all or part of a patient balance from a previous day, they are posted to the patient account on the day they are received and deposited. The day sheet usually includes a deposit slip that can be created as each payment is entered. At the end of the day, the day is closed (i.e., no further transactions are allowed for that day). To be complete, the day sheet includes not only transactions from patients seen but also any checks received in the mail that day (Procedure 44-4).

In addition, the day sheet has columns labeled "distribution" that can be used by the practice to itemize charges under several headings, commonly by the physician who generated the charge. However, it can also be used to track the type of procedure performed.

At the bottom of the day sheet is a section used to check for the correctness of the entries. In this area the daily totals are checked, as well as the monthly and year-to-date totals, which are carried forward from sheet to sheet. The process of calculating and comparing various figures on the day sheet is called **proof of posting.** The totals on a day sheet are often entered first in pencil. After the totals of each proof agree, a pen is used to rewrite all totals. Once the figures for the day are accepted, no changes are made to the day sheet (Procedure 44-5).

When a medical billing program is used, the day sheet can be printed at the end of the day. Most computer programs allow the day to be closed (so that additional entries cannot be entered using that date). Usually only one day sheet can be printed for a given date. This prevents later alterations to the financial records. If an account must be corrected at a later time, any adjustments are entered on a new screen dated the day the correction is made. The original entry should never be altered after the day is closed.

Text continued on p. 1043

BOX 44-1 Common Terminology Used in Relation to Entering Charges and Payments

Account balance: The amount remaining in the account after all entries have been totaled.

Accounts receivable control: A summary of all unpaid accounts.

Adjustment: An entry to change an account balance that is not a charge for services or a payment, often a discount.

Credit: An entry that reduces an account balance, usually a payment.

Credit balance: The balance on an account when payments exceed charges.

Day sheet: The record of daily financial transactions (daily journal in a pegboard accounting system).

Debit: An entry that increases an account balance, usually a charge.

Disbursements: Money paid out.

Invoice: A bill or written statement describing a purchase or service and the amount due.

Journal: The original record of financial transactions that identifies the accounts to which they belong.

Ledger: A card, book, or computer database in which financial transactions are recorded.

Payables: Amounts owed to others.

Posting: Recording financial transactions or transferring information from one record to another.

Proof: Validation of calculations.

Receivables: Amounts of money owed by others.

ROA (received on account): Designation used for payments that reduce the amount owed but are not payment in full.

Trial balance: A method of checking the accuracy of calculations of accounts.

From Hunt SA: *Saunders fundamentals of medical assisting,* St. Louis, 2007, Saunders.

What Would You Do? What Would You *Not* Do?

Case Study 2

When posting charges and payments for a new patient named Linda Harris, Maria notices that the physician has written in an amount for the patient's office visit that is $15.00 less than the usual charge for the service. The physician has also written an amount for a flu shot that was given that is $10.00 less than the usual charge. Maria notices that the patient has paid $75.00 on the account, which is about half the amount of the bill. In Maria's office the usual charge for every procedure is entered for every patient. On the rare occasions when charges are reduced, any reduction is posted as a write-off. ■

Figure 44-4. Day sheet. (Courtesy Bibbero Systems, Inc., Petaluma, Calif., [800] 242-2376; www.bibbero. com.)

PROCEDURE 44-1   Completing a Patient Charge Slip

Outcome Prepare an itemized charge slip for a patient using a fee schedule.

Equipment/Supplies

- Blank charge slip
- Patient information form or computer data
- Daily patient schedule
- Calculator
- Fee schedule

1. Procedural Step. Before the patient is seen by the physician, complete the top part of an itemized charge slip with the information requested including the patient's name, date of birth, insurance, insurance group, and subscriber numbers and the name of the subscriber (insured person). This may be done manually from information on a ledger card or computer account, by attaching a label printed by the computer, or by printing charge slips using the computer billing program.
Principle. Complete information about the patient and his or her insurance facilitates the billing process.
Example:

Western Medical Center
109 River Street
Western, OH 44770-0421
(490) 555-6464

Richard Warner, MD
Maria Gomez, MD
TAX ID 52-XX63777

PATIENT NAME AND ADDRESS	BIRTHDATE	SUBSCRIBER NAME	MD NAME	TODAY'S DATE
DARLA SISSLE 10 MAPLE STREET WESTERN, OH 44770	2 / 17 / 52	DARLA SISSLE	WARNER	6 / 26 /08
	ACCOUNT #	INSURANCE COMPANY	INSURANCE PHONE #	TIME
	1015	SHHMO	(490) 565-2000	10:00 AM
TELEPHONE NO. (490) 220-1156		INSURANCE ID # 21-58624	GROUP/PLAN # 8300099	SEX MALE ☐ FEMALE X

Top part of charge slip.

2. Procedural Step. Before the patient is seen by the physician, enter the patient's previous balance on the bottom of the charge slip.

Principle. The patient's account balance includes the previous balance plus new charges minus any payment made at the time of the visit.
Example:

		RETURN APPOINTMENT		BALANCE DUE	
☐ 786.50 Chest Pain	☐ 487.1 Influenza	_____ Days		Total Charge	$
☐ 250.01 Diabetes I	☐ 564.1 Irritable Bowel Syndrome	1 Weeks		Amount Paid	$
Uncomplicated	☐ 464.0 Laryngitis, Acute	_____ Months		Previous Bal	$ 35.00
☐ 250.00 Diabetes II	☐ Laryngopharyngitis, acute	_____ PRN		Balance Due	$
Uncomplicated	☐ 454.9 Leg Varicose Veins				

Enter previous balance on charge slip.

3. Procedural Step. Using the fee schedule, fill in the charges on the charge slip by writing the fee for each service provided beside the line containing the correct code and procedure name (if the physician has not already done so).
Example:

√	DESCRIPTION	CPT	FEE	√	DESCRIPTION	CPT	FEE	√	DESCRIPTION	CPT	FEE
	OFFICE VISIT				**IMMUNIZATIONS**				**PROCEDURES**		
	NEW PATIENT				Imm. admin, one	90471		√	EKG w// interpretation	93000	65--
	Problem Focused	99201			Imm. admin, each add'l	90472			Spirometry	94010	
	Exp. Prob. Focused	99202			Influenza < 3	90657			Inhalation treatment	94640	
	Detailed	99203			Influenza 3 and >	90658			Remove skin tag < 15	11200	
	Comp/ Mod MDM	99204			Medicare code	G0008			Cerumen removal	69210	
	Comp./ High MDM	99205			Varicella	90716			Wart destruction < 14	17110	
	ESTABLISHED PATIENT				DTaP	90700			I & D abscess	10060	
	Minimal / Nurse Visit	99211			Td adult	90718					
	Problem Focused	99212			Rubella	90706					
√	Exp. Problem Focused	99213	65--		MMR	90707			**OTHER**		
	Detailed	99214			Hep B Child	90744					
	Comprehensive	99215			Hep B Adult	90746					
	Post-op Exam	99024	0.00		IPV	90713					

Enter charges on charge slip.

Continued

PROCEDURE 44-2

PROCEDURE **44-1**   Completing a Patient Charge Slip—cont'd

4. Procedural Step. Complete the remainder of the charge slip by entering the total charges and payment made, and then calculate the new balance. The new balance is the sum of the total charges and previous balance minus any payment.

5. **Procedural Step.** Complete other information requested on the charge slip, such as the place of service and check number and/or method of payment.

Principle. The information on the charge slip must be complete and accurate because it will be used to post the charges and payment to the day sheet and patient ledger.

Example:

5

		RETURN APPOINTMENT		BALANCE DUE	
☐ 786.50 Chest Pain	☐ 487.1 Influenza	_____ Days		Total Charge	$ 130.00
☐ 250.01 Diabetes I	☐ 564.1 Irritable Bowel Syndrome	___1___ Weeks		Amount Paid	$ 20.00
Uncomplicated	☐ 464.0 Laryngitis, Acute	_____ Months		Previous Bal	$ 35.00
☐ 250.00 Diabetes II	☐ Laryngopharyngitis, acute	_____ PRN		Balance Due	$ 145.00
Uncomplicated	☐ 454.9 Leg Varicose Veins				

Enter totals on charge slip.

PROCEDURE **44-2**   Posting Charges to the Patient Ledger

Outcome Using the information from the completed charge slip, post charges to a patient ledger.

Equipment/Supplies

- Patient charge slip
- Patient ledger
- Fee schedule
- Pen or computer

1. Procedural Step. If using a manual system, post the charges from a completed patient charge slip on the patient ledger using one line for one day's services. Place the total charge for the service in the column labeled charges. If using a computer program, post the first charge on the first line of the transaction entry screen. For most computer programs, entering the procedure code will prompt the computer to automatically generate the correct charge for the patient's insurance.

2. Procedural Step. If using a computer system, post each additional charge on a new line.

3. **Procedural Step.** If using a manual system, enter the total charge in the balance column. If using a computer system, save your work after all charges have been posted.

Example:

3

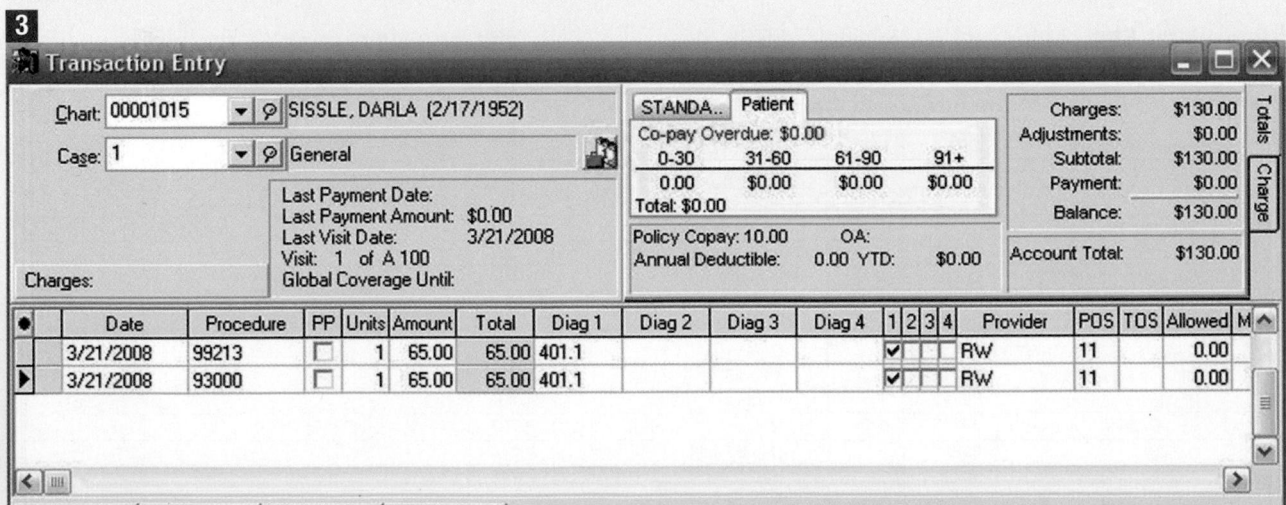

Transaction entry screen. (Screenshot used by permission of MCKESSON Corporation. All Rights Reserved. © MCKESSON Corporation 2008.)

PROCEDURE 44-3   Posting Payments and/or Adjustments

Outcome Post payments and/or adjustments to a patient account.

Equipment/Supplies

- Patient ledger card or computer
- Check or cash from the patient or check from the insurance carrier

- Calculator
- Stamp with restrictive endorsement
- Stamp pad

1. Procedural Step. When a payment has been made, locate the patient account in the computer or select the patient ledger card.
Principle. Both payments received at the patient visit and checks received in the mail must be entered to the correct patient account.

2. Procedural Step. Compare the amount of the payment against the total amount owed.
Principle. The total amount owed will be the balance due and charges for new services.

3. Procedural Step. If using a manual system, post the payment from a completed patient charge slip on the patient ledger on the same line as the day's charges. If it is a check, record the number of the check. If using a computer program, post the payment on the same screen as the charges from the day's visit. Use the appropriate payment code for cash or check when entering the payment.

3

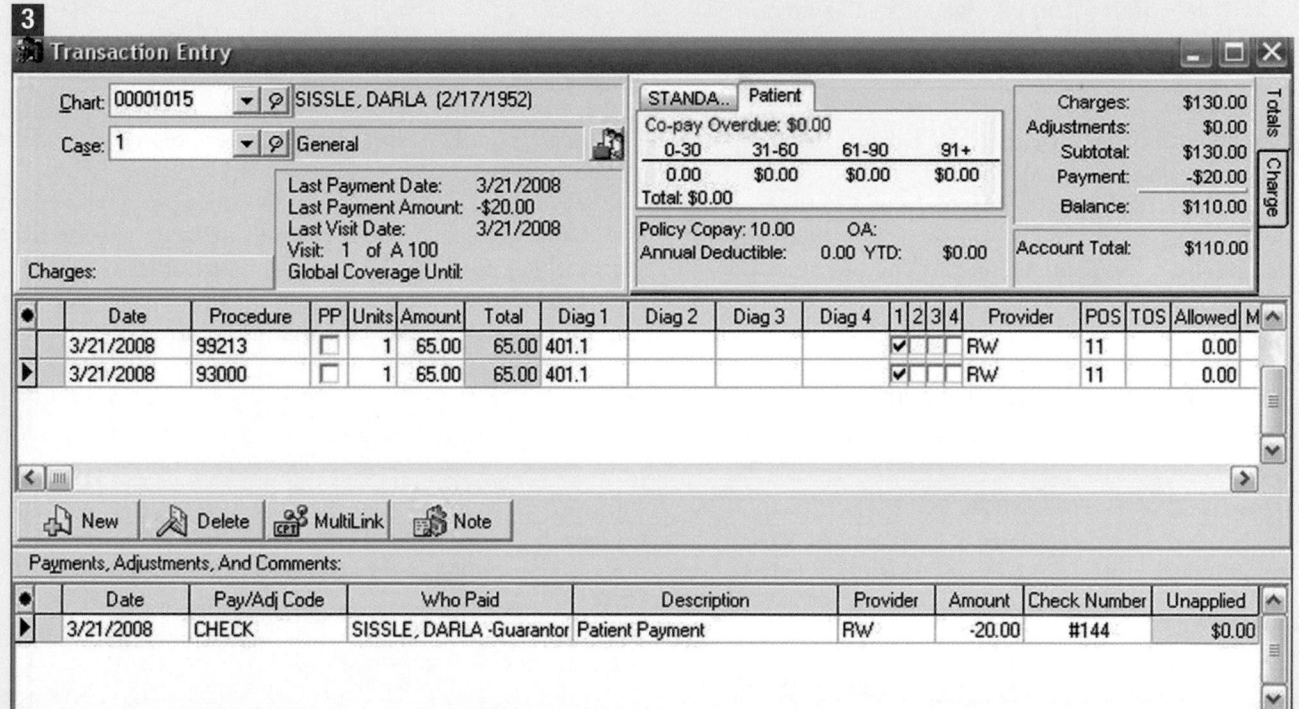

Transaction entry screen. (Screenshot used by permission of MCKESSON Corporation. All Rights Reserved. © MCKESSON Corporation 2008.)

4. Procedural Step. If posting an insurance payment, use a new line on a ledger card and a new transaction entry screen in a computer program.
Principle. All payments are posted using the date of posting. In the case of insurance payments, this is not the same as the date of service.

5. Procedural Step. Post the amount received as a payment. If using a computer program, use the code for an insurance payment.

6. Procedural Step. Enter the amount excluded by the insurance company as a credit adjustment. On a ledger card, enter in the adjustment column. If using a computer program, use the code for write-off or insurance write-off and the program will automatically deduct the amount.

Example: The statement from the insurance company shows that the insurance company paid $75.00 on the claim for Michael Lee. It excluded $25.00, which must be entered as a credit adjustment or write-off. The patient is expected to pay a copayment of $20.00.

Continued

PROCEDURE 44-3 Posting Payments and/or Adjustments—cont'd

6

UNITED WESTERN BENEFIT
1220 SIXTH STREET
WESTERN RIDGE, OH 45770

FOR SERVICES PROVIDED BY: WESTERN MEDICAL CENTER

Name of Insured: Michael Lee

Patient/ Service	Service Date(s)	Total Charge	Excluded Amounts	Patient Copayment	Plan Paid Amount
Office Visit	03/07/08	$ 65.00	$15.00 EAC	$20.00	$45.00
Electrocardiogram	03/07/08	$ 55.00	$10.00 EAC		$30.00
Total		**$120.00**	**$25.00**	**$20.00**	**$75.00**

EAC: This amount exceeds the allowable charge for the service. The provider is prohibited by law from billing the patient for this amount.

Insurance explanation of benefits.

7. **Procedural Step.** Calculate the balance. (A computer program does all calculations.)
Example: The insurance payment of $75.00 has been entered as an insurance check (INS). The excluded amount has been entered on a second line as a write-off (WO). The computer program will calculate the patient balance.

8. **Procedural Step.** Endorse the check using a stamp containing the practice name, the statement "For deposit only," and the number of the checking account.
Principle. This type of endorsement only allows the bank to deposit the check and prevents anyone from cashing the check or using it in any other way.

9. **Procedural Step.** Place cash or the processed check in the designated drawer or money box for later deposit.

7

Payments, Adjustments, And Comments:

Date	Pay/Adj Code	Who Paid	Description	Provider	Amount	Check Number	Unapplied
3/18/2008	INS	STANDARD HEALTH HMO		RW	-75.00		$0.00
3/18/2008	WO		Insurance Adjustment	RW	-25.00		$0.00

Apply   New   Delete   Note

Transaction entry screen. (Screenshot used by permission of MCKESSON Corporation. All Rights Reserved. © MCKESSON Corporation 2008.)

PROCEDURE 44-4 Recording a Patient's Visit on the Day Sheet

Outcome Post charges and payments on a day sheet.

Equipment/Supplies

- Day sheet or accounts receivable record
- Day sheet from the previous day
- Charge slips
- Ledger cards (optional)
- Checks
- Pencil
- Pen

1. Procedural Step. Prepare the day sheet by reviewing the appointment schedule. Place the day sheet on the pegboard and date the day sheet and deposit slip. If the office records month-to-date figures manually on the day sheet, copy the month-to-date totals from the day sheet of the previous day into the boxes labeled "TOTALS PREVIOUS PAGE" at the bottom of the day sheet. Copy the previous day's totals from the day sheet of the previous day on the line for the total of the previous day in Columns A-E. Enter the previous day's total accounts receivable on the first line of the month-to-date arithmetic proof box. (This box may be called "Accounts Receivable Control.") The day sheet may also have a box for a year-to-date arithmetic proof. If so, copy the figure for the accounts receivable first of the month on the first line. (This box may be called "Accounts Receivable Proof.") This amount is the same for each day of a given month.

Principle. All day sheets and deposit slips must be dated. Although it is fairly common to complete a day sheet each day and proof the daily totals, most modern medical offices rely on the computer billing program to provide month-to-date financial reports. The accounts receivable for the first of the month does not change because it represents the amount owed to the practice when the month began. This amount is used as a control to verify totals if an arithmetic proof is done manually.

Example: Copy amounts from columns A-E of the previous day in the correct column at the bottom of the sheet on the line labeled "TOTALS PREVIOUS PAGE."

Copy the amount of the Accounts Receivable End of Day from the arithmetic posting proof of the previous day into the box labeled "Accounts Receivable Previous Day."

FEE		PAYMENT		ADJUST-MENT		NEW BALANCE		OLD BALANCE			
										TOTALS THIS PAGE	31
3,948	00	3,221	00	309	00	2,733	00	2,315	00	TOTALS PREVIOUS PAGE	32
										TOTALS MONTH TO DATE	33
COLUMN A		COLUMN B		COLUMN C		COLUMN D		COLUMN E			

MONTH FROM LINE 31
ACCOUNTS RECEIVABLE PROOF

Accts Receivable Previous Day	11,496.00
Plus Column A	
Sub-Total	
Minus Column B	
Sub-Total	
Minus Column C	
Accts Receivable End of Day	

Box 2
Enter totals previous page and enter accounts receivable previous day.

2. Procedural Step. If using a complete pegboard accounting system, lay a bank of patient receipts on the pegs so that the top receipt lines up with the first line of the day sheet. If patients are given separate receipts or one copy of the charge slip as an itemized receipt, this step is not necessary.

3. Procedural Step. As each patient completes his or her appointment, enter information on the top blank line in ink including the name of the patient, the professional services provided (either abbreviations or procedure codes), the fee, payment, any adjustment,

new balance, and old balance. If using a complete pegboard system, the charge slip and patient ledger card will be filled out at the same time as the entry is made on the day sheet. This happens automatically because the information is transferred from the charge slip to the patient ledger and day sheet when the top of the charge slip is completed. If using a computerized billing system, the charge slip is completed first and the information is then transferred to the day sheet and entered into the patient's computer account.

Continued

PROCEDURE 44-4   Recording a Patient's Visit on the Day Sheet—cont'd

Principle. The day sheet is the journal of original entry, which is a running record of charges and payments made during the day.

4. **Procedural Step.** Complete the columns on the right side of the day sheet or accounts receivable record manually according to office policy by entering information tracked by the practice. This may include entering charges and payments for each physician in the practice or it may include entering information about specific procedures performed.

Principle. This enables a practice to accumulate data about the financial activity of each physician or about specific procedures. If a computer billing program is used, this type of information can be tracked through the report features of the program.

5. **Procedural Step.** Record payments received in the mail on the day sheet and patient ledger when the mail is processed. Be sure to include insurance adjustments as needed.

Principle. Payments made at the completion of the visit are posted at the same time and using the same date as the charges. Payments made through the mail are posted using the date they are received.

6. **Procedural Step.** Record all payments on the deposit slip when they are received or processed. The deposit slip can be totaled at the end of the day and used as the itemization for the deposit (see Procedure 44-7). A record can be made for the practice by filling out a duplicate deposit slip or by photocopying the deposit slip when it is complete.

Principle. It is more efficient to enter checks on the deposit slip when they are received.

Example: Two transactions on 11/24/2008 are as follows:

1. Michael Lee is seen as a patient for an office visit (99213) and an electrocardiogram (93000). He has no previous balance. He pays a copayment of $20.00 by check (#282). The charge is $65.00 for the office visit and $65.00 for the electrocardiogram. His total charges are $130.00.
2. A check from Sharon Smith's insurance company is received. The check is for $25.00. The excluded amount (write-off) is $8.00. Her previous balance was $42.00. After the insurance payment and adjustment, she owes $10.00.

6 **JOURNAL OF DAILY CHARGES, PAYMENTS AND DEPOSITS**

	DATE	PROFESSIONAL SERVICE	FEE		PAYMENT		ADJUST-MENT		NEW BALANCE		OLD BALANCE		PATIENT NAME
1	11/24/2008	99213, 93000, ch # 282	130	00	20	00			130	00	0		Michael Lee
2	11/24/2008	Ins pay, write-off			25	00	8	00	10	00	42	00	Sharon Smith

Entering charges and payments.

PROCEDURE 44-5   Balancing the Day Sheet

Outcome Verify the accounts receivable daily by balancing the day sheet entries.

Equipment/Supplies

- Day sheet with all transactions for one day
- Calculator
- Pencil
- Pen

1. **Procedural Step.** Make sure that all entries have been entered for the given day. Patient names can be checked against the appointment book, as well as copies of charge slips.

Principle. Entries cannot be added after a day sheet has been proofed, or results will be inaccurate.

2. **Procedural Step.** Add up each column with a calculator and place the total in pencil in the bottom row labeled "TOTALS THIS PAGE."

Example:

2 FEE		PAYMENT		ADJUST-MENT		NEW BALANCE		OLD BALANCE			
1,254	00	922	00	85	00	582	00	335	00	TOTALS THIS PAGE	31
3,948	00	3,221	00	309	00	2,733	00	2,315	00	TOTALS PREVIOUS PAGE	32
										TOTALS MONTH TO DATE	33
COLUMN A		COLUMN B		COLUMN C		COLUMN D		COLUMN E			

Entering totals this page.

Principle. Changes can be made more easily if totals are made in pencil and the proofs are calculated to be sure the day sheet balances before entering the totals in pen.

3. Procedural Step. Enter the total amount from each column in the correct box of the daily arithmetic proof and add and subtract the amounts as directed.

Principle. The arithmetic proof verifies that the columns of the day sheet have been totaled accurately. Accuracy in bookkeeping is necessary for financial audits and accounting.

Example:

3	DAILY FROM LINE 31 ARITHMETIC POSTING PROOF	
Column E	335.00
Plus Column A	1,254.00
Sub-Total	1,589.00
Minus Column B	922.00
Sub-Total	667.00
Minus Column C	85.00
Equals Column D	582.00

Box 1

Daily proof.

4. Procedural Step. Add the totals from the current day to totals from the previous day and enter in pencil on the line marked "Totals Month to Date." (If the figures have not yet been entered from the previous day's day sheet by the person who prepared the day sheet for the current day, they can be transferred from the day sheet of the previous day at this time.)

Example:

4 FEE		PAYMENT		ADJUST-MENT		NEW BALANCE		OLD BALANCE				
1,254	00	922	00	85	00	582	00	335	00	TOTALS THIS PAGE	31
3,948	00	3,221	00	309	00	2,733	00	2,315	00	TOTALS PREVIOUS PAGE	32
5,202	00	4,143	00	394	00	3,315	00	2,650	00	TOTALS MONTH TO DATE	33
COLUMN A		COLUMN B		COLUMN C		COLUMN D		COLUMN E			

Entering totals month to date.

5. Procedural Step. Enter the amounts from each column in the correct box of the accounts receivable proof and add and subtract the amounts as directed. This adds the amounts from the current day to the amounts from the previous day.

Example:

5	MONTH FROM LINE 31 ACCOUNTS RECEIVABLE PROOF	
Accts Receivable Previous Day	11,496.00
Plus Column A	5,202.00
Sub-Total	16,698.00
Minus Column B	4,143.00
Sub-Total	12,555.00
Minus Column C	394.00
Accts Receivable End of Day	12,161.00

Box 2

Monthly proof.

6. Procedural Step. If it is office policy, complete the year-to-date proof using the month-to-date totals. The total for the accounts receivable at the end of the day should equal the total for the accounts receivable at the end of month to date. Instead of completing this proof manually, the office may compare totals with a computer report.

7. Procedural Step. When the day sheet balances, rewrite all totals with a pen. Once the day sheet is complete, it must not be altered. If mistakes have occurred, they must be corrected by making adjustments on a subsequent day.

Principle. The day sheet represents the official record of charges and payments for a single day. Once accepted, it is completed in ink so that it cannot be altered at a future date.

BANKING ACTIVITIES

If the medical practice is to pay its bills, including salaries for medical assistants and other employees, it must have money in the bank. Part of the responsibility of the individual who handles the office's financial management is maintaining the practice's bank accounts.

Types of Accounts

Businesses such as medical practices will generally have one or more of the following types of bank accounts—checking, savings, or money market accounts.

Checking Account

A checking account is an account in which the money held can be drawn by simply writing a check against the funds available. Many banks allow businesses to earn interest on their checking accounts as long as a certain amount of money remains in the account (the minimum balance). The minimum balance can range from as little as $500 to as much as $2500. Interest is the payment the bank makes to the owner of the money on deposit for the privilege of being able to use the depositor's money to make loans to other bank customers.

If the checking account balance falls below the minimum, the account does not earn interest and there is usually a monthly service charge and a charge for each check written against the account for the entire monthly reporting period in which the balance was below the minimum.

A practice that does not want to maintain a minimum balance can open a checking account that pays no interest and has no monthly maintenance fees. Sometimes a bank will waive the minimum balance in the practice's checking account if the practice agrees to keep a higher minimum balance in either a savings account or a money market account.

Savings Account

A practice may want to keep cash that is not necessary to pay expenses in a savings account, which usually earns interest at a slightly higher rate than an interest-bearing checking account. A savings account does not have any check-writing privileges, but money can be withdrawn or transferred to the checking account if necessary.

Money Market Account

A money market account offers features of both savings and checking accounts. Money market accounts usually require a fairly high minimum balance (often $2500). However, they may earn interest at the money market rate—the rate at which major corporations lend to or borrow from one another for 10- to 30-day periods.

Money market accounts let the owner draw a specified number of checks per month without a processing fee. They often require checks to be for at least $500.

A medical practice might want to maintain a money market account in order to hold money for regular but infrequent expenses, such as quarterly, semiannual, or annual payments for malpractice insurance; licenses for physicians and other licensed professionals on the staff; or dues to the state, county, or local medical association or chamber of commerce.

Checks

Types of Checks

Checks are slips of paper used by a checking account owner to authorize payments to a third party (**payee**) for the amount of money written on the check. Paying by checks allows the medical practice to maintain a permanent record of the payments it makes for goods and services.

In addition to the checks from the practice's checkbook or money market account, the practice may have occasion to ask its bank to prepare a cashier's check to assure the payee (person or company being paid) that funds are available. A **cashier's check** is a check drawn on the bank itself rather than on an individual account. Because the bank assumes liability for payment of the check, a cashier's check is considered more reliable than the check of an individual or business. This might be the case if the office were purchasing a large piece of equipment for which the seller is unwilling to accept a simple business check. The bank may also guarantee a personal or business check by withdrawing the funds from the checking account at the time the check is issued. This is called a **certified check.**

Check Format

At the top of each check toward the right, under the check number, is a fractional number that identifies the bank on which the check is drawn. This ABA number, which is assigned by the American Bankers' Association, designates the federal reserve bank zone, the state or territory, and the unique identification number for the bank on which the check is drawn. Across the bottom of checks is a set of numbers called the **MICR line** written in magnetic ink. When checks are processed and "cleared" for payment from the issuing bank to the account of the individual making the deposit, this set of numbers is read by a magnetic ink character recognition (MICR) system. The MICR line contains the **ABA routing number (**the unique number of the bank), the account number, and the check number. Other information that is usually printed on a check includes the name and address of the account holder and the name of the bank.

Business Checkbook with Stubs

One type of business checkbook that is commonly used has three checks to a page with check stubs on the left on which to record the same information that is recorded on the check when it is written (Figure 44-5). The checks and matching stubs are preprinted in order. In addition, the stubs have room in which to write in the amount of deposits made; the stubs therefore act as a running checkbook ledger.

Computer-Generated Checks

A number of business accounting software programs will generate checks and immediately post the payment to the accounts payable ledger. To use these systems, the practice will need to buy compatible blank checks for computer printing. The software can also generate the fractional bank number and MICR numbers or they may be preprinted on the check forms.

Pegboard System for Check Writing

In addition to entering charges, a write-it-once or pegboard system can be used to write checks and create a check register at the same time. The check overlays the accounts payable ledger on the pegboard; and the "pay to the order of" and "amount" lines are copied from the check to the underlying check register (Figure 44-6).

Figure 44-5. A business checkbook is often arranged with three checks per page and check stubs to record transactions. (From Hunt SA: *Saunders fundamentals of medical assisting*, St. Louis, 2007, Saunders.)

Online Payment

The Internet has made it possible to pay bills online either as a single payment or every month. This is becoming an increasingly popular method with suppliers, who create online accounts and accept payments directly using a pay-by-computer system.

Because some businesses still do not accept on-line payment, a medical practice will still need to write or print some checks, especially if the practice handles its own payroll. Some practices may do all of their bill paying to regular suppliers, medical associations, liability insurance carriers, and other creditors on-line, and have their payroll checks written by an outside service provider, so checks are only written occasionally.

Preparing a Check

Checks are produced on watermarked paper to make it difficult for people to erase and then overwrite part of the check. The bank has the right not to honor a check with erasures, overwrites, or other alterations. Minor corrections may be accepted if initialed by the person who signs the check. This protects the account holder from having people

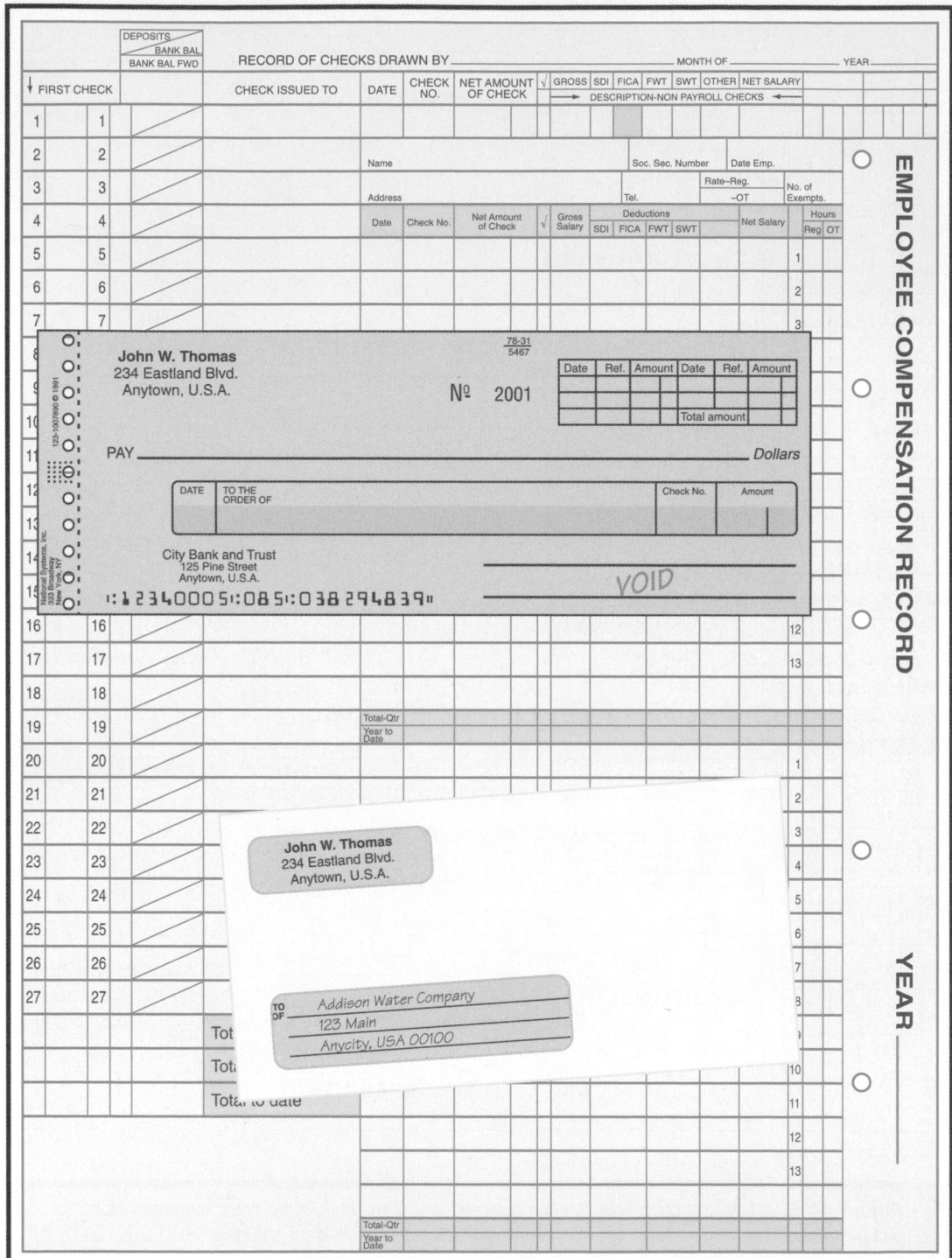

Figure 44-6. Pegboard check writing system. (Courtesy Bibbero Systems, Inc., Petaluma, Calif. [800] 242-2376. Fax [800] 242-9330.)

to whom checks are written cross out the amount and write in a larger amount. However, this also makes it important that checks be written carefully.

Most checks have at least one memo line—a line on which to write the purpose of the check. If the check is for payment of a bill or invoice, the invoice number or the account number for that particular vendor would go on the memo line.

If a mistake is made on a check, the medical assistant should write "void" on the check and check stub. The voided check should not be destroyed. It should be filed with bank statements and other account records so that it is available for the practice's auditors. When writing a check, the medical assistant should begin the amount in numbers immediately after the printed dollar sign and write the amount in words at the left side of the check. Legally, the amount in words is accepted as the amount for which the check is written if there is a discrepancy. After all of the checks for a particular period (week or month) have been written, they are attached to the supporting invoices and placed in a folder or envelope on the desk of the physician who is to sign the checks that week. In many practices, two physicians have check-signing privileges so that one can sign if the other is on vacation. Also, in some practices, checks exceeding a certain amount (e.g., $500, $1000) must be signed by two people; this is often a provision of that part of the practice's general liability insurance policy that covers employee theft (Procedure 44-6).

Bank Deposits

Preparing a Bank Deposit

Every time a deposit is made at the bank, it must be recorded on a deposit slip. A deposit slip is an itemized listing of the cash or checks being deposited. Deposit slips used to itemize checks are found at the far right side of the day sheet (Figure 44-7). A deposit slip preprinted with the account number will be found in the back of the practice's checkbook. Deposit slips may also be created and printed using a computer accounting program. This allows for deposits to be entered in the computer records for the office's checking account. When making a deposit, the amount of the total cash being deposited is written on the cash line, with the total of the checks on the check line. An itemized listing of the checks being deposited must be included with the

---

What Would You Do? What Would You *Not* Do?

Case Study 3
On January 4, Leonard Simpson paid $10.00 by check as a copayment at the time of an office visit. At the end of the day when Maria was preparing the daily deposit, she noticed that the date on Mr. Simpson's check was January 4 of the previous year instead of the current year. ■

Highlight on Check Security Features

Because of the prevalence of color copiers, many security features are built into the paper used to print checks. The paper usually has a watermark that cannot be photocopied and/or invisible florescent fibers that can be viewed under black light. The paper should have erasure protection so that the background color fades if writing or printing is altered. The paper of the check may also have a chemical stain that reacts if chemicals are used to alter information. A word, such as "nonnegotiable" or "void," may appear if the check is passed through a photocopier or treated with chemicals. Various parts of the check usually have also been treated in a special way so that they will not be reproduced if the check is photocopied. The border and endorsement line usually include microprinting that will not be reproduced if the check is photocopied. ■

---

deposit. The numerator of the fractional bank number (e.g., 94-72) should be entered on the deposit slip in the column labeled "bank number" to identify each check (Figure 44-8; Procedure 44-7).

Endorsing Checks

Each check being deposited must have an endorsement on its back. An endorsement authorizes a bank to cash or deposit the check. Endorsements are of several types.

Blank Endorsement

A simple signature of the party to whom the check was written. Once a check has been signed, it can be cashed by anyone holding the check.

Special Endorsement

The endorsement begins with a statement of the party to whom the check should be paid (usually using the words, "Pay to the order of ...") followed by the signature of the party to whom the check was written.

Restrictive Endorsement

The endorsement begins with instructions that specify how the check can be paid out (e.g., "For deposit only") followed by the signature of the party to whom the check was written. The bank must follow the instructions.

This type of endorsement can be entered on a check using a stamp approved by the bank that includes the words "for deposit only," the name of the physician or medical practice, and the bank account number. All checks received in the medical office should be stamped with the restrictive endorsement before deposit.

Making a Deposit

Deposits can be made in person or by using the night deposit box, usually located near the bank's front door. The night deposit box may require a key or personal identification number (PIN) code, which is supplied by the bank to customers who use it. (This prevents tampering or unauthorized use of the deposit slot.) Electronic technology now permits electronic readers to read the deposit bag's serial number, or there may be a radio frequency identification (RFID) tag in the deposit bag similar to the devices used for mass transit passes, parking passes, and inventory control.

Reconciling a Bank Statement

Reconciling a bank statement means making sure that the balance in the checkbook and the balance on the bank statement equal each other after adjusting for checks that were written but have not yet cleared through the bank and deposits recorded after the statement period ended.

Each month the bank will send the practice a statement of account activity or the practice may access this statement online. The account balance at the end of the statement period will almost always be different from the account balance in the office's checking account ledger.

BANK DEPOSIT DETAIL

BANK NUMBER	BY CHECK OR PMO	BY COIN OR CURRENCY	CREDIT CARD
TOTALS			

CURRENCY	
COIN	
CHECKS	
CREDIT CARDS	
TOTAL RECEIPTS	
LESS CREDIT CARD $	
TOTAL DEPOSITS	
DEPOSIT DATE: _____ FIRM: _____	

Figure 44-7. Bank deposit slip of the type found on the right side of a pegboard day sheet. (Courtesy Bibbero Systems, Inc., Petaluma, Calif. [800] 242-2376. Fax [800] 242-9330.)

Memories *from* Externship

Maria Hernandez: There was only one doctor in the office where I did my externship, and in that office, they used both a manual system to record patient accounts and a computer system. The office manager had been in charge for many years, and she said that she didn't trust the computer. Every morning we set up the pegboard by placing a day sheet on the bottom and receipts above. The receipts had carbon strips so that anything written would be duplicated on the layer below. As each patient checked out, we placed his or her ledger card between the receipt and the day sheet so that the next open line was directly above the next open line on the day sheet. The ledger cards we used were made of a special kind of carbonless paper called *NCR paper. NCR* stands for "no carbon required." When we filled in the date and charges on the receipt, it automatically was copied on the ledger card and then on the day sheet. The challenges were to be sure all three forms were lined up correctly and also to be sure to apply enough pressure with the pen. The other big challenge was to add up the entries on the day sheet at the end of the day and make sure that everything balanced. The office manager said that sometimes it would take a long time to find and fix every mistake. I don't think there are very many offices left that record patient accounts this way, but I am glad I saw how it was done. It makes me appreciate how useful the computer is in managing office finances. ■

Prepare for Success

There are several reasons for this discrepancy. First, it usually takes about a week from the time the statement period ends until the office receives the statement, during which time more checks have been written. Second, checks written near the end of the statement period usually will not have cleared the account when the period ends. Third, some vendors and others do not promptly deposit or cash checks; thus, some checks will not clear the account for a month or more. Fourth, bank charges are added to the statement for such things as checks returned for insufficient funds, per-check fees, and lockbox fees. Finally, interest may accrue on the balance during the month.

For this reason, it is important to reconcile the bank statement with the office's checkbook as a double-check of the arithmetic used by those who have written checks. Most banks have a preprinted reconciling page on the back of the statement. This form makes it possible to take the statement period-end balance, subtract from it the dollar amount of checks that have been written since the end of the period, subtract any bank charges, add the dollar amount of checks that have not cleared, and add any interest earned to get a true balance. This true balance should match the balance in the office's checking-account ledger (Figure 44-9; Procedure 44-8).

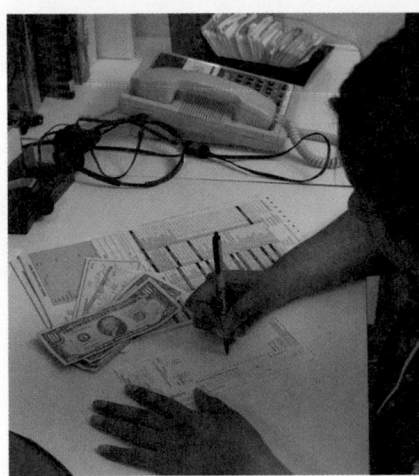

Figure 44-8. Medical assistant preparing a bank deposit.

THIS WORKSHEET IS PROVIDED TO HELP YOU BALANCE YOUR ACCOUNT

1. Go through your register and mark each check, withdrawal, Express ATM transaction, payment, deposit or other credit listed on this statement. Be sure that your register shows any interest paid into your account, and any service charges, automatic payments, or Express Transfers withdrawn from your account during this statement period.

2. Using the chart below, list any outstanding checks, Express ATM withdrawals, payments or any other withdrawals (including any from previous months) that are listed in your register but are not shown on this statement.

3. Balance your account by filling in the spaces below.

ITEMS OUTSTANDING		
NUMBER	**AMOUNT**	
TOTAL	$	

ENTER

The NEW BALANCE shown on this statement_____$

ADD

Any deposits listed in your register $
or transfers into your account $
which are not shown on this $
statement.   + $ _____

                      TOTAL

CALCULATE THE SUBTOTAL_____$

SUBTRACT

The total outstanding checks and withdrawals from the chart at left_____-$

CALCULATE THE ENDING BALANCE

This amount should be the same as the current balance shown in your check register_____$

Figure 44-9. Bank statement reconciliation form. (From Hunt SA: *Saunders fundamentals of medical assisting,* St. Louis, 2007, Saunders.)

PROCEDURE 44-6 Writing a Check

Outcome Write checks to pay bills for a medical office and record them in the checkbook or check register.

Equipment/Supplies

- Checks with check register or check stubs
- Monthly bills to be paid
- Pen

1. **Procedural Step.** Organize bills to be paid by opening envelopes and/or arranging invoices. Use a pen to prepare a check for each bill or invoice.
   Principle. This prevents alterations after the check has been written.
2. **Procedural Step.** Write the date on the line that says "Date."
   Principle. The date identifies when the check was written. Banks have specific policies that specify how long the check is valid.
3. **Procedural Step.** Write the name of the payee on the line of the check that says "Pay to the order of."
4. **Procedural Step.** Write the amount of the check in numbers in the box next to the dollar sign. When writing the numbers, use a decimal between the number of dollars and the number of cents.
   Example: $1,568.42
5. **Procedural Step.** Write the amount of the check in words on the line below the name of the payee. Begin writing at the beginning of the line. When writing the words, remember that "and" is only used before the number of cents. Numbers like 25 contain a hyphen when written in words (e.g., twenty-five). Write the number of cents as a fraction over 100. Draw a line from the end of the fraction to the word "dollars."
   Example: One thousand five hundred sixty-eight and 42/100————————DOLLARS
   Principle. Writing the amount in numbers, as well as words, helps prevent alteration of the amount of the check.
6. **Procedural Step.** Write the invoice number, account number, and/or purpose of the check on the line marked "for" or "memo."
   Principle. If the check is separated from the payment slip, this helps the payee identify what the check is for. It may also assist in record keeping after the check is returned by the bank.
7. **Procedural Step.** Record the date, check number, payee, amount of the check, and reason the check was written on the check stub in the checkbook or in the check register.

Principle. A record is kept of every check that is written.

8. **Procedural Step.** Subtract the amount of each check from the balance on the check stub or in the check register. If completing a check stub, enter and add any deposits since the previous check and add them to the previous balance. Then subtract the amount of the check and enter the new balance. Write the new balance on the stub of the check below in the box labeled "Balance carried forward."
   Principle. Keeping a running balance makes it possible to determine easily how much money is present in the checking account.
   Example: Completed check stub for a check to D&D Medical Supply.

8

	1837	
DATE 3/12/08		
TO D & D Med. Supply		
FOR Invoice #JTS006		
BALANCE BROUGHT FORWARD	4,482	21
DEPOSITS		
BALANCE	4,482	21
AMT. THIS CHECK	1,000	00
BALANCE CARRIED FORWARD	3,382	21

Filling out a check stub.

9. **Procedural Step.** If you make a mistake, draw a single line through the mistake, correct the error, and initial the correction.

10. **Procedural Step.** If the check cannot be used, write the word "Void" across the check and enter the word "Void" in the check register. Place the voided check in the folder where accounts payable records are kept.

    Principle. Keeping voided checks instead of destroying them facilitates accurate record-keeping and provides proof that the check was voided.

11. **Procedural Step.** Prepare an envelope to mail the payment or use a window envelope supplied by the vendor.

12. **Procedural Step.** Clip the prepared check to the envelope with the payment slip, and place it in the designated place for review and signature by the physician authorized to sign office checks.

PROCEDURE 44-7 Preparing a Bank Deposit

Outcome Prepare a bank deposit.

Equipment/Supplies

- Account deposit slip
- Deposit slip itemization record from the day sheet (optional)

- Cash and checks received as payments
- Calculator or adding machine
- Bank deposit envelope or bag

---

1. **Procedural Step.** Obtain an account deposit slip and place today's date on it. If the deposit slip from a day sheet is used, write the name of the medical practice and the bank account number at the top.

    Principle. The date, practice name, and account number must appear on the deposit slip so that the bank can credit the deposit correctly.

2. **Procedural Step.** Write the amount of currency and coins on the correct lines and place the total on the line that says "Cash."

3. **Procedural Step.** Stamp each check with the restrictive endorsement and write the amount of each check on the Bank Deposit detail with the numerator of the fractional ABA number. This information may have already been recorded on the deposit slip of the day sheet, which can be used as itemization.

    Principle. A reference number for each check allows the bank to verify individual items If questions arise.

4. **Procedural Step.** Total all the checks and place that total on a deposit slip in the box for checks.

5. **Procedural Step.** Total the cash and total amount of checks for the total amount of the bank deposit. The total amount of this deposit should be equal to the amount in the Payments column on the day sheet or accounts receivable record for the given day.

6. **Procedural Step.** Make a copy of the deposit slip if a duplicate deposit record has not been made when creating the day sheet.

    Principle. The office should keep a copy of the checks and cash included in a deposit in case there are questions at a later date.

7. **Procedural Step.** Place the cash, checks, and deposit slip in a bank envelope or bank deposit bag and take or send it to the bank.

8. **Procedural Step.** Record the amount of the deposit on the accounts payable record and in the check register or on the check stub nearest to the date of deposit.

    Principle. This provides information on the amount of money in the checking account against which checks can be written.

9. **Procedural Step.** File the bank deposit receipt and copy of the bank deposit detail in a labeled file folder.

    Principle. All bank records must be saved for a period of time for tax and accounting purposes.

PROCEDURE 44-7

PROCEDURE 44-8 Reconciling a Bank Statement

Outcome Reconcile a bank statement.

Equipment/Supplies

- Monthly bank statement
- Checkbook and check stubs or check register
- Pen
- Calculator

1. **Procedural Step.** Open the current bank statement and locate the ending balance and the list of checks and deposits.

   Principle. Reconciling a bank account necessitates comparing the bank statement to the checkbook record of deposits and checks written for the same time period.

2. **Procedural Step.** Locate the same time period in the checkbook record of deposits and checks.

3. **Procedural Step.** Check the checkbook register against the bank statement and place a checkmark against each check and deposit that is recorded on the bank statement.

4. **Procedural Step.** Note those checks and deposits in your record that have not cleared the bank (i.e., do not appear on the statement).

   Principle. There are several days from the bank closing date on the statement until the statement is received in the office or practice. During that period, additional checks could be written and deposits made.

5. **Procedural Step.** Note any additional charges, such as service charges, ATM charges, or charges for returned checks. If there are additional charges, include them in the check register or on a check stub.

6. **Procedural Step.** Note any credits, such as interest. Include them in the check register or on a check stub and calculate the new balance.

   Principle. To calculate the correct balance, it is necessary to include any charges or credits that do not already appear in the check ledger.

7. **Procedural Step.** Calculate the balance using a bank statement reconciliation form:
   a. starting with the bank's ending balance,
   b. adding any deposits listed on your check register to that ending balance not listed on the bank statement, and
   c. subtracting any outstanding checks from that subtotal.

   The balance on the bank statement should equal the current balance in the check register or on the last check stub.

8. **Procedural Step.** If the balance does not equal, recheck all calculations in the check ledger. If the check register still does not balance with the bank statement and you suspect an error, contact the bank.

OTHER FINANCIAL ACCOUNTS

In addition to taking money in, a practice pays money out. Some of this is done on a regular basis, taking care of weekly or biweekly salaries, mortgage or rent, equipment leases, and utilities. Other payments are made in relation to specific invoices for materials or equipment.

Unless a bill is paid immediately when presented, it becomes part of the accounts payable (money owed by the business). A complete bookkeeping system notes each month any outstanding accounts payable, as well as the **disbursements** (payments) made during the month.

In addition, many offices keep a **petty cash** account, a small amount of cash available for everyday expenses. Again, petty cash must be recorded.

Accounts Payable or Record of Cash Disbursements

The record of cash disbursements is called the *cash disbursement journal,* as shown in Figure 44-10. In a one-write or

pegboard system, cash disbursements are automatically recorded at the time each check is written out. In a computerized bookkeeping system, the cash disbursement journal is also automatically updated, or posted, when a check is drawn. In a single- or double-entry system, the cash disbursement journal must be separately maintained by hand.

Each line of the cash disbursement journal has columns to record information about payments. Usually there are also columns to track expenses by categories. These features are also found in computer accounting programs (Figure 44-10).

Petty Cash

Petty cash is the cash kept on hand to pay for small, miscellaneous items, such as tips for a delivery, postage due, reimbursement to a staff member for parking at a meeting, or even a box of Girl Scout cookies for the office break room.

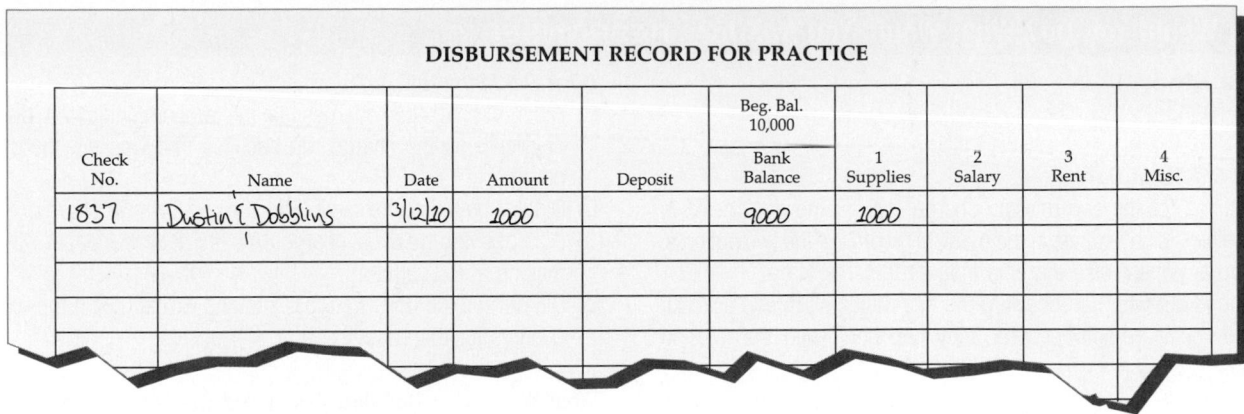

Figure 44-10. Cash disbursement journal. (From Hunt SA: *Saunders fundamentals of medical assisting,* St. Louis, 2007, Saunders.)

A check for a predetermined amount—usually $75 to $100—is drawn to cash to establish the petty cash account. It is important to keep each office account separate. Thus, cash should never be taken from any patient payment and put into petty cash. The petty cash account should always be funded via a check drawn on the practice's checking account.

A petty cash journal should be located near the cash box so that each disbursement can be recorded. Also, a pad of petty cash receipts should be available so that a receipt can be filled out each time a person receives money from the petty cash account. When the amount in the petty cash account decreases, a new check is drawn in the amount that will return the petty cash fund to the original starting balance.

Like any account, the petty cash account should be balanced on a regular basis. Staff members may need periodic reminders to fill out receipt forms every time they remove funds from petty cash.

MEDICAL PRACTICE and the LAW

Medical offices are susceptible to embezzlement (stealing money or assets of a business) by employees. The American Academy of Family Physicians reports that in a study of community health clinics, more than 40% experienced some kind of financial crime in the previous 5 years. Medical assistants should be aware of measures that may be in place to reduce the incidence or impact of embezzlement. They should understand that measures to prevent fraud are also measures to ensure the financial health of the medical office as a business. These measures should not be interpreted as evidence that the employees are not trusted.

- Medical offices should check a candidate's references and job history carefully before hiring the candidate.
- The power to sign checks should be controlled, and all checks should be reviewed carefully. A signature stamp should not be allowed for signing checks.
- Job rotation should be encouraged, and employees should take earned vacations. Fraud is more easily spotted when different individuals handle financial transactions.

- Fidelity bonding is a type of insurance purchased by a business to provide reimbursement if embezzlement occurs. The medical office may purchase a blanket policy that covers all employees or a policy for specific individuals or positions within the office. This type of insurance may be part of the overall insurance plan for the medical office. Bonding deters illegal activity because bonding companies are known to prosecute perpetrators to the full extent of the law.
- Because cash is more difficult to keep track of than checks, receipts should be issued for all cash collected using either a receipt book that makes a carbon copy or immediate entry to the computer billing program. Cash receipts should be accounted for on a daily basis.
- Employees should be encouraged to report any suspicious activity of other employees. Unfortunately, it is often a trusted employee with several years of service who has the best knowledge of the weaknesses of the financial systems of a medical office.

What Would You Do? What Would You *Not* Do? RESPONSES

Case Study 1
Page 1034

What Did Maria Do?

❑ Looked for the two missing charge slips at the front desk, in the physician's office, in the medical records of the two patients, and anywhere else that she thought they might be.

❑ Found out who had checked the two patients out and asked if they could remember what they had done with the missing charge slips.

❑ If Maria was unable to find the charge slips, she created new ones using the information from the day sheet.

❑ Verified that she had charged the patient for the correct services using the medical record and/or by checking with the physician who saw the two patients.

❑ Made a note of the numbers of the two missing charge slips so that they could be voided if they were found at a later time.

What Did Maria Not Do?

❑ Did not assume that the charge slips would turn up eventually and could be entered at that time.

❑ Did not leave the day "open" because she knew that two charge slips were missing.

❑ Did not assume that she knew what the charges should be based on the reason for each patient's visit.

What Would You Do/What Would You *Not* Do? Review Maria's response and place a checkmark next to the information you included in your response. List the additional information you included in your response.

_____

_____

_____

_____

Case Study 2
Page 1035

What Did Maria Do?

❑ Looked at the medical record and asked other staff members to determine why Linda Harris had been given a reduced rate. Possible reasons include a discount for cash payment or professional courtesy.

❑ If she could not determine the reason using other means, Maria asked the physician what the reason for the discount was.

❑ Entered the charges for Linda Harris to the computer at the usual rate. On a separate line she entered an adjustment of $25.00 ($15.00 for the office visit and $10.00 for the flu shot). She identified the reason for the adjustment (e.g., cash payment, professional courtesy) using the correct computer code.

❑ Also entered the amount of the patient's payment to the patient's account.

What Did Maria Not Do?

❑ Did not enter the charges as the amount indicated by the physician on the charge slip because that was not the office policy.

❑ Did not guess at the reason for the reduction in charges.

❑ Did not enter the usual charges into the patient account without making an adjustment.

❑ Did not tell the physician that she had written down the wrong charges for the patient.

What Would You Do/What Would You *Not* Do? Review Maria's response and place a checkmark next to the information you included in your response. List the additional information you included in your response.

_____

_____

_____

Case Study 3
Page 1047

What Did Maria Do?

❑ Contacted Leonard Simpson by telephone to tell him that he had used the incorrect date on his check.

❑ Either arranged to have Mr. Simpson send or drop off a new check. When the new check arrived, Maria returned the check with the incorrect date to Mr. Simpson.

❑ Might also have arranged for Mr. Simpson to come to the office, change the date on the check, and initial the correction.

❑ Waited until the new check arrived to post the payment to Mr. Simpson's account and deposit the check.

❑ Corrected the charge slip and the day sheet to remove the payment from that day.

What Did Maria Not Do?

❑ Did not try to deposit the check with the incorrect date.

❑ Did not alter the date and put her own initials by the correction.

❑ Did not post the payment to Mr. Simpson's account until the new check arrived.

What Would You Do/What Would You *Not* Do? Review Maria's response and place a checkmark next to the information you included in your response. List the additional information you included in your response.

_____

_____

_____

_____

TERMINOLOGY REVIEW

ABA routing number A nine-digit number that identifies a bank printed at the beginning of the magnetic ink character recognition line at the bottom of a check. It also appears in fractional form at the top right of the check under the check number.

Accounting Systematic recording and reporting of financial transactions.

Accounts payable The outstanding bills of a business, such as a medical office.

Accounts receivable Total amount owed to a business for goods and services.

Accrual basis of accounting Accounting method in which income is entered at the time of sale or provision of service.

Adjustment A change to a patient account that is neither a charge nor a payment.

Assets In accounting, a combination of property owned and money owed to a business.

Bookkeeping The process of recording financial transactions and keeping financial records.

Cash basis of accounting Accounting method in which income is entered when payment is received.

Cashier's check A check drawn on a bank instead of an individual account.

Certified check A check on an individual account that a bank assumes responsibility for, usually by withdrawing funds to cover the check from the checking account at the time the check is certified.

Charge slip A form used to keep track of charges and payments at the time of a patient visit.

Credit A posting that is subtracted from an account balance.

Day sheet The record of daily transactions in the pegboard or "write-it-once system" and also in computer medical billing programs.

Debit A posting that is added to an account balance.

Disbursements Money paid out.

Fee schedule List of charges (fees) for specific procedures that may be performed in a medical office.

Ledger A book, card, or computer account used to record financial transactions.

Liabilities In accounting, the amount owed by a business to creditors.

MICR line A line of numbers containing the ABA transit routing number and the account number that appears at the bottom left of a check. These numbers are read by a magnetic ink character recognition (MICR) system.

Payee The person to whom a check is made out.

Petty cash A cash account kept in a business office to pay for incidentals, such as postage due and other small items.

Proof of posting A process of calculation to verify that calculations on a day sheet are internally consistent and all totals are correct.

Reconciling Making sure that two financial records agree, such as a bank statement and bank balance.

Superbill An itemized charge slip usually also containing diagnosis codes and procedure codes required for insurance billing.

ON THE WEB

For Information on Centers for Medicare and Medicaid Services (CMS):

Physician Center: www.cms.hhs.gov/center/physician.asp

Physician Fee Schedule for Medicare: www.cms.hhs.gov/PhysicianFeeSched

 PREPARE FOR CERTIFICATION Visit the Evolve site at http://evolve.elsevier.com/Bonewit/today/ to actively Prepare for your Certification.

 Check out the Companion CD bound with the book to access additional interactive activities.

45

Medical Coding

CAAHEP COMPETENCIES

Administrative Competencies
Process Insurance Claims
- Perform procedural coding.
- Perform diagnostic coding.

General Competencies
Legal Concepts
- Demonstrate knowledge of federal and state health care legislation and regulations.

ABHES COMPETENCIES

Administrative Duties
- Apply managed care policies and procedures.
- Perform diagnostic coding.

Financial Management
- Implement current procedural terminology and ICD-9 coding.

established patient
modifier
morphology (mor-FAWL-uh-gee)
NEC
neoplasm (NEE-oh-plasm)

new patient
NOS
panel
surgical package

Introduction to Coding

For hundreds of years, medical researchers have been interested in collecting statistics related to health and disease, including the number of individuals who contract certain diseases and the number of deaths caused by those diseases. To facilitate this undertaking, it was necessary for physicians to agree on a system to classify diseases and procedures. Lists of symptoms and diseases had existed in various countries for many years, but the first comprehensive disease classification system in the United States was published in 1869 by the American Medical Association as the American Nomenclature of Disease. (The word *nomenclature* means what things are called; in essence, this book was a dictionary of diseases.)

Turning a classification system into a coding system requires systematic replacement of names with numbers or combinations of numbers and letters. This allows information to be standardized. Numbers or combinations of numbers and letters can be easily managed and manipulated by computers.

PROCEDURE CODING

Procedure codes are a means to classify the type of care given to patients. The three main reasons for developing what have come to be called *procedure codes* are:

1. To justify medical services by correlating procedures to diagnosis
2. To collect statistics about the outcome and effectiveness of treatments
3. To help physicians and hospitals set fees based on the amount of time and skill required to provide a specific service

In 1966 the American Medical Association published the first edition of the *Current Procedural Terminology* (CPT) coding system. The original version focused primarily on surgical procedures and was one of many attempts to translate medical and surgical procedures into numerical codes.

The fourth edition, which is currently in use, was first published in 1977 and is updated annually. It became the standard for insurance billing in the early 1980s, when it was used it as the basis for a Medicare procedure coding system, the Healthcare Common Procedure Coding System (HCPCS), pronounced "hick-picks." The first level of HCPCS codes (95% to 98% of codes used for Medicare Part B) includes the current CPT codes. In addition, there are additional HCPCS codes for procedures, injections, and durable medical equipment covered by Medicare Part B that are not included in the CPT system.

Each medical office must purchase updated versions of the code books and/or computer files containing *International Classification of Diseases, Ninth Revision, Clinical Modification* (ICD-9-CM), CPT, and HCPCS codes every year. The CPT codes are available only from the American Medical Association, but ICD-9-CM and HCPCS codes can be purchased from several publishers and are also available at some locations on the Internet.

CPT CODING

The CPT manual provides both a narrative description and a five-digit code for each procedure or service a physician or other licensed provider may perform for a patient. There must be documentation in the medical record to support the use of any procedure code used in billing the patient. When entering codes on insurance claims, the five-digit code is sufficient for most procedures. A **modifier** is an addition to a procedure code that indicates unusual circumstances related to the procedure, such as a more extensive procedure or two procedures performed in the same session.

The two-digit modifier can be added to the main code after a hyphen. The modifier can also be written as an separate five-digit code for electronic billing. The five-digit modifier always begins with "099" and ends with the two digits of the modifier (Table 45-1).

Sections of the CPT Manual

The fourth revision of *Current Procedural Terminology* (CPT) is currently used for procedure coding. It is divided into six sections, each of which defines the procedures and services provided for specific types of medical services. The six sections, and the range of codes for each, are as follows:

- Evaluation and Management   99201 to 99499
- Anesthesia   00100 to 01999
- Surgery   10021 to 69990
- Radiology   70010 to 79999
- Pathology and Laboratory   80047 to 89356
- Medicine   90281 to 99607

Table 45-1 Selected CPT Modifiers Used in the Medical Office

(See the *Current Procedural Terminology* manual, Appendix A, for a complete list of modifiers.)

Modifier	Description
-21	Prolonged Evaluation and Management Services
-22	Increased Procedural Services (not used for E/M services)
-26	Professional Component
-32	Mandated Service
-47	Anesthesia by Surgeon (not including local anesthesia)
-50	Bilateral Procedure—This code is added to the second (bilateral) procedure performed at the same operation
-51	Multiple Procedures (performed at the same session)
-52	Reduced Services
-54	Surgical Care Only—This code is used when another physician provides preoperative and postoperative care
-55	Postoperative Management Only
-56	Preoperative Management Only
-57	Decision for Surgery (added to an E/M code when the physician makes the decision for surgery during an E/M visit)
-58	Staged or Related Procedure by the Same Physician During the Postoperative Session
-59	Distinct Procedural Service
-90	Reference (Outside) Laboratory
-91	Repeat Clinical Diagnostic Laboratory Test
-92	Alternative Laboratory Platform Testing
-99	Multiple Modifiers

E/M, Evaluation and Management.

In each annual update of the CPT, new codes may be added for new procedures, old codes may be dropped for procedures no longer in use, and modifications may be made to current procedures. A darkened circle in front of a code indicates that the code is new. A darkened triangle in front of the code indicates that the description for the code has been changed or modified (Figure 45-1). The medical assistant must familiarize himself or herself with the important revisions each year when the new codes are published.

The main body of the CPT manual is organized by section, then subsection, subheading, and finally category, each providing a finer level of detail. The back of the manual contains an alphabetic index of procedures. The most common procedures performed in a given office are usually found on the charge slip and in the computer billing program.

Evaluation and Management

The Evaluation and Management (E/M) section contains codes for office visits provided by primary care practitioners and specialists. E/M codes cover the service-oriented, rather than the procedure-oriented, parts of medical care. It is important to determine where the service was provided when selecting the correct E/M code.

Although procedures are fairly easy to define—for instance, incision and drainage of a cyst—the amount of service provided by a physician during a routine visit is more difficult to describe. One physician may consider 20 minutes an appropriate amount of time for a routine visit, whereas another may consider 30 minutes the minimum amount of time to spend with a patient. One physician may focus strictly on the problem the patient presents with, whereas another may want to examine the patient more completely, especially if he or she has not been seen for several months.

The codes in the E/M section attempt to link reimbursement to the completeness of the examination and the amount of skill required to manage the patient's problems. Unfortunately, this tends to limit the physician's discretion to practice in his or her own style. If the patient does not have well-defined, complex medical problems, the visit is reimbursed as uncomplicated, no matter how much time the physician spends with the patient.

When determining the proper code for E/M services, the medical assistant must consider a number of factors.

1. For coding purposes, the patient is either an **established patient** (one who has been seen in the previous 3 years) or a **new patient** (one who has not had services performed by any provider in the medical office in the previous 3 years). There are separate groups of codes for each type of patient. New patients are expected to take longer to examine and are reimbursed at a higher rate.

2. There are separate groups of codes, depending on where the service is provided and whether the physician is the patient's primary care provider or a consultant. A medical service could have been provided in the office, in a nursing home, in a hospital to a patient who has been admitted, or in a hospital emergency department.

3. The level of service depends primarily on three key factors:
   - The extent of the history (number of body systems discussed)
   - The extent of the physical examination (number of body systems examined)
   - The complexity of medical decision making

   As secondary factors, the following may be considered:
   - Coordination of care
   - Counseling
   - The nature of the patient's problem
   - The amount of time spent with the patient

When coding for E/M services, it is important to have documentation that supports the code chosen. Often, the physician or other primary care provider checks the appropriate box on the encounter sheet at the time of the patient visit. Other times, the medical assistant may ask the physician about the level of service immediately after the visit (Figure 45-2). The medical assistant may also have to review

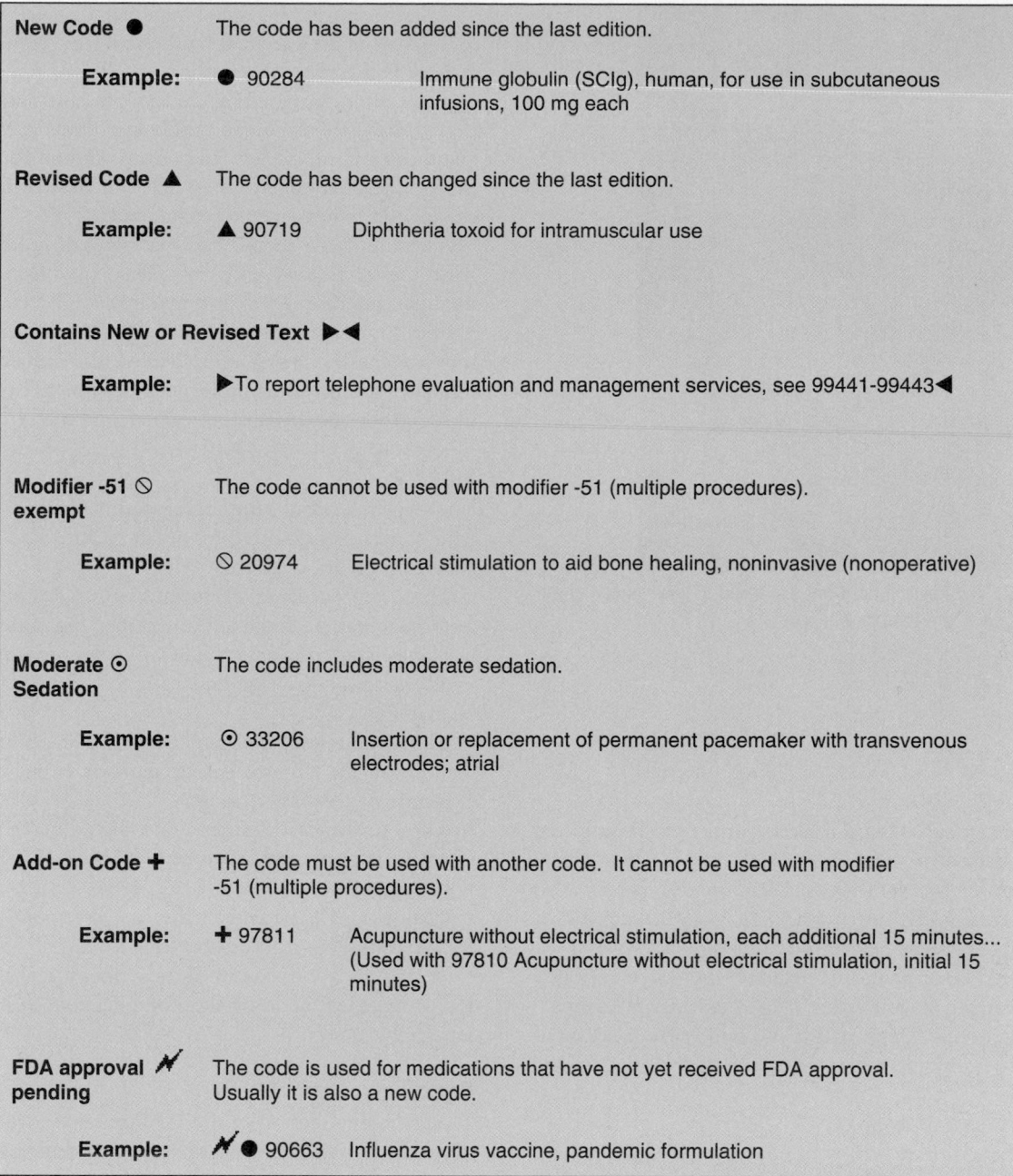

New Code ●   The code has been added since the last edition.

    Example: ● 90284   Immune globulin (SCIg), human, for use in subcutaneous infusions, 100 mg each

Revised Code ▲   The code has been changed since the last edition.

    Example: ▲ 90719   Diphtheria toxoid for intramuscular use

Contains New or Revised Text ▶◀

    Example: ▶To report telephone evaluation and management services, see 99441-99443◀

Modifier -51 ⊘ exempt   The code cannot be used with modifier -51 (multiple procedures).

    Example: ⊘ 20974   Electrical stimulation to aid bone healing, noninvasive (nonoperative)

Moderate ⊙ Sedation   The code includes moderate sedation.

    Example: ⊙ 33206   Insertion or replacement of permanent pacemaker with transvenous electrodes; atrial

Add-on Code ✚   The code must be used with another code. It cannot be used with modifier -51 (multiple procedures).

    Example: ✚ 97811   Acupuncture without electrical stimulation, each additional 15 minutes... (Used with 97810 Acupuncture without electrical stimulation, initial 15 minutes)

FDA approval 𝒩 pending   The code is used for medications that have not yet received FDA approval. Usually it is also a new code.

    Example: 𝒩 ● 90663   Influenza virus vaccine, pandemic formulation

Figure 45-1. Symbols that appear in the *2008 Current Procedural Terminology* code manual.

the medical record when completing the insurance claim and decide which of the categories is supported by the physician's progress note. All of the key components must meet or exceed the stated level of care to qualify for a particular level of E/M service.

Medical History

History taking consists of four levels: (1) problem focused, (2) expanded problem focused, (3) detailed, and (4) comprehensive:

- A problem-focused history is one that addresses the chief complaint, with a brief history of the illness or problem.

- An expanded problem-focused history addresses the chief complaint, a brief history of the present illness or problem, and a review of systems that have to do with the chief complaint.
- A detailed history addresses the chief complaint, an extended history of the present illness, and a review of body systems, including other systems beyond those related to the chief complaint. Family history is also reviewed as it relates to the present problem.
- A comprehensive history includes a chief complaint; an extended history of the present illness; a review of all body systems, especially those directly related to the problem; and a complete family history.

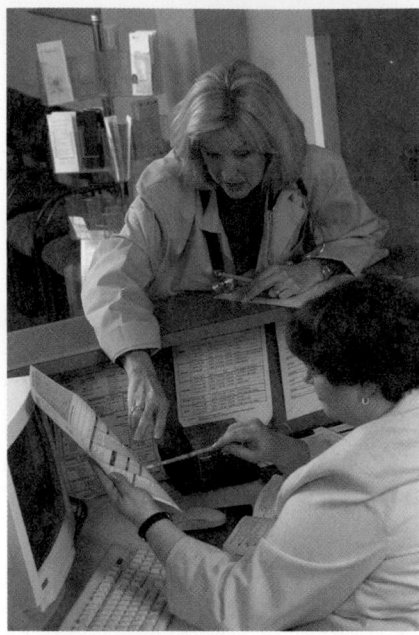

Figure 45-2. The medical assistant may need to question the physician about services provided to a patient.

Physical Examination

- A problem-focused examination is limited to the affected body system or organ.
- An expanded problem-focused examination is related to the affected body system, as well as other organs or systems that might be symptomatic.
- A detailed examination includes the affected body systems or organs and other related systems or organs.
- A comprehensive examination is a multisystem examination, or a complete examination of one system.

Medical Decision Making

- Medical decision making can be straightforward or have a low, moderate, or high level of complexity.

If a patient has one problem, medical decision making is usually straightforward. When a patient presents with multiple problems, especially if they are causing severe or life-threatening symptoms, the decision-making process is more complex. For example, if a new patient presents with poorly controlled diabetes mellitus type 1, fever, and a low white blood count, the decision-making process for the physician would be highly complex.

Anesthesia

Anesthesia is the administration of a drug that causes a total or partial loss of sensation. Anesthesia can be administered to provide analgesia (absence of pain) for a patient during a surgical procedure, wound closure, removal of a foreign body, childbirth, or for a diagnostic test, including radiology, as well as for therapeutic radiology.

Anesthesia can be general, regional, or local. CPT codes for anesthesia are specified by the anatomic region affected, as well as the type of anesthesia provided. Anesthesia services are often provided by the time, in hours and minutes, that the anesthetist or anesthesiologist was present. Local anesthesia by infiltration (the most common form of anesthesia used in the medical office) is included with the procedure and is not given a separate code.

The anesthesia section has two types of modifiers: standard modifiers and physical status modifiers. Standard modifiers are those used throughout the CPT code manual; physical status modifiers indicate the patient's condition at the time anesthesia was administered. Patient condition can influence the level of complexity of administering anesthesia in the proper dose over the proper time frame.

Surgery

The surgery section is the largest section of the CPT manual. This section is organized by organ systems and within the systems by types of procedures.

Surgical procedures are coded as a surgical package. The term **surgical package** indicates that the code covers all services related to a surgery. The following areas are included in the surgical package and cannot be coded (or billed) separately:

- One evaluation/management visit that occurs after the decision for surgery has been made either on the day before or the day of surgery
- Local or topical anesthesia or a digital nerve block
- Immediate postoperative care
- Writing orders
- Evaluating the patient in the recovery room
- Typical follow-up postoperative care

If complications occur during the surgery or during follow-up, treatment of the complications can be coded separately.

Radiology

The radiology section of the CPT manual includes radiology, nuclear medicine, diagnostic ultrasound, and radiation oncology.

Most standard radiologic procedures are found in the diagnostic radiology subsection, including plain x-ray films, computed tomography (CT or CAT), magnetic resonance imaging (MRI), magnetic resonance angiography (MRA), and standard angiography. The codes for diagnostic radiology correspond to the anatomic site of the radiographic image, starting with the head and moving down. Some codes indicate a single view, whereas others indicate multiple views.

Pathology and Laboratory

The pathology and laboratory section of the CPT manual is organized by the type of tests performed, such as individual tests, panels, or assays. A **panel** is a group of laboratory tests, usually ordered together for diagnosis or screening, such as a cardiac panel (a group of tests ordered for a patient with cardiac symptoms). To use a panel code, each test in the panel must have been done. Additional or other tests are coded separately.

Different codes are used for laboratory tests performed by automated equipment and tests performed manually. When coding for a medical office, the medical assistant must be sure that patients are only charged for tests actually performed in the office (e.g., a dipstick urinalysis). If the medical assistant draws blood to be sent to an outside laboratory, the medical office charges the patient for the venipuncture (using the code 36415), but the laboratory bills separately for the diagnostic tests. The office does not charge separately for collecting urine and throat specimens if they are sent to an outside laboratory for processing.

Pathology testing, such as Pap tests and biopsies, are usually done by a special laboratory. The medical office charges for the visit or surgery where the specimen is collected, but the laboratory usually bills for the actual specimen testing.

Medicine

The medicine section of the CPT manual gives the proper codes for noninvasive diagnostic and treatment services, many of which are performed in the offices of primary care physicians and specialists. (Invasive services, those that enter a body cavity, generally fall in the surgical section). The medicine section is organized according to body system.

A number of highly specialized types of testing and treatment, ranging from electrocardiograms (ECGs) to ophthalmologic tests, are found in the medicine section. In addition, the medicine section contains the codes for immunizations and infusion therapies, including chemotherapy.

Codes for procedures from this section that are performed frequently (e.g., ECGs in the office of an internist or cardiologist) are usually found on the charge slip and in the medical billing software. In the office of a pediatrician or family practitioner, the codes for all standard immunizations are found on the charge slip.

When a medical procedure is performed infrequently, the physician usually writes it in on the charge slip, and the medical assistant may need to look up the code for billing. In the case of injections, it is important to identify the current code for the specific immunization or medication if it is listed in the CPT manual. Injections are coded separately, and many drugs given by injection do not have specific codes. Injections are identified by the route given (i.e., subcutaneous, intramuscular, intravenous). (Injections do have specific codes for Medicare, which are discussed in the following section.) The medication name should be included with the documentation sent to the insurance company. Note that there are different codes for injections of antibiotics and injections of other medications.

Looking Up CPT Codes

The first step in coding a procedure is to look up the procedure in the alphabetic index at the back of the CPT manual. The medical assistant should never code directly

Putting It All into Practice

My name is **John Grant,** and I am a certified medical assistant. I work for a group of family practice physicians, and we have two offices. I am responsible for entering almost all of the information from the charge slips into the computer. We have found that there is more consistency if one person is responsible for this task. Our physicians usually see patients in the office, but all of our physicians also visit their patients if they are hospitalized, visit patients in nursing homes, and sometimes see patients in the hospital emergency department in the evenings and on weekends. Each time a patient is seen in the office, a charge slip is filled out, and the physician checks beside the correct box for the type of visit. Our charge slips have the E/M codes on the slip so that we can distinguish between new and established patients, as well as levels of care provided. We also have all the codes for well visits and Medicare preventative services on the charge slip. When the physicians see patients in the hospital or in nursing homes, they fill out a log sheet we developed in the office so that we can be sure that we bill patients for all services and use the correct code for each service provided. In addition, I have to be sure that the correct place of service code is entered because insurance companies will reject a claim if the place of service does not match the service provided. For example, if I use the code 99281 for an emergency department visit, I have to be sure to use the place of service code 23 (emergency room-hospital).

I also look up and enter diagnosis codes. The most common diagnosis codes are found on our charge slips, but the physician often writes in a diagnosis that is not on the slip or even in the computer. The diagnosis has to correspond to the service, and sometimes the physician forgets to enter all of a patient's conditions on the charge slip. In those cases, I have to review the medical record to find the specific diagnosis that justifies a procedure. Coding is complicated, but in the long run it saves time to spend time making sure that the codes are entered correctly when the charges are entered. Otherwise, our insurance claims are rejected, and we spend a lot of time fixing mistakes and resubmitting claims. ∎

Prepare for Success

from the index because it does not contain descriptions of the code and may result in use of an incorrect code.

It may be necessary to look up the procedure in several ways to locate the correct code. Looking under the name of the procedure, the anatomic location, and sometimes the diagnosis is important. Several pieces of information may be significant when choosing the correct code for a procedure:

- Location
- Size of lesion or repair
- Method of performing the procedure, test, or surgery
- Number of minutes allotted for a treatment (e.g., acupuncture)
- Complexity of the procedure or service

It is important to review information from the patient's medical record carefully before choosing the code that best describes the service. The CPT manual itself contains information at the beginning of each section entitled "Guidelines" to help locate the current codes. In addition to specifying which code to use for what kind of service, there are general guidelines about what substantiating documentation must be submitted in order for the claim to be approved for payment.

Information about modifiers is contained in Appendix A with directions about how to use the modifiers. Appendix B is a summary of additions, deletions, and revisions from the previous year's manual. When the new manual is published, the medical assistant may not be able to find a code that has been used in the past. Appendix B provides a fast way to find out if the code has been deleted, changed, or included in another procedure.

Clinical examples of different codes are given in Appendix C. Reading these can be very helpful in learning how to decide what code to use, especially for E/M codes.

The CPT manual contains several other appendices with specific lists or codes or information that the medical assistant should become familiar with (Procedure 45-1).

What Would You Do? What Would You *Not* Do?

Case Study 1

When John is entering patient charges from the charge slips he finds one charge slip on which the physician has checked the code for an expanded problem-focused office visit (99202) for a new patient named Peter Miller. John notices that the patient for whom he has a charge slip has other transactions in the computer from a previous visit about 12 months before the current visit. ■

PROCEDURE **45-1** Looking Up a CPT Code

Outcome Look up the proper CPT code for a procedure.

Equipment/Supplies

- Patient's medical record
- Charge slip
- CPT manual

1. **Procedural Step.** Find the name of the procedure to look up and information about the procedure (if necessary) using the patient's charge slip and/or medical record.
   Principle. The charge slip usually identifies the procedure(s) performed, but the medical record may be necessary to identify the appropriate level of service.
2. **Procedural Step.** For E/M services, identify if the patient is a new patient or an established patient.
   Principle. Different codes are used for new patients and established patients.
3. **Procedural Step.** For E/M services, identify if the patient was seen in the medical office or at another location, such as the hospital, emergency department, or nursing home.
   Principle. Different E/M codes are used depending on the location where the patient was seen. The coding and billing for visits provided by a physician to a hospitalized patient, nursing home resident, or patient in the emergency department are often done by staff at the physician's medical office.
4. **Procedural Step.** Using the index at the back of the manual, locate the section in which the category of codes will be found. You may need to look for the name of the procedure, the diagnosis, the type of patient, the location of service, or the location of the lesion.
   Examples:

A. To locate an initial office visit for a new patient, look in the index under New Patient, Initial Office Visit (99201-99205) or under Evaluation and Management, Office and Other Outpatient (99201-99215).
B. To locate the code for a rapid strep test, look under *Streptococcus,* Group A, Direct Optical Observation (87880).
5. **Procedural Step.** Look in the manual at the code or range of codes to read the description and determine the correct code. Do not code from the index.
   Principle. You cannot be sure that you have identified the correct code without reading the description of the code. You may also find additional information in the section to help you code properly.
6. **Procedural Step.** If the service is unusual or does not seem to fit the description of the code completely, check the list of modifiers for the section of the manual to see if a modifier is necessary.
   Example:
   A patient has presented with an abscess of the left upper arm, which required incision and drainage again today.
   1: In the index, you look up Abscess, Arm, Upper, Incision and Drainage. It refers you to codes 23930-23035.

Index*:

Abscess
(lines deleted)
Arm, Lower 25028
Excision.......................... 25145
Incision and Drainage................ 25035
Arm, Upper
Incision and Drainage...........23930-23935
Auditory Canal, External 69020

2: When you look at those codes, you see that these codes refer to deep abscesses.

Codes*:

Incision	
	(For incision and drainage procedures, superficial 10040-10160)
23930	Incision and drainage, upper arm or elbow area; deep abscess or hematoma
23931	bursa

3: You review the medical record and determine that the physician called the lesion a *subcutaneous abscess*.

4: For superficial abscesses, you are referred to codes 10040-10160. The code 10060 (incision and drainage of abscess: simple or single) appears to describe the procedure most accurately. Because the patient came for an office visit specifically for treatment of the abscess and no other E/M services were provided, you do not charge for a separate office visit.

Codes*:

Incision and Drainage	
	(For excision, see 11400, et seq)
10040	Acne surgery (leg, marsupialization, opening or removal of multiple milia, comedones, cysts, pustules)
10060	Incision and drainage of abscess (eg, carbuncle, suppurative hidradenitis, cutaneous or subcutaneous abscess, cyst, furuncle, or paronychial); simple or single
10061	complicated or multiple

7. **Procedural Step.** Enter the correct code(s) on the charge slip, encounter form, and if applicable in the patient's record in the computer so that it can be used for insurance billing.

Principle. Reimbursement is made by insurance companies based on the codes submitted. They must be accurate and reflect the service or procedure performed. In the example given earlier, the insurance company might refuse to pay for the service (as already provided) without the modifier, which indicates that it is in fact a repeat service of a procedure performed by another physician.

PROCEDURE 45-1

*© *Current Procedural Terminology, 2008, Standard Edition,* American Medical Association. All rights reserved.

HEALTHCARE COMMON PROCEDURE CODING SYSTEM

Level I and Level II Codes

Level I codes are identical to the AMA CPT codes and modifiers as discussed earlier. They are used for most procedures performed in the medical office.

Level II codes use a five-digit alphanumeric coding system and designate specific services and equipment. Level II codes are used primarily for items and services that do not have CPT codes. Examples of items with Level II codes include supplies, materials, specific medications, ambulance services, and some procedures. For example, if a patient is given a pair of metal underarm crutches after a cast is applied, the HCPCS code E0114 would be used to bill Medicare for the crutches. Level II codes are updated annually by the Centers for Medicare and Medicaid Services (CMS). Most commercial insurance companies also accept Level II codes for covered items or services.

Looking Up HCPCS Codes

The process for locating accurate HCPCS Level II codes is almost the same as that for looking up CPT codes (Procedure 45-2). The medical assistant should first locate the item or service in the index at the back of the HCPCS manual. A single code or code range may be found in the index, but the medical assistant should always find the complete description in the list of codes before making a final selection. The codes consist of one letter followed by four numbers, and they are arranged alphabetically by the initial letter and then numerically by the four digits. Codes marked ◆ are not valid for Medicare. They are used for Medicaid billing. When billing for specific medications given to patients in the office, the medical assistant should be sure to identify the code that contains the dose given if there is more than one code for the same medication. For example, there are three codes for injections of penicillin G benzathine:

PROCEDURE 45-2   Looking Up a HCPCS Code

Outcome Look up the proper HCPCS code for a service or piece of equipment.

Equipment/Supplies

- Patient's medical record
- Charge slip
- HCPCS manual

1. **Procedural Step.** Refer to the charge slip or the patient's medical record to locate the service, supplies, or equipment requiring a HCPCS code.
   Principle. The charge slip usually identifies the procedure(s) performed, but the medical record may be necessary to identify more detail about the service, supplies, and so on.

2. **Procedural Step.** Using the index at the back of the manual, locate the section in which the category of codes will be found.

3. **Procedural Step.** Find the code or code range by locating first the initial letter (arranged alphabetically) and then the four-digit number (arranged numerically). Read the description and determine the correct code. Do not code from the index.
   Principle. You cannot be sure that you have identified the correct code without reading the description of the code. You may also find additional information in the section to help you code properly.

4. **Procedural Step.** Check to be sure that the code is valid for the patient's insurance.

Principle. Some HCPCS codes are valid for Medicaid but not Medicare.

5. **Procedural Step.** Enter the correct code(s) on the charge slip, encounter form, and if applicable in the patient's record in the computer so that it can be used for insurance billing.
   Principle. Reimbursement is made by insurance companies on the basis of the codes submitted. They must be accurate and reflect the service or procedure performed.

Example:

1: To locate the code for an injection of diphenhydramine hydrochloride 25 mg, look up the drug in the index. (This medication may be given intramuscularly for an allergic reaction.) The code given for diphenhydramine hydrochloride is J1200.

2: Look for the code in the list of codes first under J, then under 1200. The entry J1200 states that this code covers injections up to 50 mg. It would therefore be the correct code for the example provided earlier.

J0560	Injection, penicillin G benzathine, up to 600,000 units
J0570	Injection, penicillin G benzathine, up to 1,200,000 units
J0580	Injection, penicillin G benzathine, up to 2,400,000 units

If a patient had been given penicillin G benzathine 1,800,000 units, the correct code to select would be J0850.

ICD-9-CM CODING

In addition to coding procedures, it is also necessary to code diagnoses. Diagnostic coding was originally developed to fulfill four purposes: track disease processes, classify the causes of death, collect data for medical research, and evaluate hospital service utilization.

In 1948 the World Health Organization (WHO) published the first edition of the *International Classification of Diseases,* which assigned numbers to specific diseases. This system was developed so that more accurate statistics could be collected about how often diseases and accidents occurred

What Would You Do? What Would You *Not* Do?

Case Study 2

While entering charges for Joan Drysdale, a 72-year-old patient with Medicare insurance, John sees that the patient was charged for an intramuscular injection (90772) of methylprednisolone in addition to the office visit (99213). No other charges are listed on the charge slip. John needs to enter the charges and codes for this patient so that Medicare can be billed. ■

---

and were treated. The system proved to be useful for health care review and insurance claims processing.

The WHO has revised the *International Classification of Diseases* several times since then. For insurance coding and review of medical records, a clinical modification tool was developed to better collect and compile data about specific diseases, conditions, and medical services for healthy individuals. The acronym for this coding system is ICD-9-CM, which stands for *International Classification of Diseases, Ninth Revision, Clinical Modification.* The ICD-9-CM became the system of choice for diagnostic coding after

1989, when it began to be required on all Medicare Part B insurance claims forms.

The tenth edition (ICD-10) was published in 1993 by the WHO. It is used extensively in other parts of the world, but its acceptance in the United States has been delayed. Because the ICD-9-CM is the basis for hospital billing in the United States, it requires extensive planning and review to develop the ICD-10-CM and implement the change to its acceptance. It will include several features, such as the following:

- More extensive information related to ambulatory care and managed care encounters
- An expansion of injury codes
- New combination diagnosis and symptom codes to decrease the need for two codes
- An added sixth and seventh digit for some conditions
- Increased ability to locate and choose specific codes

An updated version of the ICD-10-CM was released in July 2007, but currently an implementation plan and date has not been set.

Today, it is necessary to use ICD-9-CM coding for diagnosis to have an insurance claim approved for reimbursement. If the proper ICD code and coding format is not used, many insurance companies will reject a claim because the patient's diagnosis does not justify the procedures done for the patient. ICD-9-CM coding is required by government-financed programs, such as Medicare and Medicaid, as well as most private insurance companies.

ICD-9-CM Manual

The ICD-9-CM manual has three volumes. Volume 1 contains a tabular list of diseases, arranged numerically by disease classification. Volume 2 contains an alphabetic listing of diseases. Volumes 1 and 2 are used primarily in physicians' offices. In many handbooks, the index (Volume 2) is placed first and is followed by the tabular list of diseases (Volume 1). Volume 3, which has both a numeric tabular listing and an alphabetic listing of procedures, is primarily used in hospitals.

Format of ICD-9-CM Codes

ICD-9-CM codes consist of three digits (from 001 to 999) that can be preceded by a letter and/or followed by a decimal point plus one or two additional digits. Digits after the decimal point make a given diagnosis more specific. They are arranged in numeric order. Following the numeric codes are codes that begin with certain letters.

Numeric Codes (001-999.9)

Numeric codes are arranged beginning with infectious diseases and followed by diseases or conditions related to individual body systems. For example, the first section of the tabular list (001-139) consists of infectious and parasitic diseases. The three-digit number for salmonella infections is 003, but this number cannot be used to code the disease. When coding a patient's diagnosis, the medical assistant should try to find a code with a decimal point followed by

either one or two digits. Three-digit codes are less specific and, in most cases, not accepted. It is important to find the code that most exactly matches the diagnosis given by the physician. Zeros before the code and after the decimal point must always be included. If a code with two digits after the decimal is available, it should be selected.

In order to select the most specific and correct code, the medical assistant should not code from the index but always from the tabular list. As an example, assume that the physician lists the patient's diagnosis as *salmonella gastroenteritis.* If the medical assistant looks under *"Salmonella,"* the general code is given as 003.9. If the medical assistant looks in the tabular list, a more specific code (003.0) is easily located. In this case, the correct code could be found if the medical assistant looked in the index under *"Gastroenteritis, salmonella."*

Codes for Individuals Who Do Not Have a Disease or Injury

Codes that begin with the letter V (so-called V codes) follow the numeric codes. They identify factors influencing health status or an encounter with health services when there is no disease or injury, such as to receive an immunization. If a patient schedules an office visit because he or she has a family history of diabetes, the code V18.0 is used. The medical history alone justifies periodic examinations. V codes are used primarily for physical examinations, well-baby and well-child visits, and visits during pregnancy.

E codes cover external causes of injury or poisoning, such as injury due to collision of a motor vehicle with another motor vehicle. E codes are used in combination with other diagnosis codes to give more information about the cause of a medical problem. As an example, an open wound of the cheek without complications is given the code 873.41. In addition, an E code may be assigned to identify the cause of the wound (e.g., E 828.2, an accident to the rider of an animal, such as a horse riding accident). E codes facilitate the collection of statistics about causes and severity of injuries.

M codes describe **morphology** (structure and form) of neoplasms. A **neoplasm** is an abnormal growth or tumor. M codes, which are primarily used for statistical tracking, are included in Appendix A of the ICD-9-CM manual.

Using the Index (Volume 2)

The first step in coding a patient's diagnosis is to find the diagnosis in the alphabetic index. Some terms in the index may indicate that the diagnosis requires a fifth digit (placed in the second position, after the decimal point). Even though the categories of the fifth digit subclassification may be listed in the index, the medical assistant should never code directly from the index without looking up the code in the tabular list. The index does not contain the same detail as the tabular list of diseases.

The medical assistant must always keep in mind that insurance companies will be using the diagnosis code to pay

Memories *from* Externship

John Grant: My externship was performed in a large clinic where I spent some time in several departments. I was placed in the medical records department for 4 days, and I didn't understand why I needed to be there for such a long time. I was surprised to learn that this department was not only responsible for filing and taking care of the medical records, but they also did a considerable amount of coding. They taught me to look up diagnosis codes one day, and I spent all morning and part of the afternoon doing this. They gave me a stack of referral forms and told me to look up and write the diagnosis code on each form. If I couldn't find it or if I wasn't sure, I should put the form to one side so that someone could help me later. I was told to find the diagnosis in the index, and then look up the best code in the tabular list. I had had some practice in school, so this wasn't completely new to me. I have to admit that my pile of codes I was sure of was smaller than the pile I had questions about. I never realized that coding could be so complicated. There were some I couldn't find at all and others where I just couldn't decide what the best code was. For example, I couldn't find "unequal arm length due to old fracture." Later I found out that this would be 736.89 Deformity (acquired); arm or leg not elsewhere classified. This experience really helped me understand how to think of other words to try to look up diagnosis codes in the index. ▪

Prepare for Success

Figure 45-3. A sample of *International Classification of Diseases, Ninth Revision, Clinical Modification* codes. (From Buck C: *Saunders 2008 ICD-9-CM*, St. Louis, 2008, Saunders.)

for services. If the diagnosis codes are incorrect or incomplete, the insurance carrier may refuse to pay for the services provided.

To find the diagnosis in the tabular list, the medical assistant may look under the main word of the patient's diagnosis. It is also possible to start from the anatomic location of the medical problem. A code must be identified for each diagnosis.

During the period when the physician is still trying to determine exactly what the patient's diagnosis is, symptoms may be listed on the charge sheet. These should be coded exactly as written. If the physician writes "rule out" or "R/O" with a diagnosis or condition, that condition may *not* be used for coding (Figure 45-3).

Examples

1. If the progress note describes the patient's problem as "recurrent right shoulder pain, rule out bursitis," the code can be located in the index under: pain, joint, shoulder (region) (719.41). If the medical assistant looks up shoulder, the following instruction is given: "see condition."
2. If the patient's diagnosis is given on the charge slip as diabetic neuropathy, the medical assistant should look in the index under diabetes (diabetic), neuropathy. The

primary code is listed as 250.6 and 357.2 is listed in parentheses. The medical assistant should look up both codes as part of the process of selecting the correct code. The same information can also be located by looking under neuropathy, diabetic.

Using the Tabular List (Volume 1)

Once a code or range of codes has been identified, the medical assistant should find the correct section and determine the best code to match the information on the patient's charge slip or in the medical record. It is important to look at the additional information given relating to the diagnosis.

In the tabular list, the medical assistant should always look for the most specific code possible, remembering that the code must be supported by the information in the medical record. See Figure 45-4 for conventions used for the ICD-9-CM.

Selecting the Correct Fifth Digit

Certain codes require a fifth digit added after the subcategory code. Use of the fourth and fifth digits is not optional.

Abbreviations

NOS means "not otherwise specified." It is used only when a more specific code cannot be identified.

NEC means "not elsewhere classifiable." It is used when the medical record indicates that more information is available but a more specific code cannot be found.

Punctuation

[ ]   Brackets are used to identify synonyms or alternative wording, as in diabetes type I [juvenile type].

( )   Parentheses used around words in a subcategory identify what are called *nonessential modifiers*, words that may occur in the diagnosis but are not required. For example, hypertension (arterial) (primary) (essential) (systemic). The parentheses mean that all of the following would be covered by the same diagnosis code: hypertension, arterial hypertension, primary hypertension, essential hypertension, and systemic hypertension.

:   A colon is used after an incomplete term. It means that one of the following modifiers must be used with the term; for example, bronchitis NOS:

> catarrhal
> tracheobronchitis NOS
> with tracheitis NOS.

Symbols may vary depending on the publication. The following may be indicated:

New codes

Revised codes

Codes that are not a principle diagnosis

Codes that require additional digit(s)

Nonspecific codes

Figure 45-4. Conventions used for the *International Classification of Diseases, Ninth Revision, Clinical Modification* code manual.

If the diagnosis is diabetes mellitus, for example, a fifth digit is always required. The use of the fifth digit varies for each category where it is required, and it is necessary to review the instructions carefully before choosing the fifth digit.

If a certain code may not be used for a condition (usually a similar or related condition), the word "excludes" is placed in a box under the code and the correct code is identified. If the code cannot be used as a primary diagnosis, instructions are given to code the underlying disease first.

When the tabular list is examined, it can be seen that the category for pain in a joint is 719.4, and a fifth digit is required. As noted earlier, the fifth digit is added as the second digit after the decimal point. The medical assistant should select the most specific digit from the table of possible fifth digits. For codes 719.4, the possible fifth digits are as follows:

0   site unspecified
1   shoulder region
2   upper arm
3   forearm
4   hand
5   pelvic region and thigh
6   lower leg
7   ankle and foot
8   other specified sites
9   multiple sites

What Would You Do? What Would You *Not* Do?

Case Study 3

When entering charges for Michael Drew, a 56-year-old patient, John sees that the physician has checked the following diagnosis code: 250.90 Diabetes 1 with unspecified complications. Just below the code, the physician has written "with diabetic polyneuropathy." John needs to enter the charges and codes into the computer so that this patient's insurance can be billed. ■

The digits 0, 8, and 9 should only be used if one of the other digits does not match the diagnosis given by the physician. If the patient has pain in the left shoulder, the correct code would be 719.41.

If the medical assistant looks up the code 357.2 for polyneuropathy (multiple nerve dysfunction) in diabetes, instructions are given to code the underlying disease, diabetes mellitus, first. If the patient has the secondary condition, it is important to include both diagnoses because the specific treatment given may be related to the secondary diagnosis (which cannot be used independently) (Procedure 45-3).

PROCEDURE 45-3   Looking Up an ICD-9-CM Code

Outcome Look up the proper ICD-9-CM code for a patient's diagnosis.

Equipment/Supplies

- Patient's medical record
- Charge slip
- ICD-9-CM manual

1. **Procedural Step.** Refer to the patient's charge slip and/or medical record to identify the diagnosis. In the medical record, the physician may use the term "impression" or "diagnosis."
   Principle. The charge slip usually identifies the diagnosis, but the medical record may be necessary for additional information to select the correct code.

2. **Procedural Step.** Decide on the key word or phrase to look for the code in the index of diseases (Volume 2).

3. **Procedural Step.** Locate the key word and look for the body part or other distinguishing factors. Identify the possible code number(s).

4. **Procedural Step.** Locate the number(s) in the tabular list (Volume 1).
   Principle. You cannot be sure that you have identified the correct code without looking at the tabular list. You may also find additional information in the tabular list to help you code properly.

5. **Procedural Step.** Review the information given in the tabular list and select the four-digit code or five-digit code that most correctly corresponds to the information on the charge slip and/or in the medical record. When there is a list of possible fifth digit codes, select the most specific digit to use as a fifth digit.
   Principle. Reimbursement may be linked to selection of the correct fifth digit.

6. **Procedural Step.** Enter the correct code(s) on the charge slip, encounter form, and if necessary in the computer billing program so that it can be used for insurance billing.
   Principle. Reimbursement is made by insurance companies based on the codes submitted. Diagnosis codes must be accurate and justify the service provided.

   Example:
   1: To locate the code for a patient with the diagnosis "chest pain, possibly angina pectoris," first locate pain, then chest in the list of diseases (Volume 2). You will find entries similar to the following:

Index*:

Pain(s)	
	chest (central) 786.50
	atypical 786.59
	midsternal 786.51
	musculoskeletal 786.59
	noncardiac 786.59
	substernal 786.51
	wall (anterior) 786.52

2: Look up the code 786.50 in the tabular list (Volume 1).*

786.5 Chest pain
  786.50 Chest pain, unspecified
  786.51 Precordial pain
  786.52 Painful respiration
     Pain:
        anterior chest wall
        pleuritic
        pleurodynia
  Excludes: *epidemic pleurodynia (074.1)*
  786.59 Other
        Discomfort in chest
        Pressure in chest
        Tightness in chest

The code 786.5 may be marked with a symbol that indicates a fifth digit is required (depending on the code manual). After reviewing all the codes in the category, it is clear that 786.50 Chest pain, unspecified corresponds best to the diagnosis given by the physician. It is not permissible to select a code with words that are not found in the physician's diagnosis.

*Buck C: *Saunders 2008 ICD-9-CM,* St. Louis, 2008, Saunders.

MEDICAL PRACTICE and the LAW

When medical codes are misused in order to obtain a higher level of reimbursement than is allowed, the process is called *upcoding*. Under Section 231 of the Health Insurance Portability and Accountability Act, nearly all federal health care programs can levy fines and penalties for failure to adhere to compliance with regulations for using correct codes on claims for reimbursements. A pattern or practice of upcoding can result in large fines, and ignorance of correct procedure is not considered a defense. Medicare analyzes claims to identify atypical billing and may follow up with a more detailed analysis when a pattern has been identified for a specific provider.

Some physician offices have contracted for independent review in order to identify coding and billing errors. After such a review, it may be found that in some cases codes do not reflect a high enough level of service, resulting in lower levels of reimbursement than are justified. An independent review can also discover cases where the codes used on claims would result in charges that are higher than the level of service provided. Based on this information, the medical office can improve its coding procedures to maximize income without risking fines or other legal proceedings. ■

What Would You Do? What Would You *Not* Do? RESPONSES

Case Study 1
Page 1062

What Did John Do?
❑ Double-checked the medical record to find out if the charge slip was filled out for the correct Peter Miller and to find out if the patient had been seen before.
❑ Charged the patient correctly as an established patient if it turned out that he had been seen by any practitioner in the practice within the past 3 years.
❑ Filled out a new charge slip if it turned out from reviewing the medical record that Peter Miller was in fact a new patient with a different birth date and address.
❑ Checked with the physician to find out if he had checked the wrong box on the charge slip.

What Did John Not Do?
❑ Did not just assume that whatever box the physician checked was correct.
❑ Did not enter a charge for a new patient if the patient was in fact an established patient.
❑ Did not tell the physician to be more careful in the future when filling out the charge slip.

What Would You Do/What Would You *Not* Do? Review John's response and place a checkmark next to the information you included in your response. List the additional information you included in your response.

_____
_____
_____
_____

Case Study 2
Page 1064

What Did John Do?
❑ Entered the charge for the office visit using the appropriate CPT code in the computer.

❑ Looked up the Medicare code for methylprednisolone in the HCPCS Level II manual, where he noted that the correct code depends on the dose given.
❑ Checked the medical record to identify the dose of methylprednisolone given to the patient and selected the correct HCPCS code from that information.

What Did John Not Do?
❑ Did not assume that all the correct codes were found on the charge slip.
❑ Did not guess at the dose of methylprednisolone because he knew what dose the physician usually gave.
❑ Did not assume that he could save time by asking the physician what dose was given.
❑ Did not bother the physician with the details of this coding situation.

What Would You Do/What Would You *Not* Do? Review John's response and place a checkmark next to the information you included in your response. List the additional information you included in your response.

_____
_____
_____
_____

Case Study 3
Page 1067

What Did John Do?
❑ Checked the ICD-9-CM manual to read all codes for diabetes mellitus and locate the most specific code (or codes) for diabetes type 1 with diabetic neuropathy. He found that the code 250.61 indicates diabetes type I with neurologic manifestations.
❑ Checked the ICD-9-CM manual to determine if an additional code is necessary for diabetic polyneuropathy. He found that the code 357.2 is used for polyneuropathy due to diabetes.
❑ Entered 250.61 as the first diagnosis (primary) and 357.2 as the second diagnosis (secondary).

Continued

What Would You Do? What Would You *Not* Do? RESPONSES—cont'd

What Did John Not Do?
❑ Did not assume that the code on the charge slip was the best code for the patient's condition.
❑ Did not rely on his memory for the best code(s) for this condition.
❑ Did not bother the physician with the details related to this coding situation.
❑ Did not code from the alphabetic index of the ICD-9-CM manual.

What Would You Do/What Would You *Not* Do? Review John's response and place a checkmark next to the information you included in your response. List the additional information you included in your response.

_____
_____
_____
_____

TERMINOLOGY REVIEW

Established patient A patient who has been receiving services from the same medical practice on a regular basis.

Modifier An addition to a *Current Procedural Terminology* code that indicates unusual circumstances related to the procedure, such as a more extensive procedure or two procedures performed in the same session.

Morphology The study of structure and form.

NEC A diagnosis code that is not elsewhere classified.

Neoplasm Abnormal growth or tumor.

New patient For billing purposes, a patient who has not received services during the previous 3 years from a physician in a medical practice.

NOS A diagnosis code that is not otherwise specified.

Panel A group of diagnostic tests done in one machine at the same time.

Surgical package Surgical services usually covered by a single procedure code that includes a preoperative visit, postoperative care, and local anesthesia (if applicable).

ON THE WEB

For Information on CPT Code Information:

CPT—American Medical Association: www.ama-assn. org

CPT codes for CLIA Waived Laboratory Tests: www.cms. hhs.gov/CLIA/downloads/CR4305.waivedtbl.pdf

For Information on ICD-9 and ICD-10 Codes and Information:

ICD-9—National Center for Health Statistics: www.cdc. gov/nchs/datawh.htm#International%20Classification

ICD-10—National Center for Health Statistics: www. cdc.gov/nchs/about/otheract/icd9/abticd10.htm

ICD-9—Centers for Medicare and Medicaid Services: www.cms.hhs.gov/ICD9ProviderDiagnosticCodes/ 05_CDROM.asp#TopOfPage

ICD-10—Centers for Medicare and Medicaid Services: www.cms.hhs.gov/ICD10/01_Overview.asp

 PREPARE FOR CERTIFICATION Visit the Evolve site at http://evolve.elsevier.com/Bonewit/today/ to actively Prepare for your Certification.

 *Check out the **Companion CD** bound with the book to access additional interactive activities.*

46

Medical Insurance

CAAHEP COMPETENCIES

Administrative Competencies
Process Insurance Claims
- Apply managed care policies and procedures.
- Apply third-party guidelines.
- Perform procedural coding.
- Perform diagnostic coding.
- Complete insurance claim forms.

General Competencies
Legal Concepts
- Demonstrate knowledge of federal and state health care legislation and regulations.

ABHES COMPETENCIES

Administrative Duties
- Apply computer concepts for office procedures.
- Apply managed care policies and procedures.
- Perform diagnostic coding.
- Complete insurance claim forms.

Financial Management
- Implement current procedural terminology and ICD-9 coding.
- Analyze and use current third-party guidelines for reimbursement.

KEY TERMS

assignment of benefits
benefit
birthday rule
capitation
carrier
CHAMPVA
coinsurance
coordination of benefits
copayment
crossover claim
deductible
diagnosis-related groups (DRGs)
explanation of benefits (EOB)
fee-for-service insurance
fiscal intermediary
guarantor

indemnity
managed care
Medicaid
Medicare
premium
primary care provider
primary insurance
reimbursement
resource-based relative value scale (RBRVS)
secondary insurance
signature on file (SOF)
subscriber
TRICARE
usual, customary, and reasonable (UCR)
workers' compensation

Introduction to Health Insurance

The growth and change in the structure of health insurance has affected American health care since the end of World War II. When industrialized countries like Canada and many countries in Western Europe were introducing government-provided health care, the United States was turning primarily to the private market to provide insurance coverage for Americans.

Today, despite the variety of health insurance plans and opportunities to obtain health insurance, many Americans still do not have health insurance. Market-based, regulatory, and legislative measures have failed to solve this problem.

HISTORY OF HEALTH INSURANCE

Health insurance had its beginnings in accident insurance, which was first sold in the mid-1800s. In exchange for a monthly payment by a customer, the insurance company agreed to replace lost income due to accident, and later due to a few specific illnesses, such as smallpox, diphtheria, typhoid, and scarlet fever.

In the 1930s a group of Dallas school teachers made an arrangement with Baylor Hospital to have any necessary hospital care provided in exchange for monthly premiums. This arrangement was the precursor to the Blue Cross and Blue Shield programs, which were incorporated as not-for-profit companies in each state. These programs provided

fee-for-service insurance. In this type of plan, the amount of payment for covered services is based on the amount charged for the services provided. Insurance may cover the total amount charged or a percentage of the total, depending on the patient's insurance plan. Other insurance companies began to offer health insurance using similar models. Labor unions began to negotiate for health insurance as an employee benefit that was not taxed as income in the same way as an increase in wages.

During World War II, Henry Kaiser created clinics in California to provide both in-patient and out-patient care for the workers in his shipyards. These clinics later opened themselves to other employers and individuals and became the Kaiser Permanente program. The employer paid a fixed amount per worker over a stated period of time for all necessary medical care. This method of payment is called **capitation,** and this type of health insurance is called a *prepaid health plan.* For many years Kaiser Permanente was the country's largest health maintenance organization (HMO). The philosophy behind the HMO movement was a belief that health care costs could be lowered if members were restricted to specific providers and facilities. Covered services also included preventative medical care in the hope of preventing conditions that would be expensive to treat. Over time, the HMO model broadened from one in which physicians were salaried employees and worked in a central facility to one in which HMOs contracted with private physicians in each community.

By the 1960s, many larger and even medium-sized businesses were providing company-paid health insurance benefits as a fringe benefit instead of increasing wages or salary. Health care costs began to increase faster than the general rate of inflation, with physicians beginning to earn large incomes. But certain groups of Americans—most notably the poor, elderly, and permanently disabled—were unable to obtain medical insurance through employment.

The federal government created two programs to try to close these large gaps in medical coverage. One was **Medicare,** the health insurance program for the elderly, disabled, and those with end-stage kidney disease. Medicare is paid for with federal taxes paid by employers and workers. The second government insurance program was **Medicaid,** the health insurance program for low-income individuals and families. The Medicaid program has different names in different states, and it is administered by each state. The federal government pays for the majority of required care and a smaller percentage of optional care, such as dental care, while the states pay for the rest. Each state sets its own criteria of eligibility for the Medicaid program.

Many senators, congresspersons, and physicians were against Medicare and Medicaid at the beginning, calling it "socialized medicine." But there were precedents for the government's involvement in paying for medical care. The Veterans Administration (VA) offered medical care for life for any man or woman who had seen active duty in the military, provided he or she wished to use the VA facilities. In addition, the Civilian Health and Medical Program of the Uniformed Services (CHAMPUS) program was developed to provide medical care at government expense for dependent spouses and children of active-duty military personnel. Today the former CHAMPUS program is called **TRICARE** (because there are three different plans). A companion program, Civilian Health and Medical Program of the Veterans Administration **(CHAMPVA),** covers dependent spouses and children of military veterans with service-connected disabilities.

At the beginning of the twenty-first century, American society is still trying to resolve insurance issues. Recently a prescription drug benefit has been added to the Medicare program. Some states, such as Massachusetts, have passed laws requiring residents to have medical insurance. There has also been a movement to expand health care insurance to children living in homes with incomes too high to be eligible for Medicaid but too low to afford private insurance. Low-wage workers often do not get health insurance through their employers or have insurance only for themselves and not their dependents. The State Children's Health Insurance Program (SCHIP), established in 1997, is overseen by the Centers for Medicare and Medicaid Services (CMS) but managed by the individual states. This program is reviewed every 10 years. A bill to reauthorize this program was passed in December 2007 but vetoed by the President on December 12, 2007, because he did not believe it met the needs of the individuals for whom it was intended.

OBTAINING HEALTH INSURANCE

Individuals and families have basically three ways to obtain health insurance coverage: through a group plan, by purchasing an individual policy, or through one of the government plans described earlier.

Most group plans are available through an employer. Larger employers generally have several different plans available. Often, they will pay the full cost of the lowest-priced plan for the employee, with the employee paying for coverage for other family members, or to purchase a more expensive plan.

Unionized workers often have very good health insurance because this has been a focus of much contract negotiation, especially in years when employers were unable to pay large wage increases.

Many small business owners can purchase insurance through group plans sponsored by the local chamber of commerce or a trade organization. Individuals sometimes have access to group plans through professional associations, or even college alumni associations. The self-employed are allowed to deduct a portion of their health insurance costs from their business income, as companies do.

As part of the process of gaining the right to sell health insurance in a particular state, most insurance plans are required to offer individual policies to individuals or families who are not covered under a group plan. An open-enrollment period usually occurs at least once per year for individuals to purchase coverage. Discussion has occurred at the federal level about allowing individuals or families who purchase their own insurance to claim a tax credit, or a larger tax deduction, for the cost.

Taxpayer-funded, or government, health insurance is usually provided as an entitlement when other conditions are met. For instance, when an individual reaches age 65, he or she is entitled to Medicare benefits if he or she has worked for at least 10 years in Medicare-covered employment. However, the individual must still file an application because the benefits do not begin automatically. An individual must meet other criteria for other government health insurance programs.

PAYING FOR HEALTH INSURANCE AND HEALTH CARE

The amount of money paid by the consumer to purchase health insurance is called the **premium.** This premium can be paid monthly, quarterly, semiannually, or annually. All or part of the premium may be paid by the person enrolled in the insurance plan or by the employer. In exchange for the payment of a premium, the insurance company or managed care plan agrees to provide payment for specific services provided by physicians, hospitals, laboratories, and other health care providers. The amount of money paid for a service covered by health insurance is called a **benefit.**

When the premium is paid by a person's employer, even if the employee is responsible for part of the cost, that premium is often paid with before-tax dollars. This means that the amount of the premium paid by the employer is not included in the amount of wages reported for the employee. The employee's portion may also be deducted before tax is calculated.

Depending on the type of insurance policy, a patient may have to make certain payments for medical services. Traditional, fee-for-service insurance plans and some managed care plans have a **deductible,** an amount of money that must be paid for services provided to an individual or a family member in a group plan every calendar year before any insurance payments. After the deductible is met, the patient may be required to pay a percentage of the allowed charge or a fixed fee every time service is received. If the patient is responsible for a specific percentage of the allowed charges (such as 20%), the patient portion is called **coinsurance.** An example of an insurance plan with coinsurance is Medicare Part B. If the patient is required to pay a fixed dollar amount every time he or she obtains medical services or fills a prescription, it is called a **copayment.**

FACTORS AFFECTING INSURANCE REIMBURSEMENT
Primary, Secondary, and Tertiary Insurance

If a person is covered by more than one insurance policy, the insurance to which the insurance claim is sent first is called the **primary insurance.** When the patient is the **subscriber,** the individual named on the insurance certificate, that insurance is the primary insurance. Insurance held by another subscriber (such as a spouse) that provides additional insurance coverage would be **secondary insurance.** If a third type of insurance also covers the patient, that insurance would be tertiary insurance. As a general rule, private insurance must be billed before government insurance, and Medicaid is always the last insurance to be billed.

Coordination of Benefits

Many households have two working adults, both of whom are covered under separate employer health benefits. **Coordination of benefits** is a term for the rules insurance companies use to coordinate the payments for medical services so that no provider is paid more than 100% of the charge for any service provided.

Coordination of benefits can become complex because each state writes its own rules and some policies have no coordination of benefits provisions. In addition, some individuals—especially those who work for large corporations with many offices or plants across the country—are often covered by insurance written outside of the state in which they live.

If both members of a couple have insurance with coordination of benefits provisions, the following rules apply.

1. If the employee who holds the policy is the patient, his or her insurance is the primary insurance for any services obtained. The spouse's or partner's insurance becomes the secondary insurance and can only be used to pay for any portion of the charge not covered by the primary insurance.

2. If a child is the patient, in most states the "birthday rule" applies. Under the **birthday rule,** the primary insurance for the child of parents who both have a family health plan is the insurance belonging to the working adult whose birthday comes first in the year. The insurance of the adult whose birthday is later is the secondary insurance.

3. When the patient is a child of divorced parents, the rules can get somewhat complicated. If a court has decreed that one parent is the "responsible party," that parent's policy provides the primary insurance. A responsible party ruling is often made in cases of joint custody, although the responsible party can also be a noncustodial parent. If no court ruling is in place, the custodial parent's policy is primary if the custodial parent has remarried. If there is no court ruling in place and the custodial parent has not remarried, the birthday rule remains in effect.

Coordination of benefits issues can be avoided if individuals in households with two working adults make modifications in their benefits. In order to reduce premium costs, some employers allow employees to take cash instead of health insurance if the family already has insurance. In cases where the company covers the complete cost for individual but not family coverage, only the husband or the wife needs to pay for family coverage. Of course, available plans should be compared for cost and benefits when deciding which policy to extend to family coverage.

4. If the patient is a Medicare recipient who also is covered by an employer's policy, the employer's policy is the primary insurance and Medicare is the secondary insurance. Patients with Medicare may also have supplemental insurance to cover what would normally be a patient responsibility. These plans, which are clearly defined as Medicare supplemental insurance, are considered secondary insurance.

Assignment of Benefits

Assignment of benefits allows the medical provider to bill the insurance company and receive payments directly, rather than having the patient pay for the service, then file for **reimbursement** with the insurance company. The patient must sign a form allowing the insurance company to pay the physician directly. This authorization is usually part of the new patient information form.

In many instances, however, if the physician or other medical provider agrees to accept assignment of benefits, he or she cannot bill the patient for any portion of the charge not paid by the insurance company except the deductible and copayment or coinsurance.

TYPES OF INSURANCE

Several different types of health insurance are currently available. When learning about insurance, it is helpful to learn the characteristics of different types of insurance, although the medical assistant may also be responsible for finding out more specific information related to individual insurance plans.

Fee-for-Service Plans

Traditionally private insurance plans provided payment, either to the physician or to the patient, for each medical service provided. These traditional plans are called *fee-for-service plans* or *indemnity plans*. The term **indemnity** means an obligation to compensate an individual for loss or damage. Until the late 1980s, fee-for-service plans dominated the health care industry. They were provided through private insurance companies and also through the Blue Cross and Blue Shield plans, which were established in each state as not-for-profit, quasi-governmental agencies. Since the late 1980s, the percentage of individuals covered under traditional fee-for-service plans has steadily decreased. Fee-for-service plans usually have a deductible, and the insurance pays for a percentage of the allowed charges (commonly 80%).

The insurance company determines the allowed charge in two ways.

Putting It All into Practice

My name is Sandra O'Keefe, and I am a registered medical assistant. I work in the office of three dermatologists. With the advances in laser technology, there are many new procedures for removing spider veins, birthmarks, scars, hair, and tattoos. We also do Mohs micrographic surgery, a technique that removes skin cancers one layer at time with immediate tissue analysis. Using this technique the physicians can be sure that all malignant cells have been removed while taking a minimum of healthy tissue.

Billing in our office is somewhat complicated because many of the procedures are not covered by insurance. In general, insurance companies will pay for procedures that are medically necessary, like removal of skin cancers. They do not cover procedures that are strictly cosmetic, such as removal of spider veins (small varicose veins on the skin). Then there are some procedures that sometimes are covered by insurance and sometimes are not, such as the removal of birthmarks on the face.

When a procedure is medically necessary, we have to obtain preauthorization from the patient's insurance company and sometimes we need to provide documentation for the insurance company to review before they give their approval. When a procedure is not covered, we have to be sure that the patient is willing to pay for it and knows how much it will cost. We can help arrange for the patient to obtain financing in order to pay for the procedure over a period of time.

Our physicians accept several different types of insurance including government plans, managed care plans, and traditional insurance plans. When patients are covered by managed care plans, we have to be sure that they have the proper referrals to cover each office visit, as well as the procedure. In some cases, the insurance covers a consultation visit but the proposed treatment plan is not approved, and then the patients must decide about paying for any recommended procedure themselves. We do our best to complete all of the paperwork to obtain insurance coverage for our patients, but we are limited by the rules of each insurance company. ∎

Prepare for Success

What Would You Do? What Would You *Not* Do?

Case Study 1

Diane Bennett is a 35-year-old woman who has come to the office for treatment of a lesion on her neck. She has been referred from her primary care physician for up to three visits for consultation, diagnostic studies, and treatment. She is seen by one of the dermatologists in the practice who recommends that the lesion be removed surgically in the office with a biopsy. During this visit, the patient tells the physician that she has two other lesions she would like to have removed, one on her arm and one on her abdomen. The physician inspects the lesions and asks Sandra to contact the patient's managed care plan for authorization to treat the additional lesions. The patient says, "My physician gave me a referral to be treated by you. What's the problem? If these lesions need to be removed, I don't want any delay." ∎

1. Through a fee schedule. A fee schedule says the insurance company will pay the specified percentage of a particular amount for a particular procedure. Any additional charges are the patient's responsibility.
2. Through service benefits, which define covered services, but not the exact payments. Under service benefit plans, the insurance company will agree to pay the specified percentage of charges that are **usual, customary, and reasonable (UCR)** for the procedure and the state or region of the country it was performed in. The usual fee is the amount that a physician usually charges or charges most often. The customary fee is the amount charged by physicians in the same specialty in the same geographic area (usually the 90th percentile amount of the charges of all physicians in the area. A reasonable fee meets the two criteria described earlier or is justifiable if there are special circumstances. Based on statistics kept by the insurance company, the fee actually charged by the physician is reviewed. The insurance company's payment is based on its own determination of what is UCR.

Under a traditional fee-for-service plan, a patient can make an appointment with any doctor, in any specialty, he or she wishes, and the insurance will pay the designated amount for the services. Some plans do have lists of approved providers for whom they pay 100 percent of charges and only pay a percentage of charges for other providers (similar to a preferred provider organization [PPO], discussed in more detail later in the chapter).

Managed Care Plans

HMOs were introduced around the time of World War II, when the Kaiser plan was formed. They have evolved into many forms. Both private insurance companies and government insurance plans offer HMOs, as well as other types of managed care plans. The various HMO models and their descendents, collectively, are known as **managed care.** This term is used in two ways: It describes the movement to control health care costs while improving preventative care and is a general term for insurance programs reimbursing care provided in this way. Managed care plans negotiate reimbursement amounts and limit patients to those providers and facilities with whom they have contracts.

Most insurance plans today involve some form of managed care. The patient's care is managed by the insurance plan in several ways:

1. Each patient chooses one physician as a **primary care provider,** a physician who provides most of the patient's care and also determines what other medical services the patient requires.
2. Care may be restricted to providers, laboratories, and hospitals that have accepted the insurance plan's fee schedule or capitation payment plan.
3. The patient may or may not have access to providers and services outside the insurance plan. If there are tiers of providers, the patient must usually pay more for services obtained outside the plan. In addition, the patient may be subject to balance billing if he or she seeks service from a provider who is outside the managed care plan. This means that the patient must pay the difference between the amount allowed by insurance and the amount charged for services.
4. The insurance plan may require referrals from a primary care provider for services including consultations with specialists, therapy such as physical therapy or speech therapy, care outside of the medical office, and some diagnostic tests. The primary care provider functions as a "gatekeeper" to limit and approve access to specialty services. (The process of referrals is discussed in detail in Chapter 40.)
5. The insurance plan usually requires preauthorization for surgery and other procedures from the insurance plan itself.

Health Maintenance Organization Models

In the original HMO concept, all medical care was provided for 1 year for a fixed premium, with no deductibles or coinsurance. The patient was only responsible for a fixed amount for each visit or prescription (copayment).

HMOs have always practiced preventive medicine, on the theory that much of the cost of medical care can be eliminated through routine care by primary care providers. To reduce the cost of specialty care, primary care providers including physicians, nurse practitioners, and physician assistants act as "gatekeepers," seeing patients first for nearly all illnesses and referring them to specialists only when necessary. HMOs are usually incorporated and regulated in one state. They are subject to regulation requiring more comprehensive quality assurance programs than other types of insurance. Medical record audits allow the HMO to check the records of any physician's patients to make sure the physician is not performing unnecessary procedures or ordering unnecessary tests.

Each HMO works in its own way, and each one has a procedure book for providers. The medical assistant should familiarize himself or herself with the various requirements of each particular HMO, including such things as whether a referral to a specialist must be in writing or can be given over the telephone. Each precertification and some referrals must be authorized by the HMO, and the authorization number should be noted on all of the certification or referral paperwork.

The medical assistant must also know which laboratory can do laboratory work and where patients can be referred for diagnostic follow-up. Most HMOs have contracts with a limited number of laboratories and/or medical facilities and will pay only for services provided by an approved facility.

Staff Model Health Maintenance Organization

The staff model HMO hires its physicians directly and pays them a salary for providing health care to members. The patient can receive care only at plan facilities. This type of plan was more common when the HMO movement first began and is rare today.

Network Health Maintenance Organization

The network model HMO contracts with various group practices for services to its members. Typically, the physicians also see patients who have other types of insurance. The HMO members must be referred to in-network providers if possible. Out-of-network coverage is allowed only in cases of emergency or urgent services.

Other Managed Care Models

Health care plans that are regulated by state and federal laws as insurance plans instead of HMOs may still maintain many features of managed care. Depending on the state, there may be separate regulatory agencies.

Preferred Provider Organization

A PPO provides coverage for in-network and out-of-network services to its members, but there is a financial incentive to use in-network services. These plans usually have deductibles and coinsurance. The patient may be required to pay a percentage of in-network costs, but they must usually pay a higher percentage of out-of-network costs.

Exclusive Provider Organization

An exclusive provider organization (EPO) is similar in structure and operation to a PPO, but its members must receive all health care services only within the network in order for them to be covered. If a member receives health services outside the network, the cost will not be covered by insurance. In this way, the EPO is similar to an HMO, but its legal structure is different because it is regulated as an insurance plan and not an HMO.

Independent Practice Association

The physicians of an independent practice association (IPA) work independently in the community but formally organize a physician association. They are paid from funds collected from subscribers of the health plan minus administrative costs, marketing and sales costs, and other overhead costs. IPAs often have a "hold back"—a portion of the agreed fee that is not paid to the physicians until after the end of the association's fiscal year, when the association determines if it has earned a profit or had financial losses. This way, the association requires member physicians to share some business risk.

Point-of-Service Plans

The point-of-service (POS) plan combines an in-network plan that is regulated as an HMO with an out-of-network plan that is regulated as an insurance plan. Members receive two certificates, one for an HMO for services provided by in-network providers and one for an indemnity carrier for out-of-network services. The POS plan functions as a combination of an HMO and a PPO. Members have a higher financial obligation when they seek out-of-network services. When they remain within the network, their only financial obligation is a copayment each time they seek service.

Government Plans

Medicare

Medicare is a federally funded plan administered by the CMS. It pays for health care services for the following individuals:

- Retired individuals older than 65 who are on Social Security
- Retired railroad employees and some retired federal employees
- Individuals who have been permanently disabled for 2 years
- Blind individuals
- Individuals with chronic renal disease who require dialysis or kidney transplant
- Kidney donors

The Medicare plan has several parts. Medicare Part A provides coverage of hospitalization services. Medicare Part B covers physician and other provider services. Together these two parts make up what is called the *Original Medicare Plan*. The patient's Medicare card identifies what type of coverage the patient has (Figure 46-1). Medicare Part C was introduced in 1997 to provide more choice in the types of available plans. Several Medicare Advantage Plans, including managed care plans and fee-for service plans, replace the Original Medicare Plan if recipients choose them. Medicare Part D was passed in 2003 and went into effect in 2006. It adds a prescription drug benefit to the Original Medicare Plan and Medicare Advantage Plans that did not include this benefit.

Individuals 65 and older on Social Security, those younger than 65 but who collect Social Security disability benefits, and those who receive railroad retirement benefits are automatically enrolled in Medicare Part A. There is no premium for participation in Medicare Part A. The first day of each hospital admission is not paid by Medicare; this is the Part A deductible. Medicare Part A is funded through a tax paid by working individuals on all of their earned income.

Anyone eligible for Medicare Part A may also obtain Part B coverage. However, they must apply and pay a premium to obtain Medicare Part B or to enroll in one of the Medicare Advantage Plans. Former federal employees, who receive federal employee pensions rather than Social Security and are not covered by Medicare Part A, can purchase Medicare Part B coverage.

Medicare claims are handled by insurance companies that contract with CMS. A different **fiscal intermediary** (insurance company that contracts to review and pay Medicare claims) processes claims in each state. The amount of payment for any service is standardized nationally.

Payment for hospitals for claims under Part A is based on **diagnosis-related groups (DRGs),** a system that classifies patients according to the diagnosis, treatment, and length of hospital stay. The patient is assigned a DRG based on the primary diagnosis, and the payment made by Medicare to a hospital is determined by the DRG rather than the length of time the patient remains in the hospital.

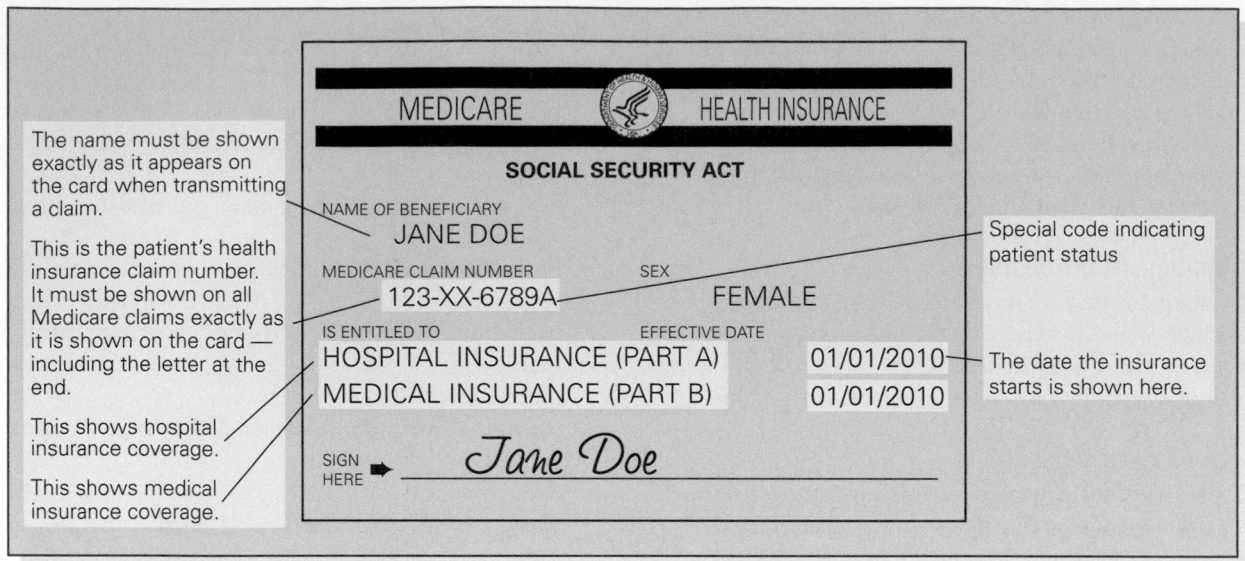

The name must be shown exactly as it appears on the card when transmitting a claim.

This is the patient's health insurance claim number. It must be shown on all Medicare claims exactly as it is shown on the card — including the letter at the end.

This shows hospital insurance coverage.

This shows medical insurance coverage.

MEDICARE ⬤ HEALTH INSURANCE

SOCIAL SECURITY ACT

NAME OF BENEFICIARY
JANE DOE

MEDICARE CLAIM NUMBER   SEX
123-XX-6789A   FEMALE

IS ENTITLED TO   EFFECTIVE DATE
HOSPITAL INSURANCE (PART A)   01/01/2010
MEDICAL INSURANCE (PART B)   01/01/2010

SIGN ➡ *Jane Doe*
HERE

Special code indicating patient status

The date the insurance starts is shown here.

Figure 46-1. Identification card for Medicare. (From Fordney M: *Insurance handbook for the medical office,* ed 10, St. Louis, 2008, Saunders.)

Since 1992, payments for services under Part B have been based on a **resource-based relative value scale (RBRVS)** developed by researchers at Harvard University. This system establishes relative value units for each procedure based on the amount of work involved, overhead expenses, and cost of malpractice insurance. The amount Medicare pays for each relative value unit is then adjusted annually; it is also adjusted for different geographic areas (because overhead and malpractice cost may vary). An annual fee schedule is available online for identifying the amount Medicare pays for specific procedures.

If a physician participates in the Medicare program, the office must bill for the patient, accept assignment of benefits, and accept Medicare's determination of the allowable charge for the service. Under Part B, after paying an annual deductible of $135 (for 2008), the patient is responsible for 20% of the allowable charge.

If a physician does not participate in the Medicare program, usually he or she does not accept assignment of benefits but collects the bill from the patient up to a limiting charge (percent limit on fees above the fee-schedule amount) set by legislation.

Many patients purchase additional insurance (known as *Medicare supplemental* or *Medigap insurance*) that covers the annual deductible and 20% coinsurance for Part B, as well as the charge for the first day of a hospital stay (the deductible for Part A). Patients in most Medicare Advantage plans do not need supplemental insurance. Some patients may also be covered by employment plans after retirement. In this case, Medicare is the primary insurance and the Medigap or employment retiree plan is secondary. If a person continues to work after 65 and obtains insurance through employment, that insurance is the primary insurance for that individual and Medicare is the secondary insurance.

Medicaid

Medicaid, formally Title XIX (Title 19) of the 1965 amendments to the Social Security laws, provides for the federal government to give each state a grant to be used toward care of low-income residents. Along with the federal government's basic funding comes an obligation for the states to provide basic health care. States may add coverage for other care to their Medicaid laws but must pay for most of those costs, with the federal government paying a portion. The name of the Medicaid program, as well as procedures for gaining access to it, varies from state to state.

A patient's Medicaid eligibility must be checked at every office visit. In many states patients have a Medicaid card similar to a credit card with a magnetic stripe (Figure 46-2). The medical assistant uses a machine similar to a credit card reader to verify the patient's eligibility as was discussed in Chapter 37.

Physicians may agree or decline to provide services to Medicaid patients. If they agree to treat Medicaid patients, physicians must agree to accept the state's payment for services, without billing patients for any difference between the state's payment and the actual charge.

Adults and children receiving basic welfare grants from a state are automatically eligible for Medicaid. Also, the children in many working households are eligible for Medicaid benefits if the parents' pay is low enough to put the family below the poverty line or if employee-provided medical insurance covers only the employed parent.

In addition to paying for medical services, Medicaid also covers the cost of long-term nursing home care for poor elderly and disabled individuals. Because nursing home care is so expensive, 20% of Medicaid beneficiaries—the elderly poor living in nursing homes—account for 70% to 80% of the cost of the Medicaid program.

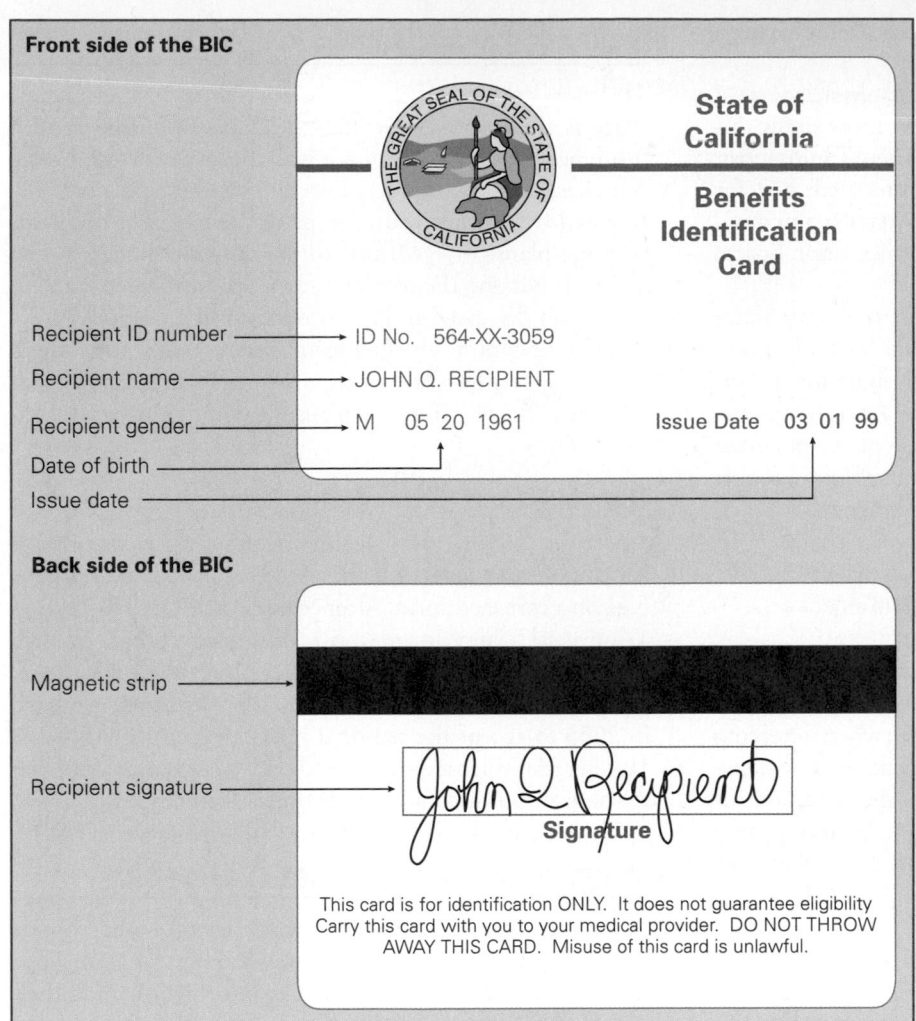

Front side of the BIC

THE GREAT SEAL OF THE STATE OF CALIFORNIA

State of
California

Benefits
Identification
Card

Recipient ID number ———→ ID No.   564-XX-3059

Recipient name ———→ JOHN Q. RECIPIENT

Recipient gender ———→ M   05 20 1961   Issue Date   03 01 99

Date of birth

Issue date

Back side of the BIC

Magnetic strip ———→

Recipient signature ———→   *John Q Recipient*
                              Signature

This card is for identification ONLY. It does not guarantee eligibility
Carry this card with you to your medical provider. DO NOT THROW
AWAY THIS CARD. Misuse of this card is unlawful.

Figure 46-2. Plastic identification card for Medi-Cal (Medicaid). (From Fordney M: *Insurance handbook for the medical office,* ed 10, St. Louis, 2008, Saunders.)

If a patient has both Medicare and Medicaid insurance, Medicare is the primary insurance. After processing, it will automatically be sent to Medicaid. For this reason, it may be called a **crossover claim**—a claim that automatically crosses over from Medicare to Medicaid.

State Children's Health Insurance Plan

In 1998 the federal government provided funding for states to establish SCHIP to further assist children whose parents cannot afford insurance for them. These programs are administered and partially funded on a state-wide basis. In some states eligible children are enrolled in the state's Medicaid plan. The medical assistant should familiarize himself or herself with the state requirements for this plan.

Workers' Compensation

Workers' compensation insurance covers lost wages and the cost of medical treatment for workers injured on the job or who fall ill due to workplace hazards or disease. Each state has its own workers' compensation program. The cost of workers' compensation insurance is paid by employers. The premium for a given employer depends on how many previous employees have made claims under workers' compensation.

Workers are required to make a prompt claim for workers' compensation coverage after an accident or the onset of an illness. In many states, the employer and the insurance company issuing the policy have the right to choose the physician who treats the patient.

If a patient visits his or her regular primary care physician and says the illness or injury is workplace related, the medical assistant should check promptly with the employer to verify that the employee has made a report and that the care will be covered by the company's workers' compensation plan.

If a patient of the medical practice is seen for a workers' compensation case, separate medical and financial records should be established for that patient. Laws require that requests for medical records for compensation cases must contain only information associated with the work-related injury. If a workers' appeal board needs work-related injury records, it is important that no other medical information about the patient be released.

For a workers' compensation case, the physician must file a Physician's First Report of Injury. In most states this must be done within 72 hours of the patient's initial visit for a workplace injury. Four copies are prepared: one for the employer's compensation insurance **carrier** (company), one for the employer, one for the state compensation board, and one for the patient's medical record.

In addition to the report, the physician submits a statement of services to the insurance carrier. The physician must sign all forms because a stamped signature is not accepted for workers' compensation cases. As in most government programs, the physician must accept the payment provided as payment in full. The physician submits a report and a statement monthly until care is completed.

Insurance Plans for Dependents of Members of the Armed Services and Veterans

CHAMPUS was established by the federal government in 1966 to provide health benefits for the dependent spouses and children of active military personnel when receiving care from civilian physicians and health facilities. The name has been changed to TRICARE with the addition of managed care services because there are three plans available to members of the armed services: TRICARE Standard (formerly CHAMPUS), TRICARE Prime, and TRICARE Extra.

TRICARE Standard benefits are available to dependent spouses and children of active-duty military personnel, dependent spouses and children of military personnel who died while on active duty, and military retirees (and their dependents) who are not old enough to be eligible for Medicare.

TRICARE Prime is an HMO-type plan with optional participation. In addition to the services covered by TRICARE Standard, it includes preventive and primary care services. There is an annual enrollment fee for families whose member of the armed forces is not on active duty. Some physicians are contracted to provide service to TRICARE beneficiaries at discounted rates to TRICARE Prime members.

TRICARE Extra allows an individual to seek care from a network provider on a visit-by-visit basis, receiving a discount on medical services provided and a lower copayment than when using TRICARE Standard.

In 1973 the federal government created CHAMPVA to provide both inpatient and outpatient medical benefits for the dependent spouses and children of veterans who have suffered total, permanent, service-connected disabilities and for surviving spouses and children of veterans who have died as a result of those service-connected disabilities. The nearest VA Medical Center determines eligibility and issues an identification card, but the CHAMPVA-covered patients are allowed to choose their own physicians and other medical service providers.

INSURANCE CLAIM FORMS

The most commonly used insurance form in the medical office is the CMS-1500. This form began as the Health Insurance Claim Form, which was approved for use by the American Medical Association in 1975. It was gradually accepted by various insurance plans for payment of claims by those plans. In 1990 this form was revised and printed in red. It became the required form for Medicare claims in 1992. It is discussed in greater detail in the next section.

Another commonly used form is the UB-04 form, which is used by hospitals and other institutions to submit paper insurance claims. It has replaced the old UB-92 (CMS-1450) form.

The CMS-1500 (8/05) Claim Form

Since the 1950s, the Health Insurance Association of America has sought to have all medical insurance claims filed on a common form. After considerable work to develop a universal claim form, most insurance companies will accept the CMS-1500 form, either alone or as an attachment to the company's own form. This form was updated in 2005 to accept the national provider identifier (NPI), a 10-digit identifier required for all health care providers that replaces all previous identification (ID) numbers.

COMPLETING THE INSURANCE CLAIM FORM

In the medical office, the medical assistant usually prepares insurance claims using a computer billing program. The medical assistant must know what information should be included so that each claim form can be reviewed before printing or submitting the claim electronically (Figure 46-3; Procedure 46-1).

Carrier Information

The name and address of the insurance company to which the claim will be sent is printed in the top section of the insurance claim form. This address should be entered without punctuation except for the hyphen in the ZIP + 5 code.

Patient and Insured Information

Patient Information

The patient section contains the patient's basic demographic information. This includes the patient's name, address, date of birth, and sex, as well as the patient's signature allowing the physician's office to release medical information to the insurance company for purposes of verifying the services provided.

It also identifies whether the physician accepts assignment of benefits, which is authorized by the patient's signature. Instead of asking patients to sign every insurance claim, the phrase **signature on file** or the abbreviation **SOF** is often used to indicate that the office maintains a copy of the patient's signature authorizing submission of the claim.

Figure 46-3. The CMS-1500 claim form (8/05 revision).

PROCEDURE 46-1

What Would You Do? What Would You *Not* Do?

Case Study 2

Daniel Litton is a 14-year-old new patient who has an appointment with one of the dermatologists in the office. He is brought to the office by his mother, who helps him fill out the new patient information form. In the section for insurance information, his mother indicates that he is covered by family insurance plans through both his father and his mother. His mother says, "I hope you will bill my insurance for him because I have better coverage for things like this." ▪

Subscriber and Insurance Information

This part of the insurance claim form includes the following information about the subscriber (sometimes called the *insured,* or the *guarantor*): the subscriber's name, address, and relationship to the patient. (In medical billing programs, **guarantor** is a term for individuals with financial responsibility who are not patients.) In addition, for employer-sponsored plans, the employer's name is listed. The subscriber has an ID number. In a family plan, other family members may use the same number or the basic ID number, followed by a one- or two-digit number, such as 2 or 02 for the spouse and succeeding numbers for the children. For a group plan there is also a group number that is common to all members who obtain insurance from that employer or through that group.

If there is insurance in the name of a second party, this is also included on the claim form with the appropriate information about the insurance policy and ID (policy) and group numbers. On every claim form, information must be included to identify whether the claim relates to a work injury, auto accident, or other accident. This helps the

Table 46-1 Place of Service Codes Used for Billing in the Medical Office

Code	Place of Service
11	Office
12	Home
21	Inpatient hospitalization
22	Outpatient hospitalization
23	Emergency room—hospital
24	Ambulatory surgical center
25	Birthing center
36	Military hospital or clinic
31	Skilled nursing facility
32	Nursing facility
33	Custodial care facility

From Hunt SA: *Saunders fundamentals of medical assisting,* St. Louis, 2007, Saunders.

insurance company identify which insurance is responsible for covering the claim.

Physician Information

The information about the medical service provided is filled in the lower half of the insurance claim form. In addition to information about the medical problem, the *International Classification of Diseases, Ninth Revision, Clinical Modification* code for each diagnosis (up to four) is listed. Each procedure must be linked to a primary diagnosis code to justify the procedure. On the lower lines, information about each procedure is given, including the date of service, place of service, pointer to the procedure code, charge for the service, number of units being billed, and ID number for the provider of each service. See Table 46-1 for a list of codes commonly used for place of service when billing from the medical office.

PROCEDURE 46-1 Completing/Reviewing the CMS-1500 Insurance Claim Form

Outcome Complete or review a CMS-1500 insurance claim form.

Equipment/Supplies

- Patient information
- Patient account or ledger
- Copy of the patient's insurance card or computer patient information screen

- Insurance claim form
- Computer with medical billing program
- Printer

1. Procedural Step. Assemble information needed to prepare an insurance claim, including a claim form, information about the patient, the patient account or ledger, a copy of the patient's insurance card, or insurance information.

2. Procedural Step. Enter or review information as required on the CMS-1500 form according to the following information. If paper claims will be submitted to be scanned by optical character recognition, use only capital letters and do not use commas, dollar signs, or other punctuation.

Principle. Most insurance companies use optical scanning to digitize information on paper claims, and the equipment works best following the guidelines outlined earlier.

3. **Procedural Step.** In the carrier section, enter or validate the name and address of the insurance company to which the claim will be sent using the following format:

Line 1: Name of carrier
Line 2: First line of address
Line 3: Second line of address (if needed)
Line 4: City [space] State [space] ZIP

Example:

3 line address: STANDARD HEALTH CARE
                    1500 SUMMIT AVENUE
                    WESTERN XY 45000

4 line address: STANDARD HEALTH CARE
                    SUITE 620
                    1500 SUMMIT AVENUE
                    WESTERN XY 45000

4. **Procedural Step.** Complete or review the patient and insured information of the claim form.

Box 1—The type of insurance is indicated with an X. Only one box can be marked. Insurance obtained through employment is a Group Health Plan.

Box 1a—The ID number of the individual who is insured as shown on the insurance card.

Box 2—The patient's last name, first name, and middle initial (separated by spaces).

Box 3—The patient's date of birth in the format MM DD YYYY and the patient's sex (M or F) marked with an X.

Box 4—The name of the insured using the format last name, first name, middle initial (separated by spaces). If the patient and the insured are the same, this box does not have to be completed.

Box 5—The patient's mailing address beginning with the street. Use the two-letter state code. Do not use commas, periods, or other punctuation in the address with the exception of the hyphen in a nine-digit ZIP code. Do not use a hyphen or space as a separator in the telephone number. Complete this box if Box 4 is completed.

Box 6—An X in the box that defines the patient's relationship to the insured (i.e., person whose name is on the insurance policy). The choices include self □ spouse □ child □ other □.

Box 7—The insured's mailing address beginning with the street. Use the two-letter state code. Do not use commas, periods, or other punctuation in the address with the exception of the hyphen in a nine-digit ZIP code. Do not use a hyphen or space as a separator in the telephone number. Complete this box if Box 4 is completed.

Box 8—The boxes that best describe the patient's marital status and employment status are checked.

If the patient has insurance through the employer, assume that he or she is employed. If the patient is a college student (older than 18), it is important to determine if he or she is a full-time student. The choices include single □ married □ other □ and employed □ full-time student □ part-time student □.

Box 9—If there is secondary insurance, the insured's name using the format described for Box 4.

Box 9a-d—If there is secondary insurance, the subscriber policy (ID) or group number, subscriber date of birth, sex, employer, and insurance plan name.

Box 10a-c—Information related to the cause of the patient's condition(s). The correct boxes are checked (yes or no) to answer the questions. If the patient's condition is caused by an automobile accident, the state where the accident occurred is identified using the correct two-letter code.

Box 11—The insured's policy group or FECA number.

Box 11a-d—If the patient is the insured, only box 11d must be completed. The insured's date of birth in the format MM DD YYYY and the insured's sex (M or F) marked with an X. The insured's employer and insurance plan name. An X is used in the correct box to indicate if there is additional insurance (yes or no). If "yes" is selected, Box 9a-d is filled out.

Box 12—If the office has on file the patient's signature on a similar permission form, the initials "SOF" or the words "Signature on File" are placed in this box. Otherwise, the patient must sign and date the form.

Box 13—If the office has on file the patient's signature on a similar permission form, the initials "SOF" or the words "Signature on File" are placed in this box. Otherwise, the patient must sign and date the form.

Continued

PROCEDURE 46-1

PROCEDURE 46-1 Completing/Reviewing the CMS-1500 Insurance Claim Form—cont'd

4

1. MEDICARE	MEDICAID	TRICARE CHAMPUS	CHAMPVA	GROUP HEALTH PLAN	FECA BLK LUNG	OTHER	1a. INSURED'S I.D. NUMBER	(For Program in Item 1)
(Medicare #)	(Medicaid #)	(Sponsor's SSN)	(Member ID#)	(SSN or ID)	(SSN)	(ID)		

2. PATIENT'S NAME (Last Name, First Name, Middle Initial) | 3. PATIENT'S BIRTH DATE MM DD YY   SEX   M ☐ F ☐ | 4. INSURED'S NAME (Last Name, First Name, Middle Initial)

5. PATIENT'S ADDRESS (No., Street) | 6. PATIENT RELATIONSHIP TO INSURED   Self ☐ Spouse ☐ Child ☐ Other ☐ | 7. INSURED'S ADDRESS (No., Street)

CITY | STATE | 8. PATIENT STATUS   Single ☐ Married ☐ Other ☐ | CITY | STATE

ZIP CODE | TELEPHONE (Include Area Code) ( ) | Employed ☐ Full-Time Student ☐ Part-Time Student ☐ | ZIP CODE | TELEPHONE (Include Area Code) ( )

9. OTHER INSURED'S NAME (Last Name, First Name, Middle Initial) | 10. IS PATIENT'S CONDITION RELATED TO: | 11. INSURED'S POLICY GROUP OR FECA NUMBER

a. OTHER INSURED'S POLICY OR GROUP NUMBER | a. EMPLOYMENT? (Current or Previous) ☐ YES ☐ NO | a. INSURED'S DATE OF BIRTH MM DD YY   SEX M ☐ F ☐

b. OTHER INSURED'S DATE OF BIRTH MM DD YY   SEX M ☐ F ☐ | b. AUTO ACCIDENT?   PLACE (State) ☐ YES ☐ NO | b. EMPLOYER'S NAME OR SCHOOL NAME

c. EMPLOYER'S NAME OR SCHOOL NAME | c. OTHER ACCIDENT? ☐ YES ☐ NO | c. INSURANCE PLAN NAME OR PROGRAM NAME

d. INSURANCE PLAN NAME OR PROGRAM NAME | 10d. RESERVED FOR LOCAL USE | d. IS THERE ANOTHER HEALTH BENEFIT PLAN? ☐ YES ☐ NO *If yes*, return to and complete item 9 a-d.

READ BACK OF FORM BEFORE COMPLETING & SIGNING THIS FORM.
12. PATIENT'S OR AUTHORIZED PERSON'S SIGNATURE I authorize the release of any medical or other information necessary to process this claim. I also request payment of government benefits either to myself or to the party who accepts assignment below.

SIGNED _____ DATE _____

13. INSURED'S OR AUTHORIZED PERSON'S SIGNATURE I authorize payment of medical benefits to the undersigned physician or supplier for services described below.

SIGNED _____

PATIENT AND INSURED INFORMATION

Patient and insurance information section.

5. Procedural Step. Complete the physician or supplier information using information from the patient charge slip.

Principle. If incomplete or incorrect information about primary and secondary insurance plans is given, the claim will be denied.

Boxes 14-16—Not usually required for Medicare, Medicaid, TRICARE, CHAMPVA, and most private insurance. If they must be filled in, the dates are obtained from the patient's medical record and/or the physician.

Box 17—Name of the physician who referred the patient.

Box 17a—Non-NPI number of the referring physician. The qualifier is entered from the table below (following "Box 17b") in the first section to identify the type of number. For Medicare and Medicaid, the NPI number must be used after May 23, 2008.

Box 17b—If the referring physician has an NPI number, the 10-digit number is entered in this box instead of completing box 17a.

Two-digit qualifiers for use in fields 17A, 24I, 24J, 32B, and 33B if the NPI number is not known:

0B	State license number
1B	Blue Shield provider number
1C	Medicare provider number
1D	Medicaid provider number
1G	Provider UPIN
1H	CHAMPUS ID number
EI	Employer's ID number
G2	Provider commercial number
LU	Location number
N5	Provider plan network ID number
SY	Social Security number (This may not be used for Medicare.)
X5	State industrial accident provider number

Box 18—If the patient's claim is for a hospitalization, either a visit or surgery performed when the patient was hospitalized, the dates of hospitalization. Otherwise, the box is left blank.

Box 19—Left blank unless instructed by a specific insurance carrier to use this box for information specific to that carrier.

Box 20—"No" is usually checked. If the office paid for outside laboratory services that are not itemized on one of the lines in Box 24, "yes" is checked.

Box 21—The ICD-9-CM code for up to four diagnoses. Use the most specific code possible. Leave a space for the period on the form.

Box 22—Left blank unless the claim is a Medicaid resubmission, when the code and original reference number are entered.

Box 23—Left blank unless a referral, preauthorization, or precertification number was assigned by the insurance company.

6. **Procedural Step.** Enter information in Box 24 on lines 1-6 for each procedure that is being billed to the insurance company. For more than six procedures, complete an additional CMS-1500 form.

Box 24A—The date service began under the "From" section in the format MM DD YYYY in the unshaded area. If the service occurred on one day only, the "To" section is left blank; otherwise, the date service ended.

Box 24B—The code for the place of service from Table 46-1.

Box 24C—This box is usually left blank. For some carriers, a "Y" is placed in this box if the service is an emergency service.

Box 24D—The CPT or HCPCS code and modifier(s) (if any) in the unshaded area.

Box 24E—The number(s) (from 1 to 4) that point to ICD-9-CM code(s) in Box 21 that justify the procedure. Only one digit can be used in this box for Medicare claims.

Box 24F—The charges in the unshaded area, leaving a space between the number of dollars and the number of cents instead of using a decimal point.

Box 24G—If charging for more than one of the same procedure (e.g., visits to a hospitalized patient on 3 consecutive days), the number of units of the procedure charged in the unshaded area. Otherwise, the number 1.

Box 24H—Left blank unless the patient is enrolled in the Medicaid program for early, periodic, screening, diagnosis, and service (EPSDT).

Box 24I—The shaded area is used to enter the qualifier from the table provided earlier (see Step 5) for a provider ID number other than the NPI number.

Box 24J—The ID number of the provider of the service. If the 10-digit NPI number is used, it is entered in the unshaded area. If another ID number is used, it is entered in the shaded area.

7. **Procedural Step.** Complete the remaining boxes on the CMS-1500 form.

Box 25—The tax ID number. If the Social Security number of an individual physician is used, box "SSN" is checked. If the employer ID number of a group practice is used, box "EIN" is checked.

Box 26—The patient account number. The box is left blank if there is no patient account number. Hyphens should not be used in this box.

Box 27—If the physician accepts assignment of benefits, an X is placed in the "yes" box. If assignment of benefits is not accepted, an X is placed in the "no" box.

Box 28—The total charges with a space between the number of dollars and the number of cents.

Box 29—The amount paid toward the covered charges, including any copayment. If the amount is zero, the box is left blank.

Box 30—The balance due with a space between the number of dollars and the number of cents.

Box 31—SOF, Signature on File, or the physician's legal signature including credentials and the date.

Box 32—The name, address, city, state, and ZIP code of the facility where the services were provided without punctuation. If services were provided at the same address as the billing address, this box, as well as 32a and 32b, can be left blank.

Box 32a—The 10-digit NPI number of the service facility location.

Box 32b—Another ID number for the service facility location beginning with the qualifier from the table provided earlier (see Step 5).

Box 33—The name, address, and telephone number of the physician group or supplier of services without punctuation. The telephone number is entered to the right of the title of the field without a hyphen. A hyphen is used in a nine-digit zip code after the fifth digit.

Box 33a—The 10-digit NPI number of the physician group or supplier of services.

Box 33b—Another ID number for the physician group or supplier of services beginning with the qualifier from the table provided earlier (see Step 5).

8. **Procedural Step.** Submit claim according to office policy. Copy a paper form before mailing, and keep the copy in an insurance claims file.

Continued

PROCEDURE 46-1 Completing/Reviewing the CMS-1500 Insurance Claim Form—cont'd

7

14. DATE OF CURRENT: MM DD YY ◄ ILLNESS (First symptom) OR INJURY (Accident) OR PREGNANCY(LMP)
15. IF PATIENT HAS HAD SAME OR SIMILAR ILLNESS. GIVE FIRST DATE MM DD YY
16. DATES PATIENT UNABLE TO WORK IN CURRENT OCCUPATION FROM MM DD YY TO MM DD YY

17. NAME OF REFERRING PROVIDER OR OTHER SOURCE
17a.
17b. NPI
18. HOSPITALIZATION DATES RELATED TO CURRENT SERVICES MM DD YY FROM TO MM DD YY

19. RESERVED FOR LOCAL USE
20. OUTSIDE LAB? $ CHARGES [ ] YES [ ] NO

21. DIAGNOSIS OR NATURE OF ILLNESS OR INJURY (Relate Items 1, 2, 3 or 4 to Item 24E by Line)
1. |___.___
2. |___.___
3. |___.___
4. |___.___
22. MEDICAID RESUBMISSION CODE ORIGINAL REF. NO.
23. PRIOR AUTHORIZATION NUMBER

24. A. DATE(S) OF SERVICE			B. PLACE OF SERVICE	C. EMG	D. PROCEDURES, SERVICES, OR SUPPLIES (Explain Unusual Circumstances)		E. DIAGNOSIS POINTER	F. $ CHARGES	G. DAYS OR UNITS	H. EPSDT Family Plan	I. ID. QUAL.	J. RENDERING PROVIDER ID. #
From MM DD YY	To MM DD YY				CPT/HCPCS	MODIFIER						
1												
2												
3												
4												
5												
6												

PHYSICIAN OR SUPPLIER INFORMATION

25. FEDERAL TAX I.D. NUMBER [ ] SSN [ ] EIN
26. PATIENT'S ACCOUNT NO.
27. ACCEPT ASSIGNMENT? (For govt. claims, see back) [ ] YES [ ] NO
28. TOTAL CHARGE $
29. AMOUNT PAID $
30. BALANCE DUE $

31. SIGNATURE OF PHYSICIAN OR SUPPLIER INCLUDING DEGREES OR CREDENTIALS (I certify that the statements on the reverse apply to this bill and are made a part thereof.)
SIGNED   DATE
32. SERVICE FACILITY LOCATION INFORMATION
a.   b.
33. BILLING PROVIDER INFO & PH # ( )
a.   b.

Provider and supplier section.

SUBMITTING INSURANCE CLAIMS

Paper Claims

The CMS-1500 form is printed in red to facilitate optical scanning when paper forms are submitted. Claim forms can be purchased from medical office supply companies. For efficient processing, it is recommended to use all capital letters and no punctuation, to be sure that all information is within the required box, and to proofread for typographical errors that might cause the claim to be rejected. The medical assistant must be sure that the insurance company accepts paper claims. (Although there are some exceptions, in general, Medicare and Medicaid now require that all claims be submitted electronically.)

If the office submits claims by mail, the frequency of submission depends on the size of the office, the number of personnel devoted to processing claims, and the number of patients seen who are covered by any particular insurance plan. Submission is usually done daily or weekly.

Electronic Claims

Electronic submission speeds things up enormously. Submission is instantaneous, instead of taking a few days to move through the mail. The office may submit insurance claims directly to the insurance company or submit them to a clearinghouse that processes the data and submits it to the appropriate carrier. The procedure for submission depends on the computer software used by the office or clearinghouse. Insurance company personnel cannot make errors inputting the information into the company's computer system because the transmission is computer to computer.

Faster delivery and faster and more accurate processing means faster reimbursement. If electronic claim submission is coupled with electronic payment from the company to the practice's operating account, the entire turnaround time from submission to money in the bank can be days instead of weeks.

Regardless of how claims are submitted, an insurance claims log needs to be kept, either manually or by computer.

TRACKING INSURANCE REIMBURSEMENT

Reimbursement is the payment received by the medical practice from the insurance company for the services performed.

Types of Reimbursement

Two basic types of insurance reimbursement exist: capitation and fee-for-service.

Under capitation, the primary care physician receives a monthly, quarterly, semiannual, or annual payment from the managed care insurance company. Specialists are usually not paid by capitation. The reimbursement per patient may vary depending on age and sex, but it does not depend on the amount of care the patient receives.

As discussed earlier, capitation moves some of the risk away from the managed care company and onto the primary care physician who treats the patient, and most physicians prefer other payment methods. In most circumstances, there will be enough healthy patients who cost the physician less to treat than the amount being paid by the company to make up for the few sick patients who cost more to treat.

Under fee-for-service reimbursement, the physician is reimbursed for each treatment or procedure performed. In this case the only difference between traditional fee-for-service insurance and managed care is that managed care companies often negotiate a fee schedule that is lower than traditional indemnity plans.

Using a Claims Register

A record of every insurance claim filed should be kept using an insurance claims register. An insurance claims register can be kept either manually or on the computer (Figure 46-4).

What Would You Do? What Would You *Not* Do?

Case Study 3

Maria Santos, a 33-year-old woman, has been seen in the office for a physical examination. When reviewing insurance claims in the computer before submission, Sandra notices that the name of the insured on the claim for Maria Santos is Jose Santos, and his date of birth is the same as her date of birth. Sandra also notices that in box 8, there is an X beside the word "Employed." ∎

Memories *from* Externship

Sandra O'Keefe: My externship was done in the office of a single gynecologist in a medium-size city. Although the office had a computer billing program, we submitted most of the insurance claims on paper. After I had been at the office for several weeks, the office manager started having me fill out some insurance claim forms by hand. Then she would have me print the forms on the computer and compare my form with the computer-generated form. She said I needed to understand how to fill out the form myself, even if I didn't usually do it, so that I would know what kind of information should be in each box. At first I found it very confusing, but after a while I began to know what to look for. For example, an insurance company will deny a claim for a Pap test if the sex of the patient is given as male. I was always glad that I had some experience with insurance, although I don't think I realized how complex it really is until I actually began to work as a medical assistant. ∎

Prepare for Success

INSURANCE CLAIM REGISTER

BLACKBURN PRIMARY CARE ASSOCIATES, PC

1990 Turquoise Drive
Blackburn, WI 54937
608-459-8857

Claim number	Service	Insurance and ID and group no	Date and amount of claim	Date and amount paid	Difference	Follow-up action

Figure 46-4. Insurance claims register. (From Hunt SA: *Saunders fundamentals of medical assisting,* St. Louis, 2007, Saunders.)

The claims register includes the claim number (the number given to the claim as part of the office's tracking system); the patient's name and insurance group or policy number; the insurance company's name; the date and amount of the claim; a column for any follow-up actions taken (by mail or telephone); the date and amount of the paid claim; and any difference between the amount submitted and the amount paid.

The medical assistant should review the claims register on a regular basis to be sure that all claims have been paid and that the insurance company has not denied services that should be covered or paid less than it should for those services. If a pattern of rejected claims is seen, the medical assistant should work together with other office staff to improve systems so that claims are not denied.

Explanation of Benefits Forms

After payment has been made by the insurance company to the physician, or if a claim is being denied, both the physician and the patient receive an **explanation of benefits (EOB)** form. Although each insurance carrier has its own form, the type of information contained on any EOB is similar, as shown in Figure 46-5. If the insurance company is denying the claim, the physician may also receive a remittance advice form, showing why the claim was disallowed.

Claims are usually denied for one of the following reasons: transposing names or numbers, incomplete information, incorrect or incomplete codes, or information that does not match codes or other information (Table 46-2).

Follow-up and Resubmission of Claims

If a claim is denied, it should be resubmitted immediately, following any advice given by the company on the remittance advice form. Any questions about a denial should be discussed with a provider relations representative at the company.

Table 46-2 Common Errors on Insurance Claim Forms

Type of Error	Example
Transposing names or numbers	Reversing the name of the patient with the subscriber (guarantor)
	Reversing the primary insurance with the secondary insurance
	Transposing numbers in one of the identification numbers
Missing information	Missing signatures or signature stamps
	Missing or inaccurate physician national provider identifier number for each service or not a physician registered with plan
	Required attachments missing (e.g., pathology report)
	Incomplete boxes
	No preapproval or preauthorization number
Inaccurate/incomplete codes	Inaccurate procedure or service codes (CPT or HCPCS)
	Missing modifier
Information does not match codes or other information	Diagnosis inconsistent with patient gender
	Diagnosis does not justify procedures performed
	Total amount of billing does not agree with services provided
	Place of service inconsistent with procedure code

From Hunt SA: *Saunders fundamentals of medical assisting*, St. Louis, 2007, Saunders.

If claims are not being paid or denied in a timely fashion, follow-up is in order. Follow-up can be made via letter or over the telephone. The claims log can be used to find all claims to any company that are becoming delinquent and include them in the follow-up call or letter.

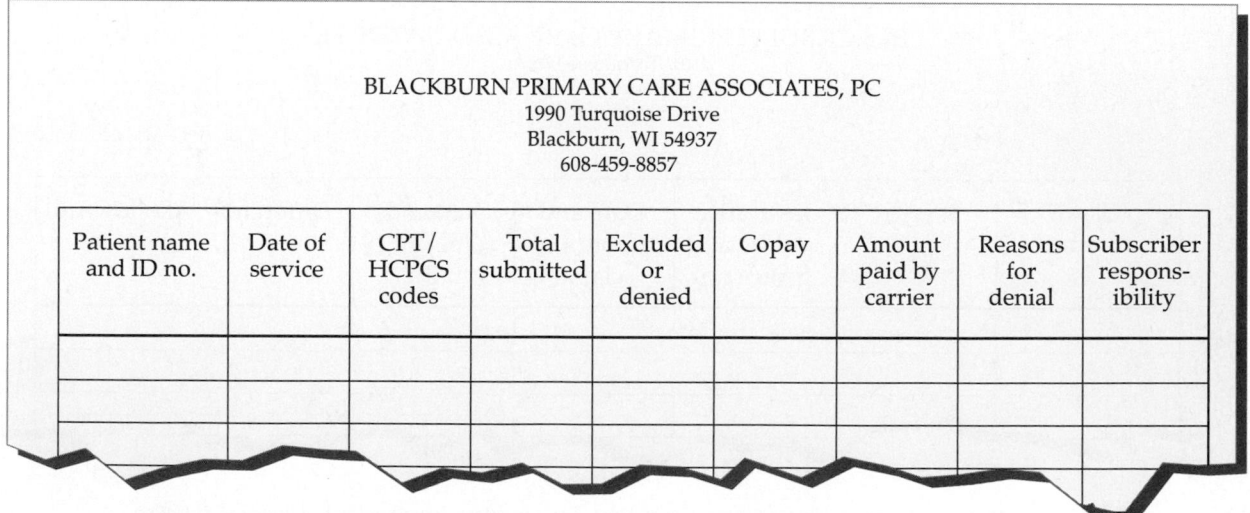

BLACKBURN PRIMARY CARE ASSOCIATES, PC
1990 Turquoise Drive
Blackburn, WI 54937
608-459-8857

Patient name and ID no.	Date of service	CPT/HCPCS codes	Total submitted	Excluded or denied	Copay	Amount paid by carrier	Reasons for denial	Subscriber responsibility

Figure 46-5. Typical information that would be contained on an explanation of benefits form. (From Hunt SA: *Saunders fundamentals of medical assisting*, St. Louis, 2007, Saunders.)

MEDICAL PRACTICE and the LAW

All parts of the Health Insurance Portability and Accountability Act of 1996 (HIPAA) affect insurance billing, but an important provision is the Transactions and Code Set Rule. This rule requires health care providers to use the same health care transactions, code sets, and identifiers for electronic transmissions.

Transaction sets for electronic data interchange (EDI) define in detail the format that must be used for electronic transmission. The EDI Health Care Claim Transaction set 837P defines the format that must be used to submit health care claim billing information electronically by medical offices or to transmit this information between and within agencies involved in the reimbursement process. Other transaction sets define the other types of information that can be exchanged electronically. They are usually referred to by the number associated with the specific transaction set.

Code sets are the codes used to identify specific diagnosis and clinical procedures on claims and encounter forms. The code sets required by HIPAA that were discussed in Chapter 45 include HCPCS codes, CPT codes, and ICD-9-CM codes. One additional code set, the National Drug Code (NDC), is used by pharmacies. It identifies the vendor (manufacturer), product, and package size of all medications recognized by the Food and Drug Administration.

The Administration Simplification Compliance Act (ASCA), which went into effect in October 2003, prohibits Medicare from paying claims unless they are submitted electronically. Small medical offices and dentists are two examples of providers that can apply for a waiver in order to continue submitting paper claims. ∎

What Would You Do? What Would You *Not* Do?   RESPONSES

Case Study 1
Page 1075

What Did Sandra Do?

❑ Explained to the patient that the original referral only authorized treatment of the lesion on the patient's neck, and the insurance company would not pay for other treatment without authorizing it.

❑ Explained that she would call the insurance company and primary care physician and take care of any required paperwork.

❑ Promised to minimize delay as much as possible.

❑ Told the patient that she would be responsible for the cost of removal if proper authorization was not obtained from her insurance company.

What Did Sandra Not Do?

❑ Did not assume that the referral covered additional lesions not specifically mentioned on the referral form.

❑ Did not assure the patient that her insurance would automatically cover the cost of removing the additional lesions.

❑ Did not schedule the removal of the additional lesions until she had received insurance authorization or the patient promised to pay for the procedure.

What Would You Do/What Would You *Not* Do? Review Sandra's response and place a checkmark next to the information you included in your response. List the additional information you included in your response.

_____
_____
_____
_____

Case Study 2
Page 1082

What Did Sandra Do?

❑ Explained to Daniel's mother that there are rules governing coverage of children when both parents have insurance plans that cover their children.

❑ Asked Daniel's mother for her birth date and her husband's birth date.

❑ Explained to Daniel and his mother that usually children are covered by the insurance of the parent whose birth date comes first in the year.

❑ Asked Daniel's mother which insurance plan covered her children for their ordinary medical care.

What Did Sandra Not Do?

❑ Did not promise to send the insurance claim to the carrier the mother preferred unless it was the primary insurance carrier.

❑ Did not tell the mother not to worry because she would take care of it.

❑ Did not tell Daniel's mother that it was her responsibility to find out which insurance was the primary insurance.

What Would You Do/What Would You *Not* Do? Review Sandra's response and place a checkmark next to the information you included in your response. List the additional information you included in your response.

_____
_____
_____
_____

Continued

What Would You Do? What Would You *Not* Do?   RESPONSES—cont'd

Case Study 3
Page 1087

What Did Sandra Do?
❑ Checked the new patient information form to be sure that the information about the insured's name and date of birth had been entered correctly because incorrect information could lead to denial of the insurance claim.
❑ Checked the new patient information form to be sure that the patient had listed an employer.

What Did Sandra Not *Do?*
❑ Did not assume that it was just a coincidence that the husband and wife had the same date of birth.

❑ Did not assume that a few errors on the insurance claim form would not matter.
❑ Did not assume that the information in the computer would always be correct.

What Would You Do/What Would You *Not* **Do?** Review Sandra's response and place a checkmark next to the information you included in your response. List the additional information you included in your response.

_____
_____
_____
_____

↻ TERMINOLOGY REVIEW

Assignment of benefits Authorization for insurance reimbursement to be made to the provider of health service rather than the insured individual.

Benefit The amount of money paid for a covered service under a health insurance plan.

Birthday rule If both parents of a child have a family health plan, the insurance plan of the parent whose birthday comes earlier in the year is defined as the primary insurance plan covering the child. The insurance of the other parent becomes secondary insurance.

Capitation A method of paying for insurance in which a fixed amount is paid to the provider per member for a specific time period regardless of the amount of care provided.

Carrier An insurance company.

CHAMPVA A government health insurance program that covers dependents of military veterans with service-connected disabilities.

Coinsurance A percentage of the allowed charge for health services, which the patient is responsible for paying.

Coordination of benefits Rules followed by insurance companies so that no claim is reimbursed at more than 100% of the charges.

Copayment A fixed amount of money that the patient must pay for any health care service.

Crossover claim An insurance claim for an individual who is covered by Medicare and Medicaid. After review by the Medicare fiscal intermediary, the claim is automatically sent to Medicaid.

Deductible An amount of money that an insured person must pay annually before health services are covered by the insurance plan.

Diagnosis-related group (DRG) A system to determine Medicare reimbursement for a hospital stay on the basis of the patient's diagnosis.

Explanation of benefits (EOB) A statement issued by the insurance company explaining reimbursement for specific procedures.

Fee-for-service insurance Insurance reimbursement that is directly related to the services provided and the amount charged by the provider.

Fiscal intermediary An insurance company that contracts to review Medicare claims for the Centers for Medicare and Medicaid Services.

Guarantor A person with financial responsibility for a bill who may or may not also be a patient.

Indemnity An obligation to provide compensation for loss or damage.

Managed care A movement in health care based on reducing health care costs while providing quality care. The term may be used for the techniques used to reduce costs or for the companies that pay for the care provided.

Medicaid The government insurance program for low-income individuals and families that is funded both by the federal government and each individual state.

TERMINOLOGY REVIEW—cont'd

Medicare The federal health insurance program that provides insurance coverage for the elderly, permanently disabled, and individuals with end-stage kidney disease.

Premium An amount of money paid in a given period to purchase health insurance.

Primary care provider The physician chosen by a patient to provide general medical care and also to determine and authorize additional medical services the patient may require.

Primary insurance The insurance company that must be billed first for any individual.

Reimbursement The amount paid for a procedure by insurance.

Resource-based relative value scale (RBRVS) A system to establish the Medicare fee schedule for Medicare Part B based on the service provided and the geographic location of the provider.

Secondary insurance Insurance that an individual has in addition to primary insurance.

Signature on file (SOF) An indication on the insurance claim form that the signature of the patient is maintained by the medical office to authorize submission of insurance claims.

Subscriber The person named on an insurance certificate.

TRICARE A government insurance plan that provides medical care to spouses and dependents of individuals on active duty in the military. Formerly this program was called *CHAMPUS*.

Usual, customary, and reasonable (UCR) A system for establishing the amount an insurance company will pay for a procedure. The reasonable charge is set by the insurance company on the basis of a physician's usual (most frequent) charge for the procedure and the customary charge of other physicians in the same geographic area.

Workers' compensation An insurance program that covers lost wages and health care costs of workers injured on the job or who suffer from work-related illnesses.

 ON THE WEB

For Information on Centers for Medicare and Medicaid Services (Medicare, Medicaid, and SCHIP):

Centers for Medicare and Medicaid Services: www.cms.gov

For Information on CHAMPVA:

U.S. Department of Veterans Affairs: www.va.gov/hac/forbeneficiaries/champva/champva.asp

For Information on CMS-1500 form—National Uniform Claim Committee:

National Uniform Claim Committee: www.nucc.org

For Information on TRICARE:

TRICARE Management Activity: www.tricare.mil

For Information on U.S. Department of Labor—Workers' Compensation:

U.S. Department of Labor: www.dol.gov/dol/topic/workcomp

 PREPARE FOR CERTIFICATION Visit the Evolve site at http://evolve.elsevier.com/Bonewit/today/ to actively Prepare for your Certification.

Check out the *Companion CD* bound with the book to access additional interactive activities.

47

Billing and Collections

LEARNING OBJECTIVES

1. Describe the process of billing and collections.
2. Describe problems that can occur when patients pay by check.
3. Explain how to adjust patient accounts for an overpayment and process a refund.
4. Develop a collection system.
5. Identify past due accounts and the actions needed.
6. Describe the information to include in a collection letter.
7. Identify legal requirements that affect collections for the medical office.
8. Describe special circumstances affecting collections in the medical office.

PROCEDURES

Process patient bills.
Post a "not sufficient funds" check.
Post an overpayment.
Process a refund.

Create and examine an accounts receivable aging record.
Write a collection letter.

Post a collection agency payment.

CHAPTER OUTLINE

Introduction to Billing
Billing Cycle
Billing Process
Billing Problems
  Problems with Checks
  Overpayments and Refunds
Account Aging
  Accounts Receivable Aging Records/Reports
  Examining Accounts for Those Overdue

Collection Activities
  Past Due Accounts
  Collection Letters
  Credit Agreements
  Truth in Lending Agreements
  Policy for Patients with Outstanding Balances
  Other Collection Techniques and Special Circumstances

CAAHEP COMPETENCIES

Administrative Competencies
Perform Bookkeeping Procedures
- Perform billing and collection procedures.
- Process credit balance.
- Process refunds.
- Post NSF checks.
- Post collection agency payments.

General Competencies
Legal Concepts
- Demonstrate knowledge of federal and state health care legislation and regulations.

ABHES COMPETENCIES

Administrative Duties
- Apply computer concepts for office procedures.
- Perform billing and collection procedures.
- Process credit balance.
- Process refunds.
- Post NSF funds.
- Post collection agency payments.

Financial Management
- Use manual and computerized bookkeeping systems.
- Manage accounts payable and receivable.
- Maintain records for accounting and banking purposes.

account aging
balance due
bankruptcy
claim message
collection agency

credit balance
overdraft
skip
truth in lending

Introduction to Billing

If patients have insurance, a bill is not usually sent to the patient until after the insurance company has paid. If the patient is covered by a managed care policy, the copayment is usually collected at the time of the visit, and a bill may not be necessary. Often, however, the patient has a deductible and/or coinsurance, and a bill must be sent to the patient.

If a patient visit will not be covered by insurance, most physicians' offices request that payment be made at the time a medical service is provided. Many medical offices also accept payment by credit card, which makes payment at the time of service possible and convenient for many patients. However, a number of patients still need to make arrangements to pay for their medical services over a period of time. In this case, the office must establish an account for the patient and send periodic bills. These bills are usually generated by a computer software program. The bill is then placed in a window envelope and sent to the patient. Even if the patient's account is being paid by capitation, a billing record is usually kept for that patient, showing the amount of charges and payments.

The billing for physician offices that are affiliated with a hospital or large health group is usually done from a central location, and office employees are only responsible for posting charges. Patients and insurance companies make payments to the central office. Other offices may contract with an outside billing service. The medical assistant should understand the billing process, however, because efficient billing maximizes revenue for the medical practice.

BILLING CYCLE

Bills can be sent to patients every 2 weeks, monthly, or at any regular period, such as once every 3 months (quarterly). The time between bills is called the *billing cycle*. A bill sent out at the end of a cycle will show the **balance due** (the amount of money owed) at the beginning of the cycle, any payments made during the billing cycle, any new charges for new services that occurred during the billing cycle, and the balance due at the end of the cycle.

Patient accounts are often divided into equal parts, usually alphabetically. Each week a different section of the patient accounts is billed. For instance, on the first week of the month, patients with a last name beginning with the letters A-E may be billed; the second week, F-L; the third week, M-S; and the fourth week, T-Z. The same cycle is followed each month. Dividing the bills in this way makes more efficient use of staff time because billing is spread out over the month instead of all occurring in 1 week.

BILLING PROCESS

Bills can be produced manually using a typewriter and billing form, but in almost all medical offices they are produced from a computer billing program. If an outside billing service is used, the service can either send a paper record of all of the bills sent out at the end of each cycle or can transfer billing information from its computer to the office's computer, linking the information into the patient's financial record and the office's bookkeeping software.

At regular intervals, patient financial accounts should be examined and the accounts that must be billed should be processed. Billing insurance companies and billing patients are both straightforward transactions. However, the medical assistant should be aware of some special situations. A patient may have been treated for a final illness just before dying. In this case, any charges will have to be billed to the patient's estate. (Billing an estate is discussed in more detail at the end of this chapter.)

A patient may be a minor who sought treatment without his or her parent's knowledge. When minors are brought to a physician by a parent or guardian for treatment, the parent or guardian acknowledges that he or she is the responsible party for financial purposes. However, if a minor is treated without the parent's knowledge, the minor is responsible for fees as well. Minors older than age 12 may give consent for certain kinds of treatment including treatment for STDs, HIV testing, and treatment of drug or alcohol abuse. Because of confidentiality, the physician may not try to collect payment from the parent or guardian.

A patient may have a credit agreement with the practice, which allows the patient to pay bills off over time, along with interest on the balance due. This is important because, in such situations, even though an outstanding balance may become old, it should not be considered delinquent and sent out of the office for collection (Procedure 47-1).

PROCEDURE 47-1

Putting It All into Practice

My name is Christa Wilson, and I have been working in the office of three physicians for the past 5 years. There are three medical assistants, and we all assist the physicians during office hours, but I am responsible for most of the billing. We do weekly billing in our office using an alphabetic system. The first week of the month we send out statements for patients whose last names begin with the letters A-F, the second week G-L, etc. By the end of the month, every patient with an outstanding balance has received a statement, and we begin again. I am also responsible for posting payments received in the mail. Every month, we run an aging report, and I analyze it to see which accounts are overdue. Our computer program lets us add written messages to the statements, but we don't have a color printer, so I prefer to use colored stickers for accounts that are older than 60 days because I think they are more likely to get the patient's attention. If there is a balance due from a patient after 90 days, I always follow up with a telephone call. When I first started making these calls, I used to get very nervous, but I have gotten accustomed to it now. I always try to stay calm and keep my cool. I have found that in most cases, there is a financial problem that makes it difficult for the individual or family to keep up with its debts. I try to work with our patients so that they pay something each month and remind them not to "forget" about their copayments. Eventually we do collect most of the money that is owed to us, and we feel that part of the reason is that we stay on top of our billing. ∎

Prepare for Success

PROCEDURE **47-1**   Processing Patient Bills

Outcome Process patient bills.

Equipment/Supplies

- Computer
- Patient accounts
- Window envelopes
- Paper or statement forms

1. **Procedural Step.** Locate patient accounts in the computer database.
2. **Procedural Step.** Identify patient accounts with an outstanding balance for which insurance payments have been made.
   Principle. Patients are usually not billed until insurance payments have been received.
3. **Procedural Step.** Print patient statements using the office patient statement form. This may be printed from the computer program, or statement forms may be loaded in the printer.
4. **Procedural Step.** Make sure that statements have printed correctly.

5. **Procedural Step.** Fold statements so that the patient name and address will be visible through the window in the envelopes.
   Principle. The patient name and address should print on the statement in a position such that it can be used as the mailing address for the statement.
6. **Procedural Step.** Insert statements in envelopes. Be sure that the name and address are visible.
7. **Procedural Step.** Place postage on envelopes and mail statements.

BILLING PROBLEMS

Problems with Checks

From time to time, the office may encounter a problem either with a check it has written or with one that has been written to the office by a patient.

Insufficient Funds in the Office Account

It is illegal to write a check for more than the amount of money in the account. However, this occasionally happens because of an arithmetic error in calculating the balance while writing checks or because of failure to reconcile a bank statement. If the office's account accidentally becomes overdrawn, the bank may refuse to honor any check written after the account is overdrawn. In this case, the check will be returned to the person or company that deposited it marked NSF (not sufficient funds) in the payer's account to cover the check. A check on an account without adequate funds to cover it is called an **overdraft**.

It is a good practice to have overdraft protection for any office checking account. In the event that a check is written against an account without adequate funds, money to cover the check (usually in increments of $100.00) will automatically be transferred from another office account, such as a savings account. There may be a small charge each time this service is used.

Stopping Payment

From time to time, it may become necessary to ask the bank to stop payment on a check. A check might have been lost and a new check issued, or there may be a dispute between the practice and a vendor about a purchase or a previous payment. Banks charge a fee for stopping payment, so this practice should be used sparingly.

Insufficient Funds in a Patient Account

The bank may not honor a check deposited by the practice because the patient's account has insufficient funds. If a check is returned marked NSF, do not hesitate to call the patient and tell him or her of the problem. This may be the first of many checks that are being returned, and it is important for the person to find out why he or she is writing checks against insufficient funds. The bank usually charges fees both to the individual who wrote the check and to the medical office that tried to deposit the check. The amount of the NSF check must be added back to the balance owed by the patient as a positive adjustment that increases the amount owed. The fee charged by the bank is also added to the patient's balance, either as a separate fee or as part of the adjustment. As an example, assume that the patient paid a copayment of $20.00 at the time of the visit. The bank returned the check for insufficient funds and charged the medical office checking account a $15.00 fee. The medical assistant would charge the patient's account $35.00 to cover both the amount of the returned check and the additional fee charged by the bank. Most offices have a sign posted in the waiting room notifying patients of the additional charge for each returned check (Procedure 47-2).

Overpayments and Refunds

If the total of patient payments and insurance payments exceed the allowed charge, it is called an *overpayment*. This might happen, for example, if a patient thought that he had not yet paid his annual deductible, when in fact he had. After posting all the payments, the balance on the account will be a negative number, or **credit balance,** indicating that the medical office owes money to the patient. Sometimes a small credit balance is left in place when a patient has a visit scheduled in the near future because new charges will be applied. Usually, however, the medical assistant will process a refund for the patient. The amount of the refund is posted to the patient's account, bringing the account balance to zero. The medical assistant sends a letter and a check to the patient with a brief explanation about the overpayment (Procedures 47-3 and 47-4).

What Would You Do? What Would You *Not* Do?

Case Study 1

The bank returns a check from a patient for NSF. The amount on the check is $10.00, and the bank includes a notice that the practice will be charged $15.00. Christa makes a telephone call to the patient, and she asks the patient to send the office a replacement check in the amount of $25.00. The patient becomes very upset. She says, "The bank will charge me the fee for the returned check, not you. All you have to do is send the check through again. There is money in the account now because I deposited my paycheck yesterday. You can't charge me a fee for this. You are just trying to make money out of this situation." ■

PROCEDURE **47-2**   Posting an NSF Check

Outcome Post a check returned for NSF.

Equipment/Supplies

- Computer
- Patient accounts
- Returned check
- Day sheet (optional)
- Calculator

1. **Procedural Step.** When the NSF check has been received, locate the patient account in the computer database. If using a day sheet, label the first open line with the name of the patient whose check was returned and enter the old balance in the *old balance* column.
2. **Procedural Step.** Create a new billing for the patient and post the returned check using the code for NSF check or Adjustment—charge and entering the amount of the check. If using a day sheet, write "NSF check returned by bank" and the check number in the *professional service* column. Place the amount of the check in the *adjustment* column in parentheses to indicate that the amount is a debit adjustment (i.e., added to the patient's balance). Add the amount to the old balance and enter it in the *new balance* column.

   Principle. The amount of the returned check must be added to return the patient balance to the amount before the check was deducted.

Continued

PROCEDURE 47-2   Posting an NSF Check—cont'd

3. **Procedural Step.** Post the amount charged by the bank as a charge using the code for a returned check fee. Record the total of the amount of the fee charged by the office for any returned check as a charge (fee). If recording on a day sheet, post the charge for the fee charged by the bank in the *fee* column. Add the amount to the old balance and record in the *new balance* column.

    Principle. The bank fee is a new charge to the patient's account. Depending on office policy, the amount charged for the NSF check may be considered a fee or a debit adjustment.

4. **Procedural Step.** If using a computer program, be sure that the box indicating that insurance should be billed is *not* checked.

    Principle. Insurance is not responsible for the charge for a returned check.

5. **Procedural Step.** When totaling the columns of the day sheet at the end of the day, subtract any debit adjustment from the total of all credit adjustments.

6. **Procedural Step.** Notify the patient by telephone or letter that the check was returned and a fee has been charged. If sending a letter, enclose a patient statement with the letter showing the total amount of the returned check and the fee.

    Example: Estelle Jordan's check for $15.00 was returned by the bank marked NSF. The bank also charged a fee of $15.00.

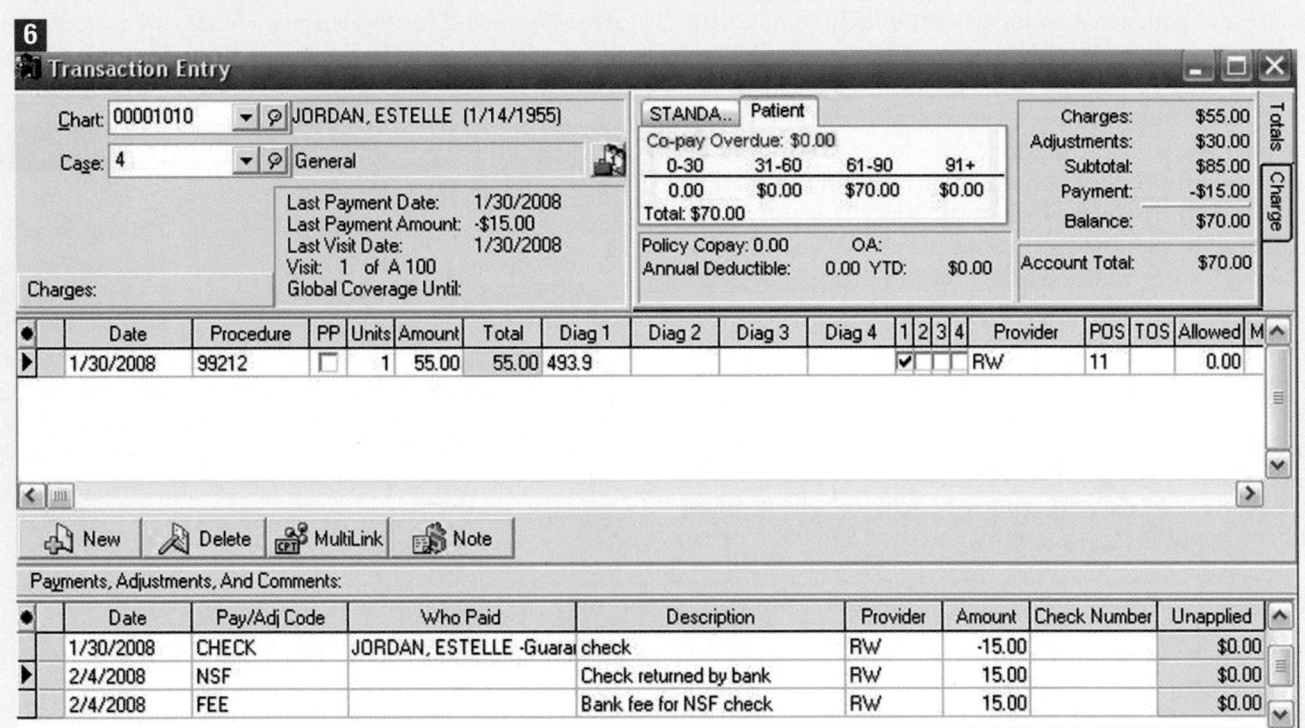

The NSF check and bank fee are posted to the patient's account. (Screenshot used by permission of MCKESSON Corporation. All Rights Reserved. © MCKESSON Corporation 2008.)

PROCEDURE 47-3   Posting an Overpayment

Outcome Post an overpayment.

Equipment/Supplies

- Computer
- Patient accounts
- Payment check(s)
- Day sheet
- Office policy manual
- Calculator

1. **Procedural Step.** When a payment has been made, locate the patient account in the computer. If using a day sheet, enter the patient's name on a new line and enter the previous balance in the *old balance* column.
   Principle. Both insurance payments and patient payments must be entered in the correct patient account.

2. **Procedural Step.** Compare the amount of the payment against the total amount owed.
   Principle. The total amount owed will be the balance due and charges for new services.

3. **Procedural Step.** Even if the payment is greater than the charges, post the payment to the computer system using the correct code (i.e., patient payment, check, insurance payment) and link to the visit for which the payment is made. If using a day sheet, post the payment on the line with the patient's name in the *payment* column.

4. **Procedural Step.** If an overpayment has occurred, note that the account balance in the computer is preceded by a minus sign. This means that the medical office owes the patient money. On the day sheet, subtract the amount of the payment from the patient's previous balance and record in the *new balance* column. Place a negative number in parentheses. When totaling the *new balance* column at the end of the day, subtract any negative number from the total instead of adding it.
   Principle. A negative balance is indicated in accounting by enclosing it in parentheses. Care must be taken when totaling columns on a day sheet to subtract a negative number from the total.

5. **Procedural Step.** Take steps to clear the balance from the system according to your office policy. If the patient has another appointment scheduled, the negative balance may be carried for a short time. In most cases, a refund should be issued promptly (see Procedure 47-4).
   Principle. Office policy guidelines indicate the proper management of a credit balance in a patient account.

PROCEDURE 47-4 Processing a Refund

Outcome Process a refund.

Equipment/Supplies

- Computer
- Patient accounts
- Payment check(s)
- Day sheet
- Office policy manual
- Calculator

1. **Procedural Step.** Locate the patient account in the computer. If using a day sheet, enter the patient's name on a new line and enter the amount of the credit balance in the *old balance* column.
   Principle. All financial transactions must be entered in the correct patient account.

2. **Procedural Step.** Calculate the amount to be refunded (usually the amount of the negative balance).

3. **Procedural Step.** Create a new transaction for the patient in the computer account and choose "Refund" for the code. If using a day sheet, write "Refund for Overpayment" in the *professional service* column.

4. **Procedural Step.** Enter the amount of the refund in the "Amount" box of the transaction screen, and verify that the patient balance becomes zero. On the day sheet, record the amount of the refund in the *adjustment* column. Add this number to the patient's old balance (a negative number) so that the new balance becomes zero, and enter zero in the *new balance* column.
   Example: The patient Darla Sissle paid $50.00 on her account followed by an insurance payment of $55.00, resulting in an overpayment of $15.00. A refund was issued for $15.00.

5. **Procedural Step.** Write a check for the refund amount including the date, amount in numbers, and amount in words on the line below. Leave the signature line blank.
   Principle. The medical assistant is generally not authorized to sign checks for the medical office.

6. **Procedural Step.** Record the check number, date, payee, and reason for the check on the check stub in the checkbook or in the check register.

7. **Procedural Step.** Subtract the amount of the check from the balance in the check register.

8. **Procedural Step.** Write a letter informing the patient of the refund, and prepare an envelope.

9. **Procedural Step.** Sign the letter and your title, or obtain the physician signature depending on office policy.

10. **Procedural Step.** Leave the check, letter, and envelope in the correct place to obtain an authorized signature on the check.

Continued

PROCEDURE 47-4

PROCEDURE 47-4   **Processing a Refund—cont'd**

4

WESTERN MEDICAL CENTER
Patient Account Ledger
As of 4/19/2008

Entry	Date	POS	Description	Procedure	Document	Provider	Amount
00001015	DARLA SISSLE				(490)220-1156		
	Last Payment: -50.00	On: 4/19/2008					
1	3/21/2008	11		99213	0804190000	RW	65.00
2	3/21/2008	11		80051	0804190000	RW	25.00
6	3/30/2008	11	Ins payment	INS	0804190000	RW	-55.00
9	4/19/2008	11	Patient payment	CHECK	0804190000	RW	-50.00
10	4/19/2008	11	Refund	REFUND	0804190000	RW	15.00
	Patient Totals						**0.00**
	Ledger Totals						**0.00**

Verify that the patient's account balance becomes zero. (Screenshot used by permission of MCKESSON Corporation. All Rights Reserved. © MCKESSON Corporation 2008.)

ACCOUNT AGING

Account aging is the process of determining how long specific accounts/balances have been outstanding.

Accounts Receivable Aging Records/Reports

An accounts receivable aging record should be created to identify accounts that are overdue. Accounts are aged in 30-day intervals. Figure 47-1 shows a sample accounts receivable aging record (see also Procedure 47-5).

Examining Accounts for Those Overdue

An account is considered overdue if it is not paid within 30 days of the date billed unless there is an outstanding credit agreement. Accounts for which all the charges are from the previous billing period are considered current (0 to 30 days). Overdue accounts are categorized as 30 to 60 days, 60 to 90 days, and longer than 120 days.

An account with an outstanding balance after 120 days requires collection activity, such as sending the account out to a collection agency or writing a demand letter informing the account holder that a lawsuit will be brought if the account is not brought up to date. Most of the time, the balance of medical office accounts is small enough to permit legal action in small claims court. (Small claims court is discussed in more detail at the end of the chapter.)

Enter credits in parentheses ( ) and subtract when totaling columns and P

ACCOUNTS RECEIVABLE AGING RECORD

Name			As of Date	Prepared by					Page of Page	
NO.	ACCOUNT NAME	Insurance Information		Date of Last Payment	Current 1 to 30 days	31 to 60 days	61 to 90 days	91 to 120 days	121 days and over	TOTAL
		Date Claim Filed	Amount of Claim							
	Amounts brought forward									
1	Mary Smith			8/8/10	120					120 -
2	John Payne			7/6/10		250 -				250 -
3	Jack Desmonde			5/25/10			500			500 -
4	Jill Jayne			4/2/10		80 -				180 -
5										

A

Figure 47-1. Sample accounts receivable aging record: **A,** prepared by hand; **B,** prepared by computer. (From Hunt SA: *Saunders fundamentals of medical assisting,* St. Louis, 2007, Saunders.)

Blackburn Primary Care Associates
Patient Aging

NAME	CURRENT 0 - 30	PAST 31 - 60	PAST 61 - 90	PAST 91 - 120	PAST over 120	Total Balance
Mary Smith Last Payment on 08/08/10	$120.00					$120.00
John Payne Last Payment on 07/06/10		$250.00				$250.00
Jack Desmonde Last Payment on 05/25/10			$500.00			$500.00
Jill Jayne Last Payment on 04/02/10		$80.00		$100.00		$180.00
Report Aging Totals Percent of Total Aging	$120.00 11.4%	$330.00 31.4%	$330.00 47.6%	$100.00 9.5%		$1,050.00 100.0%

B

Figure 47-1, cont'd.

PROCEDURE 47-5

What Would You Do? What Would You *Not* Do?

Case Study 2
A patient calls the office to say that she has received her bill, and it does not show a payment of $10.00 that she made in cash at the time of the visit. The patient is upset, and she says, "I knew I shouldn't pay cash, because now I can't prove that I made that payment. I don't see why you can't keep accurate records." Christa asks the patient if she received a receipt for the cash payment. The patient says, "How do you expect me to remember that? This happened over a month ago." ∎

PROCEDURE 47-5   Creating an Accounts Receivable Aging Record

Outcome Create and examine an accounts receivable aging record.

Equipment/Supplies

- Computer
- Patient accounts
- Accounts receivable aging record analysis form (optional)
- Office policy manual
- Pen

1. **Procedural Step.** Using the reports function of the computer billing program, create an aging report for patients and for insurance companies. It is also possible to create such a report manually using individual patient ledgers.
   Principle. In a computerized billing system, the computer program can generate the report of all overdue accounts.

2. **Procedural Step.** Review the accounts on the report and mark the proposed action for each account according to your office policy.
   Principle. Efforts to collect outstanding accounts should become increasingly more active as the account ages. Office policy may vary in respect to specific actions.

3. **Procedural Step.** Mark all accounts that are less than 31 days old "No Action Needed."
   Principle. Accounts that are less than 31 days old are considered current.

4. **Procedural Step.** Mark bills with unpaid insurance claims that are older than 31 days "Follow up with insurance."
   Principle. Patients usually do not pay on bills with outstanding insurance claims until they find out how much the insurance will pay. These bills, if overdue, need to be followed up with the insurance company.

5. **Procedural Step.** Mark accounts that are 31 to 60 days old, according to office policy. For example, a

Continued

note may be attached to the statement saying, "Payment is now due." It may be possible to include payment notices in the computer program so that they print on the statement automatically if the account is overdue.

6. **Procedural Step.** Mark accounts that are 61 to 90 days old, according to office policy. For example, a note may be attached to the statement saying, "Payment of this bill is now overdue. Please pay the balance or contact the office."

7. **Procedural Step.** Mark accounts that are 91 to 120 days old, according to office policy. It may be office policy to place a telephone call to the patient at this point to discuss the account. Follow up with a letter confirming any agreement made.

8. **Procedural Step.** For accounts older than 120 days, review previous collection attempts. Unless there are known circumstances that warrant a delay in collection activity, send a collection letter stating that if

payment is not received by a certain date the account will be given to a collection agency or pursued in small claims court (depending on the procedure used by the office to collect delinquent accounts).
Principle. After 120 days without activity, especially if the person owing money has been contacted by telephone and letter, it is unlikely that the bill will be paid without more aggressive collection measures.

9. **Procedural Step.** Record all action taken beside each account on the report.
Principle. This provides a written record of actions taken and results of telephone conversations.

10. **Procedural Step.** Write follow-up letters to document in writing any agreements made during telephone conversations. Place a copy in the patient's medical record.
Principle. A written record of verbal communications regarding bills and payments provides evidence in case further legal action is necessary.

COLLECTION ACTIVITIES

Many people who owe money have every intention of paying their bill but are unable to do so in the short term because of some emergency. As accounts age, it is appropriate to increase the forcefulness of any message to the patient that the account is overdue. Patients should always be invited to call the office and make arrangements to pay over time if they have had a true emergency. Sometimes, it is medical bills themselves that are piling up, especially in the case of a patient with a chronic illness who does not have any or adequate insurance.

Patients are also encouraged to discuss accounts for which insurance payment is expected but delayed. By working with the insurance company, the patient can more easily determine whose responsibility the bill is.

Past Due Accounts

Messages encouraging payment of the bill (often called **claim messages**) can be attached to bills or included in the billing envelope. Some computer programs will print a message on the bill itself.

A bill that is 60 days overdue should be accompanied by a claim message reminding the patient that the bill is overdue. Many offices use a series of messages that become more forceful as time passes without payment.

Bills that are 90 days overdue should be followed up with a telephone call. By contacting patients directly, the medical assistant can determine why there is no activity related to the account. The medical assistant must be careful to follow legal guidelines when discussing accounts with patients.

The Fair Debt Collection Practices Act of 1966 identifies activities that are permitted and not permitted when contacting individuals who owe money. Most states also have debt collection laws with which the medical assistant should be familiar.

Collection Letters

Bills that are aged 120 days should either be accompanied by or followed up by a collection letter, such as the one seen in Figure 47-2. When writing a collection letter, the medical assistant should gather information related to the account before composing the letter. The recipient should be clearly informed about what action is expected, as well as the deadline for action. The letter should not threaten legal action or transfer to a collection agency unless the office is prepared to follow through.

Each medical office has its own policy about who should sign a collection letter. In many offices, the medical assistant signs the letters. In other offices there may be an office manager or billing specialist, or each physician may prefer to sign letters to his or her own patients (Procedure 47-6).

If the collection letter does not receive a response, another letter should be sent stating either that the account is being turned over to a collection agency (a company that collects overdue bills for other companies) or that a lawsuit will be filed in small claims court if the account is not paid by a certain date. This letter should also ask the patient to find a new health care provider and ask the patient to request that his or her medical records be forwarded to that provider.

Highlight on Guidelines for Telephone Collections

Things to Do

1. A creditor (person or company who is owed money) may contact the person who owes money by telephone during reasonable hours. The medical assistant should gather accurate information before placing the telephone call about an overdue account:
   a. Who owes the money?
   b. How much money is owed?
   c. How long has the money been owed?
   d. Is there any insurance claim pending?
   e. Has the insurance company processed the claim and/or made any payment?
2. A creditor may take measures to locate a person but may not divulge that he or she is trying to collect a bill to anyone other than the person who owes money. The medical assistant should ask to speak with the patient or the person responsible for the account when placing the call.
3. A creditor may not misrepresent himself or herself in order to trick the person who owes money into taking the call. After asking for the person responsible for the account, the medical assistant should identify himself or herself and the office or physician.
4. A creditor may not harass or intimidate a person who owes money. The medical assistant should speak calmly and professionally. The conversation should include a discussion of the different options for payment, including full payment, partial payment, and monthly installments. If possible, the medical assistant should obtain a verbal commitment for a date and amount of at least a first payment and/or a payment plan.
5. Although a verbal agreement is legally binding, a written agreement is easier to enforce if legal action becomes necessary. It is important to follow up any verbal agreement with a letter referring to the conversation and the agreement. If an arrangement was established for monthly payments, a truth-in-lending statement must be included, even if the patient will not pay interest.
6. Although it is not permitted to harass the patient, the medical assistant may contact him or her again if payments are not made as agreed. Often, the knowledge that attention is being paid to the account will encourage the patient to adhere to the repayment schedule.

Things Not to Do

1. A creditor should not call too early in the day or too late at night.
2. A creditor should not divulge to employers, neighbors, or other third parties that he or she is trying to collect a bill from the patient.
3. A creditor should not threaten.
4. A creditor should not end the conversation on vague terms.
5. A creditor should not call repeatedly. ∎

Blackburn Primary Care Associates, PC
1990 Turquoise Drive
Blackburn, WI 54937

04/02/10

Dear Patient,

Your account in this office is more than 120 days overdue. We have made previous attempts with you to set up a mutually agreeable payment schedule but you have not as yet followed through on your commitment. This will be your final notice. If you do not contact this office within 7 days of receipt of this letter we will have no choice but to turn over this account to the collection agency. Please contact this office if you wish to avoid collection activity.

Yours truly,

Joanne Hughes, MD

Figure 47-2. Sample collection letter. (From Hunt SA: *Saunders fundamentals of medical assisting,* St. Louis, 2007, Saunders.)

As in any case where the physician ends a relationship with a patient, the letter should be sent Certified Mail, with a Return Receipt requested. The letter should allow the patient at least 2 weeks to arrange to find another health care provider.

Credit Agreements

Credit agreements are documents that allow patients to set up a schedule to pay off their bills as long as they make the specified monthly payments. If a patient decides independently to pay his or her bill in installments (i.e., without discussing it with the medical office), no credit agreement is necessary. If the office and patient make an agreement regarding installment payments, even if no interest is charged, the agreement must be in writing. An interest charge is often added to the balance due at the end of each billing cycle when a written agreement exists.

A credit agreement with a medical office is a type of revolving credit, like a department store or gasoline company charge card. As long as the monthly minimum is paid, the account is considered in good standing.

Truth in Lending Agreements

Because a credit agreement is a type of revolving credit, it falls under federal and state government fair lending practices. Thus, a truth in lending statement must be supplied to the patient when the agreement is made. **Truth in lending** refers to the legal requirement to disclose the terms of a loan to borrowers so that they can understand them.

This truth in lending statement includes facts about such things as the maximum amount the patient may charge to the account, the interest rate, how the interest is computed (i.e., average daily balance, or balance at the end of the billing period), and how the minimum monthly payment is computed (i.e., percentage of outstanding balance). Figure 47-3 shows a sample credit agreement.

Policy for Patients with Outstanding Balances

Most medical offices insist that a patient close out any current balance due before writing a credit agreement with that patient. If the practice has had trouble collecting bills from a patient in the past, it may write the credit agreement for a lower maximum balance. But the practice cannot

Blackburn Primary Care Associates, PC
1990 Turquoise Drive
Blackburn, WI 54937
608-459-8857

Federal Truth in Lending Statement

Patient _____

Address _____

1. Fee for service of _____

2. Amount down _____

3. Amount financed _____

4. finance charge _____

5. total of payments 3 + 4 _____

6. number of payments _____

7. amount of each payment _____

Total no. of payments _____ payable over _____ monthly installments

In the amount of $_____. The first payment is due _____.

Date _____ Signed _____

Figure 47-3. Sample credit agreement. (From Hunt SA: *Saunders fundamentals of medical assisting,* St. Louis, 2007, Saunders.)

charge a different interest rate or compute the minimum payment in a different way for different patients depending on past payment history.

Other Collection Techniques and Special Circumstances

Tracing "Skips"

Occasionally, a bill is returned to the medical office from the post office with the notation "address unknown." This may be an innocent mistake—the result, perhaps, of an incorrect address on file or the patient's failure to notify the office after moving. On the other hand, it may be a deliberate attempt to "skip out" on their bill and the bills of other professionals and/or merchants.

A potential **"skip"** (account for which no billing information is available) should be followed up immediately. The first step is to call the patient's phone number: He or she may have moved within the same town and still have the same telephone number or may have had the phone company use a "new number" message to forward calls.

If there is no new number listed, the next step is to call the patient's place of business and ask to speak with the individual. The medical assistant can also try to get in touch with the person by contacting professional associations, unions, or other organizations with which the person is associated.

The medical assistant should never tell a third party that an individual owes money to the medical office, only that he or she wishes to speak with the person. Also, it is illegal to call a third party more than once in an attempt to trace a skip unless that person asks the medical assistant to call back. For example, the medical assistant may speak with a third party where the individual with an overdue account works, and that third party might ask the medical assistant to call back at the end of the day when he or she is not so busy.

Another way to attempt collection is to send a letter by Registered or Certified Mail, with a Return Receipt requested, to the individual at the old address. Even if the person did not ask the post office to forward all mail, he or she may have asked for certain types of mail to be forwarded. In this case, the letter should be placed in a plain envelope, with just the return street address and no office name. This minimizes the chances that the individual will refuse to accept the mail.

The medical office may also use one of several Internet resources to trace skips. These services usually charge a fee. The more information the office has about the individual, the more likely it is that the individual can be located.

If all of these efforts fail, the bill should be turned over to a collection agency used by the office as soon as possible. A **collection agency** is a firm that is in the business of collecting outstanding accounts. Most collection agencies handle far more "skips" than individual medical offices do and sometimes use other, more aggressive techniques. The sooner the collection agency receives the account, the better chance it has to collect the bill.

Sending Accounts to a Collection Agency

Collection agencies are in business specifically to collect accounts that have "aged out." This means that by the time a collection agency receives a delinquent account, the business such as a medical office has given the person who owes the money fair warning that the bill is overdue, and that a professional collector is going to become involved.

Each state has specific laws under which collection agencies must work. These laws define when collection agency personnel can call, what they can say, and what other tactics they can use to collect the bill.

Collection agencies generally charge between 20% and 40% of the amount they collect. They are not allowed to "cut a deal" with a patient and accept less than full payment unless the medical office has agreed to the arrangement for payment.

If a patient's account is in collection, usually the office has a policy not to see the patient unless the current charges are paid in full at the time of the visit. Other offices notify patients in writing that they will not be seen by any physician in the office until their outstanding balance has been collected.

When an account is turned over to a collection agency, the patient balance in the computer system is often adjusted to zero. The amount owed by the patient can still be seen clearly in the patient ledger, but the current balance is zero. This prevents bills to the patient from being generated, and the account no longer appears as overdue on account aging reports. The medical assistant should become familiar with the exact procedure used in his or her medical office. The medical office makes no further attempts at collection, and any payments received from the patient are sent directly to the collection agency. When a payment for the patient's account is received from a collection agency, it should be recorded on the daily ledger. In addition, it should be posted to the account for which it was collected. The patient's account balance, which is usually zero, is first increased (as a positive or debit adjustment) by the amount of the payment. Then the payment is posted as a payment, bringing the current account balance back to zero (Procedure 47-7).

Small Claims Court

Small claims courts exist in each state. They are special sessions of the local district court that deal only with civil lawsuits involving small amounts of money. Most small claims lawsuits involve disputes over payments. Each state has its own rules for the maximum claim that can be brought in small claims court. This maximum amount runs from about $1,500 in some states to as much as $15,000 in others.

The question for a medical practice when choosing to use the court system is always whether it will sacrifice more in "good will" than it will gain in money if the collection is successful. Many offices bring suits in court only after a patient has left the practice without paying a bill in full. Furthermore, winning a judgment in small claims court is only the first step. The office must still collect the judgment.

Small claims courts are set up to reduce the legal fees for those seeking to collect relatively small amounts of money. Because there is no lawyer, the plaintiff (an individual or business) must represent himself or itself. The office manager or medical assistant might have to assume this duty if the office uses small claims court to try to collect on patient accounts. A collection agency cannot represent the office.

The clerk of the court has all of the documents necessary to file a small claim and can usually walk a first-time claimant through the process, explaining how to fill out the forms and which documentation to submit to back up the claim. Only the defendant can appeal a small claims court judgment; for the plaintiff, a negative judgment is final.

Billing an Estate

Patients do sometimes die without having paid their medical bills in full. In this instance, the office will have to collect the balance due from the estate. Estates fall into an area of the law known as *probate*, and probate law is administered by a special section of the court system in each state.

It is not appropriate to send a bill to a deceased patient's estate immediately after the death while the family is grieving; however, the bill should be sent within 30 days. The bill should be sent to "The Estate of" the patient at the patient's address rather than to a family member or other individual unless that person has made a written promise to cover the deceased's medical costs.

If the deceased patient had a will, it usually has a provision that the costs of the patient's final illness be paid by the estate outside of the probate process. In such a case, the bill will probably be paid promptly. The will should be filed within 30 days, and the clerk of the probate court should then be able to furnish you with the name of the executor or administrator (the person responsible for handling the estate's business dealings). An itemized final bill should then be sent to this individual by Certified Mail with a Return Receipt requested.

If the patient did not have a will, the medical practice's bill will be put in with other creditors' bills and paid only when payment is approved by the probate court and the administrator appointed by the court.

Bankruptcy

Bankruptcy laws are federal laws, meaning that they apply equally regardless of the state in which the bankrupt person lives. **Bankruptcy** is a means for an individual or business to "get out from under" a crushing load of debt, either by reorganizing the debt or by liquidating assets and dividing the funds among all of the creditors.

Individuals file for personal bankruptcy either under Chapter 7 or Chapter 13 of the bankruptcy code.

A Chapter 7 bankruptcy is a liquidation of assets. Under such a bankruptcy, only secured creditors will be paid from the proceeds from the sale of any assets. If the bankrupt patient had a credit agreement, the medical office is a secured creditor. But if the office is merely trying to collect a bill, the office is an unsecured creditor and will not receive payment.

A Chapter 13 bankruptcy is an "Adjustment of Debts" bankruptcy. In such a bankruptcy, the debtor (patient) pays a particular amount determined by the bankruptcy court to the court-appointed trustee, who then distributes the money to creditors. The debtor, if he or she has a regular income, can be required to make payments from that income into the trustee account for 3 years, and the trustee makes payments to creditors under payment plans he or she works out.

During the period the debtor is under the jurisdiction of the bankruptcy court, no creditor may try to collect a debt outside the bankruptcy process. However, a medical office can demand payment in full for any additional service it provides to a patient from whom it is collecting old debts under a bankruptcy agreement.

Memories *from* Externship

Christa Wilson: During my externship, I observed billing activities and I was allowed to assist in some ways. For example, I got a lot of practice at making sure that all bills printed correctly, checking each bill to make sure that there was an outstanding balance and that the insurance had already paid, and folding the bills to place them in window envelopes. The computer system used by the office where I did my externship printed the bills with an itemized statement of all activity on the account. The patient was expected to pay the balance on the bottom line of the statement. Sometimes patients called the office because they didn't understand what amount to pay. They usually spoke to the medical assistant at the office. I noticed that she was always polite and professional when she spoke to patients. The office also taught me how to post patient payments that were sent by check. I have to say I did not realize how important good billing practices are until my externship. I was grateful that I had experience at an office with a smooth-running system. ▪

Prepare for Success

What Would You Do? What Would You *Not* Do?

Case Study 3

On the day that Judith Mason is scheduled for an appointment, Christa notices that she has an outstanding balance of $58.00 from charges that were incurred 4 months ago. It is office policy that patients with a balance over 120 days are not seen until the balance has been paid. ▪

PROCEDURE 47-6 Writing a Collection Letter

Outcome Write a collection letter.

Equipment/Supplies

- Accounts aging report
- Computer
- Patient accounts
- Letterhead stationery
- Envelope
- Printer

1. Procedural Step. After the accounts receivable aging record has been created, determine which accounts need a letter. In general, this will be the accounts that are 90 to 120 days old.

Principle. A letter is usually sent after reminders and a telephone call have been made to collect an outstanding account balance.

2. Procedural Step. Review each account for the amount due, how long it has been due, any previous activity, and special situations. If the account is due from the estate of a deceased patient or insurance, or if there is a known reason why delayed payment is acceptable, do not take action on the account.

Principle. There may be circumstances that justify the delay in payment.

3. Procedural Step. Otherwise, prepare a letter for each outstanding account. The letter should state clearly the amount of the outstanding balance, the date that the charges were incurred, the service provided, and the amount paid by insurance. It should also describe any previous conversations and/or agreements. The letter should clearly state that the outstanding balance is due and identify the date by which it is expected to be paid (usually in 10 days).

Principle. Even though the bill is overdue, the recipient of the letter is given a reasonable amount of time to respond to this letter.

4. Procedural Step. Enter the typed signature as indicated by office policy (the medical assistant, office manager, billing specialist, or physician). If you do not sign the letter yourself, place the name of the authorized individual on the written signature line and prepare a reference line using your own initials.

Principle. The letter should be signed by a person who is authorized by the medical practice to collect outstanding accounts.

5. Procedural Step. Prepare an envelope.

6. Procedural Step. Obtain the written signature on the letter.

7. Procedural Step. Place a copy of the letter in the patient's medical record. Place a notation that a letter was sent on the aging report and in the computer account if possible. You may also file a copy of the letter in a collection follow-up file.

Principle. Future activity to collect on the account should be based on a review of your current activity.

8. Procedural Step. Place the letter in the envelope and mail the letter.

PROCEDURE 47-7 Posting a Collection Agency Payment

Outcome Post a collection agency payment.

Equipment/Supplies

- Computer
- Patient accounts
- Payment check(s)
- Day sheet
- Office policy manual
- Calculator

1. Procedural Step. When a payment has been made from a collection agency, locate the patient account in the computer.

Principle. All financial transactions must be entered to the correct patient account.

2. Procedural Step. Be sure that the patient's balance was adjusted to zero at the time the account was sent to collection. On the day sheet, label the first open line with the name of the patient whose check was returned and enter zero in the *old balance* column.

Principle. It is standard procedure to write off the patient balance when an account is sent to collection. This decreases the total accounts receivable accounts by an amount that the medical office does not expect to be able to collect.

Continued

PROCEDURE **47-7**   Posting a Collection Agency Payment—cont'd

PROCEDURE 47-7

3. Procedural Step. Create a new transaction for the patient and select the code for reverse collection. Enter the amount of the check and verify that the computer shows a positive patient balance after this entry.

Principle. The reverse collection code is used to increase the patient's balance before entering the payment.

4. Procedural Step. On the day sheet, enter the amount of the collection agency check in the *adjustment* column. The amount should be written in parentheses because it is a debit adjustment.

Principle. The patient balance, which has previously been adjusted to zero, must be increased to the amount of the collection agency check before posting the actual payment. In the computer, selecting the correct code automatically increases the patient balance. When using a day sheet, an adjustment must be added to the patient balance.

5. Procedural Step. When totaling the adjustment column of the day sheet, subtract the debit adjustment from the total of the credit adjustments.

6. Procedural Step. Enter the amount of the check in the *new balance* column. This figure is obtained by adding the adjustment to the previous balance of zero. If using a day sheet, on a new line enter "Collection Agency Payment" in the *professional service* column.

7. Procedural Step. In the computer, on a new line, select the code for collection agency payment and enter the amount of the collection agency check.

8. Procedural Step. Verify that the patient balance returns to zero in the computer account.

9. Procedural Step. On a new line of the day sheet, enter the patient's name and enter the amount of the collection agency check in the old balance column.

10. Procedural Step. Enter "Collection Agency Payment" in the *professional service* column of the day sheet.

11. Procedural Step. Enter the amount of the check in the *payment* column of the day sheet.

12. Procedural Step. Enter zero in the new balance column of the day sheet after subtracting the payment from the previous balance.

Principle. After posting the collection agency payment, the patient's balance should again be zero.

Example: The account of Robert Ricigliano, which was adjusted to zero when the account was turned over for collection, is increased to $25.00 using the code for reverse collection. Then a collection agency check for $25.00 is posted to the account leaving a zero balance.

12

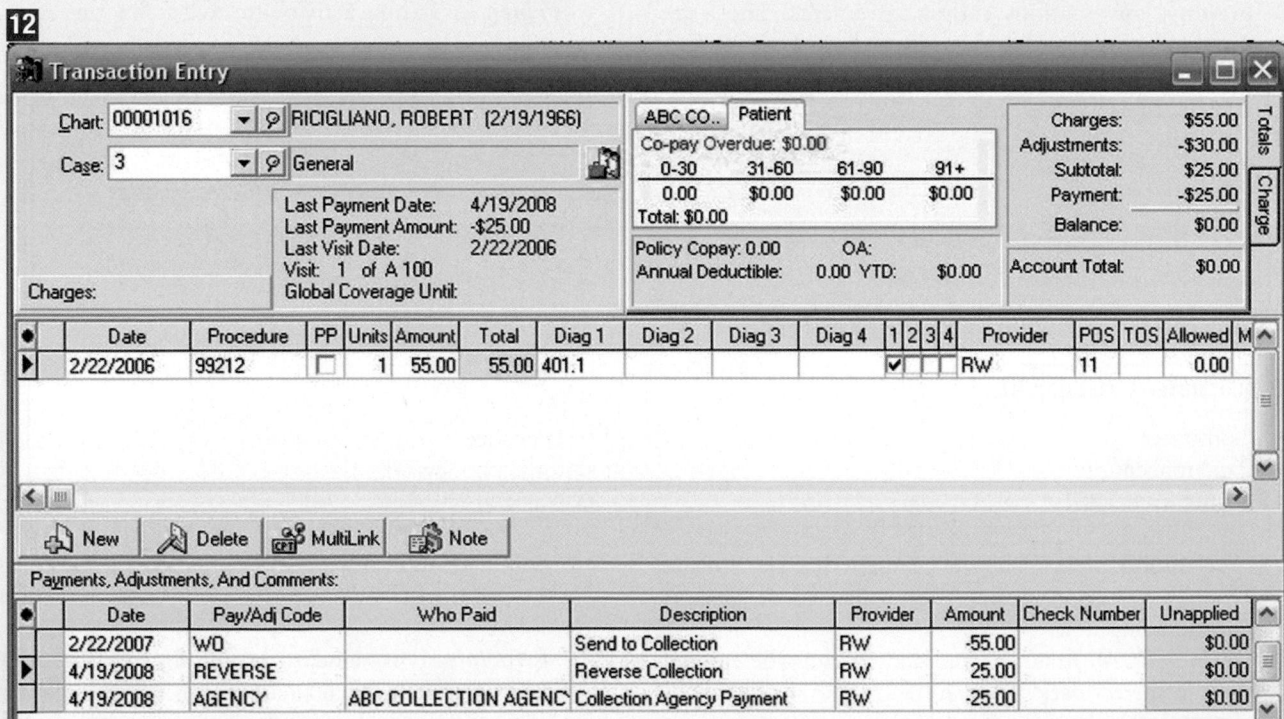

There is a zero balance after posting the collection agency check. (Screenshot used by permission of MCKESSON Corporation. All Rights Reserved.
© MCKESSON Corporation 2008.)

MEDICAL PRACTICE *and the* LAW

Several laws affect credit and collection activities.

Equal Credit Opportunity Act

This federal law prevents discrimination when offering credit based on:

a. Sex, marital status, race, national origin, religion, age
b. The fact that applicant receives public assistance income
c. The fact that applicant has exercised rights under consumer credit laws

An applicant must be informed if credit is denied and has 60 days to request, in writing, the reason for denial of credit.

Fair Debt Collection Practices Act

This is a federal law that requires the fair treatment of debtors and prevents unfair debt collection measures, including harassment, false statements, and threats.

The debt collector may not make frightening, verbally abusive, or threatening calls.

The debt collector may not call before 8 AM or after 8 PM.

The debt collector may not threaten action that cannot legally be taken or is not intended to be taken.

Federal Truth in Lending Act

Installment agreements of more than four payments (or fewer if interest is charged) must be written. The Federal Truth in Lending Act is administered by the Federal Trade Commission. It requires creditors to provide applicants with a form disclosing in a clear and obvious way all finance charges and terms.

Fair Credit Reporting Act

This act requires credit bureaus to supply correct and complete information to businesses to use in evaluating a person's application for credit, insurance, or employment.

Bankruptcy Abuse Prevention and Consumer Protection Act of 2005

This revision of federal bankruptcy laws attempts to make it more difficult for individuals to file for bankruptcy under Chapter 7, where most of the debts are forgiven by establishing a means test to determine if individuals are able to pay some of their debts. It also makes the process of filing for bankruptcy more difficult and expensive. Debtors are still able to file for bankruptcy under Chapter 13. ▪

What Would You Do? What Would You *Not* Do? RESPONSES

Case Study 1
Page 1095

What Did Christa Do?

❑ Reassured the patient that the situation is upsetting, but it can happen sometimes.
❑ Explained that most banks charge both the account of the individual who writes a check against an account with insufficient funds, as well as the account where the check was deposited.
❑ Suggested that the patient might want to consider overdraft protection.
❑ Explained politely that the office was only recovering its out-of-pocket expenses and was not, in fact, charging an additional fee.

What Did Christa Not Do?

❑ Did not get angry or raise her voice.
❑ Did not imply that the patient was trying to avoid payment or was a bad money manager.
❑ Did not make statements like, "This better not happen again!" or "How do you expect us to pay our bills if our patient's checks bounce?"

What Would You Do/What Would You *Not* Do? Review Christa's response and place a checkmark next to the information you

included in your response. List the additional information you included in your response.

_____
_____
_____
_____

Case Study 2
Page 1099

What Did Christa Do?

❑ Told the patient that she would check the receipt book, then went through the duplicate receipts of the day of the patient's visit.
❑ If a copy of the receipt for a cash payment was found, told the patient and entered the payment into the patient's account.
❑ If no copy of the receipt was found, explained to the patient that it is office policy to issue a receipt for any cash payment from a book where a duplicate is made automatically.
❑ If no copy of the receipt was found, suggested tactfully that the patient may not remember this specific visit, and perhaps she was unable to pay her copayment that day or forgot to pay it.
❑ If the patient continues to insist that she paid cash, offered to discuss the matter with the office manager or physician.

Continued

What Would You Do? What Would You *Not* Do?   RESPONSES—cont'd

What Did Christa Not Do?

❏ Did not get angry at the patient or raise her voice.

❏ Did not say that unless the patient could show her a receipt, the office would automatically assume that she had not paid.

❏ Did not accuse the patient of trying to get out of paying the copayment.

What Would You Do/What Would You *Not* Do? Review Christa's response and place a checkmark next to the information you included in your response. List the additional information you included in your response.

_____

_____

_____

_____

Case Study 3
Page 1104

What Did Christa Do?

❏ Attempted to contact Ms. Mason by telephone to inform her of the office policy so that the patient could be prepared to settle her outstanding bill.

❏ If the patient could not be contacted before the appointment, took her to a private room when she arrived at the office to discuss her account.

❏ Strongly encouraged Ms. Mason to settle the account by check or credit card before she was seen by the physician.

❏ If Ms. Mason stated that she could not pay the balance on that day, left the final decision about whether she would be seen to the physician because the patient had not been informed of the office policy before coming to the office.

What Did Christa Not Do?

❏ Did not take the sole responsibility to tell the patient that if she did not pay, under no circumstances would she be seen by the physician.

❏ Did not raise her voice or get angry with Ms. Wilson.

❏ Did not discuss Ms. Wilson's financial matters where others could overhear the conversation.

What Would You Do/What Would You *Not* Do? Review Christa's response and place a checkmark next to the information you included in your response. List the additional information you included in your response.

_____

_____

_____

_____

TERMINOLOGY REVIEW

Account aging The process of finding out how long specific account balances have been outstanding.

Balance due Total amount owed.

Bankruptcy Legal process by which the debts of an individual or business are resolved if they cannot be paid.

Claim message Messages encouraging payment of a bill, usually attached to or printed on the monthly statement.

Collection agency A firm that is in the business of collecting overdue accounts.

Credit balance A patient account that is a negative balance (i.e., money is owed by the medical office), usually due to an overpayment.

Overdraft A check (or draft) that exceeds the amount of funds in a bank account.

Skip Account for which no billing information is available.

Truth in lending Legal requirement to disclose the terms of a loan in terms that the borrower can understand.

ON THE WEB

For Information on the Federal Trade Commission: Federal Trade Commission: www.ftc.gov

 PREPARE FOR CERTIFICATION Visit the Evolve site at http://evolve.elsevier.com/Bonewit/today/ to actively Prepare for your Certification.

 Check out the Companion CD bound with the book to access additional interactive activities.

48

The Medical Assistant as Office Manager

LEARNING OBJECTIVES

1. Describe routine maintenance activities in the medical office.
2. Identify methods of fire protection for the medical office and its records.
3. Describe an efficient system of maintaining equipment inventory lists and operator manuals.
4. Maintain administrative and clinical equipment.
5. Describe the process of obtaining new equipment.
6. Explain procedures for taking inventory.
7. Describe an effective method for ordering, receiving, and storing supplies.
8. Explain how to manage office payroll.
9. Describe factors that create a professional environment.
10. Describe the medical assistant's role in orienting and training new employees.
11. Manage the physician's professional schedule and travel schedule.
12. Differentiate between medical office policies and procedures.
13. Create and/or revise medical office policies and procedures as needed to promote smooth office functioning.
14. Locate community resources to assist patients and medical office staff.
15. Describe how incident reports should be used to protect the medical office.
16. List types of liability protection for physicians, the medical office, and medical assistants.
17. Describe the various components of risk management in the medical office.

PROCEDURES

Perform routine maintenance of equipment.

Take a supply or equipment inventory.

Locate community resources.

CHAPTER OUTLINE

Introduction to Medical Office Management
Maintaining the Office
  Administrative Area
  Examination and Treatment Rooms
  Waiting Room
Routine Maintenance
  Temperature and Ventilation
  General Cleaning
  Cleaning Cabinets and Drawers
  Miscellaneous Tasks
  Security Systems
  Fire Protection
Maintaining Equipment
  Inventory
  Monitoring Equipment Function and Readiness for Use
  Service Contracts
  Service Calls

New Equipment Purchases
Supplies
  Supply Inventory
  Restocking
  Ordering Supplies
  Receiving Supplies
Creating an Environment for Teamwork
  Staff Meetings
  Orienting and Training Employees
Preparing Payroll
  Deductions
  Employer Obligations
  Preparing Payroll Checks
Managing Physician and Employee Schedules
  Professional Schedule
  Making Travel Arrangements

CAAHEP COMPETENCIES

General Competencies
Legal Concepts
- Demonstrate knowledge of federal and state health care legislation and regulations.

Patient Instruction
- Identify community resources.

Operational Functions
- Perform an inventory of supplies and equipment.
- Perform routine maintenance of administrative and clinical equipment.

ABHES COMPETENCIES

Administrative Duties
- Locate resources and information for patients and employers.
- Manage physician's professional schedule and travel.

Legal Concepts
- Maintain licenses and accreditation.
- Monitor legislation related to current health care issues and practices.
- Perform risk management procedures.

Office Management
- Maintain physical plant.
- Operate and maintain facilities and perform routine maintenance of administrative and clinical equipment safely.
- Inventory equipment and supplies.
- Evaluate and recommend equipment and supplies for practice.
- Maintain liability coverage.

Instruction
- Orient and train personnel.

Financial Management
- Process employee payroll.

KEY TERMS

back order
depreciation
gross pay
inventory
invoice
minutes
net pay
per diem
policy
procedure

purchase order (PO)
reorder point
risk management
salary
service contract
Social Security tax (FICA)
vendor
warranty
W-4

Introduction to Medical Office Management

The medical assistant performs many tasks that promote the smooth running of the medical office. These tasks include maintaining the physical space, taking inventory, ordering supplies, monitoring programs such as risk man-agement and employee safety programs, orienting new employees, and processing employee payroll. The responsibility for these management functions may be primarily that of the medical assistant in a small office, or primarily that of an office manager in a larger setting. Office management always provides the basis for effective patient care, and its importance cannot be overestimated.

MAINTAINING THE OFFICE

In many medical practices, a medical assistant assumes responsibility for maintaining the physical space of the medical office and performing general maintenance. Heavy cleaning and equipment repair is usually not performed by office staff, but rather by contractors. Thus, the medical assistant is also responsible for managing the relationship between the office and contractors or vendors of services, as well as medical, pharmaceutical, and office supply companies.

Administrative Area

When sitting at the front desk, the medical assistant must be able to effectively and efficiently answer two or three incoming calls, as well as to greet patients and handle paperwork.

Depending on the size of the administrative area, supplies and equipment for correspondence and billing may be stored in this area, including stationery, envelopes, billing forms, and coding reference books. In addition to the telephone (discussed in detail in Chapter 39), the reception area usually contains a personal computer, which may be freestanding or attached to the office's computer network. Materials for creating new patient folders should also be at hand if a paper medical record system is used.

The administrative area needs to have enough room to perform the required activities without the patient files and other papers becoming mixed up, and it must also allow the medical assistant to maintain patient confidentiality (Figure 48-1).

Again, depending on the size of the office, business operations will either take place in the front office close to the reception area or in a separate area in the office. In the business office are the rest of the pieces of equipment necessary for administering the office, including the photocopy machine, fax machine, and postage meter/electronic mailing system. In small offices, an all-in-one printer/copier/fax may be used.

Patient billing records are available either in hard-copy files in the business office or on the computer. If computers

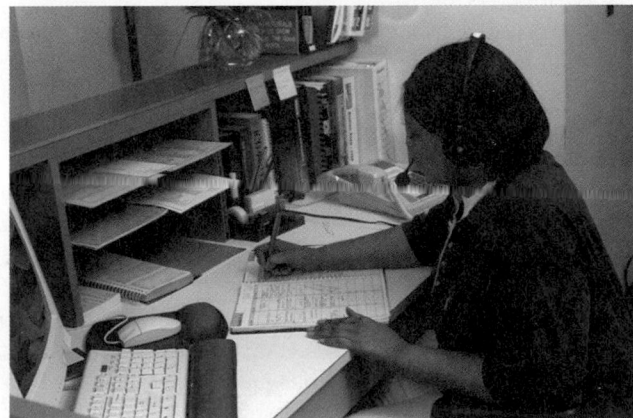

Figure 48-1. Well-organized front office.

are used to print multiple-copy charge slips, the printer may be a dot-matrix type, with the ability to handle continuous-feed forms, which have little holes along each side and ride along a tractor. For bills and documents, a laser printer or ink jet printer is usually used.

The medical assistant should be familiar not only with the office equipment's operation, but also with the maintenance responsibilities, such as reloading paper and adding toner or printer cartridges. In addition, the medical assistant may need to follow the terms of any maintenance agreements when scheduling maintenance or repairs.

Many offices also have a paper shredder for disposing of confidential documents. Although medical records must be maintained indefinitely, old telephone logs, old payroll records, canceled checks more than 7 years old, and minutes of practice management meetings should all be shredded rather than simply thrown away in the wastebasket or in a wastepaper-recycling bin. Shredded paper can still be recycled, and there is no danger that sensitive personal or business information will be seen by anyone who should not have access to it.

Examination and Treatment Rooms

Each examination or treatment room also needs approximately 100 square feet of floor space to hold an examination or treatment table, cabinets and countertop, patient chair and physician stool, and a small surface for the physician to write on. The room should be laid out so that a physician and medical assistant can move freely about the room. Equipment and supplies should be within easy reach or stored in drawers or cabinets easy to reach.

Each examination or treatment room needs to have a sink, as well as soap and paper towel dispensers. Hand sanitizer may be in a wall-mounted or freestanding dispenser. The examination room must also contain a wall-mounted rigid container for the disposal of sharps, such as needles, scalpel blades, or other objects that might puncture a plastic bag. Biohazard waste baskets with a biohazard plastic liner for materials that contain body fluids, such as blood, mucus, or pus, are located either in each examination room or in the hall. Containers for hazardous waste must be covered, except when adding waste. A foot pedal to open the cover facilitates use. The examination room usually contains an ordinary wastebasket for used paper towels and table paper.

For safety reasons, examination rooms should not contain syringes, needles, or medication samples. Cleaning materials and chemical solutions should never be stored under the counter in an examination room, especially if it is used for children.

Waiting Room

The waiting room makes a first impression on a new patient. It must be neat and welcoming. The waiting room needs two to four chairs for each physician in the office at one time, current magazines, and a table or magazine stand to hold them. If the practice sees children, some toys should be available in a separate play area. One person should be assigned to tidy up the waiting room a couple of times during the day.

A waiting room should have signs that inform patients about office policies. The signs depend on the policy of the individual office. Common signs include the following:

- No smoking
- Copayments are expected at the time of service (or some other language regarding the expectation of payment)
- Credit cards that are accepted
- No eating or drinking
- A charge will be added for returned checks to cover any bank fees
- Patients will be charged for cancelled appointments unless at least 24-hour notice is given

Some offices have a display rack with health information brochures. Brochures are available from government agencies, public agencies, and many companies. With the approval of the physician(s), these brochures are often provided to help educate patients about health promotion and disease prevention.

Sometimes there is a television or DVD player in the waiting room. In some practices, health information videos are playing. Other practices have a radio tuned to an easy-listening station or a CD player with quiet pop or light classical music. The medical assistant may need to turn on this equipment at the beginning of the day.

ROUTINE MAINTENANCE

Depending on the size of the office, many if not most routine maintenance activities are undertaken by staff. These include controlling the temperature, cleaning cabinets and drawers, changing light bulbs and replacing batteries in battery-powered equipment, turning the security system on and off, making sure fire protection equipment is in working order, and some daily cleaning. In all activities, medical assistants and other staff must be sure to protect themselves and patients from hazards and injury. Good body mechanics should be used to move supplies and equipment and when cleaning, as well as when working with patients. The workplace should be arranged to minimize strain during all routine and maintenance activities.

Temperature and Ventilation

The reception area and examination rooms should be kept at a comfortable temperature. People who are ill are sensitive to cold and drafts. The reception and patient waiting areas and examination rooms should be about 70°F to 72°F. The temperature in treatment rooms, the laboratory, and physicians' offices should be about 68°F to 70°F. A room used for procedures or minor surgery can be kept a little cooler because the physician and medical assistant will be wearing gowns, masks, and hair covers.

Ventilation is also important. Keeping air circulating is important both to dissipate odors and to allow germs to escape from the office atmosphere.

Putting It All into Practice

My name is Kelsey Whitman, and I am a registered medical assistant. I usually work in one of the satellite offices of a large medical group that includes primary care providers and medical specialists. The office where I usually work was formerly a house. They are planning to close it next spring, tear it down, and build a modern office building. Even though there are some disadvantages to the current setting, it has a lot of charm. The waiting room and three small examination rooms are on the first floor with the physicians' office, and we use the rooms upstairs for storage, a break room, and meeting rooms. I have a small office upstairs, but I never have time to sit in it. Usually we have only one physician in the office. I work with one other medical assistant, but since I have been in the practice longer, I am responsible for making sure that everything runs smoothly. I have to go to meetings at the main office once a month for a staff meeting. The meetings are held once a month late on Wednesday afternoon. We discuss issues affecting all work areas. We have also been reviewing some of the procedures done by medical assistants to be sure that every medical assistant in every office does things the same way. The other medical assistant will be going out for maternity leave in a few weeks, and we have been interviewing for a replacement. After an initial screening interview, I have been asked to talk to three applicants, to give them a tour of our office, and to give my feedback about how they might fit into this setting. One of the applicants seemed like a real team player, and I hope they hire her. It is so important for everyone to be able to work well together. ■

Prepare for Success

General Cleaning

Larger offices may contract for cleaning services, or office cleaning may be included in the monthly rent, especially in buildings that are dedicated to medical offices. Contracted cleaning is usually done one or two times a week, so even if the major cleaning is contracted out daily, cleaning tasks still must be performed.

Daily cleaning includes tidying up all areas of the office—reception and waiting rooms, administrative space, physicians' offices, examination and treatment rooms, and the laboratory.

Sinks should all be toweled dry, and rest rooms should be checked to make sure ample toilet and facial tissue, soap, and paper towels are available. Any spills or puddles on the floor of the rest room should be mopped up using gloves as needed.

Waste containers and recycling containers should be checked daily and emptied as needed. Biohazard sharps containers should be checked daily and replaced when they are three-quarters full. The plastic liners of biohazard waste containers should be changed as needed. Contracted

Highlight on Ergonomics and Worker Safety

A typical working day in a medical office puts a lot of physical stress on personnel. Bending, lifting, reaching, squatting, having a telephone stuck in the crook of the neck, and repeatedly using a typing keyboard put stress on the body. The human body was not designed by nature to perform such activities so frequently.

Common causes for disabling workplace injury include the following:

- Overexertion injuries caused from excessive lifting, carrying, or pulling an object
- Falls either on the same level or from a higher to lower level
- Injuries caused by bending, tripping, slipping without falling, or attempting to avoid falling
- Repetitive strain injuries
- Being struck by or struck against an object

Ergonomics

The word *ergonomics* comes from the Greek root *ergon,* which means "work." Ergonomics is the study of maximizing work efficiency by adapting the work environment for optimal physical and mental function. For example, office seating should be designed to provide maximum support for the back and computer keyboards should be positioned to reduce repetitive motion injuries to the hands, wrists, and arms. But ergonomics does not have to be high tech; it can be as simple as placing a small footstool at the side of an examining table, not only so the patient can step up before sitting on the table, but also so the doctor, who stands and performs examinations for hours a day, can rest a foot there and take pressure off his or her lower back. Ergonomics can also affect selection of shelving and storage units to minimize strain when storing items or removing them from storage.

Posture and Body Mechanics

Maintaining good posture can reduce backache and fatigue. The spine is a flexible stack of small bones called *vertebrae*. The back gets its flexibility because vertebrae are connected by fibrous ligaments containing gelatin-like tissue, called *disks*. To increase the strength of the back and neck, there are two primary curves in the spine, the cervical curve at the neck and the lumbar curve at the lower back.

The human head should sit above the pelvis, supported by the spine. People have a tendency to lean forward, both when walking and when sitting. This bad posture places extra strain on the back and neck muscles and causes excess muscle tension. Over time, the vertebrae are pulled out of position and lose flexibility.

Using good body mechanics, varying activities, and avoiding muscle strain can help prevent injuries from repetitive motion or overexertion.

Preventing Falls

Most workplace injuries from falls occur in the service industry, not in manufacturing. Several measures can be implemented in the medical office to prevent personnel (as well as patients) from tripping and falling. Good lighting, preventing clutter in walkways, closing drawers, cleaning spills promptly, and emphasizing safety can reduce the likelihood of falls. Medical assistants should wear sturdy shoes and avoid walking too fast, carrying items that block vision, and failing to pay attention to their surroundings. ∎

---

cleaning services will usually not empty biohazard waste containers because they contain regulated medical waste. The medical assistant must handle biohazard waste containers carefully to prevent an exposure incident. The OSHA Bloodborne Pathogen Standard outlines specific actions to take when handling regulated medical waste. These are outlined in Chapter 17.

If the office staff must do more intense cleaning, this should be done at least weekly. These tasks include mopping linoleum floors and vacuuming carpets, cleaning the glass at the reception area, polishing furniture and accessories, dusting, and thoroughly cleaning the rest rooms.

It is important to try to avoid a "medical smell" in the office. This is done by maintaining proper ventilation, as well as by cleaning up spills and accidents immediately, using light or unscented air fresheners in rest rooms and examination rooms, and keeping disinfectants and cleaning materials closed tightly when not in use and out of patients' reach.

Cleaning Cabinets and Drawers

Storage cabinets, drawers, and bookcases are cleaned less frequently, often on a day when the physician or some of

What Would You Do? What Would You *Not* Do?

Case Study 1

Jean Highsmith has brought her 1-year-old twins, Scott and Lucy, to the medical office because they have been fussy and tugging at their ears. In the waiting room, she puts the twins on the floor to play with the toys while they are waiting. When Kelsey is able to take them to an examination room, she notices that the twins, who also have runny noses, have been chewing on some of the plastic toys in the waiting room. She notices that Mrs. Highsmith has left used tissues on one of the examination room tables. After a few minutes, Mrs. Highsmith comes to the examination room door holding a child under each arm, and tells Kelsey that Scott has thrown up a little on the examination room table. ∎

the physicians in the practice are absent so that the room is not in use.

Whether cleaning an open set of bookshelves or a closed cabinet with shelving or drawers, the process is essentially the same.

First, if possible, all the items are removed from the bookcase or cabinet and placed on a table. If there are too many items, at least two shelves should be emptied at a time. The medical assistant should always work from the top of the shelving or cabinet so that dirt and dust will not fall on shelves that have already been cleaned.

For metal cabinets or shelving, the shelf is washed with warm water and soap, rinsed, and dried thoroughly. Wooden bookcases should be washed with extreme care or cleaned with furniture cleaner rather than soap and water.

The medical assistant should check labels on all items before putting them back on shelves. This is a good time to check for the expiration date on supplies and make a list of any items that need to be ordered or restocked from the general supply area to the cabinet. Outdated supplies must be disposed of properly (Figure 48-2).

Miscellaneous Tasks

Among the miscellaneous tasks that have to be performed daily are rearranging the waiting room chairs and replacing magazines in their racks (as well as toys if toys are available); cleaning mirrors in the rest rooms and examination rooms; and cleaning the tops, fronts, and undersides of cabinets and paper towel dispensers. Toys must be cleaned and disinfected on a regular basis, because they can harbor microorganisms.

The medical assistant may be responsible for replacing light bulbs in gooseneck lamps and other special lighting. Ceiling lighting is usually a responsibility of the maintenance staff employed by the building owner. If the space is owned by the practice, this may be a staff responsibility or may be covered by the cleaning/maintenance contract with an outside service.

Figure 48-2. Well-organized supply cabinet.

Security Systems

A medical office maintains a number of different security systems.

First, if the office is entered from a corridor in an office building, the building owner or office condominium association most likely has an electronic security system for the building itself.

Second, regardless of whether the office is entered from a corridor or directly from the outside, the practice should maintain an electronic security system against break-ins to the office itself.

The office's security/safety alarm system is monitored by an alarm company and may or may not also be tied to the local police and fire departments. Whether or not the system is tied into police and fire, the alarm company will call the practice's liaison to the company whenever the alarm goes off.

This designated person is often the practice administrator or "managing partner." However, two or three people are always listed as backups in case the liaison is not available.

Third, various places within the office require another layer of security. Medication cabinets—with all medications and prescription pads inside—should be locked, and a limited number of people should have keys to the medication cabinet lock. The laboratory, physicians' private offices, medical records cabinet or room, and business office are other areas that often have a lock and limited access.

If controlled substances are stored in the office, they should be "double-locked" (in a locked drawer within a locked cabinet). Two separate keys should open the two different locks.

Fire Protection

Fire protection for the building is the responsibility of the landlord or office condominium association. But fire protection for the contents of the office is the responsibility of office staff.

Many states require sprinklers in commercial and office buildings. Some states that require sprinklers for larger office buildings do not require them for smaller offices, such as a physician's office that has been converted from a house.

In addition to the health hazards smoking presents, there are also potential fire hazards related to smoking. Smoking should not be permitted in a physician's office, and signs advising patients and visitors that the office is a smoke-free environment should be clearly posted in the waiting area.

Exits should be clearly marked, and an emergency evacuation map should be posted near the door to the waiting room. Lighted exit signs should be tested by shutting off the lights in the room; bulbs should be replaced if necessary.

In a large office or free-standing clinic, there may be fire doors at certain points in corridors. These doors are designed to contain any fire on one side of the door from going into another area of the building. Fire doors should never be propped open but should be allowed to shut to their naturally closed position.

Fire extinguishers should be positioned in each room near the exit. These fire extinguishers are important not so much for putting out a fire but for giving a person in the room the ability to clear an exit path. They are placed near the door so that the fire does not get between the person and the exit. There should always be a fire extinguisher within a 50-foot travel distance of flammable liquids that are stored in containers.

Whenever possible, records should be stored in fire-resistant file cabinets. If the office uses a physical system to back up computer files (instead of a network or Internet system), the back-up drives should be stored in a fire-resistant file cabinet or fire-resistant box-type safe. It is always preferable to store a copy at another location.

Smoke detector laws vary by state, in terms of how many must be in an office and where they must be placed. In many buildings, smoke detectors are wired into the building's security and safety alarm system and are tied to the sprinkler system.

If the office has battery-operated smoke detectors, these should be tested monthly by pressing the test button. Batteries should be changed every 6 months, and the date should be noted on the detector.

MAINTAINING EQUIPMENT

Every physician's office has a number of pieces of equipment, both for medical purposes and business purposes. The medical assistant who manages the office is responsible for relationship management with the individuals or companies that sell and maintain the equipment, as well as with those who provide supplies for the equipment.

Inventory

An **inventory** is a detailed list of items in stock or in the possession of an individual or business. An equipment inventory lists each piece of equipment, the serial number, the date it was purchased, the length of the warranty, the name of the provider who services it, the manufacturer's suggested service schedule, and the last date of service. The office may also maintain a log validating maintenance and repair for larger pieces of equipment, such as computers and copiers.

An inventory is important for two reasons.
1. Tax consequence: Larger pieces of medical and office equipment are depreciated over 5 years, whereas smaller pieces of equipment and supplies can be fully deducted as an expense in the year in which they are purchased. (**Depreciation** is a name for the accounting methods used to account for the anticipated useful life of a piece of equipment and its loss of value over time.)
2. Theft or damage: In case of theft or damage, an inventory is necessary to make a complete report to the police and/or claim to the office's insurance company.

Operation manuals for the equipment can be stored centrally with the inventory list, or each manual can be stored with the piece of equipment for which it is used. Many pieces of equipment come with a plastic pouch on the side of the item or storage unit in which manuals and maintenance schedules can be kept.

Monitoring Equipment Function and Readiness for Use

The medical assistant should always be on the lookout for equipment problems, especially problems that could lead to a dangerous situation. All instruments should be checked when preparing them for sterilization. Before machines are used, the medical assistant should look for frayed wires, bent or damaged instruments, and machines that are not functioning properly.

Office machines should be dusted or wiped with a damp cloth regularly following manufacturers' guidelines. Batteries, fluids, paper, toner, or other supplies should be replaced as needed. If there is a maintenance log for the piece of equipment (e.g., the autoclave log, copier log), the medical assistant should document any maintenance (Procedure 48-1).

The decision whether to repair or replace a piece of equipment will usually be made taking several factors into account:
- The age of the piece of equipment
- How expensive a new piece of equipment is
- The level of use the equipment gets
- Whether the manufacturer still produces parts for repair
- If any important features have been added to newer models of the equipment

If there is no service contract for the piece of equipment and the decision is made to repair it, a repair service must be located and a repair arranged. The manufacturer usually has a list of authorized repair services by region. In larger organizations, a purchase order is usually necessary for an equipment repair.

Emergency equipment must always be ready for use. Because it may be required only once in a long time, this equipment must be checked at least monthly and more often in many larger facilities. The contents of the emergency box or crash cart (discussed in detail in Chapter 35) should be checked for completeness by a designated person, who will initial a form to verify the presence of each item on the checklist.

Oxygen tanks are checked at the same time as emergency equipment. They should be sent to be refilled when the level falls to a predetermined level. Expiration dates of emergency medications are checked at the same time.

Service Contracts

Most pieces of medical office equipment are purchased with a service contract. A **service contract** is an agreement that provides for repair calls over a specific time period after the manufacturer's warranty expires. A **warranty** is a promise by the manufacturer to repair or replace defective parts in an item during a specific time period. The service calls in a service contract may be free or have a specified charge, depending on the contract. Contracts usually call for larger pieces of equipment to be serviced at the physician's office. Smaller pieces of equipment often have a two-price contract: one price if the item is brought to a service center for repair and another price if repair is carried out on site.

Service Calls

Before calling in a service technician, the medical assistant should check the equipment thoroughly. A plug accidentally removed from a socket or a disconnected wire is often the cause of what seems like a machine breakdown.

If there is a service contract, all necessary routine maintenance should be performed in the office or scheduled for a technician to perform it.

The medical assistant should keep a record of all service calls, the reason the call was made, the response, whether there was a service charge, and the suggested follow-up.

New Equipment Purchases

Although the physicians in the practice or the clinic administrator may be responsible for purchasing equipment, the medical assistant may be asked to help research options.

Manufacturers are glad to send information about the piece of equipment in question. Many companies now have websites that can be browsed to see product features and costs. Some sites even have video demonstrations. A demonstration can often be arranged.

Some practices look for used equipment or furniture. Companies that sell equipment from a number of manufacturers often have used equipment in inventory. Used equipment can also be found from physicians who are buying new equipment or retiring. Before purchasing a piece of used equipment, it is recommended to be sure that the manufacturer still supports the product (i.e., manufactures replacement parts so that it can be repaired).

The medical assistant may be asked to research the "lease vs. buy" decision, whether to purchase the equipment or lease it over a period of time. Most medical and office equipment can be leased. Leasing and buying each have advantages and disadvantages, mostly in terms of tax treatment. The practice lawyer should be consulted on this decision. Laboratory equipment may be provided at a reduced cost or for a low monthly lease depending on the number of tests performed, so it is important to compare options among different companies.

When new equipment is received in the office, it is a good idea to note replacement part numbers, such as bulbs, batteries, and cartridges, and add them to the supply-ordering system.

PROCEDURE 48-1   Performing Routine Maintenance of Equipment

Outcome Perform equipment maintenance and document on equipment maintenance log.

Equipment/Supplies

- Piece of equipment to be maintained
- Cloth for dusting
- Maintenance log sheet

- Supplies necessary for the piece of equipment (e.g., paper, batteries, toner, fluids)

---

1. **Procedural Step.** Locate the piece of equipment to be checked.
2. **Procedural Step.** Check all electrical cords and plug to ensure there is no fraying or malfunction.
   Principle. Frayed electrical cords are a potential fire hazard and can cause electrical shocks.
3. **Procedural Step.** Check the piece of equipment for cracks, dents, or other damage; obvious impairment; or malfunction.
4. **Procedural Step.** Check any keyboard or keypad for cracks, faded numbers, or letters or other impairment.
5. **Procedural Step.** Dust or clean the outside or case of the piece of equipment according to manufacturer's directions.
   Principle. Dust can interfere with correct function of the machine.
6. **Procedural Step.** Check leads and other wires or other tubing.

7. **Procedural Step.** Check or change batteries, fluid, toner, or other essential components.

Add paper to the photocopier as needed.

8. Procedural Step. Schedule any required maintenance if appropriate.

9. Procedural Step. Fill out the equipment maintenance log.

Example:

Equipment description:	BESTCOPY OFFICE PHOTOCOPIER		
Serial Number:	266XXX49500	Model Number:	6500AA

Date:	Action Taken/Comments:	Initials
5/26/10	Machine checked, glass cleaned, toner added.	SH, CMA (AAMA)
5/30/10	Streaks on copies, service call arranged. Technician cleaned drum.	SH, CMA (AAMA)
6/2/10	Machine checked, glass cleaned.	SH, CMA (AAMA)

SUPPLIES

A busy medical office goes through an enormous amount of supplies—both clinical and administrative—in a month. Managing the purchase and stocking of supplies is a task that often falls to a medical assistant.

The number of supplies that can be ordered at one time is dependent on the amount of storage space in the office. A practice can usually get a better price by ordering large amounts, but many offices are limited in the amount they can store. Sometimes it is possible to get extra storage space in the basement of the building where space is being rented.

Also, many physicians receive discounts on supplies by virtue of membership in some sort of a buying group or independent practice organization. Other practices are beginning to move toward website-based purchasing of medical supplies. The savings to suppliers from their customers ordering over the Internet can sometimes be so large that they offer enormous discounts.

It is important to develop a good system of tracking supplies, usage, and storage capacity. In this way, reordering is not done too early when there is no room or too late when the practice may actually run out of important supplies.

When planning a new office or office move, it is important to plan for adequate supply-storage space.

Supply Inventory

A supply inventory is a listing of all the supplies regularly used in the office. This inventory can be kept in a notebook with a separate page for each supply, or it can be a set of cards—one for each supply item. Notebook pages or cards can be grouped either by the type of supply (e.g., surgical disposable, photocopier) or by the supplier.

The supply list should contain the following information:

1. The item's name
2. Any specific size used
3. The usual supplier

4. The cost per a standard quantity (i.e., $3.50 per 100) if known
5. The **reorder point,** which is a number that identifies when the number of items remaining is low enough that it must be reordered. The reorder point is calculated by determining the number of items used per day or week and the number of days or weeks it takes for an order to be received. For instance, if the office uses 100 pairs of gloves per day, there are 50 pairs in each box, and it takes 5 working days to receive a new order of gloves, the reorder point would be when fewer than 15 boxes (750 gloves) are in the supply room (7½ days' worth).
6. The quantity ordered each time

Figure 48-3 shows a sample supply inventory. Information related to specific items is often maintained on cards or a sheet with the items ordered (Figure 48-4).

The card usually contains additional information about order dates and dates of receipt, initialed by the person who placed and/or received the order.

Most offices routinely order supplies on a monthly basis. Some supplies are routinely reordered each ordering period, but others are ordered only on an "as needed" basis. For these items, the medical assistant may check the supply closet and generate a list of needed supplies. Computerized inventory record-keeping can be maintained on a spreadsheet (Procedure 48-2).

Even if the office has been using the same supplier for a long time, it is a good practice to check other suppliers at least annually to see if a better relationship can be established. This might involve discounts for the volumes purchased, faster delivery, better prices overall, or an availability of more product from one supplier than is currently available. If a new supplier has offered a better price, the medical assistant should always give the current supplier the opportunity to "meet or beat" the current offer. An established relationship is a known quantity in terms of delivery reliability and overall quality of the relationship. When items are ordered repeatedly from the same supplier, the medical

ITEM NAME	SUPPLIER	ITEM #	COST	REORDER AT	# TO ORDER
Bandages & Dressings					
nonsterile sponges 2" x 2"	H Medical	XY 2544	$3.50/pkg/200	5 pkg	10 pkg
nonsterile sponges 4" x 4"	H Medical	XY 7812	$8.25/pkg/200	5 pkg	10 pkg
sterile sponges 4" x 4"	H Medical	XY 5540	$22.00/box/00	2 box	5 box
non-sterile conforming bandage 2"	Winscott	49J265	$5.25/pkg/12	10 pkg	10 pkg
non-sterile conforming bandage 4"	Winscott	49J266	$8.62/pkg/12	10 pkg	10 pkg
paste bandage 4"	Winscott	57J381	$4.10 each	10	10
					10

Figure 48-3. Sample supply inventory. (From Hunt SA: *Saunders fundamentals of medical assisting,* St. Louis, 2007, Saunders.)

Figure 48-4. Form for inventory control. (Courtesy Patterson Office Supplies, Champaign, Ill.)

office is usually billed instead of having to pay in advance for the supplies.

When storing supplies in the main supply area, supplies with the expiration date closest to the current date should be placed at the front of the area so that they are used first. New supplies are stored behind the older supplies.

Restocking

Moving supplies from the central supply area to the place where they will be used is called *restocking*. Examination rooms should be restocked once or twice daily. General supplies in administrative areas are usually restocked weekly. The photocopy and fax machines may need paper daily, depending on the volume of work done.

Ordering Supplies

A supply order is created by combining the list of supplies that are routinely ordered with the items that have been "flagged" using the inventory control system. When this list is complete, the supplier for each item must be identified and orders for that supplier created. Most offices will try to have one or two suppliers for clinical supplies and one or two for administrative supplies. Medications may be purchased from the same company as the one used for clinical supplies or from a pharmaceutical supplier.

Supplies are usually ordered in one of four ways: by telephone, fax, mail, or online (Figure 48-5). Even when using the telephone or computer, it is important to print or maintain a paper record of the transaction to reconcile against

Figure 48-5. Supplies may be ordered using a catalog order form.

receipt of the supplies and for proper accounting. If ordering by fax, it is a good idea to make a follow-up phone call to make sure the fax has come through clearly and that the order-entry person at the supply house has no questions.

Fax or mail order purchases are submitted on a form listing the item, item number, amount, color, etc. This form may be unique to the office or an order form supplied by the **vendor,** the company that sells the supplies or equipment. A **purchase order (PO)** is the form used to order supplies and the order itself. In many organizations it includes a tracking number (often called a *PO number*). This number is used to reconcile receipt of supplies and payment of the invoice.

When the vendor cannot ship the item immediately, the item is said to be on **back order.** The order should be flagged to be sure it arrives when promised. A back-ordered item is usually not billed until it is shipped.

In some states, ordering of medications, needles, and sterile solutions requires an authorization from a physician and a copy of the physician's state medical license for purchase. For purchase of controlled substances, such as narcotics, a physician authorization and a copy of the physician's federal Drug Enforcement Administration certificate is necessary.

What Would You Do? What Would You *Not* Do?

Case Study 2

Kelsey accepts a delivery of a large box of supplies from UPS at a time when the office is especially busy. She places the box in the supply room and continues with her work. Toward the end of the day, she realizes that she has not opened the delivery. She goes to the supply room and opens the outer box. Inside, there are boxes and packages of dressings, bandages, tape, tissues, gauze squares, and other items. Kelsey has an appointment, and she is anxious to finish up so that she can leave the office. ∎

Receiving Supplies

Different suppliers ship their supplies in different ways, including using the U.S. Postal Service, a large national package delivery company like United Parcel Service (UPS) or FedEx Ground, or a local courier service.

Most delivery services will ask for a signature to confirm that the delivery was made. When supplies are received, they should immediately be brought to the storage room. At the first convenient opportunity, the packing slip should be inspected and reconciled with the order to make sure all items have been received or that items that are to be received in a separate delivery are noted on the packing slip. If the packing slip is incorrect, the missing items should be noted and the supplier notified.

The packing slip should be clipped to the order form. When all items have been received, the order form with all the packing slips attached should be marked all items received and placed in the accounts payable folder. If the order was not prepaid, the **invoice** (itemized bill for items that have not been prepaid) should arrive within a few days of delivery of the final items on the order.

Once the contents of a shipping box have been placed in storage, the box should be discarded. It is not recommended to keep boxes or cartons used for shipping because they may be dirty and can harbor insects or rodents.

PROCEDURE 48-2   Taking a Supply or Equipment Inventory

Outcome Take a supply or equipment inventory.

Equipment/Supplies

- Inventory list
- Notebook or cards
- Items to inventory
- Pen

1. Procedural Step. Obtain a list of items in inventory—either on a written or computer-generated inventory list, inventory notebook, or box of inventory cards.
Principle. The process of taking an inventory includes validating the presence or absence of a given set of items.

2. Procedural Step. Check each item in the inventory record against the items present in all areas of the medical office. For equipment, validate serial numbers. For supplies, consider the supplies on hand in both examination rooms and storage, checking expiration dates and disposing of those that are expired.

Continued

PROCEDURE **48-2** Taking a Supply or Equipment Inventory—cont'd

Principle. Expired items should be thrown away and not counted as part of the inventory. The point of taking inventory is to keep track of the number of items on hand that can be used.

Check the number of supplies on hand.

3. Procedural Step. For an equipment inventory, make every effort to locate each piece of equipment on the list and validate that it is in working condition. Docu-

ment if the item is missing or needs repair. For a supply inventory, check the number of supplies on hand against the number listed as the reorder point. If the number of items on hand is close to the reorder point, flag the item as one that needs to be reordered per the custom of your office.

4. Procedural Step. Check that the information on the inventory card or list is correct and complete. There should be a serial number for equipment and a description of the size, color, and price, as well as the usual supplier for supplies.

Principle. You will need this information when replacing equipment or reordering supplies.

5. Procedural Step. Be sure that your storage space is tidy, that items can be found when needed, and that supplies are arranged so that those with the oldest expiration date are at the front of the storage shelf.

Principle. Supplies are useless unless they can be found. Supplies with the oldest expiration date should be used first.

6. Procedural Step. Place inventory cards, computer printout sheet, or inventory book in the proper location for follow-up, including placing orders or updating computer information and storage until needed again.

CREATING AN ENVIRONMENT FOR TEAMWORK

An environment that supports teamwork is one in which people are willing to help each other out, but are also willing to allow each individual to display her or his particular expertise. The medical assistant may help set the tone for teamwork by showing respect for each employee and his or her skills and pitching in to help orient new employees or anyone who needs a little assistance during an especially busy time.

Staff Meetings

In a busy office where each person is performing specialized tasks, regular staff meetings can also promote teamwork. These meetings should occur often enough—weekly or, at most, monthly—so that situations in need of correction can be dealt with quickly. The medical assistant may be responsible to schedule and/or lead these meetings.

The staff meeting should be used to share information or work through changes in office practice or procedures, discuss ways to improve patient satisfaction and office performance, and encourage staff to take advantage of opportunities to improve skills. Some skill improvement efforts can take place in the form of training sessions in the office on new equipment or computer systems. Others can be opportunities to attend off-site seminars and workshops.

When planning a meeting, a written agenda (list of specific items of business to be covered) assists in focusing the meeting and ensuring that all important business is considered in an organized way. One person should be assigned the task of taking **minutes** (a record of the meeting's proceedings).

Written minutes are valuable because they assist individuals who attended a meeting to follow up on suggestions and decisions. The agenda should be prepared in advance, but except for a large, formal meeting, it need not be circulated until the meeting begins. Minutes, however, should be circulated. They should be distributed as soon as possible after the meeting, although they are not usually formally approved until the beginning of the next meeting.

Orienting and Training Employees

A new employee will be required to provide documentation in order to be added to the office payroll. All employees must have a Social Security number and complete an I-9 (Employment Eligibility Verification) form before they can begin working. The medical assistant may be responsible for reviewing the Social Security card and/or documents that establish identity and eligibility to work in the United States. Information about obtaining or replacing a Social Security card or changing the name on a Social Security card is available from the Social Security Administration.

Before the end of the first withholding period, a new employee must fill out a W-4 form, which identifies the number of exemptions claimed for proper income tax withholding. This form is updated annually, and the current version can be obtained from the Internal Revenue Service (IRS) website. An employee can submit a new form any time that his or her status changes; for example, if the employee gets married or has a child. If the employee elects to claim fewer exemptions than he or she is legally entitled to, the medical office will withhold more money from the employee's paycheck. Individuals claim fewer exemptions to be sure that adequate funds are withheld to cover their income tax liability.

A photocopy of any licenses or certificates should also be obtained from a new employee. All documents should be placed in the employee's personnel file.

Working with New Employees or Medical Assisting Students

The medical assistant may be asked to participate in the orientation and training of a new medical assistant. This usually involves explaining physician preferences and working with the new employee to be sure that he or she understands how all procedures should be performed. The office may have a check-off list where the new employee must demonstrate each skill or task before being allowed to perform it without supervision. If a new employee is not familiar with a specific piece of equipment, such as the model of electrocardiograph or spirometer, the medical assistant may be responsible for training the new employee how to use it. A similar process is used when the office accepts medical assisting students for externship. The medical assistant must allow a medical assisting student to observe each procedure and then perform it with supervision until the medical assistant can perform the procedure correctly without supervision (Figure 48-6).

PREPARING PAYROLL

Preparing a payroll is an increasingly complex task. Consequently, many offices—even those that have long done their own payroll—are switching to outside payroll services. Whether or not payroll is done in the office, files are kept on all employees.

Payroll records for individual employees include the following:

- Name, address, Social Security number, and occupation
- The employee's withholding allowance certificate (**W-4**), which is used to calculate the amount withheld for federal income taxes
- Dates of employment
- Record of hours worked, wages paid, annuity, and pensions
- Record of all payroll deductions

These records must be kept for at least 4 years and be available for review by the IRS.

Figure 48-6. Medical assistants may need to help medical assisting students during their externship.

Employees may fill out time cards to report the hours worked, or they may punch in and out using a time clock. Most medical assistants are paid by an hourly rate. In this case the **gross pay,** the amount of money earned before any deductions, is calculated by multiplying the number of hours worked times the hourly rate. Some office employees may receive a **salary,** a fixed amount paid on a regular basis that does not depend on the number of hours worked. In this case the gross pay is the predetermined amount.

Deductions
Income Taxes

Employers are required to withhold federal income taxes based on the amount paid to an employee and the number of withholding allowances the employee claims. The IRS publication *Employer's Tax Guide* contains detailed information including tables to determine the amount to withhold.

Social Security and Medicare

Social Security tax (called *FICA* after the Federal Insurance Contributions Act) funds the national program of retirement benefits into which all workers pay 6.2% of the first $102,000 in income (for 2008). In addition 1.45% of all employee wages are withheld for Medicare taxes, and the employer must pay an additional 1.45%.

State Taxes

Most states require employers to withhold state income tax based on the amount earned and the number of withholding allowances reported for the state (which may be different from the federal W-4 allowances).

Employer Obligations

The employer is required to deposit withheld income taxes, as well as employee and employer Social Security and Medicare taxes, following the schedule outlined in the IRS Employer's Tax Guide.

The employer is required to provide each employee with two copies of form W-2, the Wage and Tax Statement, by January 31. This form is used by the employee to complete his or her personal income tax forms. State income taxes are usually included on this form.

Unemployment Tax

Federal unemployment tax (FUTA) is paid by the employer on the first $7000.00 of income at a rate of 6.2% (for 2008). The money, which must be deposited quarterly, is used to pay unemployment compensation for workers who have lost their jobs. States also require employers to pay unemployment tax for their employees, and a few states also require employers to withhold an unemployment tax from their employees.

Preparing Payroll Checks

If the payroll is being done in the office, the individual who does the payroll must gather time sheets or time cards if they are used; calculate wages, taxes, and other deductions for each employee; prepare the checks; and record five items of information in the payroll record for each employee:

1. Total wages for the pay period (gross pay)
2. Federal, state, and (sometimes) local income taxes, as well as Social Security and Medicare taxes
3. Other deductions, such as health insurance, uncovered medical expenses, dependent care, and retirement savings
4. **Net pay,** or take-home pay (pay after deductions)
5. Gross pay, or total pay, from January 1 to the end of the pay period being recorded

Before calculating wages, time sheets or time cards should be reviewed for accuracy. (If a time clock is used, the exact time of clocking in and clocking out is recorded.) If the payroll is being managed by a service outside the office, the supervising medical assistant is only responsible for collecting time sheets and transmitting to the payroll agency each employee's gross pay for the pay period.

MANAGING PHYSICIAN AND EMPLOYEE SCHEDULES

Professional Schedule

In addition to the medical office appointment schedule, physicians must be scheduled for other responsibilities related to patient care. In a group practice, one physician must always be on call (i.e., available to take telephone calls from patients and make arrangements so that urgent and emergency health care needs of patients will be met). Physicians in solo practice often collaborate with other physicians in their community to provide this service. The medical office usually develops a standard schedule, but individual physicians must be assigned to cover each on-call time period. After the schedule has been arranged, physicians usually must work with each other if they want to switch or change days.

If the medical practice has satellite offices, physicians must be assigned times to see patients in the main office and in the other offices. If possible, coverage must be coordinated so that there is at least one physician in the satellite office every day. A master schedule is usually created, but variations occur depending on time of year and circumstances. For example, sometimes satellite offices are closed during holiday or vacation periods.

In many practices the physicians make nursing home visits. In addition to scheduled blocks of time for these visits, there must also be a plan to provide urgent care if a nursing home resident becomes ill. Some physicians always see their own patients, and in other practices, there is one physician who is responsible for nursing home patients on a given day.

Other staff members must also be scheduled to provide coverage in both the primary office and any satellite offices. Usually employees must submit requests for days off, changes to the regular schedule, and vacation in writing. Depending on the size of the office, the medical assistant or office manager may be responsible for creating the work schedule for staff other than the physicians. When one of the medical assistants or other staff calls in sick, efforts must be made to find a replacement. The medical office often has contact with medical assistants or other employees who will work ***per diem,*** a Latin term meaning "per day" or "by the day." *Per diem* employees do not have a fixed schedule. They may be given a weekly schedule depending on office needs, and, in addition, they may be called on a day when extra help is required. The office may also use an employment agency to obtain temporary employees, especially if one of the regular medical assistants is unable to work for an extended period of time.

Making Travel Arrangements

Office staff and physicians may travel to workshops or lectures in order to obtain continuing education. Physicians, medical assistants, and other professional staff may require continuing education units (CEUs) in order to maintain a license or certification. In addition, physicians may travel to meetings of local or national organizations to attend meetings and/or present lectures or workshops.

The medical assistant may need to perform several tasks related to travel arrangements:

- Arranging or rearranging the office schedule to cover for the individual who will be traveling
- Submitting a conference or workshop registration
- Arranging room accommodations
- Making airplane reservations and sometimes arranging airport transportation

Conference or workshop registrations can usually be made using the Internet if there is an office credit card that can be used to secure these arrangements. Otherwise, registrations can be sent in with a check. Airline reservations

Memories *from* Externship

Kelsey Whitman: The office where I did my externship was in a physician office building next to the local hospital. It was a very clean, modern office, and I learned so much there. There were two physicians specializing in internal medicine.

At the beginning of the day, we got everything ready for the patients. We made sure the waiting room was tidy, stocked every examination room, and turned on the CD player so that patients could listen to music. The office closed for an hour at noon, and after the morning patients had left, we checked the waiting room, picked up the magazines, and made sure there was no trash on the tables. In the afternoon, it was my job to go through the examination rooms and make sure that all items were restocked. While I was on my externship, one of the physicians went on vacation for a week, and we used that time to clean all the drawers and cabinets in the examination rooms. We took everything out and cleaned each area with soap and water. We found expired supplies at the back of the cabinets, and we had to discard them. It was a lot of work, but when we were done, everything seemed much better organized. Before my externship, I didn't realize the amount of work it is to keep everything looking neat and professional in a medical office. ■

Prepare for Success

and hotel reservations can be made using the Internet or by telephone, and payment or reservation is usually made with a credit card. There is often a special room rate available at one or more hotels for large conferences. The office may also use a travel agent to make hotel and airline reservations. A car rental may also need to be arranged.

For travel to local meetings, staff may be able to submit the number of miles traveled and receive reimbursement from the medical office.

PROVIDING RESOURCES FOR STAFF AND PATIENTS
Office Policy and Procedure Manuals
Medical Office Policies

Effective management of the medical office requires activities to meet all legal requirements and to maintain a high standard of patient care. A guiding principle for management of the office is called a **policy.**

Often an organization formulates its own statements (written policies) to help it adhere to laws or regulations and practice ethically. For example, a medical office might have written policies regarding sexual harassment, confidentiality, patient rights, and honest and ethical billing, to name just a few.

These are collected in a policy manual, which can easily be reviewed by employees and regulatory agencies. It is the responsibility of the manager to review existing policies and implement changes if necessary.

If a policy needs to be reviewed, it is usually discussed in a staff meeting and a draft of the revision is circulated for review among office staff. Once there is consensus about the revision, the revised policy is accepted and the revised version is placed in all copies of the policy manual. The date of acceptance and/or revision should be clearly indicated on each policy. A new policy may be necessary, especially when new federal legislation is passed, such as the HIPAA laws. A new policy is also written as a draft, circulated, discussed, and eventually accepted and added to the policy manual.

Written Procedures

In order to put policies into practice, an organization utilizes procedures. A **procedure** is a description of the steps to handle a specific situation or perform a certain task. Written procedure manuals are common in large organizations, but they can also benefit smaller medical offices, for several reasons.

They are excellent resources for new employees. They can also provide guidelines and information when a long-term employee suddenly becomes unavailable, either by changing jobs or becoming ill. They encourage office staff to reflect on the methods used to accomplish tasks and examine the reasons for specific actions.

Regular review of procedures is necessary to be sure that they are up to date and conform to changes in legal regulations and/or improvements in technology. There may be separate procedure manuals for clinical procedures and administrative procedures.

Procedures that facilitate proper functioning of every area of the office should be available. New procedures should be written when they are missing or when new equipment or different supplies have changed how things are done. It is helpful to add photographs, especially of tray setups or supplies and equipment needed for special procedures. The medical assistant may oversee the job of setting the schedule to review or create procedures, obtaining written or verbal input from those who actually carry out the tasks, and finalizing the written procedures. Like policies, each procedure should be dated. Procedure manuals throughout the office should be kept up to date.

After the procedure manual has been created, all personnel, especially new staff members or those with questions, should be encouraged to use the procedure manual as a reference. It often seems easier to ask questions of coworkers with experience, but it increases independence and individual capability if staff are encouraged to refer to the written manual.

Emergency Preparedness and Evacuation Plan

In addition to being prepared for medical emergencies, which were discussed in Chapter 35, the office should have an emergency action plan in place to respond to a fire, natural disaster, or emergency situation affecting the entire office. OSHA requires almost every business to have a written emergency evacuation plan to guide employees during an office emergency.

The written plan must include the following:
• A means of reporting emergencies
• Evacuation procedures and emergency escape routes

- Procedures to account for all employees after an evacuation
- Specific assignments for employees to follow to assist the injured or disabled
- The names and titles of individuals responsible for additional information about the plan

Usually a map is created from a floor plan showing clearly marked escape routes and exits. It is important to identify procedures for different types of emergencies and to clarify situations when employees should evacuate as opposed to situations when it is preferable to shelter in place. Responsibilities for individual employees must be clearly delineated, including identifying when selected individuals stay to shut down operations or use fire extinguishers.

Most organizations are also preparing plans for community emergencies or disasters, including natural phenomena (e.g., tornadoes, floods), epidemics, and nuclear accidents. There is an emergency management agency in each state to notify the public about and respond to emergencies that affect large areas of the state. Most communities also have emergency action committees or agencies.

Locating Community Resources

The medical assistant can be helpful to patients by identifying community resources to meet patient health needs (Procedure 48-3). The medical office may keep a list of local organizations with telephone numbers or other contact information in the following areas:

- Support for alcoholism or addiction
- Support for caregivers of individuals with decreased mental or physical function
- Adult day care
- Visiting nurse and homemaker services
- Legal aid
- Local civic organizations including services for children, families, elders, and the homeless
- Local board of health
- Hospital-sponsored rehabilitation, weight control, smoking cessation programs
- Immunization clinics
- CPR and first aid training

National organizations focus on many diseases. Most will provide information, and some have local chapters or can refer patients to local organizations. The medical assistant can be helpful by assisting the patient to search the Internet for these organizations. Many hospitals also have extensive programs related to specific diseases or conditions, and the medical assistant should become familiar with those in his or her locality, especially those sponsored by the hospital with which the practice physicians are affiliated. The hospital newsletter is a good source of information on new programs for patients. See Appendix C for the national contact information of some community resources.

What Would You Do? What Would You *Not* Do?

Case Study 3

Ellen Pritchard has brought her mother, Elizabeth Brown, a 76-year-old widow, to the office for a physical examination. Kelsey notices that Ellen looks upset at the check-out desk after Mrs. Brown has been seen by the physician. Kelsey asks Ellen if anything is the matter. Ellen says, "I'm worried about my mother. She has lost weight, and I don't think she is eating properly. She lives alone, and I help her as much as I can, but lately I'm not sure it's enough. I don't know what to do." ■

PROCEDURE 48-3 Locating Community Resources

Outcome Locate appropriate community resources.

Equipment/Supplies

- Local telephone book
- Office list of community resources
- Computer
- Local hospital newsletter(s)
- Library access
- Local newspapers
- Pen
- Notepad

1. **Procedural Step.** Research local sources to identify community agencies with resources to assist patients. Potential sources of information include the library, local newspapers, local cable TV stations, local telephone book, local hospital newsletters, and the Internet.
   Principle. Familiarity with local agencies improves the medical assistant's ability to provide useful information about community resources to patients.
2. **Procedural Step.** As resources are identified, create a list including pertinent information about the resource:

name, services available, address, telephone number, website address, contact name or information, and other useful information. The list may be created using pen and paper, but it should be transferred to a word processing file for ease of duplication.

3. **Procedural Step.** Once the document file has been substantially completed, group resources by subject and/or age group served. Alphabetize resources within each group.

Principle. Arranging lists in alphabetic order facilitates finding specific information and avoids any impression of favoritism or recommending one agency more than another.

4. **Procedural Step.** When the list is complete, save and print copies as needed.

5. **Procedural Step.** Ask the office physicians to review and approve the list.
   Principle. Any referral made by a medical office should have the approval of the practice physicians.

6. **Procedural Step.** Update the list when information changes, when a new resource is identified, and on a periodic basis to be sure information is accurate.

7. **Procedural Step.** Use the list to make appropriate recommendations to patients either in response to patient questions or when instructed to by one of the office physicians.

RISK MANAGEMENT

Risk management is the process of assessing risk and putting in place policies and procedures that minimize it. Often, the focus of risk management activities is on avoiding lawsuits. Risk in a medical office comes in a number of forms.

Minimizing Risk of Injury or Illness

Physical risk involves the risk of injury or illness to employees, patients, and vistors. Business risk also exists: the risk of reduced patient visits because of poor "customer relations." Any medical office seeks to minimize these risks and prevent lawsuits that may result from injuries related to patient care or an accident in the office.

The medical assistant or office manager is often responsible for maintaining the risk management program, in close consultation with the physician or the managing partner among the physicians. In larger clinics or hospitals, there may be a full-time risk manager or risk management may be a part of the duties of one of the clinic's top administrators. Policies and procedures are designed by the physicians and the office's top administrator, who work closely with an attorney, an insurance professional, and a risk management professional. When a new policy is adopted, a copy is given to each employee covered by the policy. Policy and procedure manuals, once developed, should be accessible to all employees when questions arise.

Incident Reports

Whenever something happens in the office for which the office could be considered liable, an incident report should be filled out. An incident can be as simple as a staff member or patient tripping over a chair, or it could be as serious as a staff member sticking himself or herself with a needle that has just been used to give an injection.

The incident report should be initiated by the staff member who is injured or who is closest to the patient or visitor when he or she is injured. A supervisor should review the report before giving it to the individual who manages the risk management program.

Incident report forms vary widely, but usually ask for the following information.

- Date and time that the incident occurred
- Name and identifying information of the individual(s) involved
- Address, building, and room number where the incident occurred
- Description of how the incident occurred and exactly what occurred
- Complete description of any injury or potential injury
- Name(s) and identifying information for any witnesses
- Name and contact information for the person in the organization to whom the incident was reported
- Date of receipt/follow-up by supervisor

Incident reports should always be filled out if a patient, employee, or visitor slips or falls, if a medication error is made, if blood is drawn from the wrong patient, if the number of surgical instruments counted after a procedure does not match the number counted before the procedure, or if an employee is stuck with a needle.

Any witnesses to the incident should be asked for their name, address, and phone number so that the office's insurance provider can call and investigate the incident further if necessary. The report should be dated and signed by the person filling it out. A physician and/or supervisor's signature also goes on the form, according to the office's policy for incident reports.

Liability Coverage

Every office should have adequate insurance protection against liability, both professional liability (commonly called *malpractice*) and liability for any accident that might occur in the office.

Professional liability insurance covers a medical professional for patient claims that diagnostic procedures, tests, or treatments either caused an injury or failed to detect an existing medical condition that should have been detected using good medical practice.

Some physicians purchase insurance in their own name only and have professional staff members purchase their own professional liability policies. If this is the case, the medical assistant can purchase a professional liability policy through a professional organization, such as the American Association of Medical Assistants.

PROCEDURE 48-3

In other cases, a practice purchases professional liability insurance for the entire staff. If this is the case, every professional staff member should be named on the policy.

The office should also have adequate insurance to cover property damage to the office because of fire, storm, or flooding (similar to homeowner insurance). In addition, the practice should have adequate coverage against personal injury sustained on the office's property by a patient or employee. Many patients are ill and/or fragile, and a fall can occur at any time. The policy should cover any injury sustained on the property controlled by the practice. If the practice is in an office building, the public hallways are the responsibility of the landlord or medical office condominium association. If the office is in a free-standing building, the practice is responsible for any occurrences that happen on walkways, in the parking lot, or other outdoor areas up to the public road or sidewalk.

MEDICAL PRACTICE and the LAW

If an injury occurs in the medical office, it is usually necessary for the injured person to prove negligence in order to be compensated for the injury.

1. The medical office and its employees can be sued by patients and visitors to the office for accidental injuries that occur anywhere on the premises. Injury that is not a result of professional activity is covered by the office's general liability insurance policy. For example, if any individual other than an employee slips and falls on a wet floor in the office and is injured, the medical office would be legally liable.

2. A patient who is injured as a result of medical treatment might initiate a lawsuit for professional negligence (malpractice). For example, a patient might be accidentally burned from a hot pack that was too hot or left on too long. This type of lawsuit would be covered by professional liability insurance.

In a second category of injuries, liability is assumed and negligence does not have to occur.

1. Injury from defective equipment falls under the category of product liability. For example, a machine might suddenly create sparks and injure anyone near it. Provided that the office staff was using the equipment correctly and had maintained the equipment according to the manufacturer's directions, the manufacturer would be liable for any injury.

2. An injury to office employees while on the job is covered by mandatory workers' compensation insurance paid for by the employer. ■

What Would You Do? What Would You *Not* Do? RESPONSES

Case Study 1
Page 1113

What Did Kelsey Do?
❑ Put the twins in an examination room as soon as possible.
❑ Asked Mrs. Highsmith to place the used tissues in the waste basket before taking the twins to the examination room. Then she provided hand sanitizer for Mrs. Highsmith.
❑ As soon as possible, put on disposable gloves and removed the plastic toys that the twins had had in their mouths so that they could be cleaned before other children played with them.
❑ When told that Scott Highsmith had thrown up a little, put on disposable gloves, used paper towels to absorb as much liquid as possible, and then promptly cleaned and disinfected the surrounding area.
❑ Reassured Mrs. Highsmith that children are ill sometimes and cleaning up is all in a day's work.
❑ Noted the color and amount of vomit so that she could inform the physician.

What Did Kelsey Not Do?
❑ Did not ask Mrs. Highsmith to prevent the twins from playing with any toys because they had colds.
❑ Did not tell other mothers in the waiting room that they might not want to let their children play with the toys until they could be disinfected.

❑ Did not wait to perform routine cleaning until the lunch break or after office hours.
❑ Did not tell another staff member or Mrs. Highsmith to clean up when Scott vomited.

What Would You Do/What Would You *Not* Do? Review Kelsey's response and place a checkmark next to the information you included in your response. List the additional information you included in your response.

_____

_____

_____

_____

Case Study 2
Page 1119

What Did Kelsey Do?
❑ Checked the number of each type of item against the packing slip to be sure the order was complete. Made a notation if any items were missing.
❑ Placed all the items in their assigned storage area, either that night or the next day. Placed newer items behind older items.
❑ When placing items into storage, checked items on the shelves to be sure that none of them had expired.

What Would You Do? What Would You *Not* Do? RESPONSES—cont'd

❑ If any items were missing or backordered, made a notation on the packing slip. Then she placed the packing slip in the accounts receivable folder to indicate that the order was received.
❑ Removed the shipping box to the designated area for trash.

What Did Kelsey Not Do?

❑ After opening the large box, did not leave the office before checking the packing slip. Another staff member might assume that the individual who opened the box had also checked the contents.
❑ Did not just stack the items on shelves in the storage room randomly because she was in a hurry.
❑ Did not discard the packing slip after checking the order.
❑ Did not keep the shipping box because it might be dirty or harbor pests.

What Would You Do/What Would You *Not* Do? Review Kelsey's response and place a checkmark next to the information you included in your response. List the additional information you included in your response.

_____
_____
_____
_____

Case Study 3
Page 1124

What Did Kelsey Do?

❑ Encouraged Ellen to reach out and find out if there were services that could help her mother.

❑ While Mrs. Brown was present, included her in the conversation.
❑ If speaking to Ellen privately was an option, offered understanding of how difficult it is to know what to do when a parent begins to be less able to function independently.
❑ Offered to help Ellen find resources for delivered meals or homemaking services in the community.
❑ Referred Ellen to local agencies that provide elder services.
❑ Offered to ask the physician if a referral to a visiting nurse would be appropriate.

What Did Kelsey Not Do?

❑ Did not exclude Mrs. Brown from the conversation or treat her like a child.
❑ Did not push Mrs. Brown or Ellen to accept her suggestions, but rather just offered information.
❑ Did not promise that the physician would make specific referrals.

What Would You Do/What Would You *Not* Do? Review Kelsey's response and place a checkmark next to the information you included in your response. List the additional information you included in your response.

_____
_____
_____

TERMINOLOGY REVIEW

Back order A term used for items ordered that cannot be shipped immediately, usually because they are out of stock.

Depreciation Accounting methods to respond to the loss of value of a property or piece of equipment over time.

Gross pay The total amount earned in a time period by an employee before any deductions.

Inventory A detailed list of items in stock or in possession of an individual or business.

Invoice An itemized bill for items that have not been prepaid.

Minutes A written record of the proceedings of a meeting.

Net pay The actual amount of money paid directly to an employee after taxes and other deductions have been taken out.

Per diem A term used for employees who do not have a fixed schedule but are scheduled by the day according to office needs.

Policy A guiding principle for the management of a medical office or business.

Procedure A list of the steps to handle a certain situation or perform a certain task.

Purchase order (PO) The form used to order supplies, as well as the order itself.

Reorder point A number on a supply inventory that indicates when a specific item should be reordered to be sure that the supply will not run out before the new order is received.

Risk management The process of assessing risk and putting policies and procedures in place to minimize it.

Continued

TERMINOLOGY REVIEW—cont'd

Salary A fixed amount of money paid on a regular basis that does not depend on the number of hours worked.

Service contract An agreement that provides for service for a piece of equipment after the warranty expires.

Social Security tax (FICA) A tax of 6.2% collected from employees to fund the Social Security program, which provides benefits to retired workers.

Vendor A company from whom supplies or equipment is purchased.

Warranty A promise by the manufacturer to repair or replace defective parts in an item during a specific time period.

W-4 The form used to claim allowances for federal income tax reporting.

ON THE WEB

For Information on U.S. Government Forms Related to Payroll and Employment:

I-9 form (United States Citizen and Immigration Services): www.uscis.gov/files/form/I-9.pdf

Internal Revenue Service: www.irs.gov

  W-2 (Wage and Tax Statement)

  W-4 form (for employee withholding)

  Withholding tax tables

  Form 941 (employer's quarterly tax return)

  Form 940 (employer's annual federal unemployment [FUTA] tax return)

Social Security Administration: www.ssa.gov/pgm/popular.htm

Obtain a Social Security number

Apply for a replacement Social Security card

For Information on Disaster Planning:

CDC Emergency Preparedness: www.bt.cdc.gov/preparedness

Citizen Corps: http://www.citizencorps.gov

Homeland Security Community and State Information: www.ready.gov/america/local

For Information on OSHA Evacuation Plans and Procedures:

OSHA Evacuation Plans: www.osha.gov/SLTC/etools/evacuation/index.html

PREPARE FOR CERTIFICATION   Visit the Evolve site at http://evolve.elsevier.com/Bonewit/today/ to actively Prepare for your Certification.

CD Check out the **Companion CD** bound with the book to access additional interactive activities.

49

Obtaining Employment

LEARNING OBJECTIVES

1. Describe the process for locating potential employers when looking for a job.
2. Discuss the steps in preparing a resumé.
3. Describe how to write a cover letter.
4. Differentiate between information placed on a resumé and information required in an employment application.
5. Explain how to provide potential employers with a resumé by mail, using a fax, or using Internet resources.
6. Prepare to answer questions commonly asked in a job interview.
7. Describe measures to prevent job burnout.
8. Identify two professional organizations to which a medical assistant may belong.
9. Identify benefits of joining a professional organization.
10. Discuss why lifelong learning is vital for a medical assistant after graduation.

CHAPTER OUTLINE

Introduction to Obtaining Employment
Successful Job Hunting
  Setting Goals
  Identifying Potential Employers
Tools for a Job Search
  Preparing a Resumé
  Writing a Cover Letter
  Sending the Resumé
  Filling Out an Employment Application
  Applying for Employment Using the Internet
Getting the Job
  Interview Techniques
  Follow-up after an Interview

Lifelong Learning
  Staying Current
  Avoiding Burnout
  Professional Organizations and Peer Support
  Continuing Education Units
Planning for Job Advancement or Career Change
  Advancing to Management
  Upgrading Technical/Clinical Skills
  Transferring Skills

CAAHEP CONTENT

Professional Components
- Job readiness
- Workplace dynamics

ABHES CONTENT

Career Development
- Job search, professionalism, and success
- Goal setting, time management, employment opportunities

- Resumé writing, interviewing techniques, and follow-up
- Dress for success

KEY TERMS

burnout
continuing education unit (CEU)
cover letter

networking
resumé

Introduction to Obtaining Employment

After graduating from a medical assisting program, most medical assistants must begin the search for their first job. Sometimes the medical office where the graduate did an externship asks the student to stay on as an employee. When this happens, it eases the transition from student to employed medical assistant. Because a student cannot count on this, it is important for the new graduate to see the process of learning how to seek employment as just another skill that must be mastered.

Finding a job involves more than simply answering a few newspaper advertisements or responding to one or two help-wanted notices on the school's career bulletin board. To find the right job, a medical assisting graduate needs to put time and effort into the job-hunting process.

SUCCESSFUL JOB HUNTING

Successful job hunting has two parts. The first is setting appropriate goals; the second is identifying potential employers where those goals might be met.

Setting Goals

Setting goals means identifying the ideal job for a medical assistant's current circumstances. The medical assistant should ask herself or himself the following questions:

- Do I want to work full-time or part-time?
- In what area of the country or region do I want to work?
- Do I want to work in a city? In the suburbs? In the country?
- Do I have a preference about the size of the organization where I would be happy?
- Am I interested in working in a particular medical specialty?
- What are my particular strengths and weaknesses?
- Do I want to specialize in either clinical or administrative duties or do I want to do both?

Identifying Potential Employers

After a graduate has set goals, it is time to begin identifying potential employers. This is done by scanning newspaper or online want ads to see what kinds of positions are being advertised and looking through the Yellow Pages to see what kinds of practices are in the community where the graduate wants to work. Many large organizations post job openings internally first. The graduate should ask family or friends who work in such institutions to keep an eye on the internal posting boards.

Larger institutions also often have personnel or human resource departments that keep files of potential employees to give to physicians or department administrators who need to fill a position. When an applicant fills out an application for such a facility, that paperwork will stay on file for a period of time—usually 6 months or 1 year. After that, a new, updated application must be submitted.

During the job-hunting period, it is important to set aside some time each day to look for a job. The more opportunities a graduate explores, the better the possibility of not only finding a job but also finding the right job.

When looking for a job, it is important not to underestimate the importance of **networking,** contacting friends and acquaintances who may know of potential jobs. A personal network may include former instructors, contacts made during the medical assisting externship, classmates, and even physicians the medical assistant knows or has worked with. It is important to develop a habit of maintaining professional contacts. Staying in touch, either through occasional telephone calls, e-mails, or meeting for coffee or lunch provides opportunities to gain both support and information. A contact may call in the future when there is an opening at work or someone has asked for names of potential employees.

TOOLS FOR A JOB SEARCH
Preparing a Resumé

The primary purpose of a resumé is to obtain an interview for an open position. A **resumé** is a summary of information about a person that describes education, work experience, and other information that employers may find pertinent in deciding whether or not to hire an individual.

A resumé is often important in making a first impression on a potential employer. It must be neat, professional, and informative. Employers, who often receive several resumés for one position, use the resumé to create a list of people with the desired training and/or experience to call in for personal interviews.

A resumé should describe a medical assistant's education, experience, and skills completely, but not in an exaggerated way. If possible, the resumé should be limited to one typewritten sheet. If the resumé is more than one page, the information that is especially pertinent to the job the medical assistant is applying for should appear on the first page. If a medical assistant is applying for many different types of positions, it may be desirable to have many variations of a resumé available, each one slanted toward the requirements of certain positions.

Personal information should not be included on a resumé. Information such as marital status, children, and hobbies does not relate to a medical assistant's credentials for a position. If personal information is included, the effect is most likely to be neutral or possibly negative, providing a reason not to grant an interview. For example, the employer may be afraid that a medical assistant with two or more children may need to be absent if the children become ill.

Resumé Styles

In general, there are three styles of resumés: chronological, functional, and targeted.

A chronological resumé contains a list of formal education, with degrees and certificates earned, followed by work experience (although work experience can come before education in this style). This is the most common type of resumé for applicants with limited work experience, or those who are seeking work similar to their present work.

A functional resumé categorizes experience according to skills or abilities, some of which may be a result of activities other than paid employment (e.g., volunteer work, unpaid work). A functional resumé is useful for an individual who wants to change from one type of work to a different type of work and wants to highlight how particular skills attained in one line of work can be helpful in the new position for which he or she is applying.

A targeted resumé organizes information about an individual who has targeted a particular job opportunity in such a way as to highlight the skills and work experiences being called for in the new employment. This type of resumé often begins with an employment objective that identifies the type of position the individual is seeking.

Information to Include

The basic pieces of information needed for a resumé are personal demographics, objective, education, experience, skills, credentials, and references. A number of computer programs are available for preparing resumés. If a computer program is used, the medical assistant should be sure to personalize the resumé. It is also helpful to use some sample resumés as guides (Figures 49-1, 49-2, and 49-3). Other samples may be available from the placement office of the graduate's college or medical assisting program, as well as resumé-writing books and websites.

Personal Demographics

Personal demographics include the name, address, telephone number, and e-mail address. This information is usually placed at the top of the resumé, either centered or flush left. The identifying information should be in a larger type size, boldfaced, and/or in a different font than the body of the resumé so that it stands out. On some resumé programs, this information is in a small font, which makes it hard to see. By changing the font size, the medical assistant can personalize the resumé and make it easier to read.

Objective

The objective is a statement of the type of position the medical assistant is looking for. A medical assistant just graduating may be—even should be—flexible about the type of position being sought. If the objective is to obtain an entry-level position as a medical assistant, there may be better ways to use the limited space on a single-sheet resumé than stating this as an objective. This becomes a matter of personal preference.

A medical assistant with a more focused goal may wish to use a statement such as: "To obtain a clinical medical assisting position in an office specializing in family practice or internal medicine." A specific objective reassures the potential employer that the candidate is interested in the position he or she is trying to fill, but it can limit the positions for which the candidate will be considered.

Education

The education section includes the institutions attended and degrees or certificates received. These should be arranged in chronological order with the most recent first. At least one program should be listed with a degree, certificate, or diploma and the year it was received. Usually the high school diploma is only included if the candidate has no higher credential.

When identifying a school or program, the anticipated graduation date can be included if the resumé is prepared before the medical assistant graduates (e.g., A.S. in Medical Assisting, anticipated June 200X). After graduation, the resumé should be revised before sending it to other potential employers.

It is also appropriate to include the grade-point average (GPA) and any honors or awards received from the educational institution, such as Dean's List.

Previous Experience

In the section on previous experience the following are included:

- The job title
- Years of employment
- Employer's name
- The town and state in which the work was performed

A new graduate may wish to present information about previous experience in two sections, titled *Related Experience* and *Other Experience.* The medical assisting externship can be included under the heading *Related Experience,* but if the section is titled *Work Experience,* only paid employment should be included. Most employers do not like to see gaps in a work history, which might be due to jobs that the applicant does not wish to acknowledge. If the applicant

Susan Anderson
2314 May Avenue
West River, MU 00000
(666) 111-5555
S.Anderson@anyserver.com

EDUCATION/CERTIFICATION

2005-2007   West River Community College
A.S. Medical Assisting, June 2007

2004-2005   University of North Brook

Certified Medical Assistant: June, 2007
BLS Healthcare Provider Level 2007

RELATED EXPERIENCE

2007   **MEDICAL ASSISTING EXTERNSHIP** (160 hours)
John Smith Medical Associates, West River, MU
- Prepared patients for examination, took vital signs and charted chief complaint.
- Performed diagnostic tests including throat cultures, rapid strep test, EKG's, dipstick urinalysis
- Performed clerical duties including answering telephones, filing, writing referrals, scheduling appointments
- Data entry of patient information and insurance payments

2005-2007   **HOME HEALTH AIDE**
Medical Home Care, Newtown, MU

Performed personal care and took vital signs in private homes.

SPECIAL SKILLS

Fluent in Spanish
Keyboarding 45 wpm
Microsoft Office, MediSoft, AltaPoint EMR

OTHER EXPERIENCE

2003-2004   **CASHIER**
Fresh and Fine Supermarket, West River, MU

Responsible for checking groceries; weekend supervisor.

Figure 49-1. Sample resumé of a recent graduate. (Modified from Hunt SA: *Saunders fundamentals of medical assisting,* St. Louis, 2007, Saunders.)

has been a homemaker, it is recommended to include the years devoted to this under *Other Experience.* Any volunteer work can also be included.

For each position or type of experience, a short summary of responsibilities should be included. If the experience was in health care or medical assisting, more details should be included than for other jobs or experience. For example, more details should be included about specific responsibilities as a home health aide than as a cashier. Action verbs should be used in the description of previous experience (Figure 49-4).

When preparing the descriptions of previous experience, the medical assistant should use one of two styles consis-

tently. Either can be written in sentence form or as a list with bullets.

Describing Responsibilities Using Verbs in the Past Tense

Example in sentence form:

Measured vital signs, prepared patients for examination, posted charges and payments, sent monthly bills, etc.

Example in bullet form:
- Measured vital signs
- Prepared patients for examination
- Posted charges and payments
- Sent monthly bills

---

26 Gillian Street
West River, MU 00000
(666) 111-5555
saychelles@anyserver.com

Patricia A. Saychelles

Objective	To obtain a challenging position as a clinical medical assistant	
Education	2001-2003	West River Community College Certificate in Medical Assisting, June 2003
Related Experience	2004 to present	Family Health Care West River, MU Clinical Medical Assistant

Duties include: preparing patients for examination; taking vital signs and completing growth charts; documenting chief complaint; taking EKG's; obtaining throat cultures; fingersticks; phlebotomy; performing lab tests including rapid strep tests, dipstick urinalysis, cholesterol, and glucose; assisting with procedures such as I & D, suture insertion, suture removal; instructing patients regarding diet and exercise; stocking exam rooms

Other Experience	1992-2001	Homemaker
	1994-2000	Library volunteer West River Elementary School

Responsible for checking books in and out, reshelving, minor repairs of torn books

	1990-1992	Package Sorter United Parcel Service Newtown, MU
Other Credentials	Registered Medical Assistant; January 2003	
Activities	Member of the American Medical Technologists since 2002	
References	Available upon request	

Figure 49-2. Sample resumé of a woman who stayed home with children for several years before training as a medical assistant. (Modified from Hunt SA: *Saunders fundamentals of medical assisting,* St. Louis, 2007, Saunders.)

Describing Responsibilities Using Participle Form of the Verb

Example in sentence form:

Responsible for measuring vital signs, preparing patients for examination, posting charges and payments, sending monthly bills

Example in bullet form:

Duties included:
- Measuring vital signs
- Preparing patients for examination
- Posting charges and payments
- Sending monthly bills

Special Skills

The special skills section describes skills learned in an educational program that may not be reflected in any direct experience, or that are usually not included in a medical assisting program. Even if the externship is included in the resumé, a graduate of a medical assisting program may have special skills he or she did not use during the

John Davidson
19 Carriage Way
West River, MU 0000
(666) 111-3333
airman@anyserver.com

OBJECTIVE: Clinical medical assistant in an emergency care setting with full range of responsibilities from health care and procedures to management.

SUMMARY: More than ten years of providing professional military and civilian health care, specializing in emergency treatment, physical examination, aeromedical safety instruction and health awareness training.

1996 to present   UNITED STATES NAVY

1998-2007 Hospital Corpsman First Class (E-6). *Squadron Medical Department Representative, Naval Air Station, Harbor Bay, MU.*

Responsible for 350 personnel in all areas of world wide medical organizational deployments, including electrocardiograms, x-ray, laboratory testing, occupational and preventative medicine, personnel health care and sanitary conditions. Trained in Federal Aviation Administration (FAA) conduction of aeromedical examinations, fixed wing aircraft rescue, emergency egress procedures for jet, propeller and helicopter aircraft, and aviation life support systems. Responsible for maintaining computerized records for over 3,00 physical examinations annually.

1996-1998 Hospital Corpsman Second Class (E-5). *Squadron Medical Department Representative, Naval Air Station, Harbor Bay, MU.*

Responsible for 250 personnel for rapid deployment to naval service ships around the world. Additionally trained in rotary wing aircraft rescue and shipboard/aircraft fire fighting. Received qualifications as Medical Assistant (MA), Nursing Assistant (NA), Emergency Medical Technician (EMT), Emergency Vehicle Operator (EVO) and Emergency Medical Dispatcher (EMD)

1994-1996   **Medical Clerk,** *State Department of Corrections, West River MU*

Responsible to assist with medical care of 600 inmates involving all aspects of health care and treatment, including scheduling appointments, admission of patients to the hospital ward, maintaining health records and instruction in personal hygiene and preventative care.

OTHER CREDENTIALS:

Instructor: Emergency Medical Technician (EMT-B)
Instructor: American Heart Association BLS
Advanced Life Support (ACLS) provider

EDUCATION: Attended West River Community College from 1993-1994 taking general education courses and introductory health courses

Figure 49-3. Sample resumé of a man who received health care training in the Armed Services. (Modified from Hunt SA: *Saunders fundamentals of medical assisting,* St. Louis, 2007, Saunders.)

externship. These may include computer skills with particular programs, ability to perform specific diagnostic tests, or knowledge of or fluency in a language other than English.

Activities and Other Credentials

In the section on activities and other credentials, the medical assistant may include certification as a CMA (AAMA) or RMA, memberships in professional organizations such as the AAMA or the AMT, and any other certifications or credentials including CPR and/or first aid. Lists of unre-

lated activities, hobbies, and interests should not be included on a professional resumé.

References

Traditional resumés always included the following statement: References will be furnished on request. This statement is considered optional on a modern resumé because it is assumed to be the case. Actual references are not listed on the resumé because the goal is to be interviewed before the potential employer checks any references. After the interview, the medical assistant provides a list of references

administer	distribute	process
analyze	document	proofread
arrange	establish	propose
assist	file	purchase
authorize	instruct	reconcile
balance	list	run
calculate	log	schedule
classify	mail	send
code	measure	set up
collect	monitor	sort
compose	order	stock
contact	organize	teach
coordinate	perform	write
copy	post	
develop	prepare	

Figure 49-4. Action verbs to use on a resumé. (Modified from Hunt SA: *Saunders fundamentals of medical assisting,* St. Louis, 2007, Saunders.)

with contact information. Before using someone's name as a reference, the medical assistant should be sure to get that person's permission. It is also polite to call individuals whose names have been used so that they can be ready to receive a phone call or written request for a reference.

For references, a medical assistant who has recently graduated should choose a balance of instructors, externship supervisor, other job supervisors, or coworkers from volunteer activities. It is not recommended to use friends or family for references. Sometimes the individual who will be used as a reference gives the medical assistant a letter that can be shown to a potential employer. More often, the potential employer contacts the individual given as a reference after interviewing the candidate.

Formatting the Resumé

The resumé should be formatted with at least 1-inch margins. It is important to lay out the resumé so that it looks balanced on the page with clear sections of information. After the resumé has been created, it should be proofread carefully. Spelling and grammar errors are unacceptable.

If the resumé will be sent through the mail, it should be either a printed original or it should be professionally printed. The medical assistant should avoid sending photocopies. Acceptable paper colors include white, cream, or light gray. It makes a good impression if a stationery-weight paper is used, which is slightly heavier than ordinary printer paper. Because medical assistants work in a fairly conservative segment of the job market, it is important to avoid using colored paper, unusual type fonts, or flashy formatting for the resumé.

Writing a Cover Letter

A **cover letter** is a letter sent with a resumé that explains briefly why the resumé is being sent. The cover letter clari-

Putting It All into Practice

My name is Deanna Taylor, and I took the CMA (AAMA) examination in June of the year that I completed my medical assisting training. During the time that I was waiting for my examination results, I went on six job interviews. I was hired in my present position 3 weeks before I found out that I passed the examination. The combination of searching for my first medical assisting job and hoping that I had passed the certification examination was very stressful.

I was looking for a position in obstetrics and gynecology, but I sent a resumé for every medical assisting job that I saw. That turned out to be good because I had a much better idea of what different offices were like, and I became more comfortable in the interview itself. When I first walked through the door of the office that hired me, I felt comfortable. I knew that if I were a patient, I would trust the staff because they were friendly but professional. This office does specialize in obstetrics and gynecology, so I was lucky enough to find exactly the position I had hoped for.

I was interviewed by the practice manager, a woman who works with several medical practices affiliated with a local hospital. We discussed my experience and the position. Later she called me back for a second interview to meet with the physicians and office staff. After that, she offered me the position. I was very excited, and I have to say that it has turned out very well. I have been here for 3 years, and it seems that there is always a new challenge and something new to learn. ∎

Prepare for Success

fies whether the medical assistant is responding to an advertisement, a referral from another individual, or simply an inquiry about possible job opportunities.

If sent through the mail, the cover letter should use the format for a business letter and be printed on the same color paper as the resumé. If possible, the medical assistant should call the office to find out the name of the office manager or other individual responsible for hiring medical assistants. If sent online with a resumé, the letter should be addressed to the human resources department.

The letter should begin with the reason for writing the letter and sending the resumé. This should be followed by a brief summary of the position being sought and the candidate's qualifications for filling that position. The final paragraph should be a request for an interview.

Each cover letter should be personalized because this is the first thing the potential employer will see. Of course, it should not contain any grammar or spelling errors. The reader should be referred to the resumé for details (Figure 49-5).

The medical assistant should keep a copy of all cover letters. The results (interview, second interview, job offer) can be written on the copy or on a separate log that keeps track of responses to all letters sent out.

2314 May Avenue
West River, MU 0000
September 5, 2010

Denise Wilson, Office Manager
Medical Practice Associates
525 Main Street
West River, MU 00000

Dear Ms. Wilson:

I read your advertisement in the West River Daily Item for a medical assistant, and I would like to be considered for the position. I have an Associate in Science degree in Medical Assisting, and I have passed the certification exam given by the American Association of Medical Assistants.

The enclosed resume summarizes my education and experience. I am self-motivated, and I get along well with people. My training in medical assisting included an externship in a physician's office, and I also have experience as a home health aide. I believe that I am well qualified for the position in your advertisement.

I can be contacted at (666)111-5555 during the late afternoon and evening, and I will respond promptly to messages. I am looking forward to hearing from you so that we can schedule an interview.

Sincerely,

Susan Anderson

Susan Anderson

Enclosure

Figure 49-5. Sample cover letter. (From Hunt SA: *Saunders fundamentals of medical assisting*, St. Louis, 2007, Saunders.)

Sending the Resumé

It is recommended to send resumés in 9- × 11-inch manila envelopes so that they do not need to be folded. If using a standard No. 10 business envelope, its color and weight should match the paper used for the resumé and cover letter if possible.

Increasingly, it is possible to respond to job openings using the Internet or fax a resumé to an office. A cover letter is still recommended.

The advantage of a faxed or e-mailed resumé and cover letter is that the material arrives quickly, often within minutes of making a telephone inquiry. The disadvantage is that a fax, or a print of an e-mail, does not look as crisp or professional as a mailed resumé and cover letter.

A few days after a mailed resumé should have arrived, a job applicant may call to see if the material did, indeed, arrive. At this time it is appropriate to ask if the person doing the hiring has an idea about the time frame in which a hiring decision will be made. However, a job applicant should not call again after that, to avoid appearing too aggressive.

Filling Out an Employment Application

Most medical facilities require a completed job application in addition to providing a resumé. In large facilities, it may be necessary to complete the application before an interview is scheduled. In smaller offices, the application may be filled out at the time of the interview.

What Would You Do? What Would You *Not* Do?

Case Study 1

Deanna was supervising a medical assisting student named Andrea in her office. Andrea had been working as a cashier at a local supermarket since graduating from high school. She had never been employed in a health care setting. At the time Andrea wrote her resumé, she was finished with her externship and her graduation date was only 2 weeks away. She had had many responsibilities at the externship, but there were some skills she had learned in school, like spirometry, that they did not do where she was placed. Andrea said, "On my resumé, I put that my externship was work experience, because I have really been working here for several weeks." ■

It is important to keep a list of information needed to fill out the job application. This includes the name and address of previous employers, dates of employment, names and telephone numbers of supervisors, as well as the names, addresses, and telephone numbers of references. Any letters of reference should be brought to the interview so that the facility can make copies to attach them to the job application.

The medical assistant should answer all questions fully and truthfully on the application. If filling the application out by hand, the medical assistant should print legibly. All questions should be answered. It is not appropriate to refer the reader to the resume. If a question does not apply, the medical assistant should write N/A or Not Applicable.

If the application asks for the reason for leaving a previous position, the medical assistant should avoid making any negative statements about the employer or supervisor. Common reasons for leaving are returning to school, relocation for a spouse's job, end of a temporary position, or exploration of new career options.

Some health care facilities may require applicants for medical assisting positions to take a keyboarding test or other skills test before an interview is granted.

Applying for Employment Using the Internet

The medical assistant may utilize on online employment website (e.g., Monster.com) to create a resume, use that resume to apply for open positions, and also post the resume on the web for potential employers to view it. The resume that is created can be saved as a document file and used to apply for other positions. Many employers also advertise for medical assistants and accept applications using their own websites. When looking for employment, the medical assistant should visit the websites of potential employers, review job postings, and submit an application on-line if a suitable position is open. By networking with other students, instructors, and friends, the medical assistant can identify on-line resources that others have used successfully.

GETTING THE JOB

Interview Techniques

An employment interview provides a potential employer with an opportunity to assess a candidate's interpersonal and communication skills, as well as preparation for a position in the medical setting. The interview also provides the medical assistant with a chance to assess the potential employer. The questions asked, the flow of the discussion, and the tour of the facility helps the medical assistant decide whether the position fits appropriately with his or her work style and personality.

In order for a job to be offered, the medical assistant must do well in the interview. Often a candidate whose skills appear excellent on paper does not create a positive impression during the interview. The key for the employer is to find the person who seems to be the best fit for the position.

It is important for a medical assistant to accept any job interview offered, even if the position does not seem ideal. The more interviews a new graduate goes on, the more comfortable the job interview process becomes. It is not appropriate, however, to accept more job interviews after a position has been accepted.

Preparing for the Interview

Before the interview, the medical assistant should try to find out as much as possible about the practice or facility. Information can be obtained by talking to someone who works there or a patient of the office, if possible. The medical assistant should ask friends and other contacts if they know anyone with information about the potential employer.

Many medical offices have a website that describes the practice. The medical assistant should enter the name of the practice and/or physician(s) into a search engine. If the practice has a website, it will probably include the names of the physicians and other practitioners, the philosophy of the practice, and other background information. If the office is small, it may only be possible to locate telephone and address information. This may indicate that the office is not using as much modern technology as some other offices.

When the interview is arranged, the medical assistant should find out the name and position of the individual(s) who will be holding the interview and whether one person or a committee will conduct the interview.

The medical assistant should ask if there are any particular things that the interviewer(s) would like to know, and if any background materials should be brought to the interview.

Appearance and Behavior

As always, a professional appearance is important. A female medical assistant should wear tailored, professional-looking clothing, such as a suit or blouse and skirt, or dress slacks. Denim skirts and jeans are not appropriate for an interview. Long hair should be worn pulled back and off the collar, as

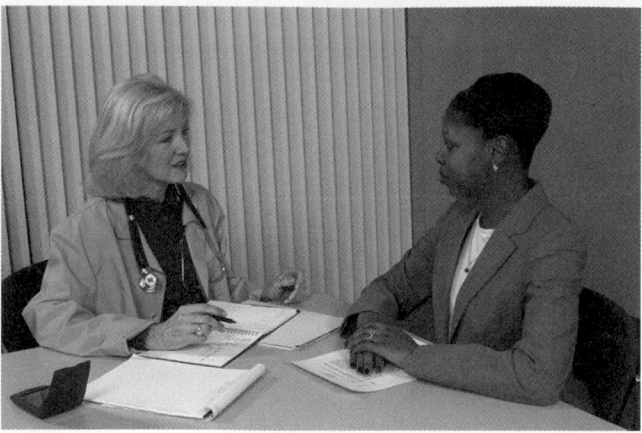

Figure 49-6. At a job interview, the medical assistant should look and act in a professional manner.

it would be when working as a medical assistant. It is recommended to avoid bulky jewelry, avoid false nails and visible piercings, and present a tailored appearance (Figure 49-6). For an interview, the medical assistant should avoid sandals or athletic shoes and never wear flip flops.

A male medical assistant should wear a suit or dress slacks and sports coat or blazer, with a dress shirt and tie. Hair, including any facial hair, should be clean and neatly trimmed.

A job applicant should never chew gum during an interview.

It is important to maintain good posture and look alert during the interview. The medical assistant should sit comfortably without slouching and avoid fidgeting or nervous habits. It is useful to have a pen and notepad handy in order to make notes. It is also helpful to write down questions that might be encountered in future interviews, in order to practice answers before the next interview.

At the same time, the medical assistant presents a better impression if he or she is relaxed and natural instead of reserved and stiff. The interviewer is looking for an individual who interacts well with patients and can make them feel at ease. If a job applicant smiles and makes conversation easily during an interview, it is likely that he or she will be comfortable with patients.

Questions That the Interviewer Should Not Ask

Interviewers are not supposed to ask questions that do not relate to the position, including marital status, number of children, and age (unless there is a legal age requirement as part of the job). If the interviewer asks a question about any of these things, the medical assistant should try to identify or respond to the underlying concern without directly refusing to answer the question.

Interviewer: "How many children do you have?"

Applicant: "Are you concerned about my ability to be dependable?"

What Would You Do? What Would You *Not* Do?

Case Study 2
When she was looking for a job, Deanna got lost on the way to an interview. The office was located about 30 minutes from her home. Deanna had allowed plenty of travel time, but she took the wrong turn off the highway and didn't realize it until she had gone almost 10 miles in the wrong direction. When she realized she was lost, she knew that backtracking would make her at least 15 minutes late. ■

Discussing Salary and Benefits

Specific salary is usually not discussed until a job is offered. But it is common for a salary range to be discussed. If the interviewer does not state the salary range, it is acceptable to ask about it as the interview is winding down. Asking about the salary range early in the interview may give the impression that money is the most important thing about the job. Failing to ask about a salary range may be interpreted as lack of interest.

It is also appropriate to ask a general question about benefits, such as how long an employee must work before becoming eligible for the benefits package and if health insurance is a benefit. It is customary not to ask specifically about vacation, sick days, and personal days until a job offer has been made.

When a position is offered, a discussion of salary and benefits helps the medical assistant make a decision about whether or not to accept the position. If the salary seems low or is less than the medical assistant currently earns, it is appropriate to ask about the specific time frame when performance will be reviewed and a raise will be possible.

Often, especially in larger facilities with rigid salary structures, a position is limited to a particular salary range. It is important to be sure that the salary is adequate to meet expenses before accepting the position. Usually an applicant can ask for 24 to 48 hours to consider a job offer.

Asking Questions

A good interviewer will ask a candidate at the end of the interview if he or she has any questions. The medical assistant may ask about who supervises the position, ask the interviewer to clarify the job responsibilities, and/or ask about the availability of training programs in-house or financial support for outside training or college courses. It is helpful to come to the interview with three or four written questions. If these were answered during the interview, the medical assistant can look over the list and say that it seems as though all his or her questions have been answered.

Determining the Timeline for Filling the Position

If the interviewer or lead interviewer in a committee does not state the employer's time frame for making a decision about filling the position, this is an important question to ask. Employers know that people must seek employment at

Highlight on Responding to Questions

Based on previous experience at interviews and suggestions from friends about their experiences, the medical assistant should try to prepare for questions the interviewer(s) will ask. Although it may seem awkward, it is helpful to practice answering sample interview questions out loud with friends, family, or a roommate. Several common interview questions and potential answers are presented in the following discussion.

1. **What can I tell you about my organization?**

   It is always important to have questions prepared. The medical assistant might ask about the history of the office or clinic and/or how long it has been in its present location. He or she should have found out how many physicians work there and what specialties are represented, but could ask how many medical assistants are employed.

2. **What was your favorite subject in school?**

   The answer is more powerful if it demonstrates enthusiasm and has some relation to the position being applied for. Math, English, science, computer courses, and medical assisting courses are good answers. If a job applicant says that poetry was her favorite subject, the interviewer may wonder if medical assisting is the applicant's real interest.

3. **Why did you choose to study medical assisting?**

   People who choose this field are usually interested in health, like people, like a job where they can be active, and believe that preventive care and early diagnosis are important components of health. This question also gives the medical assistant an opportunity to demonstrate enthusiasm and caring.

4. **What courses did you like least in school?**

   It is better if the medical assistant identifies courses that he or she found difficult (even if that does not directly respond to the question) than to give a long list of subjects that were boring. It is important to avoid looking like an individual who is uninterested in subjects that may relate to the job and also to avoid complaining or speaking negatively.

5. **What campus activities did you participate in? What did you learn from them?**

   The medical assistant can prepare by thinking of an interesting extracurricular activity he or she has participated in, even if there was not time to be a member of any club or organized activity in school. If the medical assistant worked for several hours while going to school, he or she might say so while identifying a hobby: "I worked as a cashier several hours a week in order to help pay for school, so I had to leave school right after class. But I am working with a classmate to arrange for some of our graduates to get together monthly because I think that it would be too bad to lose contact with the friends I made in school."

6. **Describe your responsibilities when you worked for XYZ company.**

   The medical assistant should identify his or her responsibilities, being sure to emphasize any promotions or leadership role. A medical assistant often has a part-time job while going to school with some extra responsibility, such as opening or closing, training new employees, or rotating to different departments. If handling money was a job responsibility, it should be mentioned because it indicates reliability.

7. **What types of problems have you encountered in your jobs? How did you handle them?**

   The medical assistant should think of an example of a problem that might occur in a medical office, such as an angry or unsatisfied customer, telephones ringing off the hook, work backing up, and being overwhelmed at first. When discussing the problem, it is important to provide a realistic solution and explain how problem solving occurred.

8. **What would your instructors or previous supervisors tell me about you if I were to call them?**

   The medical assistant should identify his or her positive attributes and practice saying them calmly, even if it seems like bragging. "They would say that I work hard, I am organized, I catch on quickly, I am good with people, I try hard to be accurate" are some examples. In an effective interview, the job applicant puts his or her best foot forward without exaggerating or distorting the truth.

9. **What are some of your weaknesses or areas you need to work on?**

   The medical assistant should think carefully about weaknesses that may be seen in some lights as positive, or weaknesses that everyone is subject to. Being a perfectionist, not liking to miss work for illness, and double-checking all work to be sure it is correct are examples of weaknesses that employers usually like. Being nervous in a new situation, becoming frustrated when there isn't enough time, and hating to see others sitting around when there is much work to do are traits common to many people. If a medical assistant is shy and reserved, this is a good opportunity to state that new situations are anxiety provoking, but that it doesn't take very long to feel comfortable and open up more.

10. **What are your long-term goals? or Where do you plan to be in 5 years?**

    The prospective employer is trying to get a sense of how long the applicant plans to stay in the position if hired. In many areas, turnover of medical assistants is rapid, but an employer would like to be able to count on at least 2 years. If the medical assistant will be returning to school within 6 months, he or she should say so and identify if part-time work would be possible at that time. ■

many facilities, and most are willing to get back to applicants who have been interviewed within a few days.

Follow-up after an Interview

The day of the interview, or the next day, the medical assistant should write a short note thanking the interviewer or committee for the opportunity to interview. This courtesy demonstrates courtesy and attention to detail. If the medical assistant has been asked to provide additional information or materials regarding a question, that material should be included (Figure 49-7).

If the interviewer has not responded by the date expected, the medical assistant may telephone to ask if the position has been filled.

LIFELONG LEARNING

The field of health care is becoming more complex all the time. It is important for every member of the health care team to constantly improve his or her skills and stay up to date on new techniques in his or her field. To provide high-quality patient care, every member of the health care team must engage in lifelong learning.

Staying Current

Medical assistants must keep their skills current. This means keeping abreast of new techniques, as well as learning how to use the latest technology.

2314 May Avenue
West River, MU 00000
September 5, 2010

Denise Wilson, Office Manager
Medical Practice Associates
525 Main Street
West River, MU 00000

Dear Ms. Wilson:

Thank you for giving me the opportunity to interview for the medical assisting position at Medical Practice Associates. After meeting with you, I believe that my skills and training would allow me to do an excellent job as your employee. In addition, this position would allow me to grow in my professional career.

I was very impressed with the organization and high quality of care given by your practice. I hope to hear from you in about a week as we discussed. Please feel free to call me at (666)111-5555 if you think of any other questions. Thank you again for your time and consideration.

Sincerely,

Susan Anderson

Susan Anderson

Enclosure

Figure 49-7. Sample letter following an interview. (From Hunt SA: *Saunders fundamentals of medical assisting,* St. Louis, 2007, Saunders.)

Administrative Skills

On the administrative side, computer software is constantly being updated. This includes operating systems and all programs used routinely in the medical office. Training to use updated versions of operating systems, word processing programs, or other general programs is often available on-line or through classes. If the office switches to an updated version of office management programs or an electronic medical record, the software company often provides training for office personnel.

Another area that requires constant updating relates to changes in coding and insurance claim submission. The medical assistant should read updates and attend classes as needed to keep skills current.

Clinical Skills

On the clinical side, it is important to learn to use new diagnostic or laboratory equipment. When a new piece of equipment is purchased, training should be arranged for all staff who will use it. The medical assistant must also stay current on new medications. Pharmaceutical representatives leave informational materials for the physician, and the medical assistant should make a point of reading this information.

Preparing for Increased Responsibility

The medical assistant may be trained to assist with special procedures. The medical assistant may be sent to an outside training program at office expense, or the physician or other staff member may provide the training. It is important to pay close attention during the training and take notes to be sure that all information is retained.

The medical assistant may also be given some responsibility to supervise other staff members. Classes or workshops in supervision, appraisal, conflict management, or other subjects may be helpful to ease this transition.

Avoiding Burnout

Burnout is a constant worry, especially for those in repetitive, high-stress jobs. **Burnout** is a term that has come to mean disillusionment with work and physical or emotional exhaustion. It is characterized by a loss of interest or enthusiasm and energy about work.

A person experiencing burnout may exhibit behavioral changes as well, including increased irritability, inability to empathize with patients, chronic fatigue, and poor relations with coworkers. Job burnout can be a precipitator for a clinical depression, and needs to be dealt with as a medical issue rather than a disciplinary problem.

Loss of enthusiasm at work may also result from factors outside the job. If an individual's life is out of balance, or if the individual is having problems with relationships within the family, he or she may not have the necessary energy to expend at work. This may appear as depression or burnout.

If a medical assistant arrives at the point where job burnout is a concern, it is important to take action. If pos-

---

What Would You Do? What Would You *Not* Do?

Case Study 3

After 6 months at the obstetrics and gynecology office where she was first hired, Deanna began to wish that she had more contact with other medical assistants to discuss job-related issues. The other medical assistants in her office seemed to be busy with their families, and they didn't socialize at all after work. Deanna wished that she knew more about new trends, new medications, and new technology. She had joined the American Association of Medical Assistants when she graduated, but there didn't seem to be an active chapter in her area. ■

---

sible, the medical assistant should reduce the hours of work, even if only for a 3- or 6-month period. Increased social activities, increased exercise, and focusing on physical and mental health can foster a more positive physical and emotional state. The medical assistant should try to find a hobby to help "decompress" from work.

Sometimes, burnout is not recognized until the problems have progressed to such a degree that professional intervention is necessary. The individual suffering severe burnout may need counseling, therapy, or a job change; and if the individual has developed a substance abuse problem, he or she may even need inpatient rehabilitation. Many large facilities have in-house employee counseling.

Professional Organizations and Peer Support

The American Association of Medical Assistants (AAMA) and the American Medical Technologists (AMT) maintain professional organizations of medical assistants. Even if a medical assistant has not obtained certification, he or she can become a member of an active chapter of one of these organizations. Through local and national meetings and workshops, medical assistants are able to enter a network of peers with whom they can share and from whom they can learn. They can also obtain insurance at reasonable cost, professional journals, and other sources of information important to the profession.

For an annual membership fee, many benefits are available, including:

1. Peer support
2. Continuing education programs
3. Legislative advocacy on issues important to medical assistants
4. Publications and/or newsletters with information related to the profession of medical assisting

Legislation Affecting Medical Assistants

Professional organizations are able to advocate for pending state and federal legislation that may affect the medical assisting profession. Changes in legislation require actions by many people. In some states, issues for medical assistants arise from actions taken by other professionals to define legally who may perform certain procedures. As a result of

Memories *from* Externship

Deanna Taylor: The biggest difference between externship and employment is that it takes more effort to stay enthusiastic about showing up every day. When I was in the externship, everything was new. I was always excited to go because it seemed like there was a new experience every day. Now that I have been working for a few years, there are many days that seem very routine. There are new experiences, but I have to remind myself to notice them. One way that I have found to stay fresh and focused is to volunteer to be on committees to gather information or to plan the implementation of new equipment or new software. For example, we purchased three new meters for glucose testing a few months ago, and I volunteered to make a poster showing how to use the meters and to work with each staff member to make sure they were doing controls correctly. I also have been taking a general business course at night for the past month. I notice things at work that I never would have before, and I am not planning to take more courses in health administration or business administration. When I was in school, all I could think of was graduating and getting a job, but now that I am a medical assistant, I realize that my career is just beginning. I realize that I am personally responsible to find a way to keep my career rewarding and satisfying. ∎

Prepare for Success

such actions, medical assistants may not take x-rays in most states, and they may not be permitted to administer injections or draw blood, depending on the state.

A future task for the medical assisting profession will be to organize and help draft legislation giving medical assistants the right to perform all skills in the workplace for which they have been trained. This can best be accomplished by working with the national professional organizations and their state chapters.

Continuing Education Units

A **continuing education unit (CEU)** is a standard measure of 10 contact hours of qualified instruction as defined by a specific profession. Most health professions require a certain amount of continuing education for licensure or certification renewal. CEUs or contact hours of instruction are required for recertification as a CMA (AAMA) or RMA. The medical assistant should keep a file with the paperwork acknowledging attendance at classes or workshops, together with the CEU credits or contact hours approved for them. With the constant change in the medical field, it is not merely important but necessary to keep skills up to date, attain new skills, and obtain new information about professional practices.

Medical assisting contact hours and CEUs can be obtained from education programs that have been approved by the particular certifying agency. These education programs may be given through the state and national organi-

zation, through other educational institutions, or through home or on-line study programs.

PLANNING FOR JOB ADVANCEMENT OR CAREER CHANGE

One of the best ways to avoid job burnout is to chart a course of career advancement.

Advancing to Management

If a medical assistant enjoys the administrative part of medical assisting, there are many opportunities to find a management position within the health care industry.

The larger the facility, the more the administrative and management tasks are broken into discrete parts, and the more management and administrative staff are in demand.

If a medical assistant is currently working in such a facility and would like to move up the management ladder, he or she should ask about the possibility of rotating through the various departments to gain experience in finance, billing, marketing, public relations, or any other department. If the medical assistant is working at a small facility or private practice, he or she should take the opportunity to learn about every job within the practice. This makes the medical assistant more versatile and more valuable as an employee. After gaining supervisory experience in a smaller facility, the medical assistant may wish to move to a larger facility.

Business courses or formal education in health administration are invaluable. A number of colleges have both bachelor's and master's degree programs in health care administration. A degree in public administration or business management would also be appropriate.

Upgrading Technical/Clinical Skills

In order to advance to a position of greater responsibility on the clinical side, it will probably be necessary to obtain more formal education. After a few years of experience, a medical assistant who wishes to remain in an outpatient setting might consider enrolling in a formal education program to become a physician's assistant, a registered nurse, a medical technologist, or an x-ray technologist.

The opportunities become broader if a medical assistant wishes to work in a hospital or rehabilitation center. The medical assistant should talk to various health professionals and explore several potential career options. Obtaining financial support for additional education may be a concern. The medical assistant must decide if financial support is available to pursue further education full-time. For most, it will be necessary to continue working either part-time or full-time at your present position. Many employers encourage education and pay all or part of an employee's education costs.

Transferring Skills

Over time, the medical assistant may have built up skills that would make it possible to find a position in a field such as computers, insurance, the pharmaceutical industry, or medical equipment sales. If a medical assistant develops a strong interest in one of these areas, he or she should develop contacts, gather information, and develop a strategy for making a lateral career move.

This discussion would also not be complete without a word about the enormous rewards that can come from teaching—transferring knowledge and abilities to others who would like to become medical assistants.

With just a medical assisting degree or certificate, a certified medical assistant may be able to get some work teaching a specific class related to medical assisting skills. A medical assistant who is interested in teaching should speak to the director of the program where he or she trained about teaching opportunities.

In order to teach full-time, in addition to maintaining certification, the medical assistant should obtain a bachelor's degree and master's degree in a health care field, or in education. Depending on the financial resources available from a spouse or partner's income, family assistance, or scholarships and loans available, this may be as a part-time or full-time student.

MEDICAL PRACTICE *and the* LAW

Under the federal Equal Opportunity Employment laws, it is illegal for a company to discriminate in hiring practices on the basis of race, sex, religion, national origin, or age. Some states also have legislation making it illegal to discriminate on the basis of sexual orientation. Under the Americans with Disabilities Act (ADA), employers must make "reasonable accommodations" to any individual with a physical or mental disability who is otherwise qualified to perform the tasks necessary in the job.

If a medical assistant believes that discrimination has occurred during the process of seeking employment or promotion, he or she should contact the U.S. Equal Employment Opportunity Commission (EEOC). A verbal contact must be made before a complaint can be filed. ∎

What Would You Do? What Would You *Not* Do?   RESPONSES

Case Study 1
Page 1137

What Did Deanna Do?
- ❑ Reminded Andrea that employers usually consider work experience to include only paid positions.
- ❑ Pointed out tactfully that putting the externship in the category of work experience might indicate unreliability or lack of knowledge to a potential employer.
- ❑ Advised Andrea to include the externship in a section on the resumé called "Related Experience."
- ❑ Offered to look over Andrea's resumé to see if she could make other helpful suggestions.

What Did Deanna Not *Do?*
- ❑ Did not tell Andrea that she was being dishonest to put the externship as work experience.
- ❑ Did not make a discouraging remark like, "That won't help you get hired."

What Would You Do/What Would You *Not* Do? Review Deanna's response and place a checkmark next to the information you included in your response. List the additional information you included in your response.

_____
_____
_____
_____

Case Study 2
Page 1138

What Did Deanna Do?
- ❑ Made sure to take the name and telephone number of the person she was going to interview with.
- ❑ When Deanna realized that she was lost, she called the individual with whom she was scheduled to interview, explained the situation, apologized, and asked if it would be better to come late or reschedule.
- ❑ At the same time Deanna asked for directions.
- ❑ Resolved always to get very clear directions before any other interview.

What Did Deanna Not *Do?*
- ❑ Did not show up 15 minutes late without making every effort to contact the individual with whom she was supposed to interview.
- ❑ Did not blame any individual for giving bad directions or failing to give directions.
- ❑ Did not act like being 15 minutes late was really not important.

What Would You Do/What Would You *Not* Do? Review Deanna's response and place a checkmark next to the information you included in your response. List the additional information you included in your response.

Continued

What Would You Do? What Would You *Not* Do? RESPONSES—cont'd

_____

_____

_____

_____

Case Study 3
Page 1141

What Did Deanna Do?

❑ Found out where there were chapters of the AAMA in her state and made a point of attending a meeting. She also looked into attending the national meeting of the organization.

❑ Asked the practice manager if there were any continuing education programs at the local hospital that she could attend.

❑ Contacted graduates from her medical assisting program and arranged to get together with graduates she had been friends with when she was in school.

❑ Looked into the possibility of establishing a local chapter of the AAMA and tried to find one or two other medical assistants who might be interested in helping her.

❑ Looked at course offerings at the local community college to see if there were any courses or continuing education programs that she might be interested in attending.

What Did Deanna Not *Do?*

❑ Did not avoid taking responsibility to meet her own needs.

❑ Did not make excuses for putting off the process of seeking helpful contacts.

❑ Did not avoid reaching out to other medical assistants.

What Would You Do/What Would You *Not* Do? Review Deanna's response and place a checkmark next to the information you included in your response. List the additional information you included in your response.

_____

_____

_____

_____

TERMINOLOGY REVIEW

Burnout Disillusionment with work and physical or emotional exhaustion.

Continuing education unit (CEU) A standard measure of 10 hours of qualified instruction or contact hours as defined by a specific profession.

Cover letter A letter sent with one or more documents (such as a resumé) to provide an explanation.

Networking Contacting acquaintances and their contacts who may know of potential jobs.

Resumé A summary of information about a person that describes education, work experience, and other information related to an individual's suitability for employment.

ON THE WEB

For Information about Job Discrimination:

U.S. Equal Employment Opportunity Commission (EEOC): www.eeoc.gov

For Information on Professional Organizations:

American Association of Medical Assistants: www.aamantl.org

American Health Information Management Association: www.ahima.org

American Medical Technologists: www.amt1.com

American Society of Phlebotomy Technicians: www.aspt.org

For Information on Writing Resumés and Cover Letters:

The OWL at Purdue University: owl.english.purdue.edu/owl/resource/681/01

Resumé Templates—Microsoft Office Online: office.microsoft.com/en-us/templates

 PREPARE FOR CERTIFICATION Visit the Evolve site at http://evolve.elsevier.com/Bonewit/today/ to actively Prepare for your Certification.

 Check out the Companion CD bound with the book to access additional interactive activities.

Medical Abbreviations

aa	of each
AA	affected area; Alcoholics Anonymous
AAA	abdominal aortic aneurysm
AAL	anterior axillary line
AAMA	American Association of Medical Assistants
Ab	abortion; antibody
ABC	airway, breathing, circulation
abd	abdomen
ABE	acute bacterial endocarditis
ABG	arterial blood gases
ABN	abnormal
ABO	a blood group system
ABP	arterial blood pressure
Abs	absent
ac	before meals (Latin, *ante cibum*)
ACLS	advanced cardiac life support
ACOA	adult child of an alcoholic
ACTH	adrenocorticotropic hormone
AD	right ear (Latin, *auris dextra*)
ADA	American Dental Association; American Diabetic Association
ADH	antidiuretic hormone
ADL	activities of daily living
ad lib	as desired
adm	admission; admit
admin	administer
AFB	acid-fast bacillus
A Fib	atrial fibrillation
AFL	atrial flutter
AFP	alpha-fetoprotein
A/G	albumin-to-globulin ratio
AGA	appropriate for gestational age
AGN	acute glomerular nephritis
AHA	American Heart Association
AI	aortic insufficiency
AICD	automatic implantable cardioverter-defibrillator
AIDS	acquired immunodeficiency syndrome
AJ	ankle jerk
AKA	above the knee amputation
AL	acute leukemia
alb	albumin
ALL	acute lymphoblastic leukemia
ALP	alkaline phosphatase
ALS	amyotrophic lateral sclerosis
ALT	alanine aminotransferase
am or a.m.	before noon; morning (Latin, *ante meridiem*)
AMA	against medical advice; American Medical Association
amb	ambulatory
AMI	acute myocardial infarction
amnio	amniocentesis
amt	amount
anes	anesthesia; anesthetist
ant.	anterior
A/O	alert and oriented
AOM	acute otitis media
AP	angina pectoris; apical pulse
APC	atrial premature complex
approx	approximately
appt	appointment
aq	water
ARC	AIDS-related complex; American Red Cross
ARD	acute respiratory distress
ARDS	acute respiratory distress syndrome
AS	left ear (Latin, *auris sinistra*)
ASA	acetylsalicylic acid (aspirin)
ASAP	as soon as possible
ASCVD	arteriosclerotic cardiovascular disease
ASD	atrial septal defect
ASHD	arteriosclerotic heart disease
ASO	antistreptolysin O; arteriosclerosis obliterans
AST	aspartate aminotransferase
ATR	Achilles tendon reflex
AU	both ears (Latin, *auris unitas*); in each ear (Latin, *auris uterque*)
aud	auditory
AVR	aortic valve replacement
A & W	alive and well
ax	axillary
BA	backache
Ba	barium

Bab	Babinski (reflex)
bas	basophil
BBB	blood-brain barrier; bundle branch block
BBT	basal body temperature
b/c	because
BC	birth control; bone conduction
BCP	birth control pills
BE	barium enema
BEA	below the elbow amputation
BG	blood glucose
bid	twice a day (Latin, *bis in die*)
bili	bilirubin
BJ	biceps jerk
BJM	bones, joints, and muscles
BK	below the knee
BKA	below the knee amputation
BLS	basic life support
BM	bowel movement
BMR	basal metabolic rate
BOM	bilateral otitis media
BP	blood pressure
BPAD	bipolar affective disorder
BPH	benign prostatic hypertrophy
BPM	beats per minute
BR	bathroom
BRB	bright red blood
BrBx	breast biopsy
BS	blood sugar; breath sounds
BSA	body surface area
BSE	breast self-examination
BSN	bowel sounds normal
BTL	bilateral tubal ligation
BUN	blood urea nitrogen
BW	birth weight
Bx	biopsy
$\bar{c}$	with
C	Celsius
C1	first cervical vertebra
C2	second cervical vertebra
Ca	calcium
CA	cancer; cardiac arrest
CAD	coronary artery disease
CAHD	coronary atherosclerotic heart disease
cal	calorie(s)
CAPD	continuous ambulatory peritoneal dialysis
caps	capsules
CAT	computerized axial tomography
cath	catheter; catheterize
CB	cesarean birth
CBC	complete blood count
CBD	common bile duct
CBF	cerebral blood flow
CBR	complete bed rest
CC	chief complaint
cc	cubic centimeter
CCU	coronary care unit; critical care unit
CD	chemical dependence

C & D	cystoscopy and dilation
CDC	Centers for Disease Control and Prevention
cerv	cervical; cervix
CF	cystic fibrosis
CFS	chronic fatigue syndrome
CGL	chronic granulocytic leukemia
CH	crown-heel (length of infant)
CHB	complete heart block
CHD	congenital heart disease; coronary heart disease
chemo	chemotherap
CHF	congestive heart failure
CHL	conductive hearing loss
Chol	cholesterol
CIS	carcinoma in situ
CK	creatine kinase
cl	chloride; chlorine
CLD	chronic lung disease
cldy	cloudy
cm	centimeter
cm^3	cubic centimeter
CMA	Certified Medical Assistant
CMV	cytomegalovirus
CNS	central nervous system
CO	cardiac output
c/o	complains of
CO_2	carbon dioxide
COPD	chronic obstructive pulmonary disease
CP	cerebral palsy
CPK	creatine phosphokinase
CPN	chronic pyelonephritis
CPR	cardiopulmonary resuscitation
CR	crown-rump (length of infant)
CRC	colorectal cancer
CRD	chronic respiratory disease
CS	cesarean section
C & S	culture and sensitivity
CSF	cerebrospinal fluid
CST	contraction stress test
CT	computed tomography
CTS	carpal tunnel syndrome
CV	cardiovascular
CVA	cerebrovascular accident
CVP	central venous pressure
CVS	cardiovascular system; chorionic villus sampling
Cx	cervix
CXR	chest x-ray
Cysto	cystoscopy
d	day
/day	per day
db	decibel
DBE	deep breathing exercise
DBM	diabetic management
DBP	diastolic blood pressure
d/c	discontinue
D & C	dilation and curettage

DD	discharge diagnosis	EBV	Epstein-Barr virus
DDD	degenerative disc disease	EC	enteric-coated
D/DW	dextrose and distilled water	ECD	esophagogastroduodenoscopy
DDx	differential diagnosis	ECF	extended care facility
D & E	dilation and evacuation	ECG	electrocardiogram
DEA	Drug Enforcement Administration	Echo	echocardiogram
del	delivery	E. coli	Escherichia coli
DES	diethylstilbestrol	ECT	electroconvulsive therapy
DI	diabetes insipidus	ED	emergency department
D & I	dry and intact	EDD	expected date of delivery
diab	diabetic	EEG	electroencephalogram
diff	differential white blood cell count	EENT	eye, ear, nose, and throat
dil	dilute	EGA	estimated gestational age
disch	discharge	elect stim	electrical stimulation
disp	dispense	ELISA	enzyme-linked immunosorbent assay
DIU	death in utero	elix	elixir
DJD	degenerative joint disease	EmBx	endometrial biopsy
DKA	diabetic ketoacidosis	EMG	electromyogram
dL	deciliter	EMS	emergency medical service
DM	diabetes mellitus	ENT	ear, nose, and throat
DNA	deoxyribonucleic acid	EOM	extraocular movement
DNKA	did not keep appointment	eos	eosinophil
DNR	do not resuscitate	ER	emergency room
d/o	disorder	ESR	erythrocyte sedimentation rate
DOA	dead on arrival	est	estimated
DOB	date of birth	ESWL	extracorporeal shock-wave lithotripsy
DOE	dyspnea on exertion	ETT	endotracheal tube
DOI	date of injury	EVAL	evaluation
DP	diastolic pressure	ex	exercise
DPT	diphtheria, pertussis, and tetanus (vaccine)	ext	extract
DR	delivery room	Ez	eczema
dr	dram		
DRE	digital rectal exam	F	Fahrenheit
DRG	diagnosis-related group	FA	fluorescent antibody
drsg	dressing	FB	foreign body
DS	double strength	FBP	femoral blood pressure
D/S	discharge summary	FBS	fasting blood sugar
DSD	dry sterile dressing	FD	fully dilated
DT	diphtheria and tetanus toxoid	FDA	Food and Drug Administration
DTaP	diphtheria and tetanus toxoids and acellular pertussis vaccine	Fe	iron
		Fe def	iron deficiency
DTR	deep tendon reflex	FEF	forced expiratory flow
DU	duodenal ulcer	FEKG	fetal electrocardiogram
DUB	dysfunctional uterine bleeding	FEV	forced expiratory volume
DUI	driving under the influence (of alcohol)	FFP	fresh frozen plasma
D & V	diarrhea and vomiting	FH	family history
DVA	distance visual acuity	FHR	fetal heart rate
DVT	deep venous thrombosis	FHT	fetal heart tones
DW	distilled water	fl	fluid
D/W	dextrose in water	flex sig	flexible sigmoidoscopy
Dx	diagnosis	FMP	first menstrual period
Dz	disease	FOB	fecal occult blood
		FOBT	fecal occult blood test
ea	each	FP	family practice
EAB	elective abortion	freq	frequent
EAC	external auditory canal	FS	finger-stick
EAM	external auditory meatus	FSH	follicle-stimulating hormone
EBL	estimated blood loss	ft	foot

FT	full term
FTND	full-term normal delivery
FTT	failure to thrive
F/U	follow-up
FUO	fever of undetermined origin
FVC	forced vital capacity
FWB	full weight bearing
Fx	fracture
g	gram
G	gravida
GA	general anesthesia; gestational age
GB	gallbladder
GC	gas chromatography; gonorrhea
GCT	glucose challenge test
GDM	gestational diabetes mellitus
gen	general
GFR	glomerular filtration rate
GH	growth hormone
GI	gastrointestinal
glu	glucose
GM	gross motor
Gm−	gram negative
Gm+	gram positive
GP	general practitioner
gr	grain
GSW	gunshot wound
gtt(s)	drop (drops)
GTT	glucose tolerance test
GU	genitourinary
G/W	glucose in water
GYN	gynecology
h	hour
H/A	headache
HAL	hyperalimentation
HAV	hepatitis A virus
HBIG	hepatitis B immunoglobulin
HBP	high blood pressure
HBsAg	hepatitis B surface antigen
HBV	hepatitis B virus
HC	head circumference
HCG	human chorionic gonadotropin
HCl	hydrochloric acid
Hct	hematocrit
HCVD	hypertensive cardiovascular disease
HD	Hodgkin's disease
HDL	high-density lipoprotein
HDN	hemolytic disease of the newborn
HEENT	head, eye, ear, nose, and throat
Hep	heparin
Hep B	hepatitis B vaccine
Hg	mercury
Hgb	hemoglobin
HGM	home glucose monitoring
HH	home health
H & H	hemoglobin and hematocrit

Hib	*Haemophilus influenzae* type b conjugate vaccine
HIV	human immunodeficiency virus
H & L	heart and lungs
HMO	health maintenance organization
H/O	history of
H₂O	water
H & P	history and physical
hpf	high-power field
HPI	history of present illness
H. pylori	*Helicobacter pylori*
HR	heart rate
HRT	hormone replacement therapy
hs	at bedtime (Latin, *hora somni*)
HSV	herpes simplex virus
ht	height
HTN	hypertension
HVD	hypertensive vascular disease
Hx	history
Hz	hertz
IA	intraarterial
IABP	intraaortic balloon pump
IBS	irritable bowel syndrome
IBW	ideal body weight
ICCU	intensive coronary care unit
ICD	International Classification of Diseases (of the World Health Organization)
ICDA	International Classification of Diseases, Adapted
ICF	intracellular fluid
ICP	intracranial pressure
ICS	intercostal space
ICU	intensive care unit
ID	intradermal
I & D	incision and drainage
IDDM	insulin-dependent diabetes mellitus
IM	intramuscular
Immuniz	immunizations
imp	impression
in	inch
I & O	intake and output
IOP	intraocular pressure
IPPB	intermittent positive-pressure breathing
IPV	inactivated polio vaccine
IQ	intelligence quotient
IU	international unit
IUD	intrauterine device
IUFD	intrauterine fetal death
IUGR	intrauterine growth rate
IV	intravenous
IVP	intravenous pyelogram
JAMA	*Journal of the American Medical Association*
jaund	jaundice
JODM	juvenile-onset diabetes mellitus

JP	Jackson Pratt (drain)	m	meter
JRA	juvenile rheumatoid arthritis	mcg	microgram
JVD	jugular venous distention	MCH	mean corpuscular hemoglobin
JVP	jugular venous pressure	MCHC	mean corpuscular hemoglobin concentration
K	potassium	MCL	midclavicular line
KCl	potassium chloride	MCV	mean corpuscular volume
kg	kilogram	MD	medical doctor; muscular dystrophy
KOH	potassium hydroxide	MDE	major depressive episode
KUB	kidney, ureter, and bladder	MDI	metered-dose inhaler
		MDR	minimum daily requirement
L	liter	med(s)	medication(s)
l	length	mEq/L	milliequivalents per liter
LA	left atrium	mg	milligram
lab	laboratory	MG	myasthenia gravis
lac	laceration	MGF	maternal grandfather
lap	laparotomy	MGM	maternal grandmother
lat	lateral	MH	marital history
LAVH	laparoscopic assisted vaginal hysterectomy	MHx	medical history
		MI	myocardial infarction
lax	laxative	min	minute
LB	lower back	ml	milliliter
lb	pound	mm	millimeter
LBBB	left bundle branch block	mm³	cubic millimeter
LBP	low back pain	mm Hg	millimeters of mercury
LBW	low birth weight	mmol	millimole
LD	lactate dehydrogenase	MMR	measles, mumps, and rubella (vaccine)
L & D	labor and delivery	MO	month old
LDL	low-density lipoprotein	mod	moderate
LE	lupus erythematosus	MODM	mature-onset diabetes mellitus
LFD	low forceps delivery	mono	mononucleosis
LFT	liver function test	MP	menstrual period
lg	large	MR	mental retardation; mitral regurgitation
LGA	large for gestational age	MRI	magnetic resonance imaging
LH	luteinizing hormone	MRM	modified radical mastectomy
liq	liquid	MS	multiple sclerosis
LLC	long leg cast	MSL	midsternal line
LLE	left lower extremity	MSU	midstream urine specimen
LLL	left lower leg	MT	medical technologist
LLQ	left lower quadrant	multip	multipara
LMP	last menstrual period	MV	mitral valve
LNMP	last normal menstrual period	MVA	motor vehicle accident
LOC	loss of consciousness	MVP	mitral valve prolapse
LOM	loss of motion	MVR	mitral valve replacement
LP	lumbar puncture		
lpf	low-power field	Na	sodium
LR	labor room	N/A	not applicable
LRQ	lower right quadrant	NaCl	sodium chloride
LS	lumbosacral	NAD	no appreciable disease; nothing abnormal detected
lt	left		
LTC	long-term care	narc	narcotic
LTM	long-term memory	NB	newborn
LUE	left upper extremity	NBS	normal bowel sounds; normal breath sounds
LUQ	left upper quadrant		
LV	left ventricle	NBW	normal birth weight
L & W	living and well	NC	no change
lymphs	lymphocytes	N/C	no complaints

NED	no evidence of disease
neg	negative
NG	nasogastric
NGT	nasogastric tube
NGU	nongonococcal urethritis
NH	nursing home
NHL	non-Hodgkin lymphoma
NI	not improved
NICU	newborn intensive care unit
NIDDM	non–insulin-dependent diabetes mellitus
NKA	no known allergies
NKDA	no known drug allergies
NL	normal limits
NMP	normal menstrual period
NMR	nuclear magnetic resonance
noct	nocturnal
non rep	do not repeat
norm	normal
NPO	nothing by mouth (Latin, *nil per os*)
NR	no refill
N/R	not responsible
NS	normal saline
NSAID	nonsteroidal antiinflammatory drug
NSR	normal sinus rhythm
NSS	normal saline solution
NST	nonstress test
NSU	nonspecific urethritis
NSVD	normal spontaneous vaginal delivery
NT	nontender
N & T	nose and throat
nullip	nullipara (never gave birth)
N & V	nausea and vomiting
NVA	near visual acuity
NVD	nausea, vomiting, and diarrhea
N & W	normal and well
NWB	non–weight-bearing
NYD	not yet diagnosed
O	oral
O$_2$	oxygen
OA	osteoarthritis
OB	obstetrics
OB/GYN	obstetrics and gynecology
obs	observed
occ	occasionally
OCD	obsessive-compulsive disorder
OCT	oxytocin challenge test
OD	right eye
O & E	observation and examination
O/E	on examination
OH	occupational history
oint	ointment
OM	otitis media
OOB	out of bed
op	operation
OP	outpatient
O & P	ova and parasites

OPV	oral polio vaccine
OR	operating room
ortho	orthopedics
OS	left eye
OT	occupational therapy
OTC	over-the-counter (nonprescription medication)
OU	both eyes; in each eye (Latin, *oculus uterque*)
OV	office visit
oz	ounce
P	pulse
PA	physician assistant; posteroanterior
PAC	premature atrial contraction
Pap	Pap test
PAT	paroxysmal atrial tachycardia
path	pathology
Pb	lead
PBI	protein-bound iodine
pc	after meals (Latin, *post cibum*)
PC	platelet count
PCC	Poison Control Center
PCV	packed cell volume
PD	Parkinson's disease
PDR	*Physician's Desk Reference*
PE	physical examination
peds	pediatrics
PEG	pneumoencephalogram; pneumoencephalography
PEN	penicillin; pharmacy equivalent name
per	by, through
peri	perineal
PERRLA	pupils equal, round, regular, react to light, and accommodation (normal)
PET	positron emission tomography
PFS	pulmonary function studies
PFT	pulmonary function test
PGF	paternal grandfather
PGH	pituitary growth hormone
PGM	paternal grandmother
pH	hydrogen ion concentration
PH	past history
pharm	pharmacy
PI	present illness
PID	pelvic inflammatory disease
PIH	pregnancy-induced hypertension
PKU	phenylketonuria
pm or p.m.	afternoon; evening (Latin, *post meridiem*)
PMB	postmenopausal bleeding
PMH	past medical history
PMN	polymorphonuclear neutrophils
PMP	past menstrual period
PMS	premenstrual syndrome
PMT	premenstrual tension
PN	progress notes
PND	paroxysmal nocturnal dyspnea

PNX	pneumothorax		RBS	random blood sugar
po or PO	by mouth (Latin, *per os*)		RCV	red cell volume
POL	physician's office laboratory		RD	respiratory distress
POR	problem-oriented medical record		RDA	recommended daily allowance
pos	positive		RDS	respiratory distress syndrome
postop	postoperative (after surgery)		RE	rectal examination
PP	postpartum		reg	regular
PPB	positive-pressure breathing		rehab	rehabilitation
PPBS	postprandial blood sugar		REM	rapid eye movement
PPD	purified protein derivative		REP	retrograde pyelogram
PPH	postpartum hemorrhage		resp	respiration
PPT	partial prothrombin time		RF	rheumatic fever
preop	preoperative (before surgery)		RG	random glucose
prep	preparation		Rh	rhesus blood factor
primip	woman bearing first child		RHD	rheumatic heart disease
prn	as the occasion arises; as needed (Latin, *pro re nata*)		RHF	right heart failure
			RI	respiratory illness
procto	proctoscopy		RLQ	right lower quadrant
prog	prognosis		RMA	Registered Medical Assistant
PROM	premature rupture of membranes		RMSF	Rocky Mountain spotted fever
prox	proximal		RNA	ribonucleic acid
PSA	prostate-specific antigen		R/O	rule out
pt	patient; pint		ROM	range of motion; rupture of membranes
Pt	patient		ROS	review of systems
PT	physical therapy; prothrombin time		RP	retrograde pyelogram
PTA	prior to admission		RQ	respiratory quotient
PTB	prior to birth		RRR	regular rate and rhythm
PTD	prior to discharge		RSV	respiratory syncytial virus
PTH	parathyroid hormone		rt	right
PTT	partial thromboplastin time		RT	radiation therapy; room temperature
PUD	peptic ulcer disease		R/T	related to
PVC	premature ventricular contraction		RTW	return to work
PVD	peripheral vascular disease		RUE	right upper extremity
PWB	partial weight bearing		RUQ	right upper quadrant
Px	physical examination		RV	right ventricle
			RVH	right ventricular hypertrophy
q	each; every (Latin, *quaque*)		Rx	prescription
q AM	every morning			
qd	every day (Latin, *quaque die*)		$\bar{s}$	without
qh	every hour (Latin, *quaque hora*)		SA	sinoatrial
q2h (q3h, q4h)	every 2 (3, 4) hours		SAB	spontaneous abortion
			SARS	severe acute respiratory syndrome
qid	four times a day (Latin, *quater in die*)		SB	sinus bradycardia; stillborn
qn	every night (Latin, *quaque noctes*)		SBE	subacute bacterial endocarditis
QNS	quantity not sufficient		SBO	small bowel obstruction
qod	every other day (Latin, *quater altera die*)		SBP	systolic blood pressure
QS	quantity sufficient		SC	subcutaneous
qt	quart		SCD	sudden cardiac death
quad	quadriplegic		schiz	schizophrenia
			SCI	spinal cord injury
R	respiration		SD	spontaneous delivery; standard deviation
RA	rheumatoid arthritis		SDH	subdural hematoma
RAF	rheumatoid arthritis factor		S/E	side effects
RAST	radioallergosorbent test		sec	second
RBC	red blood cell; red blood (cell) count		sed rate	sedimentation rate
RBC/hpf	red blood cells per high-power field		segs	segmented neutrophils
RBCV	red blood cell volume		seq	sequela

SF	scarlet fever; spinal fluid		TENS	transcutaneous electrical nerve stimulation
SG	specific gravity		TF	tube feeding; transfer factor
SGA	small for gestational age		ther	therapy
SH	serum hepatitis; social history		THR	total hip replacement
sid	once a day (Latin, *semel in die*)		TIA	transient ischemic attack
SIDS	sudden infant death syndrome		tid	three times a day (Latin, *ter in die*)
sig	write on label		tinct	tincture
sigmoid	sigmoidoscopy		TKR	total knee replacement
sl	slight		TLC	tender loving care; total lung capacity
SLC	short leg cast		TM	tympanic membrane
SLE	systemic lupus erythematosus		TMJ	temporomandibular joint
SM	simple mastectomy		TND	term normal delivery
sm	small		TO	telephone order
SNF	skilled nursing facility		tol	tolerate; tolerated
SOAP	subjective data, objective data, assessment, and plan		TOP	termination of pregnancy
			TOPV	trivalent oral poliovirus vaccine
SOB	shortness of breath		TP	total protein
sol	solution		TPM	temporary pacemaker
SOM	serous otitis media		TPN	total parenteral nutrition
SP	systolic pressure		TPR	temperature, pulse, and respiration
sp gr	specific gravity		Tq	tourniquet
SPA	suprapubic aspiration		tr	trace
spec	specimen		trig	triglycerides
spont ab	spontaneous abortion		TRUS	transrectal ultrasound
SQ	subcutaneous		TSE	testicular self-examination
SR	sustained release		TSH	thyroid-stimulating hormone
SROM	spontaneous rupture of membranes		tsp	teaspoon
ss	one half		TSP	total serum protein
Staph	*Staphylococcus*		TSS	toxic shock syndrome
STAT	immediately		TVH	total vaginal hysterectomy
STD	sexually transmitted disease		Tx	treatment
std	standard			
STM	short-term memory		U	unit
Strep	*Streptococcus*		UA	urinalysis
subcut	subcutaneous		UC	ulcerative colitis
sup	superior		U/C	urine culture
supp	suppository		UCG	urinary chorionic gonadotropin
surg	surgery		UCHD	usual childhood diseases
SV	stroke volume		UE	upper extremity
Sx	symptoms		UGI	upper gastrointestinal
Sz	seizure		ULQ	upper left quadrant
			UOQ	upper outer quadrant
T	temperature		UR	upper respiratory
T_3	triiodothyronine		URI	upper respiratory infection
T_4	thyroxine		Urol	urology
T & A	tonsils and adenoids		URQ	upper right quadrant
tab(s)	tablet(s)		US	ultrasound
TAB	therapeutic abortion		USI	urinary stress incontinence
TAH	total abdominal hysterectomy		*USP*	*United States Pharmacopoeia*
TB	tuberculosis		UT	urinary tract
TBF	total body fat		UTI	urinary tract infection
TBLC	term birth, living child		UV	ultraviolet
tbsp	tablespoon			
TBW	total body water		VA	visual acuity
TC	total capacity		VAD	vascular access device
T & C	type and cross-match		vag	vagina; vaginal
temp	temperature		VAP	vascular access port

VC	vital capacity		WBC	white blood cell; white blood (cell) count
VD	venereal disease		WC	white cell
VDRL	Venereal Disease Research Laboratory (test)		W/C	wheelchair
			WDWN	well developed, well nourished
VE	vaginal examination		wk	week
VFib	ventricular fibrillation		WN	well nourished
VH	vaginal hysterectomy		WNF	well-nourished female
VHD	valvular heart disease		WNL	within normal limits
VHDL	very-high-density lipoprotein		WNM	well-nourished male
vit	vitamin		WO	written order
VLDL	very-low-density lipoprotein		w/o	without
VO	verbal order		WR	weakly reactive
VP	venipuncture		W/U	workup
VS	vital signs			
VSD	ventricular septal defect		X	magnification
VSS	vital signs stable		XM	cross-match
VT	ventricular tachycardia		XR	x-ray
VV	varicose veins			
			y	year(s)
WB	weight bearing		yd	yard(s)
WBAT	weight bearing as tolerated		YOB	year of birth

Spanish-English Phrases

The following is a guide to help you complete the history and examination of Spanish-speaking patients. Initial questions presented are general ones used at the beginning of the examination. Questions for pain assessment follow. The remaining translations are arranged in order of the body systems. Each system's section contains basic vocabulary, questions used for history taking, and instructions that would facilitate examination. The intent of this guide is to offer an array of questions and phrases from which the examiner can choose as appropriate for assessment.

HINTS FOR PRONUNCIATION OF SPANISH WORDS

1. *h* is silent.
2. *j* is pronounced as *h*.
3. *ll* is pronounced as a *y* sound.
4. *r* is pronounced with a trilled sound, and *rr* is trilled even more.
5. *v* is pronounced with a *b* sound.
6. A *y* by itself is pronounced with a long *e* sound.
7. Accent marks over the vowel indicate the syllable that is to be stressed.

INTRODUCTORY

I am _____.	Soy _____.
What is your name?	¿Cómo se llama usted?
I would like to examine you now.	Quisiera examinarlo(a) ahora.
	Note (a) when speaking to female.

GENERAL

How do you feel?	¿Cómo se siente?
Good	Bien
Bad	Mal
Do you feel better today?	¿Se siente mejor hoy?
Where do you work?	¿Dónde trabaja? (¿Cuál es su profesión o tra-bajo?) (¿Qué hace usted?)

Are you allergic to anything?	¿Tiene usted algerias?
Medications, foods, insect bites?	¿Medicinas, alimentos, picaduras de insectos?
Do you take any medications?	¿Toma usted algunas medicinas?
Do you have any drug allergies?	¿Es usted alérgico(a) a algún médicamento?
Do you have a history of . . .	¿Padece usted enfermedad . . .
Heart disease?	del corazón?
Diabetes?	del diabetes?
Epilepsy?	la epilepsia?
Bronchitis?	de bronquitis?
Emphysema?	de enfsema?
Asthma?	de asma?

PAIN

Have you any pain?	¿Tiene dolor?
Where is the pain?	¿Dónde está el dolor?
Do you have any pain here?	¿Tiene usted dolor aquí?
How severe is the pain?	¿Qué tan fuerte es el dolor?
Mild, moderate, sharp, or severe?	¿Ligero, moderado, agudo, o severo?
What were you doing when the pain started?	¿Qué haciá usted cuando le comenzó el dolor?
Have you ever had this pain before?	¿Ha tenido este dolor antes? (¿Ha sido siempre así?)
Do you have a pain in your side?	¿Tiene usted dolor en el costado?
Is it worse now?	¿Está peor ahora?
Does it still hurt?	¿Le duele todavía?
Did you feel much pain at the time?	¿Sintió mucho dolor entonces?
Show me where.	Muéstreme dónde.
Does it hurt when I press here?	¿Le duele cuando aprieto aquí?

HEAD

Vocabulary

Head	La cabeza
Face	La cara

History

How does your head feel?	¿Cómo siente la cabeza?
Have you any pain in the head?	¿Le duele la cabeza?
Do you have headaches?	¿Tiene usted dolores de cabeza?
Do you have migraines?	¿Tiene usted migrañas?
What causes the headaches?	¿Qué le causa los dolores de cabeza?

Examination

Lift up your head.	Levante la cabeza.

EYES

Vocabulary

Eye	El ojo

History

Have you had pain in your eyes?	¿Ha tenido dolor en los ojos?
Do you wear glasses?	¿Usa usted anteojos/gafas/lentes/espejuelos?
Do you wear contact lenses?	¿Usa usted lentes de contacto?
Can you see clearly?	¿Puede ver claramente?
Better at a distance?	¿Mejor a cierta distancia?
Do you sometimes see things double?	¿Ve las cosas doble algunas veces?
Do you see things through a mist?	¿Ve las cosas nubladas?
Were you exposed to anything that could have injured your eye?	¿Fue expuesto a cualquier cosa que pudiera haberle dañado el ojo?
Do your eyes water much?	¿Le lagrimean mucho los ojos?

Examination

Look up.	Mire para arriba.
Look down.	Mire para abajo.
Look toward your nose.	Mírese la nariz.
Look at me.	Míreme.
Tell me what number it is.	Dígame qué número es éste.
Tell me what letter it is.	Dígame qué letra es ésta.

EAR, NOSE, AND THROAT

Vocabulary

Ears	Los oídos
Eardrum	El tímpano
Laryngitis	La laringitis
Lip	El labio
Mouth	La boca
Nose	La naríz
Tongue	La lengua

History

Do you have any hearing problems?	¿Tiene usted problemas de oir?
Do you use a hearing aid?	¿Usa usted un audífono?
Do you have ringing in the ears?	¿Le zumban los oídos?
Do you have allergies?	¿Tiene alergias?
Do you use dentures?	¿Usa usted dentadura postiza?
Do you have any loose teeth, removable bridges, or any prosthesis?	¿Tiene dientes flojos, dientes postizos, o cualquier prostesis?
Do you have a cold?	¿Tiene usted un resfriado/resfrío?
Do you have sore throats frequently?	¿Le duele la garganta con frecuencia?
Have you ever had a strep throat?	¿Ha tenido alguna vez infección de la garganta?

Examination

Open your mouth.	Abra la boca.
I want to take a throat culture.	Quiero hacer un cultivo de la garganta.
This will not hurt.	Esto no le va a doler.

CARDIOVASCULAR

Vocabulary

Heart	El corazón
Heart attack	El ataque al corazón
Heart disease	La enfermedad del corazón
Heart murmur	El soplo del corazón
High blood pressure	Alta presión

History

Have you ever had any chest pain?	¿Ha tenido alguna vez dolor de pecho?
Where?	¿Dónde?
Do you notice any irregularity of heartbeat or any palpitations?	¿Nota cualquier latido o palpitación irregular?
Do you get short of breath?	¿Tiene usted problemas con la respiración?
When?	¿Cuándo?
Do you take medicine for your heart?	¿Toma medicina para el corazón?
How often?	¿Con qué frecuencia?
Do you know if you have high blood pressure?	¿Sabe usted si tiene la presión alta?
Is there a history of hypertension in your family?	¿En su familia, se encuentran varias personas con alta presión?
Do you take medicine for high blood pressure?	¿Toma medicina para la presión alta?
How often?	¿Con qué frecuencia?
Are any of your limbs swollen?	¿Están hinchados algunos de sus miembros?
Hands, feet, legs?	¿Manos, pies, piernas?

How long have they been swollen like this?

¿Desde cuándo están hinchados así?
(¿Qué tanto tiempo tiene usted con esta hinchazón?)

Examination

Let me feel your pulse.

Déjeme tomarle el pulso.

I am going to take your blood pressure now.

Le voy a tomar la presión ahora.

RESPIRATORY

Vocabulary

Chest	El pecho
Lungs	Los pulmones

History

Do you smoke?	¿Fuma usted?
How many packs a day?	¿Cuántos paquetes al día?
Have you any difficulty in breathing?	¿Tiene dificultad al respirar?
How long have you been coughing?	¿Desde cuándo tiene tos?
Do you cough up phlegm?	¿Al toser, escupe usted flema(s)?
What is the color of your expectorations?	¿Cuándo usted escupe, qué color es?
White/Green	Blanco/Verde
Do you cough up blood?	¿Al toser, arroja usted sangre?
Do you wheeze?	¿Le silba a usted el pecho?

Examination

Take a deep breath.	Respire profundo.
Breathe normally.	Respire normalmente.
Cough.	Tosa.
Cough again.	Tosa otra vez.

GASTROINTESTINAL

Vocabulary

Abdomen	El abdomen
Intestines/bowels	Los intestinos/las entrañas
Liver	El hígado
Nausea	Náusea
Gastric ulcer	La úcera gástrica
Stomach	El estómago, la panza, la barriga
Stomachache	El dolor de estómago

History

What foods disagree with you?	¿Qué alimentos le caen mal?
Do you get heartburn?	¿Suele tener ardor en el pecho?
Do you have indigestion often?	¿Tiene indigestión con frecuencia?
Are you going to vomit?	¿Va a vomitar (arrojar)?
Do you have blood in your vomit?	¿Tiene usted vómitos con sangre?
Do you have abdominal pain?	¿Tiene dolor en el abdomen?

How are your stools?	¿Cómo son sus defecaciones?
Are they regular?	¿Son regulares?
Have you noticed their color?	¿Se ha fijado en el color?
Are you constipated?	¿Está estreñido?
Do you have diarrhea?	¿Tiene diarrea?

GENITOURINARY

Vocabulary

Genitals	Los genitales
Penis	El pene, el miembro
Kidney	El riñón
Urine	La orina

History

Have you any difficulty passing water?	¿Tiene dificultad en orinar?
Do you pass water involuntarily?	¿Orina sin querer?
Do you have a urethral discharge?	¿Tiene secreción de la uretra?
Do you have burning with urination?	¿Tiene ardor al orinar?

ANUS, RECTUM, AND PROSTATE

Vocabulary

Abdomen	El abdomen
Intestines/bowels	Los intestinos/las entrañas
Nausea	Náusea
Stomach	El estómago, la panza, la barriga
Stomachache	El dolor de estómago
Urine	La orina

History

Are you going to vomit?	¿Va a vomitar (arrojar)?
Do you have abdominal pain?	¿Tiene dolor en el abdomen?
How are your stools?	¿Cómo son sus defecaciones?
Are they regular?	¿Son regulares?
Have you noticed their color?	¿Se ha fijado en el color?
Are you constipated?	¿Está estreñido?
Do you have diarrhea?	¿Tiene diarrea?
Have you any difficulty passing water?	¿Tiene dificultad en orinar?
Do you have a urethral discharge?	¿Tiene secreción de la uretra?
Do you have burning with urination?	¿Tiene ardor al orinar?

MUSCULOSKELETAL

Vocabulary

Ankle	El tobillo
Arm	El brazo
Back	La espalda
Bones	Los huesos

Elbow	El codo
Finger	El dedo
Foot	El pie
Fracture	La fractura
Hand	La mano
Hip	La cadera
Knee	La rodilla
Leg	La pierna
Muscles	Los músculos
Rib	La costilla
Shoulder	El hombro
Thigh	El muslo

History

Did you fall, and how did you fall?	¿Se cayó, y cómo se cayó?
How did this happen?	¿Cómo sucedio esto?
How long ago?	¿Cúanto tiempo hace?

Examination

Raise your arm.	Levante el brazo.
Raise it more.	Más alto.
Now the other.	Ahora el otro.
Stand up and walk.	Párese y camine.
Straighten your leg.	Enderece la pierna.
Bend your knee.	Doble la rodilla.
Push	Empuje
Pull	Jale
Up	Arriba
Down	Abajo
In/out	Adentro/afuera
Rest	Descanse
Kneel	Arrodíllese

NEUROLOGIC

Vocabulary

Brain	El cerebro
Dizziness	El vértigo, el mareo
Epilepsy	La epilepsia
Fainting spell	El desmayo
Unconsciousness	La insensibilidad (inconsciente)

History

Have you ever had a head injury?	¿Ha tenido alguna vez daño a la cabeza?
Do you have convulsions?	¿Tiene convulsiones?
Do you have tingling sensations?	¿Tiene hormigueos?
Do you have numbness in your hands, arms, or feet?	¿Siente entumecidos las manos, los brazos, o los pies?
Have you ever lost consciousness?	¿Perdió alguna vez el sentido? (inconsciente)
For how long?	¿Por cuánto tiempo?
How often does this happen?	¿Con qué frecuencia ocurre esto?

Examination

Squeeze my hand.	Apriete mi mano.
Can you not do it better than that?	¿No puede hacerlo más fuerte?
Turn on your left/right side.	Voltéese al lado izquierdo/al lado derecho.
Roll over and sit up over the edge of the bed.	Voltéese y siéntese sobre el borde de la cama.
Stand up slowly. Put your weight only on your right/left foot.	Párese despacio. Ponga peso sólo en la pierna derecha/izquierda.
Take a step to the side.	Dé un paso al lado.
Turn to your left/right.	Doble a la izquierda/derecha.
Is this hot or cold?	¿Está frío o caliente esto?
Am I sticking you with the point or the head of the pin?	¿Le estoy pinchando con el punto o la cabeza del alfiler?

ENDOCRINE AND REPRODUCTIVE

Vocabulary

Genitals	Los genitales
Uterus	El útero, la matríz
Vagina	La vagina

History

Have you had any problems with your thyroid?	¿Ha tenido alguna vez problemas con el tiroides?
Have you noticed any significant weight gain or loss?	¿Ha notado pérdida o aumento de peso?

Women:

How old were you when your periods started?	¿Cuántos años tenía cuando tuvo la primera regla?
How many days between periods?	¿Cuántos dias entre las reglas?
When was your last menstrual period?	¿Cuándo fue su última regla?
Have you ever been pregnant?	¿Ha estado embarazada?
How many children do you have?	¿Cuántos hijos tiene?
When was your last Pap smear?	¿Cuándo fue su última prueba de Papanicolau?
Would you like information on birth control methods?	¿Quiere usted información sobre los métodos del control de la natalidad?
Do you have a vaginal discharge?	¿Tiene secreción vaginal?

From Seidel M, Ball J, Dains J et al: *Mosby's guide to physical examination,* ed 6, St. Louis, 2006, Saunders.

Community Resources for the Medical Assistant

PROFESSIONAL ORGANIZATIONS RELATED TO MEDICAL ASSISTING

AHDI (Association for Healthcare Documentation Integrity): www.ahdionline.org
4230 Kiernan Avenue
Suite 130
Modesto, CA 95356
(800) 982-2182

AHIMA (American Health Information Management Association): www.ahima.org
233 N. Michigan Avenue
21st Floor
Chicago, IL 60601-5800
(312) 233-1100

American Association of Medical Assistants: www.aama-ntl.org
20 North Wacker Drive
Suite 1575
Chicago, IL 60606-2963
(312) 899-1500

American Medical Technologists: www.amt1.com
10700 West Higgins Road
Suite 150
Rosemont, IL 60018
(847) 823-5169

American Society of Phlebotomy Technicians, Inc.: www.aspt.org
P.O. Box 1831
Hickory, NC 28603
(828) 294-0078

American Society of Podiatric Medical Assistants: www.aspma.org
2124 South Austin Boulevard
Cicero, IL 60804
(708) 863-6303

Joint Commission on Allied Health Personnel in Ophthalmology: www.jcahpo.org
2025 Woodlane Drive
St. Paul, MN 55125-2998
(651) 731-2944

ORGANIZATIONS THAT PROVIDE CPR CERTIFICATION

American Heart Association: www.americanheart.org
7372 Greenville Avenue
Dallas, TX 75231
See website to identify CPR training sites.

American Red Cross: www.redcross.org
2025 E Street NW
Washington, DC 20006
See website to locate local CPR training sites.

ACCREDITING AGENCIES

Accreditation Association for Ambulatory Health Care: www.aaahc.org
(Accredits ambulatory care organizations)
5250 Old Orchard Road
Suite 200
Skokie, IL 60077
(847) 853-6060

Accrediting Bureau of Health Education Schools: www.abhes.org
(Accredits various health education programs including medical assisting programs)
7777 Leesburg Pike
Suite 314
N. Falls Church, VA 22043
(703) 917-9503

Commission on Accreditation of Allied Health Education Programs: www.caahep.org
(Accredits health education programs including medical assisting programs)
1361 Park Street
Clearwater, FL 33756
(727) 210-2350

Joint Commission: www.jointcommission.org
(Accredits health care organizations and programs including physician offices)
One Renaissance Boulevard
Oakbrook Terrace, IL 60181
(630) 792-5000

AGENCIES OF THE UNITED STATES GOVERNMENT

Centers for Disease Control and Prevention: www.cdc.gov
1600 Clifton Road
Atlanta, GA 30333
(404) 498-1515

Centers for Medicare and Medicaid Services: www.cms.gov
7500 Security Boulevard
Baltimore, MD 21244
See website for telephone numbers for specific services and locations.

Drug Enforcement Administration: www.dea.gov
Mailstop: AES
2401 Jefferson Davis Highway
Alexandria, VA 22301
See website for telephone number of nearest DEA office.

Food and Drug Administration: www.fda.gov
5600 Fishers Lane
Rockville, MD 20857-0001
(888) 463-6332

National Institutes of Health: www.nih.gov
9000 Rockville Pike
Bethesda, MD 20892
(301) 496-4000
See website for specific institutes and services.

Occupational Safety and Health Administration: www.osha.gov
(U.S. Department of Labor)
200 Constitution Avenue NW
Washington, DC 20210
(800) 321-6742

U.S. Department of Health and Human Services: www.dhhs.gov
200 Independence Avenue SW
Washington, DC 20201
(877) 696-6775

See *On the Web* at the end of each chapter for websites related to individual diseases or conditions.

Glossary

Abandonment Failure to continue to provide medical care to a patient without proper notification.

ABA routing number A nine-digit number that identifies a bank printed at the beginning of the MICR line at the bottom of a check. It also appears in fractional form at the top right of the check under the check number.

Abortion The termination of a pregnancy before the fetus reached the age of viability (20 weeks).

Abrasion A wound in which the outer layers of the skin are damaged; a scrape.

Abscess A collection of pus in a cavity surrounded by inflamed tissue.

Absorbable suture Suture material that is gradually digested by tissue enzymes and absorbed by the body.

Absorption The passage of digestive end products from the gastrointestinal tract into the blood or lymph.

Accommodation Mechanism that allows the eye to focus at various distances, primarily achieved by changing the curvature of the lens.

Account aging The process of finding out how long specific account balances have been outstanding.

Accounting Systematic recording and reporting of financial transactions.

Accounts payable The outstanding bills of a business, such as a medical office.

Accounts receivable Total amount owed to a business for goods and services.

Accreditation Credit or recognition for maintaining certain standards by a regional or national organization.

Accrual basis of accounting Accounting method in which income is entered at the time of sale or provision of service.

Acronym A word formed from the first letters in a name.

Act A bill or measure that has become law. Often refers to legislation with several parts.

Acting out Translating unconscious emotions into inappropriate behavior.

Action potential A nerve impulse; a rapid change in membrane potential that involves depolarization and repolarization.

Active listening Paying close attention to a speaker without thinking of anything else.

Active record The medical record of a patient who has been seen within a time frame specified by the office (usually 2 to 3 years).

Active transport Membrane transport process that requires cellular energy.

Adenohypophysis Anterior portion of the pituitary gland.

Adjustment A change to a patient account that is neither a charge nor a payment.

Adnexal Adjacent.

Adolescent An individual 12 to 18 years old.

Adventitious sounds Abnormal breath sounds.

Adverse reaction An unintended and undesirable effect produced by a drug.

Aerobe A microorganism that needs oxygen to live and grow.

Afebrile Without fever—the body temperature is normal.

Agglutination The aggregation or uniting of separate particles into clumps or masses; the clumping of blood cells.

Allergen A substance that is capable of causing an allergic reaction.

Allergy An abnormal hypersensitivity of the body to substances that are ordinarily harmless.

ALU (arithmetic/logic unit) The part of the CPU that executes the program's instructions by performing mathematic computations and logical operations.

Alveoli Microscopic dilations of terminal bronchioles in the lungs, where diffusion of gasses occurs; air sacs in the lungs.

Ambulation Walking or moving from one place to another.

Ambulatory Able to walk, as opposed to being confined to bed or a wheelchair.

Ambulatory care Medical care that is provided on an outpatient basis. The patient is able to come to the facility providing care and return home after receiving services.

Amenorrhea The absence or cessation of the menstrual period. Amenorrhea occurs normally before puberty, during pregnancy, and after menopause.

Amphiarthrosis (*pl.* **amphiarthroses**) A slightly movable joint.

Amplitude Refers to amount, extent, size, abundance, or fullness.

Ampule A small sealed glass container that holds a single dose of medication.

Anaerobe A microorganism that grows best in the absence of oxygen.

Anaphylactic reaction A serious allergic reaction that requires immediate treatment.

Anatomic position Standard reference position for the body.

Anemia A condition in which there is a decrease in the number of erythrocytes or amount of hemoglobin in the blood.

Annotate To underline or highlight important words and phrases in correspondence.

Antagonist A muscle that has an action opposite to the prime mover.

Antecubital space The space located at the front of the elbow.

Antibody A substance capable of combining with an antigen, resulting in an antigen-antibody reaction.

Anticoagulant A substance that inhibits blood clotting.

Antigen A substance capable of stimulating the formation of antibodies.

Antipyretic An agent that reduces fever.

Antiseptic An agent that inhibits the growth of or kills microorganisms.

Antiserum (*pl.* **antisera**) A serum that contains antibodies.

Anxiety A vague unpleasant emotion of fear or dread often accompanied by restlessness or nervousness.

Aorta The major trunk of the arterial system of the body. The aorta arises from the upper surface of the left ventricle.

Apnea The temporary cessation of breathing.

Application software Software designed to accomplish a specific task (e.g., word processing); also called *application program* and *software program.*

Approximation The process of bringing two parts, such as tissue, together through the use of sutures or other means.

Arbitration A formal process where the parties to a dispute agree to submit to the decision of a neutral party.

Arrector pili Muscle associated with hair follicles.

Arrhythmia An irregular heart rhythm; also termed *dysrhythmia.*

Artifact Additional electrical activity picked up by the electrocardiograph that interferes with the normal appearance of the electrocardiogram cycles.

Asepsis Free from infection or pathogens; the actions practiced to make and maintain an area or object free from infection or pathogens.

Assets In accounting, a combination of property owned and money owed to a business.

Assignment of benefits Authorization given by the patient to allow the insurance company to make payments directly to the health care provider instead of to the patient.

Assumption of risk A defense to a lawsuit that establishes the plaintiff assumed the risk of whatever caused the injury.

Atherosclerosis Buildup of fibrous plaques of fatty deposits and cholesterol on the inner walls of the coronary arteries.

Atrioventricular valve Valve between an atrium and a ventricle in the heart.

Attending physician The physician responsible for the care of a hospitalized patient.

Atypical Deviation from the normal.

Audiometer An instrument used to measure hearing.

Auscultation The process of listening to the sounds produced within the body to detect signs of disease.

Autoclave An apparatus for the sterilization of materials, using steam under pressure.

Autoimmune disease A condition in which the body's immune system produces antibodies that attack the body's own cells. The cause is unknown.

Automated method (*for testing laboratory specimens*) A method of laboratory testing in which the series of steps in the test is performed by an automated analyzer.

Autonomy Ability to make independent decisions without constraint or coercion from others.

Axilla The armpit.

Bacilli (*sing.* **bacillus**) Bacteria that have a rod shape.

Back order A term used for items ordered that cannot be shipped immediately, usually because they are out of stock.

Backup A duplicate copy of a program or data kept for reference in case the original is damaged, lost, or destroyed.

Balance due Total amount owed.

Bandage A strip of woven material used to wrap or cover a part of the body.

Bankruptcy Legal process by which the debts of an individual or business are resolved if they cannot be paid.

Barcode clear zone The area on the lower right-hand corner of a card or letter, which is left clear for the postal barcode to be printed.

Bariatrics The branch of medicine that deals with the treatment and control of obesity, and diseases associated with obesity.

Baseline The flat horizontal line that separates the various waves of the electrocardiogram cycle.

Beneficence Acting in the best possible way; performing good deeds.

Benefit The amount of money paid for a covered service under a health insurance plan.

Bilirubin An orange-colored bile pigment produced by the breakdown of heme from the hemoglobin molecule.

Bilirubinuria The presence of bilirubin in the urine.

Bill A law proposed by a legislative body.

Biopsy The surgical removal and examination of tissue from the living body. Biopsies are generally performed to determine whether a tumor is benign or malignant.

Birthday rule If both parents of a child have a family health plan, the insurance plan of the parent whose birthday comes earlier in the year is defined as the primary insurance plan covering the child. The insurance of the other parent becomes secondary insurance.

Bladder catheterization The passing of a sterile catheter through the urethra and into the bladder to remove urine.

Blocked Times in the appointment matrix when physicians are not available to see patients.

Blood antibody A protein in blood plasma that is capable of combining with its corresponding blood antigen to produce an antigen-antibody reaction.

Blood antigen A protein present on the surface of red blood cells that determines a person's blood type.

Body language Communication that is expressed through facial expressions, body position, muscle activity, and other nonverbal means.

Bookkeeping The process of recording financial transactions and keeping financial records.

Bounding pulse A pulse with an increased volume that feels very strong and full.

Brace An orthopedic device used to support and hold a part of the body in the correct position to allow functioning and healing.

Bradycardia An abnormally slow heart rate (less than 60 beats per minute).

Bradypnea An abnormal decrease in the respiratory rate of less than 10 respirations per minute.

Brain stem The portion of the brain, between the diencephalon and spinal cord, that contains the midbrain, pons, and medulla oblongata.

Braxton Hicks contractions Intermittent and irregular painless uterine contractions that occur throughout pregnancy. They occur more frequently toward the end of pregnancy and are sometimes mistaken for true labor pains.

Bronchial tree The bronchi and all their branches that function as passageways between the trachea and the alveoli.

Buffy coat A thin, light-colored layer of white blood cells and platelets that lies between a top layer of plasma and a bottom layer of red blood cells when an anticoagulant has been added to a blood specimen.

Burn An injury to the tissues caused by exposure to thermal, chemical, electrical, or radioactive agents.

Burnout Disillusionment with work and physical or emotional exhaustion.

Byte A unit of computer storage capacity. One byte is approximately equal to one character.

Call in times Blocks of time when a physician accepts telephone calls from patients.

Canthus The junction of the eyelids at either corner of the eye.

Capillary action The action that causes liquid to rise along a wick, tube, or gauze dressing.

Capitation A set payment provided by managed care insurance per patient per month regardless of the amount of service the patient receives.

Cardiac arrest A condition in which the heart has stopped beating or beats too irregularly to circulate blood effectively through the body.

Cardiac cycle A complete heartbeat consisting of contraction and relaxation of both atria and both ventricles.

Carrier An insurance company.

Case law Law established by decisions of previous court cases.

Cash basis of accounting Accounting method in which income is entered when payment is received.

Cashier's check A check drawn on a bank instead of an individual account.

Celsius scale A temperature scale on which the freezing point of water is 0° and the boiling point of water is 100°; also called the *centigrade scale*.

Cerebellum Second largest part of the human brain, located posterior to the pons and medulla oblongata, and involved in the coordination of muscular movements.

Cerebrum The largest and uppermost part of the human brain; concerned with consciousness, learning, memory, sensations, and voluntary movements.

Certificate of need A regulatory mechanism to ensure that new or expanded health care services will meet the needs of the community.

Certified check A check on an individual account that a bank assumes responsibility for, usually by withdrawing funds to cover the check from the checking account at the time the check is certified.

Cerumen Ear wax.

Ceruminous gland A gland in the ear canal that produces cerumen or ear wax.

Cervix The lower narrow end of the uterus that opens into the vagina.

CHAMPVA A government health insurance program that covers dependents of military veterans with service-connected disabilities.

Charge slip A form used to keep track of charges and payments at the time of a patient visit.

Charting The process of making written entries about a patient in the medical record.

Chemoreceptor A sensory receptor that detects the presence of chemicals; responsible for taste, smell, and monitoring the concentration of certain chemicals in body fluids.

Chemotherapy The use of chemicals to treat disease. *Chemotherapy* is most often used to refer to the treatment of cancer using antineoplastic medications.

Chondrocyte Cartilage cell.

Chronic Existing over a long period of time.

Chyme The semifluid mixture of food and gastric juice that leaves the stomach through the pyloric sphincter.

Cilia Slender, hairlike projections that constantly beat toward the outside to remove microorganisms from the body.

Civil law Law that regulates relationships and interactions between individuals and groups.

Claim message Messages encouraging payment of a bill, usually attached to or printed on the monthly statement.

Clinical diagnosis A tentative diagnosis of a patient's condition obtained through the evaluation of the health history and the physical examination, without the benefit of laboratory or diagnostic tests.

Cloning Producing genetically identical cells or individuals artificially.

Closed questions Questions that anticipate a yes/no or short answer.

Clustering Scheduling similar types of patients or examinations on the same day or part of the day.

Coagulation The process of blood clotting.

Cocci (*sing.* **coccus**) Bacteria that have a round shape.

Coinsurance A percentage of the allowed charge for health services, which the patient is responsible to pay.

Collagenous fibers Strong and flexible connective tissue fibers that contain the protein collagen.

Collate To assemble the pages of a document in numerical order.

Collection agency A firm that is in the business of collecting overdue accounts.

Colonoscopy The visualization of the entire colon using a colonoscope.

Colposcope A lighted instrument with a binocular magnifying lens used to examine the vagina and cervix.

Colposcopy Examination of the cervix using a colposcope (a lighted instrument with a magnifying lens).

Common law Unwritten body of law based on general custom.

Comparative negligence A defense to a lawsuit that establishes a percentage of responsibility for injury by the plaintiff.

Compress A soft, moist, absorbent cloth that is folded in several layers and applied to a part of the body in the local application of heat or cold.

Computer An electronic machine that has the ability to process data according to a program in order to produce a desired result.

Computer system All of the hardware and software components making up the computer.

Conduction The transfer of energy, such as heat, from one object to another by direct contact.

Conduction myofibers Cardiac muscle cells specialized for conducting action potentials to the myocardium; part of the conduction system of the heart; also called *Purkinje fibers.*

Consultation report A narrative report of an opinion about a patient's condition by a practitioner other than the attending physician.

Contagious Capable of being transmitted directly or indirectly from one person to another.

Contaminate To soil or to make impure. An aseptic object is contaminated when it touches something that is not clean.

Contingency A condition that must be met before a contract is binding.

Continuing education unit (CEU) A standard unit of measure on continuing education for professionals defined as 10 contact hours of participation.

Contrast medium A substance that is used to make a particular structure visible on a radiograph.

Contributory negligence A defense to a lawsuit that establishes any responsibility for injury by the plaintiff.

Controlled substance A drug that has the potential for addiction or abuse.

Control unit The part of the CPU that directs and coordinates the processing functions of the computer.

Contusion An injury to the tissues under the skin that causes blood vessels to rupture, allowing blood to seep into the tissues; a bruise.

Convection The transfer of energy, such as heat, through air currents.

Conversion Changing from one system of measurement to another.

Coordination of benefits Rules followed by insurance companies so that no claim is reimbursed at more than 100% of the charges.

Copayment A fixed amount of money that the patient is responsible to pay at each visit.

Cover letter A letter sent with one or more documents (such as a resumé) to provide an explanation.

CPU (central processing unit) The "brain" of the computer housed in the main unit that interprets and executes the instructions that operate the computer. The CPU consists of the control unit and the ALU.

Crash cart A specially equipped cart for holding and transporting medications, equipment, and supplies needed for performing lifesaving procedures in an emergency.

Credit A posting that is subtracted from an account balance.

Credit balance A patient account that is a negative balance (i.e., money is owed by the medical office), usually due to an overpayment.

Crepitus A grating sensation caused by fractured bone fragments rubbing against each other.

Crime An offense in violation of a law that prohibits or requires certain behavior.

Criminal law Law that regulates offenses against the public welfare.

Crisis (pertaining to fever) A sudden falling of an elevated body temperature to normal.

Critical item An item that comes in contact with sterile tissue or the vascular system.

Cross-index To file under one unit and use a guide or card filed under another unit that refers to the primary filing location.

Crossover claim An insurance claim for an individual who is covered by Medicare and Medicaid. After review by the Medicare fiscal intermediary, the claim is automatically sent to Medicaid.

Cryosurgery The therapeutic use of freezing temperatures to destroy abnormal tissue.

Cubic centimeter (cc) The amount of space occupied by 1 milliliter (1 ml = cc).

Culture The propagation of a mass of microorganisms in a laboratory culture medium.

Culture medium A mixture of nutrients in which microorganisms are grown in the laboratory.

Cyanosis A bluish discoloration of the skin and mucous membranes.

Cytokinesis Division of the cytoplasm at the end of mitosis to form two separate daughter cells.

Cytology The science that deals with the study of cells, including their origin, structure, function, and pathology.

Data Raw, unorganized facts about subject matter presented to the computer for processing.

Data processing The changing of raw facts or data into usable information following a three-part sequence: input, processing, output.

Day sheet The record of daily transactions in the pegboard or "write it once system" and also in computer medical billing programs.

DEA number A registration number assigned to physicians by the Drug Enforcement Administration for prescribing or dispensing controlled drugs.

Debit A posting that is added to an account balance.

Decontamination The use of physical or chemical means to remove, inactivate, or destroy pathogens on a surface or item to the point where they are no longer capable of transmitting infectious particles; the surface or item is rendered safe for handling, use, or disposal.

Deductible An amount of money that an insured person must pay annually before health services are covered by the insurance plan.

Defendant The person or group against whom an action is brought in a court of law.

Denial Failure to acknowledge the reality of a situation.

Depreciation Accounting methods to respond to the loss of value of a property or piece of equipment over time.

Dermis Inner layer of the skin that contains the blood vessels, nerves, glands, and hair follicles; also called *stratum corium.*

Detergent An agent that cleanses by emulsifying dirt and oil.

Diagnosis The scientific method of determining and identifying a patient's condition.

Diagnosis-related group (DRG) A system to determine Medicare reimbursement for a hospital stay based on the patient's diagnosis.

Diagnostic procedure A procedure performed to assist in the diagnosis, management, and treatment of a patient's condition.

Diapedesis The process by which white blood cells squeeze between the cells in a vessel wall to enter the tissue spaces outside the blood vessel.

Diaphysis The long straight shaft of a long bone.

Diarthrosis (*pl.* diarthroses) Freely movable joint characterized by a joint cavity; also called a *synovial joint.*

Diastole Relaxation phase of the cardiac cycle; opposite of systole.

Diastolic pressure The point of lesser pressure on the arterial wall, which is recorded during diastole.

Diencephalon Part of the brain between the cerebral hemispheres and the midbrain; includes the thalamus, hypothalamus, and epithalamus.

Differential diagnosis A determination of which of two or more diseases with similar symptoms is producing a patient's symptoms.

Diffusion Movement of substances from a region of high concentration to a region of low concentration.

Digital image A picture stored in the compute in the form of pixels.

Dilation (of the cervix) The stretching of the external os from an opening a few millimeters wide to an opening large enough to allow the passage of an infant (approximately 10 cm).

Disbursements Money paid out.

Discharge summary report A brief summary of the significant events of a patient's hospitalization.

Disinfectant An agent used to destroy pathogenic microorganisms but not their spores. Disinfectants are usually applied to inanimate objects.

Dislocation An injury in which one end of a bone making up a joint is separated or displaced from its normal anatomic position.

Documentation A written set of instructions accompanying an application program, designed to assist the user in understanding how to operate the program. Examples include the user manual, help screens, and reference cards.

Do not resuscitate (DNR) A medical order signed by a physician that relieves health care personnel from the obligation to resuscitate a patient who stops breathing or whose heart stops.

Dose The quantity of a drug to be administered at one time.

Double booking Scheduling two patients for the same appointment time.

Drug A chemical used for the treatment, prevention, or diagnosis of disease.

Drug Enforcement Administration (DEA) The federal agency that enforces the Controlled Substances Act of 1970.

DSL (digital subscriber line) Technology that allows digital signals to be transmitted over telephone lines at high speed even if the telephone line is also being used for voice transmission.

Duplex To produce double-sided copies by storing images from both sides of the original in the memory of a photocopier.

Duty Commitment to act in a certain way.

Dysmenorrhea Pain associated with the menstrual period.

Dyspareunia Pain in the vagina or pelvis experienced by a woman during sexual intercourse.

Dysplasia The growth of abnormal cells. Dysplasia is a precancerous condition that may or may not develop into cancer.

Dyspnea Shortness of breath or difficulty in breathing.

Dysrhythmia An irregular rhythm; also termed *arrhythmia.*

ECG cycle The graphic representation of a heartbeat.

Echocardiogram An ultrasound examination of the heart.

Ectocervix The part of the cervix that projects into the vagina and is lined with stratified squamous epithelium.

EDD Expected date of delivery, or due date.

Edema The retention of fluid in the tissues, resulting in swelling.

Effacement The thinning and shortening of the cervical canal from its normal length of 1 to 2 cm to a structure with paper-thin edges in which there is no canal at all. Effacement occurs late in pregnancy, during labor, or both. The purpose of effacement along with dilation is to permit the passage of the infant into the birth canal.

Ego defense mechanism Unconscious mental process that offers psychological protection.

Elastic fibers Yellow connective tissue fibers that are not particularly strong, but can be stretched and will return to their normal shape when released.

Electrocardiogram (ECG) The graphic representation of the electrical activity of the heart.

Electrocardiograph The instrument used to record the electrical activity of the heart.

Electrode A conductor of electricity that is used to promote contact between the body and the electrocardiograph.

Electrolyte A chemical substance that promotes conduction of an electrical current.

Electronic health record (EHR) An individual patient's health record in digital format. Also called an *electronic medical record.*

Electronic medical record (EMR) A medical record that is stored on a computer. Also called an *electronic health record.*

E-mail The exchange of information from one computer to another using telecommunication.

Emancipated minor A person younger than the age of 18 with the rights of an adult, including the ability to consent to medical care.

Embezzlement Fraudulent appropriation of funds or property of an employer or client.

Embryo The child in utero from the time of conception to the beginning of the first trimester.

Emergency medical services (EMS) system A network of community resources, equipment, and personnel that provides care to victims of injury or sudden illness.

Empathy Objective awareness and sensitivity to the feelings and emotions of others.

Empirically Learned from observation or experiment.

Endocervix The mucous membrane lining the cervical canal.

Endocrine gland Gland that secretes its product directly into the blood; opposite of exocrine gland.

Endoscope An instrument that consists of a tube and an optical system that is used for direct visual inspection of organs or cavities.

Enema An injection of fluid into the rectum to aid in the elimination of feces from the colon.

Engagement The entrance of the fetal head or the presenting part into the pelvic inlet.

Enteral nutrition The delivery of nutrients through a tube inserted into the gastrointestinal tract.

Enunciation The act of speaking clearly and concisely.

Epidermis Outermost layer of the skin.

Epiphyseal plate The cartilaginous plate between the epiphysis and diaphysis of a bone; responsible for the lengthwise growth of a long bone.

Epiphysis The end of a long bone.

Erythema Reddening of the skin caused by dilation of superficial blood vessels in the skin.

Erythrocyte Red blood cell.

Erythropoiesis The process of red blood cell formation.

Erythropoietin A hormone released by the kidneys that stimulates red blood cell production.

Established patient A patient who has been receiving services from the same medical practice on a regular basis.

Etiquette Rules of socially acceptable behavior; manners.

Eupnea Normal respiration. The rate is 16 to 20 respirations per minute, the rhythm is even and regular, and the depth is normal.

Evacuated tube A closed glass or plastic tube that contains a premeasured vacuum.

Exhalation The act of breathing out.

Exocrine gland Gland that secretes its product to a surface or cavity through ducts; opposite of endocrine gland.

Expected date of delivery (EDD) Projected birth date of the infant.

Explanation of benefits (EOB) A statement issued by the insurance company explaining reimbursement for specific procedures.

External os The opening of the cervical canal of the uterus into the vagina.

External respiration Exchange of gases between the lungs and the blood.

Externship A work experience that is required in an educational program and usually unpaid.

Exudate A discharge produced by the body's tissues.

Fahrenheit scale A temperature scale on which the freezing point of water is 32° and the boiling point of water is 212°.

False negative A test result denoting that a condition is absent when it is actually present.

False positive A test result denoting that a condition is present when it is actually absent.

Familial Occurring or affecting members of a family more frequently than would be expected by chance.

Fasting Abstaining from food or fluids (except water) for a specified amount of time before the collection of a specimen.

Fax Transmission of scanned, printed material using telephone lines.

Febrile Pertaining to fever.

Fee-for-service A means of payment for health care in which each service provided is reimbursed in full or in part.

Fee-for-service insurance Insurance reimbursement that is directly related to the services provided and the amount charged by the provider.

Fee schedule List of charges (fees) for specific procedures that may be performed in a medical office.

Fee splitting The practice of sharing fees with colleagues, especially for making referrals.

Felony A serious crime punishable by death or imprisonment.

Fetal heart rate The number of times per minute the fetal heart beats.

Fetal heart tones The sounds of the heartbeat of the fetus heard through the mother's abdominal wall.

Fetus The child in utero from the third month after conception to birth; during the first 2 months of development, it is called an *embryo*.

Fever A body temperature that is above normal; synonym for *pyrexia*.

Fibroblast An immature cell from which connective tissue can develop.

Fidelity Faithfulness.

Filing system The way in which records are arranged. Common filing systems in the medical office include alphabetic, numeric, subject, or chronological.

Firewall A system that protects a computer network from unauthorized access by users on its own network or another network such as the Internet.

First aid The immediate care that is administered to an individual who is injured or suddenly becomes ill before complete medical care can be obtained.

Fiscal intermediary An insurance company that contracts to review Medicare claims for the Centers for Medicare and Medicaid Services.

Fixed appointment scheduling An appointment scheduling method in which each patient is given a different, specific appointment time. Also called *stream scheduling*, *time-specified scheduling*, or *single booking*.

Floppy disk A portable storage device consisting of flexible Mylar plastic disk coated with a magnetically sensitive material. The disk is encased in a square plastic jacket that protects it from damage.

Fluoroscope An instrument used to view internal organs and structures directly.

Fluoroscopy Examination of a patient with a fluoroscope.

Forceps A two-pronged instrument for grasping and squeezing.

Formulary A list of prescription drugs covered or preferred by a managed care insurance company.

Fracture Any break in a bone.

Fraud Intentional deception resulting in injury or loss.

Frenulum linguae The midline fold that connects the undersurface of the tongue with the floor of the mouth.

Full block style A letter format where all parts of the letter are left justified.

Fundus The dome-shaped upper portion of the uterus between the fallopian tubes.

Furuncle A localized staphylococcal infection that originates deep within a hair follicle. Also known as a *boil*.

Gametes Sex cells: sperm and ova.

Gauge The diameter of the lumen of a needle used to administer medication.

Gene therapy Giving patients new genes or parts of genes to treat a disease or condition.

Genetic engineering Making, altering, or repairing genetic material.

Gestation The period of intrauterine development from conception to birth; the period of pregnancy. The average pregnancy lasts about 280 days, or 40 weeks, from the date of conception to childbirth.

Gestational age The age of the fetus between conception and birth.

Gigabyte (GB) A unit of computer storage capacity. One gigabyte is equal to a little more than a billion bytes or 1000 megabytes.

Glomerular capsule Double-layered epithelial cup that surrounds the glomerulus in a nephron; also called *Bowman's capsule*.

Glycogen The form in which carbohydrate is stored in the body.

Glycosuria The presence of sugar in the urine.

Glycosylation The process of glucose attaching to hemoglobin.

Gonads Primary reproductive organs; organs that produce the gametes: testes in the male and ovaries in the female.

Grammar The study of accepted rules used to create meaning in a language.

Gross pay The total amount earned in a time period by an employee before any deductions.

Guarantor A person with financial responsibility for a bill who may or may not also be a patient.

Gynecology The branch of medicine that deals with diseases of the reproductive organs of women.

Hand hygiene The process of cleansing or sanitizing the hands.

Hard copy Printed output from a computer.

Hard disk A storage device consisting of one or more rigid, nonflexible platters coated with a magnetically sensitive material and encased in a permanently sealed, air-tight container.

Hardware The physical devices making up a computer system (e.g., main computer unit, keyboard, monitor, printer).

Hazardous chemical Any chemical that presents a threat to the health and safety of an individual coming into contact with it.

HDL cholesterol A lipoprotein, consisting of protein and cholesterol, that removes excess cholesterol from the cells.

Health care proxy A legal document that names an agent to make decisions about a person's medical care if he or she becomes unable to make his or her wishes known.

Health history report A collection of subjective data about a patient.

Health insurance Purchase of protection for covered services related to health care.

Hematology The study of blood and blood-forming tissues.

Hematoma A swelling or mass of coagulated blood caused by a break in a blood vessel.

Hematopoiesis Blood cell production, which occurs in the red bone marrow; also called *hemopoiesis.*

Hemoconcentration An increase in the concentration of the nonfilterable blood components in the blood, such as red blood cells, enzymes, iron, and calcium, as a result of a decrease in the fluid content of the blood.

Hemocytoblast A stem cell in the bone marrow from which the blood cells arise.

Hemoglobin The iron-containing pigment of erythrocytes that transports oxygen in the body.

Hemoglobin A_{1C} Compound formed when glucose attaches or glycosylates to the protein in hemoglobin.

Hemolysis The breakdown of erythrocytes with the release of hemoglobin into the plasma; the breakdown of blood cells.

Hemophilia An inherited bleeding disorder caused by a deficiency of a clotting factor needed for proper coagulation of the blood.

Hemostasis The arrest of bleeding by natural or artificial means.

Hierarchy Classified according to rank or importance.

Histology Branch of microscopic anatomy that studies tissues.

Holistic Considering the whole; in medicine considering the entire person when providing health care.

Home health care The provision of medical and nonmedical care in a patient's home or place of residence.

Homeostasis The state in which body systems are functioning normally and the internal environment of the body is in equilibrium; the body is in a healthy state.

Hormone A substance secreted by an endocrine gland.

Hospice Palliative service provided for patients whose life expectancy is less than 6 months. Services may be provided in the patient's home, nursing home, or special hospice facility.

Human anatomy Study of body shape and structure and the relationships of its parts.

Human physiology Study of the functions of living organisms and their parts.

Hyperglycemia An abnormally high level of glucose in the blood.

Hyperopia Farsightedness.

Hyperpnea An abnormal increase in the rate and depth of respiration.

Hyperpyrexia An extremely high fever.

Hypertension High blood pressure.

Hyperventilation An abnormally fast and deep type of breathing usually associated with acute anxiety conditions.

Hypoglycemia An abnormally low level of glucose in the blood.

Hypopnea An abnormal decrease in the rate and depth of respiration.

Hypotension Low blood pressure.

Hypothermia A body temperature that is below normal.

Hypoxemia A decrease in the oxygen saturation of the blood. Hypoxemia may lead to hypoxia.

Hypoxia A reduction in the oxygen supply to the tissues of the body.

Immune globulin A blood product consisting of pooled human plasma containing antibodies.

Immunity The resistance of the body to the effects of a harmful agent, such as a pathogenic microorganism and its toxins.

Immunization (active, artificial) The process of becoming immune or of rendering an individual immune through the use of a vaccine or toxoid.

Impacted Wedged firmly together so as to be immovable.

Inactive record The medical record of a patient who has not been seen within the past 2 to 3 years, or some other time frame specified by a given medical office.

Incision A clean cut caused by a cutting instrument.

Incubate To provide proper conditions for growth and development.

Incubation period The interval of time between the invasion by a pathogenic microorganism and the appearance of first symptoms of the disease.

Indemnity An obligation to provide compensation for loss or damage.

Indexing units Pieces of information used to identify a correct filing location.

Induration An area of hardened tissue.

Infant A child from birth to 12 months of age.

Infection The condition in which the body, or part of it, is invaded by a pathogen.

Infectious disease A disease caused by a pathogen that produces harmful effects on its host.

Infiltration The process by which a substance passes into and is deposited within the substance of a cell, tissue, or organ.

Inflammation A protective response of the body to trauma and the entrance of foreign matter. The purpose of inflammation is to destroy invading microorganisms and to repair injured tissue.

Information Data that have been processed into a usable form by the computer.

Informed consent 1. Agreement to a medical procedure based on understanding of the procedure and its possible consequences and effects. 2. Consent given by a patient for a medical procedure after being informed of the nature of his or her condition, the purpose of the procedure, an explanation of the risks involved with the procedure, alternative treatments or procedures available, the likely outcome of the procedure, and the risks involved with declining or delaying the procedure.

Infusion The administration of fluids, medications, or nutrients into a vein.

Inhalation The act of breathing in.

Inhalation administration The administration of medication by way of air or other vapor being drawn into the lungs.

Initiative The ability to begin or carry through on a plan of action independently.

Inoculate To introduce microorganisms into a culture medium for growth and multiplication.

Inpatient A patient who has been admitted to a hospital for at least one overnight stay.

Input 1. (noun) Data that have been entered into the computer. 2. (verb) The transfer of data to the computer for processing.

Input device A device for entering data into the computer (e.g., keyboard, mouse, scanner).

Inscription The part of a prescription that indicates the name of the drug and the drug dosage.

Insertion The end of a muscle that is attached to a relatively movable part; the end opposite the origin.

Inspection The process of observing a patient to detect signs of disease.

Instillation The dropping of a liquid into a body cavity.

Insufflate To blow a powder, vapor, or gas (e.g., air) into a body cavity.

Intercostal Between the ribs.

Internal os The internal opening of the cervical canal into the uterus.

Internal respiration Exchange of gases between the blood and tissue cells.

Interval The length of a wave or the length of a wave with a segment.

Intradermal injection Introduction of medication into the dermal layer of the skin.

Intramuscular (IM) injection Introduction of medication into the muscular layer of the body.

Intravenous (IV) therapy The administration of a liquid agent directly into a patient's vein, where it is distributed throughout the body via the circulatory system.

Inventory A detailed list of items in stock or in possession of an individual or business.

In vitro Occurring in glass. Refers to tests performed under artificial conditions, as in the laboratory.

In vivo Occurring in the living body or organism.

Invoice An itemized bill for items that have not been prepaid.

Irrigation The washing of a body canal with a flowing solution.

Ischemia Deficiency of blood in a body part.

Judgmental Making judgments about what is good or bad based on personal opinion.

Juxtaglomerular apparatus Complex of modified cells in the afferent arteriole and the ascending limb/distal tubule in the kidney; helps regulate blood pressure by secreting renin; consists of the macula densa and juxtaglomerular cells.

Keratinization Process by which the cells of the epidermis become filled with keratin and move to the surface where they are sloughed off.

Ketonuria The presence of ketone bodies in the urine.

Ketosis An accumulation of large amounts of ketone bodies in the tissues and body fluids.

Kilobyte (KB) A unit of computer storage capacity. One kilobyte is equal to 1024 bytes (characters).

Korotkoff sounds Sounds heard during the measurement of blood pressure that are used to determine the systolic and diastolic blood pressure readings.

Laboratory test The clinical analysis and study of materials, fluids, or tissues obtained from patients to assist in diagnosing and treating disease.

Laceration A wound in which the tissues are torn apart, leaving ragged and irregular edges.

Larceny Stealing another person's property or money without violence.

LDL cholesterol A lipoprotein, consisting of protein and cholesterol, that picks up cholesterol and delivers it to the cells.

Ledger A book, card, or computer account used to record financial transactions.

Left justified Lines of type that begin at the left margin of a document.

Length (recumbent) The measurement from the vertex of the head to the heel of the foot in a supine position.

Letterhead A sheet of stationery preprinted with information about a business, including name, address, telephone number, and other information.

Leukocyte White blood cell.

Leukocytosis An abnormal increase in the number of white blood cells (greater than 11,000 per cubic millimeter of blood).

Leukopenia An abnormal decrease in the number of white blood cells (less than 4500 per cubic millimeter of blood).

Liability Legal responsibility. In accounting, liabilities are the amount owed by a business to creditors.

License Official permission to perform an activity or practice a profession.

Licensure The process by which the state examines qualifications and gives permission to an individual or organization to engage in a profession or business.

Ligate To tie off and close a structure, such as a severed blood vessel.

Lipoprotein A complex molecule consisting of protein and a lipid fraction, such as cholesterol. Lipoproteins transport lipids in the blood.

Litigation The process of taking a lawsuit through the courts.

Living will A legal document that specifies the kind of medical treatment a patient wants or does not want if he or she becomes incapacitated.

Load The articles that are being sterilized.

Local anesthetic A drug that produces a loss of feeling and an inability to perceive pain in only a specific part of the body.

Lochia A discharge from the uterus after delivery that consists of blood, tissue, white blood cells, and some bacteria.

Maceration The softening and breaking down of the skin as a result of prolonged exposure to moisture.

Macrophage Large phagocytic connective tissue cell that functions in immune responses.

Mainboard The primary circuit board of the main computer unit, which allows all of the computer components to communicate with each other.

Main computer memory The part of the CPU that is responsible for temporarily storing information until it is needed for processing by the computer. Main memory in a microcomputer is known as *RAM.*

Malaise A vague sense of body discomfort, weakness, and fatigue that often marks the onset of a disease and continues through the course of the illness.

Malfeasance A crime or wrongdoing that is illegal or contrary to official obligation.

Malpractice Negligence by a professional.

Managed care A system that manages the delivery of health care with the intention of controlling costs.

Manometer An instrument for measuring pressure.

Manual method A method of laboratory testing in which the series of steps in the test method is performed by hand.

Mast cell A connective tissue cell that produces heparin and histamine.

Material safety data sheet (MSDS) A sheet that provides information regarding a chemical, its hazards, and measures to take to prevent injury and illness when handling the chemical.

Matrix A rectangular or linear arrangement of numbers or information.

Mayo tray A broad, flat metal tray placed on a stand and used to hold sterile instruments and supplies when it has been covered with a sterile towel.

Mechanoreceptor A sensory receptor that responds to a bending or deformation of the cell; examples include receptors for touch, pressure, hearing, and equilibrium.

Mediation Negotiation by a third party to help two parties resolve a dispute.

Medicaid A federal and state insurance program for low-income patients. The Medicaid program has a different name in each state.

Medical asepsis Practices that are employed to reduce the number and hinder the transmission of pathogens.

Medical impressions Conclusions drawn by the physician from an interpretation of data. Other terms for impressions include *provisional diagnosis* and *tentative diagnosis.*

Medical practice management program A program that provides instructions to the computer for performing medical practice management procedures.

Medical record A written record of the important information regarding a patient, including the care of the individual and the progress of the patient's condition.

Medical record format The way a medical record is organized. The two main types of medical record format are the source-oriented record and the problem-oriented record.

Medical records management Activities related to the creation, management, use, and disposition of patient medical records.

Medicare The federal health insurance program that provides insurance coverage for the elderly, permanently disabled, and individuals with end-stage kidney disease.

Megabyte (MB) A unit of computer storage capacity. One megabyte is equal to a little more than 1 million bytes or 1000 kilobytes.

Meiosis Type of nuclear division in which the number of chromosomes is reduced to one half the number found in a body cell; results in the formation of an egg or sperm.

Melanin A dark brown or black pigment found in parts of the body, especially skin and hair.

Melena The darkening of the stool caused by the presence of blood in an amount of 50 ml or greater.

Memo (memorandum) A form of communication within a company that is usually short and limited to one subject.

Meniscus The curved surface on a column of liquid in a tube.

Menopause The permanent cessation of menstruation, which usually occurs between the ages of 45 and 55.

Menorrhagia Excessive bleeding during a menstrual period, in the number of days or the amount of blood or both. Also called *dysfunctional uterine bleeding* (DUB).

Mensuration The process of measuring the patient.

Mesentery Extensions of peritoneum that are associated with the intestine.

Metabolism The total of all biochemical reactions that take place in the body; includes anabolism and catabolism.

Metered mail Mail for which the postage has been applied using a postage meter.

Metrorrhagia Bleeding between menstrual periods.

MICR line A line of numbers containing the ABA transit routing number and the account number that appears at the bottom left of a check. These numbers are read by a magnetic ink character recognition (MICR) system.

Microbiology The scientific study of microorganisms and their activities.

Microcomputer A small general purpose computer that relies on a tiny microprocessor chip to perform its processing functions.

Microorganism A microscopic plant or animal.

Micturition The act of voiding urine.

Minutes A written record of the proceedings of a meeting.

Misdemeanor A less serious crime, punishable by a fine or imprisonment for less than 1 year.

Misfeasance Performing a legal act in an improper way.

Mitosis Process by which the nucleus of a body cell divides to form two new cells, each identical to the parent cell.

Modified block style A format for business letters where the date line, complimentary close, and printed signature line are on a tab at the center or right justified and all other parts of the letter are left justified.

Modified wave scheduling An appointment system that has some fixed appointments and some appointment times during which patients are seen in order of arrival.

Modifier An addition to a Current Procedural Terminology code that indicates unusual circumstances related to the procedure, such as a more extensive procedure or two procedures performed in the same session.

Morphology The study of structure and form.

Motor unit A single neuron and all the muscle fibers it stimulates.

Mucous membrane A membrane lining body passages or cavities that open to the outside.

Multigravida A woman who has been pregnant more than once.

Multipara A woman who has completed two or more pregnancies to the age of fetal viability regardless of whether they ended in live infants or stillbirths.

Myelin White, fatty substance that surrounds many nerve fibers.

Myopia Nearsightedness.

NEC A diagnosis code that is not elsewhere classified.

Needle biopsy A type of biopsy in which tissue from deep within the body is obtained by the insertion of a biopsy needle through the skin.

Negative feedback A mechanism of response in which a stimulus initiates reactions that reduce the stimulus.

Negligence Failure to act (or refrain from acting) as a reasonably prudent person in similar circumstances.

Neoplasm Abnormal growth or tumor.

Nephron The functional unit of the kidney, consisting of a renal corpuscle and a renal tubule.

Net pay The actual amount of money paid directly to an employee after taxes and other deductions have been taken out.

Networking Contacting acquaintances and their contacts who may know of potential jobs.

Neurilemma The layer of Schwann cells that surrounds a nerve fiber in the peripheral nervous system and, in some cases, produces myelin; also called *Schwann's sheath*.

Neuroglia Supporting cells of nervous tissue; cells in nervous tissue that do not conduct impulses.

Neurohypophysis Posterior portion of the pituitary gland.

Neuromuscular junction The area of communication between the axon terminal of a motor neuron and the sarcolemma of a muscle fiber; also called a *myoneural junction.*

Neuron Nerve cell, including its processes; conducting cell of nervous tissue.

Neurotransmitter A chemical substance that is released at the axon terminals to stimulate a muscle fiber contraction or an impulse in another neuron.

New patient For billing purposes, a patient who has not received services during the previous 3 years from a physician in a medical practice.

Nociceptor A sensory receptor that responds to tissue damage; pain receptor.

Nonabsorbable suture Suture material that is not absorbed by the body and either remains permanently in the body tissue and becomes encapsulated by fibrous tissue or is removed.

Noncompliant Failing to adhere to recommendations or a treatment regimen.

Noncritical item An item that comes into contact with intact skin but not mucous membranes.

Nonfeasance Failing to perform an act that should have been performed, resulting in injury.

Nonintact skin Skin that has a break in the surface. It includes, but is not limited to, abrasions, cuts, hangnails, paper cuts, and burns.

Nonmalfeasance Ethical concept requiring that an action do no harm, or do less harm than good.

Nonpathogen A microorganism that does not normally produce disease.

Nonverbal Communication that occurs without words such as through body posture or facial expression.

Normal flora Harmless, nonpathogenic microorganisms that normally reside in many parts of the body but do not cause disease.

Normal range *(for laboratory tests)* A certain established and acceptable parameter or reference range within which the laboratory test results of a healthy individual are expected to fall.

Normal sinus rhythm Refers to an electrocardiogram that is within normal limits.

NOS A diagnosis code that is not otherwise specified.

No-show A patient who does not keep a scheduled appointment.

Nullipara A woman who has not carried a pregnancy to the point of fetal viability (20 weeks of gestation).

Objective symptom A symptom that can be observed by an examiner.

Obstetrics The branch of medicine concerned with the care of a woman during pregnancy, childbirth, and the postpartal period.

Occult blood Blood in such a small amount that it is not detectable by the unaided eye.

Oliguria Decreased or scanty output of urine.

Oogenesis Process of meiosis in the female in which one ovum and three polar bodies are produced from one primary oocyte.

Open questions Questions that could have a variety of answers and encourage a personal response.

Operating system A type of system software that performs tasks required by the computer to operate itself.

Ophthalmoscope An instrument for examining the interior of the eye.

Opportunistic infection An infection that results from a defective immune system that cannot defend the body from pathogens normally found in the environment.

Optical disc A storage device consisting of a flat, round portable disk that stores data using laser technology.

Optical drive A device installed in a drive bay on the main computer unit that uses a laser to read an optical disc or write onto (burn) an optical disc.

Optimum growth temperature The temperature at which an organism grows best.

Oral Spoken; pertaining to the mouth.

Oral administration Administration of medication by mouth.

Origin The end of a muscle that is attached to a relatively immovable part; the end opposite the insertion.

Orthopedist A physician who specializes in the diagnosis and treatment of disorders of the musculoskeletal system, which includes the bones, joints, ligaments, tendons, muscles, and nerves.

Orthopnea The condition in which breathing is easier when an individual is in a sitting or standing position.

Osmosis Diffusion of water through a selectively permeable membrane.

Osteoblast Bone-forming cell.

Osteochondritis Inflammation of bone and cartilage.

Osteoclast Cell that destroys or resorbs bone tissue.

Osteocyte Mature bone cell.

Osteomyelitis Inflammation of the bone as a result of bacterial infection.

Osteon Structural unit of bone; haversian system.

Otoscope An instrument for examining the external ear canal and tympanic membrane.

Out guide A cardboard or plastic card to insert in a file when a medical record is removed.

Output 1. (noun) Information that has been generated by the computer. 2. (verb) The transfer of processed data back to the user.

Output device A device that transfers processed data to the user (e.g., computer monitor, printer).

Ovarian cycle Monthly cycle of events that occur in the ovary from puberty to menopause; occurs concurrently with the uterine cycle.

Ovarian follicle An oocyte surrounded by one or more layers of cells within the ovaries.

Overdraft A check (or draft) that exceeds the amount of funds in a bank account.

Oxyhemoglobin Hemoglobin that has combined with oxygen.

Pager An electronic device that notifies the recipient to receive a message or return a telephone call.

Palliative treatment Therapy that reduces the effects of disease or condition but does not remove the disease itself.

Palpation The process of feeling with the hands to detect signs of disease.

Panel A group of diagnostic tests done in one machine at the same time.

Paper-based patient record (PPR) A medical record in paper form.

Paraphrasing A restatement of the words of another, often to clarify meaning.

Parenteral Taken into the body through the piercing of the skin barrier or mucous membranes, such as through needlesticks, human bites, cuts, and abrasions. Administration of medication by injection.

Passive transport Membrane transport process that does not require cellular energy.

Pathogen A disease-producing microorganism.

Patient An individual receiving medical care.

Payee The person to whom a check is made out.

PDA (personal digital assistant) A portable handheld computing device with access to various reference tools, such as a drug reference, calculator, and address book.

Pediatrician A physician who specializes in the care and development of children and the diagnosis and treatment of children's diseases.

Pediatrics The branch of medicine that deals with the care and development of children and the diagnosis and treatment of children's diseases.

Percussion The process of tapping the body to detect signs of disease.

Percussion hammer An instrument with a rubber head, used for testing reflexes.

Per diem A term used for employees who do not have a fixed schedule but are scheduled by the day according to office needs.

Perimenopause Before the onset of menopause, the phase during which a woman with regular periods changes to irregular cycles and increased periods of amenorrhea.

Perinatal Relating to the period shortly before and after birth.

Perineum The external region between the vaginal orifice and the anus in a female and between the scrotum and the anus in a male.

Peristalsis Rhythmic contractions of the intestine that move food along the digestive tract.

Peroxidase (as it pertains to the guaiac slide test) A substance that is able to transfer oxygen from hydrogen peroxide to oxidize guaiac, causing the guaiac to turn blue.

Petty cash A cash account kept in a business office to pay for incidentals, such as postage due and other small items.

pH The degree to which a solution is acidic or basic.

Phagocytosis Cell eating; a form of endocytosis in which solid particles are taken into the cell.

Pharmacology The study of drugs.

Phlebotomist A health professional trained in the collection of blood specimens.

Phlebotomy Incision of a vein for the removal of blood; the collection of blood.

Photoreceptor A sensory receptor that detects light; located in the retina of the eye.

Physical examination An assessment of each part of a patient's body to obtain objective data about the patient that assists in determining the patient's state of health.

Physical examination report A report of the objective findings from the physician's assessment of each body system.

Physiologic Pertaining to body processes.

Pinocytosis Cell drinking; a form of endocytosis in which fluid droplets are taken into the cell.

Pixels (picture elements) Dot locations on a computer screen that can be lit up as needed to display images.

Plaintiff The person or group that makes the complaint in a lawsuit.

Plasma The liquid part of the blood, consisting of a clear, yellowish fluid that comprises approximately 55% of the total blood volume.

Plicae circulares Circular folds in the mucosa and submucosa of the small intestine.

Poison Any substance that causes illness, injury, or death if it enters the body.

Policy A guiding principle for the management of a medical office or business.

Polycythemia A disorder in which there is an increase in the red blood cell mass.

Polyuria Increased output of urine.

Position The relation of the presenting part of the fetus to the maternal pelvis.

Postage meter A machine that automatically stamps a piece of mail with the correct postage.

Postal bar code A series of vertical bars of two lengths, which represent the delivery address of a piece of mail. The barcode facilitates automated sorting of mail.

Postexposure prophylaxis (PEP) Treatment administered to an individual after exposure to an infectious disease to prevent the disease.

Postoperative After a surgical operation.

Postpartum Occurring after childbirth.

Preadmission testing (PAT) A series of diagnostic tests done before surgery to establish the patient's health status and identify any potential problems that may occur during surgery.

Preauthorization Permission from a patient's insurance company for a test, procedure, or surgery. Usually the insurance company issues a preauthorization number, which must be communicated to the laboratory or hospital that will be billing for the test or procedure.

Preeclampsia A major complication of pregnancy, the cause of which is unknown, characterized by increasing hypertension, albuminuria, and edema. If this condition is neglected or not treated properly, it may develop into eclampsia, which could cause maternal convulsions and coma. Preeclampsia generally occurs between the twentieth week of pregnancy and the end of the first week postpartum.

Premium An amount of money paid in a given period to purchase health insurance.

Prenatal Before birth.

Preoperative Preceding a surgical operation.

Presbyopia A decrease in the elasticity of the lens that occurs with aging, resulting in a decreased ability to focus on close objects.

Preschool child A child 3 to 6 years old.

Prescription An order to a pharmacist to dispense a supply of medication.

Presentation Indication of the part of the fetus that is closest to the cervix and is delivered first. A cephalic presentation is a delivery in which the fetal head is presenting against the cervix. A breech presentation is a delivery in which the buttocks or feet are presented instead of the head.

Pressure point A site on the body where an artery lies close to the surface of the skin and can be compressed against an underlying bone to control bleeding.

Preterm birth Delivery occurring between 20 and 37 weeks of gestation regardless of whether the child was born alive or stillborn.

Primary care provider The physician chosen by a patient to provide general medical care and also to determine and authorize additional medical services the patient may require.

Primary insurance The insurance company that must be billed first for any individual.

Prime mover The muscle that is mainly responsible for a particular body movement; also called *agonist*.

Primigravida A woman who is pregnant for the first time.

Primipara A woman who has carried a pregnancy to fetal viability (20 weeks of gestation) for the first time, regardless of whether the infant was stillborn or alive at birth.

Printing speed The number of pages per minute (ppm) generated by a printer.

Privilege A special immunity that protects against legal liability.

Problem Any patient condition that requires further observation, diagnosis, management, or patient education.

Problem-oriented medical record (POMR) A system for arranging information within the medical record based on patient problems.

Procedure A list of the steps to handle a certain situation or perform a certain task.

Processing The manipulation and reorganization of data according to the instructions in a program.

Profile Numerous laboratory tests providing related or complementary information used to determine the health status of a patient.

Prognosis The probable course and outcome of a patient's condition and the patient's prospects for a recovery.

Program A set of instructions organized in a logical step-by-step sequence, which tells the computer how to perform a specific function.

Projection Experiencing one's own emotions as those of another.

Proof of posting A process of calculation to verify that calculations on a day sheet are internally consistent and all totals are correct.

Proofread To identify and correct errors in a document.

Proprioception The sense of body position and movements.

Proprioceptor A type of mechanoreceptor located in muscles, tendons, and joints; provides information about body position and movements.

Proteinuria The presence of protein in the urine.

Prudent Using care or common sense.

Puerperium The period of time, usually 4 to 6 weeks after delivery, in which the uterus and the body systems are returning to normal.

Pulse oximeter A computerized device consisting of a probe and monitor used to measure the oxygen saturation of arterial blood.

Pulse oximetry The use of a pulse oximeter to measure the oxygen saturation of arterial blood.

Pulse pressure The difference between the systolic and diastolic pressures.

Pulse rhythm The time interval between heartbeats.

Pulse volume The strength of the heartbeat.

Puncture A wound made by a sharp pointed object piercing the skin.

Purchase order (PO) The form used to order supplies, as well as the order itself.

Quality control The application of methods to ensure that test results are reliable and valid and that errors are detected and eliminated.

Quickening The first movements of the fetus in utero as felt by the mother, which usually occurs between the sixteenth and twentieth weeks of gestation and is felt consistently thereafter.

Radiation The transfer of energy, such as heat, in the form of waves.

Radiograph A permanent record of a picture of an internal body organ or structure produced on radiographic film.

Radiography The taking of permanent records (radiographs) of internal body organs and structures by passing x-rays through the body to act on a specially sensitized film.

Radiologist A physician who specializes in the diagnosis and treatment of disease using radiant energy, such as x-rays, radium, and radioactive material.

Radiology The branch of medicine that deals with the use of radiant energy in the diagnosis and treatment of disease.

Radiolucent Describing a structure that permits the passage of x-rays.

Radiopaque Describing a structure that obstructs the passage of x-rays.

RAM (random-access memory) The main computer memory of a microcomputer, which is used to temporarily store items until needed by the computer for processing. Also known as *main computer memory.*

Read The transfer of information from a storage device, such as a hard disk, to computer memory.

Reciprocity Automatic issuing of a license in one state to the holder of a license in another state.

Reconciling Making sure that two financial records agree, such as a bank statement and bank balance.

Referral Recommendation that a patient receive additional medical services. For patients with managed care insurance, a referral must be accompanied by a written form that specifies the nature of the service and the number of visits that have been authorized.

Reflecting Expressing the meaning and emotion of another's words back to the person.

Refraction The deflection or bending of light rays by a lens.

Refractive index The ratio of the velocity of light in air to the velocity of light in a solution.

Refractometer *(clinical)* An instrument used to measure the refractive index of urine, which is an indirect measurement of the specific gravity of urine.

Regulated medical waste (RMW) Medical waste that poses a threat to health and safety.

Reimbursement The amount paid for a procedure by insurance.

Renal threshold The concentration at which a substance in the blood that is not normally excreted by the kidneys begins to appear in the urine.

Renal tubule Tubular portion of the nephron that carries the filtrate away from the glomerular capsule; site where tubular reabsorption and secretion occur.

Reorder point A number on a supply inventory that indicates when a specific item should be reordered to be sure that the supply will not run out before the new order is received.

Reservoir host The organism that becomes infected by a pathogen and serves as a source of transfer of the pathogen to others.

Residency A program to provide training in a medical specialty to a physician who has finished medical school.

Resident flora Harmless, nonpathogenic microorganisms that normally reside on the skin and usually do not cause disease. Also known as *normal flora.*

Resistance The natural ability of an organism to remain unaffected by harmful substances in its environment.

Resolution The number of horizontal and vertical pixels in a display device, such as a computer screen.

Resource-based relative value scale (RBRVS) A system to establish the Medicare fee schedule for Medicare Part B based on the service provided and the geographic location of the provider.

Respiratory membrane Any surface in the lungs where diffusion occurs; consists of the layers that the gases must pass through to get into or out of the alveoli.

Respondeat superior A legal doctrine making an employer liable for the negligent acts of employees.

Resumé A summary of information about a person that describes education, work experience, and other information related to an individual's suitability for employment.

Reverse chronological order Arrangement of documents with the most recent document on top or in the front, which means that the oldest document is on the bottom or at the back of a section or file.

Right A claim that is expected to be honored.

Right-justified Type that is aligned with the right margin of a document.

Risk factor Anything that increases an individual's chance of developing a disease. Some risk factors (e.g., smoking) can be avoided, but others cannot (e.g., age, family history).

Risk management Processes to protect a health care facility from the risk of legal action.

Routine test Laboratory test performed routinely on apparently healthy patients to assist in the early detection of disease.

Rugae Longitudinal folds in the mucosa of the stomach.

Salary A fixed amount of money paid on a regular basis that does not depend on the number of hours worked.

Saltatory conduction Process in which a nerve impulse travels along a myelinated nerve fiber by jumping from one node of Ranvier to the next.

Sanitization A process to remove organic matter from an article and to reduce the number of microorganisms to a safe level as determined by public health requirements.

SaO₂ (saturation of arterial oxygen) Abbreviation for the percentage of hemoglobin that is saturated with oxygen in arterial blood.

Scalpel A surgical knife used to divide tissues.

School-age child A child 6 to 12 years old.

Scissors A cutting instrument.

Sebaceous cyst A thin, closed sac or capsule that contains fatty secretions from a sebaceous gland.

Sebaceous gland An oil gland of the skin that produces sebum or body oil.

Secondary insurance Insurance that an individual has in addition to primary insurance.

Segment The portion of the electrocardiogram between two waves.

Seizure A sudden episode of involuntary muscular contractions and relaxation, often accompanied by a change in sensation, behavior, and level of consciousness.

Self-actualization The fulfillment of each individual's potential.

Semiblock style A letter format in which the date line, complimentary close, and printed signature line are on a tab at the center or right justified, all paragraphs are indented five to eight spaces, and the other parts of the letter are left justified.

Semicritical item An item that comes into contact with nonintact skin or intact mucous membranes.

Semilunar valve Valve between a ventricle of the heart and the vessel that carries blood away from the ventricle; also pertains to the valves in veins.

Sensory adaptation Phenomenon in which some receptors respond when a stimulus is first applied but decrease their response if the stimulus is maintained; receptor sensitivity decreases with prolonged stimulation.

Sequela (*pl.* sequelae) A morbid (secondary) condition occurring as a result of a less serious primary infection.

Sequential-access memory Computer memory in which all stored data must be searched sequentially from beginning to end to locate the desired information.

Serum The clear, straw-colored part of the blood (plasma) that remains after the solid elements have been separated out of it.

Service contract An agreement that provides for service for a piece of equipment after the warranty expires.

Shock The failure of the cardiovascular system to deliver enough blood to all the vital organs of the body.

Sigmoidoscope An endoscope that is specially designed for passage through the anus to permit visualization of the rectum and sigmoid colon.

Sigmoidoscopy The visual examination of the rectum and sigmoid colon using a sigmoidoscope.

Signatura The part of a prescription that indicates the information to print on the medication label.

Signature on file (SOF) An indication on the insurance claim form that the signature of the patient is maintained by the medical office to authorize submission of insurance claims.

Simplified letter style A letter format in which all elements are left justified. The greeting is replaced by a subject line in all capital letters. The complimentary close and typed signature are replaced by a typed signature in all capital letters.

Single booking An appointment scheduling method in which each patient is given a different, specific appointment time. Also called *stream scheduling* or *fixed appointment scheduling.*

Skip Account for which no billing information is available.

Smartphone A cell phone with computer capabilities.

Smear Material spread on a slide for microscope examination.

Soak The direct immersion of a body part in water or a medicated solution.

SOAP format A method of organization for recording progress notes. The SOAP format includes the following categories: *s*ubjective data, *o*bjective data, *a*ssessment, and *p*lan.

Social Security tax (FICA) A tax of 6.2% collected from employees to fund the Social Security program, which provides benefits to retired workers.

Soft copy The visual display of information on the display screen of a computer monitor.

Software A general term for the programs or instructions that tell a computer what to do.

Sonogram The record obtained with ultrasonography.

Sorter A device that facilitates putting papers or records in alphabetic or numeric order.

Sound card A circuit board connected to the mainboard that converts computer audio output into electronic signals. The electronic signals are then sent to speakers that convert them into sound.

Source-oriented medical record (SOMR) A system for arranging information within the medical record based on the types of services that were performed.

Special keys Keys that issue commands to the computer to perform specific functions on the information displayed on the screen.

Specific gravity The weight of a substance compared with the weight of an equal volume of a substance known as the *standard*. In urinalysis, the *specific gravity* refers to the measurement of the amount of dissolved substances in the urine compared with the same amount of distilled water.

Specimen A small sample of something taken to show the nature of the whole.

Speculum An instrument for opening a body orifice or cavity for viewing.

Spermatogenesis Process of meiosis in the male in which four spermatids are produced from one primary spermatocyte.

Spermiogenesis Morphologic changes that transform a spermatid into a mature sperm.

Sphygmomanometer An instrument for measuring arterial blood pressure.

Spirilla (*sing.* spirillum) Bacteria that have a spiral or curved shape.

Spirometer An instrument for measuring air taken into and expelled from the lungs.

Spirometry Measurement of an individual's breathing capacity by means of a spirometer.

Splint Any device that immobolizes a body part.

SpO₂ (saturation of peripheral oxygen) Abbreviation for the percentage of hemoglobin that is saturated with oxygen in arterial blood as measured by a pulse oximeter.

Spore A hard, thick-walled capsule formed by some bacteria that contains only the essential parts of the protoplasm of the bacterial cell.

Sprain Trauma to a joint that causes injury to the ligaments.

SSL (Secure Sockets Layer) A protocol for managing secure transmission of data over the Internet by means of encryption.

Standard of care Level of appropriate care required of a health professional.

Statute of limitations A law limiting the time period for beginning a lawsuit.

Statutory law Law enacted by a legislative body.

Stem cells Cells that have the capacity to develop into various types of body tissue.

Sterile Free of all living microorganisms and bacterial spores.

Sterilization The process of destroying all forms of microbial life, including bacterial spores.

Stethoscope An instrument for amplifying and hearing sounds produced by the body.

Storage capacity The maximum amount of information that a device can hold measured in bytes.

Storage device A device that permanently stores information for later retrieval by the computer.

Strain An overstretching of a muscle caused by trauma.

Stream scheduling An appointment scheduling method in which each patient is given a different, specific appointment time. Also called *fixed appointment scheduling, time-specified,* or *single booking.*

Subcutaneous (SC) injection Introduction of medication beneath the skin, into the subcutaneous or fatty layer of the body.

Subcutaneous layer Below the skin; a sheet of areolar connective tissue and adipose tissue beneath the dermis of the skin; also called *hypodermis* or *superficial fascia.*

Subjective symptom A symptom that is felt by a patient but is not observable by an examiner.

Sublingual administration Administration of medication by placing it under the tongue, where it dissolves and is absorbed through the mucous membrane.

Subpoena A court order for a witness to appear and give testimony.

Subpoena *duces tecum* A court order to produce documents or records.

Subscriber The person named on an insurance certificate.

Subscription The part of a prescription that gives directions to the pharmacist and usually designates the number of doses to be dispensed.

Sudoriferous gland A gland in the skin that produces perspiration; also called *sweat gland.*

Summarizing Expressing the most important points of a conversation or written document.

Superbill An itemized charge slip usually also containing diagnosis codes and procedure codes required for insurance billing.

Supernatant The clear liquid that remains at the top after a precipitate settles.

Superscription The part of a prescription consisting of the symbol Rx (from the Latin word *recipe,* meaning "take").

Suppuration The process of pus formation.

Suprapubic aspiration The passing of a sterile needle through the abdominal wall into the bladder to remove urine.

Surfactant A substance, produced by certain cells in lung tissue, that reduces surface tension between fluid molecules that line the respiratory membrane and helps keep the alveolus from collapsing.

Surgical asepsis Practices that keep objects and areas sterile or free from microorganisms.

Surgical package Surgical services usually covered by a single procedure code that includes a preoperative visit, postoperative care, and local anesthesia (if applicable).

Surname Last name or family name of an individual terminal digit filing.

Susceptible Easily affected; lacking resistance.

Sutures Material used to approximate tissues with surgical stitches.

Swaged needle A needle with suturing material permanently attached to its end.

Sympathy Feeling the same emotions as another.

Symptom Any change in the body or its functioning that indicates a disease might be present.

Symptomatic treatment Therapy for symptoms of a disease or condition that does not remove the disease itself.

Synapse The region of communication between two neurons.

Synarthrosis (*pl.* synarthroses) An immovable joint.

Synergist A muscle that assists a prime mover but is not capable of producing the movement by itself.

System software A group of programs that control or maintain the operations of a computer.

Systole Contraction phase of the cardiac cycle; opposite of diastole.

Systolic pressure The point of maximum pressure on the arterial walls, which is recorded during systole.

Tab A projection of a folder that extends beyond the top or side of the folder.

Tachycardia An abnormally fast heart rate (greater than 100 beats per minute).

Tachypnea An abnormal increase in the respiratory rate of more than 20 respirations per minute.

Target tissue A tissue (cells) that responds to a particular hormone because it has receptor sites for that hormone.

Template A standard form to which additional information can be added as needed.

Terminal digit filing A chronological filing system that uses the last number or number group as the first indexing unit.

Thermolabile Easily affected or changed by heat.

Thermoreceptor A sensory receptor that detects changes in temperature.

Thready pulse A pulse with a decreased volume that feels weak and thin.

Threshold stimulus Minimum level of stimulation that is required to start a nerve impulse or muscle contraction; also called *liminal stimulus.*

Thrombocyte One of the formed elements of the blood; functions in blood clotting; also called *platelet.*

Tickler file A chronological file containing reminders of things to be done.

Time-specified scheduling An appointment scheduling method in which each patient is given a different, specific appointment time. Also called *stream scheduling, fixed appointment scheduling,* or *single booking.*

Tissue Group of similar cells specialized to perform a certain function.

Toddler A child 1 to 3 years old.

Topical administration Application of a drug to a particular spot, usually for a local action.

Tort An injury or wrong against a person or property that does not involve breach of contract.

Toxemia A condition that can occur in pregnant women that includes preeclampsia and eclampsia. If preeclampsia goes undiagnosed or is not satisfactorily controlled, it could develop into eclampsia, characterized by convulsions and coma.

Toxin A poisonous or noxious substance.

Toxoid A toxin (poisonous substance produced by a bacterium) that has been treated by heat or chemicals to destroy its harmful properties. It is administered to an individual to prevent an infectious disease by stimulating the production of antibodies in that individual.

Transcription The process of changing verbal dictation to typed or printed form.

Transfusion The administration of whole blood or blood products through the intravenous route.

Transient flora Microorganisms that reside on the superficial skin layers and are picked up in the course of daily activities. They are often pathogenic but can be removed easily from the skin by sanitizing the hands.

Triage The process of separating patients by the urgency of their need for care.

TRICARE A government insurance plan that provides medical care to spouses and dependents of individuals on active duty in the military. Formerly this program was called *CHAMPUS.*

Trimester Three months, or one third, of the gestational period of pregnancy.

Truth in lending Legal requirement to disclose the terms of a loan in terms that the borrower can understand.

Tympanic membrane A thin, semitransparent membrane between the external ear canal and the middle ear that receives and transmits sound waves. Also known as the *eardrum.*

Ultrasonography The use of high-frequency sound waves (ultrasound) to produce an image of an organ or tissue.

Urinalysis The physical, chemical, and microscopic analysis of urine.

User The individual using the computer.

Usual, customary, and reasonable (UCR) A system for establishing the amount an insurance company will pay for a procedure. The reasonable charge is set by the insurance company based on a physician's usual (most frequent) charge for the procedure and the customary charge of other physicians in the same geographic area.

Uterine cycle Monthly cycle of events that occur in the uterus from puberty to menopause; also called the *menstrual cycle;* occurs concurrently with the ovarian cycle.

Utilization review Assessing medical services to determine whether they are appropriate, necessary, and of high quality.

Vaccine A suspension of attenuated (weakened) or killed microorganisms administered to an individual to prevent an infectious disease by stimulating the production of antibodies in that individual.

Vendor A company from whom supplies or equipment is purchased.

Venipuncture Puncturing of a vein.

Venous reflux The backflow of blood (from an evacuated tube) into a patient's vein.

Venous stasis The temporary cessation or slowing of the venous blood flow.

Ventilation Movement of air into and out of the lungs; breathing

Veracity Truthfulness.

Verbal Using words to communicate.

Vertex The top of the head.

Vial A closed glass container with a rubber stopper that holds medication.

Video card A circuit board connected to the mainboard that converts computer video output into electronic signals. The electronic signals are then sent to the monitor, where they are converted into text and images that can be viewed by the user.

Voice mail A method for delivery, storage, and retrieval of telephone messages that is built into the telephone system.

Void To empty the bladder.

Vulva The region of the external female genital organs.

W-4 The form used to claim allowances for federal income tax reporting.

Warranty A promise by the manufacturer to repair or replace defective parts in an item during a specific time period.

Wave scheduling A method of scheduling appointments in which several patients are given the same appointment time and seen in the order in which they arrive.

Webcam Small video camera attached to a computer that allows video to be transmitted on the Internet.

Wheal A small raised area of the skin.

Workers' compensation An insurance program that covers lost wages and health care costs of workers injured on the job or who suffer from work-related illnesses.

Wound A break in the continuity of an external or internal surface caused by physical means.

Write The transfer of information from computer memory to a storage device, such as a hard disk.

ZIP code A five-digit code that identifies the post office to which a given piece of mail is to be delivered.

ZIP + 4 code A more detailed mailing code consisting of the original five-digit ZIP code followed by a hyphen and four additional digits. These digits identify a specific geographic segment within the delivery area.

Index

A

AAMA. *See* American Association of Medical Assistants (AAMA).
Abandonment, 44b, 45, 56
Abdomen, 400t
Abdominal wall, 140–141, 140t
Abduction, 137t
ABHES. *See* Accrediting Bureau of Health Education Schools (ABHES).
ABO blood groups, 209–210, 210t
ABO blood typing, 482, 800
Abortion, 38
Abrasions, 537, 537f, 837f, 838
Absorbable sutures, 541–542, 542f
Absorbed poisons, 844
Absorption, 241
Abuse, reporting of, 38b, 52
Accommodation, 177, 177f
Account aging, 1098–1099f, 1099–1100b
Accounting, 1030. *See also* Practice finances.
Accounts receivable aging records, 1098–1099f, 1099–1100b
Accreditation, voluntary, 54
Accrediting Bureau of Health Education Schools (ABHES), 23
Accrual basis of accounting, 1030
Accu-Chek Advantage glucose meter, 795–797, 796f, 797–799b
Acetylcholine, 132–133, 155, 156t
Acne, 104b
Acquired immune deficiency syndrome (AIDS), 6, 289–290b, 294b
ACTH. *See* Adrenocorticotropic hormone (ACTH).
Acting out, 69
Action potentials, 154, 154f, 155f
Active listening, 61, 62, 63t
Active records, 989
Active transport, 87t, 89–90
Acupuncture, 17, 18f
Acute illness, 377
Acute otitis media, 425b
ADA. *See* Americans with Disabilities Act (ADA).
Addison's disease, 192
Address standards, 1020, 1021b, 1021t, 1022, 1022f, 1023b
Adduction, 137t
Adenocarcinoma, 93b
Adenoma, 93b, 189b
Adhesion, 100b
Adhesive skin closures, 547–548, 548–552b, 548f
Adipose tissue, 97, 97f, 104b
Adjustments to patient accounts, posting, 1034–1035, 1035b, 1039–1040b
Administration of medication, 573–574, 634b
   allergy testing and, 620–624, 623f, 623t, 624f, 625–626b
   charting of, 893

Administration of medication *(Continued)*
   classification of drugs and, 578–579, 579–585t
   controlled drugs and, 588, 590–591t
   converting units of measurement, 588, 589t
   drug nomenclature and, 574, 578
   drug references in, 574, 575–577f
   factors affecting drug action, 597
   guidelines for preparation and, 598
   intravenous therapy in, 628–632, 628f, 630f, 631f
   legal issues in, 574, 632b
   medication records and, 596–597, 596f
   oral administration in, 598, 599–600b
   parenteral administration in. *See* Parenteral administration.
   prescriptions and, 589, 592–595, 592f, 593t, 594b, 595b
   routes of, 574
   systems of measurement for, 585–588, 586b, 587b, 588t
Administrative areas, 1111, 1111f
Administrative responsibilities, 29–30, 29f, 30f
Adolescents, immunizations for, 515t
Adrenal medulla, 188t, 192, 193f
Adrenal (suprarenal) glands, 188t, 191–192, 192f, 193f
Adrenocorticotropic hormone (ACTH), 188t, 189f, 190
Advance directives, 40–42, 41b, 41f, 50b
Adventitia, 228, 228f
Adventitious sounds, 352
Adverse reactions, 597
Aerobic exercise, 349b
Aerobic respiration, 133, 135f
Afferent neurons, 150, 152, 152t
Afferent (sensory) division, 148, 151f
Aging
   circulatory system and, 210b
   nervous system and, 169b
   reproductive system and, 264b
   respiratory system and, 223b
   the senses and, 183b
   skeletal system and, 116b
   of skin, 109b
   website information on, 699b
AIDS. *See* Acquired immune deficiency syndrome (AIDS).
Albinism, 106
Albumins, 205, 205t
Alcohol abuse, 635b
Alcohol-based hand rubs, 270–271, 270b, 270f, 274–275b
Aldosterone, 188t, 191–192, 248
Allergens, 620, 621b
Allergic reactions
   to drugs, 597, 621b
   to insect stings, 621b, 844–845, 845f
Allergic rhinitis, 622t

Page numbers followed by *f* indicate figures; *t*, tables; *b*, boxes.